A Practical Guide to
Contemporary
Pharmacy Practice

THIRD EDITION

A Practical Guide to

Contemporary Pharmacy Practice

THIRD EDITION

Judith E. Thompson, RPh, MS

Clinical Associate Professor Emeritus
School of Pharmacy
University of Wisconsin–Madison
Madison, Wisconsin

With CD/audiovisuals by **Lawrence W. Davidow, RPh, PhD**
Director, Pharmacy Skills Laboratories
Department of Pharmacy Practice
The University of Kansas
Lawrence, Kansas

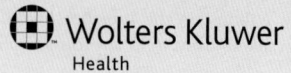
Wolters Kluwer | Lippincott Williams & Wilkins
Health

Philadelphia • Baltimore • New York • London
Buenos Aires • Hong Kong • Sydney • Tokyo

Acquisitions Editor: John Goucher
Managing Editor: Meredith Brittain
Marketing Manager: Allison Noplock
Associate Production Manager: Kevin P. Johnson
Designer: Teresa Mallon
Compositor: Aptara Inc.

Third Edition

Library of Congress Cataloging-in-Publication Data

Thompson, Judith E.
  A practical guide to contemporary pharmacy practice / Judith E. Thompson, with CD/audiovisuals by Lawrence W. Davidow.—3rd ed.
      p. ; cm.
  Includes bibliographical references and index.
  ISBN 978-0-7817-8396-5 (alk. paper)
  1. Pharmacy—Outlines, syllabi, etc. 2. Pharmacy—Handbooks, manuals, etc. I. Davidow, Lawrence W. II. Title.
    [DNLM: 1. Drug Compounding—Handbooks. 2. Pharmaceutical Preparations—administration & dosage—Handbooks. 3. Pharmacy—methods—Handbooks. QV 735 T473p 2009]
  RS98.T47 2009
  615'.1—dc22
                                                                                                            2008043846

DISCLAIMER

    Care has been taken to confirm the accuracy of the information present and to describe generally accepted practices. However, the authors, editors, and publisher are not responsible for errors or omissions or for any consequences from application of the information in this book and make no warranty, expressed or implied, with respect to the currency, completeness, or accuracy of the contents of the publication. Application of this information in a particular situation remains the professional responsibility of the practitioner; the clinical treatments described and recommended may not be considered absolute and universal recommendations.
    The authors, editors, and publisher have exerted every effort to ensure that drug selection and dosage set forth in this text are in accordance with the current recommendations and practice at the time of publication. However, in view of ongoing research, changes in government regulations, and the constant flow of information relating to drug therapy and drug reactions, the reader is urged to check the package insert for each drug for any change in indications and dosage and for added warnings and precautions. This is particularly important when the recommended agent is a new or infrequently employed drug.
    Some drugs and medical devices presented in this publication have Food and Drug Administration (FDA) clearance for limited use in restricted research settings. It is the responsibility of the health care provider to ascertain the FDA status of each drug or device planned for use in their clinical practice.

To purchase additional copies of this book, call our customer service department at **(800) 638-3030** or fax orders to **(301) 223-2320.** International customers should call **(301) 223-2300.**

Visit Lippincott Williams & Wilkins on the Internet: http://www.lww.com. Lippincott Williams & Wilkins customer service representatives are available from 8:30 am to 6:00 pm, EST.

To our students, with gratitude for the joys, the challenges, and the potential they bring to our profession and the patients we serve.

Preface

The goal of *A Practical Guide to Contemporary Pharmacy Practice*, from its beginning, has been to provide a succinct, easy-to-use, current, and very functional handbook on the practice of pharmacy. The third edition continues in this tradition. This edition has been written at this particular time because various pharmacy organizations and agencies have recently developed and published new practice standards, and a practical guide should contain the most current information and recommended procedures. In addition, students, pharmacists, pharmacy technicians, and pharmacy educators who have used this book offered suggestions for features or content that would make this text even more valuable to users. Some of the features added or augmented with this edition include the following:

- Creation of a separate and more comprehensive section (Part 6, Sterile Dosage Forms and Their Preparation, composed of Chapters 32 through 35) on sterile dosage forms and their preparation, with emphasis on new standards and processes in *USP* Chapter ⟨797⟩, Pharmaceutical Compounding—Sterile Preparations.
- Expanded discussion of medication errors, together with prescribing and dispensing practices that have been shown to improve patient medication safety.
- Inclusion of processing tools such as master control and compounding records, standard operating procedures, and quality control tests that are now standards of practice because they can improve our compounded preparations and reduce errors.
- Addition of a chapter (Chapter 7) containing instruction on proper use of metric (SI) symbols and units of measurement, temperature and density conversions, use of significant figures, and basic methods for pharmaceutical calculations.
- Patient cases with the sample compounded prescription orders and parenteral preparation medication orders to show typical situations and problem solving to meet special therapeutic and patient needs.
- Acknowledgment of the increasingly important roles of pharmacy technicians in the practice of pharmacy.
- Addition of a section (Part 7) on the important specialty area of veterinary pharmacy practice.
- Expansion of the companion CD that does such a great job of "show-and-tell."
- Color photographs that better illustrate techniques and materials.

As I prepared the materials for this edition, I was continually amazed at the rapid pace with which practice guidelines and standards are revised and updated; even as this text was going into production, I was making adjustments and revisions to reflect new releases of information. To aid the reader in coping with this fact of modern professional life, I have included whenever possible reference source information and Internet site addresses. The Internet sites for government agencies and professional organizations are rich sources of current information, and I strongly encourage you to check these sites on a regular basis. In addition, the United States Pharmacopeia has recognized the importance of developing current practice standards for pharmacists and now publishes this information in a special volume for pharmacists. This *USP Pharmacists' Pharmacopeia* is available in print with electronic updates.

Because pharmacy has become increasingly complex and specialized, and because we wanted you to have the most current actual practice information and examples, this edition of the *Practical Guide* is more of a collaborative effort than previous editions have been. The following sections of the book were written or revised by a number of contributing authors, all writing in their area of specialty:

- Chapter 5, Drug Utilization Review and Medication-Use Evaluation, and Chapter 6, Patient Counseling, revised by Karen Kopacek: As a clinical assistant professor and the director of the pharmacotherapy laboratories at the University of Wisconsin (UW) School of Pharmacy, Ms. Kopacek is responsible for the teaching of patient assessment, counseling, and therapy management and monitoring. She has been honored multiple times with awards for teaching excellence. She also maintains clinical practices in cardiac and cardiothoracic intensive care units and in an outpatient cardiac rehabilitation and heart transplant clinic.
- Part 4, Pharmaceutical Excipients (Chapters 15 through 24) and Part 8, Compatibility and Stability (Chapter 37), revised by Melgardt de Villiers: Dr. de Villiers: is an associate professor (CHS) in the Division of Pharmaceutical Sciences at the UW School of Pharmacy, where he lectures and directs a two-semester course in drug delivery systems laboratories. With teaching and research experience in this area and a PhD degree in pharmaceutics, he has the special expertise to revise these chapters.
- Chapter 32, General Principles of Sterile Dosage Form Preparation, and Chapter 35, Total Parenteral Nutrition: New Chapter 32 was written, and Chapter 35 was revised, by Gordon Sacks. Dr. Sacks is a clinical professor and Chair of the Pharmacy Practice Division at the UW School of Pharmacy. He is certified in Nutrition Support Pharmacy by the Board of Pharmaceutical Specialties and maintains an active practice in parenteral and enteral nutrition at UW Hospitals and Clinics. In 2001, he received the Distinguished Nutrition Support Pharmacist Award.
- Chapter 34, Parenteral Preparations, revised by Mary Swandby: Ms. Swandby has worked in sterile preparation production in either hospital or home infusions practices for more than 25 years. From 1996 through 2006, she held supervisory and management roles at Chartwell Midwest Wisconsin, a partnership between Chartwell Home Therapies and UW Hospitals and Clinics, where she had major responsibility for JCAHO and *USP* ⟨797⟩ compliance processes. She is currently Clinical Pharmacy Specialist–Drug Information at Dean Health Systems, including clinical pharmacist duties in the infectious disease, infusion, and oncology clinics.
- Chapter 36, Veterinary Pharmacy Practice, a new chapter written by Gigi Davidson: Ms. Davidson is currently director of clinical pharmacy services at the North Carolina State University College of Veterinary Medicine, where she has been practicing veterinary pharmacy for 25 years. She was awarded the Diplomate status in the International College of Veterinary Pharmacy in 2000 and currently serves on two USP Expert Committees, Compounding Pharmacy and Veterinary Medicine.

Students, pharmacists, and pharmacy technicians all praised the CD that was developed by Lawrence Davidow and included with the second edition of the *Practical Guide*. As we know, a picture (and even more, a slide show) is worth a thousand words. We have included a CD-ROM icon ⊙ throughout the text to direct readers to related exercises, images, or other content on the CD-ROM. Dr. Davidow also provided many of the images found in the second edition. For this third edition, Dr. Davidow has revised and created new material for his CD, and he has added some new text photographs (including ten color images), which make these even more valuable tools. Dr. Davidow has a perfect and unique background and skill set for this work: He has a BS degree in Pharmacy, a PhD degree in Pharmacology, is the director of Pharmacy Skills Laboratory at the University of Kansas, has kept in close contact with professional practice, has written and reviewed material for APhA's *Handbook of Nonprescription Drugs* and the NAPLEX exam, and has extensive background and experience in computer-based technology and photography. As a thoughtful and knowledgeable collaborator, Larry has also provided helpful insight and counsel for the text portion of this edition, and I thank him for this.

I also wish to express my appreciation to my colleagues and former students who have generously given their time, advice, and assistance for all three editions of the *Practical Guide*. I wish to especially acknowledge the following people:

My colleagues and fellow committee members on the USP Pharmacy Compounding Expert Committee, including Loyd Allen, Mary Ann Kirkpatrick, Graham Nairn, Lawrence Trissel, Mark

Klang, Lawson Kloesel, Gigi Davidson, Lisa Ashworth, Robin Bogner, Claudia Okeke, Rick Schnatz, and Shawn Becker.

Mary Ann Kirkpatrick and her students at Shenandoah University School of Pharmacy, for reading and offering suggestions on a variety of chapters as I was determining what features are most useful to pharmacy students. Dr. Kirkpatrick has been a leader in setting standards for pharmacy compounding and has been a friend and mentor to me and to many faculty members who teach in this area. She has contributed her advice and expertise for numerous parts of this book.

Paul Trusten, a fellow pharmacist and public relations director at the U.S. Metric Association, for his advice and assistance with the material on the metric (SI) system.

Colleague and former student Tom Heckenkamp, owner of Pharmaceutical Balances Systems, for reading and critiquing Chapter 14, Selection and Use of Weighing and Measuring Equipment.

Physician Kenneth Felz and pediatric pharmacist Brian LaRowe, for their help with case studies, and Robert Schwartz, a model pharmacist and teacher, for sharing his community pharmacy experience in writing many of the original sample compounded prescriptions and patient consults.

Jeanine Mount, professor of social and administrative sciences at the UW School of Pharmacy, and L.D. King, executive director of the International Academy of Compounding Pharmacists, for their assistance with current issues on pharmaceutical law.

Joni Mitchell, program assistant for pharmaceutical sciences at the UW School of Pharmacy, and a master with language, word processing, and equation software, for helping me with these aspects of writing this book.

Bonnie Fingerhut, laboratory supervisor of the Drug Delivery Teaching Laboratories at the UW School of Pharmacy, for her help with making and testing many of the formulations in this book. Bonnie and I began working together in 1976 at Spring Green Pharmacy and, in our 30-plus years of working together became best friends as well as a professional team that epitomizes the successful pharmacist–pharmacy technician relationship.

UW emeritus professors Kenneth Connors and George Zografi, who have been my pharmaceutical mentors for nearly 40 years. They have generously shared their time and expertise, and I am deeply indebted to them.

Lippincott Williams & Wilkins managing editors Meredith Brittain and Elizabeth Connolly, for their guidance and support with this project.

Many of my former students researched and tested formulations described in this book and offered helpful suggestions on content. I wish to particularly acknowledge Susan Stein, John Dopp, Michael Brown, Tom Heckenkamp, MaryAnn Steiner, Matthew Loring, Rachel Thomas, Kevin Favro, Jenna Bakkum, Eileen Cobb, Tait Waege, Ronald Popp, Matthew Chambers, Susan Kruel, Deborah Schmitt, Alisha Hahn, Karen Hansen, Jim Grogan, Kimberly Buckfinck, and Tony Bridgeman.

Finally, I wish to thank my family—my husband, Wayne; my children, grandchildren, brother, and sister; and my mom. They have encouraged and supported me and shown great patience with me as I have written and rewritten "the book."

Judith E. Thompson
Madison, Wisconsin

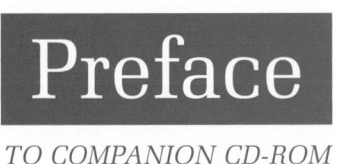

Preface

TO COMPANION CD-ROM

I began using Judy Thompson's book, *A Practical Guide to Contemporary Pharmacy Practice*, in 1998 for teaching laboratory courses at the University of Kansas. I chose this textbook because it was well written and organized, with many prescription examples. Over the years, I have asked students their opinion of the *Practical Guide*, and they have collectively praised it. Some students commented that they felt overwhelmed by the depth of subject matter and struggled with trying to visualize compounding procedures from only a written description. Because of limited class time, I needed some way outside of class to address these student needs. To accomplish this, Robert Emerson, the lab coordinator, and I began to develop a multimedia CD-ROM that would be used as a companion to the *Practical Guide*. The CD-ROM companion was developed to (1) enhance reading comprehension by providing study guides for key chapters of the text, (2) encourage student self-assessment by quizzing on basic concepts, and (3) help students visualize compounding procedures using a narrated slide show. We chose a slide show format because it has a step-by-step feel, and high-resolution images taken at very close range best illustrate the compounding process. In addition to developing these slide shows, we reviewed calculations, product labeling, and pharmacist documentation. A CD-ROM icon 📀 appears in the text whenever additional related content is available on the CD-ROM.

Use of the CD-ROM in lab has been a positive experience. It allows us to make better use of class time because students are better prepared, ask intelligent clarifying questions before beginning procedures, and feel more confident about what they are doing.

For the third edition of this textbook, the CD-ROM was revised to include much more content to support the earlier chapters of the textbook, including those discussing processing the prescription, prescription labeling, patient counseling, and an enlarged section on calculations review.

I owe many thanks to Judy Thompson for her help in determining what should be included on the CD-ROM as well as her assistance in revising and reviewing the content. I am also indebted to Robert Emerson for his help with the original CD-ROM and to Donna Coffman for her assistance in revising the CD-ROM for the third edition. A debt of gratitude is owed to Sandy Urish for her exceptional administrative assistance. I am also very thankful for the support of my wife, Clarissa, and daughter, Abigail, while completing this project. Lastly, I thank all of my former students who supported and encouraged these efforts despite suffering through failed auto-starts, incompatible Web browsers, and no sound. They have reminded me of the value of patience and perseverance.

Lawrence W. Davidow
Lawrence, Kansas

Contents

Contents

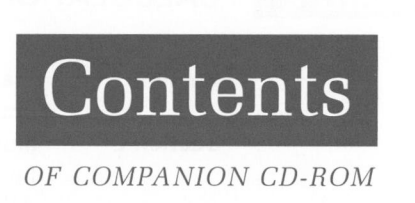

Contents
OF COMPANION CD-ROM

Note: The parts in this Table of Contents correspond to the parts in the book's Table of Contents. There are no CD contents for Parts 4, 7, and 8.

PART 6   STERILE DOSAGE FORMS AND THEIR PREPARATION

Part 1

Processing the
Prescription

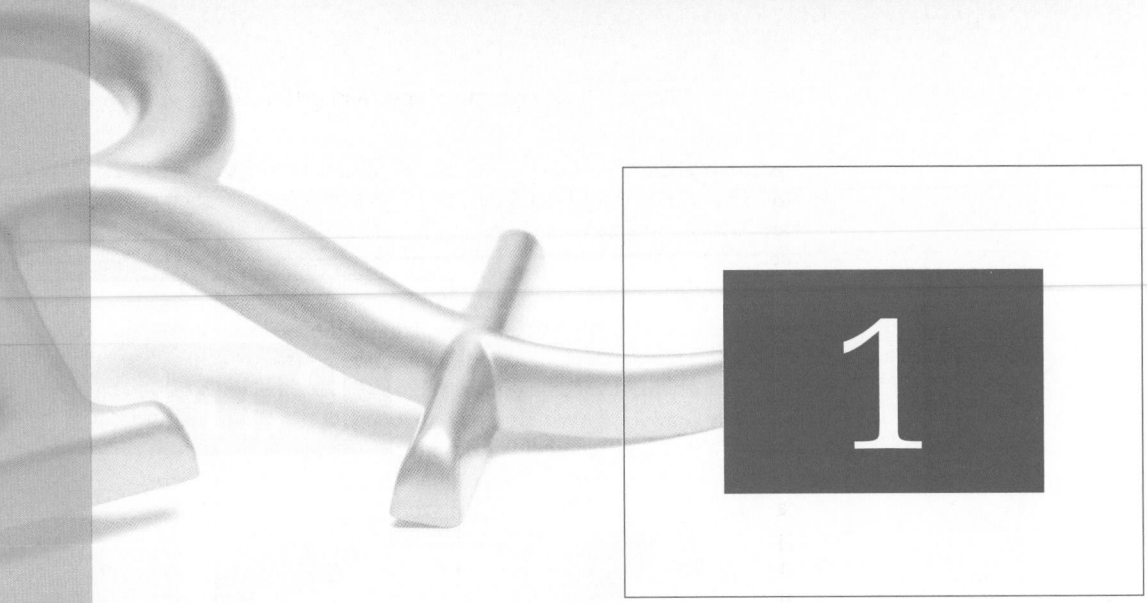

Prescription and Medication Drug Orders

I. **INTRODUCTION AND DEFINITIONS**

A. The starting point for furnishing drug therapy to patients is the prescription or medication drug order. When discussing required and recommended elements of these drug orders and identifying both authorized personnel and safe and effective procedures for handling the various phases of the drug order process, it is essential to have some basic definitions.

B. The definitions given in this section are taken from the *Model State Pharmacy Act of the National Association of Boards of Pharmacy*. The National Association of Boards of Pharmacy (NABP) publishes a Model State Pharmacy Act and model rules for various areas of pharmacy practice. Although states are encouraged to use these in formulating individual state laws, each state is free to enact its own laws and administrative codes regulating the practices of pharmacy and medicine. To learn the specific definitions and legal requirements for the state where you are practicing, consult the applicable state statutes. The *Model State Pharmacy Act* and the *Model Rules of the National Association of Boards of Pharmacy* are revised and updated frequently; a current copy is available on their Internet Web site at http://www.nabp.net, Accessed December 2007.

C. **Definitions:** Because the language for these definitions has been carefully chosen by the NABP, most definitions given here are direct quotes from the 2007 Model Act. (Note that the Act uses uppercase beginning letters for all words or terms that are given specific definitions in the Act.)

    1. The **Practice of Pharmacy** is defined in Section 104 of the NABP Model Act as follows:

> The "Practice of Pharmacy" means the interpretation, evaluation, and implementation of Medical Orders; the Dispensing of Prescription Drug Orders; participation in Drug and Device selection; Drug Administration; Drug Regimen Review; the Practice of Telepharmacy within and across state lines; Drug or Drug-related research; the provision of Patient Counseling; the provision of those acts or

services necessary to provide Pharmacist Care in all areas of patient care, including Primary Care and Collaborative Pharmacy Practice; and the responsibility for Compounding and Labeling Drugs and Devices (except Labeling by a Manufacturer, Repackager, or Distributor of Non-Prescription Drugs and commercially packaged Legend Drugs and Devices), proper and safe storage of Drugs and Devices, and maintenance of required records. (1)

2. **Dispensing:** "The interpretation, evaluation, and implementation of a Prescription Drug Order, including the preparation and Delivery of a Drug or Device to a patient or patient's agent in a suitable container appropriately labeled for subsequent Administration to, or use by, a patient" (2).

3. **Pharmacist:** "An individual currently licensed by this State to engage in the Practice of Pharmacy" (3).

4. **Pharmacy Technician:** "Personnel registered with the Board [of Pharmacy] who may, under the supervision of the Pharmacist, assist in the pharmacy and perform such functions as assisting in the Dispensing process; processing of medical coverage claims; stocking of medications; cashiering but excluding Drug Regimen Review; clinical conflict resolution; prescriber contact concerning Prescription Drug Order clarification or therapy modification; Patient Counseling; Dispensing process validation; prescription transfer; and receipt of new Prescription Drug Orders" (4). It is important to note that not all states have registration of pharmacy technicians, and individual states differ with respect to the scope of allowed activities for pharmacy technicians and the required level of supervision by the pharmacist. Therefore, it is essential that you consult state statutes and/or applicable regulations for your practice site.

5. **Certified Pharmacy Technician:** "Personnel registered with the Board [of Pharmacy] who have completed a certification program approved by the Board and may, under supervision of a Pharmacist, perform certain activities involved in the Practice of Pharmacy, such as receiving new Prescription Drug Orders; prescription transfer; and Compounding but excluding Drug Regimen Review; clinical conflict resolution; prescriber contact concerning Prescription Drug Order clarification or therapy modification; Patient Counseling; and Dispensing process validation." (5) As is the case for pharmacy technicians, not all states have registration of certified pharmacy technicians; furthermore, some states that register such personnel do not make a legal distinction, including allowed activities, between pharmacy technicians and certified pharmacy technicians. Because states differ with respect to the scope of allowed activities of certified pharmacy technicians, it is essential to obtain this information by consulting the state statutes or applicable regulations where you are practicing.

6. **Practitioner:** "An individual currently licensed, registered, or otherwise authorized by the appropriate jurisdiction to prescribe and Administer Drugs in the course of professional practice" (4). In most cases the "appropriate jurisdiction" is the state, but the federal government has such authority for federal facilities such as military bases and veterans' hospitals and clinics. Traditionally practitioners have included medical and osteopathic doctors, dentists, and veterinarians, but now others such as podiatrists, physician assistants, and nurse practitioners may also be given authority to prescribe and administer drugs. For more specifics on this topic, see the information on prescribing authority in section II of this chapter.

7. **Prescription Drug** or **Legend Drug:** "A Drug which is required by any applicable Federal or State law or rule to be Dispensed pursuant only to a Prescription Drug Order or is restricted to use by Practitioners only" (4). The term "Legend Drug" comes from the legend that is required on the manufacturer or distributor's label on containers of such drugs. The legend states "Caution: Federal law prohibits dispensing without a prescription," "Caution: Federal law restricts this drug to use by, or on the order of, a licensed veterinarian," "Rx only," or a similar phrase.

8. **Prescription Drug Order:** "A lawful order from a Practitioner for a Drug or Device for a specific patient, including orders derived from Collaborative Pharmacy Practice, that is communicated to a Pharmacist in a licensed Pharmacy" (4). The terms "prescription drug order," "prescription order" and "prescription" are used interchangeably by health care workers and the public. The slang terms "Rx" and "script" are also sometimes used by pharmacists, technicians, and other health care workers. These various terms are most commonly used to describe drug orders for ambulatory patients (also referred to as "outpatients") who get their prescribed medications from retail or clinic pharmacies. The terms "medication order" and "chart drug order" are often used when referring to drug orders for persons who are patients in hospitals, nursing homes, or other institutional settings. These patients are referred to as "inpatients."

9. **Medical Order:** "A lawful order of a Practitioner that may or may not include a Prescription Drug Order" (6).

10. **Chart Order:** "A lawful order entered on the chart or a medical record of an inpatient or resident of an Institutional Facility by a Practitioner or his or her designated agent for a Drug or Device" (7). A chart order is considered a prescription drug order if it contains the usual elements of a prescription drug order, such as the name of the patient, date of the order, name, strength, and dosage form of the prescribed drug, directions for use, and name or signature of the prescriber (7).

11. **Compounding:** "The preparation of Components into a Drug product (1) as the result of a Practitioner's Prescription Drug Order or initiative based on the Practitioner/patient/Pharmacist relationship in the course of professional practice, or (2) for the purpose of, or as an incident to, research, teaching, or chemical analysis and not for sale or Dispensing. Compounding also includes the preparation of Drugs or Devices in anticipation of receiving Prescription Drug Orders based on routine, regularly observed prescribing patterns" (7).

12. **Collaborative Pharmacy Practice Agreement:** A written and signed agreement between a pharmacist and licensed practitioner that allows the pharmacist to initiate or modify a patient's drug regimen within the guidelines of an agreed protocol for the purpose of drug therapy management (7,8). Collaborative Pharmacy Practice Agreements are often used by pharmacists and physicians or other practitioners to manage patients with specific disease states such as diabetes or asthma or intense drug therapy such as anticoagulation.

II.   ISSUING AND RECEIVING DRUG ORDERS

A. Prescribing authority

1. As described earlier in the definition of "practitioner", state statutes regulate which licensed health care providers may prescribe and administer drugs in that state. In federal facilities, such as military or veterans' hospitals and clinics, the federal government stipulates who has this authority.

2. Medical and osteopathic doctors, podiatrists, dentists, and veterinarians have traditionally been the practitioners given authority to prescribe drugs; however, many states now also give this authority to optometrists, nurse practitioners, physician assistants, psychologists, and/or pharmacists. In the later cases, certain restrictions may apply. For example, such practitioners may be required to possess advanced degrees or to pass special certification exams, or they may be restricted to prescribing only under the supervision of a licensed physician or under a limited, established protocol, such as a collaborative pharmacy practice agreement. It is the duty of pharmacists to stay informed about laws regulating current prescribing authority for health professionals in their practice area.

3. In all cases, practitioners are restricted to prescribing within the scope of their practice and for a legitimate medical purpose (9). For example, veterinarians can prescribe only for animals; dentists are limited to prescribing medications required by their dental patients for their dental problems, and so on.

4. An institutional facility, such as a hospital or nursing home, may further restrict who may prescribe for patients in that facility.

5. If allowed by the appropriate jurisdiction, practitioners may delegate to a designated agent certain portions of the physical act of writing or transmitting the prescription order.

B. Transmitting and receiving prescription drug orders

1. Pharmacists are the individuals authorized to receive prescription drug orders. In some states, certified pharmacy technicians are allowed to perform this function, provided there is a system in place that allows the pharmacist to review the prescription drug order as transmitted to the technician (9).

2. There are several methods allowed for transmitting prescription drug orders from practitioner to pharmacist:

   a. **Written** prescription drug orders may be used for any legal drugs, including controlled substances in Schedules II through V (9,10). See Chapter 3 of this book for additional information on prescription drug order regulations for controlled substances.

   b. In most states, orders by **electronic** transmission, facsimile or fax, and e-prescribing are acceptable for legal drugs and for controlled substances in Schedules III through V. Under certain prescribed circumstances, these methods may also be used for controlled substances in Schedule II (9,10). See applicable state statutes and federal laws for your practice area for regulations on transmitting prescription orders electronically.

    c. Verbal orders, including both face-to-face and telephone voice communication, are allowed for legal drugs and controlled substances in Schedules III through V. As with electronic orders, under certain prescribed circumstances, verbal orders may also be used for controlled substances in Schedule II (9,10). See applicable state statutes, federal laws, and Chapter 3 of this book for additional information on these regulations for controlled substances.

    (1) Traditionally it was the rule that verbal orders be "reduced to writing" immediately after receiving the order. With electronic record-keeping systems, this rule has been broadened; the NABP *Model Rules for the Practice of Pharmacy* now state that orders transmitted verbally or electronically "shall be immediately reduced **to a form** [emphasis added] by the Pharmacist or Certified Pharmacy Technician that may be maintained for the time required by laws or rules" (9).

    (2) Because verbal orders may easily be misunderstood, they are one source of medication errors. For this reason, current practice standards discourage the use of verbal orders except in urgent situations (11,12). Recent standards state that the person receiving the order **record and "read back"** [emphasis added] the complete order (11–13).

    d. Both written and verbal orders have been one source of medication errors. For this reason, various health care organizations have been working to establish for this area of practice standards that will minimize errors and ensure greater safety for patients. These standards and recommendations are discussed in section VI of this chapter.

III. OUTPATIENT PRESCRIPTION DRUG ORDERS

A. In addition to regulating who may prescribe and who may receive and process prescription drug orders, state statutes also spell out what information is required on these drug orders and what must be kept in records of dispensing.

B. Required information on prescription drug orders

    1. The information given in this section concerning recommended legal requirements for prescription drug orders comes from that section of the *Model State Pharmacy Act of the National Association of Boards of Pharmacy* entitled *Model Rules for the Practice of Pharmacy* (9). The NABP recommended elements are outlined below and are illustrated in Figures 1.1 and 1.2 and on the CD that accompanies this book. To learn the specific legal requirements for the state where you are practicing, consult the applicable state statutes. For the samples in Figures 1.1 and 1.2, the information printed in blue simulated handwriting type denotes those items that are normally entered on the prescription order by the prescriber. Those elements on the samples that are printed in black simulated handwriting are added by the pharmacist at the time of dispensing and are described in section D.

    a. Full name and address of the patient

    Note: If the patient is an animal, the full name is generally considered to include the animal's name, species, and owner.

CONTEMPORARY PHYSICIANS GROUP PRACTICE
20 S. PARK STREET, TRITURATE, WI 53706
TEL: (608) 555-1333 FAX: (608) 555-1335

℞ #   *123456*

NAME *John Doe*   **DATE** *00/00/00*

ADDRESS *123 N. Main Street*

℞   **RUGBY LABS**   *J.Thompson 00/00/00*

        Amoxicillin Capsules 250 mg   *#30*

    Sig: i cap tid for 10 days.

REFILLS <u>NR</u> 1 2 3 4 5   *Linus Ashman*   **M.D.**

             DEA NO. _____

FIGURE 1.1. PRESCRIPTION ORDER FOR A GENERIC DRUG PRODUCT.

CONTEMPORARY PHYSICIANS GROUP PRACTICE
20 S. PARK STREET, TRITURATE, WI 53706
TEL: (608) 555-1333 FAX: (608) 555-1335

℞ #   *123457*

NAME *Jane Doe*   **DATE** *00/00/00*

ADDRESS *123 N. Main Street*

℞   *J. Thompson 00/00/00*

                    Tylenol w/ Codeine   No. 3 Tablets #30

       Sig: i tab q 4-6 hr prn severe pain

REFILLS NR 1 2 3 4 5   *Lysander Coupe*   **M.D.**

NOTE: No red "C" – Record   **DEA NO.** *AC 3936199*

KEPT ELECTRONICALLY

FIGURE 1.2. PRESCRIPTION ORDER FOR A BRANDED, CONTROLLED SUBSTANCE DRUG PRODUCT.

  b. Date of issue
  c. Name and address of the prescriber
  d. Name, strength, dosage form, and quantity of the drug product prescribed
  e. Directions for use
  f. Refills authorized, if any
     Note: Accepted interpretation of refill, or lack of refill, information may be specified in state law. Common interpretations include the following:
     (1) For drug products available only on prescription, the absence of refill information usually means zero refills are authorized.
     (2) The number of allowed refills for controlled substances is specified in both state and federal law. Information on this topic can be found in Chapter 3 of this book and in the applicable laws.
     (3) The designation "prn" refills for prescription medications that are not controlled substances is limited to authorizing refills for 1 year, or other specified time period, from the date of issue.
  g. Prescriber's signature (written orders)
  h. For controlled substances, the following additional requirements apply:
     (1) DEA registration number of the prescriber
     (2) The **prescriber's signature is required** on all prescription orders for **Schedule II** drugs; however, most states allow oral or electronic transmission, including voice-telephoned prescription orders, for **Schedule II** medications in emergency situations, provided the quantity prescribed is limited and a written, signed document is received within a specified period, usually 7 days. Other federal restrictions on oral and electronic prescriptions for Schedule II drugs are covered in more detail in Chapter 3 of this book. Also, because the most stringent law (i.e., federal or state) always applies, check your current state statutes for the standard at your practice site.
2. Missing information
  a. If the prescriber neglects to include a required element, such as the patient address, the pharmacist may ascertain the missing information from pharmacy records or by asking the patient, the prescriber, or the agent of the patient or prescriber. The prescriber must be consulted concerning missing information on the drug, strength, quantity, or directions for use.
  b. The omission of some items of information by the prescriber, such as the date of issue on an order for a controlled substance, may render the order invalid.
3. Brand-generic substitution
  a. All states and the District of Columbia have laws that either allow or require pharmacists to substitute lower-priced generic products for brand-name products unless the prescriber or patient prohibits this (14). Accommodation for the state laws governing this practice is often found on the prescription document. For example, there may be check-off boxes wherein

the prescriber indicates "Brand medically necessary," "Do not substitute," "Dispense as written," "May use generic," or "Substitution Permitted." (For some examples of formats, see the sample prescription orders on the CD accompanying this book.)

    b. Regulations of generic substitution are complex and vary greatly from state to state. Furthermore, some private and government health insurance programs have policies with regard to the use of generic products, and patients and prescribers may be required to agree to these policies as a condition for participation in the program. It is important to be knowledgeable about the applicable generic substitution laws, regulations, and policies for your patients.

C. Essential activities before preparing the prescription

    1. When the patient or the caregiver hands the prescription order to the pharmacist (or, if permitted, to the certified pharmacy technician), the pharmacist should ask for information needed in preparing the prescription and label. For example, does the patient have any drug allergies; does he or she want a generic product for a prescribed branded product; can the patient or caregiver open child-resistant safety closures; can the patient swallow prescribed tablets or capsules; can the patient or caregiver read labels in English, etc. This information should be noted on the prescription order and may be added to the patient's medication profile record. More information on this part of the patient consultation process can be found in Chapter 6 of this book.

    2. Before filling the prescription order, the pharmacist must also review the prescription order for appropriateness of drug, dose, and dosing schedule. The pharmacy's medication profile record for the patient must be checked for such things as drug allergies, therapeutic duplication, drug-drug interactions, and drug-disease interactions. An example of a medication profile record is shown, and use of this type of record is illustrated on the CD that accompanies this book; it is also discussed in Chapter 5.

D. Records of dispensing

    1. At the time of dispensing a prescription, the pharmacist must make a record of the dispensing.

    2. The NABP Model Rules recommend that this information be kept by pharmacies for 5 years (15), and some other authorities suggest that it be kept for at least the time of state and federal statute of limitations. This period varies with the type of offense alleged, with 2 years from the date of injury for civil negligence suits and up to 5 or 6 years for felony offenses (16).

    3. It is recommended that, because the prescription order is a legal document, information on it should be written in ink or indelible pencil or be typed. The ink requirement is specified in the law only for legal requirements on prescription orders for controlled substances in Schedule II, but the use of ink is prudent practice for information recorded on all prescription orders.

    4. The elements listed below and printed in black simulated handwriting on the samples in Figures 1.1 and 1.2 are the items recommended or required for inclusion in the dispensing record (15). Some of these items are now kept by pharmacies in their computer system and, if recorded in this way, it is not required that they be entered directly on the hard copy of the prescription document. Some dispensing computer systems print a "sticker" that has the required information, and this can be attached to the front or back of the prescription order document.

        a. Quantity dispensed, original and all refills, if different from that prescribed

        b. Dispensing pharmacist's identification

        c. Date of dispensing

        d. Retrieval designation (e.g., serial number of the prescription order)

        e. Brand name or manufacturer of manufactured drug products prescribed generically
           Note: In Figure 1.1, the prescriber ordered amoxicillin. At the time of dispensing, the pharmacist specified the manufacturer of the brand dispensed (Rugby Labs in this example).

        f. Record of all refills

        g. For controlled substances, additional dispensing records are required to permit the identification and retrieval of prescription orders for controlled substances. These requirements are part of the federal Controlled Substances Act of 1970, described in more detail in Chapter 3 of this book.

    5. Additional information is kept by some pharmacies either directly on the prescription document or in their computer system. Examples include lot numbers and expiration dates of the products dispensed. This information is useful for getting in touch with affected patients in cases of drug product recalls from manufacturers and the U.S. Food and Drug Administration (FDA).

IV.   INPATIENT MEDICATION ORDERS

A. Inpatient medication orders are used to order medications for persons who are patients in hospitals, nursing homes, or other institutional settings. In this case, rather than using individual prescription drug order forms, these orders are entered into the patient's chart or medical record together with all other practitioner orders for such things as nursing care, laboratory tests, x-rays, and the like. Some sample inpatient medication orders are given in Figure 1.3 and on the CD that accompanies this book.

B. Although there are no legal requirements for information to be included on medication orders for inpatients, there are recommendations for good practice. Some institutions have written requirements in their policy and procedure manuals.

C. The items listed here are those recommended for medication orders in the *ASHP Technical Assistance Bulletin on Hospital Drug Distribution and Control* that is published by the American Society of Health-System Pharmacy (ASHP) (17). (Available on the ASHP Internet site, http://www.ashp.org/, Accessed December 2007.)

1. Patient name

2. Patient location (i.e., room and bed number)

3. Date and time of order

4. Name (generic) of medication

5. Dosage with quantity expressed (when possible, in the metric system)

6. Route of administration

7. Frequency of administration

8. Signature of prescriber for written orders; for verbal orders, the document states that the order as taken by the pharmacist or nurse should be immediately reduced to writing and should be countersigned by the prescriber within 48 and, if possible, 24 hours.

MEDICAL CENTER HOSPITAL
TRITURATE, WISCONSIN 53706

PATIENT ORDERS

PATIENT NAME   *David John*

HISTORY NUMBER   *120579*   **ROOM NUMBER**   *430*

WEIGHT   *125 lb*   **HEIGHT**   *5' 9"*

AGE   *62 y.o.*

ATTENDING PHYSICIAN   *R. Farrell*

DATE	TIME	ORDERS
00/00/00	1300	10,000 units Heparin Sodium in 250 mL N.S. Infuse IV over 4 hr.
		R. Farrell M.D.
		J. Thompson 0/00/00
00/00/00	1600	Penicillin G K IM Inj. Give 200,000 units stat then 100,000 units q 4 hr.
		R. Farrell M.D.
		J. Thompson 0/00/00
00/00/00	1400	Morphine sulfate 10 mg and Atropine sulfate 0.4 mg Injection Give IM On call for surgery at 0800 on 00/00/00.
		R. Farrell M.D.
		J. Thompson 0/00/00

FIGURE 1.3. INPATIENT MEDICATION ORDERS.

D. Other items recommended for the medication order include the patient's identification number (sometimes called the patient history number) and the date and time and initials of personnel who transcribe the order to the nursing and/or pharmacy records that are used to furnish and administer the medication to the patient.

V. RECORDS FOR COMPOUNDED DRUG ORDERS

A. Compounding records are essential quality control devices for this special type of prescription drug order. They make it easier for the pharmacist or technician who is preparing a refill of the prescribed drug preparation to make an identical preparation, they minimize errors and facilitate tracking if there are problems with a compounded preparation, and they enable the pharmacist to make appropriate alterations in the formulation based on feedback from the patient about the acceptability of the preparation.

B. **Compounding records**
1. Traditionally, especially when compounding was done infrequently, pharmacists recorded information concerning compounding components, amounts, and procedures directly on the prescription drug order.
2. Current standards recommend recording this information on separate control and/or formula sheets that are cross-referenced on the prescription drug order or electronic record of dispensing. Recommendations for records of compounding can be found in (a) *Good Compounding Practices Applicable to State Licensed Pharmacies*, which is part of the *Model State Pharmacy Act of the National Association of Boards of Pharmacy* (18); (b) *ASHP Technical Assistance Bulletin on Compounding Nonsterile Products in Pharmacies* (available on the ASHP Internet site, http://www.ashp.org/ under Practice and Policy Resources, Accessed December 2007); and (c) *USP/NF* chapters ⟨795⟩ Pharmaceutical Compounding–Nonsterile Preparations, ⟨797⟩ Pharmaceutical Compounding–Sterile Preparations, ⟨1075⟩ Good Compounding Practices, and ⟨1163⟩ Quality Assurance in Pharmaceutical Compounding. This topic is discussed in detail in Chapter 12 of this book, and multiple examples of prescription orders with compounding records that comply with these recommendations are given in the dosage form chapters.
3. Since some states may have specific recordkeeping requirements for compounded prescriptions, consult the applicable state laws or regulations for the state in which you practice.

VI. RECOMMENDED PRACTICES TO PREVENT MEDICATION ERRORS IN DRUG ORDERS

A. Medication errors have long been recognized as a major problem in providing safe and effective medication to patients. Though the problem was brought into the national spotlight in 1999 with the Institute of Medicine report, *To Err Is Human*, such organizations as the Institute for Safe Medication Practices (ISMP) and United States Pharmacopeia (USP) have had long-standing initiatives to learn about and reduce medication errors (19,20). Progress in reducing medication errors is considered essential to ensuring the five basic "rights" of patients in receiving drug therapy: the right drug in the right dose by the right route of administration to the right patient at the right time.

B. **Medication Errors Reporting (MER) Program and National Coordinating Council for Medication Error Reporting and Prevention (NCC MERP)** In 1991, the USP and the ISMP founded the Medication Errors Reporting (MER) Program to monitor and learn about the causes of medication errors. Then, in 1995, recognizing that medication errors were both a serious and interdisciplinary problem, USP and ISMP, together with 13 national health care organizations, founded the National Coordinating Council for Medication Error Reporting and Prevention (NCC MERP), a public/private group of national organizations with the purpose of using an interdisciplinary and collaborative approach to reducing medication errors in health care delivery (21). The Council (expanded to 23 organizations by 2007) maintains an Internet Web site at http://www.nccmerp.org with the latest recommendations that this interdisciplinary group has developed. The NCC MERP has three main objectives: understanding, reporting, and preventing medication errors (21).

C. **Recommendations to improve written prescription and medication orders** One project of the NCC MERP has been to develop recommendations to foster safer prescription writing. Originally written in 1996 and revised in 2005, they are summarized here (22). (Updates are published on the NCC MERP Internet site.)
1. **All written prescription or medication orders must be legible, and verbal orders should be minimized.** In reviewed reports of the USP MER Program, illegible handwriting on prescription and

Table 1.1	POTENTIALLY DANGEROUS AND ERROR-PRONE MEDICAL ABBREVIATIONS AND SYMBOLS		
ABBREVIATION/SYMBOL	**INTENDED MEANING**	**POSSIBLE MISINTERPRETATION**	**WRITE INSTEAD**
@	at	Misread as the number 2	"at"
> and <	greater than and less than	Confused for one another	"greater than" and "less than"
μg	microgram	Misread as mg (milligram)	"mcg" or "microgram"
/ (slash mark)	per; divided by (in a fraction)	Misread as the number 1; in a fraction (4/5), misinterpreted as a decimal point (4.5)	"per" (for fractions, write four-fifths or the decimal equivalent (0.8))
&	and	Misread as a number 2 or 4	"and"
+	plus; and	Misread as a number 4	"plus" or "and"
°	hour	Misread as a number zero	"hour"
×5d	times or for 5 days	Misinterpreted as times or for 5 doses	"for 5 days"
Abbreviations for drug names	Various	Confuse for another drug with a similar name	Write out drug name
Apothecary symbols	Various	Confusion over the meaning, e.g., minim misinterpreted as mL, dram misread as a number 3	Use metric units
AU, AS, AD	both ears, left ear, right ear	Misinterpreted as OU (both eyes), OS (left eye) OD (right eye)	"both ears," "left ear," "right ear"
cc	cubic centimeter	Misread as "u" (unit)	"mL"
D/C	either discontinue or discharge	Confused for one another	"discontinue" or "discharge"
HS or hs	bedtime or half-strength	Confused for one another	"bedtime" or "half-strength." For bedtime, specify "for one dose" or "nightly"
IU*	International unit	Misread as IV or the number 10	"International Unit"
MS, MSO$_4$, or MgSO$_4$*	Either magnesium sulfate or morphine sulfate	Confused for one another	"magnesium sulfate" or "morphine sulfate"
"Naked" decimal point (.5 mg)*	0.5 mg	Decimal point is not seen with 10-fold overdose	Write 0.5 mg or 500 mcg
Numbers at or above 1,000 without commas, e.g., 10000, 1000000	10,000, 1,000,000	Misread number of zeros with a 10-fold error in amount	Use commas for numbers at or above 1,000
Omitting spaces between drug name, strength, and unit, e.g. Propranolol20mg or Propranolol 20mg	Propranolol 20 mg	Misread as Propranolol 120 mg or Propranolol 200mg (last "l" in drug name read as a one; "m" in mg read as a zero)	Place adequate space between drug name, strength, and unit of measure
OU, OS, OD	both eyes, left eye, right eye	Misinterpreted as AU (both ears), AS (left ear) AD (right ear)	"both eyes," "left eye," "right eye"
qhs	nightly at bedtime	Misread as qhr (every hour)	"nightly at bedtime"
Q.D., QD, q.d., or qd*	daily	Misread as qid (four times daily) or qod (every other day)	"daily"

Table 1.1	POTENTIALLY DANGEROUS AND ERROR-PRONE MEDICAL ABBREVIATIONS AND SYMBOLS *(Continued)*		
ABBREVIATION/SYMBOL	**INTENDED MEANING**	**POSSIBLE MISINTERPRETATION**	**WRITE INSTEAD**
Q.O.D., QOD, q.o.d., or qod*	every other day	Misread as qid (four times daily) or qd (daily)	"every other day"
SC, SQ, or sub q	subcutaneous	Misinterpreted as sublingual; "q" misinterpreted as "every"	"subcut" or "subcutaneously"
SID (veterinary practice)	once a day	Misread as 5ID (5 times a day)	"daily"
TIW	3 times a week	Misinterpreted as three times a day or two times a week	"3 times weekly"
Trailing zero after decimal point (5.0 mg)*	5 mg	Decimal point is not seen with 10-fold overdose	5 mg
U or u*	unit	Misread as a zero with a 10-fold overdose	"unit"

*On the JCAHO Do Not Use list.
Source: Documents published by USP, NCC MERP, JCAHO, FDA, and ISMP.[22–28]

medication orders was a widely recognized cause of medication errors. Verbal orders are considered to be so potentially problematic that the NCC MERP has published an additional set of recommendations specifically addressing this topic (see section D that follows). Because of the inherent difficulty in reading individual handwriting and miscommunication with verbal orders, the Council has encouraged progress toward direct, computerized medication and prescription order entry systems.

2. **Prescribers should avoid the use of abbreviations.** Both for drug names and Latin directions for use. The abbreviations that the NCC MERP found to be particularly dangerous are included in the list of potentially dangerous and error-prone abbreviations given in Table 1.1. Additional information on this topic is given below in section E on medical abbreviations.

3. **All prescriptions and medications orders should be written using the metric system.** Excepted are those therapies that use standard units, such as insulin and some vitamins and antibiotics. The apothecary and avoirdupois systems were singled out as archaic systems using symbols easily misinterpreted. Furthermore, these older systems often require conversions and calculations that provide an additional and unnecessary potential for error.

4. **Prescribers should provide the age and, when appropriate, weight of the patient.** This information, especially for pediatric and geriatric patients, can aid the pharmacist, nurse, or other health care provider in checking appropriateness of drug and dose. Generally, this information is not written on the prescription order, but it should be available on the pharmacy's medication profile record for patients or, for inpatients, their chart record.

5. **The prescription or medication order should include the drug name, metric weight or concentration, and dosage form.** The pharmacist should check with the prescriber if any information is missing or questionable.

6. **A leading zero should always precede a decimal point in quantities less than 1, and a trailing zero should never be used after a decimal point.** That is, in the leading zero case, write 0.25 mg, not .25 mg, because if the decimal point is not seen, 25 mg would be given rather than the desired 0.25 mg. In the trailing zero case, write 250 mg, not 250.0 mg because, once again, if the decimal point is not seen, a tenfold dose error would occur.

7. **Prescription and medication orders should include, when possible, a notation of purpose of the medication.** This gives the provider of the medication a useful double-check for the appropriateness of the drug and dose. The Council recognized that there may be instances in which

confidentiality issues warrant the omission of this information. However, if this information is not written on the order, the pharmacist should always discretely ask the patient about the intended use of the medication. This provides an important safeguard, especially for drugs that have names that look or sound alike.

8. Prescribers should not use imprecise instructions, such as "Take as directed" or "Take as needed." Even if the patient has been given more exact verbal instructions, these may be forgotten or misinterpreted. Precise directions for use also aid the pharmacist in checking the appropriateness of the dose and in providing a useful medication consultation to the patient. When written orders are vague, the pharmacist should check with the prescriber (22).

D. **Recommendations for verbal orders** As discussed previously in this chapter, verbal orders may easily be misunderstood and have been one source of medication errors. Eliminating miscommunications of this sort is one of the National Patient Safety Goals as set by the Joint Communication on Accreditation of Healthcare Organizations (JCAHO or The Joint Commission). National Patient Safety Goals have been published yearly since 2003 and are available on The Joint Commission Internet site. The NCC MERP also developed a document addressing this issue, "Recommendations to Reduce Medication Errors Associated with Verbal Medication Orders and Prescriptions" (12). The following gives a brief synopsis of the recommendations; for a complete review of the topic, visit the NCC MERP Internet site.

1. Verbal orders should be used only in urgent situations when written or electronic orders are not practicable.
2. Health care organizations, including pharmacies and prescriber's offices, should analyze their use of verbal orders and develop policies for their safe and appropriate use.
3. Health care organizations should foster an environment in which it is acceptable for pharmacists and nurses to ask questions of prescribers about verbal orders, and any questions should be resolved before giving the prescribed medication to the patient.
4. Because antineoplastic agents have narrow safety margins, verbal orders should never be permitted for these drugs.
5. All of the usual required elements of a written prescription order should be given with the verbal order.
6. When possible, the person receiving the order should write it down and then read the order back to the prescriber. This recommendation mirrors that in the JCAHO 2007 Patient Safety Goals (13). In addition, the NCC MERP document recommends the following:
   a. The drug name should be verified either by spelling, by giving both the brand and generic name, or by giving the indication for use.
   b. If there is any possibility for misunderstanding, numbers in doses should be verified (e.g., say "thirty milligrams, that is three zero milligrams," to distinguish that number from 13 milligrams).
   c. Abbreviations should not be used (e.g., say "one tablet four times daily" rather than "one tablet qid").
7. The order should be immediately written down in the patient's chart or on a prescription drug order, and the order should be signed or initialed by the person taking the order.
8. For inpatient orders, the verbal order should be reviewed and signed by the prescriber as soon as possible (12). [The ASHP recommends that this be done in 48 or, if possible, 24 hours (17).]

E. **Medical abbreviations and symbols**

1. As can be seen in Figures 1.1 through 1.3 and in the various examples in this book and the accompanying CD, many abbreviations and symbols are used in writing prescription and medication orders.
2. Appendix A gives a very brief list of some commonly used abbreviations with a longer list on the CD that accompanies this book. For a more complete compilation, consult one of the published books of medical abbreviations, such as *Medical Abbreviations: 24,000 Conveniences at the Expense of Communications and Safety*, by Dr. Neil M. Davis or one of the free Internet sites, such as Global RPh Inc (http://www.globalrph.com/abbrev.htm), Accessed December 2007. An Internet search using the words "Medical Abbreviations" will give you numerous other current sources of this information.
3. The use of this sort of shorthand, while perhaps time-saving for the writer, has been widely criticized because of the possibility of confusion or misinterpretation with resulting errors

when furnishing medications to patients. Various health care organizations, such as the NCC MERP, JCAHO, ISMP, USP, and FDA, have monitored this source of medication errors and have actively discouraged the use of problematic abbreviations. Each of these organizations has published and/or posted (on their Internet site) lists of abbreviations considered to be potentially dangerous or error-prone.

4. The Joint Commission has published and posted on its Internet site a list of **prohibited** abbreviations; institutions that it accredits must show good faith and progress toward eliminating the use of these abbreviations in their facilities. The Joint Commission also requires facilities to formulate and publish a list of abbreviations, acronyms, symbols, and dose designations that are not to be used in the organization (11,13,23).

5. A list of problematic abbreviations is given in Table 1.1. More complete lists can be found on the Internet Web sites of the NCC MERP (22), JCAHO (23), ISMP (24,25), USP (26), and FDA (25,27,28). The CD that accompanies this book has some practice activities with prescription orders that contain potentially dangerous abbreviations.

F. **Sound-alike, look-alike drug names** Drug products that have names that look and/or sound alike have also been recognized as potential sources of medication errors.

1. Confusion over medications with similar names, written or spoken, was reported to account for a significant number (15%–25%) of all reports to the USP MER Program (12,29,30).

2. Although the FDA and pharmaceutical manufacturers make a concerted effort to avoid and eliminate this problem through the careful selection of both brand and generic names for drugs, problems still exist. In an effort to provide more visual differentiation of the established names of particularly problematic drug pairs with look-alike names, the FDA has asked manufacturers of these drugs to use "Tall Man" letters on their labels. An example would be vin-BLAStine and vinCRIStine (31).

3. Lists of drugs with similar names—look-alike and sound-alike drug pairs—are available. It is helpful for prescribers, pharmacists, and pharmacy technicians to be familiar with those drug names that have caused confusion so that special caution is used when dealing with these medications.

   a. The USP periodically publishes a current list of drug names that have caused confusion as reported to the MER Program (29,30 32). A copy of the most current list can be printed from the USP Web site by accessing issues of *USP Quality Review* that are archived under Patient Safety, Newsletters.

   b. The journal *Hospital Pharmacy* also periodically publishes wall charts that list look-alike or sound-alike drug names. These charts can be purchased through their Internet Web site at http://www.factsandcomparisons.com/Products, Accessed May 2007.

   c. Similar lists are published and posted on the Internet Web sites of The Joint Commission and the ISMP. The CD that accompanies this book has some practice activities with prescription orders that contain some sound-alike/look-alike drug names.

4. Confusion with look-alike/sound-alike drug names has been found to be aggravated by the following factors (32):

   a. Illegible handwriting on prescription or medication orders

   b. Lack of information or incomplete knowledge of drug names or products, especially newly available products with which pharmacists, nurses, or technicians are not yet familiar

   c. Similar packaging, labeling, or product strengths

   d. Dispensing software systems that employ computerized drug product lists that make incorrect selection of a product with a similar name more likely. This is exacerbated by the fact that most dispensing software systems use mnemonics, several letter abbreviations for long drug names (e.g., CPZ for chlorpromazine), that can easily be confused or used incorrectly for another drug name.

5. Mix-ups of drug products with names that look or sound alike can be minimized by the following practices:

   a. Being familiar with error-prone drug pairs from lists of sound-alike/look-alike drugs

   b. Determining from the prescriber or patient the therapeutic intent of the product prescribed

   c. Encouraging prescribers to indicate both the generic and brand names on prescription orders for drug products with confusing names

   d. On pharmacy shelves, stocking drug products with confusing names or strengths in such a way that they are separated or well-marked so as to alert pharmacy staff to exercise special caution in product selection

   e. Providing patients with consultations that include the brand and generic names and the therapeutic use of the product (11)

G. **Tracking and analyzing medication errors** In order to track, monitor, and analyze the incidence of medication errors from a systems viewpoint, health care professionals are encouraged to report medication errors or potential errors to one of the organizations that are collaborating to develop and maintain a national database on medication errors. There are several ways that the reporting can be done easily.

1. The USP operates two medication error–reporting programs, the MER Program and MedMARx. Each program can be accessed on the Internet through the USP's Web site at www.usp.org.

   a. The MER Program, operated in cooperation with the ISMP, is a spontaneous, voluntary reporting program that health care professionals can use to report medication errors to the USP. This can be done directly, online through the USP's Web site or by printing a report form from the Web site and mailing or faxing the report to the USP. Practitioners can also report by calling toll-free anytime: 1-800-23-ERROR. There is also a link to this program through the ISMP's Web site at www.ismp.org. Practitioners who report medication errors through this program are assured of confidentiality and may, if preferred, make their report anonymously. USP and ISMP staff members review these reports for any possible general patient safety concerns. Information from the reports is sent to the FDA and to the manufacturers of the drug product involved. The information is then added to the MER database for analysis of error type and cause.

   b. MedMARx is an internet-accessible program that enables participating hospitals to anonymously report and track medication errors for the purpose of internal quality improvement. The information is also entered into the USP's national database for analysis. Summary reports of information submitted through the MedMARx system have been available through the USP's Web site.

2. The FDA operates the MedWatch Program for the voluntary reporting of adverse events, product problems, and product use errors. This program is intended primarily for serious events, such as those that could cause permanent impairment, hospitalization, or death. Reports can be made through the FDA Internet site at http://www.fda.gov with a link to MedWatch.

3. The FDA also operates a voluntary drug problem–reporting program for veterinary products. Reports can be made through the FDA Internet site at http://www.fda.gov/cvm/ADEFAQs.htm.

REFERENCES

1. Model State Pharmacy Act and Model Rules of the National Association of Boards of Pharmacy. National Association of Boards of Pharmacy, Mount Prospect, IL, 2007; 1–2.
2. Model State Pharmacy Act and Model Rules of the National Association of Boards of Pharmacy. National Association of Boards of Pharmacy, Mount Prospect, IL, 2007; 6.
3. Model State Pharmacy Act and Model Rules of the National Association of Boards of Pharmacy. National Association of Boards of Pharmacy, Mount Prospect, IL, 2007; 14.
4. Model State Pharmacy Act and Model Rules of the National Association of Boards of Pharmacy. National Association of Boards of Pharmacy, Mount Prospect, IL, 2007; 14–15.
5. Model State Pharmacy Act and Model Rules of the National Association of Boards of Pharmacy. National Association of Boards of Pharmacy, Mount Prospect, IL, 2007; 4.
6. Model State Pharmacy Act and Model Rules of the National Association of Boards of Pharmacy. National Association of Boards of Pharmacy, Mount Prospect, IL, 2007; 12.
7. Model State Pharmacy Act and Model Rules of the National Association of Boards of Pharmacy. National Association of Boards of Pharmacy, Mount Prospect, IL, 2007; 4.
8. Pharmacist Scope of Practice. American College of Physicians–American Society of Internal Medicine. Ann Intern Med. 2002; 136: 84.
9. Model State Pharmacy Act and Model Rules of the National Association of Boards of Pharmacy. National Association of Boards of Pharmacy, Mount Prospect, IL, 2006; 78.
10. 21 CFR § 1306.11 and 1306.21.
11. Look-alike/sound-alike drug list updated for 2006–2007, JCAHO, Oakbrook Terrace, IL, 2007; 12–13. http://www.jointcommission.org/PatientSafety/NationalPatientSafetyGoals/. Accessed December 2007.
12. NCC MERP Recommendations to Reduce Medication Errors Associated with Verbal Medication Orders and Prescriptions, Feb. 24, 2006. http://www.nccmerp.org/council/council2001-02-20.html. Accessed December 2007
13. 2007 National Patient Safety Goals, JCAHO, Oakbrook Terrace, IL, 2007. http://www.jointcommission.org/PatientSafety/National PatientSafetyGoals/. Accessed December 2007.
14. Parker RE, Martinez D, Covington TR. Drug Product Selection—Part 1: History and Legal Overview. Am Pharm 1991; 31:72.
15. Model State Pharmacy Act and Model Rules of the National Association of Boards of Pharmacy. National Association of Boards of Pharmacy, Mount Prospect, IL, 2006; 88.
16. Fink JL, III, Vivian JC, Bernstein IBG, eds. Pharmacy law digest, 39th ed. St. Louis: Facts and Comparisons, Inc., 2004; 46.
17. American Society of Hospital Pharmacists. ASHP technical assistance bulletin on hospital drug distribution and control. Am J Hosp Pharm. 1980; 37: 1097–1103.
18. Model State Pharmacy Act and Model Rules of the National Association of Boards of Pharmacy. National Association of Boards of Pharmacy, Mount Prospect, IL, 2007; 207–216.
19. About ISMP. http://www.ismp.org/about/. Accessed December 2007.

20. USP Quality Review No. 67. Rockville, MD: The United States Pharmacopeial Convention, Inc., June 1999.
21. About NCC MERP. http://www.nccmerp.org/. Accessed December 2007.
22. NCC MERP Recommendations to Enhance Accuracy of Prescription Writing, June 2, 2005. http://www.nccmerp.org/council/council1996-09-04.html. Accessed December 2007.
23. Official "Do Not Use" Abbreviations List. http://www.jointcommission. org/PatientSafety/DoNotUseList/. Accessed March 2007.
24. Error-Prone Abbreviations List. http://www.ismp.org. Accessed December 2007.
25. ISMP and FDA Campaign to Eliminate Use of Error-Prone Abbreviations. http://www.ismp.org/tools/abbreviations. Accessed December 2007.
26. USP Quality Review No. 80. Rockville, MD: The United States Pharmacopeial Convention, Inc., July 2004.
27. FDA and ISMP Launch Campaign to Reduce Medication Mistakes Caused by Unclear Abbreviations. http://www.fda.gov/bbs/topics/NEWS/2006/NEW01390.html.
28. Medication Errors. http://www.fda.gov/cder/drug/MedErrors.
29. USP Quality Review No. 66. Rockville, MD: The United States Pharmacopeial Convention, Inc., May 1999.
30. USP Quality Review No. 76. Rockville, MD: The United States Pharmacopeial Convention, Inc., Mar. 2001.
31. Errors, FDA Consumer Magazine, July-Aug 2005. http://www.fda.gov/fdac/features/2005/405_confusion.html. Accessed February 2007.
32. USP Quality Review No. 79. Rockville, MD: The United States Pharmacopeial Convention, Inc., Apr. 2004.

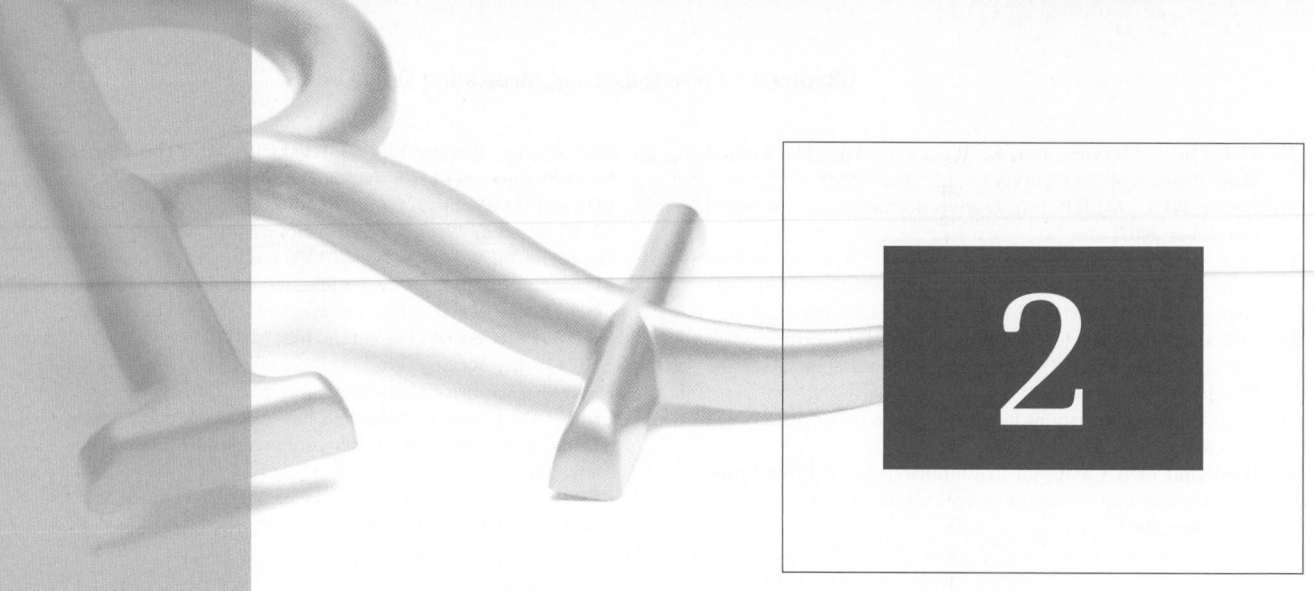

Labeling Prescriptions and Medications

I. DEFINITIONS

A. The terms "labeling" and "label" are defined differently for manufactured drug products and for products dispensed by the pharmacist to a patient on a prescription order.

B. Labeling and labels for manufactured drug products

    1. For manufactured drug products, both the Federal Food, Drug, and Cosmetic Act and the *United States Pharmacopeia* (*USP*) define and differentiate the terms "labeling" and "label" as follows. The term "labeling" is used for all labels and other written, printed, or graphic matter both upon the immediate container of a drug product or in any package or wrapper in which it is enclosed, except any outer shipping container. The term "label" designates just that part of the labeling that appears upon the immediate container (1,2).

    2. Labeling and labels of manufactured drug products are strictly controlled by the U.S. Food and Drug Administration (FDA).

C. Labeling and labels for dispensed drug products

    1. The NABP *Model State Pharmacy Act* defines the terms "label" and "labeling" for the purpose of pharmacist dispensing of drug products to patients as follows:

        a. Label: "A display of written, printed, or graphic matter upon the immediate container of any Drug or Device" (3).

        b. Labeling: "The process of preparing and affixing a label to any Drug container exclusive, however, of the Labeling by a Manufacturer, packer, or Distributor of a Non-Prescription Drug or commercially packaged Legend Drug or Device" (3).

    2. The information on the labels of prescription drug containers dispensed to ambulatory patients is regulated by both state and federal laws. These regulations also apply to drug containers dispensed to inpatients who will self-administer their drugs.

3. Information on labels for drug products that will be administered by health professionals, such as physicians or nurses, to inpatients in such facilities as hospitals and nursing homes is not specified in federal law. At one time, this label information was also not regulated by state laws; rather, various health care organizations recommended label and labeling standards for inpatient drugs. More recently, the NABP's *Model Rules for the Practice of Pharmacy* have recommended that state laws specify the required elements for labels on drug products for inpatients. Consult the applicable state laws for your practice area for regulations on dispensed drug product labels for inpatients.

II. LABELS FOR OUTPATIENT PRESCRIPTION ORDERS

A. **Required information on labels for outpatient prescriptions**
1. The Federal Food, Drug, and Cosmetic Act requires that drug products dispensed on prescription order be labeled with "the name and the address of the dispenser, the serial number and the date of the prescription or of its filling, the name of the prescriber, and, if stated in the prescription, the name of the patient, and directions for use and cautionary statements, if any, contained in such prescription" (4).
2. State laws have additional requirements for outpatient prescription labels. The pharmacist must label the dispensed drug product with those items specified in the federal law plus any additional state requirements.
3. As with prescription drug orders, the NABP *Model Rules for the Practice of Pharmacy* contain recommendations for state statutes on required items of information for the prescription product label (5). These are listed below and are illustrated in the label examples shown in Figures 2.1 and 2.2. The labels correspond to the prescription orders given in Figures 1.1 and 1.2 of Chapter 1. Additional samples are given on the CD that accompanies this book and in the prescription examples in the dosage forms chapters of the book. For the specific standards for your practice site, consult the applicable state law.
   a. Name and address of the pharmacy that dispensed the drug
   b. Name of the patient; if the patient is an animal, the species of animal and the owner's name
   c. Name of the prescriber
   d. Directions for use as given on the prescription order
   e. Date dispensed
   f. Cautionary statements, if any
   g. Serial number of prescription
   h. Name or initial of the dispensing pharmacist
   i. Name (proprietary or generic) and strength of drug product dispensed; special requirements with regard to the name of the product may apply if an equivalent drug product is dispensed (i.e., generic substitution for a branded product)
   j. Name of the manufacturer or distributor of the product dispensed
   k. The beyond-use date of the product (5)

PRACTICAL PHARMACY
425 S. CHARTULAE STREET
TRITURATE, WI 53706
(608) 555-1200 FAX: (608) 555-1210

℞ 123457   Pharmacist: JET   Date: 00/00/00
John Doe   Dr. Lysander Coupe
Take one tablet every four to six hours as needed for severe pain

Tylenol w/Codeine No. 3 Tablets

Mfg: McNeil Labs   Quantity: 30
Refills: 1

Discard after: 00/00/00

PRACTICAL PHARMACY
425 S. CHARTULAE STREET
TRITURATE, WI 53706
(608) 555-1200 FAX: (608) 555-1210

℞ 123456   Pharmacist: JET   Date: 00/00/00
John Doe   Dr. Linus Ashman
Take one capsule three times daily for ten days.

Amoxicillin 250 mg. Capsules

Mfg: Rugby Labs   Quantity: 30
Refills: 0

Discard after: 00/00/00

FIGURE 2.1. PRESCRIPTION LABEL FOR A GENERIC DRUG PRODUCT.

Auxiliary Labels: May Cause Drowsiness; Alcohol and Operating Car or Machine Warning
Federal "Do Not Transfer" label

FIGURE 2.2. PRESCRIPTION LABEL FOR A BRANDED, CONTROLLED SUBSTANCE DRUG PRODUCT.

Note: Some dispensing software automatically puts a 1-year beyond-use date on the label. The pharmacist or pharmacy technician must verify that this date is within the expiration date given on the container of the product dispensed. For more information on expiration and beyond-use dates, see Chapter 4 of this book.

4. Although most of the previously mentioned elements are fairly standard from state to state, there is considerable variation in state regulations governing the required label information when dispensing equivalent drug products (i.e., generic substitution for a branded or proprietary product). The NABP's Model Rules recommend the use of the word "INTERCHANGE" or the letters "IC" on labels when an equivalent product is dispensed (5). Some states require just the generic name or the name given the generic product by the generic manufacturer or distributor; other states want words to the effect of "generic name equivalent to brand name." This is an attempt to inform the patient without infringing on company trademarks, such as brand names. It would not be legal to label one company's product with another company's brand name.

5. For controlled substances in Schedules II through IV, the following auxiliary label is required: "Caution: Federal law prohibits the transfer of this drug to any person other than the patient for whom it was prescribed."

6. Some states have additional requirements for the label. Examples include quantity dispensed, number of refills, and date of the original prescription drug order. It is the duty of each pharmacist to be informed about the specific legal requirements for labels on dispensed drug products for the state in which he or she is practicing.

B. Computerized dispensing software, created for a national market, is now used extensively for generating prescription labels. Although label software may include additional nonrequired information, it is important that pharmacists ensure that, at a minimum, all label elements required by their state law are included in the dispensing software package purchased for their practice.

C. Three of the labeling requirements merit additional discussion: (i) directions for use, (ii) name of the product/dosage form/ingredients, and (iii) strength or quantity of product or ingredients.

1. **Directions for use**

   a. The directions for use should be written in clear, concise English using terminology that the general public (including patients with minimal education) understands. Avoid such abbreviations as BP, GI, and SOB and medical terms that the patient may not understand. For patients who do not speak English, be certain that they understand how to use their medication. Some dispensing software programs have options for labels in languages (e.g., Spanish) in addition to English. For complex dosage forms, such as inhalers, use a combination of the standard dispensing label, printed product instructions, with picture illustrations if available, and, when appropriate, demonstration of dosing techniques by the pharmacist. For more information on this topic, see Chapter 6 of this book.

   b. Although the directions for use should be as close as possible to those on the prescription order, the pharmacist may—and in fact should—clarify indefinite instructions as long as the intent of the prescriber is not changed.

   c. Vague labeling instructions, such as "Take as directed" or "Take as needed," are not sufficient directions for use. They assume that the patient was given adequate additional oral instructions and that he or she had a correct interpretation and understanding of these instructions. Furthermore, such instructions rely on both the short-term and long-term memory of the patient. If vague instructions are given on the prescription order, the pharmacist should consult the prescriber for more specific instructions (6).

   d. Directions for use should be in complete sentences. The following format is a useful template for most circumstances.

Verb	Quantity	Dosage Form	Route	Frequency	Modifiers
Take	one	capsule	by mouth	three times a day	for 10 days.

   e. **Verb:** Use easily understood verbs, such as take, give, apply, insert, place, use, and put. Avoid outdated terms, such as "instill," unless you are certain the patient understands. For topical administration, the adverbs "topically" or "locally" are sometimes used, but these are optional and can be confusing to the patient. For example, what does it mean to "apply locally"?

   f. **Quantity:** Quantities are usually expressed as numbers, but they may also be descriptive adverbs, such as "lightly" or "in a thin layer."

      (1) Numbers, when part of the directions for use, should be spelled out whenever possible. This is a safety feature. Because the numbers are next to each other on the keyboard, it would be easy to type a "2" when a "3" is desired. A typing error made in spelling the number, such as tjree for three, would be detected easily, and the patient would not confuse the misspelling with another number.

(2) Fractions should also be written out, such as one-half or one-quarter rather than ½ or ¼.

(3) If numbers must be used, avoid trailing zeros (e.g., use 1 rather than 1.0) and "naked" decimal points (e.g., type 0.5 rather than .5) as described in section VI in Chapter 1.

g. Dosage form: Examples include tablets, capsules, suppositories, lotions, and drops.

(1) For oral liquids, the dosage form may be expressed as milliliters (mL) or common equivalents, such as teaspoonful or tablespoonful. Volume doses, such as teaspoons, should be written with the suffix "ful" (e.g., teaspoonful). Teaspoonfuls is the preferred plural of teaspoonful but, according to *Webster's New Collegiate Dictionary*, teaspoonsful is also acceptable.

(2) If the prescription is for a bulk powder, specify "level" (e.g., level teaspoonful).

(3) To avoid dosing errors, many pharmacists will include metric volumes along with household measurement terms, such as "Take one teaspoonful (5 mL) by mouth..."

h. Route of administration: The route of administration should be specified in most cases, including eye, ear, nose, rectum, vagina, and urethra.

(1) For topical skin preparations, the route of administration is often given as "affected area."

(2) For tablet and capsule medications given by mouth, the route is usually understood from the directions and is not required unless the prescriber has specifically written this in the directions for use. The words "by mouth" should always be included if there is any possibility of confusion. For example, the directions for use of an oral liquid antibiotic used for an ear infection should specify "by mouth" because otherwise the patient might think it should be put in the ear. Some states require the route of administration to be specified in all cases, including oral products.

(3) Specialty capsules and tablets that are used by routes of administration other than oral require specific labeling. For this reason, the *USP* states, "The label of any form of Capsule or Tablet intended for administration other than by swallowing intact bears a prominent indication of the manner in which it is to be used" (1).

i. Frequency: This refers to how often a patient should take or use the medication. This can be expressed as a number of times per day (e.g., once a day, two times a day, etc.) or hourly frequency (e.g., every eight hours, every four to six hours, etc). Some medications may need to be given at more specific times. For example, a prescription may state to take a drug one hour before each meal; another may state more specifically to take at 8 AM and at 1 PM.

j. Modifiers: Modifying phrases can be added for numerous purposes.

(1) As a safety feature, it is now highly recommended that whenever possible, the directions for use include the therapeutic intent of the medication (e.g., "for high blood pressure"). This is especially useful for patients who are on multiple medications. Of course, patient confidentiality concerns must always be respected.

(2) Modifiers are also used to affect the frequency of administration. The common modifier "as needed" is used frequently with pain medication prescriptions, such as "every four to six hours as needed for pain." Another example is stating that the medication should be taken for a certain number of days such as "for ten days." This is common for antibiotic prescriptions when the prescriber wants to ensure that the patient will complete the full course of treatment.

(3) Some prescribers will also include some patient education statements, such as "with food or meals" to help their patients avoid such side effects as stomach upset.

2. Names of products/dosage forms/ingredients

a. Recommended formats for identifying drug dosage forms are (i) name of the drug—route of administration—dosage form (e.g., Calcium Carbonate Oral Suspension, Cefazolin Ophthalmic Solution, Miconazole Topical Powder, etc.) and (ii) name of drug—dosage form (e.g., Digoxin Tablets, Diltiazem HCl Extended Release Capsules, and the like) (7). The first method has the advantage that it is specific and unambiguous with regard to the route of administration.

b. For manufactured products, when permitted by the applicable state law, prescriptions may be labeled either with the generic name or the brand name of the product dispensed, as long as the legal standard for trademarks is followed. As stated earlier under section A on required elements for prescription labels, there is considerable variation from state to state on label requirements for clear and full disclosure when dispensing equivalent drug products.

c. For branded combination products or official USP products or preparations with set formulations, the brand name or the official name of the product is sufficient because the ingredients are specified in the official or brand formula. An example of such a branded product would be Bactrim tablets, which contain Sulfamethoxazole 400 mg and Trimethoprim 80 mg. An example of an official *USP* preparation with a set formula is Salicylic Acid Collodion USP, which contains 10% Salicylic Acid in Flexible Collodion.

d. If a generic version of a fixed combination is dispensed, NABP Model Rules suggest use of USP official pharmacy equivalent names (PENs); however, in June 2002, the USP Expert Committee on Nomenclature and Labeling voted to remove PENs from the *USP* (8), and the organization has discontinued publishing lists of PENs. An example of a PEN was Co-spironozide Tablets for the combination of Spironolactone and Hydrochlorothiazide Tablets. The Expert Committee thought that these abbreviated names could cause confusion and might lead to medication errors. In the absence of official PENs, the NABP recommends that the pharmacist use professional judgment, "secundum artem," in labeling the active ingredients in combination products (5).

e. For prescription labeling, when the salt form is identified, chemical symbols for the common inorganic salts are permitted: HCl for hydrochloride, HBr for hydrobromide, Na for sodium, and K for potassium. However, by *USP* convention, when sodium or potassium appears at the beginning of a drug name, as for example sodium nitroprusside, the word rather than the chemical symbol is used (1).

f. The labeling of active ingredients and components of compounded preparations is discussed in section IV on labels for compounded preparations.

3. Strength or quantity of ingredients

a. When possible, the metric system of measurement should always be used.

b. For individual dosage forms (e.g., tablets, capsules, divided powders, lozenges, suppositories), the strength is expressed as a metric weight (or, when applicable, units) of each active ingredient per dosage unit (1).

c. For oral liquids and oral bulk powders, label either

(1) The quantity of active ingredient per standard volume (e.g., Amoxicillin Oral Suspension 250 mg per 5 mL [5 mL is the volume of a standard household teaspoon] or Digoxin Oral Solution 50 mcg per mL) or

(2) The quantity of active ingredient(s) per dosage volume specified in the directions for use on the label. For example, with directions of "Take one tablespoonful one hour after each meal," the label may specify the quantity of active ingredient as Calcium Carbonate Oral Suspension 20 mg per mL, 100 mg per 5 mL, or 300 mg per tablespoonful and/or per 15 mL.

d. The content of electrolytes for replacement therapy should be stated in milliequivalents (mEq) of the electrolyte(s). The metric weight or percentage concentration of the ingredient(s) providing the electrolyte should also be given (1). For example, potassium chloride capsules could be labeled as Potassium Chloride Capsules 10 mEq (800 mg). An example for a liquid product is Potassium Chloride Oral Solution 10%, 20 mEq per 15 mL.

e. It is recommended as a safety feature that labels for phosphorus supplements include the number of millimoles of phosphorus and the number of milliequivalents of potassium and/or sodium. For example, K-Phos Neutral Tablets would be labeled K Phos Neutral (phosphorus 8 mmol, potassium 1.1 mEq, and sodium 13 mEq) (9).

f. For topical products and preparations:

(1) The concentration usually is expressed as a percent using the conventions for percentage measurement as set down in the *USP* and described in Chapter 8 of this book.

(2) Some topical, ophthalmic, and otic products, particularly those containing antibiotics, are labeled in units or milligrams of active ingredient per gram of solid or semisolid or per milliliter of liquid product.

(3) Some drug preparations that are used in very dilute concentrations have traditionally been labeled in ratio strength. While this is acceptable, this practice has been discouraged because of possible confusion with that format. If using the ratio strength format, be sure to use commas for numbers of 1,000 or above.

g. The content of alcohol in a liquid dosage form should be stated as a percentage v/v of C_2H_5OH (1).

III.   LABELS FOR INPATIENT DRUG ORDERS

A. Required information on labels for drug products and preparations dispensed to inpatients

1. There are no federal legal requirements for labels on drug products dispensed to inpatients.

2. Although many states also do not have legal requirements for labels on dispensed drug products for inpatients, The *NABP Model Rules for the Practice of Pharmacy* does address this issue and gives recommendations for state statutes in this area of pharmacy practice (5). The Model Rules divide labeling of drug products for these patients into three types: (i) labels for single-unit packages, (ii) labels for multiple-dose containers, and (iii) labels for parenteral products and preparations. These three label types assume that the drug product is not in the possession of the patient until time of administration and that it will be administered to the patient by an appropriate health care professional in the facility. For drugs that are self-administered by inpatients, the label elements for outpatients apply.

a. The label for single-unit or unit-dose packages should include the following:

(1) Name (proprietary or generic) of the drug product

(2) Route of administration, unless oral

(3) Strength and, if applicable, volume of the product, expressed when possible in the metric system

(4) Control number and expiration date

(5) If repackaged, identification (name or license number) of the repackager

(6) Special storage conditions, if needed (5)

b. If a multiple-dose distribution system is used, the container should be labeled with the following:

(1) Identification of the dispensing pharmacy

(2) Patient's name

(3) Date of dispensing

(4) Name (proprietary or generic) of the drug product

(5) Strength, expressed when possible in the metric system (5)

c. Label information for parenteral products is briefly addressed by the *NABP Model Rules for the Practice of Pharmacy* (5). A more complete list of label recommendations has been published by the American Society for Health-System Pharmacists (10). The following list is a combination from both sources with the NABP recommendations starred (*). Sample labels using the elements from this list are illustrated in Figures 2.3 through 2.5, which correspond to the inpatient medication orders given in Figure 1.3 of Chapter 1. Some information listed below is optional on the label if it is easily retrieved from a preparation control log.

(1) For patient-specific preparations: the patient's name* and any other appropriate patient identification (e.g., location, identification or history number)

(2) Control or lot number*

(3) Bottle sequence number or other system control number*

(4) All solution names* and volumes*

(5) All additive names,* quantities,* and concentrations (when applicable)

(6) Date of preparation* (and time, when applicable)

(7) Beyond-use date* (and time, when applicable)

(8) Prescribed administration regimen, when appropriate (including infusion rate* and route of administration)

(9) Appropriate auxiliary labeling (including precautions*)

(10) Storage requirements

(11) Identification (e.g., initials) of the responsible pharmacist and, if applicable, the technician making the preparation

(12) Device-specific instructions (when appropriate)

(13) Any additional information, in accordance with state and federal requirements (5, 10)

David John   H.N. 120579   Rm 430   ℞ 105124

Morphine SO$_4$ 10 mg, Atropine SO$_4$ 0.4 mg per 2 mL

This syringe contains 0.1 mL excess for priming

On call for surgery at 0800 00/00/00   Give IM

Prepared 0700 00/00/00 JET   Control #000000-1

Do not use after 0900 00/00/00

FIGURE 2.3. PATIENT-SPECIFIC SYRINGE LABEL.

Control # 000000-2   Prepared: 00/00/00 1700 JET

Penicillin G K 200,000 units per mL   For IM use

Do not use after 00/02/00 1700

This syringe contains 0.1 mL excess for priming

Refrigerate, Do not freeze

FIGURE 2.4. BATCH-PREPARED SYRINGE LABEL.

```
┌─────────────────────────────────────────────┐
│                                               │
│             MEDICAL CENTER HOSPITAL           │
│             Triturate, Wisconsin 53706        │
│                                               │
│   David John    Rm 430            Bottle #1   │
│                                               │
│                                               │
│   History Number:. 120579     Control # 000000-3 │
│                                               │
│                                               │
│             Heparin Na 10,000 units           │
│                                               │
│                                               │
│   IN:  Sodium Chloride Injection 0.9%   250 mL │
│                                               │
│                                               │
│   Infuse           over 4 hours               │
│                    at 62 mL/hr                │
│                    10 drop/min using 10 drop/mL IV set │
│                                               │
│                                               │
│   Date/Time prepared:   00/00/00   1400   By: JET │
│   Do not use after:   00/01/00   1400   Checked: BJF │
│   Refrigerate; Do not Freeze                  │
│                                               │
└─────────────────────────────────────────────┘
```

FIGURE 2.5. PATIENT-SPECIFIC IV ADMIXTURE LABEL.

B. The following are additional guidelines for labeling pharmacy-prepared parenteral preparations:

1. Labels for parenteral preparations should be affixed on the container (e.g., syringe, or intravenous [IV] bag) such that the contents can be inspected, the volume can be identified, and the capacity markings can easily be read. Prior to administration, the preparation should always be inspected and verified by the nurse or other practitioner who is administering the parenteral preparation.

2. For large-volume parenterals, the name, type of solution, and lot number on the manufacturer's label should be visible. The pharmacy-prepared label should be positioned so that it can be read as the preparation is being administered. For example, the label should be upright when the IV is hanging. An exception to this rule would be for IV bags or syringes that are enclosed in infusion devices.

3. Abbreviations, such as KCl for potassium chloride, are permissible on labels for parenteral preparations because these labels are intended to be read by health professionals who are knowledgeable about such abbreviations.

4. When possible, the metric system of measurement should be used for additives. Exceptions include units for such drugs as heparin, insulin, and some antibiotics and milliequivalents (mEq) or millimoles (mmol) for certain electrolytes.

5. **For injections, the concentration,** not just the quantity of the drug, **must be specified** on the label. For example, "Atropine SO_4 0.4 mg" is not sufficient labeling for a syringe. The label must give a concentration, such as "Atropine SO_4 0.4 mg per mL." This is necessary because the person giving the dose to the patient must verify the dose and volume at the time of administration. It is recommended that the concentration be given as the quantity of active ingredient per specified volume in milliliters of one dose. This makes verification easier for the person administering the dose.

6. When excess volume is added to a syringe to allow for priming a needle or administration set prior to administration of the preparation, the label should state this fact (e.g., "This syringe contains 0.1 mL excess to prime needle"). Because desired priming volume may vary by institution, by nursing unit within an institution, by drug solution to be administered, and by route of administration (e.g., intramuscular [IM] versus IV), the pharmacist should always verify the desired priming volume when preparing syringes. Some drug solutions require larger priming volumes to allow for priming of IV tubing used to administer the drug solution; this information must be stated clearly and boldly on the label because not including the needed priming volume for this procedure would result in a significant dosage error.

7. For IV additives, the strength of the additive is not given as a concentration. The preparation is labeled with both the name and quantity of the additive and the name, concentration, and volume of the large-volume parenteral (e.g., KCl 20 mEq in Dextrose 5% Injection 250 mL).

IV. LABELS FOR COMPOUNDED DRUG PREPARATIONS

A. Labels for dispensed compounded drug preparations should include the same elements of information as are required by state and federal laws for dispensed manufactured products. These are discussed in sections II and III of this chapter. The labels for these compounded preparations require some modifications; these are discussed here.

B. The section of the label that gives the name of the manufacturer or distributor should indicate that the preparation was compounded. The International Academy of Compounding Pharmacists also suggests the following wording for labels on preparations compounded for ambulatory patients: "This medicine was compounded in our pharmacy for you at the direction of your prescriber" (11).

C. Because compounded formulations are customized for individual patients, the label needs to identify the names and quantities of the active ingredients in the preparation.

1. For official *USP* formulations, when the **name(s) and quantity(s)** of all ingredients are specified in the official monograph, the official name of the preparation is sufficient because the formulation information is given in the official compendium and is accessible to the patient, prescriber, or other health care professionals when needed. Two examples of such official preparations include Coal Tar Ointment USP and Cocaine and Tetracaine Hydrochlorides and Epinephrine Topical Solution USP.

2. For official *USP* formulations, when the **name(s)** of ingredients are specified in the official monograph but the quantity of the active ingredient(s) varies, the official name of the preparation plus the quantity of active ingredient must be included on the label of the dispensed preparation. One example would be Hydralazine Hydrochloride Oral Solution USP; the monograph gives a choice of a 0.1% and a 1% solution, so the strength must also be included on the label. In this case, the monograph also states that the concentration in mg per 5 mL be stated on the label (12).

3. For all other dispensed compounded preparations for ambulatory patients, the names and quantities of all active ingredients should be included on the label. Trivial names, such as Magic Mouthwash, Brompton's Cocktail, and TAC solution, unless combined with the names and quantities of the active ingredients, should not be used because there are many different formulations with same name.

4. In some cases, it is advisable to include the names and, when feasible, quantities of inactive ingredients on the label. Examples include ingredients known to cause hypersensitivity reactions, such as preservatives like Benzalkonium Chloride and Thimerosal, and such solvents as Peanut Oil and Castor Oil.

5. The content of alcohol in a compounded liquid dosage form should be stated as a percentage v/v of C_2H_5OH (1).

V. AUXILIARY LABELS

A. Auxiliary labels are placed on drug product containers to give the patient, caregiver, or health care provider important information needed for storing or using the product. Auxiliary labels may be used to clarify directions, provide additional instructions, or reinforce directions given on the regular label. They are not to be used as a substitute for consultation with the patient.

B. Although some labels are absolutely required (e.g., Shake Well labels for dispersed systems such as emulsions and suspensions), in most cases the pharmacist must exercise professional judgment in deciding what, if any, auxiliary labels to use. If the container has too many labels, the truly important information may not be as obvious and may be overlooked.

 C. Common auxiliary labels and some recommended uses are given here. Examples are also shown on the CD that accompanies this book and in the prescription examples given in the dosage form chapters (Chapters 25–35).

1. Labels to ensure proper preparation, storage, and disposal

a. **Shake Well** Required on all liquid dispersed systems, such as suspensions and emulsions, unless specific product labeling instructs otherwise. For example, some protein or peptide suspensions are unstable to shaking and have instructions to gently agitate before use. Shaking of some insulin suspensions may result in air bubbles or foam, so it is recommended that the bottle be "rolled" between the fingers to uniformly redisperse the suspensions particles.

    b. Keep in the Refrigerator, Do Not Freeze Required on products that are chemically unstable at room temperature (e.g., many reconstituted antibiotics) and on products that are physically unstable at room temperature (e.g., cocoa butter suppositories). It is recommended for parenteral preparations that have been manipulated (e.g., IV additives and liquids drawn into syringes in the pharmacy) and are not being used immediately, especially those that do not contain a preservative.

    c. Do Not Use After Required on all manipulated parenteral preparations, reconstituted antibiotics and liquids, compounded preparations, other products known to have limited stability, and all dispensed drug products when required by state law. Even when not required by state law, this label is recommended on all dispensed products so that patients do not retain old, unused prescription products that may no longer have their desired potency. This information is now often printed directly on the prescription label by dispensing software.

    d. Refrigerate, Shake Well, Discard After Used to avoid multiple auxiliary labels when all three messages (**a**, **b**, and **c** above) are required, such as on most reconstituted antibiotic suspensions.

    e. Protect from Light Required for parenteral products that are photosensitive, such as sodium nitroprusside, furosemide, and some phenothiazines. This label is especially important when the immediate container for these products is not amber or opaque. It is appropriate labeling for all photosensitive drugs.

    f. Keep out of the Reach of Children May be used for any drug product container but is required for drug containers without safety closures.

    g. Cancer Chemotherapy, Dispose of Properly Required for containers of cytotoxic drug products.

2. Labels to ensure proper route of administration.

    a. External Use Only Recommended on external use products, especially those that would potentially be dangerous if ingested.

    b. Route of Administration Labels Examples include, "For the Eye," "For Rectal Use," and "For Inhalation Use Only." These labels are especially important when there is any possibility of confusion about the route of administration for the dosage form (e.g., capsules containing drugs for use in an inhaler).

3. Warning labels about potential adverse drug reactions

    a. May Cause Drowsiness; Alcohol and Operating Car or Machinery Warnings Used for adult ambulatory patients. Required for all Schedule II narcotics and other medications, such as some muscle relaxants, that may cause significant drowsiness. Recommended on other narcotics, antianxiety agents, tranquilizers, long-acting barbiturates, sedating anticonvulsants, antihistamines and antidepressants, and any other medication that may cause drowsiness. The use of this label on products prescribed as sleeping aids is a matter of professional judgment.

    b. May Cause Drowsiness Used for pediatric patients and nonambulatory adults with the same recommendations as for a above.

    c. Avoid Sun Exposure Required on drugs that cause photosensitivity reactions, such as tetracyclines, sulfonamides, griseofulvin, nalidixic acid, thiazides, and phenothiazines.

    d. May Cause Discoloration of Urine or Feces Recommended for drugs that discolor urine or feces, such as methylene blue, nitrofurantoin, and phenazopyridine.

4. Warning labels about potential drug–drug and drug–food interactions.

    a. Do Not Drink Alcohol Required for medications that give a disulfiram reaction, such as disulfiram, metronidazole, and chlorpropamide. Recommended with hypnotic drugs or others in which the additive central nervous system effect may be hazardous and on drug products that interact adversely with alcohol. Oral explanation should also be given.

    b. Do not Take with Dairy Products, Antacids . . . Required for tetracycline products to prevent inactivation of the drug by polyvalent ions. Recommended for enteric-coated products because milk products and antacids may cause premature dissolution of the enteric coating in that they create a basic pH in the stomach.

    c. Do not Take Aspirin Required on warfarin-type anticoagulants

5. Labels to ensure appropriate dosing considerations.

    a. Take with Food Recommended for drugs that cause stomach upset when this effect may be decreased by taking the medication with food. Examples of medications in this group include nitrofurantoin, valproic acid, oral nonsteroidal anti-inflammatory drugs (NSAIDs), and aspirin.

    b. Take on an Empty Stomach Recommended for drugs, such as tetracycline and ampicillin, that have decreased absorption or increased destruction in the stomach when taken with food. For some drugs, the desirability of improved absorption must be weighed against the adverse effect of stomach upset when a drug is taken on an empty stomach. This requires appropriate patient consultation by the pharmacist.

    c. Take with a Full Glass of Water Recommended for sulfonamides to decrease the likelihood of crystalluria, for expectorants to enhance viscosity reduction of bronchial secretions, for bulk laxatives to increase stool bulk and decrease the likelihood of compaction, and for irritating drugs, such as potassium supplements, oral NSAIDs, chloral hydrate, certain antibiotics, and theophylline products.

    d. Finish all this Medication Recommended as a compliance aid for antibiotics and anti-infectives, especially when a specific time course is not given in the directions for use

6. Labels to meet legal requirements or recommendations.

    a. Caution: Federal Law Prohibits Transfer of this Drug to Another Person Required by law on all outpatient drug containers for controlled substances in Schedules II through IV.

    b. This Prescription May be Refilled X Times Unless required by state laws, this is an optional label informing the patient of the number of refills. This information is now often printed directly on the prescription label by dispensing software.

REFERENCES

1. General Notices. 2008 USP 31/NF 26. Rockville, MD: The United States Pharmacopeial Convention, Inc., 2007;11.
2. 21 USC §321 (k) and (m)
3. Model State Pharmacy Act and Model Rules of the National Association of Boards of Pharmacy. National Association of Boards of Pharmacy, Mount Prospect, IL, 2007; 11.
4. 21 USC § 353(b)(2)
5. Model State Pharmacy Act and Model Rules of the National Association of Boards of Pharmacy. National Association of Boards of Pharmacy, Mount Prospect, IL, 2007; 82–83.
6. Sitowitz J, Roberts, SB. Danger of "as directed" instructions. Am J Health-Syst Pharm 2001; 58:1657.
7. Chapter ⟨1121⟩. 2008 USP 31/NF 26. Rockville, MD: The United States Pharmacopeial Convention, Inc., 2007;605–606.
8. Pharmacy Equivalent Names (PEN Names). USP Expert Committee Nomenclature and Labeling, Abbreviated summary of discussions, recommendations, and actions on June 27–28, 2002, Rockville, MD, EC NL Letter 21, p. 155.
9. Cohen MR. ISMP medication error report analysis. Hosp Pharm 2002; 37: 593.
10. ASHP technical assistance bulletin on quality assurance for pharmacy-prepared sterile products. Am J Hosp Pharm 2000; 57: 1156.
11. IACP Recommended Labeling for Medications Compounded for Human Use. IACP, January 2006. http://www.iacprx.org/Labeling, Accessed December 2007.
12. 2008 USP 31/NF 26. Rockville, MD: The United States Pharmacopeial Convention, Inc., 2007;Official Monographs.

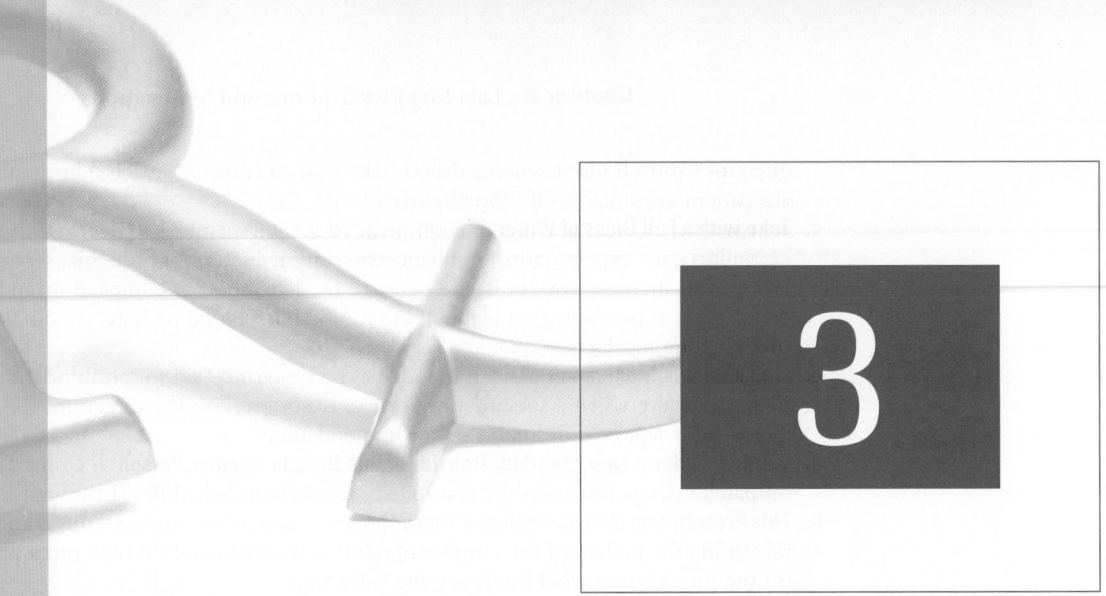

3

Controlled Substances

I.

LEGAL JURISDICTION FOR CONTROLLED SUBSTANCES

Controlled substances are regulated by both federal and state laws.

A. **Federal laws**

1. The original U. S. federal law regulating addictive substances was the Harrison Narcotics Act of 1914. Because, at that time, the distribution and sale of narcotics was controlled through the use of a tax on narcotic drug products, this law was enforced by the Bureau of Internal Revenue in the Department of the Treasury. In 1968, through an administrative reorganization, enforcement was transferred to the newly created Bureau of Narcotics and Dangerous Drugs (BNDD) in the Department of Justice (1,2).

2. By 1970, in addition to the Harrison Narcotics Act, there were many diverse federal laws regulating drugs considered to be addictive and/or dangerous. As a result, a comprehensive new law, the Federal Comprehensive Drug Abuse Prevention and Control Act of 1970 (Public Law 91-513), was passed. The Controlled Substances Act of 1970 is Title II of this law; it went into effect on May 1, 1971. It remains the primary federal law regulating all aspects, from manufacturing through distribution to dispensing, administration and use, of drugs that have the potential for abuse or psychological or physical dependences (2,3). The law can be found in Chapter 13 of Title 21 of the United States Code (USC).

Note: The USC contains the general and permanent laws of the United States. It is divided into approximately 50 broad subject areas with title names and numbers. For example, Title 2 deals with Congress, Title 12 with Banks and Banking, Title 29 with Labor, and Title 21 with Food and Drugs. The general title subjects are further subdivided into chapters so that Title 21 has Chapter 9, which contains the Federal Food, Drug, and Cosmetic Act, whereas the laws in Chapter 13 are those that deal with Drug Abuse and Prevention. Title 21, Chapter 13 contains the provisions of the Controlled Substances Act (CSA) and its amendments. The latest version of the text of the USC can be accessed on the Internet through the U.S. Government Printing Office Web site: www.access.gpo.gov. This site has a selection for access to government information that provides a list with links to various important public documents, such as the USC. You can purchase printed copies of the documents through this site, but it also provides selected documents online in text and/or pdf formats.

3. Since 1973, the CSA has been under the jurisdiction of the Drug Enforcement Administration (DEA) in the Department of Justice. The DEA was created in 1973 by merging the BNDD (in the Department of Justice) with the Drug Investigation arm of the U.S. Customs Service (in the Department of the Treasury). This was to be a "superagency" that would coordinate all federal efforts related to narcotic and dangerous drug enforcement, including domestic drug abuse, diversion, and international smuggling of illicit drugs into the United States. The DEA was put in the Department of Justice so it would have ready access to the robust investigative resources of the Federal Bureau of Investigation (FBI) (2).

4. The DEA regulations that spell out the provisions and applications of the CSA (21 USC § 801 and following) can be found in Title 21 of the Code of Federal Regulations (CFR). As with the USC, the latest revision the CFR can be accessed on the Internet through the U.S. Government Printing Office Web site given earlier. The applicable information can be found in 21 CFR §1300 and following. In accessing the text, you will be required to request each part of the regulation separately (e.g., 21CFR1300, 21CFR1301, 21CFR1302, and so on), but the first section, 1300, contains a useful table of contents.

5. In the 1990s, it was recognized that there was a growing problem nationally with drug abuse of the Schedule II drug methamphetamine (also known as "speed" or "crank"). In addition to being a less expensive alternative to cocaine, methamphetamine was easier to obtain; the drug can be synthesized in "home labs" (often referred to as clandestine labs) using readily available precursors, such as ephedrine, pseudoephedrine, and phenylpropanolamine, which at that time were noncontrolled, nonprescription drugs used legitimately for coughs, colds, and congestion. As a result, in October 1996, the U.S. Congress passed the Comprehensive Methamphetamine Control Act of 1996. The purpose of this law was to restrict access to the precursor drugs and the solvents and chemicals used to make methamphetamine (2). This effort was further strengthened when the Combat Methamphetamine Epidemic Act of 2005 (Title VII of the USA PATRIOT Improvement and Reauthorization Act of 2005, Public Law 109-177) was signed into law in March 2006 (4).

B. **State laws**
   1. All states have laws and regulations that are similar to those described previously, but states may have provisions that are stricter than those in the federal acts.
   2. Pharmacists must follow the most stringent regulations, federal or state, which apply for their practice site.

C. The information given in this chapter is a brief synopsis of the federal regulations of controlled substances that affect general dispensing activities of pharmacists. Other areas of regulation for controlled substances, such as security requirements, inventory requirements, disposal of controlled substances, and narcotic treatment programs, are beyond the scope of this text.
   1. For more complete information on this subject, consult the applicable sections of the Code of Federal Regulations (21 CFR §1300 and following), the USC (21 USC. § 801 and following), current state pharmacy practice acts, reference books on pharmacy law, and Internet Web sites on the subject. Because the laws and regulations are frequently changed and updated, it is important to check current laws and regulations.
   2. The DEA Diversion Control Program maintains an excellent resource for pharmacists, pharmacy students, and pharmacy technicians to assist them in understanding and complying with the provisions of the CSA. Called the *Pharmacist's Manual*, it is available in print or on the Internet at http://www.deadiversion.usdoj.gov/pubs/manuals/pharm2/index.htm, Accessed December 2007. The *Pharmacist's Manual* explains the applicable regulations in very understandable language and includes tables that give easy comparisons for requirements for the various classes.

II.   DEFINITIONS

A. In understanding the regulations regarding controlled substances, it is useful to have the definitions of certain terms as specified by 21 USC § 802 and 21 CFR § 1300. The definitions that follow give the basic sense of these terms as found in these laws and regulations; in most cases, the definitions are paraphrased to simplify some of the legal language and to eliminate some of the redundancy. Some definitions are included here because their use in the CSA differs from the usual meaning of the terms.

B. **Definitions**

1. **Controlled substances** are drugs or other substances or immediate precursors that are specified in schedules I through V of the CSA (5). They are substances that have been deemed to have the potential for abuse or psychological or physical dependence and include narcotics, depressants, stimulants, anabolic steroids, and hallucinogens. Descriptions of Schedules I through V with examples of drugs in each schedule are given in section IV of this chapter. A complete list of drugs and substances, by schedule, is published in 21 CFR § 1308.

2. **Narcotics** include opium, opiates, coca leaves, cocaine, ecgonine, and any of their salts, derivatives and isomers, and compounds, mixtures, and preparations of these substances (5). CFR §1300.1 gives a long list of narcotics drugs, including codeine, morphine, hydrocodone, hydromorphone, and oxycodone (6).

3. **Depressant or stimulant substances** are barbiturates, amphetamines, lysergic acid, and any of their salts, derivatives, and isomers plus any drugs or substances designated by the Attorney General to have the potential for abuse because of their depressant, stimulant, or hallucinogenic effect (5). Examples of drugs that have been added to the original list by the Attorney General include the benzodiazepines, such as alprazolam and diazepam, the depressants methaqualone and gamma hydroxybutyric acid, and the stimulant drug methylphenidate.

4. **Marihuana** includes all parts of the *Cannabis sativa* plant, including the seeds and extracted resins and all compounds, salts, derivatives, mixtures, and preparations of the plant (5).

5. **Anabolic steroids** are drugs or hormonal substances chemically and pharmacologically related to testosterone (6). 21 CFR § 1300.1 gives approximately two pages of listed substances in this group.

6. **List I Chemicals** are drugs or chemicals specified by the Attorney General as precursor chemicals that are used in the illegal manufacture of controlled substances. They include the drugs ephedrine, pseudoephedrine, and phenylpropanolamine, which are precursors used in the synthesis of methamphetamine; and ergotamine and ergonovine, which can be used to make lysergic acid diethylamide and similar hallucinogens (5).

7. **List II Chemicals** are chemicals designated by the Attorney General that are used in the illegal manufacture of controlled substances. They include solvents, such as acetone, ethyl ether, and toluene; and oxidizing and reducing agents, such as potassium permanganate and iodine (5).

8. **Scheduled listed chemical products** are products that (i) contain ephedrine, pseudoephedrine, or phenylpropanolamine and (ii) have been approved for nonprescription (over-the-counter) distribution by the Federal Food, Drug, and Cosmetic Act (4).

9. In this Act, the term **person** is not limited to an individual but includes businesses, corporations, government agencies, associations, and other legal entities (6).

10. An **individual practitioner** is a physician, dentist, veterinarian, or other individual who is registered or licensed by the appropriate jurisdiction (usually the state) to dispense controlled substances in the course of his or her professional practice. It does not include pharmacists, pharmacies, or institutional practitioners (6).

11. An **institutional practitioner** is a hospital or other entity (but not an individual) that is registered or licensed by the appropriate jurisdiction to dispense controlled substances. It does not include pharmacies (6). It is interesting that CFR subdivides practitioners as shown here, whereas the USC just defines the word "practitioner" and has a broader definition that includes pharmacies and also scientists who use controlled substances in research and teaching (5).

12. A **mid-level practitioner** is an individual other than a physician, dentist, veterinarian, or podiatrist who is licensed by their jurisdiction (e.g., state government) to dispense controlled substances. Examples include nurse practitioners, nurse midwives, nurse anesthetists, and physician assistants (6). Specific privileges and restrictions on prescribing by mid-level practitioners are defined by each state.

13. The term **dispenser** includes practitioners (as defined earlier) and pharmacies and pharmacists who dispense controlled substances (6).

14. The term **pharmacist** has the usual meaning, but it also includes pharmacy interns working under the supervision of a pharmacist (6).

III.   DEA REGISTRATION

A. The CSA uses the medium of registration to regulate all aspects of narcotics, stimulants, depressants, hallucinogenic drugs, anabolic steroids, and chemicals used to illegally manufacture controlled substances (3). To aid government officials in administering and enforcing the controlled substance regulations, all importers and exporters, manufacturers, distributors, researchers, practitioners, pharmacies, hospitals, and teaching and research institutions that handle controlled substances must register with the DEA. In fact, 21 CFR § 1301.13 lists ten different classes of registrants.

B. Upon registration, these parties are issued DEA registration numbers.
   1. Registrants must record their DEA numbers on all documents that they use for the transfer or distribution of controlled substances up to the ultimate consumer.
   2. DEA numbers are unique, nine-character numbers that are computer-generated to contain check digits that help pharmacists identify invalid registration numbers and fraudulent prescription orders for controlled substances.

C. Practitioners, hospitals, clinics, retail pharmacies, and teaching institutions are included in the registration class "Dispensing or Instructing." This class uses DEA application form 224 for initial registration and 224a for renewal, which is required every 36 months (7).

D. Prescribers of controlled substances
   1. Individuals who are registered with the DEA to prescribe controlled substances include the individual practitioners and mid-level practitioners as described in the section above on definitions.
   2. The DEA registration number of the prescriber must appear on any outpatient prescription order for a controlled substance.
   3. Many dispensing software packages automatically check for invalid registration numbers when new prescription orders for controlled substances are entered into the computer. The pharmacist or pharmacy technician may also manually check for an invalid DEA registration number on a prescription order by using the following steps.

Example 3.1   DEA # AD5426817

1. The first digit should be a letter: A, B, or F for prescribers and dispensers, M for midlevel practitioners, and P for distributors.
2. The second digit is usually a letter, specifically, the first letter of the registrant's last name. In the foregoing case, if the prescriber's last name is Jones, the second letter of a valid DEA number would be J, so the example DEA number would be invalid. If the registrant is a business with a name that starts with a number, such as "5th Avenue Pharmacy," the second digit should be the number "9."
3. The third through the eighth positions of the DEA number contain numbers that are used to calculate the number in the ninth position, the check digit.
   a. Add the first, third, and fifth digits: $5 + 2 + 8 = 15$.
   b. Add the second, fourth, and sixth digits and multiply this sum by 2: $4 + 6 + 1 = 11 \times 2 = 22$.
   c. Add the two results: $15 + 22 = 37$.
   d. The far right-hand digit of this check number should be the same as the ninth digit of the DEA number. In this example, both numbers are "7," so the DEA number is a valid number.

E. Dispensers of controlled substances
   1. Though prescribers register as individuals, dispensers, such as pharmacists, do not. A pharmacist who is dispensing controlled substances is considered an agent of a registered pharmacy.
   2. Pharmacies that order, receive, handle, and dispense controlled substances must be registered with the DEA and must have a DEA registration number.
   3. The pharmacy's DEA number is required when the pharmacy orders controlled substances from manufacturers or distributors (8). The number is imprinted on the special DEA form 222,

which (or their electronic equivalent) are required for ordering controlled substances in Schedule I or II.

A. Controlled substances are divided into five classes, Schedules I through V, based on their potential for abuse. Drugs in Schedule I have the highest abuse potential and no accepted medical use; Schedule V drug products have the lowest abuse potential. The CSA also allows for certain non-narcotic scheduled substances, when in combination with other therapeutic agents, to be excluded from any schedule. To be excluded, the drug product must have a very low potential for abuse. Furthermore, it must be designated by the FDA as lawfully sold over the counter (i.e., without a prescription), and the manufacturer must apply for and receive permission from the DEA for exclusion of the product from any schedule (9).

B. A brief but representative list of drugs and drug products in the various schedules is given in this section. For an official list of all drugs and drug products in Schedules I through V, see 21 CFR § 1308.11–1308.15. In professional practice, the easiest way to determine the schedule of a drug product is to look at the drug package; the CSA requires that the schedule symbol (e.g., C-II, C-III, and the like) be imprinted on the label of the manufactured product container (10).

1. **Schedule I**
   a. High potential for abuse; unique in that the substances in this schedule have been deemed to have no accepted medical use in the United States and to lack acceptable safety even under medical supervision (11). Therefore, drugs and substances in this class cannot be prescribed, dispensed, or administered. DEA does allow research with these substances, but this requires a special permit and registration (12).
   b. Examples of drugs in Schedule I include (13) the following:
      (1) The narcotic heroin and more than 70 other listed narcotics
      (2) The hallucinogenic drugs lysergic acid diethylamide (LSD), mescaline, peyote, psilocybin, methylene dioxymethamphetamine (MDMA or "Ecstasy")
      (3) Marihuana (marihuana has been used for the treatment of nausea and vomiting associated with chemotherapy and to improve appetite in AIDS patients. Though laws allowing the medical use of marihuana have been passed by some states, it is not permitted under federal law.)
      (4) Depressants such as methaqualone and gamma hydroxybutyric acid (GHB)

2. **Schedule II**
   a. High potential for abuse but with accepted medical use in the United States; abuse potential that can lead to severe psychological or physical dependence (11). Drugs in Schedule II are treated more stringently than those in Schedules III through V.
   b. Examples of drugs in Schedule II include (14) the following:
      (1) All narcotics, such as codeine, morphine (e.g., MS Contin), meperidine (e.g., Demerol), hydromorphone (e.g., Dilaudid), methadone (e.g., Dolophine), oxycodone (e.g., Oxycontin), and fentanyl (e.g., Duragesic), when not combined with another therapeutic agent.
      (2) Certain potent narcotic agonists even when in combination products, such as oxycodone and acetaminophen tablets (e.g., Percocet) and powdered opium with belladonna suppositories.
      (3) Codeine, morphine, and several other narcotic combination products may be in Schedules II, III, or V, depending on the amount of the narcotic in the product. These levels are listed under Schedules III and V following.
      (4) Cocaine
      (5) Stimulants, such as amphetamine (e.g., Dexedrine and Adderall), methamphetamine (e.g., Desoxyn), and methylphenidate (e.g., Ritalin)
      (6) Short-acting barbiturates, such as amobarbital (e.g., Amytal), pentobarbital (e.g., Nembutal), and secobarbital (e.g., Seconal), except when in combinations or in suppository form (they are then in Schedule III) and certain other depressants, such as glutethimide.

3. **Schedule III**
   a. Less potential for abuse than drugs in Schedules I and II; accepted medical use in the United States; abuse potential that can lead to moderate or low physical dependence or high psychological dependence (11).
   b. Examples of drugs in Schedule III include (15) the following:
      (1) Specified narcotics combined with other therapeutically active nonnarcotic drugs wherein the amount of narcotic is restricted to a given level. Several common examples

are given here. When the quantity of narcotic exceeds the given amount, the product is in Schedule II.

- **(a)** Codeine or dihydrocodeine in combination with one or more nonnarcotic drugs wherein the maximum amount of codeine or dihydrocodeine is 90 mg per unit or 18 mg per mL (90 mg per 5 mL) (e.g., Tylenol with Codeine tablets, Synalgos-DC)
- **(b)** Hydrocodone or ethylmorphine in combination with one or more nonnarcotic drugs wherein the maximum amount of hydrocodone or ethylmorphine is 15 mg per unit or 3 mg per mL (15 mg per 5 mL) (e.g., Vicodin, Lortab, Hycotuss Expectorant)
- **(c)** Morphine in combination with one or more nonnarcotic drugs wherein the maximum amount of morphine is 0.50 mg per mL (2.5 mg per 5 mL) or per g
- **(d)** Opium in combination with one or more nonnarcotic drugs where the maximum amount of opium is 5 mg per mL (25 mg per 5 mL) or per g (e.g., Paregoric USP)

- **(2)** All barbiturates alone or in combination not listed in another schedule. Examples include injectable thiopental, which is used for anesthesia; short-acting barbiturates, such as amobarbital, pentobarbital, and secobarbital when in combinations or in suppository form; and some intermediate-acting barbiturates, such as butabarbital.
- **(3)** Certain specified stimulants, such as benzphetamine (e.g., Didrex) and phendimetrazine (e.g., Bontril)
- **(4)** Anabolic steroids, such as testosterone, unless excepted or listed in another schedule

4. Schedule IV

- **a.** Lower potential for abuse than drugs in Schedule III; relative to drugs in Schedule III, abuse of drugs in this class may lead to limited physical or psychological dependence (11). From a control and regulation standpoint, drugs in this schedule are treated essentially the same as are products in Schedule III.
- **b.** Examples of drugs in Schedule IV include (16) the following:
  - **(1)** Specified sedative/hypnotics, such as phenobarbital, chloral hydrate, meprobamate, and zolpidem (e.g., Ambien)
  - **(2)** Benzodiazepines, such as alprazolam (e.g., Xanax) and lorazepam (e.g., Ativan)
  - **(3)** Propoxyphene when formulated into a drug product, alone or in combination (e.g., Darvon-N)
  - **(4)** Certain stimulants, such as phentermine (e.g., Ionamin) and diethylpropion (e.g., Tenuate)
  - **(5)** Miscellaneous substances such as pentazocine (e.g., Talwin)

5. Schedule V

- **a.** Lowest potential for abuse among the controlled substance drugs (11). Drug products in this schedule have low amounts of designated narcotics always in combination with one or more nonnarcotic medicinal agents (17). Most are either cough suppressants or antidiarrheal agents.
- **b.** Examples of drugs in Schedule V include (17) the following:
  - **(1)** Narcotic drugs in combination with other therapeutic agents when the amount of the narcotic does not exceed the specified level. Most commonly, the examples given here are used therapeutically as cough suppressants.
    - **(a)** Codeine not more than 2 mg per mL (10 mg per 5 mL) or per g (e.g., Guiatuss AC)
    - **(b)** Dihydrocodeine or ethylmorphine not more than 1 mg per mL or per g
  - **(2)** The following combination medications, usually used as antidiarrheals, when the amount of the narcotic does not exceed the specified level:
    - **(a)** Opium not more than 1 mg per mL or per g
    - **(b)** Not more than 2.5 mg of diphenoxylate HCl with not less than 25 mcg of atropine sulfate per dosage unit (e.g., Lomotil)

V. REQUIREMENTS FOR PRESCRIPTION ORDERS FOR CONTROLLED SUBSTANCES

- **A.** The federal requirements for prescription orders for controlled substances are given in this section. These are the requirements as of the April 1, 2006 revision of 21 CFR § 1300. Because these regulations change from time to time, it is best to access the most up-to-date revision. As described at the beginning of this chapter, this can be done on the Internet through the U.S. Government Printing Office site. State-controlled substance laws may add additional requirements. Furthermore, federal and state laws concerning required elements for all prescription orders also apply. For information on these laws, see Chapter 1, Prescription and Medication Orders.

B. All schedules Prescription drug orders for all controlled substances have the following requirements (18):

1. Date of issue
2. Full name and address of the patient
3. The drug name, strength, dosage form, quantity prescribed
4. Directions for use
   (**Note:** For states that limit prescription orders for controlled substances to a 34-day supply, the directions for use must be specific enough to ascertain that amount.)
5. Full name, address, and DEA number of the prescriber
6. For written prescription orders, the signature of the prescriber
7. When an oral order is not permitted (e.g., Schedule II), the prescription must be written with ink, indelible pencil, or typewriter. Though the order can by written by an agent of the prescriber, the registered prescriber is responsible for the prescription, and he or she must manually sign the order.

C. Schedule II Because of the greater potential for abuse, drugs in Schedule II have additional requirements.

1. In general, the dispenser must have a **written or typed prescription order, signed by the prescriber,** at the time of dispensing. However, as stated in Chapter 1, federal regulations allow oral, including voice-telephoned prescription orders, for Schedule II medications in emergency situations, with certain provisions (19):
   a. The quantity prescribed is limited to the amount needed for the emergency period.
   b. The prescription order, containing all required information except the signature, is immediately put in written form.
   c. The pharmacist makes a good-faith effort to verify that the order came from a registered practitioner if the prescriber is not known to the pharmacist.
   d. The pharmacist writes on the face of the temporary prescription the words "Authorization for Emergency Dispensing" and the date of the oral order.
   e. A written, signed document must be received within 7 days (if mailed, the postmark must be within 7 days), and the signed prescription must be attached to the temporary prescription.
2. Faxed prescriptions are permitted in nonemergency situations provided the pharmacist is given the original signed prescription order for review prior to the actual dispensing of the controlled drug. Facsimile orders without original signed prescriptions are permitted in certain practices, such as IV infusion services, long-term care, and hospice (19).
3. Refills are prohibited (20).
4. Partial filling of a Schedule II prescription is permissible, but the remaining portion may be provided only if this can be done within 72 hours.
   a. If this cannot be done, the prescriber must be notified.
   b. Exceptions are made for patients in long-term care facilities (LTCF) and for patients who are terminally ill; however, the pharmacist must record on the prescription the words "terminally ill" or "LTCF patient."
   c. At each partial filling, the pharmacist must record in the electronic record or on the back of the prescription order the date, the quantity dispensed, remaining quantity on the order, and the initials or identification of the pharmacist (21).
5. Though there is no federal limitation, some states have quantity limitations, such as a 34-day supply or 120 doses, though exceptions may be permitted in special circumstances (22).
6. The aforementioned requirements are those in CFR § 1306; because the most stringent law (i.e., federal or state) always applies, check your current state statutes for the standard at your practice site.

D. Schedules III and IV Drugs and drug products in Schedules III and IV have less potential for abuse than drugs in Schedule II. Though Schedule III substances have greater abuse potential than those in Schedule IV, drugs in these two schedules are treated essentially the same, with the same requirements and restrictions.

1. Prescription orders for these drug products may be written or given orally or transmitted by phone or fax (23).
2. Refills are permitted with a maximum of five refills or 6 months from date of the original order, whichever is first.
   a. Records of refills must be kept and may be either in writing on the prescription order or on a medication record or recorded electronically.

     b. The information that must be readily retrievable by prescription number includes name, dosage form and quantity dispensed, dates of original and refills, and identification of the pharmacist (24).

   3. In a two-file system (described in section VII), a red "C" no smaller than 1 inch in height must be applied to the lower right-hand corner of prescription orders in Schedules III, IV, and V. DEA regulations do allow waiver of the red "C" requirement for pharmacies that use electronic record-keeping systems, which permit identification by prescription number and which allow retrieval of original documents by prescriber's name, patient's name, drug dispensed, and date filled (25). Check your current state statutes to determine whether the state in which you practice has this standard.

   4. Though there is no federal limitation, some states have quantity limitations, such as a 34-day supply or 120 doses (22), but some states allow such exceptions as a 90-day supply for anticonvulsant drug products that are in Schedule IV.

  E. Schedule V

   1. Drug products in Schedule V have the lowest potential for abuse among the controlled substance drug products.

   2. There are some drug products in this Schedule that the FDA has determined may be sold without a prescription drug order. The requirements for selling these products are given in the next section.

   3. For drug products dispensed on a prescription order, most of the prescription order requirements are the same as for Schedule III and IV. One exception is the treatment of refills. The CSA gives no refill restrictions on drug products in Schedule V (24), so these are handled like nonscheduled prescriptions (i.e., a specific number of refills must be indicated, but there is no time or number limit).

VI. REQUIREMENTS FOR NONPRESCRIPTION SALES OF CONTROLLED SUBSTANCES

  A. For drug products in Schedule V that the FDA has determined may be sold without a prescription, the following CSA restrictions apply (26):

   1. May be dispensed only by a pharmacist (though the cash or credit transaction may be done by a nonpharmacist).

   2. The purchaser must be at least 18 years old, and any person, if not known by the pharmacist, must provide identification and, when appropriate, proof of age.

   3. Limitations of quantity and frequency of purchase:

     a. 240 mL (8 ounces) or 48 dosage units of an opium product per 48-hour period. (Most of these products are antidiarrheal products.)

     b. 120 mL (4 ounces) or 24 units of any other controlled substance per 48-hour period. (Most of these products are codeine-containing cough suppressants.)

   4. Special record-keeping requirements include a bound log with date of purchase, name and quantity of product, name and address of purchaser, and name or initials of the pharmacist. Some states also require the signature of the purchaser and the pharmacist.

  B. For scheduled listed chemical products (for a description of these products, see section II. Definitions), the following restrictions apply (4):

   1. Sale of these products is not limited to pharmacies or pharmacists (i.e., they may be sold in grocery or general merchandise stores or by mobile retail vendors or mail-order companies). Sellers are regulated; they must undergo training in the proper sale of these products and must self-certify to the Attorney General that they have completed the approved training.

   2. In retail settings, the products must be placed in an area that is not directly accessible to customers.

   3. Sales must be for personal use, and the purchaser must provide a photographic identification card.

   4. The seller must maintain an electronic record or a logbook of all sales of these products.

     a. The purchaser must sign the logbook and enter date and time of the purchase and his or her name and address. The seller must verify the entry and ensure that it corresponds with the information on the identification card presented by the purchaser.

     b. The seller must enter the name and quantity of the product purchased.

     c. The logbook must contain notice to purchasers about the penalties for making false statements in the logbook.

     d. The logbook must be kept for at least 2 years after the last entry.

5. Limitations of quantity and frequency of purchase:

   a. For retail distributors, the daily sales limit per purchaser is 3.6 g of ephedrine, pseudoephedrine, or phenylpropanolamine in terms of base chemical.

   Note: Because these drugs are not sold as the base chemical but rather as their salt forms, and because the labeled amount of drug per unit is in terms of the salt form, the daily limit in terms of units (e.g., tablets or capsules) is different for each drug and each salt form. For example, the daily limit of pseudoephedrine **HCl** 30 mg tablets is 146 tablets (corresponding to 4,380 mg of pseudoephedrine HCl and 3,600 mg of pseudoephedrine base), but the daily limit of pseudoephedrine **sulfate** 30 mg tablets is 155 tablets (corresponding to 4,650 mg pseudoephedrine sulfate but the same 3,600 mg pseudoephedrine base). The DEA Internet Web site contains tables that show the daily allowable amounts in terms of the number of tablets of the various drugs and strengths.

   Phenylpropanolamine: The FDA has deemed this drug to be unsafe for human use and has issued a voluntary recall of human drug products containing this ingredient. Currently, it is still available on prescription for veterinary use only.

   b. For mail order, the sales limit is 7.5 g per customer per 30-day period.

   c. All nonliquid dosage forms (e.g., tablets, capsules, gel caps, and the like) must be in two-unit blister packs (4).

VII. RECORD KEEPING FOR CONTROLLED SUBSTANCES

A. Though different restrictions apply to drug products based on their schedule, registered pharmacies must make records of both receipt and delivery of all controlled substances. These must be kept for a minimum of 2 years (25). The specifics of the inventory requirements can be found in 21 CFR § 1304.11.

B. Controlled substances must be inventoried every 2 years (27). Though a perpetual inventory is not required by DEA, there are some instances when such a record would be both practical and a good quality control procedure. One example would be for controlled substances in bulk that are used for compounding. Since the original amount of drug in the container is known, if each time drug is removed an accurate record of this amount is kept, the amount remaining in the container can easily be determined.

C. Because they have the greatest abuse potential of drugs with legitimate medical use, Schedule II drugs are singled out. Records and inventories of these drugs must be maintained separately (25). They must be ordered on special narcotic ordering forms, DEA Form 222 (28).

   1. These are triplicate forms that are ordered by the pharmacy from the DEA. They are serially numbered and come imprinted with the name and address of the pharmacy and its registration number. In November 2007, the DEA proposed a rule change to 21 CFR Part 1305 that would implement a new easier-to-use single-sheet order form that would have enhanced security features (29). The proposal was published in the November 27, 2007, *Federal Register*; consult current DEA regulations for the appropriate official form.

   2. They must be completed using ink or indelible pencil or typed, with one product item per line, and the total number of lines used must be listed on the bottom of the form. The name and address of the supplier to whom the order is addressed must also be written or typed on the form.

   3. The form must be dated and signed by the pharmacist who has been authorized by the DEA to sign such forms for the registered pharmacy (28).

D. For drug products in the other schedules, invoices must be kept to document their receipt in the pharmacy. As indicated earlier, these must be kept for a minimum of 2 years (25).

E. Pharmacies must also follow specified record-keeping requirements for the dispensing of controlled drug products and substances.

   1. The CSA requires the following on records of dispensing (8):

      a. Name and address of the patient

      b. Date of dispensing

      c. The name, dosage form, and quantity of the product dispensed

      d. The name or initials of the dispenser

   2. Pharmacists may choose to file prescription orders for controlled substances in either a two- or three-file system as described here. These systems are designed so that scheduled prescriptions can be easily identified and retrieved. Because of the higher abuse potential for drugs in Schedule II, these prescriptions must either be kept separately or, if filed with other scheduled prescriptions, they must be easily identified (25).

    a. Three-file system:
        (1) Schedule II prescriptions orders are in one file.
        (2) Schedules III through V orders are in a second file.
        (3) All noncontrolled prescription orders are in a third file.
    b. Two-file system, Option A:
        (1) Schedule II orders are in a separate file.
        (2) Schedule III through V orders are filed with noncontrolled prescription orders. The Schedule III through V prescription orders must be distinguished from the nonscheduled prescription orders by having a 1-inch, red "C" in the bottom right-hand corner of the prescription document. This marking enables law enforcement officials, when they are inspecting the pharmacy's records, to easily distinguish the orders for the controlled prescriptions. As stated previously, DEA regulations allow waiver of the red "C" requirement for pharmacies that use electronic record-keeping systems that permit identification by prescription number and allow retrieval of original documents by prescriber's name, patient's name, drug dispensed, and date filled (25). Check your current state statutes to determine the requirements for your practice site.
    c. Two-file system, Option B:
        (1) Schedule II through V orders are filed together but separately from prescription orders for noncontrolled products. Again, the Schedule III through V prescription orders must have a 1-inch, red "C" in the bottom right-hand corner of the prescription document. This is to allow easy separation of the Schedule III through V orders from those in Schedule II. As stated earlier, the same waiver of the red "C" is allowed for pharmacies that use electronic record keeping.
        (2) Prescription orders for noncontrolled products are in a separate file.

VIII. LABELING OF PRESCRIPTIONS FOR CONTROLLED SUBSTANCES

A. The federal requirements for labeling controlled substances are given in 21 CFR § 1306, Schedule II in subsection 14 and Schedules III–V in subsection 24 (30,31). These requirements are summarized here. State laws may add additional requirements.
    1. Date of dispensing (date of initial dispensing for Schedules III, IV, and V)
    2. Pharmacy name and address
    3. Prescription identification or serial number
    4. Name of patient
    5. Name of prescriber
    6. Directions for use and cautionary statements, if any
    7. A federal transfer label is required on prescriptions in Schedules II through IV but not Schedule V. This label states:
        Caution: Federal law prohibits the transfer of this drug to any person other than the patient for whom it was prescribed (32).
B. Notice that though the federal labeling requirements for controlled substances do not require the name and strength of the drug product dispensed, these are requirements for general prescription labels in most states. See Chapter 2, Labeling Prescriptions and Medications, for general information on labeling prescriptions.

IX. OTHER REQUIREMENTS

As stated at the beginning of this chapter, the foregoing data provide an overview of requirements for handling controlled substances in the pharmacy. The specifics of registration, storage and security, inventory records, order forms, transferring of prescriptions, detoxification programs, required institutional records, and complete schedules for drug products are beyond the scope of this text. For more information refer to the current revisions of appropriate sections of the Code of Federal Regulations, the USC, state pharmacy practice acts, and/or reference books on pharmacy law.

REFERENCES

1. DEA Genealogy. http://www.usdoj.gov/dea/agency/genealogy.htm. Accessed December 2007.
2. A tradition of excellence, the history of the DEA from 1973 to 2003. http://www.usdoj.gov/dea/history.htm. Accessed December 2007.
3. Fink JL III, Vivian JC, Bernstein IBG. Pharmacy law digest, 39th ed. St. Louis: Facts and Comparisons, Inc, 2005; 127.
4. General Information Regarding the Combat Methamphetamine Epidemic Act of 2005 [Title VII of Public Law 109-177]. http://www.deadiversion.usdoj.gov/meth/index.html. Accessed December 2007.

5. 21 USC § 802.
6. 21 CFR §1300.1
7. 21 CFR §1301.13.
8. 21 CFR §1304.22.
9. 21 CFR §1308.21.
10. 21 CFR §1302.03.
11. 21 USC §812(b).
12. Pharmacist's manual, schedule of controlled substances. http://www.deadiversion.usdoj.gov/pubs/manuals/pharm2/index.htm. Accessed December 2007.
13. 21 CFR §1308.11.
14. 21 CFR §1308.12.
15. 21 CFR §1308.13.
16. 21 CFR §1308.14.
17. 21 CFR §1308.15.
18. 21 CFR §1306.05.
19. 21 CFR §1306.11.
20. 21 CFR §1306.12.
21. 21 CFR §1306.13.
22. Fink JL III, Vivian JC, Bernstein IGB. Pharmacy law digest, 39th ed. St. Louis: Facts and Comparisons, Inc, 2005; 150.
23. 21 CFR §1306.21.
24. 21 CFR §1306.22.
25. 21 CFR §1304.04.
26. 21 CFR §1306.26.
27. 21 CFR §1304.11.
28. 21 CFR §1305.11–1305.12.
29. *Federal Register*, vol. 72, No. 227/November 27, 2007/Proposed rules; 66,118-66,122.
30. 21 CFR §1306.14.
31. 21 CFR §1306.24.
32. 21 U.S.C. §825(c).

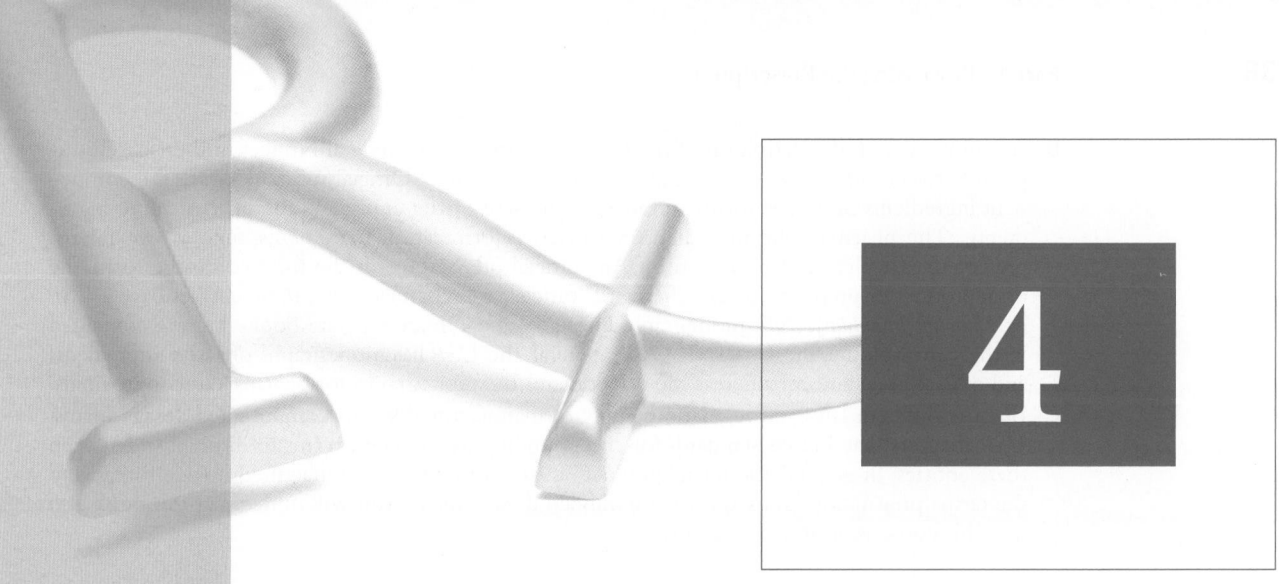

Expiration and Beyond-Use Dating

I. DEFINITIONS

A. **Expiration date:** This is the date put on the label of a drug product by the **manufacturer** or distributor of the product. The *United States Pharmacopeia* (*USP*) defines expiration date in the following way.

> The expiration date identifies the time during which the article may be expected to meet the requirements of the Pharmacopeial monograph, provided it is kept under the prescribed storage conditions. The expiration date limits the time during which the article may be dispensed or used. Where an expiration date is stated only in terms of the month and the year, it is a representation that the intended expiration date is the last day of the stated month (1).

B. **Beyond-use date:** This is the date put on the **dispensing container** by the pharmacist or pharmacy technician. According to the *USP*:
  1. "The dispenser shall place on the label of the prescription container a suitable beyond-use date to limit the patient's use of the article based on any information supplied by the manufacturer and the *General Notices and Requirements* of this Pharmacopeia. The beyond-use date placed on the label shall not be later than the expiration date on the manufacturer's container" (1).
  2. "The beyond-use date is the date after which an article must not be used" (1).

C. It should be noted that these definitions use the term "article", which is defined in the *USP* as "an item for which a monograph is provided whether an official substance or an official preparation" (2). Therefore, technically these definitions apply only to official *USP* articles. In practice, these definitions are generalized to include nonofficial drug substances, products, and preparations and nutrients and dietary supplements.

D. As can be seen in the definition of the *USP* word article, the General Notices of the *USP* distinguish between official substances and official preparations. "Official substances" are the component ingredients of dosage forms and include the active drug entity and the pharmaceutic ingredients. The pharmaceutic ingredients are inactive formulation ingredients, such as sweeteners, preservatives, tablet binders, and so on. An "official preparation" is the finished dosage form, the drug product or preparation (2). The word "official" merely means that these entities have a *USP* or *National Formulary* (*NF*) monograph. The *USP* and *NF* are separate books, but are contained in the same volume, the *USP–NF* (2). In general, the *USP* has monographs of active ingredients and official preparations; whereas the *NF* contains the monographs for pharmaceutic ingredients.

E. Because different laws and regulations apply to manufactured versus compounded dosage forms, *USP* chapters that address standards for compounding use different terms to distinguish between these entities: In general, the term "product" is used to refer to manufactured dosage forms, and the term "preparation" is used for compounded dosage forms. You will notice that this book also uses this convention for these terms.

II. REGULATION OF EXPIRATION AND BEYOND-USE DATING

A. Manufactured drug products and bulk ingredients in their original containers

1. Prior to the late 1960s, except for insulin and antibiotics, most commercial packages of drug products carried no expiration date. It was common to find drug products in prescription departments of pharmacies that were 20 to 30 years old. This gradually changed during the 1970s so that by September 28, 1978, Good Manufacturing Practice regulations required expiration dates on almost all manufactured drug products.

2. Manufactured products are covered by federal regulations because they are shipped in interstate commerce. The requirement for expiration dates on these products is found in 21CFR § 211.137. This states:

> **(a)** To assure that a drug product meets applicable standards of identity, strength, quality, and purity at the time of use, it shall bear an expiration date determined by appropriate stability testing described in Sec. 211.166.
>
> **(b)** Expiration dates shall be related to any storage conditions stated on the labeling, as determined by stability studies as described in Sec. 211.166 (3).

3. The General Notices of the *USP* contains the following statement about the requirement for expiration dates:

> The label of an official drug product, nutritional or dietary supplement product shall bear an expiration date. All articles shall display the expiration date so that it can be read by an ordinary individual under customary conditions of purchase and use (1).

4. Currently, the only exceptions for the requirement of expiration dates on manufactured drug products are for nonprescription drug products or nutritional supplements packaged in containers for sale at retail with labeling that allows no limitation of dosage, and the product must be shown to be stable (with supporting stability data) for at least 3 years under the recommended storage conditions (1,3).

5. Notice that both the *USP* and CFR requirements are for drug products, not for bulk drugs or chemicals. Though most bulk drugs and many pharmaceutic ingredients are labeled with expiration dates, some are not. When these are used in the manufacturing process, the manufacturer assays the ingredients prior to use. Because most pharmacies do not have this analytical capability, sound scientific and professional judgment and good procedures are needed when dealing with these ingredients.

a. When possible, purchase bulk ingredients labeled with expiration dates.

b. For bulk ingredients not labeled with an expiration date, label the container with the date when you received the ingredient from the supplier, and develop a reasonable written standard for the length of time the ingredient can be retained and used in compounding.

c. For all bulk ingredients, request a certificate of analysis from the supplier. These certificates give helpful information, such as expiration dates, re-test dates, or quality control release dates. If a re-test date is given, you can contact the supplier on that date to determine whether the expiration date can be extended on the basis of recent analysis conducted on that lot by the supplier. For quality control release dates, the supplier will have standard dating policies (e.g., 1 year from the quality control release date) for assurance of specifications stated on the certificate of analysis.

B. Drug products labeled, packaged, and dispensed on prescription orders

1. Because the dispensing of prescribed drug products to patients is regulated by state law, the requirements for beyond-use dates on most prescription containers are regulated by state statutes. The NABP *Model Rules for the Practice of Pharmacy* recommends that a beyond-use date be included on the prescription label (4). As a result, many states have adopted this standard. Check the regulations for the state in which you are practicing for information about requirements for labeling prescription containers with beyond-use dates.

2. As quoted earlier in the definitions section, the General Notices of the *USP* state that the dispenser (this includes both pharmacists and dispensing physicians) shall label a prescription container with a beyond-use date (1).

3. One area in which federal law has jurisdiction in regulating the labeling of prescriptions is for drug products dispensed for nursing home patients; the Code of Federal Regulations specifies that FDA and *USP* requirements be followed for prescriptions dispensed to nursing home patients in intermediate-care and skilled nursing facilities. Therefore, prescriptions for these patients must be labeled with beyond-use dates.

4. Even when it is not required by law, most pharmacists feel that the labels of all prescription containers should include beyond-use dates; they feel it is their professional responsibility to provide their patients with a date after which a medication may no longer have its labeled potency. It is well known that many patients keep any unused portion of their prescription drugs in case they need it in the future, so many households have partially used prescription drug products that could unknowingly be used well past their expiration date if the container were not labeled with a beyond-use date.

5. Many dispensing software programs automatically place a 1-year beyond-use date on all labels for prescriptions. The pharmacist or pharmacy technician must verify that this date is within the expiration date given on the container of the product dispensed. As stated in the section on definitions, when an expiration date is given with just a month and year, this means that the intended expiration date is the last day of the given month (1).

III. DIFFICULTIES IN ASSIGNING BEYOND-USE DATES

A. Assigning beyond-use dates is a complex issue because we are dealing with drug molecules with multiple reactive functional groups, various added pharmaceutic ingredients, dispensing containers and closures, and varying conditions of storage and use. Though patient safety and intended therapy are of primary importance, this must be balanced against both economic and ecological concerns; we do not want to unnecessarily discard drug products that still have their labeled potency.

B. A major stumbling block to assigning and labeling dispensed drug products with beyond-use dates has been the lack of adequate stability information available to the pharmacist. The question is, how should the pharmacist determine a valid beyond-use date without the benefit of stability studies conducted with the drug product in the dispensing container stored in the uncontrolled home environment?

C. This problem was recognized in Resolution No. 11 at the 1990 United States Pharmacopeial Convention:

> The United States Pharmacopeial Convention is encouraged to explore with the Food and Drug Administration the development of mechanisms by which reliable data and information can be generated to establish scientifically sound beyond-use dates for repackaged products (5).

D. The USP has taken the initiative to address this concern. Studies have been conducted by the USP and pharmaceutical manufacturers, stakeholder conferences have been held, and the *Pharmacopeial Forum* of the USP has been used as a medium for exchanging ideas and soliciting information from pharmacists, regulatory bodies, pharmacy professional organizations, and the pharmaceutical industry. While the process is ongoing, the current consensus can be seen in the General Notices and General Chapters of the *USP* as summarized here.

1. Manufacturers are given responsibility for providing the pharmacist with needed information to use in assigning beyond-use dates and, as indicated earlier, the dispenser is to use any information provided by the manufacturer in assigning a beyond-use date (1).

2. The *USP* states that for any article that is required to have an expiration date (which would include almost anything dispensed on a prescription order), it shall be dispensed only in, or from, a container labeled with an expiration date, and the product dispensed must be within its labeled expiration time period (1). This has implications for pharmacies that serve institutional

or long-term care facilities because unused drug products that are returned to the pharmacy should not be comingled with products that have a different (especially longer) expiration date.

3. Pharmacists are reminded to use professional judgment when using the available information for determining beyond-use dates.

    a. For products requiring reconstitution before use, the manufacturer's recommendations on the product labeling should be followed.

    b. For all other products, pharmacists are instructed to take into account the following factors:

        (1) The nature of the drug

        (2) The characteristics of the container used by the manufacturer and the expiration date on the product label

        (3) The properties of the dispensing container

        (4) The expected storage conditions for the product during the time of use, including any unusual conditions to which it may be exposed

        (5) The expected length of time that the product will be used (1)

4. For manufactured drug products, pharmacists are given default guidelines to use in assigning beyond-use dates that are based on the type of dispensing packaging used: multi-dose containers, unit-dose containers, and customized patient medication packages. These are described in the next section.

5. Pharmacists are also given guidelines for determining beyond-use dates for compounded preparations. These are described in section V.

IV. ASSIGNING BEYOND-USE DATES TO MANUFACTURED DRUG PRODUCTS DISPENSED BY THE PHARMACIST

A. Multi-dose containers

1. For prescription drug products dispensed in multi-dose containers, the *USP* allows use of the manufacturer's expiration date or 1 year from the date the drug product is dispensed, whichever is earlier (1).

    a. Remember that this is the **maximum** length allowed and that the factors given earlier must be considered, including the drug, the container, and storage conditions.

    b. The pharmacist should be conscious of the recommended storage conditions for a drug product. Many products require storage at controlled room temperature. Therefore, it is prudent to be conservative with beyond-use dates when a product is dispensed in hot weather, especially when it cannot be ensured that the product will be stored under controlled conditions. [Keep in mind that when a *USP* monograph or drug product package label specifies temperature and humidity conditions for storage and distribution, this includes shipping and mailing of dispensed products to patients (1).] Furthermore, many tablets and capsules are sensitive to moisture, and dispensing them in a prescription vial, even though it is classified as a tight container, may decrease their shelf-life, and the patient will be opening and closing the dispensing container as doses are taken, thus exposing the drug product to the atmosphere. All of these factors should be considered in assigning beyond-use dates.

    c. Though it is usually satisfactory to use the maximum allowable time when the drug product is dispensed in its original commercial container and the patient will be storing the product as directed, an exception to this would be a volatile drug like nitroglycerin. Even though this drug is dispensed in its original glass container, it will lose potency over time as the patient opens and closes the bottle to remove doses.

    d. Dispensing software packages that automatically label prescriptions with expiration dates of 1 year from the date dispensed should be used with discretion; the manufacturer's expiration date should always be consulted, and a shorter dating should be printed on the prescription label when this is warranted either by the product's expiration date or one of the factors identified earlier.

2. The *USP* specifies that the facility in which drug products are packaged and stored have a temperature that is maintained so as not to exceed a mean kinetic temperature of 25°C. Temperature records are to be kept by the pharmacy (1). An explanation and sample calculation for mean kinetic temperature are found in Chapter 7 of this book, and a discussion of *USP* storage temperatures is found in Chapter 13.

3. To adequately protect the product from humidity or moisture permeation, any plastic packaging material must provide protection better than that given by polyvinyl chloride (1). For multi-dose containers, this specification can be met by using tight containers.

B. Single-unit and unit-dose containers for nonsterile dosage forms

1. For nonsterile solid and liquid dosage forms dispensed in single-unit or unit-dose containers, the *USP* allows use of the manufacturer's expiration date or 1 year from the date the drug product is packaged in the unit container, whichever is earlier (1).

    a. Longer beyond-use dates are allowed if the product labeling allows this or if independent stability studies that have been done justify a longer dating (1).

    b. Notice that this recommendation uses the date **packaged** whereas that for multi-dose containers uses the date **dispensed**. These recommendations assume that drugs repackaged in multi-dose containers are dispensed at that time, whereas unit-dose packaging is often carried out in advance of the act of dispensing.

2. All of the other considerations stated earlier for multi-dose packaging also apply to single-unit or unit-dose packaging. Of special concern for this type of packaging is the requirement that plastic packaging materials give better moisture permeation protection than polyvinyl chloride; the dispenser must confirm that materials used for this type of packaging meet this specification.

3. **There are some additional requirements**

    a. In addition to a temperature requirement, there is a maximum relative humidity requirement for nonsterile solid and liquid dosage forms repackaged in unit containers. These products are to be repackaged and stored under conditions specified in the product monograph or, if the monograph does not specify the conditions, the conditions should be controlled room temperature with relative humidity not exceeding 60% (6).

    b. *USP* Chapter ⟨681⟩ also prohibits reprocessing of repackaged unit-dose containers. In other words, the dispenser may not remove dosage units from one unit-dose container (such as a blister card) and dispense them in another unit-dose container. However, a unit-dose container may be transferred between secondary containers (such as a unit-dose cart drawer or carrier) as long as the original expiration date is maintained (6).

C. Customized patient medication packages (6)

1. A customized patient medication package (patient med pak) is a package prepared by a pharmacist or pharmacy technician for a specific patient. It comprises a series of packets or containers that contain two or more prescribed solid oral dosage forms. It is intended as a compliance aid for the patient so that each packet or container is labeled with the day and time that the contents of that packet are to be taken.

2. The *USP* has separate recommendations for labeling of patient med paks. These can be found in the *USP*, Chapter ⟨681⟩, Repackaging into Single-Unit Containers and Unit-Dose Containers for Nonsterile Solid and Liquid Dosage Forms.

3. With regard to assigning a beyond-use date to a patient med pak, Chapter ⟨681⟩ directs that it be no longer than the shortest recommended beyond-use date for any dosage form in the patient med pak or not longer than 60 days from the date of preparation of the patient med pak and that it not exceed the shortest expiration date on the original manufacturer's bulk container for any of the dosage forms in the pak.

4. Chapter ⟨681⟩ also contains requirements for packaging materials for patient med paks: Unless there are more strict packaging requirements for any units contained in the patient med pak, the materials for these med paks must meet the specifications for Class B single-unit or unit-dose containers as described in *USP* Chapter ⟨661⟩, Containers—Plastics, and ⟨671⟩, Containers—Performance Testing. Pharmacists who repackage in single-unit, unit-dose, or patient med paks should consult the applicable chapters of the *USP* for complete information on packaging materials and storage and packaging requirements.

V. ASSIGNING BEYOND-USE DATES TO COMPOUNDED DRUG PREPARATIONS

A. The General Notices of the *USP* state that compounded drug preparations shall be labeled with a beyond-use date. Guidance for assigning beyond-use dates to extemporaneously compounded nonsterile drug preparations is given in *USP* General Notices and in Chapter ⟨795⟩, Pharmaceutical Compounding—Nonsterile Preparations. It states the following:

> The beyond-use date is the date after which a compounded preparation is not to be used and is determined from the date the preparation is compounded. Because compounded preparations are intended for administration immediately or following short-term storage, their beyond-use dates may be assigned based on criteria different from those applied to assigning expiration dates for manufactured drug products (7).

B. In applying these standards, it is important to keep in mind the general rules for assigning beyond-use dates, which state that you must take into account the nature of the drug or drugs involved, the characteristics of the preparation container, and the expected storage conditions.

C. Before compounding any drug preparation, consult the available literature for stability information.

   1. Numerous references that are available give helpful information on drug preparation stability. A partial list of these references appears in Chapter 37. If you are unable to find needed information or if you do not have access to a particular reference, you may be able to obtain the needed information by consulting with a college of pharmacy faculty member or colleague or by contacting the library at a school or college of pharmacy or a drug information service at a teaching hospital. Some companies that specialize in selling compounding supplies also maintain customer service departments that can help you with your questions. One very helpful reference, which gives specific compatibility and stability information on a large number of drugs, is *Trissel's Compatibility of Compounded Formulations*, published by the American Pharmacists Association.

   2. If information specific to the situation cannot be found, judgment of stability can be based on several factors, including structural formula of the drug, availability of similar manufactured dosage forms of the drug, and published stability information on drugs with similar chemistry. When extrapolating information from the literature, be conscious of significant differences between the study conditions and those of your preparation: containers, storage conditions, vehicles, and pharmaceutic ingredients, to name a few. Details on compatibility and stability considerations are discussed in Chapter 37.

D. When assigning a beyond-use date to a compounded preparation, you must take into consideration the expiration dates of all the ingredients used in formulating the preparation. In addition, because you are manipulating these ingredients and are usually mixing them with other drugs and pharmaceutic ingredients, the new preparation should have a shorter beyond-use date than the expiration date assigned to any of the single original ingredients. How much should you reduce the beyond-use date? There are six key factors to consider:

   1. The nature of each ingredient. For example, we know that some drugs, such as potassium chloride and calamine, are intrinsically very stable chemically, whereas others, like penicillin and aspirin, are subject to chemical decomposition.

   2. The combination of ingredients. For example, an isoniazid suspension formulated with 50% sorbitol solution is stable for approximately 3 weeks, whereas an isoniazid suspension made with sugar-base syrups is not nearly that stable (8).

   3. The final pharmaceutical dosage form. Most drugs formulated as dry powders, such as bulk powders, chartulae, or capsules, are much more stable than when these same drugs are dispensed in dosage forms that contain water, such as aqueous solutions and suspensions. Keep in mind, however, that though hard capsule shells look "dry," the material for gelatin capsule shells contains 10% to 15% water (9), so a very vulnerable drug in close contact with the capsule shell may be subject to some instability.

   4. Compounding procedures. Variation in compounding procedures and equipment used for making a formulation can affect the stability of the final preparation. For example, the physical properties of preparation uniformity and rate of sedimentation for suspensions can be altered by passing the preparation through a hand homogenizer. Use of heat during compounding can have a negative effect on the chemical properties of some ingredients in the final preparation.

   5. Packaging used for the preparation. Many drugs are sensitive to moisture and are more stable when packaged in a tight container than in a well-closed container. Other preparations need protection from light.

   6. Possible storage conditions. Most drugs with limited stability degrade more rapidly as temperatures increase. Many preparations are sensitive to high humidity. Though the pharmacist tries to control storage conditions through proper labeling and consultation with the patient, this is one variable over which control is relinquished once the preparation leaves the pharmacy.

E. As indicated earlier, *USP* Chapter ⟨795⟩ has established some basic guidelines that are useful in assigning beyond-use dates for nonsterile compounded preparations.

   1. To avoid any misinterpretations of this information, the guidelines are quoted directly here.

   > In the absence of stability information that is applicable to a specific drug and preparation, the following maximum beyond-use dates are recommended for nonsterile compounded drug preparations that are packaged in tight, light-resistant containers and stored at controlled room temperature unless otherwise indicated (see *Preservation, Packaging, Storage, and Labeling* in the *General Notices*).

For Nonaqueous Liquids and Solid Formulations—

Where the Manufactured Drug Product is the Source of Active Ingredient—The beyond-use date is not later than 25% of the time remaining until the product's expiration date or 6 months, whichever is earlier.

Where a USP or NF Substance is the Source of Active Ingredient—The beyond-use date is not later than 6 months.

For Water-Containing Formulations (prepared from ingredients in solid form)—The beyond-date is not later than 14 days for liquid preparations when stored at cold temperatures between 2° and 8° (36° and 46°F).

For All Other Formulations—The beyond-use date is not later than the intended duration of therapy or 30 days, whichever is earlier. These beyond-use date limits may be exceeded when there is supporting valid scientific stability information that is directly applicable to the specific preparation (i.e., the same drug concentration range, pH, excipients, vehicle, water content, etc.) (7).

2. To illustrate the application of the foregoing maximum default beyond-use dates, consider the following examples:

   a. The pharmacist is crushing diazepam tablets for incorporation into compounded capsules. If the bulk package of tablets has a labeled expiration date of 1 year from the date of compounding, the **maximum** possible beyond-use date for this compounded nonaqueous solid preparation would be 3 months (25% of 1 year). This assumes that the capsules will be dispensed in a tight, light-resistant container and stored at controlled room temperature.

   b. If the same situation was to occur but the compounded capsules were made using pure diazepam USP powder, the maximum beyond-use date would be 6 months. This assumes that the expiration date on the diazepam powder is longer than 6 months; if it is 6 months or less, the beyond-use date on the compounded capsules would have to be shortened appropriately. For example, if the diazepam powder had an expiration date of 4 months, the assigned beyond-use date for the compounded capsules obviously would be limited to 4 months, but a more conservative 1- or 2-month dating would be reasonable (a 1-month beyond-use date would use the usual standard of 25% of the time remaining on the bulk powder expiration date).

   c. If either crushed manufactured tablets or pure powder were used to make a diazepam aqueous oral suspension, the maximum default beyond-use date would be 14 days. This assumes that the suspension will be stored in a cold place, such as a refrigerator. In the case of diazepam, there have been numerous stability studies for compounded suspensions, and some formulations have acceptable stability for up to 60 days. If one of these specific formulations is used, the beyond-use date could be lengthened to that given in the study. A good review of these studies for diazepam is given in *Trissel's Stability of Compounded Formulations* (10).

   d. If either crushed manufactured tablets or pure diazepam powder were used to make a nonaqueous dosage form, such as diazepam suppositories or lozenges, the pharmacist would have the option to select 3 months (if using the crushed tablets just described) or 6 months (if using pure drug powder), or the 30 days or intended length of therapy guideline as recommended for "other formulations." In this case the pharmacist would have to use professional judgment in selecting an appropriate date. If heat is used in the compounding procedure for making the suppositories or lozenges, a conservative beyond-use date would be recommended. Stability studies for diazepam suppository formulations have also been reported (10).

F. Guidelines on beyond-use dates for sterile preparations are discussed in *USP* Chapter ⟨797⟩. Because of the added requirement for sterility, assigning beyond-use dates for these preparations is more complex; this is discussed in Chapter 32 of this book.

VI. SUMMARY

A. Because the subject of assigning scientifically based beyond-use dates is one that continues to be debated, it is important to be knowledgeable about the latest published standards.

   1. For all dispensing and for repackaging of drug products in unit-dose or single-unit packages, check the General Notices and specific relevant chapters of the most current *USP*.
   2. For compounded nonsterile preparations, check *USP* Chapter ⟨795⟩.
   3. For sterile preparations, check the current *USP* Chapter ⟨797⟩.

B. As professionals charged with protecting the health of their patients, pharmacists want to be sufficiently conservative in assigning beyond-use dates so that the label adequately reflects the actual potency of the product or preparation. At the same time, the dates should not be unnecessarily conservative so that patients are burdened with frequent visits to the pharmacy and drug products or preparations are wasted because items are discarded when still within labeled limits.

C. Though it has been pointed out that there is only one reported case in which a degraded drug (tetracycline) has caused human toxicity (11), it must be remembered that therapeutic failure, especially in the case of a critical drug, a critical disease, or a critical patient, caused by a subpotent drug product or preparation may be just as serious as a case of toxicity caused by a degraded drug. This should always be kept in mind when assigning beyond-use dates, and the patient should be instructed to monitor the results of the therapy.

REFERENCES

1. The United States Pharmacopeial Convention, Inc. General Notices. 2008 USP 31/NF 26. Rockville, MD: Author, 2007; 10–12.
2. The United States Pharmacopeial Convention, Inc. General Notices. 2008 USP 31/NF 26. Rockville, MD: Author, 2007; 3.
3. 21CFR § 211.137 (a), (b), and (h).
4. Model State Pharmacy Act and Model Rules of the National Association of Boards of Pharmacy. National Association of Boards of Pharmacy: Mount Prospect, IL, 2006; 74.
5. The United States Pharmacopeial Convention, Inc. Pharmacopeial Forum. Rockville, MD: Author, 1998; 24: 43–56.
6. The United States Pharmacopeial Convention, Inc. Chapter ⟨681⟩. 2008 USP 31/NF 26. Rockville, MD: Author, 2007; 258–259.
7. The United States Pharmacopeial Convention, Inc. Chapter ⟨795⟩. 2008 USP 31/NF 26. Rockville, MD: Author, 2007; 317.
8. ASHP Handbook on extemporaneous formulations. Bethesda, MD: American Society of Hospital Pharmacists, 1987; 27.
9. The United States Pharmacopeial Convention, Inc. Chapter ⟨1151⟩. 2008 USP 31/NF 26. Rockville, MD: Author, 2007; 617.
10. Trissel LA. Trissel's stability of compounded formulations, 2nd ed. Washington, DC: American Pharmaceutical Association, 2000; 121–124.
11. Drug past their expiration date. The Medical Letter. New Rochelle, NY: The Medical Letter, Inc., 2002; 44: 93–94.

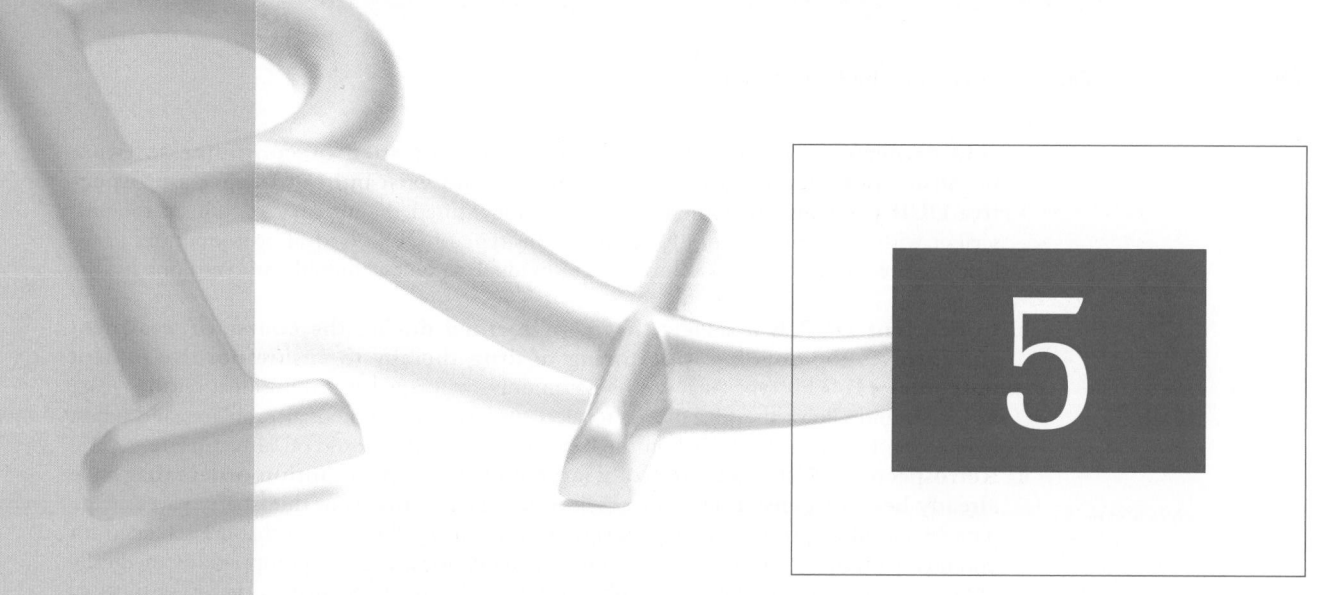

5

Drug Utilization Review and Medication-Use Evaluation

Karen Kopacek, R.Ph.

I. DEFINITIONS

A. **"Drug Utilization Review"** (DUR) is a process used to **assess the appropriateness of drug therapy** by engaging in the evaluation of data on drug use in a given health care environment against predetermined criteria and standards (1).

    1. This definition was published as part of a report called *Principles of a Sound Drug Formulary System.* The report was prepared and endorsed by a coalition of national organizations, including the Academy of Managed Care Pharmacy (AMCP), the American Medical Association, the American Society of Health-System Pharmacists (ASHP), and the United States Pharmacopeia (USP), with a primary interest in promoting rational, clinically appropriate, safe, and cost-effect drug therapy (1).

    2. There are three distinct types of DUR: prospective, concurrent, and retrospective DUR.

        a. Prospective DUR is the review that a pharmacist conducts prior to dispensing a new or refill medication. The prescription or medication order is compared with predetermined criteria to prevent or correct a potential drug-related problem before it reaches the patient. Criteria may be determined by state Medicaid programs or private-sector prescription programs (e.g., pharmacy benefit managers and managed care organizations) and is available online through the pharmacy's computer system to immediately "alert" the pharmacist to a "violation" of the criterion. **However, each pharmacist, using his or her own pharmaceutical care knowledge and professional judgment, should be**

45

able to perform a basic DUR without the assistance of computer software because a potential drug therapy problem could exist but not trigger a prospective DUR program. If a potential problem is identified, the pharmacist contacts the prescriber with recommendations for change. This type of DUR is ideal, as it identifies problems before they occur and allows for individual patient-centered interventions by the pharmacist (2).

b. **Concurrent DUR is a review that is performed during the course of treatment and involves the ongoing monitoring of drug therapy to ensure positive patient outcomes (3).** This type of DUR is commonly performed in institutional settings (e.g., hospitals) and allows the pharmacist to alert prescribers to potential problems and adjust medication therapy if necessary on the basis of ongoing diagnostic or laboratory tests.

c. **Retrospective DUR is a review of a large number of prescription orders that have already been dispensed.** Data are obtained using a pharmacy's or third-party payer's (e.g., state Medicaid or private-sector prescription programs) billing claims that are screened for potential patterns or problems, such as fraud, abuse, overuse, or inappropriate or medically unnecessary care among physicians, pharmacists, and patients. Similar to the other types of DUR, each retrospective DUR has established criteria in which to screen the data for "violations." Once a "violation" is identified, an "alert" is generated, and those practitioners involved are educated by mail or via telephone. A typical "alert" letter sent to practitioners contains the name of the patient, an introduction to the DUR program, information describing the criterion that has been "violated," literature references supporting the validity of the criterion, and a listing of the prescriptions and medical diagnoses that are exceptions to that particular DUR. This educational process is intended to minimize inappropriate prescribing in the future (4). Though the easiest and least costly to perform, retrospective DUR does not provide the pharmacist with an opportunity to modify drug therapy before it is dispensed (3). Many health care systems have shifted from the traditional retrospective DUR, with its focus on drug-specific problems, to include disease management concepts, such as evidenced-based treatment guidelines and algorithms, to ensure patient-centered, cost-effective, and clinically efficacious care (3).

B. **"Drug Use Evaluation" or "Drug Use Review"** is a process that involves the formal development, monitoring, and adjustment of objective, measurable criteria that describe the appropriate use of a drug (5). The underlying concepts of drug use evaluation (DUE) are now contained as part of the more current and broader concept of medication-use evaluation (6).

C. **"Medication-Use Evaluation"** is a performance improvement method that focuses on evaluating and improving medication use processes with the goal of optimal patient outcomes (6).

1. A medication-use evaluation (MUE) focuses on the outcome of a patient's medication therapy according to predetermined criteria. **The goal of the evaluation is to optimize medication management and improve the patient's quality of life throughout all phases of the medication-use process (6).** The medication-use *process* includes the responsibilities of prescribing, preparation and dispensing, administration, and monitoring of medications. The medication-use *evaluation* is concerned with the interrelatedness of these functions and the continuum of care.

2. A MUE can be initiated for a variety of reasons and is not restricted to the prescribing and dispensing functions of a pharmacist. It can evaluate a single medication, an entire therapeutic class of medications, various disease states or conditions, and actual or potential medication-use process problems. Reasons prompting a MUE include the following:

a. Problem-prone drugs
b. High-volume and high-cost drugs
c. High-risk medications
d. High-risk patient populations
e. New drug entities
f. New therapeutic plans

3. A MUE can be conducted in any health care setting provided the process is interdisciplinary, collaborative, and prospective and has access to comprehensive patient information.

4. The MUE is compatible with the performance improvement model. The performance improvement steps of "Plan, Do, Check, and Act" are paramount to the MUE process. The evaluation process not only provides a guide to optimize therapy management, prevent medication-related problems, control costs, and maximize patient safety, but it also provides insight into the appropriateness of the criteria used and optimal functioning of the medication-use

process. Therefore, the MUE has become an essential component of performance improvement initiatives within many health care systems.

D. **"Criteria"** are predetermined parameters of drug prescribing and use established by a DUR program for comparison to actual practice. Development of criteria is the collaborative responsibility of practitioners (e.g., physicians, pharmacists, and nurses) and administrators and is based on standards of practice and evidence-based guidelines published in the primary literature.

II. HISTORY

A. **Drug Utilization Review (DUR)**

1. DUR has been mandated by our federal and state governments for several decades and is required by organizations that seek government funding for medical services provided to Medicare and Medicaid patients.

2. The funding of health care began in the 1930s with the creation of the Social Security Act. Medicare and Medicaid came into existence in the 1960s to address the financial needs of patients in nursing facilities. In 1967, Congress authorized the first set of standards for nursing facilities. Since that time, several regulations have been adopted and amended. Though long-term care (LTC) facilities and hospitals have been under these regulations for the longest period of time, outpatient providers of care, including managed care organizations, home health care agencies, and mail order pharmacies, are also included under these regulations. Outpatient prescribing practices were brought into the review process in the 1990s with the passage of the **Omnibus Budget Reconciliation Act of 1990 (OBRA '90).**

3. OBRA '90 (42USC1396r-8) mandated the formation of DUR boards by each state for providing outpatient prescription services to state Medicaid patients. The intent of OBRA '90 was to increase patient education and promote appropriate medication use through prescribing practices, thereby controlling health care costs funded by the government.

   a. Three excerpts from the current version of OBRA '90 that are relevant to DUR requirements for pharmacists are given here (7).

      (1) . . . a State shall provide . . . for a drug use review program . . . for covered outpatient drugs in order to assure that prescriptions (i) are appropriate, (ii) are medically necessary, and (iii) are not likely to result in adverse medical results. The program shall be designed to educate physicians and pharmacists to identify and reduce the frequency of patterns of fraud, abuse, gross overuse, or inappropriate or medically unnecessary care, among physicians, pharmacists, and patients, or associated with specific drugs or groups of drugs, as well as potential and actual severe adverse reactions to drugs including education on therapeutic appropriateness, overutilization and underutilization, appropriate use of generic products, therapeutic duplication, drug-disease contraindications, drug-drug interactions, incorrect drug dosage or duration of drug treatment, drug-allergy interactions, and clinical abuse/misuse.

      (2) The State plan shall provide for a review of drug therapy before each prescription is filled or delivered to an individual receiving benefits under this subchapter, typically at the point-of-sale or point of distribution. The review shall include screening for potential drug therapy problems due to therapeutic duplication, drug-disease contraindication, drug-drug interactions (including serious interactions with nonprescription or over-the-counter drugs), incorrect drug dosage or duration of drug treatment, drug-allergy interactions, and clinical abuse/misuse.

      (3) As part of the State's prospective DUR program . . . applicable State law shall establish standards for counseling of individuals receiving benefits under this subchapter by pharmacists . . .

   b. As DUR is required by all states and in all health care settings, you should become knowledgeable about the applicable statutes requiring DUR activities for the state in which you are practicing.

4. The USP has also developed and published similar standards to be incorporated by the state DUR boards. Standards are established and enforced by the Health Care Finance Administration (HCFA), and the focus of these standards is to prevent the following:

   a. Over/under-utilization of drugs

   b. Duplication of therapy

   c. Drug-drug, drug-food, drug-disease, and drug allergy interactions

   d. Incorrect dosage or duration

   e. Clinical abuse or misuse

5. In addition to these standards, the USP adopted the *Guiding Principles Supporting Appropriate Drug Use at the Patient and Population Level* in 2001, to guide prescribers and health care systems in decisions affecting drug therapy in regard to patient care, formulary management, and reimbursement issues (8). Appropriate drug use includes steps to ensure that:

    a. drug selection is optimally adjusted to the needs of individual patients;

    b. patients are appropriately monitored for the result of therapeutic intervention and adverse events;

    c. patients are adequately educated and the treatment program is communicated to all concerned;

    d. steps are taken to assure, for individual patients and for the whole population or population group under consideration, that both over and under utilization are adequately scrutinized and addressed;

    e. and necessary interventions occur when drug use is shown not be appropriate (8).

6. OBRA '90 was further revised by HCFA in 1999 to incorporate quality indicators into the review of nursing facilities. A total of 24 indicators and 11 domains were created to evaluate the quality of the health care process and outcomes of care. Though medication use can be evaluated in all domains, it is the primary focus for the specific domains of clinical management, infection control, psychotropic drug use, and quality of life indicators.

7. LTC facilities are evaluated according to the OBRA '90 regulations and the Beers Criteria (9), which was published in 1997, and were included in the revision of OBRA '90 in 1999. These criteria were incorporated to assist in the evaluation of potential inappropriateness of medication use by elderly patients in LTC facilities. The criteria are categorized according to high and low severity levels and identify specific medications as well as disease and medication combinations that could be inappropriate.

B. Medication-Use Evaluation (MUE)

1. MUE is a concept more recent than that of either DUE or DUR. The *ASHP Guidelines on Medication-Use Evaluation* was approved in 1996 (6) and adopted to replace the *ASHP Guidelines on the Pharmacist's Role in Drug-Use Evaluation* published in 1987 (5).

2. Unlike DUR, MUE is not mandated by government regulations. However, health care systems seeking accreditation by appropriate agencies or organizations (e.g., The Joint Commission) are subjected to an evaluation of the MUE process.

3. MUEs satisfy The Joint Commission's Medication Management Standards for hospital accreditation (10). The Joint Commission recognizes that safe medication management systems should address a hospital's medication-use *processes,* which includes medication selection, ordering and transcribing, preparing and dispensing, administration, and monitoring. A successful medication management system continuously *evaluates* these processes using MUE principles to improve the quality of patient care by

    a. reducing practice variation, errors, and misuse;

    b. monitoring medication management processes with regard to efficacy, quality and safety;

    c. standardizing equipment and processes across the hospital to improve the medication management system;

    d. using evidence-based good practices to develop medication management processes;

    e. managing critical processes associated with medication management to promote safe medication management throughout the hospital . . . (10)

III.   PROFESSIONAL STANDARDS OF PRACTICE

The current codes of ethics and standards of practice endorsed by the American Pharmacists Association (APhA), the ASHP, the NABP, the AMCP, and other pharmacy associations address the issue of the pharmacist's responsibility for conducting DUR and MUE.

A. The APhA *Code of Ethics for Pharmacists* discusses this issue in a general sense in the following statements:

1. "Pharmacists are health professionals who assist individuals in making the best use of medications."

2. ". . . a pharmacist promises to help individuals achieve optimum benefit from their medications, to be committed to their welfare, and to maintain their trust" (11).

B. The ASHP has adopted and published several documents that speak to the responsibility of the pharmacist in this area of practice.

1. The most current guidelines for evaluating the medication-use process are contained in the *ASHP Guidelines on Medication-Use Evaluation* (6).

2. A second document, the *ASHP Statement on Pharmaceutical Care*, states that pharmaceutical care "merits the highest priority in all practice settings (12)." In providing this type of service, ASHP identifies a major function of the pharmacist to be the identification, resolution, and prevention of drug-related problems caused by untreated indications, improper drug selection, sub-thera-peutic dosage, failure to receive medication, over-dosage, adverse drug reactions, drug interac-tions, and medication use without indication.

C. Section 3 of the NABP *Model Rules for the Practice of Pharmacy* defines the elements that should be covered by a pharmacist conducting a prospective DUR (13):

> **A Pharmacist shall review the patient record and each Prescription Drug Order for**
> **(1)** known allergies;
> **(2)** rational therapy contraindications;
> **(3)** reasonable dose, duration of use, and route of Administration, considering age, gen-der, and other patient factors;
> **(4)** reasonable directions for use;
> **(5)** potential or actual adverse Drug reactions;
> **(6)** Drug-Drug interactions;
> **(7)** Drug-food interactions;
> **(8)** Drug-disease interactions;
> **(9)** therapeutic duplication;
> **(10)** proper utilization (including over- or under-utilization), and optimum therapeutic outcomes; and
> **(11)** abuse/misuse. [Emphasis added]
>
> "Upon recognizing any of the above, the Pharmacist shall take appropriate steps to avoid or resolve the problem which shall, if necessary, include consultation with the Practitioner (13).

D. The AMCP is a professional association of pharmacists who serve patients and the public by the pro-motion of rational drug therapy through the application of managed care principles, with the objec-tive of ensuring appropriate health care outcomes for all individuals. In the position paper *Concepts in Managed Care Pharmacy Series: Pharmaceutical Care*, the pharmacist's role in pharmaceutical care and DUR are clearly defined (14). Though this paper is intended for those pharmacists working in man-aged care settings, the core activities are applicable to all pharmacists and include the following:
1. Assess patient therapy.
2. Develop systems to maximize safety (prevent/minimize adverse drug events).
3. Educate patients about medications.
4. Provide oversight of therapy management and monitoring initiatives.

IV. MEDICATION PROFILE RECORDS

A. Comprehensive and accurate patient medication profile records are necessary tools in performing any form of DUR or MUE. In order to perform prospective DUR well, the pharmacist must have access to information concerning the patient's medical history, current diagnosis, past and present medication use, laboratory values, and lifestyle. Some of this information can be found on the patient's medication profile in a community pharmacy or the medical chart in a hospital, ambulatory clinic, or LTC facility. Needed information not on the profile or in the chart should be obtained from the patient, caregiver, or prescriber.

B. The NABP *Model Rules for the Practice of Pharmacy* addresses the issue of recommended patient records systems for pharmacies. It is important to note that the Model Rules recommend that these patient records be kept for not less than 5 years from the date of the last profile entry (13).

C. The following list identifies information that should be available in a patient's medication profile and reviewed by the pharmacist when performing a prospective DUR. Some of the items for inclusion on medication profile records maintained by pharmacists are required by the NABP Model Act (13), whereas others are required by law in some states. Be sure to check the applica-ble laws for the state in which you practice.
1. Patient identification information: full name, address, telephone number, date of birth, and gender
2. Patient medical history: allergies, adverse drug reactions, idiosyncrasies, history of chronic con-ditions and medical and surgical events, use of drug products or devices (either prescription, over-the-counter, or herbal/dietary supplements) that are not in the dispensing record. If there are none, this should be indicated.
3. Other useful patient information: height, weight, occupation, any additional helpful information, such as inability to use safety closures or swallow tablets or capsules
4. Information on third-party payers insurance: or medical assistance

5. **Information for each prescription order dispensed:**
   a. Drug product information: name (generic and/or brand), strength, and dosage form
   b. Quantity dispensed
   c. Directions for use: should identify dose, frequency and route of administration, and, if not treating a chronic lifetime condition, duration of use
   d. Therapeutic indication or the diagnosis related to the prescription order
   e. Supplemental information and warnings (e.g., administration instructions)
   f. Prescriber identification and contact information
   g. Retrieval designation assigned to the prescription order
   h. Date of dispensing for initial fill and all renewals
   i. Identification of dispensing pharmacist
6. Pharmacist comments relevant to the individual's drug therapy

V.   ELEMENTS FOR PROSPECTIVE DRUG UTILIZATION REVIEW

When a new or refill prescription or medication order is presented to the pharmacist, the following elements of a prospective DUR should be considered when evaluating the medication for potential drug-related problems (15,16).

A. **Accuracy and completeness of the prescription or medication order** Is there any information missing from the prescription that you should confirm with the patient, caregiver, or prescriber prior to dispensing the medication?

B. **Allergies or adverse events** Is the patient allergic to or intolerant of any treatments currently being taken or used in the past?

C. **Appropriateness of the medication selected**
   1. Is the medication selected for this patient the most efficacious to treat his or her condition?
   2. Could the patient's condition be refractory to this medication?
   3. Is this medication the safest option for this patient?
   4. Does this patient have any contraindications for using this medication (e.g., pregnancy or lactation, kidney or liver impairment/failure, age, other medications or medical conditions)?
   5. Would non–drug therapy be indicated as initial treatment?

D. **Appropriateness of the medication regimen prescribed**
   1. Are the *dose, frequency, and duration or length of therapy* appropriate for the following:
      a. The patient's medical condition being treated
      b. The patient's characteristics (e.g., age, gender, race, pregnancy, or lactation)
      c. The patient's height and weight (if applicable)
      d. The patient's kidney or liver function
      e. The patient's baseline laboratory values (if available)
      f. The patient's other medical conditions
   2. Is the *formulation and route of administration* appropriate for this patient?
      a. Is the patient able to self-administer or use the medication appropriately?
      b. Can the patient swallow solid dosage forms?
      c. Is this formulation appropriate to treat this patient's condition?

E. **Potential or actual drug adverse effects**
   1. What are the potential adverse effects of this drug?
   2. Are any of the patient's current symptoms or medical conditions possibly drug-induced?
   3. If unavoidable, does the patient need additional therapy (drug or non-drug) to tolerate these adverse effects?

F. **Potential drug interactions**
   1. Are there any clinically significant *drug-drug* interactions?
   2. Are there any clinically significant *drug-disease* interactions?
   3. Are there any clinically significant *drug-food* interactions?
   4. Are there any clinically significant *drug-laboratory value* interactions (if applicable)?
   5. What is the patient's usual consumption of alcohol?
   6. Is the patient's current use of social drug problematic?

G. **Therapeutic duplication**
   1. Is the patient already receiving therapy (drug or non-drug) to treat this condition?
   2. Is synergist therapy (e.g., another medication, dietary restrictions, lifestyle changes) recommended with this medication?

H. **Proper utilization and optimum therapeutic outcomes**
   1. **For a *new* prescription or medication order:**
      a. Does the patient understand the purpose of this medication?
      b. Will the patient be able to take this medication as prescribed?
      c. Will the cost of the medication pose a financial barrier to the patient adhering to use?
      d. What are the anticipated clinical outcomes from the use of this medication?
   2. **For a *refill* prescription or medication order:**
      a. Is the patient using this medication for a condition that no longer exists?
      b. Does the patient forget to take this medication or prefer not to?
      c. Does the patient not understand the purpose and directions for use, or is he or she unable to administer the medication?
   3. Does the patient require any adherence or educational tools to prevent over- or under-utilization of this medication?
   4. Is the medication available for the patient to use?
I. **Abuse or misuse** Is the patient addicted to or using this medication for recreational purposes?

VI. WHAT TO DO WHEN A PROBLEM IS IDENTIFIED

A. When working with patients and other health professionals concerning a drug therapy problem always be tactful and professional. No matter what the problem (including over-utilization, failure to adherence to prescribed therapy, illogical prescribing, etc.), approach a patient, caregiver, and health care provider with the assumption that there is a good reason or a logical explanation for the prescribed therapy or the present course of action.

B. **Considerations:**
   1. What is the severity or clinical relevance of the problem? This must be considered because it will determine your course of action.
   2. There is a potential problem with *a new prescription or medication order.*
      a. Dispense the medication as written. For example: There may be a drug interaction, but no special precautions are necessary or it can be accommodated with appropriate patient education on the use of the medication and/or monitoring.
      b. A change in therapy is required, and the prescriber should be contacted.
         (1) *Briefly* identify the patient by name and describe his or her medical condition and the medication(s) involved.
         (2) *Briefly* describe the problem and your recommendations to correct or minimize the problem. Provide a reference source for your information if applicable.
         (3) Have suggestions ready for alternatives.
         (4) If the problem cannot be resolved to your satisfaction, you may decide to not dispense the medication. You should fully inform the patient of your concerns and actions on his or her behalf and document your intervention.
   3. There is a potential problem with *current existing therapy.*
      a. If the problem is over- or under-utilization of a current medication:
         (1) Talk with the patient or caregiver. Remember to be tactful as there may be a logical reason for the suspected overuse or non-adherence.
         (2) You may need to alert the patient's prescriber so that together you can work with the patient to solve the problem.
         (3) Document the intervention.
      b. If the problem is a *new adverse event* as a result of current therapy:
         (1) Get detailed information from the patient about the adverse reaction: what happened, when, specific circumstances, and other medications (prescription, over-the-counter, and herbal/dietary supplements) he or she is currently taking.
         (2) Discuss the problem with the patient's physician:
            (a) *Briefly* identify the patient by name and describe his or her medical condition and the medication(s) involved.
            (b) *Briefly* describe the problem and your recommendations. Provide a reference source for your information if applicable.
            (c) Have suggestions ready for alternatives.
         (3) Document the intervention.
         (4) If this is a serious adverse event, report it to the FDA. Report forms, including both on-line and printed forms that can be mailed or faxed, are available on the FDA Web site at www.fda.gov under the MedWatch system.

REFERENCES

1. The United States Pharmacopeial Convention, Inc. Principles of a sound drug formulary system. www.usp.org/hqi/patientSafety/resources/soundFormularyPrinciples.html Accessed December 2007.

2. The U.S. Pharmacopeia Drug Utilization Review Advisory Panel. Drug utilization review: Mechanisms to improve its effectiveness and broaden its scope. J Am Pharm Assoc 2000; 40: 538–545.

3. Academy of Managed Care Pharmacy. *Concepts in managed care pharmacy series: Drug use evaluation.* Accessed December 2007.

4. Hennessy S, Bilker WB, Zhou L, et al. Retrospective drug utilization review, prescribing errors, and clinical outcomes. JAMA 2003; 290: 1494–1499.

5. American Society of Health Systems Pharmacists. ASHP guidelines on the pharmacist's role in drug use evaluation. Am J Hosp Pharm 1988; 45: 385–386.

6. American Society of Health-System Pharmacists. ASHP guidelines on medication-use evaluation. Am J Health-Syst Pharm 1996; 53: 1953–1955.

7. 42USC1396r-8.

8. Council of Experts Information Executive Committee. Guiding principles supporting appropriate drug use at the patient and population level. Statement of scientific policy. United States Pharmacopeia Convention, Inc., March 12, 2001. http://www.usp.org/pdf/EN/patientSafety/pSafetyDrugGuidPrinc.pdf Accessed December 2007.

9. Beer NH Explicit criteria for determining potentially inappropriate medication use by the elderly: An update. Arch Int Med 1997; 157: 1531–1536.

10. The Joint Commission on Accreditation of Healthcare Organizations. Comprehensive accreditation manual for hospitals: The official handbook. Oakbrook Terrace, IL, 2008.

11. American Pharmaceutical Association. Code of ethics for pharmacists. Adopted by the membership of the American Pharmaceutical Association, Washington, DC, October 27, 1994.

12. American Society of Health-System Pharmacists. ASHP statement on pharmaceutical care. Am J Health-Syst Pharm 1993; 50: 1720–1723.

13. National Association of Boards of Pharmacy. Model rules for the practice of pharmacy. Park Ridge, IL: National Association of Boards of Pharmacy, 2007; 83.

14. Academy of Managed Care Pharmacy. Concepts in managed care pharmacy series: Pharmaceutical care. Accessed December 2007.

15. Galt K. Developing clinical practice skills for pharmacists. Bethesda, MD: American Society of Health-System Pharmacists, 2006: 170–172.

16. Cipolle RJ, Strand LM, Morely PC. Pharmaceutical care practice: The clinician's guide, 2nd ed. New York: McGraw-Hill, 2004: 171–200.

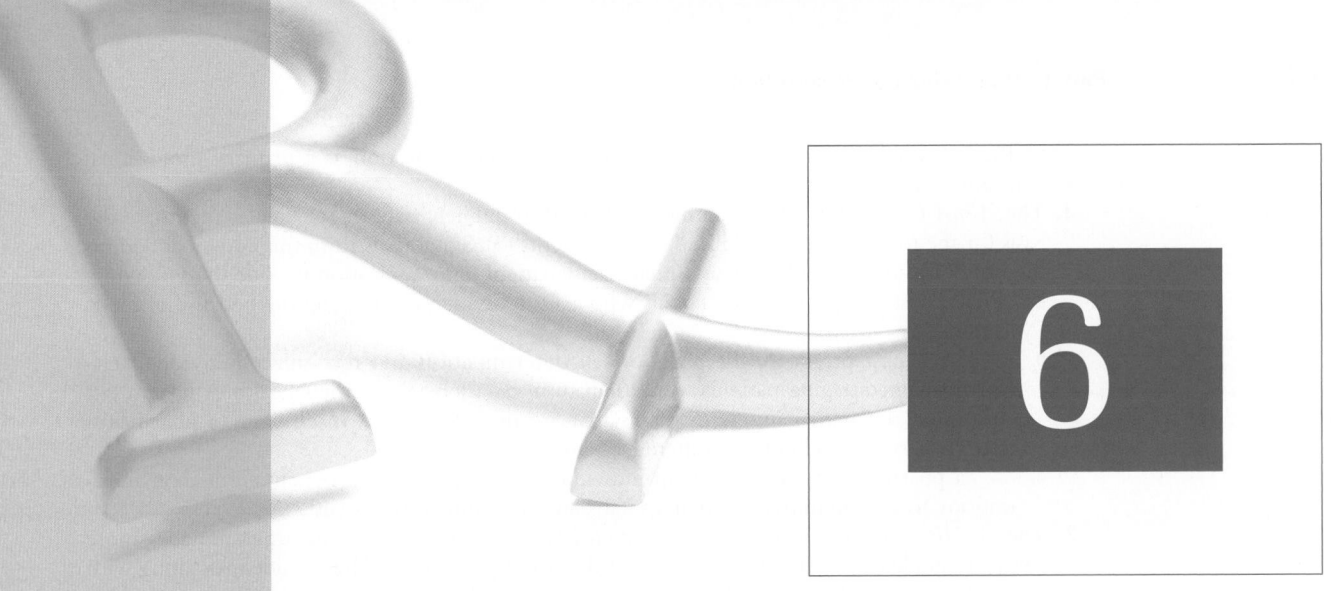

6

Patient Counseling

Karen Kopacek, R.Ph.

I. PROFESSIONAL STANDARDS OF PRACTICE

A. Though it may seem that talking with a patient about his or her medications is a normal function of the pharmacist, this has not always been true. From the 1940s until the late 1960s, ethical codes for pharmacists advised them against discussing medications with their patients. There was concern that a pharmacist could disrupt the patient-physician relationship if he or she discussed topics such as therapeutic indications, side effects, and precautions with a patient. To illustrate the evolution in standards of practice concerning the level of patient interactions with the pharmacist, compare the following excerpt from the American Pharmacists Association (APhA) code of ethics published in 1952 to a recent definition of pharmaceutical care written decades later:

1. **1952:** "The pharmacist does not discuss the therapeutic effects or composition of a prescription with a patient. When such questions are asked, he suggests that the qualified practitioner (physician or dentist) is the proper person with whom such matters should be discussed" (1).

2. **1998:** "Pharmaceutical care is a patient-centered practice in which the practitioner (pharmacist) assumes responsibility for a patient's drug-related needs and is held accountable for this commitment" (2).

Notice how the role of the pharmacist has shifted from holding a limited discussion with the patient concerning the use of a prescription medication to working cooperatively with the patient, in coordination with other health care providers (including the physician), to address all the patient's health care needs.

B. The current codes of ethics and standards of practice promulgated by the APhA, the American Society of Health-System Pharmacists (ASHP), the American Association of Colleges of Pharmacy

(AACP), and other pharmacy associations promote patient education as a primary professional responsibility of pharmacists.

1. The *APhA Code of Ethics* is a document intended to publicly state the principles that form the basis for the roles and responsibilities of pharmacists (3). Statements from this code that address the issue of patient consultation and pharmacist-patient communication include the following:

   a. "Pharmacists are health professionals who assist individuals in making the best use of medications."

   b. "A pharmacist promotes the right of self-determination and recognizes individual self-worth by encouraging patients to participate in decisions about their health. A pharmacist communicates with patients in terms that are understandable. In all cases, a pharmacist respects personal and cultural differences among patients."

   c. ". . . a pharmacist promises to help individuals achieve optimum benefit from their medications, to be committed to their welfare, and to maintain their trust."

2. The *ASHP Guidelines on Pharmacist-Conducted Patient Education and Counseling* provides more complete guidelines for the pharmacist on this area of practice (4). These guidelines, along with the *APhA Code of Ethics,* should be recommended reading for pharmacy students and pharmacists in all practice settings. The first paragraph in the introductory "Purpose" section emphasizes the influential role the pharmacist has in achieving better patient outcomes and improving the quality of life of each patient:

   > Providing pharmaceutical care entails accepting responsibility for patients' pharmacotherapeutic outcomes. Pharmacists can contribute to positive outcomes by educating and counseling patients to prepare and motivate them to follow their pharmacotherapeutic regimens and monitoring plans. The purpose of this document is to help pharmacists provide effective patient education and counseling.

II.   STATE LAW

A. Because professions such as pharmacy, medicine, and law are regulated by state laws, the legal responsibilities of these professionals vary from state to state. As part of their pharmacy practice acts, individual states have implemented pharmacist consultation requirements.

B. To provide more uniformity of regulation from state to state, the National Association of Boards of Pharmacy (NABP) mandated patient counseling and endorsed the development of model regulations in 1990. *The Model Rules for the Practice of Pharmacy* includes a section addressing patient consultation and lists specific elements for counseling (5).

1. Section 3 of the *Model Rules for the Practice of Pharmacy* states that

   > Upon receipt of a Prescription Drug Order and following a review of the patient's record, a Pharmacist shall personally initiate discussion of matters which will enhance or optimize Drug therapy with each patient or caregiver of such patient.

   The pharmacist is encouraged to consult with the patient or caregiver in person but may use the telephone, if necessary. The Model Rules further state that alternative means of communication, such as information leaflets, pictogram labels, or video programs, shall be used to supplement (not replace) the discussion when appropriate.

2. The elements (or matters) recommended in the Model Rules for discussion with patients include the following:

   (a) The name and description of the Drug;

   (b) the dosage form, dose, route of Administration, and duration of Drug therapy;

   (c) intended use of the Drug and expected action;

   (d) special directions and precautions for preparation, Administration, and use by the patient;

   (e) common severe side or adverse effects or interactions and therapeutic contraindications that may be encountered, including their avoidance, and the action required if they occur;

   (f) techniques for self-monitoring Drug therapy;

   (g) proper storage;

   (h) prescription refill information;

   (i) action to be taken in the event of a missed dose; and

   (j) Pharmacist comments relevant to the individual's Drug therapy, including any other information peculiar to the specific patient or Drug (5).

3. To further emphasize the importance of patient consultation, Section 6 of the Model Rules identifies the following as an act of unprofessional conduct on the part of a pharmacist or pharmacy: "Attempting to circumvent the Patient Counseling requirements, or discouraging the patient from receiving Patient Counseling concerning their Prescription Drug Orders" (6).

C. Though the NABP may recommend model pharmacy practice legislation, it is up to individual state governments to introduce and pass recommended legislation. States may and do customize such rules for their own purposes. Because all states have now codified requirements for patient counseling by pharmacists, consult the pharmacy practice act for the state in which you are practicing to determine the specific requirements of your state law on patient counseling.

III.   FEDERAL LAW

A. If regulation of professional practice is left to the states, how does the federal government get involved? The federal government has a vested interest in keeping medical costs under control, particularly when it has to pay the bill. In 1990, the 101st Congress included in the Omnibus Budget Reconciliation Act (OBRA '90) provisions aimed at controlling escalating medical costs for entitlement programs. Under OBRA '90, pharmacists are held responsible for patient counseling and are required to perform a drug utilization review. This was the result of a series of studies issued by the Office of the Inspector General for the Department of Health and Human Services. These studies found that pharmacists who monitor drug therapy and help patients to use their medications appropriately were providing valuable medical services and ultimately reducing the costs of providing medical care (7–9). Though OBRA '90 technically covered patients receiving care through various Medicaid programs, all states have now passed regulations that expand these services to all patients. Refer to Chapter 5 for more information on OBRA '90 requirements for drug utilization review.

B. An excerpt from OBRA '90 (42USC1396r-8) that is relevant to patient consultation requirements for pharmacists is given here (10). Note the similarity between the NABP's Model Rules and the OBRA '90 recommended elements that a pharmacist should discuss with a patient.

> (I) The pharmacist must offer to discuss with each individual receiving benefits under this subchapter or caregiver of such individual (in person, whenever practicable, or through access to a telephone service which is toll-free for long-distance calls) who presents a prescription, matters which in the exercise of the pharmacist's professional judgment (consistent with State law respecting the provision of such information), the pharmacist deems significant including the following:
>> (aa) The name and description of the medication.
>> (bb) The route, dosage form, dosage, route of administration, and duration of drug therapy.
>> (cc) Special directions and precautions for preparation, administration and use by the patient.
>> (dd) Common severe side or adverse effects or interactions and therapeutic contraindications that may be encountered, including their avoidance, and the action required if they occur.
>> (ee) Techniques for self-monitoring drug therapy.
>> (ff) Proper storage.
>> (gg) Prescription refill information.
>> (hh) Action to be taken in the event of a missed dose.
>
> (II) A reasonable effort must be made by the pharmacist to obtain, record, and maintain at least the following information regarding individuals receiving benefits under this subchapter:
>> (aa) Name, address, telephone number, date of birth (or age) and gender.
>> (bb) Individual history where significant, including disease state or states, known allergies and drug reactions, and a comprehensive list of medications and relevant devices.
>> (cc) Pharmacist comments relevant to the individual's drug therapy.

Nothing in this clause shall be construed as requiring a pharmacist to provide consultation when an individual receiving benefits under this subchapter or caregiver of such individual refuses such consultation (10).

IV.   GENERAL GUIDELINES FOR PATIENT COUNSELING

There are many excellent journal articles, books, and programs available to pharmacy students and pharmacists on the subject of patient education and counseling. The sections that follow in this chapter provide a basic introduction to this subject. Though this information is written primarily from the point of view of a patient receiving counseling in a community pharmacy, the principles can be easily applied to any practice setting.

A. **Appropriate physical environment** Discussion with patients or caregivers about health, pharmacotherapy, and other medical issues is a private activity. This aspect of patient counseling is critical and should be respected no matter what the practice site is—hospital room, clinic, busy community pharmacy, or drive-up window. Some means of conducting this activity in a confidential, semiprivate area away from other people is required by the Health Insurance Portability and Accountability Act of 1996 (HIPAA). If the environment precludes privacy (e.g., a drive-up window), the pharmacist should either request that the patient come into the pharmacy or make arrangements to talk about relevant issues by telephone.

B. Before you prepare the prescription The consultation process begins not when you transfer the prescription to the patient but as you receive the prescription order from the patient or the agent of the patient.

1. **Input from the patient**
   a. Ask the patient or caregiver if there is any information you should have before preparing the prescription. For example, has the prescriber given the patient any special instructions? Can the patient open child-resistant safety closures? What about language barriers; can the patient read labeling in English?
   b. An issue of increasing relevance is that of third-party coverage for prescription medications. Some plans have formulary restrictions concerning which medications will be covered at varying costs to the patient. Patients may need help in understanding that a formulary restriction does not imply that they cannot obtain a prescribed medication, but it may mean that the patient has to pay more for the medication or the pharmacy may need prior-authorization prior to dispensing it. These can be complex issues, especially for patients, so explanations and discussions should take place in an atmosphere of patience and mutual respect.
   c. If the prescription order is for a branded product, check if a generic equivalent can legally be dispensed. If so, does the patient want a generic product? What are the implications with respect to therapy, cost to the patient, third-party coverage, and co-payments?

2. **Drug utilization review**
   a. Perform the normal prospective drug utilization review of the patient's medication record as described in Chapter 5. Are there any contraindications to the new therapy, any therapeutic duplication with current medications, or drug-drug interactions?
   b. Look not only for problems with the new prescription but also review the patient's complete drug therapy regimen. Issues to monitor for include the following:
      (1) Do there appear to be problems with adherence to or over-utilization of existing therapy?
      (2) Does this patient need reinforcement on the importance and benefits of taking his or her medication as prescribed or advice on strategies to improve adherence?
      (3) Would a dosing aid, such as a pill reminder box, a tablet splitter, or a pocket pill box, be helpful?

C. Delivery of prescription to the patient
1. It is helpful to give the patient an estimate of the length of time the consultation will require. Recognize the patient's right to refuse counseling. Most patients are appreciative of your professional advice and counsel; however, circumstances may exist that interfere with a complete consultation. For example, a patient may be very ill and wants or needs to get home. Perhaps the patient is a sick child, and the parent or caregiver is not in a position to be attentive to your counseling. In cases like this, you may want to give only the essential information and offer to call the patient or caregiver later for a more complete consultation. Patients who are in pain or other distress are most likely unable to concentrate on what you are saying. When they have returned to the familiar surroundings of their home and have experienced some relief, they are better able to understand you and remember what you have told them.
2. Maintain a professional, sincere attitude. Use a professional, friendly, relaxed, and sincere demeanor. This attitude should help put the patient at ease and foster an atmosphere that encourages the patient to ask questions.
3. Use language appropriate to the needs and level of understanding of the patient. Avoid technical medical terms and jargon unless you are talking with a fellow health care provider. At the same time, do not "talk down" to the patient. Many patients are very knowledgeable; assessing their level of understanding is essential to a good consultation. Listening to the patient and using open-ended questions will help you to assess the patient's level of knowledge and understanding.
4. The pharmacist's role in promoting the right of self-determination for patients is explicitly stated in the *APhA Code of Ethics,* so it is essential that pharmacists inform their patients about both the positive and negative aspects of drug therapy. However, necessary precautions to warn the patient or caregiver about should be disclosed in a tactful way. Consider how you would feel about taking a medication if your pharmacist informed you that you may cough up blood, stop breathing, or go into convulsions while taking it. Would you want to take such a medication?

5. Pay close attention to the patient's body language. Watch the patient's face for feedback. Do the eyes indicate that you are being understood? Does the patient appear to be interested in what you are saying, or have you obviously lost contact?

6. Be aware of cultural differences among patients. If you work with patients who have different cultural backgrounds from your own, make it a point to learn about cultural issues that will help you in communicating most effectively with these patients.

V.   ELEMENTS FOR PATIENT COUNSELING

Guidelines published by several agencies and organizations provide the pharmacist with a list of elements (or topics) to discuss when providing patient consultations. Following are some suggestions on how to cover these topics when preparing your consults using the Consultation Prep Form found in Figure 6.1. If you are unsure as to how to phrase a question or begin discussing on a particular topic, Figures 6.2 and 6.3 include expanded consultation skill checklists for new prescriptions and refill medications.

A. Introduction

1. Establish a relationship with patient

   a. Introduce yourself to the patient if he or she is not known to you.

   b. Find out whether you are talking directly with the patient, a family member, or some other agent of the patient. You may want to find out how the patient prefers to be addressed. Some patients prefer being called by their first names, whereas others may be offended by such familiarity. This is also your opportunity to get an initial sense of the patient's level of understanding.

2. Intent and duration of consult

   a. Offer to spend a few minutes with the patient to give advice on the effective use of the prescribed medication and to answer any questions.

   b. If the use and monitoring of the medication is complicated and needs an extended consult, be honest with the patient about this. He or she may want to be told the essentials with an agreed time in the future for a more complete conversation.

   c. Again, be sensitive to patients who are obviously ill. They may need a brief consult with a follow-up phone call.

3. Data gathering

   a. If the patient is new to your pharmacy, document the following information into the patient's record: **name, address, telephone number(s), date of birth (or age), and gender.** Other personal information that may be beneficial to have on record includes height and weight, especially for those medications that require dosing based on body weight or body surface area.

   b. **Prior medical history to document includes acute or chronic disease state(s), known allergies, any adverse drug reactions, and a comprehensive list of medications that covers prescription medications, over-the-counters, and herbal or dietary supplements.** Screen the patient for required vaccinations; many community pharmacies offer influenza clinics during the fall and winter months, and this can be a way to identify potential patients to provide this service to.

   c. It is not unprofessional for the pharmacist to ask about alcohol or tobacco use, as these substances have been linked with chronic medical conditions and interact with certain medications. However, you should use tact when asking a patient about alcohol consumption or tobacco use, as he or she may be hesitant to discuss this with you. Be clear with the patient why this information is important for you to know and remain professional and nonjudgmental. If the patient currently uses or recently quit using tobacco products, this may offer the opportunity for you to provide information on tobacco cessation or support his or her current cessation efforts.

   d. In some cases, asking the patient about family history can be important for assessing his or her risk for developing chronic illnesses, such as cardiovascular disease.

   e. If the patient is picking up a refill prescription, verify the current information documented in your medication record and enter any updates.

B. Administration

1. Patient knowledge assessment

   a. Assess the patient's current understanding of the prescribed medication and the medical condition it is intended to treat by using open-ended questions. **What did the prescriber tell the patient about this medication? Does the patient know the medication's name(s) and it's indication for use? Did the prescriber instruct the patient on**

how to take or use the medication and for how long? What is the patient to expect from this therapy?

b. Ask the patient if he or she has ever taken this medication or has received a similar one in the past. If so, what was the result? Has the patient ever had either an unusual or allergic reaction to a medication of this type?

c. If the prescription is a refill, ask questions to determine the effectiveness of the therapy. Rather than simply asking if the patient has any questions, find out whether he or she thinks that the medication is "working." How is the patient feeling? Is he or she experiencing any side effects? What time(s) of day are the doses being taken? Are there problems with adherence to the prescribed frequency owing to work or home schedules or with other medications he or she is also taking?

2. **Name of medication, indication, and mechanism of action**
   a. From the patient assessment, you should have a sense about the patient's current understanding of the medication. Therefore, avoid repeating information that the patient already knows unless you need to stress important issues concerning administration.
   b. **It is absolutely essential to establish with the patient the name, dosage, and therapeutic indication of the medication being dispensed.** This is an important safeguard in preventing a medication error by dispensing the wrong medication or dosage to the patient. Many drug names look or sound alike but have entirely different indications for use.
   c. Discuss how the medication is expected to work or treat his or her medical condition. Again, avoid using technical medical terms and jargon unless you are talking with a fellow health care provider. This information will help to stress the importance of taking the medication as prescribed and assist the patient in monitoring for the effectiveness of treatment.

3. **Directions for use**
   a. When discussing the directions for use on the prescription label with the patient, use the **"show and tell"** method.
      (1) Open the prescription vial and "show" the tablets or capsules to yourself and the patient. This provides you with an opportunity to check that the correct medication is in the container. You may want to pour a few doses into the vial cap, but avoid spilling or touching the medication. Another important benefit of "showing" the medication to the patient or caregiver prior to dispensing is to assess the patient's ability to swallow the capsule or tablet. If the drug is too large for the patient to easily swallow or should not be chewed, cut, or crushed, you will need to discuss other alternatives with the patient and prescriber.
      (2) Then review the prescription label and read back or "tell" the instructions to the patient. "Show and tell" is also important when dispensing refill medications, as the patient can confirm if the drug in the prescription vial is the same one they have been taking.
   b. Also review when the patient should begin taking the new medication. Did the prescriber indicate that the medication should be started immediately upon filling the prescription or at a future date and time? If no advice was provided, the pharmacist should use his or her professional judgment or contact the prescriber for this information.

4. **Special instructions**
   a. Give any special instructions, such as taking on an empty stomach, swallowing tablets whole, or separating the medication's administration from other drugs the patient is also taking. Check that the appropriate auxiliary labels have been placed on the prescription vial or bottle to emphasize special administration instructions.
   b. If you have a special dosage formulation, such as an inhaler, ophthalmic drops, injections, or suppositories, make sure that the patient knows how to use the product. In some cases, you may need to demonstrate the use of the product, especially inhalers or injections. Leaflets or visual aids should be provided to the patient; these are extremely helpful, as the multiple steps involved in using a device correctly can be difficult to remember until they have been reinforced by the patient's continued use of the product.
   c. Stress whether the medication should be carried with the patient for emergency use. A short-acting beta-agonist inhaler for asthma attacks, sublingual nitroglycerin tablets for chest pain, or injectable epinephrine for severe allergies should be available for use at all times and does not help the patient if the medication is stored at home with his or her other medications.
   d. Reinforce any applicable lifestyle changes recommended by the prescriber. Many medications for chronic illnesses require that the patient adjust his or her diet (e.g., low salt, low fat) and exercise regimen or lose weight.

5. Missed dose instructions

   a. Help the patient to establish clear, specific guidelines for deciding when, and whether, to skip or double forgotten doses.

   b. Offer strategies to aid adherence with therapy and supply a dosing aid, such as a pill reminder box, medication chart, or a pocket pill box if appropriate.

6. Anticipated length of therapy

   a. Patients need to know whether medications should be taken only when needed, on a scheduled basis until all the medication is gone, indefinitely, or until told to discontinue by their prescriber.

   b. If the anticipated length of therapy is unclear, the pharmacist should contact the prescriber to clarify this information for the patient.

C. Drug interactions, precautions/side effects, and monitoring therapy

   1. Potential drug interactions What are the important drug interactions that the patient should be made aware of? Though the patient may not have any drug interactions at this time, an interacting medication may be started at a later date, or the patient's medication profile may not be currently up to date. Provide information on potential drug, food, or disease interactions and how to avoid them (e.g., separate from dairy products) or manage the interaction if unavoidable in the future.

   2. Precautions and side effects Communicating about precautions and side effects is probably the area of greatest difficulty for pharmacists. How much should I say? What are the most important issues? Will I scare the patient if I talk about possible serious side effects? As discussed previously, current philosophy concerning drug therapy holds that patients have the right to self-determination; that is, they should be given full information about proposed therapy so that they can make informed decisions about their own health care.

   a. Some drugs have many potential side effects that range in clinical significance from minor to severe. Rather than read off a list of all potential side effects, begin your discussion by emphasizing the more common side effects. If you are unsure which ones are more common, refer to a tertiary drug information source that indicates the incidence of side effects as percentages.

   b. Distinguish between those side effects that may be annoying, but of no clinical harm and those that require contacting the prescriber. For example, a dry cough may occur during lisinopril therapy. While not life-threatening, this side effect can be annoying to the patient or those around him or her. The patient should be instructed to contact the prescriber if this occurs and becomes bothersome. However, throat or tongue swelling accompanied with difficulty in breathing (symptoms of angioedema) is a serious, potentially life-threatening side effect of lisinopril therapy that requires immediate medical attention.

   c. If a side effect can be minimized by timing of administration (e.g., taking the medication with food) or will diminish over time (e.g., headache from nitroglycerin therapy), communicate this information to the patient.

   d. If a side effect occurs or persists, provide the patient with information on appropriate steps to take. Patients should be instructed not to stop a medication on their own without first talking with the prescriber or the pharmacist. Some medications can be immediately discontinued, whereas others may require the patient to taper the dosage before stopping.

   3. Monitoring of therapy

   a. Monitoring of therapy can range from encouraging the patient to see the prescriber for follow-up checks or lab work to giving instructions on how to watch for signs of improvement or sharing warning signals of potential drug toxicity. Provide a time frame during which the patient will know whether the therapy is working. This will obviously vary with each medication and the condition it is being used to treat.

   b. You may want to recommend that the patient use a diary to record medication administration, side effects, improvements in symptoms, lab values, or the date/time of last episode. This tool can be helpful to monitor the medication's efficacy and improve overall adherence with therapy.

D. Storage instructions These instructions are given in many tertiary resources, such as the *USP/DI* and the Prescribing Information (or product package insert from the manufacturer) that accompanies the medication. The usual instructions are to keep out of the reach of children, in a place at controlled room temperature (68°–77°F), and away from high humidity.

E. Refills

   1. Are refills authorized? If so, how many are there? How should the patient order refills?

   2. Are there any special circumstances? For example, if the patient is seriously ill and taking a Schedule II pain medication, be sure you give information on how he or she can get more medication. It is not appropriate to say that there are no refills with this medication.

F. Verify patient understanding of information

1. Ask open-ended questions to verify that the patient understands all necessary information, but do this in a pleasant way; you obviously do not want to sound like you are quizzing the patient. Try to determine your patient's understanding in a way that puts the responsibility for any missed or inadequate communication on yourself rather than on them. You may want to say, "I know we have covered a lot of information. So that I am sure I didn't forget any important points, please tell me how you are going to take this medication."

2. To supplement (not replace) information provided during the consultation, you should also provide written information or a drug monograph for each medication being picked up by the patient to answer any questions that may arise during therapy. Many computer programs, pharmaceutical companies, and tertiary sources provide drug information written specifically for consumers and several offer monographs in other languages.

G. Closure Prior to the patient's or caregiver's leaving your pharmacy, provide him or her with a phone number, along with the days and hours a pharmacist would be available, to contact for questions or concerns. If applicable, this would also be an appropriate moment to establish a date, time of day, and phone number you could contact to follow-up with the patient on how the therapy is working.

VI.   ASSESSMENT OF PATIENT CONSULTATIONS

To aid you in evaluating your consultation skills and help monitor your progress, an assessment tool is shown in Figure 6.4. This sample form is used by pharmacy preceptors and clinical faculty to evaluate the patient consultations of pharmacy students in their clerkships and internships. You might want to ask a friend or family member to use this tool in evaluating your skills as you practice this aspect of professional practice.

Name _____

Date _____

Complete the following form to aid you in preparation for your drug consult. You may list important information in a short answer or outline manner; complete sentences are not necessary.

Drug Name, Dosage, & Frequency: _____

Data Gathering: (list data that should be gathered from the patient before proceeding–indicate why it is important to <u>this</u> consult.)

Indication & Mechanism of Action:

How to Take & Duration of Therapy:
1. **First dose** (when to take, how many to take if started later in day)

2. **Administration/adherence issues** (with or without food, adherence tools to aid compliance?)

3. **Missed dose information**

4. **Storage/quantity/refills**

5. **Time to benefit**

Interactions, Side Effects, Cautions & Management:
1. **Most common adverse effects** (include management: Will effect lessen with time? Should drug be discontinued or dosage decreased? Should patient call prescriber?)

2. **Severe, but rare, adverse effects to be aware of** (and when to call prescriber)

3. **Potential drug interactions (include most common herbal, OTC & food interactions)**

FIGURE 6.1. CONSULTATION PREP FORM.
(Used with permission. University of Wisconsin School of Pharmacy, Pharmacotherapy Lab. Copyright 2007.)

Goals of Therapy & Monitoring for Efficacy/Toxicity:

Lifestyle and/or Adjunct Therapies (if appropriate):

What do you consider as the 3-5 most important points to cover with your patient?

(Data gathering, drug name, dosage & frequency are considered <u>absolutely</u> necessary–these should not be listed below.)

1.

2.

3.

4.

5.

What references were used to prepare this consult? (You should use two separate references)

1.

2.

FIGURE 6.1. (CONTINUED)

	Yes	No
1. Introduces self to patient - *Hello, I'm (name), a pharmacy student, and you are Mr/Ms (patient name or caregiver's name)?*	☐	☐
2. Identifies purpose of counseling/interaction - *I'd like to take a few minutes to talk with you about your medications to make sure you get the most benefit from them. Would that be alright?*	☐	☐
3. Gathers pertinent patient data (allergies, adverse drug reactions, current medications, assess what patient knows, etc.) - *First, to make sure our records are up to date, I need to ask a few questions about your health conditions and any current medication use. (Collect/verify information in patient's medical record, including allergies, adverse drug reactions, etc.)* - *Is there anything else you'd like to mention?*	☐	☐
4. Medication name and dose - *Your prescription today is for (drug name and dose). Another name for it is (alternate name generic or brand).* - *Have you used this medication in the past? (or) Are you familiar with this medication?* - *What did Dr. (name) tell you about this medication?*	☐	☐
5. Indication and mechanism of action - *What did the prescriber say it was for (or) how it would help?* - *This medicine is a (class or use of medicine). It will help cure/control/reduce/prevent (indication) by (mechanism of action).*	☐	☐
6. How to take - *How did the prescriber tell you to take it?* - *Take _____ times a day. (Expand on when, special instructions, and verify how the patient will work it into his/her schedule or if he/she has concerns about the schedule.)* - *If a device, demonstrate proper technique to patient.* - *If you miss a dose, (instruct on what to do).* - *Your first dose can be taken (when).* - *Do you see any difficulties in taking the medication this way?*	☐	☐
7. Duration of therapy - *You should see some benefit from this medication (by when).* - *You will be taking this medication for (# of days) (or) as long as needed to manage (condition).* - *It is important to take it every day (or) only as needed for (condition).*	☐	☐
8. Interactions (drug/food/disease) - *(Explain possible interactions with current medications, foods, or conditions and how to avoid or manage.)*	☐	☐
9. Side effects and management - *Sometimes some unwanted or unexpected effects can occur when using this medication. Did the prescriber mention anything about this?* - *(Mention common side effects and how to minimize or avoid them.)*	☐	☐
10. Cautions or adverse effects and management - *Very rarely patients may experience a reaction to the medication. This probably won't happen to you, but if you notice (allergic symptoms, signs of adverse effects) let your prescriber and pharmacist know right away.*	☐	☐
11. Goal of therapy and/or self-monitoring by patient - *You should be noticing some relief / start to feel better / notice some improvement in symptoms in about (hours, days, weeks, etc.).* - *If you haven't noticed any improvements in your symptoms by then, call your prescriber or pharmacist.*	☐	☐
12. Storage instructions - *Store this medicine in a cool, dry place, away from children.* - *(Discuss applicable special storage instructions.)*	☐	☐
13. Refill instructions - *The prescriber has added (number) refills if you need them (or) so that you can continue therapy.* - *(If no refills indicated) What did the prescriber tell you to do when you finish this medication?*	☐	☐
14. Checks for patient understanding - *Do you have any concerns or questions?* - *We've covered a lot of information rather quickly. To be sure I didn't miss anything, tell me how you're going to take this medicine.*	☐	☐
15. Closure - *If you have any questions or problems, please don't hesitate to call us.* - *May I call you on (date) to see how you are doing? Would (time) be alright? (Confirm phone number, etc.)*	☐	☐

FIGURE 6.2. EXPANDED CONSULTATION SKILLS CHECKLIST—NEW PRESCRIPTION.
(Used with permission. University of Wisconsin School of Pharmacy, Pharmacotherapy Lab. Copyright 2007.)

	Yes	No
1. Introduces self to patient - *Hello, I'm (name), a pharmacy student, and you are Mr/Ms (patient's name or caregiver's name)?*	☐	☐
2. Identifies purpose of consultation/interaction - *I'd like to take a few minutes to talk with you about your refill medication to make sure you are receiving the most benefit from it. Would that be all right?*	☐	☐
3. Confirms pertinent patient data (allergies, adverse drug reactions, current medications, assess what patient knows, etc.) - *First, to make sure our records are up to date, I need to ask a few questions about your health conditions and current medication use. (Continue to collect/verify information in record, including allergies, adverse drug reactions, etc.)* - *Is there anything else you'd like to mention?* - *What has changed since the last time we saw you?* - *What concerns or questions would you like me to address today?*	☐	☐
4. Medication name and dose - *Your refill today is for (drug name and dose) or an alternative name is (generic or brand).*	☐	☐
5. Indication - *What are you taking this medication for?* - *How is the medication working to treat/control your (condition)? (Clarify previous symptoms disease improvement; obtain specific objective measurements and confirm goals.)* - *What are you doing to monitor your (condition)? (List appropriate monitoring tools. Offer to check specific objective measurements, i.e. blood pressure, heart rate, blood glucose.)*	☐	☐
6. How to take - *How have you been taking this? (If a device, ask patient to demonstrate.)* - *What difficulties have you had taking the medication this way?* - *What do you do if you miss a dose?*	☐	☐
7. Side Effects - *What kinds of problems are you having with this medication? (Probe for specific side effects.)*	☐	☐
8. Disease Monitoring - *When is your next follow-up with your health care practitioner? (Expand on disease-specific issues: lifestyle, monitoring tools, and goal.)*	☐	☐
9. Storage Instructions - *How have you been storing this medication? (Store in a cool, dry place, away from children; confirm any special storage instructions.)*	☐	☐
10. Refill Instructions - *You have (number) refills remaining.* - *(If no refills remain) When did the prescriber say that you would finish this medication? (or) How long did the prescriber want you to remain on this medication?*	☐	☐
11. Closure - *Any other concerns?* - *(Summarize main points.)* - *(Offer written/contact information if needed.)*	☐	☐

FIGURE 6.3. EXPANDED CONSULTATION SKILLS CHECKLIST—REFILL MEDICATION.
(Used with permission. University of Wisconsin School of Pharmacy, Pharmacotherapy Lab. Copyright 2007.)

Student: _____   Evaluator: _____

Drug Name: _____

CONTENT AREAS:	COMMENTS
Gathers Pertinent Patient Data • introduces self • purpose/time of consult • name • current medications (Rx, OTC, other remedies) • allergies/ADR • prior medical history • social history • family history	
Medication Name and Indication • brand/generic name • indication • mechanism of action • show and tell	
How to Take and Duration of Therapy • dosing regimen • administration issues/route • first dose • duration • missed dose • time to benefit	
Interactions, Side Effects, Cautions and Their Management • common and severe side effects • cautions • managing side effects • drug interactions	
Goals of Therapy and Self-Monitoring • goals of therapy • monitoring techniques • follow-up with prescriber • non-drug therapy	
Closure • storage • refills • summarizes material • checks for understanding • addresses patient's concerns	

Process:

	Poor	Marginal	Good	Very Good	Excellent
Audible	☐	☐	☐	☐	☐
Uses lay language	☐	☐	☐	☐	☐
Correct use of terms	☐	☐	☐	☐	☐
Puts patient at ease	☐	☐	☐	☐	☐
Maintains eye contact	☐	☐	☐	☐	☐
Asks open-ended questions	☐	☐	☐	☐	☐
Well-paced	☐	☐	☐	☐	☐
Consult tailored to patient-specific needs	☐	☐	☐	☐	☐
Did not overly rely on notes	☐	☐	☐	☐	☐

Additional Comments:

FIGURE 6.4. PATIENT CONSULTATION EVALUATION FORM.
(Used with permission. University of Wisconsin School of Pharmacy, Pharmacotherapy Lab. Copyright 2007.)

REFERENCES

1. Higby GJ. Pharmacy in the American century. Pharm Times 1997; 63: 16–24.
2. Cipolle R, Strand LM, Morley PC. Pharmaceutical care practice. New York: McGraw Hill, 1998.
3. American Pharmacists Association. Code of ethics for Pharmacists. Washington, DC: Author. Last updated 2/18/05. Accessed on 9/1/07 at: http://www.pharmacist.com/AM/Template.cfm?Section=Search1&template=/CM/HTMLDisplay.cfm&ContentID=2903.
4. American Society of Health-System Pharmacists. ASHP guidelines on pharmacist-conducted patient education and counseling. Am J Health-Syst Pharm 1997; 54: 431–434.
5. National Association of Boards of Pharmacy. Model rules for the practice of pharmacy. Park Ridge, IL: Author, 2007; 86.
6. National Association of Boards of Pharmacy. Model rules for the practice of pharmacy. Park Ridge, IL: Author. 2007; 100.
7. Office of Inspector General-Office of Analysis and Inspections. The clinical role of the community pharmacist. Department of Health and Human Services. Publication OAI-01-89-89020. January, 1990.
8. Office of Inspector General-Office of Analysis and Inspections. State discipline of pharmacists. Department of Health and Human Services. Publication OAI-01-89-89160. January, 1990.
9. Office of Inspector General-Office of Analysis and Inspections. Medication regimens: Causes of noncompliance. Department of Health and Human Services. Publication OAI-04-89-89121. March, 1990.
10. 42USC1396r-8. Payment for covered outpatient drugs. Washington, DC: United States Code 2000, Suppl. 4. Accessed on 9-20-07 at: http://frwebgate1.access.gpo.gov/cgi-bin/waisgate.cgi?WAISdocID=301217408141+9+0+0&WAISaction=retrieve.

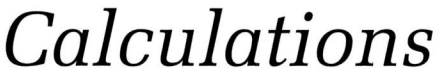

Part 2

Calculations

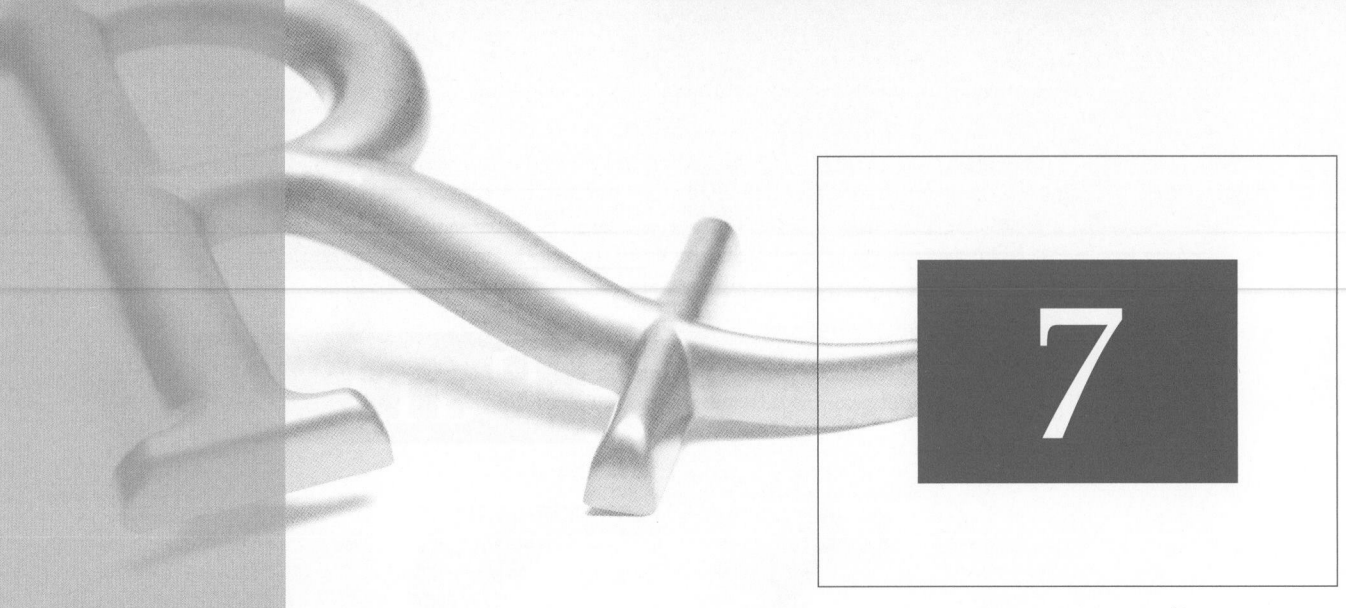

Systems of Measurement and Introduction to Pharmaceutical Calculations

I. SYSTEMS OF MEASUREMENT

Three systems of measurement are currently used in the United States: the metric or International System of Units (SI), the apothecaries' system, and the avoirdupois system. The SI or metric system is now the only system of measurement acceptable for use in pharmacy and medicine, but since both the apothecaries' and avoirdupois systems (sometimes called the *common* or *customary systems*) are used both in commerce and daily life activities, pharmacists and pharmacy technicians must be knowledgeable about all three systems. The discussion here gives a summary of the various systems; for a more detailed treatment, consult the chapter on metrology in *Remington: The Science and Practice of Pharmacy* and the guidebook and Internet Web sites referenced below.

A. Metric or International System of Units (SI)

1. The metric system was formalized in France in the late 1700s. It employs a decimal system that is both logical and easy to use. It was adopted as a legal system (although not a mandatory one) in the United States in 1866. At this time, rapid scientific and industrial development was taking place, and it became apparent that a standardized, internationally recognized system of measurement was needed. In 1875, the United States joined 20 other countries in signing the *Treaty of the Meter*, which adopted the metric system and established the International Bureau of Weights and Measures to work internationally to advance and maintain the system (1,2).

2. The original basic units of the metric system were the meter for length and the kilogram for mass. For many years, the reference standard for the meter was a platinum–iridium bar with etch marks delineating a meter; a 1-kg platinum–iridium block was used as the standard for mass. The originals were kept in a vault at the International Bureau headquarters in France, and each of the treaty member countries received two copies of the standards. The reference standards for these basic units have changed over the years as technology has advanced. Standards were desired that were based on unchanging physical characteristics of specified elements. Currently, the meter is defined as "the length of the path traveled by light in a vacuum during the time interval of 1/299,792,458 of a second" (3), with a second equivalent to 9,129,631,770 oscillations of the ^{133}Cs atom (2).

3. In 1960, the metric system was refined and the International System of Units (SI) was adopted. The initial basic units of the metric system are the same in SI, but some units were added or updated and some of the symbols and notation were slightly changed and were standardized. There are seven basic units in SI: the meter (m) for length, the kilogram (kg) for mass, the second (s) for time, the mole (mol) for amount of substance, the kelvin (K) for thermodynamic temperature, the ampere (A) for electric current, and the candela (cd) for luminous intensity (4). The international group in charge of SI is still located in France and is now called the *Conference Generale des Poids et Mesures,* or CGPM; the United States is represented on this body by the National Institute of Standards & Technology (NIST), an arm of the U.S. Department of Commerce (4). All the symbols, special names, and formulas for the basic, supplementary, and derived SI units are listed in the miscellaneous tables section of *The Merck Index.* These lists and other useful information on SI can be found in the book *Guide to the Use of the Metric System [SI Version],* which is available from the U.S. Metric Association through its Internet site (5).

4. In pharmacy and medicine, we most often need to measure or use units of length, mass, and volume.

   a. As stated previously, the basic unit of length in SI is the meter, although in pharmacy we more often use the centimeter, which is 0.01 meter (that is, 1/100 of a meter).

   b. The basic unit of volume in SI is the cubic meter (m^3), but the liter (L), although not an SI unit, is approved for use in SI for measuring liquid volume. The liter is the fundamental unit of volume used in pharmacy and medicine; it is essentially the volume of 1,000 cubic centimeters (cm^3). You will sometimes see the abbreviation "cc" used for cubic centimeter, but this notation does not follow SI conventions. Furthermore, it has been the source of medication errors (see Table 1.1 in Chapter 1) and should not be used.

   c. Although the official basic unit of mass in SI is the kilogram, the gram (g) has been used as the basic stem unit (see later). One gram is the mass of 1 cm^3 of water at 4°C. Because 1 mL (1 mL = 0.001 L) is equal to 1 cm^3, 1 mL of water also has a mass of 1 g. [Note that kilograms and grams are units of mass (not weight), even though in practice we usually use the term *weight* when we actually mean *mass*. In this text, we will use the terms weight and mass interchangeably, although technically weight is a measure of force and is mass times gravitational acceleration.]

   d. Other metric units of length, volume, and weight are achieved by applying prefixes to an appropriate stem unit: meter (m), liter (L), or gram (g). The prefix specifies a power of ten that is multiplied by the stem unit. For example, the prefix milli (m) is associated with a 10^{-3} multiple, so that a millimeter (mm) is 10^{-3} meters, a milligram (mg) is 10^{-3} grams, and a milliliter (mL) is 10^{-3} liters. Prefixes for SI units, together with their associated powers of ten and their symbols, are given in Table 7.1. Note that the letter case, capital (uppercase) letter or lowercase letter, is important; lowercase m for milli signifies 10^{-3}, whereas uppercase M for mega designates 10^6—a huge difference! Uppercase letters are used for symbols indicating powers of 10^6 and higher. Also note that, while the SI symbol for micro is the lowercase Greek letter mu (μ), this symbol should not be used when expressing doses (e.g., use mcg instead of μg), because μg can easily be misread as mg (see Table 1.1 in Chapter 1).

   e. Metric units of length, volume, and weight most commonly used in pharmacy and medicine are given in Table 7.2. In older scientific literature, you may see the unit of length, the angstrom, which uses the symbol Å; 1 Å = 10^{-10} m.

5. The U.S. Metric Association maintains an Internet site that contains information on correct usage of the SI-metric system; their *Guide to the Use of the Metric System [SI Version]* has even more complete information (4,5). Some of the basic rules are listed here, and the correct format for some of the symbols commonly used in pharmacy and medicine are listed in Table 7.3 (4,5).

Table 7.1	SI PREFIXES, VALUES, AND SYMBOLS

POWER OF TEN	PREFIX	SYMBOL
10^{18}	exa	E
10^{15}	peta	P
10^{12}	tera	T
10^{9}	giga	G
10^{6}	mega	M
10^{3}	kilo	k
10^{2}	hector	h
10	deka	da
1	no prefix (basic unit)	—
10^{-1}	deci	d
10^{-2}	centi	c
10^{-3}	milli	m
10^{-6}	micro	μ
10^{-9}	nano	n
10^{-12}	pico	p
10^{-15}	femto	f
10^{-18}	atto	a

a. The short forms for the dimension units, such as "cm" for centimeter, are called *symbols* rather than abbreviations.

b. There should always be a space between the numeric digits of a quantity and its SI symbol (e.g., "5 g" rather than "5g").

c. The symbols are never followed by periods unless a symbol is at the end of a sentence.

d. Symbols are always written in singular form but, when the word for a unit is used, the plural form is used when appropriate. For example, write "5 mL" (not "5 mLs"), but write "5 milliliters."

e. When a symbol is a compound unit, and it is a quotient of two units, that quotient may be designated with a solidus (forward slash mark, "/") or a negative exponent (e.g., g/cm^3 or g cm^{-3}). The letter "p" is not to be used for the word *per*, but per may be written out (e.g., 5 milligrams per milliliter). (Note: In pharmacy and medicine, when writing dose concentrations, the use of the solidus is not recommended because of medication errors that have

Table 7.2	METRIC MEASURES COMMONLY USED IN PHARMACY AND MEDICINE

METRIC MEASURES OF LENGTH

100 centimeters (cm) = 1 meter (m)
10 millimeters (mm) = 1 centimeter (cm)
1,000 micrometers (μm) = 1 millimeter (mm)

METRIC MEASURES OF VOLUME

1,000 milliliters (mL) = 1 liter (L)
1,000 microliters (μL) = 1 milliliter (mL)

METRIC MEASURES OF WEIGHT

1,000 grams (g) = 1 kilogram (kg)
1,000 milligrams (mg) = 1 gram (g)
1,000 micrograms (μg or mcg) = 1 milligram (mg)

Table 7.3	CORRECT SI-METRIC SYMBOLS
SYMBOL	**FOR**
m	meter
cm	centimeter
mm	millimeter
L or l	liter
mL or ml	milliliter
kg	kilogram
g	gram
mg	milligram
μg (mcg for drug orders)	microgram
h	hour
s	second
cm³ (mL for drug orders)	cubic centimeter
°C	degree Celsius
K	kelvin

Source: Correct SI-metric usage. U.S. Metric Association, http://lamar.colostate.edu/~hillger/correct.htm. Accessed May 2007.

resulted from reading it as a number one. In this text, the word *per* is used in place of the solidus in these circumstances.)

   f. As noted earlier in the example of milli (m) and mega (M), letter case is important. Some of the SI rules with regard to letter case are given here.

      (1) Metric unit **names** (such as gram, meter, kelvin) are not capitalized (unless, of course, the name is at the beginning of a sentence), even though some units, such as the basic unit kelvin and derived units such as the newton (for force) and the pascal (for pressure), are named for persons. The exception is Celsius, which is always capitalized.

      (2) Most metric **symbols** are also lowercase letters (e.g., g and m); however, in contrast to metric unit names, those symbols that are named after persons have uppercase letters (for example, the symbol for newton is N, for pascal is Pa, and for kelvin is K).

      (3) Notice in Table 7.3 that the symbol for liter may be either upper- or lowercase el (L or l, mL or ml); uppercase L is preferred in the United States, Canada, and Australia, while the lowercase letter is used in most other countries.

  6. Italics are not to be used for metric symbols (e.g., 5 g, not 5 *g*). This is because italics are often used to designate measurements in mathematical formulas: For example, in the formulas for density and specific gravity shown later in this chapter, the *m* stands for mass, not meter.

  7. Both from a patient safety viewpoint and to correctly convey information about quantities, it is important to know and use correct and current SI symbols. Two examples may help to illustrate this: At one time the abbreviation "Gm" was sometimes used as a symbol for gram, but under SI this is the symbol for gigameter; the abbreviation "gr" has sometimes been mistakenly used or misinterpreted to mean gram, but it is the symbol for the apothecaries'/avoirdupois grain, which equals 64.8 mg. The lowercase g without a period is the only acceptable symbol for gram. It is essential that all health care personnel know and use precisely the correct SI symbols.

B. Avoirdupois System

  1. The avoirdupois system is the common or customary system of weights used in commerce and households in the United States. Although the U.S. government has strongly encouraged conversion to the metric system (called *metrication*), it has been an uphill battle to get industry and the population to use and think in terms of SI or metric units. We still measure and give our body weight in terms of pounds, buy butter and meat by the pound and pasta and cereal by the ounce, and have postage for letters and packages calculated based on ounces and pounds.

Table 7.4	AVOIRDUPOIS MEASURES OF WEIGHT

437.5 grains (gr) = 1 ounce (oz)
16 ounces (7,000 grains) = 1 pound (lb)

2. The basic units of mass for the avoirdupois system are the grain, the ounce, and the pound. The avoirdupois grain has the same mass as the apothecaries' system grain (see section C, Apothecaries' System), but both the ounce and the pound are different in the two systems.

3. In the United Kingdom, Canada, and some other commonwealth countries, the British Imperial system of mass is still sometimes used. For grains, ounces, and pounds, these are the same as those comparable units in the avoirdupois system.

4. The exact conversion for mass between the metric and avoirdupois systems is 1 pound = 453.59237 grams. See Tables 7.4 and 7.7 for other equivalents and conversion factors. In Table 7.7, the designation (av) following an avoirdupois unit is used to distinguish it from the similar, but not equal, apothecaries' unit.

C. Apothecaries' System

1. Apothecaries' weight

   a. The apothecaries' system for mass is used only in pharmacy and medicine. While the use of this system of measurement is strongly discouraged, some older compounding formulas are written using the apothecaries' system, so it is important to know about it and understand how to convert apothecaries' quantities to metric equivalents.

   b. The units of mass for the apothecaries' system are the grain, the scruple, the dram (formerly spelled *drachm*), the ounce, and the pound. As stated previously, only the grain has the same mass in both the apothecaries' and avoirdupois systems (and in the British Imperial system). See Tables 7.5 and 7.7 for apothecaries' equivalents and conversion factors. In Table 7.7, the designation (ap) following an apothecaries' unit is used to distinguish it from the similar, but not equal, avoirdupois unit.

2. Apothecaries' liquid volume

   a. The apothecaries' system for liquid measurement is the common system for commerce and household use in the United States. As with the apothecaries' system of weights, it was formerly used for prescriptions and compounding formulas. It is no longer an official system for medicine and pharmacy, and its use is strongly discouraged.

   b. The units of volume for this system include the minim, the fluid dram and fluid ounce, the pint, the quart, and the gallon. See Tables 7.5 and 7.7 for the various units of measurement and equivalents.

Table 7.5	APOTHECARIES' MEASURES OF VOLUME AND WEIGHT

MEASURES OF VOLUME

60 minims $^{(m)}$ = 1 fluid dram (fl(ʒ) or (ʒ))
8 fluid drams = 1 fluid ounce (fl(ʒ) or (ʒ) or oz)
16 fluid ounces = 1 pint (pt or O)
2 pints = 1 quart (qt)
4 quarts = 1 gallon (gal or C)

(Cu)

MEASURES OF WEIGHT

20 grains (gr) = 1 scruple (ɘ)
3 scruples = 1 dram (ʒ)
8 drams = 1 ounce (ʒ̄)
12 ounces (5,760) = 1 pound (℔)

Table 7.6	**HOUSEHOLD MEASURES**

MEASURES OF VOLUME

3 teaspoonfuls (t or tsp) = 1 tablespoonful (T or tbsp)
2 tablespoonfuls = 1 fluid ounce (oz)
8 fluid ounces = 1 cup (Cu)
2 cups = 1 pint (pt)
2 pints = 1 quart (qt)
4 quarts = 1 gallon (gal)

MEASURES OF WEIGHT

16 ounces (oz) = 1 pound (lb)

MEASURES OF LENGTH

12 inches (in or ") = 1 foot (ft or ')
3 feet = 1 yard (yd)

    c. The British Imperial system of volume uses the same unit names, but these represent different quantities. Consult an appropriate reference for conversion factors if using a formula based on the British system.

D. Household and other measure

    1. The units of measurement used in the United States for cooking and daily life is a conglomerate from the avoirdupois system of weights, the apothecaries' system of volume, and a hodgepodge of drops, teaspoons, tablespoons, quarts, inches, feet, yards, and so on. See Table 7.6 for household measures and Table 7.7 for conversion equivalents.

    2. Because the teaspoon is so commonly used in the home to measure liquid medications, the *USP* has a general chapter to address this volume. Chapter ⟨1221⟩ Teaspoon states that although an American Standard Teaspoon has been established by the American National Standards Institute as containing 4.93 ± 0.24 mL, for household use this volume is taken to be 5 mL. Chapter ⟨1221⟩ directs that liquid medications formulated for oral administration by teaspoon be made on the basis of 5-mL units (6). Therefore, for purposes of dispensing medication, one teaspoonful is taken to mean 5 mL.

    3. In *USP* Chapter ⟨1101⟩ Medicine Dropper, a Pharmacopeial medicine dropper is described; the specifications state that the tip delivers between 45 mg and 55 mg of water per drop (7). Using the average of 50 mg/drop, and the density of water of 1 g/mL, this would give 20 drops/mL or 0.05 mL/drop. The *USP* chapter notes that other liquids have viscosities and surface tensions that are different from water; therefore, the same dropper would give different quantities per drop for these other liquids (7). The section on volumetric apparatus in Chapter 14 of this book describes the procedure needed to calibrate a medicine dropper before using it as a dosing device. Fortunately, we now have better and more accurate measuring devices to use or dispense with liquid medications for measuring doses.

    4. At one time, it was common practice for physicians and nurses to use apothecaries' fluid volume symbols as "abbreviations" for common measurements when writing the directions-for-use portion of a prescription or medication order. This practice is now strongly discouraged, both because the apothecaries' system is now considered obsolete and because such symbols with dual meanings are so prone to misinterpretation and error.

        a. Although a fluid dram contains only 3.69 mL, some prescribers formerly used the dram symbol (ℨ) as an abbreviation for a teaspoonful, which is 5 mL.

        b. Although a USP drop is 0.05 mL, some nurses use the minim symbol (ɱ) as an abbreviation for drop. A minim is 0.06 mL.

        c. Even more hazardous was the use of the apothecary ounce symbol (℥) as an abbreviation for 30 mL or two tablespoonfuls, and the apothecary symbol for one-half ounce (℥ss) as an abbreviation for 15 mL or 1 tablespoonful. In this case, pharmacists and physicians have mistakenly used or interpreted the (℥) symbol as an abbreviation for 1 tablespoonful, giving a dose that was either one-half or double that which was intended.

Table 7.7	CONVERSION EQUIVALENTS COMMONLY USED IN PHARMACY AND MEDICINE

CONVERSION EQUIVALENTS OF VOLUME

1 drop (gtt) = 0.05 mL
1 mL = 20 drops
1 teaspoonful = 5 mL
1 tablespoonful = 15 mL
1 mL = 16.23 minims
1 minim = 0.06 mL
1 fluid dram = 3.69 mL
1 fluid ounce = 29.57 mL
1 pint = 473 mL
1 quart = 946 mL
1 gallon = 3,785 mL

CONVERSION EQUIVALENTS OF WEIGHT

1 g = 15.432 grains
1 kg = 2.20 pounds (av)
1 grain = 64.8 mg
1 ounce (av) = 28.35 g
1 ounce (ap) = 31.1 g
1 pound (av) = 454 g
1 pound (ap) = 373 g
1 pound (av) = 7,000 grains
1 pound (ap) = 5,760 grains
1 grain (av) = 1 grain (ap)

CONVERSION EQUIVALENTS OF LENGTH

1 inch = 2.54 cm
1 m = 39.37 inches

II. INTERSYSTEM CONVERSION FOR WEIGHTS AND VOLUMES

It would seem that conversion between the different systems of measurement would be fairly straightforward. Since in pharmacy we use the metric or SI system, if we are presented with a quantity in either the avoirdupois or apothecaries' system, it seems logical to go to a table of conversion factors and use the appropriate factor to calculate its equivalent in the metric system. The problem is a bit more complex because the factor to use and the allowed degree of rounding depend on the situation. The following principles generally apply.

A. If a compounding formula, either on a prescription order or in a reference source, is written in the apothecaries' system, you must use three significant figures to convert each quantity to its metric equivalent (8). (See Table 7.7 and section V, Significant Figures, in this chapter.)

B. If a prescription order is written for a manufactured product, the amount to dispense or the strength of a dosage unit may be rounded to that which is commercially available (8).

    1. For example, if you have a prescription order for hydrocortisone 1% ointment, 1 oz, and the commercial product is 30 g, you may dispense that amount even though an avoirdupois ounce is 28.35 g and an apothecaries' ounce is 31.1 g. Likewise, if the order is written "hydrocortisone 1% ointment, 30 g," and you have a commercial product that is an avoirdupois ounce (that is 28.35, 28.4, or 28 g), you may dispense that commercial package; you do not have to add extra ointment from another tube to make exactly 30 g.

    2. Similarly, if you receive an order for a dosage unit in the apothecaries' system, you may dispense a comparable manufactured dosage unit with strength in the metric system. For example, you have an order for ferrous sulfate tablets, 5 gr (that is, 5 grains), and the product you stock is 325,

320, or 300 mg per tablet, you may dispense that product. You are not required to dispense tablets that are 5×64.8 mg = 324 mg (8).

C. If the prescription order is written for a compounded preparation with a set formula, such as Coal Tar Ointment USP, and the amount to dispense is written in one of the common systems, you may dispense the rounded metric equivalent (e.g., 30 g).

III. TEMPERATURE CONVERSIONS AND CALCULATION OF MEAN KINETIC TEMPERATURE

Three temperature units and scales are used in the world: Fahrenheit, Celsius, and Kelvin. Fahrenheit is the common system in use in the United States, but Celsius is official in the United States; it is also the common system used throughout most of the rest of the world and is used almost exclusively internationally in science. The kelvin is the basic unit of thermodynamic temperature in SI, but the degree Celsius is an accepted unit in that system.

A. Fahrenheit

1. The first modern temperature scale was developed in the early 1700s by the German physicist Gabriel Fahrenheit. As an inventor and manufacturer of precision instruments, Fahrenheit devised a temperature scale that used the degree (°) as the individual unit of measurement. He originally designed his system using three temperature points: 0° for a salt-ice-water mixture, 30° for the freezing point of pure water, and 90° for normal human body temperature.

2. As conditions were more closely defined, the scale became set with 32° as the freezing point of water and 212° as the boiling point of water at normal atmospheric pressure. This gave a span of 180° between the freezing and boiling points of water. On this refined scale, normal body temperature became 98.6°. (Temperatures, especially body temperatures for clinical purposes, are rounded to the nearest tenth degree.)

3. The symbol for the unit of measurement on the Fahrenheit scale is °F.

B. Celsius

1. Approximately 20 years after Fahrenheit introduced his temperature scale, the Swedish astronomer and physicist Anders Celsius developed what he considered to be a more convenient scale, one that would place the freezing point of water at 0° and the boiling point of water at 100°.

2. Celsius used the same measurement unit name, the degree (°), but since his temperature interval of 100° covered the same span (from freezing to boiling for water) as that for 180 Fahrenheit degrees, 1-Celsius degree equals 180/100 (9/5 or 1.8) Fahrenheit degrees.

3. The symbol for the unit of measurement on the Celsius scale is °C. Because the Celsius scale is official in the United States and is the accepted system internationally, when a degree symbol (°) is given without a C or F, the temperature is assumed to be Celsius. This convention is used in the *USP, The Merck Index,* and other scientific references.

4. Because of the 100-degree interval between the freezing and boiling of water, the Celsius system was formerly often referred to as the *centigrade system.*

C. Kelvin

1. One hundred years later, in 1848, Scottish physicist and mathematician Lord Kelvin was working on ideas related to the second law of thermodynamics and developed the concept of absolute temperature. Using the Celsius scale, thermodynamic absolute zero is −273.1°C.

2. The kelvin measurement unit is the basic SI unit for thermodynamic temperature; notice in Table 7.3 that the symbol for the kelvin unit is the capital letter K, written without a degree (°) symbol.

D. Conversions among the temperature systems

1. Even though the Celsius temperature system is a more logical and easier system to use, the Fahrenheit system remains the common or customary system used in the United States. Patients and most hospitals and clinics report clinical temperatures in °F, although some clinical guidelines now use Celsius temperatures. The scientific community uses Celsius temperatures almost exclusively, except where thermodynamic temperatures are appropriate, in which case temperatures are given as degrees kelvin (K). As a result, it is essential that pharmacists and pharmacy technicians, as well as others in the medical sciences, be able to convert among these various systems of temperature measurement.

2. Conversion between Fahrenheit and Celsius

a. The most common equations for converting between Fahrenheit and Celsius temperatures use two factors that differentiate these two systems: (i) 0°C is equal to 32°F and (ii) one Celsius degree equals 9/5 or 1.8 Fahrenheit degrees. We get the following equations.

$$°F = \frac{9}{5}°C + 32 \quad or \quad °F = 1.8 \times °C + 32$$

$$°C = \frac{5}{9} \times (°F - 32) \quad or \quad °C = 0.556 \times (°F - 32)$$

Because of the difficulty in remembering when to use the parenthesis and whether to add or subtract the 32, some people find it easier to memorize just one of the above equations and then solve for whatever temperature (°F or °C) is desired.

b. Another system of conversion was developed that simplifies the calculation. This method makes use of the fact that −40° is the same in both systems. The steps are as follows:
   (1) To the given temperature (no matter whether it is Fahrenheit or Celsius) add 40.
   (2) If the conversion is from Celsius to Fahrenheit, multiply the answer to **(1)** by 9/5; if the conversion is from Fahrenheit to Celsius, multiply the answer to **(1)** by 5/9.
   (3) Subtract 40 from the answer to **(2)**.

c. Temperatures, especially body temperature for clinical purposes, are rounded to the nearest tenth degree.

3. Conversion between °C and K is a relatively simple matter since the measurement unit in each system is the Celsius degree. As stated earlier, the kelvin scale starts at thermodynamic absolute zero, which is −273.1°C. Therefore,

$$K = °C + 273.1 \quad and \quad °C = K - 273.1$$

E. Mean Kinetic Temperature (MKT)

1. During the 1990s, there were reports of drug product degradation resulting from improperly controlled warehouse or shipment conditions (including mailing of prescription products to patients). Although the prescribed storage conditions for most drugs and drug products was the *USP*'s Controlled Room Temperature (CRT), it was understood that temperature fluctuations outside of this range were sometimes unavoidable. As a result, studies were conducted by USP and discussions and conferences were held to address this problem in a practical but scientific manner. The end result was to redefine CRT to include the concept of mean kinetic temperature (MKT). This definition of CRT is quoted here:

> *Controlled Room Temperature*—A temperature maintained thermostatically that encompasses the usual and customary working environment of 20° to 25° (68° to 77°F); that results in a mean kinetic temperature calculated to be not more than 25°; and that allows for excursions between 15° and 30° (59° and 86°F) that are experienced in pharmacies, hospitals, and warehouses. Provided the mean kinetic temperature remains in the allowed range, transient spikes of up to 40° are permitted as long as they do not exceed 24 hours. Spikes above 40° may be permitted if the manufacturer so instructs (9).

Because of this new definition of CRT, either the temperature in pharmacies (including all drug storage areas) must be consistently maintained below 25°C, or it must be monitored, the MKT must be calculated, and the temperature in these areas be adjusted and maintained in accordance with *USP* standards. This procedure and the calculations are shown here.

2. The MKT or T_k is a single calculated temperature that gives approximately the same drug product degradation as would occur if the product were subjected to various temperatures. It is calculated using an equation derived from the Arrhenius equation and gives a value that is slightly higher than a simple arithmetic mean. The equation for MKT is given in the *USP* Chapter ⟨1160⟩ Pharmaceutical Calculations and is shown here (10).

$$T_k = \frac{\Delta H/R}{-\ln\left(\dfrac{e^{-\Delta H/RT_1} + e^{-\Delta H/RT_2} + \cdots + e^{-\Delta H/RT_n}}{n}\right)}$$

where:

T_k = mean kinetic temperature in K (kelvin)
ΔH = heat of activation (83.144 kJ mol^{-1})
R = universal gas constant (0.0083144 kJ mol^{-1} deg^{-1})
T_1 = avg. temperature in K for period 1 (e.g., week)
T_n = avg. temperature in K for the nth period

	Table 7.8				**MEAN KINETIC TEMPERATURE (MKT) SAMPLE CONTROL SHEET**		
WEEK	**DATE/ TIME**	**LOW TEMP. °C**	**HIGH TEMP. °C**	**AVERAGE TEMP. T_n°C**	**AVERAGE TEMP. T_n K**	**$\Delta H/RT$**	**$e^{-\Delta H/RT}$**
1	1/01/00 0900	17	25	21	294.1	−34.0020	1.7105×10^{-15}
2	1/08/00 0900	19	27	23	296.1	−33.7724	2.1520×10^{-15}
3	1/15/00 0900	20	24	22	295.1	−33.8868	1.9193×10^{-15}
4	1/22/00 0900	22	28	25	298.1	−33.5458	2.6993×10^{-15}
5	1/29/00 0900	23	29	26	299.1	−33.4336	3.0198×10^{-15}
6–52							
Totals				117	1482.5		11.5009×10^{-15}
Means				23.4	296.5		2.3002×10^{-15}

n = the total number of storage temperatures recorded during the annual observation period (minimum of 52 weekly entries)

3. The MKT equation is used as follows. (Refer to Table 7.8 for sample data and Figure 7.1 for the associated sample calculations.)

   a. The temperature in the pharmacy or storage area is monitored and recorded. The easiest method is to use an automated recording device that gives a tracking of temperatures measured at specified intervals (e.g., every 30 minutes) or gives a high and low temperature for the period. For example, each week at the same time, the pharmacist or pharmacy technician checks the temperature monitor, notes the recorded high and low temperatures for the previous week, and calculates an arithmetic mean or average of the high and low temperature. This temperature, when expressed in K, is T_n for that week.

   b. This procedure is repeated weekly and average temperatures are calculated for a minimum of 52 equally spaced periods over a year.

   c. Using the equation given previously, the pharmacist uses the T_1 through T_n values for all weeks monitored to calculate the MKT for the storage space. Because of the numeric values for ΔH and R, the MKT equation is easier to use than it would appear. A sample calculation using data in Table 7.8 is shown in Figure 7.1.

   d. This information is used to make any necessary adjustments in the temperature-controlling equipment for the pharmacy or storage space.

   e. If the temperature in the storage space is consistently maintained below 25°C, the MKT need not be calculated.

IV. DENSITY AND SPECIFIC GRAVITY

A. Definitions

1. Density: the mass per unit volume of a substance at a given temperature (t°C) and pressure: $d^t = (m/V)^t$.

2. Specific gravity: the ratio of the weight of a substance at t°C to the weight of an equal volume of a reference substance (usually water) at t°C (11):

$$d^t_{t'} = \frac{(m/V)^t_{test}}{(m'/V)^{t'}_{water}}$$

B. Density

1. Although density may be measured and reported in any mass and volume units, it is usually given in g/cm^3. Because 1 cm^3 is essentially equal to 1 mL, density in g/cm^3 is taken to be equal numerically to the density in g/mL (12).

$$T_k = \frac{\Delta H / R}{- \ln\left(\dfrac{e^{-\Delta H/RT_1} + e^{-\Delta H/RT_2} + ... + e^{-\Delta H/RT_n}}{n}\right)}$$

(1)   The numerator of the MKT equation, $\Delta H/R$, is simply 10,000 K as can be seen here:

$$\frac{\Delta H}{R} = \frac{83.144 \text{ kJ mol}^{-1}}{0.0083144 \text{ kJ mol}^{-1} \text{ deg}^{-1}} = 10,000 \text{ deg}$$

(2)   In the denominator of the equation, the exponent of e for each time period is –10,000 divided by the temperature (in K) for that time period. For example, if the average temperature for a given week is 21 °C, the average temperature in degrees kelvin is calculated to be: 21 + 273.1 = 294.1 K (recall from the discussion in section III D, Conversions among the temperature systems, that you add 273.1 to the Celsius temperature to convert it to degrees K). The exponent of e for that week is calculated to be:

$$\frac{-\Delta H}{R T_1} = \frac{-10,000}{294.1} = -34.0020$$

(3)   With the value of the exponent known, calculating the value of e taken to that exponent is a simple matter on a hand-held calculator that has logarithmic functions: use operation key e^x and enter the number (–34.0020 in this case). For this example, the answer is 1.7105×10^{-15}.

(4)   These numbers for all the periods are then summed. An example of this is shown in Table 7.8 where, for simplicity, data for just five time periods are shown. In this case the sum is 11.5009×10^{-15}.

(5)   This sum for all the periods is then divided by the number of periods. For the example in Table 7.8, the sum 11.5009×10^{-15} is divided by 5 to give 2.3002×10^{-15}.

(6)   Using a calculator or spreadsheet program, take the -ln of this number. For this example,

$$-\ln 2.3002 \times 10^{-15} = 33.7058$$

(7)   This answer is then divided into 10,000 to get the MKT in K. In this case the MKT is 296.7 K or 23.6 °C. This calculation is shown here for this sample data.

$$T_k = \frac{10,000 \text{ deg}}{-\ln\left(\dfrac{11.5009 \times 10^{-15}}{5}\right)} = \frac{10,000 \text{ deg}}{-\ln(2.3002 \times 10^{-15})} = \frac{10,000 \text{ deg}}{33.7058} = 296.7 \text{ K} = 23.6 \text{ °C}$$

FIGURE 7.1 MEAN KINETIC TEMPERATURE SAMPLE CALCULATION.

     2. Because the density of a substance changes with temperature, the temperature of the measurement is specified (e.g., the notation d^{20} 0.987 indicates that the substance has a measured density of 0.987 g/mL at 20°C).

     3. Because the SI gram is defined as the mass of 1 cm^3 of water at 4°C, the density of water at 4°C is 1.0000000 g/cm^3 (or g/mL).

C. Specific gravity

     1. Specific gravity is easier to measure accurately than is density, so specific gravity is more often reported on specifications for bulk chemicals, in journal articles, and in references such as the USP/NF and The Merck Index.

     2. When measuring or reporting specific gravity, the temperatures of both the test substance and the reference substance (water) are specified (written, $d_{t'}^{t}$). Most often these temperatures are the same (that is, t °C = t'°C). For example, in the USP/NF monographs, the specific gravity specifications are for 25°C/25°C, unless otherwise stated in the monograph (13). This is denoted d_{25}^{25}. Whenever you see this d notation with two temperatures, it always means that this value is a specific gravity rather than a density, which has a d with one temperature. It is somewhat confusing to have the same symbol, d, used for both density and specific gravity.

3. Because specific gravity is a ratio, it has no units. However, as stated earlier, at 4°C water has a density of 1.0000000 g/mL so, when substituting this value in the equation given previously in the definition for specific gravity, the specific gravity of the test substance at t°C relative to water at 4°C (that is, d_4^t) is equal to the density of the test substance at t°C. Because of this equivalence, it is permissible to give the units of density (g/mL) to reported numeric values for specific gravity. This is particularly advantageous when using dimensional analysis in calculations that involve specific gravity.

4. In compounding, we often use published specific gravity values to convert the desired weight of a liquid to a more easily measured volume of that liquid. Since our volumetric measurements are usually limited to a precision of ±0.1 mL, it is permissible to use the reported specific gravity values interchangeably with density in such calculations without correcting for temperature differences.

5. When specific gravity is used to verify or establish the identity, purity, or concentration of a liquid, more precision is needed, and temperature should be considered. Precise specific gravity measurements can be easily made with a volumetric device known as a *pycnometer* but, in compounding situations, a syringe can be used as an improvised pyknometer. (This is illustrated with Sample Prescription 27.3 in Chapter 27, Solutions.) The measurements for both the test substance and the water should be made after the temperature of each liquid has equilibrated using a constant temperature bath. Mathematically it is easiest to make these measurements using the temperatures for the published specific gravity values in the literature. If this is not possible, consult a book on pharmaceutical analysis for the necessary equation and density values for water at various temperatures to make the necessary adjustments (11).

6. Specific gravity and density values for many liquids of interest pharmaceutically can be found in *Remington: The Science and Practice of Pharmacy*, *The Merck Index*, and *International Critical Tables of Numerical Data, Physics, Chemistry and Technology* (ICT).

D. Pharmaceutical applications for density and specific gravity
1. Checking on the identity and/or purity of purchased bulk liquid chemicals.
2. Quality control checks for compounded liquid preparations.
3. Converting between weight of a liquid and its comparable volume. This is useful in several situations: when a compounding formula gives the desired quantity of a liquid as a weight and it is more convenient to measure the volume (or vice versa); for performing both quality control and formulation functions when using an automated compounding machine (a device that measures the ingredient solutions by gravimetric rather than volumetric methods) for making parenteral nutrition solutions; for performing certain calculations for bulk liquids that have their concentrations expressed as weight-weight percents (e.g., phosphoric acid in Sample Prescription 27.3 in Chapter 27).
4. Certain clinical diagnostic applications such as urinalysis.

V. SIGNIFICANT FIGURES

A. Definitions
1. Absolute number: a number taken at its face value, that is, a counting number.
2. Denominate number: a number that specifies a quantity in terms of a unit of measurement, such as 3 in 3 g.
3. Significant figures: the figures of a number that begin with the first figure to the left that is not a zero and end with the last figure to the right that is not a zero or is a zero that is known or considered to be exact. Examples from Table 7.7 of conversion equivalents with three significant figures include the following:

1 g = 15.4 gr

1 kg = 2.20 lb (the more accurate number is 2.2046 lb, so the zero in this case is significant)

1 gr = 64.8 mg (the more accurate number is 64.799 mg)

1 oz (av) = 28.3 g (the more accurate number is 28.3495 g)

B. Significant figures express the value of a denominate number as accurately as possible or as needed for an intended purpose.
1. As indicated in the previous section on intersystem conversions, when converting compounding formula quantities from a common system (such as the apothecaries' system) of measurement to the metric equivalents, three significant figures are to be used. If conversion equivalents with more than three significant figures are known, these obviously may be used and, with

the use of calculators, the math is easily accomplished. More accurate conversion factors are given in the miscellaneous tables section of *The Merck Index* and other similar references.

2. In compounding, the number of significant figures recorded is often limited by the measuring equipment used.

   a. It would be incorrect to report that you weighed 324.9 mg of powder on either a Class III torsion balance or on an electronic balance with a readability of 1 mg, because these instruments do not measure to that degree of precision.

   b. If the dose of a liquid medication is calculated to be 0.34 mL, and you are to make eight doses, the total volume needed is 2.72 mL (8 × 0.34 mL = 2.72 mL), but it would be incorrect to report that you measured 2.72 mL in a 10-mL graduated cylinder because it would be impossible to read the volume in this device to that degree of precision. However, in cases such as this, the rounding is usually done after the mathematical operation; for example, do not round the 0.34 mL to 0.3 mL before multiplying by eight. Keep as many digits as possible until you obtain the final answer.

   c. If very precise and accurate dosing (e.g., 2.72 mL in the preceding example) is truly needed for a medication, either a more precise measuring device, such as an appropriate syringe or a micropipette, should be used or a dilution and aliquot method should be employed (see Chapter 10, Aliquot Calculations).

3. When dealing with doses for patients, two different principles may be used to determine the level of accuracy and precision in using a product or making a custom preparation: number of significant figures and degree of rounding. As you will read in Chapter 9, Evaluating Dosage Regimens, doses for patients (especially infants and children) are often in terms of milligrams per kilogram (mg/kg) of body weight or milligrams per square meter (mg/m^2) of body surface area (BSA). This often gives rise to nonstandard doses.

   a. Take, for example, the situation with mercaptopurine in sample prescription 25.6 (Chapter 25). The recommended dose is 75 mg/m^2/day in two divided doses, and the patient has a BSA of 0.57 m^2. The daily dose is calculated to be 42.75 mg (75 mg/m^2 × 0.57 m^2 = 42.75 mg) with the quantity per dose of 21.375 mg (42.75 mg/day ÷ 2 doses/day = 21.375 mg/dose). If expressing the individual dose with three significant figures, the quantity would be 21.4 mg; if using a dose rounded to the nearest milligram, the dose would be 21 mg. In this case, the dosing reference states to increase the daily dose to the nearest 25 mg, so the daily dose would be 50 mg and each individual dose would be 25 mg.

   b. When using a patient's kilogram weight to determine drug doses, there are some general rules for rounding the kilogram body weight that is calculated from the patient's weight in pounds (14).

      (1) For adults and children with body weights of more than 25 lb, round the calculated kilogram weight to the nearest kilogram (e.g., 30 lb ÷ 2.2 lb/kg = 13.6363 kg, rounded to 14 kg).

      (2) For infants and children with body weights between 6 and 25 lb, round the calculated kilogram weight to the nearest one-tenth of a kilogram (e.g., 10 lb ÷ 2.2 lb/kg = 4.545 kg, rounded to 4.5 kg).

      (3) For premature infants (whose weight is expressed in grams), round the gram weight to the nearest whole gram (e.g., 2.5 lb ÷ 2.2 lb/kg = 1.13636 kg, rounded to 1,136 g).

4. When dealing with **scientific data**, we do not want to give the impression that a reported value is more precise or accurate than its measurement method justifies. Therefore, when performing mathematical operations (such as addition and multiplication) with a measured denominate number, there are standard rules for determining the number of significant figures to report in the final answer. You have probably seen these rules in chemistry or physics textbooks. For a review of these principles and more detailed information on the subject of significant figures and rules for rounding for scientific reporting, consult an appropriate book on pharmaceutical analysis or calculations.

VI.   METHODS FOR PHARMACEUTICAL CALCULATIONS

As you know, pharmaceutical calculations are essential to the practice of pharmacy—everything from calculating doses for patients to determining amounts of ingredients to add to compounded formulations and intravenous admixtures. By this point in your education or career, you have probably developed some favorite and successful methods for doing calculations; therefore, the following section may serve as a review or may provide some new insights into using known methods of calculation for solving pharmacy-related problems. You will find that there are often several ways of approaching even the most basic calculations, so you are encouraged to access several sources, such as the CD that accompanies this book, textbooks on pharmacy calculations, and course instruction and lab manuals; then use proven methods that make sense to you because you will then be less likely to make errors. The methods shown in this section have general application to many types of problems. For calculation methods specific to a problem type or area of practice, see the applicable chapters of this book [e.g., for IV flow rates, see Chapter 34; for calculation methods (such as alligation and algebra) used specifically for dilution and concentration, see Chapter 8].

A. Ratio and proportion

1. Some pharmacy calculation texts define a ratio as a "quotient of two like numbers" and a proportion as "the expression of the equality of two ratios" (15). With these definitions, you would approach a problem using ratio and proportion in the following way.

Example 7.1

Given: You have an antibiotic suspension that is 250 mg/5 mL and a pediatric patient who needs 100 mg. You want to calculate the number of milliliters of the suspension that will contain the desired 100 mg. Using ratios of two **like** numbers, the proportion would be set up as follows:

$$\frac{250 \text{ mg}}{100 \text{ mg}} = \frac{5 \text{ mL}}{x \text{ mL}}$$

Recall that for proportions, the product of the extremes (the first and last numbers) equals the product of the means (the middle numbers), so:

$$(250 \text{ mg})(x \text{ mL}) = (100 \text{ mg}) (5 \text{ mL})$$

Solving for x:

$$x = \frac{(100 \text{ mg})(5 \text{ ml})}{250 \text{ mg}} = 2 \text{ mL}$$

One difficulty with this method is that there may be confusion when setting up the proportion: Should you put the x in the numerator or the denominator?

2. Another approach to the same basic method that some pharmacists find more intuitive is to set up an "If, then" proportion. Using the same data as given in example 7.1, you would solve this problem as shown here in example 7.2.

Example 7.2

If there is 250 mg in 5 mL (250 mg/5 mL), **then** there will be (=) 100 mg in x mL (100 mg/x mL). This proportion is set up as follows:

$$\frac{250 \text{ mg}}{5 \text{ mL}} = \frac{100 \text{ mg}}{x \text{ mL}}$$

Solving for x in the same way as in example 7.1:

$$(250 \text{ mg})(x \text{ mL}) = (100 \text{ mg})(5 \text{ mL})$$

$$x = \frac{(100 \text{ mg})(5 \text{ mL})}{250 \text{ mg}} = 2 \text{ mL}$$

Many of the sample problems in this text are solved using this second approach to ratios and proportions.

B. Dimensional analysis

1. The ratio and proportion method works quite well for relatively simple problems, but many pharmacy problems are more complex and would require that you solve multiple proportions to get the final desired answer. The dimensional analysis method works very well for these more complex problems. With this method, when you finish setting up the problem, if the units on the right side of the equals sign are the same as the desired units on the left side of the equals sign, you have done the problem correctly (provided, of course, that you label quantities with their correct units).

2. You were probably taught this method in high school chemistry or physics; while there are slight variations of this system, the end result is the same. Basically:

   a. Start by asking what are the unit(s) or dimension(s) of the answer that you are seeking.

b. Determine the necessary information, including the units, from your given problem and any needed conversion factors.

c. Arrange these factors as fractions in such a way that when you multiply the fractions, all the units cancel out except the units for your desired answer. It is easiest if you pick and arrange the first fraction on the left so that the unit of the numerator of this fraction is the same as the unit of the numerator of your desired answer.

d. When you arrange the fractions, you will have to invert some of them to be able to cancel desired units (e.g., 250 mg/5 mL may need to be written as 5 mL/250 mg). An example will make this clear.

Example 7.3

You have a pediatric patient who weighs 50 lb. Her pediatrician has prescribed cefaclor 15 mg/kg/dose to be given two times per day. You have available the oral suspension, which is 125 mg/5 mL. Calculate the desired number of milliliters for each dose.

1. Determine the unit(s) of the answer you are seeking and place them to the far right-hand side of the space for setting up your problem. Leave just enough space for your answer and just to the left of that space put an equals sign. For this example, the units of the desired answer are milliliters per dose.

$$= \text{mL/dose}$$

2. Determine the necessary information (including units) from the problem and any needed conversion factors: 125 mg cefaclor/5 mL; 15 mg/kg/dose; 50 lb; 2.2 lb/kg.

3. Arrange the needed information as multiple fractions, starting with the fraction containing mL (the numerator unit of the desired answer) in the numerator of the first fraction in the series.

$$\left(\frac{5 \text{ mL}}{125 \text{ mg}} \right) = \text{mL/dose}$$

4. Following this first fraction, arrange the others so that each of the undesired units cancels out until all you have remaining are the desired units on both sides of the equation.

$$\left(\frac{5 \text{ mL}}{125 \text{ mg}} \right) \left(\frac{15 \text{ mg}}{\text{kg/dose}} \right) \left(\frac{\text{kg}}{2.2 \text{ lb}} \right) \left(\frac{50 \text{ lb}}{} \right) = 13.6 \text{ mL/dose}$$

If you solve this problem using proportions, you will need three equations: one to convert the patient weight from pounds to kilograms, one to calculate the number of milligrams per dose from the patient weight in kilograms and the 15 mg/kg/dose, and one to determine the number of milliliters per dose from the calculated milligrams per dose and the 125 mg/5 mL. You can see why dimensional analysis makes computation of such a complex problem easier and less prone to error.

---

3. When using dimensional analysis, there are situations when you must be especially cautious about using very specific labeling of units. This is particularly true when the same basic metric units are used for two different kinds of quantities. A good example of this is the use of g/mL for both the density of a liquid and concentration of active ingredient in the liquid. Density is a physical measurement, the number of grams that 1 mL weighs, while concentration is the quantity (e.g., number of grams) of an active component per unit volume. An example may make this clearer. Concentrated hydrochloric acid (i.e., Hydrochloric Acid NF) has a density of 1.18 g/mL (that is, 1 mL of the acid weighs 1.18 g). When you assay this concentrated acid solution, you will find that each milliliter contains 0.37 g of the chemical HCl, 0.37 g/mL—the same metric units but two very different values for two different aspects of the same liquid. Sample prescription 27.3 in Chapter 27 has a sample calculation using dimensional analysis that illustrates a method for handling this phenomenon. Obviously, it is very important to carefully and explicitly attach both the correct units and descriptors to such quantities.

C. Mathematical formulas

1. For some calculations we have mathematical formulas that have been derived for specific purposes. In a case like this, fill in the required data and solve the equation. Examples include the formulas for calculating pH and acid or base concentration (see Table 18.1 in Chapter 18), equations for calculating mean kinetic temperature and for converting between Celsius and

Fahrenheit temperatures (see section III on this subject in this chapter), equations for calculating body surface area (see Chapter 9), and so on.

2. You should be able to check the validity of any formula by including the metric units and performing dimensional analysis. This is illustrated with the White-Vincent equation for isotonic volumes in Chapter 11.

REFERENCES

1. Penzes WB. Time line for the definition of the meter. National Institute of Standards and Technology, http://www.nist.gov/div821/museum/timeline.htm. Accessed May 2007.

2. Layer HP. Length—evolution from measurement standard to a fundamental constant. National Institute of Standards and Technology, http://www.nist.gov/div821/museum/length.htm. Accessed May 2007.

3. Taylor BN. NIST Special Publication 330—The international system of units (SI). Gaithersburg, MD: National Institute of Standards and Technology, 1991.

4. U.S. Metric Association. Guide to the use of the metric system [SI version]. Northridge, CA: Author, 2007.

5. U.S. Metric Association. Correct SI-metric usage. http://lamar.colostate.edu/~hillger/correct.htm2. Accessed May 2007.

6. The United States Pharmacopeial Convention, Inc. Chapter ⟨1221⟩. 2008 USP 31/NF 26. Rockville, MD: Author, 2007; 678.

7. The United States Pharmacopeial Convention, Inc. Chapter ⟨1101⟩. 2008 USP 31/NF 26. Rockville, MD: Author, 2007; 578.

8. The United States Pharmacopeial Convention, Inc. 1990 USP XVII/NF XVII. Rockville, MD: Author, 1989; inside front cover, 1881.

9. The United States Pharmacopeial Convention, Inc. General Notices. 2008 USP 31/NF 26. Rockville, MD: Author, 2007; 10.

10. The United States Pharmacopeial Convention, Inc. Chapter ⟨1160⟩. 2008 USP 31/NF 26. Rockville, MD: Author, 2007; 633–634.

11. Connors KA. A textbook of pharmaceutical analysis, 3rd ed. New York: John Wiley & Sons, 1982; 321–325.

12. The United States Pharmacopeial Convention, Inc. General Notices. 2008 USP 31/NF 26. Rockville, MD: Author, 2007; 13.

13. The United States Pharmacopeial Convention, Inc. General Notices. 2008 USP 31/NF 26. Rockville, MD: Author, 2007; 8.

14. O'Sullivan TA. Understanding pharmacy calculations. Washington, DC: American Pharmaceutical Association, 2002; 5.

15. Ansel HC, Stoklosa MJ. Pharmaceutical calculations, 12th ed. Baltimore: Lippincott Williams & Wilkins, 2006; 12–13.

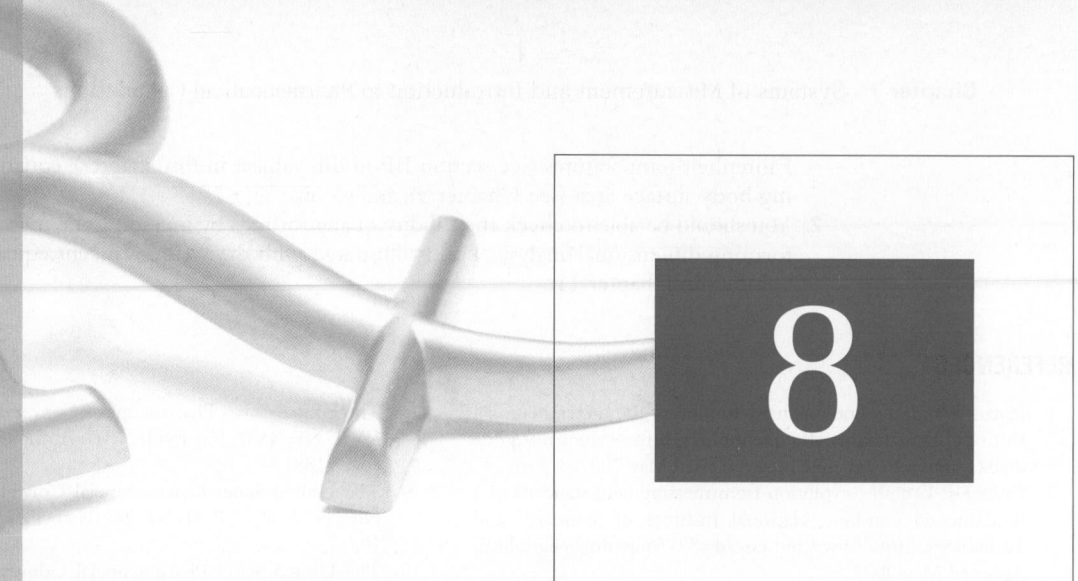

8

Quantity and Concentration Expressions and Calculations

I. INTRODUCTION

A. An essential function of pharmacy service is to ensure that patients get the intended drug in the correct amount. These are two important components of the five recognized "rights" of patients in receiving medication: the right drug in the right dose by the right route of administration to the right patient at the right time. Although providing the correct drug in the correct amount is considered a basic right of medical care, the difficulty of ensuring that it occurs for all patients 100% of the time is evident in the various studies of medical errors, including the famous 1999 Institute of Medicine report, "To Err Is Human." The health professions continue to struggle with this issue; improper dose/quantity continues to be in the top tier of causes of medication errors as reported by hospitals that are part of USP's MedMARx error reporting network (1). Although medication safety is a joint responsibility of all members of the health care team, it is clearly an area in which pharmacists and pharmacy technicians can and do play a major role.

B. Basic to providing correct doses of drugs to patients is a firm understanding of units of measurement for drugs, accepted expressions of quantity and concentration for drug products and preparations, and knowledge and skill in using this information to perform the calculations needed in providing correct and intended drug therapy. Systems and units of measurement and basic calculations techniques were presented in Chapter 7; this forms the basis for the current chapter on quantity and concentration expressions and calculations, which, in turn, will be used in Chapter 9 for calculating and evaluating appropriate doses and dosage regimens. This information will also be used in later chapters of this book when sample prescription and medication orders are evaluated. Most important, this composite information and skill set is vital to providing safe and effective therapy to patients.

C. In general, the following factors determine the accepted method for representing the quantity of a drug and the concentration of the drug in a dosage form.
   1. Accurate representation of the quantity of active moiety, a drug molecule or ion, acting at a receptor
   2. Convenience of measurement
   3. Route of administration
   4. Tradition

II. QUANTITY EXPRESSIONS AND CALCULATIONS USED IN DRUG THERAPY

A. **Metric (SI) weights and volumes**
   1. Quantities for drugs and dosage form ingredients are most often expressed as either metric weights or volumes.
   2. The metric (SI) system is described in Chapter 7, and the metric units of weight and volume most commonly used in pharmacy and medicine are given in Table 7.2 of that chapter.
   3. Chapter 14 contains information on the use of balances and volumetric apparatus to measure weights and volumes of drugs, dosage forms, and compounding ingredients. The use of this equipment is demonstrated on the CD that accompanies this book, and multiple examples of the proper use of weighing and measuring equipment are given in the dosage forms chapters in this book.

B. **Biological units of activity**
   1. Biological units of activity are used for certain natural products including insulin, heparin, and some antibiotics, vitamins, anticancer agents, biotechnology drugs, vaccines, and miscellaneous others.
   2. The units are specific to each drug or natural product with the standards set in the United States by the FDA and USP and internationally by the World Health Organization.
   3. In most cases, the standards give an accepted metric weight equivalent or range. For example, the *USP* monograph for Insulin Human USP states, "Its potency, calculated on the dried basis, is not less than 27.5 USP Insulin Human Units in each mg" (2). Sample prescription 25.3 in Chapter 25 uses nystatin powder to illustrate the conversion between units of activity and metric weight in milligrams when compounding with a drug that has its dose expressed in biological units of activity.
   4. Insulin is the most common drug with potency expressed in units. To facilitate the use and administration of insulin by patients, special syringes are available with volumes marked in units. Caution must be exercised when using these syringes because the markings are specific to a particular strength of insulin product. For example, the unit markings on a U–100 insulin syringe can be used to measure only insulin, and only U–100 insulin (that is, insulin that has a concentration of 100 units/mL).

C. **Molecules, moles, and millimoles**
   1. The most fundamental unit of active ingredient acting on a biological receptor is a drug molecule or ion. However, a molecule of a substance is too small a quantity to be pharmaceutically useful because we always deal with fairly large numbers of molecules. It is therefore convenient to measure in terms of a larger unit. Usually the unit used for this purpose is the mole (SI symbol, mol), which is Avogadro's number (6.023×10^{23}) of molecules.
   2. Because we cannot count out molecules or directly measure moles, a method is needed to equate these units with a quantity that we can measure. The molecular weight (MW) of a compound is the weight in grams of 1 mole of the compound; that is, it is the weight in grams of 6.023×10^{23} molecules. For example, the MW of water is 18.0, meaning that 18.0 g of water contains 6.023×10^{23} molecules of water. Similarly, the MW of phenobarbital is 232.2, meaning that 232.2 g of phenobarbital contains 6.023×10^{23} molecules of phenobarbital. Because elements, ions, and molecules react in integral ratios (1:1, 1:2, and so on), the mole is a more fundamentally useful unit than is the gram, but the gram offers convenience of measurement.

3. Millimole (mmol) units are often used in pharmacy and medicine rather than moles because the required quantities and concentrations of drugs are relatively small. There are 1,000 mmol/mol of a compound. The number of grams per mole (g/mol, the molecular weight) is also equal to the number of milligrams per millimole (mg/mmol); for example, 1 mmol of phenobarbital weighs 232.2 mg.

4. One example of a drug that traditionally has its dose expressed in millimoles is phosphate when administered in total parenteral nutrition (see Chapter 35). In this case, we are interested in the amount of phosphorus, the P part of the phosphate, and we need a way to get at this. One millimole of phosphate, whether in the form $H_2PO_4^{-1}$, HPO_4^{-2}, or PO_4^{-3}, contains the same amount of phosphorus, P, but all three forms have different weights (and different numbers of milliequivalents).

Examples 8.1 and 8.2 demonstrate conversions between metric and molar units.

Example 8.1

Calculate the weight in grams from moles:

You have a formula that calls for 0.5 moles of Sodium Hydroxide (NaOH). Sodium Hydroxide is available as a solid. How many grams of NaOH should you weigh? The MW of NaOH = 40.0.

$$\left(\frac{40.0 \text{ g NaOH}}{\text{mol NaOH}}\right)\left(\frac{0.5 \text{ mol NaOH}}{}\right) = 20.0 \text{ g NaOH}$$

Example 8.2

Calculate millimoles from weight in milligrams:

You have a liquid formulation that contains 600 mg of Potassium Chloride (KCl) in each teaspoonful of syrup. You want to know how many millimoles of KCl are in each teaspoonful. The MW of KCl = 74.5.

$$\left(\frac{\text{mmol KCl}}{74.5 \text{ mg KCl}}\right)\left(\frac{600 \text{ mg KCl}}{}\right) = 8 \text{ mmol KCl}$$

D. Equivalents and milliequivalents

1. When dealing with electrolytes in solution, we are at times interested in only one of the ion pair. For example, with mineral acids, we may be interested only in the number of H^+ ions in solution. We do not care about the counter ion, the Cl^-, the SO_4^{-2}, the NO_3^-, and so on. Therefore, we do not care about the weight of the acid present or the number of moles of compound present; we want to know how many moles of H^+ are present. The concept of equivalents evolved from this special need.

2. Equivalents (Eq), sometimes referred to as *combining power*, are the number of univalent counter ions needed to react with each molecule of the substance. Hydrochloric acid (HCl) has 1 Eq/mol because 1 mole of the univalent ion OH^- reacts exactly with one mole of H^+ in HCl. (Also note that one mole of Na^+ reacts exactly with one mole of Cl^- in HCl.) Sulfuric acid (H_2SO_4) contains 2 Eq/mol because 2 moles of OH^- are required to react with 1 mole of sulfuric acid. The compound $Al_2(SO_4^{-2})_3$ has 6 Eq/mol because, in aqueous solution, two Al^{+3} ions are obtained for each $Al_2(SO_4)_3$, and they would react with six univalent anions, such as six Cl^-s. The sulfate (3 SO_4^{-2}) also reacts with six univalent counter ions, such as six Na^+s.

3. The definition of equivalent depends on the particular type of reaction undergone, so it is subject to some ambiguity. The number of equivalents per mole for electrolytes with variable valence, such as phosphate and carbonate, depends on the pH of solution: For instance, Na_2HPO_4 with 2 Eq/mol is predominant at high pH, whereas NaH_2PO_4 with 1 Eq/mol predominates at lower pH. For this reason, phosphate concentration for replacement therapy is expressed in terms of millimoles rather than as milliequivalents.

4. As with moles, equivalents cannot be measured directly, so a method is needed to equate these units with a quantity that we can measure. The equivalent weight or gram-equivalent weight (Eq) of an element or compound is that weight in grams which combines chemically with one equivalent of another element or compound. The equivalent weight of HCl is its molecular weight, because this compound has 1 equivalent per mole and reacts with one equivalent of

another compound. The equivalent weight of sulfuric acid is its molecular weight divided by two because sulfuric acid has 2 equivalents per mole. The equivalent weight of aluminum sulfate is its molecular weight divided by six because there are 6 equivalents per mole. This can be expressed by the general equation:

$$\text{Equivalent Weight} = \frac{\text{Atomic or Molecular Weight of the Substance}}{\text{Number of Equivalents per Atomic or Molecular Weight}}$$

5. Milliequivalents (mEq), rather than equivalents, are often used in pharmacy and medicine because, when dosing electrolytes, we are usually dealing with small quantities. There are 1,000 mEq per equivalent. The number of equivalents per mole for a given compound equals the number of milliequivalents per millimole for that substance.

6. Electrolytes such as potassium, sodium, calcium, and chloride often are dosed in terms of milliequivalents because, from a therapeutic point of view, it is the individual ion that is of interest. Often the method of expressing the dose of an electrolyte may be a matter of tradition. For example, oral doses of calcium usually are given in terms of milligrams or grams of the compound (e.g., calcium carbonate 500 mg), whereas parenteral electrolyte replacement doses of calcium are more often expressed in terms of milliequivalents (e.g., Ca^{++} 4.6 mEq).

7. There is a trend toward expressing electrolyte doses in terms of milligrams or millimoles of the pertinent ion rather than as milliequivalents of the ion or grams or milligrams of the salt. This method has the advantage of being unambiguous, and it is the system now used internationally; equivalent (Eq) is not a recognized SI unit. As is often the case when there is a change in systems, errors of misinterpretation can occur; there have been reports of doses written in terms of milligrams of the salt (e.g., 500 mg Calcium Chloride) and interpreted and administered as milligrams of the ion (e.g., 500 mg calcium ion, which is 1,836 mg of the Calcium Chloride, nearly a fourfold overdose). Pharmacists must be **very careful** when interpreting these orders. Fortunately, product labeling and therapeutic reference books now usually give concentrations in all three systems [e.g., Calcium Chloride 10% Injection (1 g/10 mL; each milliliter of solution provides 27.2 mg or 1.36 mEq of calcium)].

Examples 8.3 through 8.5 show calculations for converting between milliequivalents and milligrams of ions and metric weights of salts.

Example 8.3

Calculate weight in milligrams of the salt from milliequivalents:

A potassium supplement tablet contains 10 mEq of KCl. How many milligrams of KCl are in each tablet? The MW of KCl = 74.5

$$\left(\frac{74.5 \text{ mg KCl}}{\text{mmol KCl}}\right)\left(\frac{\text{mmol KCl}}{1 \text{ mEq KCl}}\right)\left(\frac{10 \text{ mEq KCl}}{}\right) = 745 \text{ mg KCl}$$

Example 8.4

Calculate weight in milligrams of salt from milligrams of the ion.

A dose of calcium chloride is prescribed as 136 mg of calcium ion. How many milligrams of calcium chloride are needed for this dose? Calcium chloride is available as the dihydrate ($CaCl_2 \cdot 2H_2O$), which has a MW = 147; calcium ion has an atomic weight of 40.

$$\left(\frac{147 \text{ mg CaCl}_2 \cdot 2H_2O}{40 \text{ mg Ca}}\right)\left(\frac{136 \text{ mg Ca}}{}\right) = 500 \text{ mg CaCl}_2 \cdot 2H_2O$$

Example 8.5

Calculate milliequivalents from weight in milligrams of salt:

The powder for oral solution for a bowel-cleansing product contains 568 mg of anhydrous sodium sulfate (Na_2SO_4). How many milliequivalents of Na^+ are in this product? The MW of Na_2SO_4 = 142.

$$\left(\frac{2 \text{ mEq Na}^+}{1 \text{ mmol Na}_2SO_4}\right)\left(\frac{\text{mmol Na}_2SO_4}{142 \text{ mg Na}_2SO_4}\right)\left(\frac{568 \text{ mg Na}_2SO_4}{}\right) = 8 \text{ mEq Na}^+$$

(For an alternative way of conceptualizing and solving this problem, see the CD that accompanies this book.)

E. Osmoles and milliosmoles

1. Osmotic pressure is discussed in Chapter 11, Isotonicity Calculations. Basically, pharmaceutical solutions that come in contact with cell membranes should have the same osmotic pressure as the cell contents to prevent tissue damage and discomfort. Because osmotic pressure is a colligative property, it depends on the number of individual solute particles (ions or molecules) per given volume of solution.

2. An osmole (Osmol) is the number of moles of solute present multiplied by the number of particles per molecule obtained when the solute is dissolved in water. Nonelectrolytes, such as dextrose, do not dissociate in solution, so 1 mole of dextrose yields 1 osmole. Sodium chloride dissociates into two ions in aqueous solution, so 1 mole of sodium chloride gives 2 osmoles. Sodium sulfate (Na_2SO_4) gives three ions per molecule, so there are 3 osmoles per mole of sodium sulfate.

3. Milliosmole (mOsmol) units, rather than osmoles, are often used in pharmacy and medicine. There are 1,000 mOsmol per Osmol. The number of osmoles per mole for a given compound equals the number of milliosmoles per millimole for that substance.

4. If a drug or chemical is present in solid form as a hydrate (e.g., $MgSO_4 \cdot H_2O$), the water molecules do not count as particles because they merely become part of the solvent in aqueous solution.

Examples 8.6 and 8.7 show calculations for converting between osmole and metric units.

Example 8.6

Calculate osmoles from weight in grams:

Isotonic Sodium Chloride Solution (0.9%) has 9 grams of NaCl in each liter of solution. How many osmoles are there in each liter of solution? The MW of NaCl = 58.5.

$$\left(\frac{2 \text{ Osmol}}{\text{mol NaCl}} \right)\left(\frac{\text{mol NaCl}}{58.5 \text{ g NaCl}} \right)\left(\frac{9 \text{ g NaCl}}{\text{L}} \right) = 0.308 \text{ Osmol/L}$$

Example 8.7

Calculate milligrams from milliosmoles:

You want to add solute to a liter of water so that there are 300 mOsmol in this solution. Your source of solute is Magnesium Sulfate Heptahydrate ($MgSO_4 \cdot 7H_2O$), which has a MW = 246.5. How many milligrams of this solute should you add?

$$\left(\frac{246.5 \text{ mg } MgSO_4}{\text{mmol } MgSO_4} \right)\left(\frac{\text{mmol } MgSO_4}{2 \text{ mOsmol}} \right)\left(\frac{300 \text{ mOsmol}}{} \right) = 36{,}975 \text{ mg } MgSO_4 \cdot 7H_2O$$

III.   CONCENTRATION EXPRESSIONS AND CALCULATIONS USED IN DRUG THERAPY

A. **Concentration** gives **quantity of drug** or active ingredient **per** amount (volume or weight) of product or preparation.

1. Concentrations are used for expressing doses for all topical preparations. In this case, concentration has conceptual importance because concentration gradient is the driving force for transfer of the drug across the membrane or barrier, such as the skin.

2. Concentration also is used to express the strength of liquid systemic products—for example, amoxicillin suspension 250 mg/5 mL, or dextrose 5% injection.

3. For individual dosage units such as capsules, tablets, and suppositories, the dose is expressed as a quantity of drug rather than as a concentration. However, because pure drug is almost never dispensed, these quantities are really concentrations. For example, when the label on a bottle of acetaminophen states "Acetaminophen 500 mg," what this really means is acetaminophen 500 mg **per** tablet. Because the tablet usually contains other ingredients (e.g., pharmaceutical ingredients such as binders, disintegrants, lubricants) in addition to the acetaminophen, the tablet weighs more than 500 mg; the content could be expressed as a concentration, such as acetaminophen 500 mg per 750 mg of tablet material.

B. **Metric units of weight and volume**

Metric units for weight and volume can be combined to give expressions of concentration.

1. Weight of active ingredient per weight of product: For example, gentamicin ophthalmic ointment 3 mg per gram (also written 3 mg/g) is 3 mg of gentamicin in each 1 g of ointment.

2. Weight of active ingredient per volume of product: For example, tobramycin ophthalmic solution 3 mg per milliliter (also written 3 mg/mL) is 3 mg of tobramycin in each 1 mL of solution; amoxicillin suspension 250 mg per 5 mL (also written 250 mg/5 mL) is 250 mg of amoxicillin per 5 mL of suspension.

C. Molarity and molality

1. Molarity (M) is the number of moles of solute per liter of solution. For example, a 1 M solution of sodium hydroxide contains 1 mole of sodium hydroxide per liter of solution. Because the molecular weight of sodium hydroxide is 40.0, a 1 M solution of sodium hydroxide contains 40.0 grams of sodium hydroxide per liter of solution (40 g/L) or 40 mg/mL.

2. Molality (m) is the number of moles of solute per 1,000 grams of solvent.

3. For dilute aqueous solutions, the numeric values of molarity and molality are nearly equal. This is because water has a density of 1.0 g/mL, so one liter weighs 1,000 grams. Furthermore, for dilute solutions the quantity of solute is small and therefore takes up very little volume in the solution, and the density of the solution is also very close to 1.0 g/mL. This does not hold true for more concentrated solutions in which there is a large amount of solute and when the densities of the solvent and solution are not equal to 1.0. The example given below for Syrup NF is a good illustration of the large difference in molarity and molality for a concentrated solution.

4. Other molar concentration terms used in pharmacy include millimoles per milliliter (mmol/mL) or millimoles per liter (mmol/L).

Examples 8.8 through 8.11 show methods of converting between molar and molal concentrations and metric quantities and concentrations.

Example 8.8

Calculate molarity from grams of solute per 100 milliliters of solution:

Diluted Hydrochloric Acid NF contains 10 g of HCl in 100 mL of solution. Calculate its molarity. The MW of HCl = 36.5.

$$\left(\frac{\text{mol HCl}}{36.5 \text{ g HCl}}\right)\left(\frac{10 \text{ g HCl}}{100 \text{ mL}}\right)\left(\frac{1{,}000 \text{ mL}}{\text{L}}\right) = 2.74 \text{ mol/L} = 2.74 \text{ } M$$

Example 8.9

Calculate the grams of solute needed for a desired volume of M solution:

You want to make 500 mL of a 3 M solution of NaOH. How many grams of NaOH do you need? The MW of NaOH = 40.0.

$$\left(\frac{40.0 \text{ g NaOH}}{\text{mol NaOH}}\right)\left(\frac{3 \text{ mol NaOH}}{\text{L}}\right)\left(\frac{0.5 \text{ L}}{}\right) = 60.0 \text{ g NaOH}$$

Example 8.10

Calculate the molarity and the molality of a solution from its weight/volume concentration and the density of the solution.

Syrup NF contains 850 g of sucrose in 1,000 mL of solution. The solution has a density of 1.3. The MW of sucrose = 342.

Molarity (M) of the solution:

$$\left(\frac{\text{mol sucrose}}{342 \text{ g sucrose}}\right)\left(\frac{850 \text{ g sucrose}}{1{,}000 \text{ mL solution}}\right)\left(\frac{1{,}000 \text{ mL solution}}{\text{L}}\right) = 2.49 \text{ mol/L} = 2.49 \text{ } M$$

Molality (m) of the solution:

Because molality is based on kilograms of solvent, to calculate the molality of the solution, we first must calculate the weight of the solution using its density and then use this information to calculate the weight in kilograms of the solvent, water.

Weight of 1 L of solution:

$$\left(\frac{1.3 \text{ g solution}}{\text{mL solution}}\right)\left(\frac{1{,}000 \text{ mL solution}}{\text{L}}\right) = 1{,}300 \text{ g solution/L solution}$$

Remembering that weights are additive:

$$\text{grams of solute} + \text{grams of solvent} = \text{grams of solution}$$

$$850 \text{ g sucrose} + x \text{ g of water} = 1{,}300 \text{ g of solution/L}$$

$$x \text{ g of water} = 1{,}300 \text{ g solution} - 850 \text{ g sucrose} = 450 \text{ g water/L solution}$$

Calculation of molality of the solution:

$$\left(\frac{\text{mol sucrose}}{342 \text{ g sucrose}}\right)\left(\frac{850 \text{ g sucrose}}{\text{L solution}}\right)\left(\frac{\text{L solution}}{450 \text{ g water}}\right)\left(\frac{1{,}000 \text{ g water}}{\text{kg water}}\right) = 5.5 \text{ mol/kg water} = 5.5 \; m$$

For those of you who like using formulas, molarity and molality can be interconverted using the formula:

$$M = m \times \textit{(solution density} - \textit{anhydrous solute concentration in g/mL)}$$

In this example, to convert from M to m, solve for m:

$$m = \frac{M}{\textit{soln density} - \textit{solute conc.}} = \frac{2.49}{1.3 - 0.85} = \frac{2.49}{0.45} = 5.5$$

Example 8.11

Calculate millimoles per liter (mmol/L) from milligrams per deciliter (mg/dL or mg%):

To conform to the international system of units, reporting of cholesterol blood plasma levels has changed from milligrams per deciliter (1 dL = 100 mL), sometimes referred to as mg%, to millimoles per liter. A patient's medical record from a former hospitalization shows a cholesterol level of 230 mg/dL. What is the equivalent of this level in mmol/L? The MW of cholesterol = 387.

$$\left(\frac{\text{mmol choles.}}{387 \text{ mg choles.}}\right)\left(\frac{230 \text{ mg choles.}}{100 \text{ mL}}\right)\left(\frac{1{,}000 \text{ mL}}{\text{L}}\right) = 5.94 \text{ mmol cholesterol/L}$$

D. Normality and milliequivalents per milliliter (mEq/mL)

1. Normality (N) is the number of equivalents per liter of solution. A 1 N solution of HCl has 1 Eq/L. Because the MW of HCl is 36.5 g and because there is 1 Eq/mol, a 1 N solution has 36.5 g of HCl per liter of solution, and a 1 N solution of HCl equals a 1 M solution of HCl. A 1 N solution of sulfuric acid also has 1 Eq/L. However, because sulfuric acid has 2 Eq/mol, a 1 N solution of sulfuric acid has 49.0 g (half the molecular weight) of sulfuric acid per liter of solution. In this case, a 1 N solution of H_2SO_4 equals a 0.5 M solution of H_2SO_4. Both solutions, 1 N HCl and 1 N H_2SO_4, provide the same number of H^+ ions in each liter of solution.

2. Other concentration terms used in pharmacy include milliequivalents per liter (mEq/L) and milliequivalents per milliliter (mEq/mL).

Examples 8.12 and 8.13 show methods of converting between concentrations in metric units and normality and mEq/mL concentrations.

Example 8.12

Calculate grams per liter from normality:

You want to make 500 mL of a 1 N solution of sulfuric acid (H_2SO_4). How many grams of H_2SO_4 do you need? The MW of H_2SO_4 = 98.1.

$$\left(\frac{98.1 \text{ g } H_2SO_4}{\text{mol } H_2SO_4}\right)\left(\frac{\text{mol } H_2SO_4}{2 \text{ Eq}}\right)\left(\frac{1 \text{ Eq}}{\text{L}}\right)\left(\frac{0.5 \text{ L}}{}\right) = 24.5 \text{ g } H_2SO_4$$

Example 8.13

Calculate milliequivalents per milliliter from grams per milliliter:

You have a pint of potassium chloride syrup that is labeled 10% (10 g KCl per 100 mL of syrup). The dose of this liquid is 1 tablespoonful (i.e., 15 mL). You want to know the number of milliequivalents of K$^+$ in each dose. The MW of KCl = 74.5.

$$\left(\frac{1 \text{ mEq K}^+}{\text{mmol KCl}}\right)\left(\frac{\text{mmol KCl}}{74.5 \text{ mg KCl}}\right)\left(\frac{1{,}000 \text{ mg}}{\text{g}}\right)\left(\frac{10 \text{ g KCl}}{100 \text{ mL}}\right)\left(\frac{15 \text{ mL}}{}\right) = 20.1 \text{ mEq K}^+$$

E. Osmolality and osmolarity

1. The concepts of osmolality and osmolarity apply to aqueous solutions in contact with biological membranes. Expressing concentrations of pharmaceutical solutions in osmolar terms is important when evaluating the appropriateness of solutions that come in contact with sensitive body membranes and tissues.

2. Osmolality is the number of osmoles per kilogram of the solvent water. For an aqueous solution of a nonelectrolyte that behaves ideally (no dissociation or association), a 1 m solution has an osmolality of 1 Osmol/kg of water. For an aqueous solution of a univalent-univalent electrolyte such as NaCl, if behaving ideally and giving two ions per molecule, a 1 m solution would have an osmolality of 2 Osmol/kg of water.

3. Osmolarity is the number of osmoles per liter of solution. For a compound that does not ionize in water, a 1 M solution has an osmolarity of 1 Osmol/L of solution. For an aqueous solution of the univalent-univalent electrolyte NaCl, if behaving ideally and giving two ions per molecule, a 1 M solution would have an osmolarity of 2 Osmol/L of solution.

4. As with molarity and molality, the numeric values for osmolality and osmolarity are very close in dilute solutions but can vary substantially with concentrated solutions. This is clearly illustrated with the 85% sucrose solution, which has calculated osmolality and osmolarity values of 5.5 Osmol/kg water and 2.49 Osmol/L of solution, respectively. It is very important to keep this difference in mind when you are given values in either osmolarity or osmolality. In pharmacy practice, osmolarity is used most frequently because we usually make pharmaceutical solutions to a volume, and we can calculate an estimate of osmolarity from the weights of the solutes, their molecular weights, and the expected number of particles per mole for each species. The values obtained from such calculations are only estimates because these calculations assume that the particles behave ideally: Electrolytes completely dissociate and do not interact with each other, and none of the particles self-associate or interact with the water molecules. In reality, solutions, especially concentrated solutions, do not behave ideally.

5. As indicated previously, the concept of osmolarity/osmolality is an important one when dealing with solutions that come in contact with sensitive body tissues.
   a. The osmolarity of a solution that is isotonic with body fluids is approximately 0.307 Osmol/L or 307 mOsmol/L.
   b. We try to match this osmolarity as closely as possible when we prepare pharmaceutical solutions that are administered parenterally or applied topically to sensitive membranes, such as the eye.
   c. For most adults, the lining of the gastrointestinal tract can tolerate highly hypertonic solutions (those of high osmolarity). In contrast, the gastrointestinal lining of neonates is sensitive to hypertonic solutions. Oral solutions for these infants should be close to 300 mOsmol/L (3,4).

6. Because of deviations from ideality, when true effective osmolarity is needed, it should be measured using an appropriate method and instrument. Unfortunately osmolarity cannot be measured directly. Osmometers (instruments that are used in hospitals and laboratories to measure the osmotic properties of biologic fluids and other solutions) measure osmolality rather than osmolarity. It is possible to calculate effective osmolarity from measured osmolality, but you must know (or can measure) the density of the solution and the concentration(s) of the solute(s) in the solution. In this case, the following equation can be used (5).

   osmolarity = (measured osmolality)
   × (solution density in g/mL − anhydrous solute concentration in g/mL)

Notice the similarity between this equation and the equation for converting between molarity and molality, which was shown example 8.10. The usefulness of this equation is somewhat limited because in many situations we are dealing with complex solutions containing multiple ingredients. For example, say you are evaluating oral liquid vehicles for use in the neonatal intensive care nursery. The specifications for the manufactured syrup vehicle Ora-Sweet give the osmolality as 3,240 mOsmol/kg. To convert this concentration to osmolarity requires that you have both the density of the syrup and the exact quantities of all the ingredients; while you could measure the density of the syrup, exact formulation ingredient information is not available to you. Fortunately, for most pharmaceutical purposes, we are most interested in an approximate osmolarity because we want to determine whether the solution has an osmolarity close to the desired 300 mOsmol/L of biologic fluids. For the example given earlier, you can easily see that both Ora-Sweet (published osmolality of 3,240 mOsmol/kg) and Syrup NF (calculated osmolarity of 2,490 mOsmol/L) are highly hypertonic and would not be acceptable for use in neonates.

Note: For more precise treatment on the subject of converting between measured osmolality and effective osmolarity, see *USP* Chapter ⟨785⟩ Osmolarity and Osmolality.

Examples 8.14 and 8.15 show methods of calculating osmolar concentrations from metric concentrations.

Example 8.14

Calculate milliosmoles per liter from grams per milliliter:

Magnesium sulfate injection is available in a concentration of 50% magnesium sulfate heptahydrate (50 g of $MgSO_4 \cdot 7H_2O$/100 mL). Calculate its concentration in milliosmoles per liter (mOsmol/L). The MW of $MgSO_4 \cdot 7H_2O$ = 246.5.

$$\left(\frac{1,000 \text{ mOsmol}}{\text{Osmol}}\right)\left(\frac{2 \text{ Osmol}}{\text{mol } MgSO_4}\right)\left(\frac{\text{mol } MgSO_4}{246.5 \text{ g } MgSO_4}\right)\left(\frac{50 \text{ g } MgSO_4}{100 \text{ mL}}\right)\left(\frac{1,000 \text{ mL}}{\text{L}}\right) = 4,057 \text{ mOsmol/L}$$

This answer corresponds closely to the calculated osmolarity of 4,060 mOsmol/L given in Trissel's *Handbook of Injectable Drugs*. This book also gives the measured osmolality of this solution as determined by freezing-point depression, 2,620 mOsmol/kg, and as determined by vapor pressure, 2,875 mOsmol/kg (6). As you can see, for this concentrated solution, the values for the calculated osmolarity and the measured osmolality are quite different.

Example 8.15

Calculate the metric weight of salt to add per liter of solution to obtain a desired milliosmoles per liter concentration.

You want to make an oral calcium supplement for a neonate. You will use calcium gluconate as the source of calcium, and you want the concentration of the solution to be 300 mOsmol/L. How many milligrams of calcium gluconate will you need to make a liter of solution? The MW of calcium gluconate = 430.4, and the formula is $Ca(gluconate)_2$, which means that each molecule of calcium gluconate gives three ions.

$$\left(\frac{430.4 \text{ mg Ca gluc.}}{\text{mmol Ca gluc.}}\right)\left(\frac{\text{mmol Ca gluc.}}{3 \text{ mOsmol}}\right)\left(\frac{300 \text{ mOsmol}}{\text{L}}\right) = 43,040 \text{ mg Ca gluc.}$$

F. Percent

1. In pharmacy and medicine, percentages are often used for expressing concentrations—for example,

    a. Active ingredients in topical products.

    b. Alcohol and some excipients, such as preservatives, in both internal and external products.

    c. Some ingredients in parenteral products.

    d. Active ingredients in dosage forms for internal use (which is less common).

2. The general meaning of *percent* is "parts in 100" (from the Latin *per centum,* meaning "per 100"). By standard pharmaceutical convention, as given in the General Notices of the *USP,* unless otherwise stated, percent has the following meanings based on the physical states of the constituents (7):

    a. *For mixtures of solids and semisolids:* percent weight in weight—that is, the number of grams of solid constituent in 100 g of solid or semisolid mixture. For example, hydrocortisone 1% ointment is 1 g hydrocortisone powder in 100 g of ointment mixture. For clarity, percent weight in weight may be written %w/w. When a *USP* monograph or a product label states a given percent with the words "by weight," this means % w/w.

    b. *For solutions or suspensions of solids in liquids:* percent weight in volume—that is, the number of grams of solid constituent in 100 mL of solution or liquid preparation. For example, dextrose 5% injection is 5 g of dextrose powder in 100 mL of solution. For clarity, percent weight in volume may be written %w/v.

   c. *For solutions of liquids in liquids*: percent volume in volume—that is, the number of milliliters of liquid constituent in 100 mL of solution or liquid preparation. For example, isopropyl alcohol 70% is 70 mL of isopropyl alcohol in 100 mL of solution. For clarity, percent volume in volume may be written %v/v.

   d. *For solutions of gases in liquids*: percent weight in volume—that is, the number of grams of gas in 100 mL of solution or liquid preparation.

3. Few major exceptions exist to these general conventions on percent. The concentrated acids and formaldehyde are two examples in this category. Some examples and guidelines concerning percent mixtures of these compounds are presented in the sections of this chapter that discuss special calculations involving these chemicals. Sample prescription 27.3 in Chapter 27 gives an example of a solution of a concentrated acid prescribed by percent.

G. Ratio strength

1. Concentrations of dilute solutions or solid mixtures are sometimes expressed as ratio strengths rather than as percents. This notation has been used for many years, probably owing to tradition but possibly because some practitioners may think it is easier to visualize a dilute concentration written as 1:10,000 rather than as the percent 0.01%.

2. The use of ratio strength notation is to be discouraged because the 1:*x* symbolism may be interpreted in two ways: the colon may be interpreted either as "qs ad" or as "plus." By standard pharmaceutical definition, the colon stands for "qs ad" (8): That is, when a ratio strength of 1:1,000 is indicated, this is interpreted as follows:

   a. *For solids in liquids:* 1 g of solute or solid in 1,000 mL of solution or liquid preparation

   b. *For liquids in liquids:* 1 mL of liquid constituent in 1,000 mL of solution or liquid preparation

   c. *For solids in solids:* 1 g of solid constituent in 1,000 g of solid mixture (8)

3. An example of a preparation with concentration expressed as ratio strength is given in sample prescription 27.1, which is for a solution of potassium permanganate in water. The prescribed concentration is 1:6,000, which is 1 g of potassium permanganate crystals in 6,000 mL of aqueous solution.

4. Not all prescribers are knowledgeable about the aforementioned conventions and may use ratio notation in a more colloquial sense. You may get prescription orders that use ratios for which the prescriber intends the colon to be interpreted as a "plus" rather than the conventional "qs ad."

Example 8.16	℞	Gentamicin ointment

White petrolatum   1:2

Dispense 30 g

Two interpretations are possible:

1. If interpreted by official convention (qs ad), this ointment would be made by weighing one part of gentamicin ointment (15 g), then qs ad to two parts total mixture (30 g ointment) with white petrolatum. In other words, there would be one part of gentamicin ointment and one part of white petrolatum for a total of two parts.

2. The alternative *plus* interpretation would mean to mix one part of gentamicin ointment (10 g) with two parts of white petrolatum (20 g) for a total of three parts (30 g).

---

   a. This ambiguity of interpretation causes no great inaccuracy if the solution or mixture is very dilute. If, however, as in the preceding example, the preparation is quite concentrated, a rather large error in product concentration would result from using the unintended interpretation. In cases such as these, consult the prescriber for clarification. Sample prescription 25.3 in Chapter 25 illustrates this process.

   b. At times, internal evidence may give you a hint as to the intention of the prescriber. For example, if 8 oz is prescribed and the ratio strength designation is 1:7, the desired interpretation of the colon is probably a plus; that is, 1 oz of component A plus 7 oz of component B to give a total of 8 oz. In contrast, if 8 oz is prescribed and the ratio strength designation is 1:8, the desired interpretation of the colon is probably a qs ad; that is, 1 oz of component A plus 7 oz of component B to give a total of 8 oz. When in doubt, consult the prescriber concerning the actual intent.

IV. METHODS OF CALCULATING QUANTITIES AND CONCENTRATIONS WHEN COMBINING OR DILUTING PREPARATIONS

In Chapter 7, three general methods of performing pharmaceutical calculations were presented: ratio and proportion, dimensional analysis, and mathematical formulas. In addition to these methods are a few techniques that are especially useful in calculating quantities and concentrations when making, evaluating, and labeling pharmacy preparations. These calculation methods are described here, and examples are provided to illustrate their use. At the end of this section, an array of problems, from simple to complex, are presented and solved using the various methods and techniques; often a combination of methods is most efficient. When performing calculations such as this, use the methods and techniques that make the most sense to you for the type of problem presented.

A. Percent: *Rate × Whole = Part*

  1. This general formula is one that you probably first learned in grade school when calculating interest on savings accounts. It provides a simple method that is very useful in performing calculations for quantities and concentrations when the concentration of the ingredient is given in percent.

  2. The most typical problem is a prescription order or formula that gives the desired concentration of the active ingredient(s) in percent (i.e., the *Rate*) and the quantity to dispense (i.e., the *Whole*) in grams or milliliters. In compounding such a preparation, the first step is to calculate the metric quantity of the prescribed active ingredient (i.e., the *Part*). All the *USP* rules for percentages (w/w, w/v and v/v) with regard to solids and liquids apply.

Example 8.17   ℞   Salicylic acid   10%

White petrolatum   qs ad   30 g

Solving for the quantity of salicylic acid:

$$Rate \times Whole = Part$$
$$10\% \times 30 \text{ g} = 0.1 \times 30 \text{ g} = 3 \text{ g}$$

One difficulty with this method is remembering how to convert the percent to a decimal—how many places and which way (left or right) to move the decimal point. It may help to recall that percent comes from the Latin *per centum*, meaning "per 100" (like the word *cent*ury for 100 years), so you can write the percent as a fraction with 100 in the denominator (e.g., 10% would be 10/100); then either perform the mathematical operation using the fraction or convert the fraction to the equivalent decimal by dividing the numerator by the denominator, $10 \div 100 = 0.1$.

  3. This basic equation may also by used to calculate a percent concentration of an ingredient from the quantity of the ingredient in grams or milliliters (the *Part*) and the quantity of the preparation (the *Whole*). This calculation is needed for labeling a preparation when the formula is written with metric quantities.

Example 8.18   ℞   Salicylic acid   3 g

White petrolatum   qs ad   30 g

Solving for the percent concentration of salicylic acid:

$$Rate \times Whole = Part$$
$$Rate \times 30 \text{ g} = 3 \text{ g}$$
$$Rate = 3 \text{ g}/30 \text{ g} = 0.1 = 10\%$$

B. Algebra

Algebra is a useful tool when you are obtaining a required ingredient from more than one source, each with a different concentration. This presents the type of situation commonly encountered in algebra of solving two equations with two unknowns. This is best described using an example.

Example 8.19   You want to make 120 mL of a solution that is 60% v/v isopropyl alcohol (IPA) in water, and you want to use a 70% IPA solution and a 30% IPA solution. How many milliliters of each will you need?

Let:
$$x = \text{the number of milliliters of 30\% solution needed}$$
$$y = \text{the number of milliliters of 70\% solution needed}$$

Assuming that the volumes are additive (no contraction with mixing),

Then:
$$x + y = 120 \text{ mL}$$

Solving for x:
$$x = 120 - y$$

Also:
$$30\% \, x + 70\% \, y = 60\% \, (120)$$

Substituting for x and solving this equation:

$$30\%(120 - y) + 70\% \, y = 60\% \, (120)$$

$$0.3 \, (120 - y) + 0.7 \, y = 0.6 \, (120)$$

$$36 - 0.3 \, y + 0.7 \, y = 72$$

$$0.4 \, y = 36$$

$$y = 90$$

$$x = 120 - y = 120 - 90 = 30$$

Measure 90 mL of 70% Isopropyl Alcohol and 30 mL of 30% Isopropyl Alcohol; combine these solutions to give 120 mL of a 60% IPA solution.

C. Alligation

1. Alligation is a method favored by many pharmacists and pharmacy technicians because it offers a technique for solving problems that require algebra, but it uses a mechanical approach, sort of a fill-in-the-blanks method. In fact, the relationships for alligation can be derived algebraically; this is explained in some books on pharmaceutical calculations (9).

2. The steps in alligation are presented and illustrated below. For easy comparison with the algebra method, this example uses the same problem and data as are used for example 8.19 shown earlier. A similar example with slightly different numbers is shown on the CD that accompanies this book.

   a. Visualize a square with boxes at each corner and one in the center:

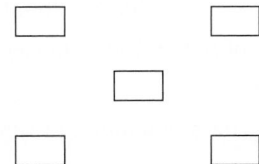

   b. In the center box, place the number of the desired concentration for your preparation: 60. (See the completed square below.)
   c. In the upper left-hand corner, place the concentration of the ingredient with the higher concentration: 70.
   d. In the lower left-hand corner, place the concentration of the ingredient with the lower concentration: 30.
   e. Subtract the desired concentration from the higher concentration and place this answer in the lower right-hand corner box: 10. This is the number of parts of the ingredient with the lower concentration.
   f. Subtract the lower concentration from the desired concentration and place this answer in the upper right-hand corner box: 30. This is the number of parts of the ingredient with the higher concentration.
   Note: Always subtract diagonally and read the resulting parts across (i.e., horizontally).

g. Add the two numbers from the right-hand corners: 10 + 30 = 40. This is the total number of parts for the preparation.

h. Use these numbers to set up the proportions for the quantities in your preparation.

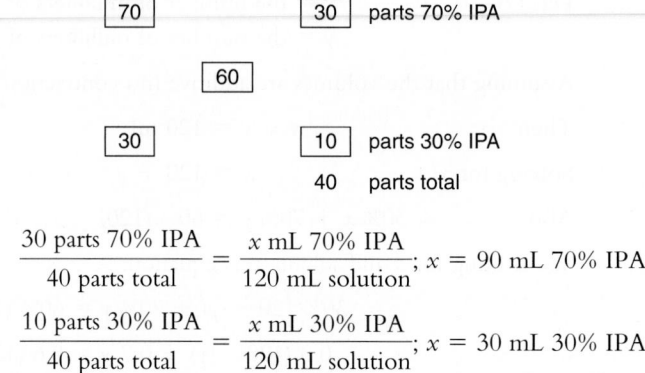

$$\frac{30 \text{ parts } 70\% \text{ IPA}}{40 \text{ parts total}} = \frac{x \text{ mL } 70\% \text{ IPA}}{120 \text{ mL solution}}; x = 90 \text{ mL } 70\% \text{ IPA}$$

$$\frac{10 \text{ parts } 30\% \text{ IPA}}{40 \text{ parts total}} = \frac{x \text{ mL } 30\% \text{ IPA}}{120 \text{ mL solution}}; x = 30 \text{ mL } 30\% \text{ IPA}$$

Measure 90 mL of 70% Isopropyl Alcohol and 30 mL of 30% Isopropyl Alcohol; combine these solutions to give 120 mL of a 60% IPA solution.

3. When using the alligation system, all concentrations entered in the boxes of the square must be expressed in a common system: That is, all must be in percents, all in milligrams per milliliter, or whatever system is most convenient for your data.

D. Sample problems

As indicated at the beginning of this section, we will conclude this discussion by presenting some typical pharmacy-related problems and showing solutions to these problems based on the various calculation methods and techniques. This discussion will start with the most basic problems and progress to more complex but typical situations.

1. Probably the simplest quantity and concentration problem is diluting pure active ingredient with pure vehicle. The example shown here is similar to example 8.17 but, in the example given here, we are dealing with liquids instead of solids and semisolids. For comparison, three calculation methods are shown for this problem.

Example 8.20

You want to make 120 mL of a 70% solution of Isopropyl Alcohol (IPA). You have available pure (100%) IPA and Purified Water USP. How many milliliters of each will you need?

By percent:

$$Rate \times Whole = Part$$

$$70\% \times 120 \text{ mL} = 0.7 \times 120 \text{ mL} = 84 \text{ mL IPA}$$

Measure 84 mL of IPA and add sufficient Purified Water to give 120 mL of solution.

By proportion:

By definition, a 70% v/v solution of IPA means 70 mL of IPA/100 mL solution. Therefore,

$$\frac{70 \text{ mL IPA}}{100 \text{ mL solution}} = \frac{x \text{ mL IPA}}{120 \text{ mL solution}}; x = 84 \text{ mL IPA}$$

Measure 84 mL of IPA and add sufficient Purified Water to give 120 mL of solution.

By dimensional analysis:

Again, by definition a 70% v/v solution of IPA means 70 mL of IPA/100 mL solution. Therefore,

$$\left(\frac{70 \text{ mL IPA}}{100 \text{ mL solution}} \right) \left(\frac{120 \text{ mL solution}}{} \right) = 84 \text{ mL IPA needed}$$

Measure 84 mL of IPA and add sufficient Purified Water to give 120 mL of solution.

---

2. Examples 8.21 and 8.22 present a slightly more complex situation because the source of the active ingredient is not pure drug or chemical.

Example 8.21

This time you want to make a 50% v/v IPA solution, but you have available only 70% IPA and Purified Water (that is, you have no pure IPA). How many milliliters of each do you need?

By alligation:

| 70 | | 50 | parts of 70% IPA |

| | 50 | | |

| 0 | | 20 | parts of Purified Water |

| | | 70 | parts total |

Using the parts information determined in the alligation square, calculate the volume of the 70% IPA needed to give the desired final solution. For example, by proportion:

$$\frac{50 \text{ parts } 70\% \text{ IPA}}{70 \text{ parts total}} = \frac{x \text{ mL } 70\% \text{ IPA}}{120 \text{ mL solution}}; x = 86 \text{ mL } 70\% \text{ IPA}$$

Measure 86 mL of 70% IPA and add sufficient Purified Water to give 120 mL of solution.

This problem can be solved in one step using dimensional analysis.

By dimensional analysis:

$$\left(\frac{100 \text{ mL } 70\% \text{ IPA}}{70 \text{ mL IPA}}\right)\left(\frac{50 \text{ mL IPA}}{100 \text{ mL soln}}\right)\left(\frac{120 \text{ mL soln}}{}\right) = 86 \text{ mL } 70\% \text{ IPA}$$

Measure 86 mL of 70% IPA and add sufficient Purified Water to give 120 mL of solution.

Example 8.22

You have a prescription order for this sterile ophthalmic solution: 6 mL of a 0.2% solution of tobramycin. You have available a 0.3% tobramycin ophthalmic solution (TOS) and sterile saline. How much of each do you need?

First, calculate the amount of drug needed in the final solution.

By percent:

$$Rate \times Whole = Part$$

$$0.2\% \times 6 \text{ mL} = 0.012 \text{ g}$$

Next calculate the volume of the available solution that gives you this amount.

By proportion:

$$\frac{0.3 \text{ g tobramycin}}{100 \text{ mL TOS}} = \frac{0.012 \text{ g tobramycin}}{x \text{ mL TOS}}; x = 4 \text{ mL TOS}$$

Measure 4 mL of the 0.3% tobramycin ophthalmic solution and qs ad 6 mL with the sterile saline solution.

Again, this problem can be solved in one step using dimensional analysis.

By dimensional analysis:

$$\left(\frac{100 \text{ mL TOS}}{0.3 \text{ g tobramycin}}\right)\left(\frac{0.2 \text{ g tobramycin}}{100 \text{ mL Rx soln}}\right)\left(\frac{6 \text{ ml Rx soln}}{}\right) = 4 \text{ mL TOS}$$

---

3. The next level of difficulty involves using two sources for the active ingredient, each source having a different concentration. This is similar to example 8.19 in which either alligation or algebra must be used. This problem occurs in practice situations, so it is important that you know how to solve a problem of this sort. The problem given here is a typical one of making a fortified ophthalmic solution by combining a commercial lower-concentration ophthalmic solution and a sterile injectable solution that has a higher concentration. For an additional discussion of this problem, see the CD that accompanies this book.

Example 8.23

You have received a medication order for 6 mL of a fortified tobramycin ophthalmic solution 1.5%. You have available the commercial products tobramycin ophthalmic solution 0.3% and tobramycin sterile injection 80 mg/2 mL. How many milliliters of each do you need to make the fortified solution?

Before using either algebra or alligation to solve this problem, remember that the concentrations of both ingredient solutions must be expressed in consistent dimensional units. In this example, it is decided to express all of the concentrations as percents by converting 80 mg/2 mL to its equivalent percent (that is, the number of grams of tobramycin per 100 mL):

$$\left(\frac{1 \text{ g}}{1{,}000 \text{ mg}}\right)\left(\frac{80 \text{ mg tobramycin}}{2 \text{ mL injection}}\right)\left(\frac{100 \text{ mL injection}}{}\right) = 4 \text{ g tobramycin in } 100 \text{ mL} = 4\%$$

By algebra:

Let: x = the number of milliliters of 0.3% solution needed

           y = the number of milliliters of 4% (the 80 mg/2 mL injection) solution needed

Assume that the volumes are additive.

Then: $x + y = 6 \text{ mL}$

Solving for x: $x = 6 - y$

Also: $0.3\% \, x + 4\% \, y = 1.5\% \, (6)$

Substituting for x and solving this equation:

$$0.3\% \, (6 - y) + 4\% \, y = 1.5\% \, (6)$$

$$0.003 \, (6 - y) + 0.04 \, y = 0.015 \, (6)$$

$$0.018 - 0.003 \, y + 0.04 \, y = 0.09$$

$$0.037 \, y = 0.072$$

$$y = 1.95 \text{ mL or } 2 \text{ mL}$$

$$x = 6 - y = 6 - 2 = 4 \text{ mL}$$

Measure 2 mL of the tobramycin injection in a syringe and transfer it to the ophthalmic solution bottle that contains 4 mL of the 0.3% solution.

By alligation:

| 4 | | 1.2 | parts of the injection |

| | 1.5 | |

| 0.3 | | 2.5 | parts of the 0.3% ophthalmic solution |

                                        3.7   parts total

Using the parts information determined in the alligation square, calculate the volume of the injection needed to give the desired final solution. For example, by proportion:

$$\frac{1.2 \text{ parts injection}}{3.7 \text{ parts total}} = \frac{x \text{ mL injection}}{6 \text{ mL final solution}}; x = 1.95 \text{ or } 2 \text{ mL injection}$$

Measure 2 mL of the injection using a syringe and transfer it to the ophthalmic solution bottle that contains 4 mL of the 0.3% solution.

4. The final problem type involves the calculation of the final concentrations of active ingredients when combining two separate products into a single preparation. This is one of the most basic and common of compounding situations; it happens each time you get a prescription order to combine two ointments or creams into a single combination preparation. It is also a very common occurrence in sterile compounding of parenteral products; for

example, in mixing two or more injection solutions in one syringe when making a preoperative sedative. This problem always involves three steps:

a. Calculate the quantity of active ingredient in the designated volume of each product.

b. Calculate the final volume of the combined preparation.

c. Calculate the concentration of each active ingredient based on the answers to steps a and b.

Example 8.24

You have an intramuscular injectable solution of edetate 200 mg/mL. You put 10 mL of it in an empty sterile vial and dilute it with 3.3 mL of procaine HCl 2% injection. What is the final concentration of the edetate in milligrams per milliliter? What is the final concentration of the procaine HCl in percent?

Edetate:

1. 200 mg/mL × 10 mL = 2,000 mg

2. 10 mL + 3.3 mL = 13.3 mL

3. 2,000 mg/13.3 mL = 150 mg/mL

Procaine HCl:

1. 2% = 2 g/100 mL   2 g/100 mL × 3.3 mL = 0.066 g

2. 10 mL + 3.3 mL = 13.3 mL

3. 0.066 g/13.3 mL = 0.005 g/mL

4. Expressing this concentration as a percent:

$$0.005 \text{ g/mL} \times 100 \text{ mL} = 0.5 \text{ g in } 100 \text{ mL} = 0.5\%$$

V. SPECIAL CALCULATIONS INVOLVING ALCOHOL USP

A. General information and conventions concerning alcohol

1. Although the word *alcohol* is a general term for organic compounds of the form R–OH, by convention, the term *alcohol*, when used without modifiers, means a solution of 95% ethanol in water. This is the result of both historical use and practicality. Alcohol has been made for centuries by fermentation, mostly for use as a beverage. It can be purified by distillation, the product of that process being the azeotropic mixture of 95% ethanol in water. This process cannot further purify it, so this is the form of alcohol that is generally available for industrial and pharmaceutical purposes. Because of its easy availability and modest cost, its chemical and physical properties, and its relative safety, alcohol has been for many years a common solvent and liquid vehicle for drugs. If you look up the solubility of a drug, it will usually state the drug's solubility in water and alcohol; the alcohol referred to here is the 95% ethanol solution. In some solubility references, alcohol is abbreviated simply "alc."

2. The General Notices of the *USP* contain the following statements about alcohol.

   a. "**Alcohol**—All statements of percentages of alcohol, such as under the heading *Alcohol content*, refer to percentage, by volume of C_2H_5OH at 15.56°. Where reference is made to "C_2H_5OH," the chemical entity possessing absolute (100%) strength is intended" (10).

   b. "*Alcohol*—Where 'alcohol' is called for in formulas, tests, and assays, the monograph article *Alcohol* is to be used" (10).

   c. "The content of alcohol in a liquid preparation shall be stated on the label as a percentage (v/v) of C_2H_5OH" (11).

3. The *USP* monograph for Alcohol USP states that it is 92.3% to 93.8% by weight and 94.9% to 96.0% by volume C_2H_5OH at 15.56° (2). The percent concentration for alcohol is generally taken to be 95% v/v of C_2H_5OH in water. Additional information on Alcohol USP and other *USP* alcohol articles is given in Chapter 15, Pharmaceutical Solvents and Solubilizing Agents.

4. In summary:

   a. When the word alcohol is written on a prescription order or in a formula, as for example, "alcohol 10 mL" or "dissolve in 5 mL of alcohol," the compounder should take the bottle of Alcohol USP (that is, 95% C_2H_5OH) off the shelf and use it. As an esteemed colleague says, when alcohol is written in milliliters, "Pour and go."

b. When the word alcohol is written with a percent, as for example, "alcohol 20%," this means 20% v/v of C_2H_5OH. If this percent is on the label of a commercial product, it means the product contains 20% v/v C_2H_5OH. If this is part of a compounding formula, it means the compounder must add the equivalent of 20% v/v C_2H_5OH. This will require some calculations, as illustrated in example 8.26.

c. Labels of products and compounded preparations are to include the content of C_2H_5OH in v/v%. For compounded preparations, this value must often be calculated based on the volume(s) of alcohol-containing ingredients added, as illustrated in examples 8.25 and 8.27.

B. Although the *USP* standards are fairly straightforward, their application can be confusing in practical situations. The examples that follow are intended to aid you in understanding how to apply the *USP* specifications when preparing compounded drug preparations. In each case, the first step is to determine the quantity (in milliliters) of alcohol needed or added, and the second step is to determine the v/v% of C_2H_5OH in the final preparation so it can be properly labeled.

Example 8.25

℞
Castor Oil	40 mL
Acacia	qs
Alcohol	15 mL
Cherry Syrup	20 mL
Purified Water qs ad	100 mL

1. Determine the quantity of alcohol needed and added:

Because the monograph article Alcohol USP is to be used when alcohol is called for in formulas, simply measure 15 mL of Alcohol USP—pour and go.

2. Determine the v/v% alcohol content for labeling:

Because alcohol is to be labeled by v/v% of C_2H_5OH, the percent concentration of C_2H_5OH in this product must be calculated. First, calculate the number of milliliters of C_2H_5OH added based on the percent and volume of the source of alcohol:

$$95\% \times 15 \text{ mL Alcohol USP} = 0.95 \times 15 \text{ mL} = 14.25 \text{ mL of } C_2H_5OH$$

Second, calculate the v/v% content of C_2H_5OH in the final preparation:

$$\frac{14.25 \text{ mL } C_2H_5OH}{100 \text{ mL preparation}} = 14.25\%$$

Example 8.26

℞
Clindamycin	1%
Alcohol	15%
Propylene glycol	5%
Purified Water qs ad	60 mL

1. Determine the quantity of alcohol needed and added:

In this prescription order, the alcohol 15% means 15% v/v of C_2H_5OH. For 60 mL of preparation, we must first calculate the quantity of C_2H_5OH needed:

$$15\% \times 60 \text{ mL} = 0.15 \times 60 \text{ mL} = 9 \text{ mL } C_2H_5OH$$

Because the normal source of C_2H_5OH is Alcohol USP, calculate the number of milliliters of Alcohol USP needed to give 9 mL of C_2H_5OH:

$$\frac{95 \text{ mL } C_2H_5OH}{100 \text{ mL Alcohol USP}} = \frac{9 \text{ mL } C_2H_5OH}{x \text{ mL Alcohol USP}}; x = 9.5 \text{ Alcohol USP}$$

Therefore, we will add 9.5 mL of Alcohol USP for this product.

2. Determine the v/v% alcohol content for labeling:

Because all labeling of alcohol is v/v% of C_2H_5OH, the alcohol content of this product would be labeled: Alcohol 15%.

Example 8.27   ℞   Guaifenesin   2.4 g

Tussend Liquid   90 mL

Cherry Syrup   qs ad   120 mL

1. Determine the amount of Alcohol needed and added:

Guaifenesin has limited solubility in water but is freely soluble in alcohol (1 g/1–10 mL). The pharmacist wants this preparation to be a solution and determines the quantity of Alcohol USP required to dissolve the 2.4 g of guaifenesin and keep it in solution★: 12 mL Alcohol USP.

2. Determine the v/v% alcohol content for labeling:

First, determine the total C_2H_5OH content of the formulation:

The content in the 12 mL of Alcohol USP:

$$95\% \times 12 \text{ mL Alcohol USP} = 0.95 \times 12 \text{ mL} = 11.4 \text{ mL}$$

The labeled alcohol content of Tussend Liquid is 5%. Therefore,

$$5\% \times 90 \text{ mL Tussend} = 0.05 \times 90 \text{ mL} = 4.5 \text{ mL}$$

The cherry syrup used is the soda fountain type and contains no alcohol.

The total quantity of C_2H_5OH in the preparation:

$$11.4 \text{ mL} + 4.5 \text{ mL} = 15.9 \text{ mL}$$

Next calculate the v/v% content of C_2H_5OH in the final formulation:

$$\frac{15.9 \text{ mL C}_2\text{H}_5\text{OH}}{120 \text{ mL preparation}} = \frac{x \text{ mL C}_2\text{H}_5\text{OH}}{100 \text{ mL preparation}}; x = 13.25 \text{ mL} = 13.25\%$$

★For a detailed discussion of solvent effects, see Chapter 37 and sample prescription 27.5 in Chapter 27. Also see the CD that accompanies this book for an additional problem involving alcohol calculations when using alcohol for its solvent effect.

VI.   SPECIAL CALCULATIONS INVOLVING CONCENTRATED ACIDS

A. Recall from the section of this chapter on percent that *USP* conventions for expressing percent concentrations of mixtures are: % w/w for solids in solids, % w/v for solids in liquids, % v/v for liquids in liquids, and % w/v for gases in liquids. Concentrated acids are unique in that often they do not follow these conventions.

   1. Irrespective of the physical state (solid, liquid, or gas) of the pure chemical, the concentrations of concentrated acid solutions (all of which are liquids) have traditionally been expressed as % w/w (Hydrochloric Acid NF is 36.5% to 38.0% by weight of the gas HCl in water; Phosphoric Acid NF is 85.0% to 88.0% by weight of H_3PO_4; Sulfuric Acid NF is 95.0% to 98.0% by weight of H_2SO_4; Glacial Acetic Acid USP is 99.9% to 100.5% by weight of $C_2H_4O_2$) (2,12).

   2. Although diluted solutions of concentrated acids are mixtures of liquids in liquids, their concentrations, as given in official monographs, are not expressed as % v/v of the concentrated acid solution in water but, depending on the concentration, are given either as % w/v or % w/w of the pure acid in water. For example, Diluted Hydrochloric Acid NF is 10% w/v of HCl in water, and Diluted Phosphoric Acid NF is 10% w/v of H_3PO_4, but Acetic Acid NF is 37% w/w of $C_2H_4O_2$ in water (12).

B. To get a better idea of the complexity and diversity of concentration expressions for concentrated acids, consider the following acetic acid descriptions and preparations. Keep in mind that the situation with most concentrated acids is made more difficult by the fact that the common name for the chemical has sometimes been used as the official name or title for a USP article, which may contain less than 100% of the pure chemical. THIS IS VERY IMPORTANT. There have been several serious and even some fatal medication errors due to incorrect prescribing or interpretation of drug orders for concentrated acids.

   1. Acetic acid is the common name for the simple organic acid with the molecular formula $C_2H_4O_2$ (sometimes written CH_3COOH).

   2. Glacial acetic acid is both the official *USP* title and the common or trivial name for acetic acid ($C_2H_4O_2$) when in pure form. It is a viscous liquid at normal room temperature and has a

density of 1.053. It got the name glacial acetic acid because it freezes at cool room temperature (16.7°C) to form a crystalline structure that resembles ice. The *USP* monograph for Glacial Acetic Acid follows the convention for concentrated acids by expressing its concentration as 99.5% to 100.5% w/w of $C_2H_4O_2$ (2).

3. Acetic Acid NF is an aqueous solution of acetic acid. This is a classic example of the same name, acetic acid, being applied to a chemical and an official solution of the chemical. The NF monograph gives its concentration as 36.0% to 37.0%, by weight of $C_2H_4O_2$ (12).

4. Diluted Acetic Acid NF is an aqueous solution made by measuring 15.8 mL of Acetic Acid NF and adding sufficient Purified Water to give 100 mL of solution. Its monograph states that its concentration is 5.7 to 6.3 g of $C_2H_4O_2$ per 100 mL of solution, or 6% w/v (12).

5. Acetic Acid Irrigation USP has its monograph concentration specified as 237.5 to 262.5 mg $C_2H_4O_2$/100 mL of solution (2). Unfortunately, but understandably, acetic acid irrigations are often prescribed by percent (the commercial product is labeled 0.25%). There have been reports of subpotent compounded preparations when the compounder used the General Notices conventions for a mixture of a liquid in a liquid and made the preparation 0.25% v/v of Acetic Acid NF in water, which gave a final concentration of 95 mg $C_2H_4O_2$/100 mL instead of the intended 250 mg/100 mL.

6. Acetic Acid Otic Solution USP contains glacial acetic acid in a nonaqueous solvent. Here the monograph just gives a range of 85% to 130% of label claim (2). Commercial products are dilute solutions (usually 2%) of acetic acid in either glycerin or propylene glycol. One might assume the percent concentration to be v/v with respect to Glacial Acetic Acid in the solvent, but it could also be w/v of the pure chemical in the chosen solvent or even w/w. This brings up the question: How should a prescription order for a similar compounded preparation be interpreted?

7. The *British Pharmacopeia* and several other pharmacopeias have similar products, but the percent strengths vary [e.g., Acetic Acid (6%) BP and Acetic Acid (33%) BP].

8. Acetic Acid 2% in Spirit Drops. The twenty-ninth edition of *Martindale The Extra Pharmacopeia* listed this product from The Royal National Throat, Nose, and Ear Hospital, London, England. From the preceding examples, one might expect this product to contain 2% w/w or 2% w/v of $C_2H_4O_2$. Neither is true. This product was formulated following the *USP* General Notices convention for a mixture of a liquid in a liquid. Its formula is given as Acetic Acid (33%) 2 mL, industrial methylated spirit 50 mL, water to 100 mL (13). This product is 2% v/v with respect to Acetic Acid (33%) BP. It is only 0.66% w/v with respect to the chemical acetic acid ($C_2H_4O_2$). Fortunately, the thirtieth and later editions of *Martindale* have recognized and addressed this problem. *Martindale* states, "The nomenclature of acetic acid often leads to confusion as to whether concentrations are expressed as percentages of glacial acetic acid ($C_2H_4O_2$) or of this diluted form. In *Martindale,* the percentage figures given against acetic acid represent the amount of $C_2H_4O_2$" (14).

C. With all these conflicting examples in mind, consider the following simple prescription order.

Example 8.28

℞   Hydrochloric Acid 10%

    Purified Water   qs ad   100 mL

How should this prescription be compounded?

Possibility #1

Make this solution 10% v/v of Hydrochloric Acid NF in water. This follows the convention in the General Notices for a mixture of a liquid in a liquid.

$$10\% \times 100 \text{ mL} = 10 \text{ mL of Hydrochloric Acid NF}$$

Procedure: Measure **10 mL** of Hydrochloric Acid NF and qs ad 100 mL with water. (Remember, of course, that we add acid to water, so add the concentrated acid to some of the water first before final qs'ing with water.)

Possibility #2

Make this solution 10% w/v with respect to the chemical HCl in water. This follows one of the conventions for dilute solutions of concentrated acids (see Diluted Hydrochloric Acid NF).

$$10\% \times 100 \text{ mL} = 10 \text{ g of HCl}$$

How would you measure this? Given that Hydrochloric Acid NF is 37.3% by weight or 37.3 g HCl/100 g of Hydrochloric Acid NF. How many grams of Hydrochloric Acid NF solution will you need for 10 g of pure HCL?

$$\frac{37.3 \text{ g HCl}}{100 \text{ g HCl NF}} = \frac{10 \text{ g HCl}}{x \text{ g HCl NF}}; x = 26.8 \text{ g HCl NF}$$

You could weigh 26.8 g of Hydrochloric Acid NF solution by taring out the weight of a beaker and pouring the NF acid solution into the beaker to a weight of 26.8 g. An easier method is to convert this weight to a volume. Conversions such as this are done using the density or specific gravity of the liquid. Hydrochloric Acid NF has a specific gravity of 1.18.

$$\frac{1.18 \text{ g HCl NF}}{1 \text{ mL HCl NF}} = \frac{26.8 \text{ g HCl NF}}{x \text{ mL HCl NF}}; x = 22.7 \text{ mL HCl NF}$$

These last two calculations also can be done in one process using dimensional analysis:

$$\left(\frac{1 \text{ mL HCl NF}}{1.18 \text{ g HCl NF}}\right)\left(\frac{100 \text{ g HCl NF}}{37.3 \text{ g HCl}}\right)\left(\frac{10 \text{ g HCl}}{}\right) = 22.7 \text{ mL HCl NF}$$

Procedure: Measure **22.7 mL** of Hydrochloric Acid NF and qs to 100 mL with water.

Possibility #3

Make this solution 10% w/w with respect to the chemical HCl in water. This follows another of the conventions for diluted solutions of concentrated acids (see Acetic Acid NF). This calculation is slightly more complex and requires the density or specific gravity of a 10% w/w solution of HCl in water. (Information such as this can sometimes be found in *The Merck Index* or *International Critical Tables*. In this case, *The Merck Index* gives the density of a 10% w/w HCl solution as 1.05 g/mL.)

First, calculate the weight of the desired 100 mL of 10% HCl solution:

$$\frac{1.05 \text{ g 10\% HCl solution}}{\text{mL 10\% HCl solution}} = \frac{x \text{ g 10\% HCl solution}}{100 \text{ mL 10\% HCl solution}}; x = 105 \text{ g 10\% HCl solution}$$

Next calculate the number of grams of HCl needed for 105 g of a 10% w/w solution:

$$\frac{10 \text{ g HCl}}{100 \text{ g 10\% solution}} = \frac{x \text{ g HCl}}{105 \text{ g 10\% solution}}; x = 10.5 \text{ g HCl}$$

Calculate the number of milliliters of Hydrochloric Acid NF that will be needed for this 10.5 g of HCl. For ease, use dimensional analysis.

$$\left(\frac{1 \text{ mL HCl NF}}{1.18 \text{ g HCl NF}}\right)\left(\frac{100 \text{ g MCl NF}}{37.3 \text{ g HCl}}\right)\left(\frac{10.5 \text{ g HCl}}{}\right) = 23.9 \text{ mL HCl NF}$$

Procedure: Measure **23.9 mL** of Hydrochloric Acid NF and qs to 100 mL with water.

As you can see, there are considerable differences in the amounts of Hydrochloric Acid NF (10 mL, 22.7 mL, 23.9 mL) depending on the interpretation, and all three methods follow accepted conventions for percents.

D. You easily can think of more complex scenarios. For example, what happens when you have a mixture of a concentrated acid in a semisolid? Consider the common example of a prescription order that calls for Lactic Acid 5% in a semisolid formulation (e.g., an ointment or cream). What does this mean? (Bear in mind that Lactic Acid USP is 87% by weight and has a specific gravity of 1.2.) For 100 g of product, would you use: 5 g of the liquid Lactic Acid USP (a % w/w interpretation with respect to Lactic Acid USP); 5 g of the chemical entity lactic acid (% w/w with respect to $C_3H_6O_3$); 5 mL of the liquid Lactic Acid USP [% v/w (is there such a thing?) with respect to Lactic Acid USP]? When you read the label of a manufactured ointment or cream containing 5% lactic acid, how is this to be interpreted?

E. It is readily apparent that there can be considerable differences in the potencies of preparations made with concentrated acids, all with the same numeric percent and each made following accepted conventions. For drug orders that are specific and unambiguous, the pharmacist need only evaluate the order for appropriateness of strength for the intended purpose. If the drug order is like the hydrochloric acid case illustrated in example 8.28 the pharmacist must consult with the prescriber. If the prescriber received the formula from a colleague or found it in a reference book or journal article, and the nonspecific percent is all that was given, more research is required to determine the safe and effective concentration for the intended purpose. As was indicated at the beginning of this discussion, this is not just of academic importance; a number of serious and harmful medication errors have been made owing to incorrect prescribing or interpretation of drug orders for concentrated acids. Unless you are certain, always check to be sure a concentration and interpretation are correct and appropriate.

VII.   SPECIAL CALCULATIONS INVOLVING FORMALDEHYDE SOLUTIONS

A. Another exception to the General Notices rules is Formaldehyde Solution USP. It is a solution of a gas in a liquid and, by the general convention as stated in the General Notices, it should have its concentration expressed as % w/v; instead, its monograph gives its concentration as % w/w (2).

B. Formaldehyde Solution USP, also known by the common name of formalin, contains not less than 36.5% or 37% (depending on container size) by weight of formaldehyde (CH_2O), with methanol present to prevent polymerization (2). *The Merck Index* states: "This soln is the full strength and also known as Formalin 100% or Formalin 40 which signifies that it contains 40 grams of formaldehyde within 100 mL of the soln" (15).

C. If one should get a prescription order requesting a given percent of formaldehyde, how is this to be interpreted?

1. If the order calls for Formaldehyde Solution 37% or Formalin 40%, it would seem logical, because of the coincidental numbers, to conclude that the prescriber really wants the full strength Formaldehyde Solution. Obviously, it is always best to check.

2. What if the order calls for Formaldehyde 10% Solution, Dispense 100 mL?

   a. One convention is the use of the word **formalin** or **formaldehyde solution** to indicate the USP solution and the term **formaldehyde** to indicate the compound CH_2O (16). With this in mind, this prescription order asking for formaldehyde 10% would require 10 g of formaldehyde (CH_2O) or 25 mL of Formaldehyde Solution (containing 40% w/v of formaldehyde) to make 100 mL of preparation.

   b. *Martindale—The Extra Pharmacopoeia* gives a different interpretation and is very clear in its explanation of the accepted interpretation for the United Kingdom. It states:

   > Formaldehyde solution is sometimes known as formalin or just formaldehyde and this has led to confusion in interpreting the strength and the form in which formaldehyde is being used. In practice formaldehyde is available as formaldehyde solution which is diluted before use, the percentage strength being expressed in terms of formaldehyde solution rather than formaldehyde (CH_2O). For example in the UK formaldehyde solution 3% consists of 3 volumes of Formaldehyde Solution (B.P.) diluted to 100 volumes with water and thus contains 1.02 to 1.14% w/w of formaldehyde (CH_2O); it is not prepared by diluting Formaldehyde Solution (*B.P.*) to arrive at a solution containing 3% w/w of formaldehyde (CH_2O). (17)

   Unfortunately, no similar statement of official interpretation for the United States is given in the *USP–NF*.

3. Although this discussion creates many questions but no satisfactory answers, it should serve to alert you to the problem and gives some possible interpretations.

VIII.   CALCULATIONS INVOLVING SALTS AND COMPOUNDS CONTAINING WATER OF HYDRATION

A. Drugs and chemicals that contain water of hydration
   When a solid drug or chemical is available in both anhydrous form and as one or more hydrates, there may be ambiguity when expressing concentrations and when calculating quantities to weigh or measure. Examples are given here for one such drug, magnesium sulfate, but the same considerations apply to any drug or chemical that is available in both anhydrous and hydrated form.

   1. The *USP* monograph Magnesium Sulfate Injection states that it "contains magnesium sulfate equivalent to not less than 93.0 percent and not more than 107.0 percent of the labeled amount of $MgSO_4 \cdot 7H_2O$" (2). In other words, when you have magnesium sulfate injection labeled 50%, it is not 50% with respect to the magnesium sulfate ($MgSO_4$), but rather 50% with respect to magnesium sulfate heptahydrate. At one time, there was some logic to labeling the injection in this manner because magnesium sulfate heptahydrate was how magnesium sulfate was available, and the *USP* monograph for magnesium sulfate recognized only this form. This is no longer true; magnesium sulfate is now readily available in both anhydrous and hydrated forms, and the *USP* monograph for magnesium sulfate now lists anhydrous, monohydrate, and heptahydrate forms. However, to make changes now in how doses and quantities and concentrations of injectable magnesium sulfate are expressed could cause confusion and could lead to wrong doses being given. Currently, parenteral doses of magnesium sulfate are given either as

metric (i.e., grams and milligrams) weight of magnesium sulfate heptahydrate or as milliequivalents of magnesium ion. Fortunately, many manufacturers of parenteral products now include both units in their labeling. For example, a premix intravenous bag of magnesium sulfate is labeled Magnesium Sulfate in Water for Injection, 40 mg/mL (0.325 mEq Mg^{++}/mL) 2 g total; Each 50 mL contains magnesium sulfate heptahydrate 2 g (equivalent to 0.325 mEq magnesium) in water for injection.

2. Now consider another example, this one for a nonparenteral dosage form. (Magnesium sulfate aqueous solutions are used orally as saline laxatives and topically as soaking solutions.)

| **Example 8.29** | R_x | Magnesium Sulfate | 25% |
| | | Purified Water | qs ad | 100 mL |

How should this prescription be interpreted?

Because of the large differences in the molecular weights of the anhydrous (120 g) versus the heptahydrate (246 g), there would be a great difference in the final concentration of magnesium sulfate in the preparation, depending on the form used. For this example, assume that the pharmacist has determined that the intent of the order is for magnesium sulfate heptahydrate. (This makes sense because the traditional form of the salt is magnesium sulfate heptahydrate, also known as Epsom salts.) If the pharmacy stocks the heptahydrate form of the chemical, the pharmacist or pharmacy technician just weighs the 25 g needed. If, however, the pharmacy only has the anhydrous form, the amount of anhydrous powder that will give an equivalent quantity of magnesium sulfate must be calculated:

$$\left(\frac{120 \text{ g MgSO}_4 \text{ anhy.}}{246 \text{ g MgSO}_4 \cdot 7\text{H}_2\text{O}} \right) \left(\frac{25 \text{ g MgSO}_4 \cdot 7\text{H}_2\text{O}}{} \right) = 12.195 \text{ g MgSO}_4 \text{ anhy.}$$

B. Salt, complex, and ester forms of drugs

1. Many drugs are available in both the free form of the drug (the active moiety) and as a salt, complex, or ester of the drug. These chemical modifications are made primarily to confer water solubility on poorly soluble organic drug molecules. When the counter ion, complex, or ester group contributes significantly to the weight of the molecule, the same problems can occur as with anhydrous and hydrate forms of a drug.

2. In some cases, the situation is even more complicated because the drug, the salt, the complex, or the ester may also contain various amounts of water of hydration. Two examples illustrate this problem:

   a. Theophylline is available as:

   theophylline, anhydrous   MW 180

   theophylline monohydrate   MW 198

   theophylline ethylenediamine 2:1(aminophylline)   MW 420

   theophylline ethylenediamine 2:1 dihydrate   MW 456

   Obviously, problems could occur with dosing and measuring this drug. In this case, the drug also has a narrow therapeutic window so that incorrectly determined amounts of this drug could have serious consequences. Fortunately, drug information references and package labeling carefully specify which dose belongs to which form of the drug, but the pharmacist must be careful in dealing with this drug.

   b. Morphine is another classic example. The official *USP* form of morphine is the sulfate salt, Morphine Sulfate (2). Although both the anhydrous and pentahydrate forms of the drug are listed in the monograph, it states that the drug content is calculated on the basis of the anhydrous salt. However, all three of the official morphine dosage forms (Morphine Sulfate Injection, Morphine Sulfate Extended-Release Capsules, and Morphine Sulfate Suppositories) have their labeled amount based on morphine sulfate pentahydrate (2). Morphine is also available as the free base, the base monohydrate, the hydrochloride salt, and several other forms (see *The Merck Index*). In contrast to theophylline, in the case of morphine, drug information references are not specific with respect to dose in terms of base/salt/hydrate form of the drug.

C. Interpretation of name/strength nomenclature for base/salt/complex/hydrate drug forms

1. The fact that there are various drug forms of the same drug might be purely academic if it were not that the multiple forms together with ambiguous drug product labeling and drug order

writing and misinterpretation can lead to medication errors. Obviously, the potential for errors with serious consequences is greatest with medications that have narrow therapeutic indices (such as the theophylline example given previously) and drugs administered parenterally. While these drugs and routes of administration require extra vigilance, all drug therapy deserves careful evaluation and interpretation. In dealing with this issue, it is important to recognize where potential problems exist with regard to proper and intended dosing of drugs based on their base/salt/complex/hydrate form.

    a. Part of the problem is the result of lack of knowledge about the various forms and the proper way to write clear and specific drug orders and labels. In example 8.29, the difficulty is not in being able to perform the rather simple base-hydrate conversion calculation but rather in (i) having a prescription order that is not sufficiently specific and (ii) not knowing that there are several forms of the drug. If the drug order in that example had been written specifically for magnesium sulfate heptahydrate, there would be no question of interpretation. Fortunately, in that example, while the drug order was not written specifically, the pharmacist knew about the various forms of magnesium sulfate and was able to ascertain the desired interpretation.

    b. A second part of the problem lies with inconsistent nomenclature with regard to drug names, strengths, and dosage. This problem has been recognized recently because of improved gathering and analysis of drug error information; organizations and agencies, particularly FDA and USP, have focused on finding a remedy for this problem. In 2005, at the USP Quinquennial meeting, one of the resolutions concerned improved standards for nomenclature and labeling (18). As a follow-up to this resolution, the USP Nomenclature Expert Committee addressed this issue with a major revision to *USP* Chapter, ⟨1121⟩ Nomenclature; the new revision was first published in *USP 31*. It is hoped that this new policy will simplify and clarify things, because content labeling formats are currently complex and inconsistent.

  2. *USP* Chapter ⟨1121⟩ Nomenclature

    a. The former *USP* nomenclature policy, known as the Salt Nomenclature Policy, held that for a drug product that employs a salt form, the monograph name or title will include the salt in that monograph title (19). The drug product strength, as given in the monograph, was sometimes (but not always) in terms of the salt form. *USP* has not always been consistent in administering this policy. For example, the drug product for Fluoxetine Capsules USP employs the hydrochloride salt, but the word *Hydrochloride* is not in the monograph title; and the labeled strength in the monograph is in terms of the base (the active moiety). On the other hand, the monograph title Erythromycin Stearate Tablets USP includes the ester name in the monograph title but, as with fluoxetine, the labeled strength in the monograph is in terms of the active moiety erythromycin.

    b. The new USP nomenclature policy states that both the names and strengths of drug products and compounded preparations formulated as salts will be stated in terms of the active moiety (20).

    c. New *USP* Chapter ⟨1121⟩ gives a rather complete definition of active moiety. In essence, an active moiety is the molecule or ion, without any appended salt, complex, chelate, hydrate, and the like, that gives the intended pharmacologic or physiologic action (20).

    d. As with all significant changes of this sort, USP will give all impacted stakeholders (in this case, practitioners, pharmacists, and the pharmaceutical industry) sufficient time to understand and comply with the new standards. Therefore, this new policy will not be official until May 1, 2013 (19,20).

    e. Furthermore, the policy will apply only to newly recognized drug products and preparations; existing *USP* monographs will not change unless the change is needed for safety reasons (20).

  3. For the foreseeable future, until consistent nomenclature is uniformly employed, it will be important to understand and correctly interpret the various formats for names, strengths, and dosages of drug products that are currently in use. The most common formats with examples are given here.

    a. Name, strength, and dosage of the product may be given in terms of the active moiety.

    Example

    Baclofen: In the dosage instructions, the 5 to 10 mg means 5 to 10 mg of the active moiety; the tablets are labeled as baclofen 10 mg, meaning 10 mg of active moiety.

    b. Name, strength, and dosage of the product may be given in terms of the salt, ester, and such of drug.

Example

Diltiazem HCl: In the dosage instructions, 60 mg means 60 mg of the salt diltiazem HCl; the tablets are labeled as diltiazem HCl 60 mg, meaning 60 mg of diltiazem salt per tablet.

c. Dosage is given in terms of the active moiety, but the name and strength of the product use mixed terminology. If the active ingredient in the product is in the form of a salt, ester, or the like, this information will either be on the label and/or it will be described in the labeling (e.g., the prescribing information or product package insert).

Examples

Erythromycin base, estolate, and stearate: All have their doses of 250 to 500 mg, meaning the active moiety; the tablets, capsules, and suspension are labeled in those terms but may use different formats to express this [e.g., either "erythromycin 250 mg (as the stearate)" or "erythromycin stearate 250 mg (as base)," both meaning that each dosage unit contains 250 mg of the active moiety].

Ondansetron HCl: In the dosage instructions, 8 mg means 8 mg of the active moiety; the tablets are labeled ondansetron 8 mg (as HCl dihydrate) and prescribing information states: Each 8-mg ondansetron tablet for oral administration contains ondansetron HCl dihydrate equivalent to 8 mg ondansetron.

d. Occasionally, the product is labeled in terms of the salt or ester and the dosage instructions are in these terms, but the product information explains the equivalence to a given quantity of active moiety.

Example

Erythromycin ethyl succinate: The tablets are labeled erythromycin ethyl succinate 400 mg, and the dosage information gives the dose in terms of 400 to 800 mg of erythromycin ethyl succinate, but the product information states that 400 mg erythromycin ethyl succinate produces the same free erythromycin serum levels as 250 mg of erythromycin bases, stearate, or estolate.

4. Compounded preparations: When drug preparations are compounded, particular care must be exercised to match the dose desired with an equivalent quantity in the unit to be administered. For example, you can verify by calculation that, with respect to an equivalent amount of active moiety, there is a 20% difference between the metric weights of ondansetron and ondansetron HCl dihydrate; hence, desiring a dose in terms of one while weighing and adding in terms of the other will give a significant dosage error. Obviously, the larger the appended salt counter ion, complex, or hydrate when compared with size of the active moiety, the greater the potential dosage error when not taking this into consideration. When the dose is in terms of the active moiety and the desired or available form of the drug is a salt, complex, ester, and/or hydrate, an appropriate conversion must be calculated to determine the amount of the available entity to weigh or measure.

Example 8.30   The pharmacy at Comprehensive Care Hospital has an order for 100 mL of ondansetron oral suspension in a concentration of 4 mg/5 mL. As indicated in the previous example, ondansetron's strength is in terms of the base, the active moiety. Usually, the pharmacy buys this oral suspension from a manufacturer, but recently it has been informed that this product will not available for several weeks. As a result, the pharmacy will compound this preparation. The active ingredient is available as ondansetron HCl dihydrate powder. Calculate the quantity of ondansetron HCl dihydrate powder (Ond. HCl · 2H$_2$O) needed for this preparation. The MW of Ond. HCl · 2H$_2$O = 365.9; the MW of Ond. base = 293.4.

$$\left(\frac{365.9 \text{ mg Ond. HCl} \cdot 2\text{H}_2\text{O}}{293.4 \text{ mg Ond. base}} \right) \left(\frac{4 \text{ mg Ond. base}}{5 \text{ mL liquid}} \right) \left(\frac{100 \text{ mL liquid}}{} \right) = 100 \text{ mg Ond. HCl} \cdot 2\text{H}_2\text{O}$$

The preparation will be labeled: Each 5 mL of ondansetron suspension contains ondansetron 4 mg as ondansetron HCl (dihydrate).

---

5. Summary

If all practitioners and pharmacists were knowledgeable about these issues, and if drug information references were always specific in labeling drug names and strengths and in expressing doses, this issue would be handled more easily. Unfortunately, many practitioners and nurses, and even some pharmacists and pharmacy technicians, do not realize that this problem exists or are unaware of its complexity or possible ramifications. Fortunately, more drug information references and product labeling are now addressing the problem by giving names, strengths, doses, and concentrations in specific terms and, when appropriate, adding doses and concentrations in unambiguous terms such as millimoles of active moiety. This will all be greatly simplified if there is a uniform use of dosage form nomenclature as recommended by USP.

REFERENCES

1. The United States Pharmacopeial Convention, Inc. Summary of information submitted to MedMARx in the year 2002: The quest for quality. Rockville, MD: Author, 2003; 14.

2. The United States Pharmacopeial Convention, Inc. 2008 USP 31/NF 26. Official USP monographs. Rockville, MD: Author, 2007.

3. White KC, Harkavy KL. Hypertonic formulas resulting from added oral medications. Am J Dis Child 1982; 136: 931–933.

4. Ernst JA, Williams JM, Glick M, et al. Osmolality of substances used in the intensive care nursery. Pediatrics 1983; 72: 347–352.

5. Murty BSR, Kapoor JN, Deluca PO. Compliance with USP osmolarity labeling requirements. Am J Hosp Pharm 1976; 33: 546–551.

6. Trissel LA. Handbook of injectable drugs, 12th ed. Bethesda, MD: American Society of Health-System Pharmacists, 2003; 868.

7. The United States Pharmacopeial Convention, Inc. General Notices. 2008 USP 31/NF 26. Rockville, MD: Author, 2007; 13.

8. Ansel HC, Stoklosa MJ. Pharmaceutical calculations, 12th ed. Baltimore: Lippincott Williams & Wilkins, 2006; 87–88.

9. Ansel HC, Stoklosa MJ. Pharmaceutical calculations, 12th ed. Baltimore: Lippincott Williams & Wilkins, 2006; 248–249.

10. The United States Pharmacopeial Convention, Inc. General Notices. 2008 USP 31/NF 26. Rockville, MD: Author, 2007; 6.

11. The United States Pharmacopeial Convention, Inc. General Notices. 2008 USP 31/NF 26. Rockville, MD: Author, 2007; 11.

12. The United States Pharmacopeial Convention, Inc. 2008 USP 31/NF 26. Official NF monographs. Rockville, MD: Author, 2007.

13. Reynolds JEF, ed. Martindale—the extra pharmacopoeia, 28th ed. London: The Pharmaceutical Press, 1982; 784.

14. Parfitt K, ed. Martindale—the complete drug reference, 32nd ed. London: Pharmaceutical Press, 1999; 1329.

15. O'Neil MJ, ed. The Merck index, 14th ed. Whitehouse Station, NJ: Merck & Co., Inc., 2006; 4233.

16. Horn DW, Osol A. Fumigation with formaldehyde. Am J Pharm 1929; 101: 742.

17. Parfitt K, ed. Martindale—the complete drug reference, 32nd ed. London: Pharmaceutical Press, 1999; 1113.

18. Standards for nomenclature and labeling, http://www.usp.org/aboutUSP/resolutions.html. Accessed July 2007.

19. General chapter ⟨1121⟩ proposed revisions, http://www.usp.org/USPNF/pf/generalChapter1121.html. Accessed July 2007.

20. The United States Pharmacopeial Convention, Inc. Chapter ⟨1121⟩. 2008 USP 31/NF 26. Rockville, MD: Author, 2007; 605–607.

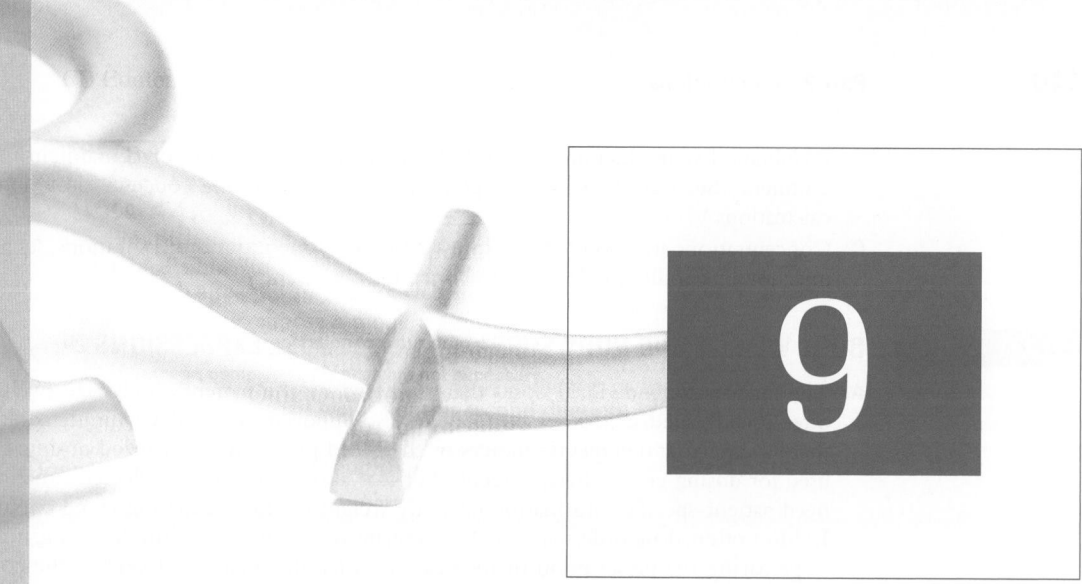

Evaluating Dosage Regimens

Introduction

Dose Formats Used in Drug Therapy

Body Weight and Body Surface Area in Dose Expressions

Dosage Regimens

Translating Dosage Regimens to Products and Directions for Use

Special Cases

I. INTRODUCTION

As stated in Chapter 8, an essential responsibility of the pharmacist is to ensure that each patient gets the correct amount of the intended drug. This function is the focus of this chapter on evaluating doses and dosage regimens. It builds on the subjects of systems and units of measurement, which were presented in Chapter 7, and on expressions of quantity and concentration, which were discussed in Chapter 8. This chapter examines the various accepted methods of expressing doses and dosage regimens and shows some sample dosing calculations. Special attention is given to patient populations and clinical statuses that require consideration of additional factors in establishing appropriate doses. In all instances of providing patients with drug products, whether they are manufactured dosage forms or preparations specially formulated by the pharmacist, the dose and dosage regimen must always be verified for accuracy and appropriateness before the product or preparation is delivered to the patient.

II. DOSE FORMATS USED IN DRUG THERAPY

A. Individual doses are expressed using one of the following formats:

1. Quantity of drug
    For example, atenolol 25 mg, NPH insulin 10 units, potassium chloride 8 mEq
    (See Chapter 8 for the various quantity expressions used for drugs in pharmacy and medicine.)
2. Quantity of drug per kilogram of patient body weight
    For example, amoxicillin 20 mg/kg, heparin 50 units/kg, potassium phosphate 1.5 mmol/kg
3. Quantity of drug per square meter of patient body surface area (BSA)
    For example, doxorubicin 70 mg/m^2 and asparaginase 7,000 units/m^2

B. For topical products and preparations, doses are expressed as concentrations. This makes conceptual sense as concentration gradient is the driving force for transfer of drug across the skin or membrane barrier. Examples include hydrocortisone 1% lotion or gentamicin 0.3% ophthalmic ointment. (See Chapter 8 for accepted methods of expressing concentrations and related sample calculations.)

C. Concentrations are also used to express doses for some intravenous solutions, such as dextrose 5% injection and sodium chloride 0.9% injection.

III.   BODY WEIGHT AND BODY SURFACE AREA IN DOSE EXPRESSIONS

A. The formats for individual doses that are based on the patient's body size (weight or BSA) are often used for pediatric doses, but they are also important when determining adult doses for drugs that have narrow therapeutic indices or that need precise individualized dosing. BSA is routinely used for dosing chemotherapy agents, but it is also used in other selected situations. Pharmacists need patient-specific information on body weight or BSA in the following circumstances.

   1. Most often, drug orders are written in terms of a quantity of drug (e.g., mg, unit, mEq). Before preparing the prescription or medication order, the pharmacist verifies the correctness of the dose. If the drug information reference gives the dose as a quantity per kilogram body weight or based on BSA, the pharmacist needs this patient information to check the prescribed dose for appropriateness.

   2. In same cases, a prescriber will write a drug order in terms of a quantity of drug per kilogram of body weight (or square meter BSA) or will prescribe a drug, such as an antibiotic for a pediatric patient, and will ask the pharmacist to dose the patient on the basis of that patient's weight. In cases like this, the pharmacist needs the patient's weight to provide the proper dose.

   3. Some types of therapy, such as chemotherapy and total parenteral nutrition, use protocols based on patient weight or BSA. In these situations, the pharmacist needs these patient dimensions to calculate the needed quantities of drugs, electrolytes, or nutrients.

B. Body weight

   1. There are two types of body weight used in calculating doses: actual body weight (ABW) and ideal body weight (IBW). In most cases, the patient's ABW is used.

   a. If the patient is an inpatient, this information can usually be found in the patient's medical chart. If the information is not in the chart, ask the nurse who is taking care of that patient; this is often necessary when evaluating orders for newly admitted patients.

   b. If this is an ambulatory or outpatient, the pharmacist or pharmacy technician can obtain this information from the prescriber's office or the patient or patient caregiver. Realize that body weight can be a sensitive issue for some patients, so it is essential to be tactful and to communicate with the patient about the purpose for this information and the importance of accurate information in establishing a correct dose.

   c. For pediatric outpatients, an initial check of dosage range can be made if the child's age is known. An estimate of the patient's body weight can be obtained from one of the percentile charts of body weight versus age. Percentile weight-height measurements based on ages for infants and children are given in Appendix C and on the CD that accompanies this book. The charts in Appendix C are also available on the Center for Disease Control and Prevention (CDC) Internet site at http://www.cdc.gov/growthcharts/. Though charts like this are handy for initial checking of dosage ranges, the dose should always be verified based on the child's ABW.

   2. For some types of therapy, dosing is based on estimated IBW, also referred to as *lean body weight* (LBW). IBW is a calculated weight based on gender, height (or length for infants and children), and, for pediatric patients, age of the patient. As the LBW name implies, this is what the person would weigh if he or she had little or no fat or adipose tissue. This weight is especially useful for dosing drugs that do not distribute into adipose tissue; drugs such as these have a smaller volume of distribution than the entire body mass (especially for obese patients who have significant adipose tissue) so that basing the dose on ABW would result in a drug blood concentration that is higher than desired. Both ABW and IBW are used for TPN therapy calculations because, though adequate nourishment is needed, it would not be desirable to maintain an overweight state using parenteral nutrition.

   3. The following equations are used to calculate estimated IBW in kilograms. For children, several methods are shown based on age or height. The last equation given for children ages 1 to 17 years is based on CDC data for the fiftieth percentile weight for children of a given age and gender. As mentioned earlier, the CDC weight/height charts are shown in Appendix C; these can be used to determine an IBW for a child of a given age by choosing the weight at the fiftieth percentile (1).

Male Adults:
$$IBW_{(kg)} = 50 + (2.3 \times \text{height in inches beyond 5 feet})$$

Female Adults:
$$IBW_{(kg)} = 45.5 + (2.3 \times \text{height in inches beyond 5 feet})$$

Children:

Children less than 5 feet tall (2):

$$IBW_{(kg)} = \frac{\text{height}^2_{(cm)} \times 1.65}{1,000}$$

Children 5 feet and taller (2)

Boys:
$$IBW_{(kg)} = 39 + (2.27 \times \text{height}_{(in)} \text{ beyond 5 feet})$$

Girls:
$$IBW_{(kg)} = 42.2 + (2.27 \times \text{height}_{(in)} \text{ beyond 5 feet})$$

Ages 1 to 17 years (1)

$$IBW_{(kg)} = 2.396e^{0.01863(\text{height})}; \text{ height is in cm.}$$

C. Body surface area (BSA)

1. Drug dosage may also be based on estimated BSA of the patient. This parameter is sometimes used for pediatric dosing and, as previously stated, many cancer drug protocols base dosage on BSA. When a dose is given in terms of drug quantity per square meter of BSA, the pharmacist must use the patient's weight and height (or length for an infant) plus either an equation or a BSA nomogram to determine a value for the patient's BSA. Though some clinicians think that BSA is a better parameter than body weight for individualizing doses for patients, this is a subject that is still debated.

2. There are numerous BSA equations and each will give a slightly (or moderately) different answer. It should be understood that BSA is not a measurement (like a height or a weight) taken of the individual patient. It is an estimate based on an equation that was developed experimentally using a selected representative patient population. The weights, heights, and BSA of these patients were measured and correlated using an equation that mathematically modeled the experimental results. The first work on BSA was published in 1916 by DuBois and DuBois (3), but numerous other studies have subsequently been conducted. For more information on BSA equations, see a book on pharmaceutical calculations or one of the Internet Web sites devoted to this issue.

3. BSA nomograms for adults and children are shown in Appendix B and are based on the equations of DuBois and DuBois (3). They are used as follows:
   a. Find the patient's weight in pounds or kilograms on the right-hand side of the nomogram.
   b. Find the patient's height in inches or centimeters on the left-hand side of the nomogram.
   c. Draw a straight line connecting these two points and read the BSA in square meters at the point where the line intersects with the middle BSA line.

4. BSA can also be calculated using one of the equations developed for that purpose. Because the various equations give slightly different BSA values, some hospitals and clinics have standardized which equation will be used in their facility; this makes it easier to check and verify doses based on BSA. The equations given below were originally published by Mosteller (4,5); they have gained favor in clinical practice because BSA calculations can be done quite easily using one of these equations and a hand-held calculator (6).
   a. Using weight in pounds and height in inches:

   $$BSA(m^2) = \sqrt{\frac{Ht(in) \times Wt(lb)}{3,131}}$$

   b. Using weight in kilograms and height in centimeters:

   $$BSA(m^2) = \sqrt{\frac{Ht(cm) \times Wt(kg)}{3,600}}$$

IV.   DOSAGE REGIMENS

A. Dosage regimens combine the name and quantity or dose of the drug with a frequency of administration or use. As with doses, dosage regimens can be written in different formats. It is extremely important for the pharmacist to be attentive when reading and checking dosage regimens, because slight changes in wording can mean significant differences in intended dosing.

B. Formats for dosage regimens

   1. Name and quantity of drug with frequency of use or administration

      For example,

         Diazepam 1 mg 3 times a day

         or

         Diazepam 3 mg per day in 3 divided doses

      Note: Use great **CAUTION** when doses are expressed in the second way because it has been misread as 3 mg/dose to be given 3 times a day rather than 3 mg total per day—in this case a threefold error! If a drug information reference gives the dosage regimen in the second format, convert it to the less error-prone first dosing format when providing information to a prescriber.

   2. Name and concentration of drug with frequency of use or application

      For example,

         Hydrocortisone Lotion 1% apply q.i.d.

   3. Name and quantity of drug per kilogram of body weight with frequency of use or administration

      For example,

         Diazepam 40 mcg per kg 3 times a day

         or

         Diazepam 120 mcg per kg per day in 3 divided doses

      Note: Again, use great caution with this equivalent expression because it has been misread and misinterpreted.

   4. Name and quantity of drug per square meter of body surface area with frequency of use or administration

      For example,

         Diazepam 1.17 mg/m^2 BSA 3 times a day

         or

         Diazepam 3.51 mg per m^2 BSA per day in 3 divided doses

      Note: Again, use great caution with this equivalent expression because it has been misread and misinterpreted.

V. TRANSLATING DOSAGE REGIMENS TO PRODUCTS AND DIRECTIONS FOR USE

A. Though we calculate doses in terms of quantity or concentration of drug, we take or administer drugs as part of a dosage form (e.g., tablets, capsules, oral or topical liquids, ointments). Therefore, once an individual dose or daily dosage regimen is determined, this must be linked to a drug product or preparation and directions for use for the patient.

B. Route of administration

   1. Before a drug product can be selected, the route of administration must be determined. Most often, the route of administration will be obvious or specified on the drug order; however, selection of route of administration is an area in which pharmacists possess special expertise and often provide advice and counsel to practitioners. Examples of common routes of administration include oral, rectal, topical, ophthalmic, otic, intranasal, inhalation, intramuscular, intravenous, and subcutaneous.

   2. The desired route of administration is determined by such factors as therapeutic indication for the drug (e.g., are we treating a systemic disorder, such as hypertension, or a topical problem like poison ivy); severity of the condition (e.g., mild poison ivy may be treated with a topical corticosteroid cream, but a severe case may require a course with an oral agent); the patient's age and status (e.g., infant versus adult, mentally conscious versus unconscious); and drug absorption and disposition factors. Often the route of administration will affect the appropriate dose range and dosage regimen. For example, dosage adjustments are commonly made for hospitalized patients when switching their drug therapy from an injectable to an oral dosage form of the drug.

C. Dosage form and strength or concentration

   1. When the drug, route of administration, and dosage regimen have been determined, a dosage form and a particular product or preparation must be selected.

   2. In choosing a dosage form, various factors must be considered. This topic is discussed in greater detail in the dosage forms chapters of this book, but a few examples are given here to illustrate some of the considerations.

a. For oral products, can the patient swallow a tablet or capsule or will oral liquid or divided powder packets be needed?

b. For topical administration, will an ointment, a lotion, or a solution provide more effective and convenient therapy?

c. For parenteral therapy, which route gives the most desirable onset of action and blood levels with the least pain and discomfort for the patient?

3. When possible, manufactured drug products should be used because they have undergone extensive testing with known bioavailability and well-established quality control. If an appropriate dosage form and/or strength are not available, alternatives, including compounded preparations, need to be considered.

4. Very often, doses are given as ranges rather than as a single quantity value; a product and directions for use must then be selected that fall within the calculated range. For example, in the next section of this chapter, a pediatric patient has a dosage range calculated for the drug diazepam of 0.76 to 3.8 mg, to be given three to four times a day. Manufactured oral dosage forms of the drug include 15-mg extended-release capsules, 2-, 5-, and 10-mg tablets, and 1 mg/mL and 5 mg/mL oral solutions. For this patient, the 2-mg tablets offer one possibility, while the two oral solutions provide both greater flexibility of dose and a convenient dosage form if this child cannot swallow tablets.

5. Pharmacy students and technicians often ask about "rules" to use in deciding whether a dose is outside the acceptable range. Unfortunately, there are no set rules that fit all situations; establishing patient-, disease-, and drug-specific acceptable doses comes with both education and experience.

VI. SPECIAL CASES

A. Pediatric patients

1. One obvious difference between adults and pediatric patients is size, but it is important to remember that infants and children are not just little adults. Their physiologic systems often are not fully developed, and this must be considered in dosing these patients. Furthermore, there are differences in metabolism and excretion capabilities as children progress from birth to adulthood. When these factors are known to be significant in drug dosing, this information is usually given in drug information references and prescribing information (product package inserts). To use this information, it is helpful to know the accepted descriptive terms for the stages of childhood. Here is a scheme in common use.

a. Neonate or newborn: birth to 1 month

b. Infant: 1 month to 1 year

c. Early childhood: 1 year through 5 years

d. Late childhood: 6 years through 12 years

e. Adolescence: 13 years through 17 years (7)

Another more recently published system has slight changes in the descriptive terms and ages for childhood through adolescence. They are early childhood, 1 year through 4 years; middle childhood, 5 years through 10 years; and adolescence, 11 years through 17 years (8).

2. Unfortunately, pediatric drug information is often limited or unavailable, and general drug information references and manufacturer prescribing information may state only that safety and efficacy have not been established for this patient population. Sometimes a literature search for case reports may provide some guidance. Because of the importance of this topic and the potential danger to infants and children caused by the absence of well-documented pediatric dosing information, the U.S. Congress enacted the 2002 Best Pharmaceuticals for Children Act, which offers incentives to pharmaceutical manufacturers to perform studies in pediatric populations (9).

3. In the absence of specific pediatric dosing information, there are general rules for calculating an infant or child's dose of medication when given the age, weight, or BSA of the patient and the normal adult dose. A variety of these rules are given in Table 9.1. **The general rules are not drug-specific and should be used only in the absence of more complete information.** It is the duty of the pharmacist to be knowledgeable about the limitations of using set formulas or rules for calculating pediatric doses. In the absence of specific pediatric dosing information, always be conservative in dosing these patients, particularly neonates and infants.

4. Sample calculations for pediatric dosing are given in Examples 9.1 through 9.5.

Table 9.1	FORMULAS FOR PEDIATRIC DOSAGE CALCULATIONS

RULE NAME	EQUATION	EXAMPLES*
Drug-specific calculation based on weight		
	$\dfrac{\text{Dose}}{\text{kg of body weight}} \times \text{Weight(kg)} = \text{Dose for child}$	$\left(\dfrac{0.04 - 0.2\text{ mg}}{\text{kg}}\right)\left(\dfrac{19.1\text{ kg}}{}\right) = 0.76 - 3.82\text{ mg}$
Drug-specific calculation based on BSA		
	$\dfrac{\text{Dose}}{\text{BSA m}^2} \times \text{BSA(m}^2) = \text{Dose for child}$	$\left(\dfrac{1.17 - 6\text{ mg}}{\text{m}^2}\right)\left(\dfrac{0.76\text{ m}^2}{}\right) = 0.89 - 4.56\text{ mg}$
General rules based on weight		
Clark's Rule	$\dfrac{\text{Weight (lbs)}}{150} \times \text{Adult dose} = \text{Dose for child}$	$\dfrac{42\text{ lbs}}{150} \times 2 - 10\text{ mg} = 0.56 - 2.8\text{ mg}$
General rule based on BSA		
	$\dfrac{\text{BSA m}^2}{1.73\text{ m}^2} \times \text{Adult dose} = \text{Dose for child}$	$\dfrac{0.76\text{ m}^2}{1.73\text{ m}^2} \times 2 - 10\text{ mg} = 0.87 - 4.39\text{ mg}$
General rules based on age		
Young's Rule	$\dfrac{\text{Age}}{\text{Age} + 12} \times \text{Adult dose} = \text{Dose for child}$	$\dfrac{5}{5 + 12} \times 2 - 10\text{ mg} = 0.59 - 2.94\text{ mg}$
Cowling's Rule	$\dfrac{\text{Age at next birthday (in years)}}{24} \times \text{Adult dose} = \text{Dose for child}$	$\dfrac{6}{24} \times 2 - 10\text{ mg} = 0.5 - 2.5\text{ mg}$
Bastedo's Rule	$\dfrac{\text{Age in years} + 3}{30} \times \text{Adult dose} = \text{Dose for child}$	$\dfrac{8}{30} \times 2 - 10\text{ mg} = 0.53 - 2.67\text{ mg}$
Dilling's Rule	$\dfrac{\text{Age (in years)}}{20} \times \text{Adult dose} = \text{Dose for child}$	$\dfrac{5}{20} \times 2 - 10\text{ mg} = 0.5 - 2.5\text{ mg}$
Fried's Rule for infants	$\dfrac{\text{Age (in months)}}{150} \times \text{Adult dose} = \text{Dose for infant}$	$\dfrac{0.5}{150} \times 25\text{ mg} = 0.083\text{ mg}$

*These examples use the data from the text on patient D.A. with the drug and dosage information for diazepam except for the final example for Fried's Rule for Infants; that example uses the data for the 2-week-old infant J.A. and dosing for captopril.

Example 9.1	**Dosing based on specific information in a drug information reference.**

D.A. is a 5-year-old boy. He weighs 42 pounds and is 43 inches tall. The prescriber wants to give diazepam to D.A. What is an acceptable dose of diazepam for D.A.?

Usual pediatric dose: Children 6 months of age and older: Oral, 1 to 2.5 mg, 40 to 200 mcg (0.04 to 0.2 mg) per kilogram of body weight, or 1.17 to 6 mg per square meter of body surface, three to four times a day, the dosage being increased gradually as needed and tolerated.

1. What is the dosage regimen of diazepam for D.A. based on the **quantity** given in the above reference?

$$1 \text{ to } 2.5 \text{ mg given 3 to 4 times a day}$$

2. What is the dosage regimen of diazepam for D.A. based on the **mg/kg** dose given in the reference?

   a. Calculation of kilogram weight of D.A.:

$$\frac{2.2\text{ lbs}}{1\text{ kg}} = \frac{42\text{ lbs}}{x\text{ kg}}; \quad x = 19.1\text{ kg}$$

   b. Calculation of dose:

$$\left(\frac{0.04 - 0.2\text{ mg}}{\text{kg}}\right)\left(\frac{19.1\text{ kg}}{}\right) = 0.76 - 3.82\text{ mg}$$

   c. Dosage regimen: 0.76 to 3.82 mg given 3 to 4 times a day.

3. What is the dosage regimen of diazepam for D.A. based on the referenced **mg/m²** BSA dose?

  a. Determine the BSA of D.A. from the pediatric nomogram found in Appendix B:

$$BSA = 0.76 \text{ m}^2$$

  b. Calculation of dose:

$$\left(\frac{1.17 - 6 \text{ mg}}{\text{m}^2} \right) \left(0.76 \text{ m}^2 \right) = 0.89 - 4.56 \text{ mg}$$

  c. Dosage regimen: 0.89 to 4.56 mg given 3 to 4 times a day

Notice that there is some variation in dosage range based on the various methods used to calculate dose. Individual patient circumstances and available dosage forms will dictate the specific milligram amount to administer. For pediatric patients, the general rule is to "start low and go slow," but there are many exceptions to this general principle and each case should be carefully considered.

Example 9.2

Dosage calculated using a normal adult dose and "rules" for pediatric doses based on the child's age, weight, and BSA.

For the following examples, diazepam doses are calculated for D.A. using one of the so-called "rules" for pediatric dosing given in Table 9.1. The numbers for the next example are based on the age/weight/height information for D.A. given in the foregoing example and on the adult dose information given for diazepam for similar therapeutic indications. This adult dose is given as:

Oral: 2 to 10 mg 2 to 4 times a day

In each case given below, the calculated dose would be given two to four times a day.

1. Using **Young's Rule**, what is the dose of diazepam for D.A. based on the normal adult dose and D.A.'s **age**?

$$\frac{Age}{Age + 12} \times Adult \ dose = Dose \ for \ child$$

$$\frac{5}{5 + 12} \times 2 - 10 \text{ mg} = 0.59 - 2.94 \text{ mg}$$

2. Using **Clark's Rule**, what is the dose of diazepam for D.A. based on the normal adult dose and D.A.'s **weight**?

$$\frac{Weight \ (lbs)}{150} \times Adult \ dose = Dose \ for \ child$$

$$\frac{42 \ lbs}{150} \times 2 - 10 \text{ mg} = 0.56 - 2.8 \text{ mg}$$

3. What is the dose of diazepam for D.A. based on the normal adult dose and D.A.'s **BSA**?

  This is based on the BSA of an "average" adult of 1.73 m².

$$\frac{BSA \ \text{m}^2}{1.73 \ \text{m}^2} \times Adult \ dose = Dose \ for \ child$$

$$\frac{0.76 \ \text{m}^2}{1.73 \ \text{m}^2} \times 2 - 10 \text{ mg} = 0.87 - 4.39 \text{ mg}$$

Notice that in each case, the doses of diazepam for D.A. are similar. As stated earlier, Table 9.1 lists several other equations for calculating pediatric doses from established adult doses. While these so-called rules may be helpful as a starting point in determining a pediatric dose in the absence of specific information, the following example shows the danger inherent in using this generalized approach.

Example 9.3

Dosing for an infant based on normal adult dose and "rules" for pediatric dosing.

J.A. is a 2-week-old infant who weighs 8 pounds. The prescriber wants to give captopril to J.A. What is an acceptable dose of captopril for J.A.?

Usual adult and adolescent dose:

Antihypertensive—Initial: Oral, 25 mg 2 or 3 times a day, the dosage being increased if necessary

Usual pediatric dose:

Newborns—Initial: Oral, 10 mcg (0.01 mg) per kilogram of body weight 2 or 3 times a day, the dosage being adjusted as needed and tolerated

1. What is the dose of captopril for J.A. based on the newborn initial **mg/kg** dose given in the drug information reference?

   a. Calculation of kilogram weight of J.A.:

   $$\frac{2.2\ \text{lbs}}{1\ \text{kg}} = \frac{8\ \text{lbs}}{x\ \text{kg}};\ x = 3.6\ \text{kg}$$

   b. Calculation of dose:

   $$\left(\frac{0.01\ \text{mg}}{\text{kg}}\right)\left(\frac{3.6\ \text{kg}}{}\right) = 0.036\ \text{mg}$$

2. Using **Clark's Rule**, what is the dose of captopril for J.A. based on the normal adult dose and J.A.'s **weight**?

   $$\frac{8\ \text{lbs}}{150} \times 25\ \text{mg} = 1.33\ \text{mg}$$

This method was not so successful—nearly 40 times the recommended dose! Notice that even when using Fried's Rule, which was specifically developed for infants, the dose of captopril is more than two times the recommended drug-specific dose for J.A.

**ALWAYS USE DRUG-SPECIFIC PEDIATRIC DOSES
WHEN THESE ARE AVAILABLE**

B. Geriatric patients

   1. Geriatric patients may require special consideration when designing dosage regimens. Often the organ systems of these patients are not functioning at top efficiency because of the aging process or disease. Because some clinical conditions, such as liver impairment and kidney dysfunction, that are important to the metabolism and elimination of drugs are more prevalent in the elderly, it is essential for the pharmacist to have medical histories of these patients. See examples 9.4 and 9.5 for sample dose adjustment calculations that are made using the results of clinical lab tests.

   2. With geriatric patients, modifications in dosing regimen are often given, when applicable, in drug information references and prescribing information.

C. Use of pharmacokinetic parameters and laboratory values to set and adjust dosage levels

   1. For some drugs and electrolytes, laboratory tests of blood levels are used to monitor established therapy and adjust doses and dosage regimens to ensure optimal drug effectiveness and avoid toxicity.

   a. In some cases, the actual drug or electrolyte blood levels are measured. Examples include digoxin, lithium, phenytoin, carbamazepine, theophylline, vancomycin, gentamicin, cyclosporine, tacrolimus, and electrolytes such as potassium, magnesium and calcium.

Example 9.4

The pharmacist has been asked to provide magnesium supplementation for a 75-kg patient whose serum magnesium is 0.5 mmol/L. The *Textbook of Therapeutics* gives a magnesium dose of 1 mEq/kg/day for patients with magnesium serum concentration <0.6 mmol/L (10). Calculate the daily dose of magnesium in milliequivalents per day for this patient.

$$\frac{1\ \text{mEq}}{\text{kg/day}} \times 75\ \text{kg} = 75\ \text{mEq/day}$$

Magnesium sulfate injection is available as the heptahydrate ($MgSO_4$ HH), MW = 246.5. Calculate the number of milligrams of $MgSO_4$ HH the patient should receive per day.

$$\left(\frac{246.5\ \text{mg MgSO}_4\ \text{HH}}{\text{mmol MgSO}_4\ \text{HH}}\right)\left(\frac{\text{mmol MgSO}_4\ \text{HH}}{2\ \text{mEq Mg}^{+2}}\right)\left(\frac{75\ \text{mEq Mg}^{+2}}{\text{day}}\right) = 9{,}244\ \text{mg MgSO}_4\ \text{HH/day}$$

Magnesium sulfate (heptahydrate) Injection is available in a concentration of 500 mg/mL. Calculate the number of milliliters of the injection that the patient should receive per day.

$$\left(\frac{\text{mL}}{500\ \text{mg MgSO}_4\ \text{HH}}\right)\left(\frac{9{,}244\ \text{mg MgSO}_4\ \text{HH}}{\text{day}}\right) = 18.5\ \text{mL/day}$$

  b. For some other drugs, doses are adjusted on the basis of indirect lab measurements. For example, dosages for anticoagulants such as heparin and warfarin are set and modified on the basis of activated partial thromboplastin time (aPTT or PTT) and international normal ratio (INR) for prothrombin time (PT). Levothyroxine doses for thyroid therapy are adjusted by monitoring thyroid stimulating hormone (TSH) and thyroxine (T4) levels.

2. For some therapeutic classes and certain patient populations, pharmacokinetic parameters are used to set or adjust dose quantities and/or dosage regimens.

  a. The most common example of this is the use of patient creatinine clearance values for adjusting the dosage regimens for drugs that are eliminated by the kidney. In this case, creatinine clearance is used as a measure of renal function, and drug toxicity is avoided in patients with impaired renal function by adjusting the dosage regimen based on this measured parameter. You will see these adjusted doses in many drug information references.

  b. Though creatinine clearance can be measured directly in a hospital or other institutional setting by collecting a 24-hour urine sample, creatinine clearance (Cl_{cr}) can be estimated using the patient's serum creatinine (SCr), a lab value that is more readily available. Several methods are be used to link these two values; the easiest uses the Cockcroft-Gault equation (11):

$$Cl_{cr} = \frac{(140 - age) \times ABW(\times 0.85 \text{ if female})}{72 \times SCr} \text{ mL/min}$$

3. More complete discussion of these topics, though extremely important, is beyond the scope of this text. However, the following example should serve to illustrate some of the principles presented in this chapter.

Example 9.5

P.F. is a 94-year-old woman who was admitted to a nursing home four months ago. She is 5-foot, 1-inch tall and weighs 108 pounds. She recently has been diagnosed with herpes zoster (shingles). Her physician has asked the pharmacist to determine an appropriate dosage regimen of valacyclovir for P.F. The drug information reference gives the following dosing information:

Adults dose for herpes zoster: 1 g 3 times a day for 7 days

Dosing interval in renal impairment:

  Cl_{cr} 30 to 49 mL/min: 1 g every 12 hours

  Cl_{cr} 10 to 29 mL/min: 1 g every 24 hours

  Cl_{cr} <10 mL/min: 500 mg every 24 hours

On a recent lab panel, P.F.'s SCr was found to be 0.8 mg/dL. Using the Cockcroft-Gault equation, calculate a Cl_{cr} for P.F. and determine an acceptable dosage regimen of valacyclovir for her.

Though the Cockcroft-Gault equation was originally developed using ABW, many clinicians now use IBW (12). Therefore, first, use the IBW equation given in section III of this chapter to calculate P.F.'s IBW:

$$\text{IBW} = 45.5 + 2.3(1) = 47.8 \text{ kg}$$

Insert this value and P.F.'s age and SCr into the Cockcroft-Gault equation and solve for Cl_{cr}:

$$Cl_{cr} = \frac{(140 - 94) \times 47.8 \times 0.85}{72 \times 0.8} = 32.4 \text{ mL/min}$$

Using this Cl_{cr} value and the dosage information given here for valacyclovir, select an appropriate dosage regimen for P.F.: She should get valacyclovir 1 g every 12 hours for 7 days. Valacyclovir is available as 500-mg and 1-g caplets. Because of P.F.'s age and possible difficulty with swallowing large caplets, the pharmacist has recommended giving two 500-mg caplets every 12 hours. If P.F. has trouble swallowing these caplets, the caplets can be crushed and given with soft food or a liquid suspension can be compounded using the caplets.

REFERENCES

1. Traub SL, Kitchen L. Estimating ideal body mass in children. Am J Hosp Pharm 1983; 40: 107–110.
2. Traub SL, Johnson CE. Comparison of methods of estimating creatinine clearance in children. Am J Hosp Pharm 1980; 37: 195–201.
3. DuBois D, DuBois EF. A formula to estimate the approximate surface area if height and weight be known. Arch Intern Med 1916; 17: 863–871.
4. Mosteller RD. Simplified calculation of body surface area. N Engl J Med 1987; 317: 1098.
5. Lam TK, Leung DT. More on simplified calculation of body surface area. N Engl J Med 1988; 318: 1130.
6. Halls SB. Body surface area calculator for medication. http://www.halls.md/body-surface-area/bsa.htm. Accessed July 2007.
7. Berkow R, ed. The Merck manual, 15th ed. Rahway, NJ: Merck & Co., Inc., 1987; 1798–1799.
8. Berkow R, Beers MH, ed. The Merck manual, 17th ed. West Point, PA: Merck & Co., Inc., 1999; 2076–2077.
9. Best Pharmaceuticals for Children Act. Public Law No. 107-109. January 4, 2002.
10. Helms RA, Quan DJ, Herfindal ET, et al. Textbook of therapeutics, 8th ed. Philadelphia: Lippincott Williams & Wilkins, 2006; 718.
11. Cockcroft DW, Gault MH. Prediction of creatinine clearance from serum creatinine. Nephron 1976; 16: 31.
12. O'Sullivan TA. Understanding pharmacy calculations; Washington, DC: American Pharmaceutical Association, 2002; 122.

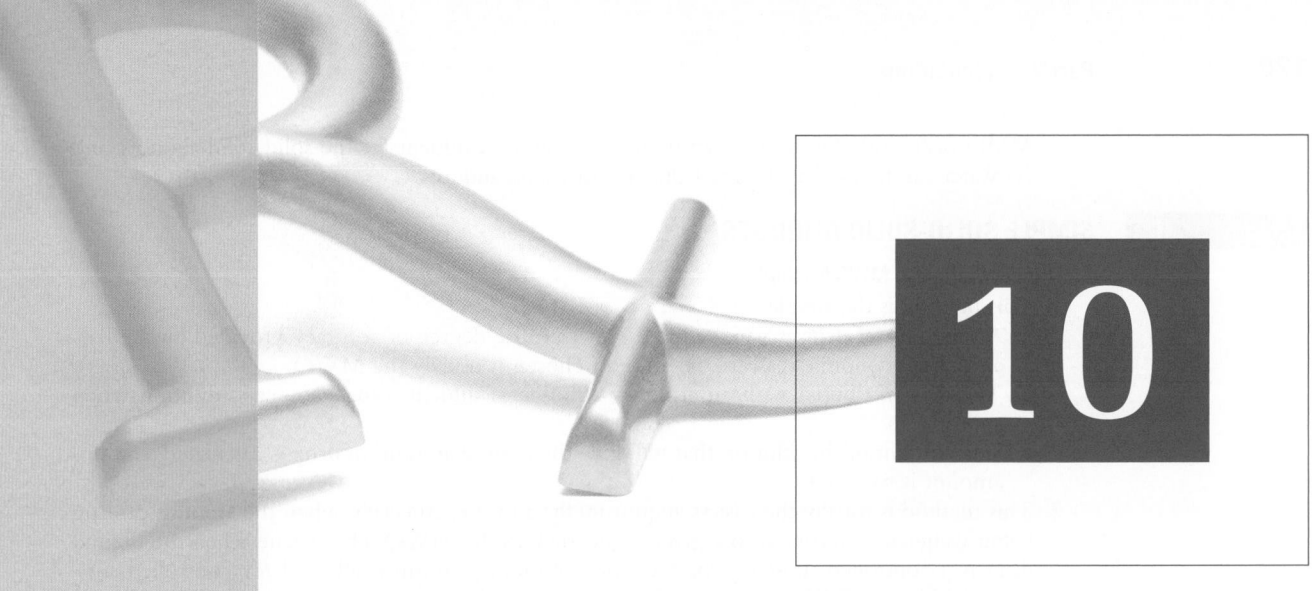

Aliquot Calculations

I.   GENERAL PRINCIPLES

A. In pharmacy we often deal with potent drug substances that require accurate measurement when preparing dosage forms for our patients. When the quantity of drug desired requires a degree of precision in measurement that is beyond the capability of the available measuring devices, the pharmacist or pharmacy technician may use the aliquot method of measurement.

B. Aliquot means "contained an exact number of times in something else." Therefore, 5 is an aliquot part of 15 because 5 is contained exactly 3 times in 15.

C. When aliquots are used in pharmacy, the general procedure is as follows:
  1. Weigh or measure an amount of the desired drug that is within the degree of accuracy provided by the measuring device.
  2. Weigh or measure a compatible, inert diluent. For solid aliquots, lactose is a common diluent. For liquid aliquots, water is used if possible, but alcohol or another pharmaceutical solvent may also be used when solubility or miscibility dictates this.
  3. Add the diluent to the drug with adequate mixing to give a homogeneous mixture or solution. In all cases when combining powders, use geometric dilution and mix thoroughly using trituration in a glass mortar. (Note: A description of geometric dilution is given in Chapter 25, Powders: the Principles of Compounding for Powders section.)
  4. Weigh or measure an aliquot part of the mixture that contains exactly the desired amount of drug.

D. How are the numbers for aliquot parts determined?
  1. Examples given later show several commonly used methods. Any method is satisfactory as long as the correct amount of drug is obtained. Use a system that makes sense to you because this usually means that there is less potential for error.
  2. Because aliquots usually are used for potent drugs, it is always best to have a colleague independently check the amounts calculated.
  3. For the examples given next, the following assumptions were made: (i) the available balance has a minimum weighable quantity (MWQ) of 120 mg; (ii) the smallest graduated cylinder available has a capacity of 10 mL with a minimum measurable quantity (MMQ) of 2 mL (20% of the capacity of the graduated cylinder); (iii) the smallest syringe or micropipette available has a

MMQ of 0.2 mL; (iv) lactose can be used as the inert diluent for the solid-solid aliquots; and (v) water can be used as the inert diluent for liquid aliquots.

II.   **SIMPLE SOLID-SOLID ALIQUOTS**

A. Aliquot Method 1: MWQ Method

1. This method is the simplest.
   a. An amount of drug is weighed that is within the degree of accuracy provided by the balance. For economic reasons, the amount chosen is usually the MWQ.
   b. The drug is diluted with an arbitrary amount of diluent using geometric dilution when appropriate.
   c. The amount of the dilution that will give the desired amount of drug is calculated, and this amount is weighed.
2. This method is usually the easiest aliquot method to use, especially when the amount of drug being weighed is restricted to a given value, such as the MWQ. This is true when the desired drug is a controlled substance because only minimum waste is allowed for controlled substances. Using the MWQ is also preferred when the drug is expensive.
3. This method is illustrated with several examples. The first example (10.1), Trial 1, starts with the basic necessary steps. Trial 1 is then analyzed, and the method is refined. Example 10.2, Trial 2, shows the results of these modifications. A final analysis is then given to show additional possibilities. The objective of presenting the method in this way is to show a pattern of possible thought processes that can be used in a general sense for developing methods of problem solving when dealing with pharmaceutical calculations.

Example 10.1   *drug/amount desired:* **codeine 20 mg**

1. Trial 1: Basic steps
   a. Weigh the MWQ of codeine: 120 mg.
   b. Weigh an arbitrary amount of lactose that is $\geq$ the MWQ: 300 mg.
   c. Mix the two powders thoroughly by triturating in a mortar.
   d. Calculate the total weight of the dilution: 120 mg + 300 mg = 420 mg.
   e. Calculate the number of milligrams of dilution that contain the desired 20 mg of codeine. By proportion:

$$\frac{120 \text{ mg codeine}}{420 \text{ mg dilution}} = \frac{20 \text{ mg codeine}}{x \text{ mg dilution}}; \quad x = 70 \text{ mg dilution}$$

   By dimensional analysis:

$$\left(\frac{420 \text{ mg dilution}}{120 \text{ mg codeine}}\right)\left(\frac{20 \text{ mg codeine}}{}\right) = 70 \text{ mg dilution}$$

   f. Weigh this calculated amount of the dilution, 70 mg, to get the desired 20 mg of codeine.
2. Analysis of Trial 1
   Analysis of these calculations reveals that some judgment is required in selecting the quantity of diluent to add to the drug. In this case, the required amount of the aliquot was calculated to be 70 mg, which is below the MWQ. The following are general guidelines for selecting the amount of diluent to use:
   a. Pick a quantity of diluent that will give aliquots that are at or above the MWQ. In this case, it is obvious that 300 mg of lactose is not enough diluent when the desired amount of drug is 20 mg. The 70 mg of the dilution, which is the amount needed to give 20 mg of codeine, is below the MWQ of 120 mg and cannot be weighed with the desired level of accuracy.
   b. When possible, pick convenient amounts of diluent to make the mathematics easy. It is always best to use simple numbers, or amounts that reduce to simple numbers, because it is then easier to spot errors. In this case, if the amount of diluent is chosen to be a multiple of 120 mg (the amount of codeine weighed), then the fraction "mg codeine/mg dilution" reduces to a simple integer that is easily multiplied times the "mg codeine" to get the desired "mg dilution." The following example illustrates this principle.

Example 10.2   Trial 2: Revised steps

1. This example is a repeat of the foregoing problem using a more "convenient" quantity of diluent that will give an aliquot $\geq$ the MWQ.

a. Weigh the MWQ of codeine: 120 mg.

b. Weigh a convenient amount of lactose (that is, a multiple of 120 mg) that will give an aliquot ≥ 120 mg, the MWQ: 600 mg is selected.

c. Add the lactose to the codeine using geometric dilution and mix the two powders thoroughly by triturating in a mortar.

d. Calculate the weight of the dilution: 120 mg + 600 mg = 720 mg.

e. Calculate the number of milligrams of dilution that contain the desired 20 mg of codeine. By proportion:

$$\frac{120 \text{ mg codeine}}{720 \text{ mg dilution}} = \frac{20 \text{ mg codeine}}{x \text{ mg dilution}}; x = 120 \text{ mg dilution}$$

By dimensional analysis:

$$\left(\frac{720 \text{ mg dilution}}{120 \text{ mg codeine}}\right)\left(\frac{20 \text{ mg codeine}}{1}\right) = 120 \text{ mg dilution}$$

f. Weigh this calculated amount of the dilution to get the desired 20 mg of codeine.

2. Analysis of Trial 2

   a. As you can see, 720 is a multiple of 120 (6 × 120 = 720), so the fraction 120/720 reduces to 1/6, and the mathematics becomes a simple matter of multiplying 20 mg of codeine by 6 to get 120 mg of dilution.

$$\frac{\overset{1}{\cancel{120}} \text{ mg codeine}}{\underset{6}{\cancel{720}} \text{ mg dilution}} = \frac{20 \text{ mg codeine}}{x \text{ mg dilution}}; x = 120 \text{ mg dilution}$$

   Even though most of us use calculators for math operations, it is important to look at the answers we get to see whether they seem reasonable. This sort of inspection is much easier if the numbers are simple.

   b. In using this method, you may wonder, What is the best way to pick the quantity of diluent so that the amount of dilution needed is at least the MWQ, but the amounts are not so large as to waste ingredients or give an aliquot that is excessively bulky? There are several ways in which this may be accomplished.

   (1) Pick any reasonable amount, do the math and, if the amount of dilution calculated is too little or too much, pick a different amount. While simple, this can be tedious.

   (2) In picking amounts, notice that the amount of diluent needed is not completely arbitrary. An inspection of the calculations given here reveals that the smaller the amount of drug needed (20 mg in this case), the larger the amount of diluent needed to give a minimum amount of dilution to weigh.

   (3) Further inspection of the equations in Trial 2 reveals that instead of picking the amount of the diluent and solving for the amount of the aliquot, you may also set up the equation by picking the amount of the aliquot and solving for the amount of the dilution. For example, if you want 120 mg for the aliquot, set up the equation as shown here:

$$\frac{120 \text{ mg codeine}}{x \text{ mg dilution}} = \frac{20 \text{ mg codeine}}{120 \text{ mg dilution}}; x = 720 \text{ mg dilution}$$

   You will need to remember that the 720 mg is the total amount of the dilution (i.e., drug plus diluent). To determine the amount of diluent, subtract the quantity of drug weighed from this total to obtain the amount of the diluent. In this case,

$$720 \text{ mg dilution} - 120 \text{ mg drug} = 600 \text{ mg diluent}$$

   (4) For pharmacists who like formulas, the formula given below may be useful:

$$\frac{\textit{Amount of drug desired}}{\textit{Amount of drug weighed}} = \frac{\textit{Amount of dilution weighed}}{\textit{Total amount of dilution}}$$

   To use this formula, fill in the desired quantities for Amount of drug desired, Amount of drug weighed, and Amount of dilution weighed. Then, solve for Total amount of dilution. In the foregoing example:

$$\frac{20 \text{ mg}}{120 \text{ mg}} = \frac{120 \text{ mg}}{x}; x = 720 \text{ mg}$$

Table 10.1	DETERMINATION OF SOLID–SOLID ALIQUOT AMOUNTS			
AMOUNT OF DRUG NEEDED (A)	AMOUNT OF DRUG WEIGHED (B)	AMOUNT OF DILUENT (LACTOSE) (C)	AMOUNT OF DILUTION (D)	DILUTION FACTOR (D) ÷ (B) (E)
60–120 mg	120 mg	120 mg	240 mg	2
30–59 mg	120 mg	360 mg	480 mg	4
12–29 mg	120 mg	1,080 mg	1,200 mg	10
3–11 mg	120 mg	4,680 mg	4,800 mg	40
1.2–2.9 mg	120 mg	11,880 mg	12,000 mg	100

As with the previous example, remember that 720 mg is the total amount of the dilution (i.e., drug plus diluent). To determine the amount of diluent, subtract the quantity of drug weighed from this total to obtain the amount of the diluent. Though formulas may simplify solving pharmaceutical calculations, the problem with using a formula is that you have to remember it—unless, of course, it is intuitive to you.

(5) You may wish to perform the calculations for aliquots for a variety of drug weights and construct a table of values such as the one shown in Table 10.1. Using a table of that type is fairly easy.

    (a) Determine the amount of drug needed: 20 mg.

    (b) Weigh 120 mg of the drug. (Notice in column (B) of Table 10.1 that this amount is always the same. This table was constructed for a Class III torsion balance, and 120 mg was chosen as the amount to weigh because that is the MWQ for that balance; a similar table using 20 mg for a typical electronic balance could also be constructed.)

    (c) Determine the weight range for the amount of drug needed from column (A), 12–29 mg, and read off the amount of lactose or other diluent from column (C), 1,080 mg. The combined weight of the drug and diluent is shown in column (D), 1,200 mg.

    (d) Calculate the amount of dilution to weigh that will contain the desired amount of drug.

$$\frac{\overset{1}{\cancel{120}} \text{ mg codeine}}{\underset{10}{\cancel{1200}} \text{ mg dilution}} = \frac{20 \text{ mg codeine}}{x \text{ mg dilution}}; x = 200 \text{ mg dilution}$$

    (e) Alternatively, you may read the appropriate dilution factor given in column (E), which in this case is 10, and multiply the dilution factor times the amount of drug needed to get the amount of aliquot to weigh.

$$10 \times 20 \text{ mg} = 200 \text{ mg}$$

When using this approach, it is always best to check the values obtained by completing a full calculation using the chosen numbers as shown in the calculation in part (d).

B. Aliquot Method 2: Dilution Factor Method

    1. This method is useful when there is more flexibility in the amount of drug that may be weighed; for example, you are not required to use the MWQ.

    2. This method consists of the following steps:

        a. The quantity of drug to be weighed is determined by multiplying the amount of drug needed by an appropriately determined factor, called the *dilution factor*.

        b. An arbitrary amount of diluent is weighed and added.

        c. The amount of dilution needed is determined by multiplying the weight of the dilution by the inverse of the dilution factor. Dilution factors are usually chosen to be whole numbers.

Example 10.3   *drug/amount desired:* **codeine 20 mg**

1. Basic steps
   a. Select a dilution factor that will give a quantity that is ≥ the MWQ. Weigh this amount. In this case, the dilution factor may be anything ≥6 because 6 × 20 = 120 mg.
   b. Weigh a convenient amount of lactose that will give an aliquot ≥MWQ: 600 mg is selected.
   c. Mix the two powders thoroughly by triturating in a mortar.
   d. Calculate the total weight of the dilution: 120 mg + 600 mg = 720 mg.
   e. Calculate the aliquot part of the dilution that contains the 20 mg of codeine by multiplying the total weight of the dilution by the inverse of the dilution factor, 1/6 in this case: 1/6 × 720 mg = 120 mg.
   f. Weigh this calculated amount of the dilution to get the desired 20 mg of codeine.
2. Analysis
   a. Once again, there is the problem of selecting an appropriate amount of diluent. Fortunately, in the foregoing example, 600 mg was sufficient to give an aliquot that is ≥ the MWQ.
   b. With this method, because the aliquot part is determined by multiplying the weight of the total dilution by the inverse of the dilution factor, the easiest way to determine the minimum amount of dilution is to set up and solve the following equation:

   $$\left(\frac{1}{dilution\ factor}\right)x = 120 \text{ mg (or desired weight of aliquot)}$$

   where x is the total amount of the dilution.
   In this sample:

   $$\left(\frac{1}{6}\right)x = 120 \text{ mg}; \ x = 720 \text{ mg}$$

   c. As was mentioned, the dilution factors chosen are usually whole numbers. This means that the only time the amount of drug weighed may be calculated to be a specified quantity, such as 120 mg, is when the weight of drug needed is a factor of that specified quantity.
   d. The Dilution Factor Method becomes more difficult when you are restricted to weighing a certain amount of drug, such as the MWQ. In this case, the dilution factor must be calculated in the following fashion:

   $$dilution\ factor \times quantity\ of\ drug\ needed = 120 \text{ mg}$$

   $$dilution\ factor = \frac{120 \text{ mg}}{quantity\ of\ drug\ needed}$$

   For the example just given, the calculated dilution factor is 6 for a needed drug quantity of 20 mg and a MWQ of 120 mg:

   $$\frac{120 \text{ mg}}{20 \text{ mg}} = 6$$

   If the amount of drug needed is 14 mg, the dilution factor is:

   $$\frac{120 \text{ mg}}{14 \text{ mg}} = 8.57$$

   The value 8.57 is a rounded value, so the subsequent calculated amounts are somewhat imprecise.
   e. Once the dilution factor is determined, the amount of the dilution can then be calculated just as was done in b.:

   $$\left(\frac{1}{8.57}\right)x = 120 \text{ mg}; \ x = 1,028 \text{ mg}$$

   For this example, 120 mg of drug and 908 mg of lactose are weighed (908 mg lactose + 120 mg drug = 1,028 mg dilution). These are triturated together, and 120 mg of the dilution is weighed to give 14 mg of drug. This should always be verified.
   By proportion:

   $$\frac{120 \text{ mg codeine}}{1,028 \text{ mg dilution}} = \frac{14 \text{ mg codeine}}{x \text{ mg dilution}} \simeq x = 119.9 \text{ mg} \simeq 120 \text{ mg dilution}$$

By dimensional analysis:

$$\left(\frac{1{,}028 \text{ mg dilution}}{120 \text{ mg codeine}}\right) = \left(\frac{14 \text{ mg codeine}}{}\right) = 119.9 \text{ mg} \simeq 120 \text{ mg dilution}$$

    f. When circumstances dictate that the dilution factor must be calculated and the calculated dilution factor is not an integer, this method becomes cumbersome. This often occurs when the amount of drug to be weighed is restricted to a specified amount, such as the MWQ, when an aliquot must be made for a controlled substance.

III. SOLID-SOLID SERIAL DILUTIONS

A. Notice in Table 10.1 that the minimum amount given in the "Amount of Drug Needed" column is 1.2 mg. This is because, as a general rule, an amount of drug requiring a dilution of greater than 100 to 1 is usually not done with a single dilution: Homogeneous mixing at this level is difficult. Furthermore, the amount of diluent needed becomes unreasonably large. When very small quantities of drug are needed (e.g., <1 mg), a serial dilution is usually used. This method is avoided when possible because the mathematics is more difficult, and it is easy to get confused.

B. Determine the necessity of a serial dilution.

Example 10.4

drug/amount desired: **hyoscine HBr 0.35 mg**

1. Notice in Table 10.1 that 0.35 mg of drug requires a dilution of greater than 100 to 1 (>12,000 mg dilution to 120 mg drug).
2. Refer back to example 10.2, the Analysis of Trial 2. Notice that there are two methods that could be used to calculate the amount of dilution needed for a single aliquot to measure 0.35 mg of drug.
   a. A calculation like that described in part b.(3) could be used:

   $$\frac{120 \text{ mg hyoscine}}{x \text{ mg dilution}} = \frac{0.35 \text{ mg hyoscine}}{120 \text{ mg dilution}}; \, x = 41{,}143 \text{ mg dilution}$$

   b. The equation given in part b. (4) could also be used:

   $$\frac{\text{Amount of drug desired}}{\text{Amount of drug weighed}} = \frac{\text{Amount of dilution weighed}}{\text{Total amount of dilution}}$$

   $$\frac{0.35 \text{ mg}}{120 \text{ mg}} = \frac{120 \text{ mg}}{x}; \, x = 41{,}143 \text{ mg dilution}$$

   The amount of dilution needed is 41,143 mg (120 mg hyoscine plus 41,023 mg of lactose). This represents a ratio of 41,023 to 120, or 342:1.

C. Perform a serial dilution.

Example 10.5

drug/amount desired: **hyoscine HBr 0.35 mg**

1. Basic steps
   a. Weigh the MWQ of hyoscine 120 mg.
   b. Weigh an arbitrary amount of lactose that is ≥ MWQ. In this case, because we need such a small quantity of drug, chose a larger quantity of lactose: 3,000 mg is selected.
   c. Thoroughly mix the two powders by triturating in a mortar. Remember to use geometric dilution.
   d. Calculate the total weight of the dilution: 120 mg + 3,000 mg = 3,120 mg dilution A.
   e. Weigh the MWQ, 120 mg, of dilution A.
   f. Calculate the number of milligrams of hyoscine that will be contained in 120 mg of dilution A. By proportion:

   $$\frac{120 \text{ mg hyoscine}}{3{,}120 \text{ mg dilution A}} = \frac{x \text{ mg hyoscine}}{120 \text{ mg dilution A}}; \, x = 4.6 \text{ mg hyoscine}$$

By dimensional analysis:

$$\left(\frac{120 \text{ mg hyoscine}}{3,120 \text{ mg dilution A}}\right)\left(\frac{120 \text{ mg dilution A}}{}\right) = 4.6 \text{ mg hyoscine}$$

g. Weigh a second amount of lactose that is ≥ MWQ. Again, because we need such a small quantity of drug, choose a moderate quantity of lactose: 3,000 mg is selected.

h. Thoroughly mix the 120 mg of dilution A with the 3,000 mg of lactose by triturating in a mortar.

i. Calculate the total weight of this second dilution: 120 mg + 3,000 mg = 3,120 mg dilution B.

j. Calculate the number of milligrams of dilution B that contains the desired 0.35 mg of hyoscine. (Remember that though you weighed 120 mg of dilution A, it contained only 4.6 mg of hyoscine.)

By proportion:

$$\frac{4.6 \text{ mg hyoscine}}{3,120 \text{ mg dilution B}} = \frac{0.35 \text{ mg hyoscine}}{x \text{ mg dilution B}}; x = 237 \text{ mg dilution B}$$

By dimensional analysis:

$$\left(\frac{3,120 \text{ mg dilution B}}{4.6 \text{ mg hyoscine}}\right)\left(\frac{0.35 \text{ mg hyoscine}}{}\right) = 237 \text{ mg dilution B}$$

k. Weigh this calculated amount of dilution B to get the desired 0.35 mg of hyoscine.

2. Analysis
   a. If the amount of dilution B is calculated to be less than the MWQ, either larger amounts of lactose may be used for the dilutions or a third dilution may be performed.
   b. If you do calculations of this sort frequently, you may wish to do an analysis like that done earlier for simple dilutions, or you may want to make a table similar to Table 10.1.

IV. SOLID-LIQUID ALIQUOTS

A. When a quantity of drug is needed that is below the MWQ and the drug is to be incorporated into a liquid preparation, such as a solution, an emulsion, or a suspension, it is usually better to make a solid-liquid aliquot. This can be done only if the drug or chemical is soluble in a suitable solvent (such as water or alcohol) that is compatible with the preparation. Solid-liquid aliquots are preferred because (i) they are easier to make—dissolving a drug in a solvent is less time-consuming than triturating a drug with a powdered diluent—and (ii) complete homogeneity of the dilution is achieved with the solutions obtained using solid-liquid aliquots, so there is not the concern about uniform mixing, which is a possible problem with solid-solid aliquots.

B. **Aliquot method 1: MWQ Method**
   This is the aliquot method that is based on measuring the MWQ of the drug, adding diluent, then calculating the amount of dilution to contain the desired quantity of drug.

Example 10.6   *drug/amount desired:* **hydromorphone HCl 8 mg**

1. Basic steps
   a. Weigh the MWQ of hydromorphone HCl: 120 mg.
   b. Check the solubility of hydromorphone HCl in the chosen solvent, water: 1 g/3 mL.
   c. Dissolve the hydromorphone in a convenient volume of water: 12 mL.
   d. Calculate the concentration of the drug in solution:

   $$120 \text{ mg}/12 \text{ mL} = 10 \text{ mg/mL}$$

   e. Calculate the number of milliliters of dilution that contain the desired 8 mg of hydromorphone.
   By proportion:

   $$\frac{10 \text{ mg hydromorphone}}{1 \text{ mL solution}} = \frac{8 \text{ mg hydromorphone}}{x \text{ mL solution}}; x = 0.8 \text{ mL solution}$$

By dimensional analysis:

$$\left(\frac{1 \text{ mL solution}}{10 \text{ mg hydromorphone}}\right)\left(\frac{8 \text{ mg hydromorphone}}{}\right) = 0.8 \text{ mL solution}$$

    f. Measure this calculated amount of the solution to get the desired 8 mg of hydromorphone.

2. Analysis

    a. When using 120 mg of the drug, 12 mL and 120 mL are convenient quantities of diluent as they give concentrations of 10 mg/mL (120 mg/12 mL) and 1 mg/mL (120 mg/120 mL), respectively. Concentrations such as these make the mathematics relatively easy.

    b. The amount of diluent chosen depends on the solubility of the drug, the amount of liquid that can be accommodated in the preparation, and the MMQ of the available measuring device.

    c. In the foregoing example, the amount of solution to be measured is 0.8 mL. This quantity can be measured accurately in a 1- or 3-mL syringe. If syringes or micropipettes are not accessible and the smallest graduated cylinder available has a capacity of 10 mL, a different aliquot would be necessary. Because the MMQ is 20% of the capacity of a graduated cylinder, 2 mL would be the MMQ for a 10-mL graduated cylinder. In this case, the drug could be dissolved in 120 mL of water, giving a concentration of 1 mg/mL. The volume needed for 8 mg would be 8 mL. Other intermediate dilutions could be used as the circumstances dictate.

C. Aliquot method 2: Dilution Factor Method

This is the aliquot method that is based on using a dilution factor, adding diluent, then using the inverse of the dilution factor to obtain the desired quantity of drug.

Example 10.7

drug/amount desired: **hydromorphone HCl 8 mg**

1. Basic steps

    a. Select a dilution factor that gives an amount that is ≥ MWQ, and weigh this amount:

$$15 \times 8 \text{ mg} = 120 \text{ mg}$$

    b. Check the solubility of hydromorphone HCl in the chosen solvent, water: 1 g/3 mL.

    c. Dissolve the hydromorphone in a convenient volume of water: 15 mL.

    d. Calculate the aliquot part of the dilution that contains the 8 mg of hydromorphone by multiplying the solution volume by the inverse of the dilution factor, 1/15 in this case: 1/15 × 15 mL = 1 mL.

    e. Measure this volume of the solution to get the desired 8 mg of hydromorphone.

2. Analysis

    a. Again, the amount of diluent chosen depends on the solubility of the drug, the amount of liquid that can be accommodated in the preparation, and the MMQ of the available measuring device.

    b. In this example the dilution factor may not be chosen at random. It must be 15 because 15 × 8 mg = 120 mg. Hydromorphone is a controlled substance that requires no extra waste. As was illustrated in the section on solid-solid aliquots, the dilution factor can be calculated using the following equation:

$$dilution\ factor = \frac{120 \text{ mg}}{quantity\ of\ drug\ needed}$$

As was illustrated in the discussion on solid-solid aliquots, this method is not as convenient when a specified weight of drug must be measured, such as 120 mg, and the amount of drug needed is not a factor of this weight. For our example, 8 is a factor of 120, so a convenient integer, 15, is calculated for the dilution factor. If the amount of drug needed were 9 mg, the dilution factor would be a less convenient 13.33.

    c. In choosing the amount of solution to make, 15 mL was chosen as a convenient volume. Any volume that is a multiple (may be a whole number or a decimal) of the dilution factor is a convenient amount. This is because the volume of the aliquot is determined by multiplying the volume of solution by the inverse of the dilution factor. Any volume that is a multiple of the dilution factor gives an aliquot that has a non-rounded volume.

    d. In the previous example, the amount of solution to be measured is 1 mL. This quantity can be measured accurately in a 1- or 3-mL syringe. If syringes or micropipettes are not accessible and the smallest graduated cylinder available has a capacity of 10 mL, a different aliquot would be necessary. As just indicated, 2 mL is the MMQ for a 10-mL graduated cylinder. In this case, the drug could be dissolved in 30 mL of water. A 1/15 aliquot needed to obtain 8 mg would then be 2 mL. Other dilutions could be used as the circumstances dictate.

V.   **LIQUID–LIQUID ALIQUOTS AND SERIAL DILUTIONS**

A. Liquid–liquid aliquots can be required of two different types of liquids: a pure liquid or a concentrated solution of a drug. Aliquots of pure liquids are relatively uncommon because few drugs are liquid in their pure state. Aliquots involving concentrated solutions are more common. Examples of both are given here.

B. Pure liquid

    1. Determine the necessity of an aliquot. Use direct volumetric measurement if appropriate equipment is available.

Example 10.8   *drug/amount desired:* **glacial acetic acid 0.2 mL**

If a 1-mL syringe or a micropipette is available, measure 0.2 mL directly. If the smallest measuring device is a 10-mL graduated cylinder, an aliquot method of measurement is needed.

---

    2. Aliquot Method 1: MMQ Method

        If appropriate equipment is not available for direct measurement, you may use an aliquot method that is based on the MMQ for your smallest measuring device.

Example 10.9   *drug/amount desired:* **glacial acetic acid 0.2 mL**

1. Basic steps

    a. The smallest volumetric device available is a 10-mL graduated cylinder.

    b. Measure the MMQ (20% of the capacity of the graduated cylinder) in a 10-mL graduated cylinder: 2 mL.

    c. Completely transfer the liquid to a graduated cylinder of adequate size: a 25-mL graduated cylinder is selected.

    d. Q.s. with water to a convenient amount: 20 mL.

        Note: In this case, because glacial acetic acid is a concentrated acid for which the normal procedure is to add acid to water, you would put some of the water in the 25-mL graduated cylinder; transfer the glacial acetic acid to the graduate, then q.s. to the final volume with water and mix well.

    e. Calculate the volume of the solution needed to give the 0.2 mL of glacial acetic acid:
By proportion:

$$\frac{2 \text{ mL gl. acetic acid}}{20 \text{ mL solution}} = \frac{0.2 \text{ mL gl. acetic acid}}{x \text{ mL solution}}; \quad x = 2 \text{ mL solution}$$

By dimensional analysis:

$$\left(\frac{20 \text{ mL solution}}{2 \text{ mL gl. acetic acid}}\right)\left(\frac{0.2 \text{ mL gl. acetic acid}}{}\right) = 2 \text{ mL solution}$$

    f. Measure this calculated amount of the solution to get the desired 0.2 mL of glacial acetic acid.

---

    3. Aliquot method 2: Dilution Factor Method

Example 10.10   *drug/amount desired: glacial acetic acid 0.2 mL*

1. Basic steps

    a. The smallest volumetric device available is a 10-mL graduated cylinder, which has an MMQ of 2 mL.

    b. Select a dilution factor that gives an amount that is ≥ MMQ for your smallest measuring device; measure this amount:

$$10 \times 0.2 \text{ mL} = 2 \text{ mL}$$

    c. Transfer the liquid to a graduated cylinder of adequate size: a 25-mL graduated cylinder is selected.

    d. Q.s. with water to a convenient amount: 20 mL.

       Note: Again with this case, because glacial acetic acid is a concentrated acid for which the normal procedure is to add acid to water, you would put some of the water in the 25-mL graduated cylinder; transfer the glacial acetic acid to the graduate, then q.s. to the final volume with water and mix well.

    e. Calculate the aliquot part of the dilution that contains the 0.2 mL of glacial acetic acid by multiplying the solution volume by the inverse of the dilution factor, 1/10 in this case:

$$1/10 \times 20 \text{ mL} = 2 \text{ mL}$$

    f. Measure this volume of the solution to get the desired 0.2 mL of glacial acetic acid.

C. Concentrated solutions

1. Determine the quantity of drug needed for the final preparation.
2. Determine whether the volume of concentrated solution needed for the desired drug quantity can be measured directly. Use direct volumetric measurement if appropriate equipment is available.

3. For concentrated solutions, if appropriate equipment is not available for direct measurement, it is easiest to use the aliquot method that is based on the MMQ for your smallest measuring device.

Example 10.11

drug/amount desired: **benzalkonium chloride 1.5 mg**

Benzalkonium chloride (BAC) is often used as a preservative for liquid preparations in a concentration of 0.01%. It is commercially available as a 17% w/v concentrated solution of BAC in water. For this example, 15 mL of an ophthalmic solution is prescribed, and 0.01% w/v BAC is desired as the preservative.

1. Calculate the quantity of BAC needed for the prescribed preparation.

$$\frac{0.01 \text{ g BAC}}{100 \text{ mL}} = \frac{x \text{ g BAC}}{15 \text{ mL}} \; ; x = 0.0015 \text{ g} = 1.5 \text{ mg BAC}$$

2. Determine whether the volume of concentrated solution needed for the desired drug quantity can be measured directly.

   By proportion:

$$\frac{17 \text{ g BAC}}{100 \text{ mL solution}} = \frac{0.0015 \text{ g BAC}}{x \text{ mL solution}} \; ; x = 0.0088 \text{ mL solution}$$

   By dimensional analysis:

$$\left(\frac{100 \text{ mL solution}}{17 \text{ g BAC}} \right) \left(\frac{0.0015 \text{ g BAC}}{} \right) = 0.0088 \text{ mL solution}$$

   The volume 0.0088 mL is too small to measure, even with a syringe. An aliquot method must be used.

3. MMQ aliquot method

   a. Measure the MMQ in a 1 mL syringe: 0.2 mL.

   b. Calculate the amount of BAC in the 0.2 mL:

     By proportion:

$$\frac{17 \text{ g BAC}}{100 \text{ mL solution}} = \frac{x \text{ g BAC}}{0.2 \text{ mL solution}} \; ; x = 0.034 \text{ g} = 34 \text{ mg BAC}$$

     By dimensional analysis:

$$\left(\frac{17 \text{ g BAC}}{100 \text{ mL solution}} \right) \left(\frac{0.2 \text{ mL solution}}{} \right) = 0.034 \text{ g} = 34 \text{ mg BAC}$$

   c. From the quantity calculated here, determine a convenient volume of solution for the dilution: 34 mL is selected.

d. Transfer the 0.2 mL of concentrated BAC to an appropriate sized graduated cylinder (e.g., 50-mL) and q.s. with water to the volume determined in c. : 34 mL. Mix well.

e. Calculate the concentration of the drug in the diluted solution:

$$34 \text{ mg}/34 \text{ mL} = 1 \text{ mg/mL}$$

f. Calculate the volume of the solution needed to give the 1.5 mg of BAC:
By proportion:

$$\frac{1 \text{ mg BAC}}{1 \text{ mL solution}} = \frac{1.5 \text{ mg BAC}}{x \text{ mL solution}} ; x = 1.5 \text{ mL solution}$$

By dimensional analysis:

$$\left(\frac{1 \text{ mL solution}}{1 \text{ mg BAC}}\right)\left(\frac{1.5 \text{ mg BAC}}{}\right) = 1.5 \text{ mL solution}$$

g. Measure this calculated amount of the solution to get the desired 1.5 mg of BAC.

4. Analysis
   a. The mathematics is easiest if the amount of the aliquot solution is chosen to give a convenient concentration of the drug in solution. This is done by first calculating the amount of drug or chemical in the measurable volume of the concentrate and then matching the volume of the aliquot solution to this quantity. In this case, the measurable volume of 0.2 mL of the BAC concentrate gives 34 mg of BAC. Therefore, 34 mL was chosen for the aliquot volume to give a convenient concentration of 1 mg/mL. Convenient numbers such as these make it easier to check you answers to be sure that they are reasonable.
   b. Once again, the amount of diluent chosen depends on the amount of liquid that can be accommodated in the final preparation and the measuring devices available.

Example 10.12

One of the most common uses for liquid-liquid aliquots is the preparation of dilute solutions of antibiotics and some other drugs for skin tests and desensitization procedures. The appendix section of the *Drug Information Handbook* contains a number of these protocols. A typical example for penicillin skin test preparation is given here.

You are asked to prepare a multidose vial containing 20 penicillin G skin tests, each with a concentration of 10 units/0.1 mL. You have available a vial of reconstituted penicillin G 100,000 units/mL and a vial of Sterile Water for Injection. Prepare the needed vial of skin tests.

1. Calculate the quantities needed for the desired preparation.
   a. Calculate the number of units of penicillin G (Pen G) needed for the multidose vial.

$$\frac{10 \text{ units}}{1 \text{ test}} = \frac{x \text{ units}}{20 \text{ tests}} ; x = 200 \text{ units}$$

   b. Calculate the final volume of the drug solution desired for the skin tests.

$$\frac{0.1 \text{ mL}}{1 \text{ test}} = \frac{x \text{ mL}}{20 \text{ tests}} ; x = 2 \text{ mL}$$

2. Determine whether the desired quantity of drug solution can be measured directly. Do this by calculating the volume of the reconstituted Pen G solution needed to give 200 units of Pen G.

$$\frac{100{,}000 \text{ units Pen G}}{\text{mL reconst'd soln}} = \frac{200 \text{ units Pen G}}{x \text{ mL reconst'd soln}} ; x = 0.002 \text{ mL}$$

   This is a volume too small to measure with available syringes.

3. MMQ aliquot method
   a. From the reconstituted Pen G vial, withdraw the MMQ with a 1-mL syringe: 0.2 mL.
   b. Calculate the number of units of Pen G contained in this volume.

$$\frac{100{,}000 \text{ units Pen G}}{1 \text{ mL}} = \frac{x \text{ units Pen G}}{0.2 \text{ mL}} ; x = 20{,}000 \text{ units Pen G}$$

   c. Inject this volume into an empty 20-mL sterile vial.
   d. Add to the vial a volume of Sterile Water for Injection that gives a convenient volume (i.e., a volume that does not exceed the capacity of the vial and that gives a concentration of Pen G

that is convenient for calculation): 19.8 mL Sterile Water for Injection is added to give a total volume of 20 mL.

$$20,000 \text{ units Pen G}/20 \text{ mL} = 1,000 \text{ units Pen G}/\text{mL}$$

e. Calculate the volume of this solution that will give the desired 200 units of Pen G.

$$\frac{1,000 \text{ units Pen G}}{1 \text{ mL}} = \frac{200 \text{ units Pen G}}{x \text{ mL}} ; x = 0.2 \text{ mL}$$

Notice that with the convenient volume selected, this value can be easily checked by inspection.

f. Withdraw this volume (0.2 mL) and transfer to a fresh empty sterile vial; then add 1.8 mL of Sterile Water for Injection. This gives the desired multidose vial with 200 units/2 mL (i.e., 20 skin tests each with a concentration of 10 units/0.1mL).

4. Analysis
   a. If the volume calculated just now in e. is still below the MMQ, a third dilution will be required.
   b. Often for dilutions such as this, some mathematical manipulation of quantities and volumes is required. As always, start with a quantity at or near the MMQ and pick diluent volumes that give convenient concentrations.
   c. Finally, because the mathematics can sometimes be complex, have a colleague verify your answer.

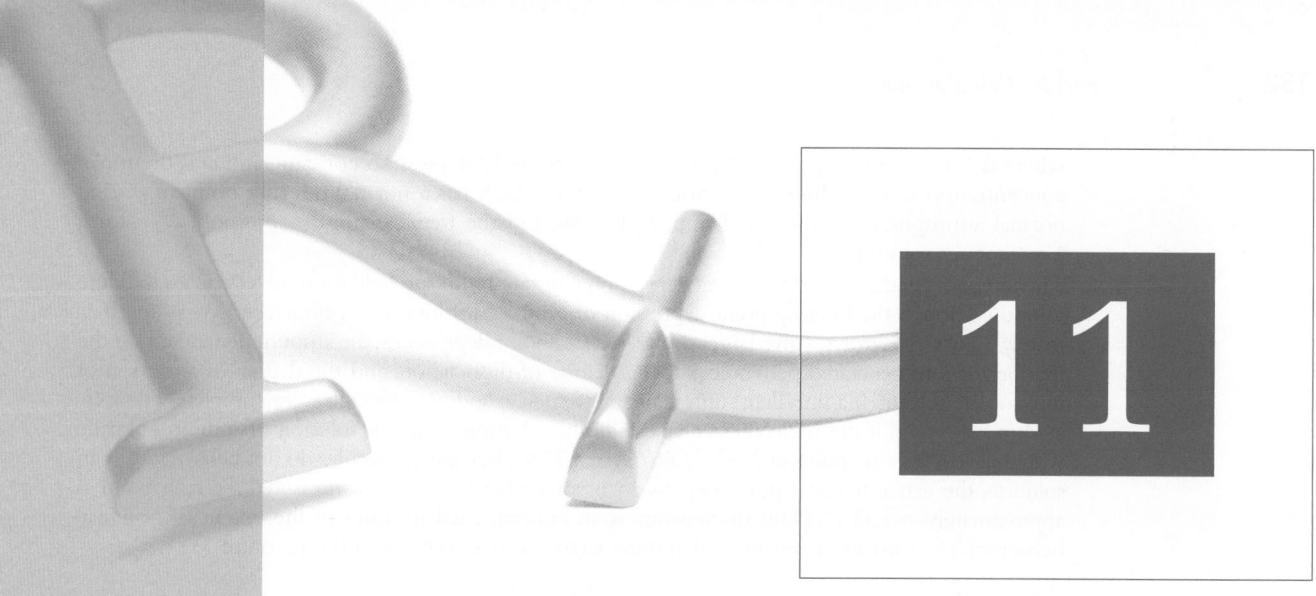

11

Isotonicity Calculations

I. **GENERAL PRINCIPLES**

A. Pharmaceutical solutions are sometimes applied to the sensitive membranes of the eye or nasal passages, or they may be injected into muscles, blood vessels, organs, tissue, or lesions. These solutions should be adjusted to have approximately the same osmotic pressure as that of body fluids because solutions that have the same osmotic pressure as cell contents do not cause a net movement of fluid into or out of the cells and therefore do not cause tissue damage or discomfort when placed in contact with cells. Solutions that exert the same osmotic pressure are called *isoosmotic*; solutions that exert the same osmotic pressure as a body fluid are termed *isotonic*, meaning of equal tone.

B. Osmotic pressure, like vapor pressure lowering, freezing point depression, and boiling point elevation, is a colligative property. Colligative properties depend not on the weight or the nature of the solute present in solution but only on the **number of solute particles** per given volume of solution. For example, one mole of dextrose (180 grams), when dissolved in one liter of solution, has the same effect on the osmotic pressure as does one mole per liter of sucrose (342 grams). Both of these substances are nonelectrolytes, and one mole of each gives an equal number of solute particles (Avogadro's number—6.02×10^{23}) when dissolved in water. In contrast, one mole of a univalent–univalent electrolyte, such as sodium chloride (58.5 grams), has twice the effect on osmotic pressure when dissolved in a liter of water because each sodium chloride gives two particles, an Na^+ ion and a Cl^- ion, when this salt is dissolved in water.

C. For pharmaceutical solutions, though we are interested in the changes in osmotic pressure caused by dissolved drugs and chemicals, we usually measure changes in freezing point caused by these substances. This is because osmotic pressure is difficult to measure directly, whereas freezing points are determined rather easily. Because both osmotic pressure and freezing point depression are colligative properties, freezing point depression can be used as a measure of change in osmotic pressure caused by dissolved drug or solute.

D. The fundamental expression relating freezing point depression and concentration of solute in solution is given by the equation

$$\Delta T_f = K_f m$$

where ΔT_f is the freezing point depression, K_f is the molal depression constant, and m is the molal concentration of the solute in solution. For water, which has a normal freezing point of $0°C$ at normal atmospheric pressure of 1 atm, K_f is 1.86, and the freezing point depression, ΔT_f, for a 1 m aqueous solution is $1.86°C$.

E. The foregoing equation and the molal depression constant hold true only for nonelectrolytes in dilute solution. Though the freezing point depression of a 1-molal solution of a nonelectrolyte is approximately $1.86°C$, electrolytes give larger molal freezing point depressions, the amount dependent on the number of ions generated per molecule, the degree of dissociation, and the degree of attraction of ions for the solvent. If a univalent–univalent solute such as sodium chloride were completely dissociated in water and if the molecules behaved ideally, a 1-molal aqueous solution of sodium chloride would have a freezing point of $2 \times -1.86° = -3.72°C$. Because molecules do not behave ideally in solution, the actual freezing point depression is somewhat less, and the measured freezing point is approximately $-3.35°C$. (This discrepancy is an experimental measure of the extent of nonideal behavior.) The van't Hoff equation takes these factors into account with the equation

$$\Delta T_f = iK_f m$$

where i, the van't Hoff factor, is the ratio of the colligative effect produced by a given concentration of electrolyte divided by the effect observed for the same concentration of nonelectrolyte.

F. This expression has been further modified for the dilute aqueous solutions encountered at isotonic concentrations to give the useful equation:

$$\Delta T_f = L_{iso}\, c$$

where c is the molar (rather than the molal) concentration of solute in aqueous solution and L_{iso} is the experimentally determined iK_f, the molar freezing point depression at isotonic concentration of the various ionic types (e.g., nonelectrolytes, univalent-univalent electrolytes, univalent-divalent electrolytes). Table 11.1 gives average L_{iso} values for various ionic types (1). The foregoing equation and the values in Table 11.1 can be used to estimate freezing point depression for solutes in aqueous solution for which there are no published values of freezing point depression for that solute.

G. Known concentrations of various drugs and chemicals have been dissolved in water and the freezing points of the solutions measured. These values have been published, and the table in Appendix D gives values for many common drugs; more complete tables of values can be found in *Remington: The Science and Practice of Pharmacy,* and in the miscellaneous tables section in the back of the 13th edition of *The Merck Index.* For more information on this subject, consult a book on physical pharmacy such as *Martin's Physical Pharmacy and Pharmaceutical Sciences* or the applicable chapters in *Remington: The Science and Practice of Pharmacy.*

II. FREEZING POINT DEPRESSION METHOD

A. Scientists have accurately measured the freezing points of the two critical body fluids, blood and tears, and have found these to be approximately the same: $-0.52°C$. For drug solutions to be isotonic with these fluids, they must have this same freezing point.

B. As stated, the freezing point depressions of many drugs in various concentrations in water have been measured and published in tables such as those shown in Appendix D, where the values in the column marked $\Delta T_f^{1\%}$ are the freezing point depressions in degrees Celsius of 1% solutions of the drug or chemical in water. Because freezing point depression is additive, pharmacists can use these data to calculate the amount of solute to add in making isotonic solutions (i.e., in making solutions with the same freezing point as blood or tears). This method of adjusting the tonicity of solutions using freezing point depression is shown next. The values for the example are taken from Appendix D.

C. Basic steps of the freezing point depression method
  1. Note or determine the percent concentration of the drug in the prescribed solution.
  2. Read from Appendix D the freezing point depression caused by a 1% concentration of the drug in solution.
  3. Calculate the freezing point depression caused by the prescribed concentration of drug in solution.
  4. Subtract this from the desired freezing point depression of $0.52°$.
  5. Decide on an appropriate solute for adjusting the tonicity of the solution.
  6. Using the table, determine the freezing point depression caused by a 1% concentration of this solute in solution.
  7. Calculate the concentration of this solute needed to give the remaining freezing point depression.
  8. Calculate the weight of solute in grams needed for the desired quantity of solution.

Table 11.1	AVERAGE L_{iso} VALUES BY IONIC TYPE (1)	
IONIC TYPE	**AVERAGE L_{iso} VALUE**	**EXAMPLES**
Nonelectrolytes: Substances that do not dissociate in aqueous solution	1.9	Sucrose, dextrose, camphor, glycerin
Weak electrolytes: Substances that dissociate very slightly in solution	2.0	Weak acids, such as boric acid and citric acid, amine bases such as ephedrine and codeine
Divalent-divalent electrolytes: Substances that dissociate into two ions, the anion polyvalent	2.0	Magnesium sulfate, zinc sulfate
Univalent-univalent electrolytes: Substances that dissociate into two ions, the anion univalent	3.4	Sodium chloride, silver nitrate, cocaine hydrochloride, pilocarpine hydrochloride, penicillin V potassium
Univalent-divalent electrolytes: Substances that dissociate into three ions, the anion polyvalent	4.3	Atropine sulfate, sodium carbonate, dibasic sodium phosphate (Na_2HPO_4), physostigmine sulfate
Divalent-univalent electrolytes: Substances that dissociate into three ions, the anion univalent	4.8	Calcium chloride, calcium gluconate, zinc chloride, magnesium chloride
Univalent-trivalent electrolytes: Substances that dissociate into four ions, the anion polyvalent	5.2	Sodium citrate, potassium citrate
Trivalent-univalent electrolytes: Substances that dissociate into four ions, the anion univalent	6.0	Aluminum chloride, ferric chloride
Tetraborates	7.6	Sodium borate, potassium borate

Example 11.1   Ŗ   Atropine sulfate   2%

Make isotonic with boric acid

Purified Water   qs ad   15 mL

1. Note or determine the percent concentration of the drug in the prescribed solution: 2%.
2. Read from Appendix D the freezing point depression caused by a 1% concentration of the drug in solution: 0.07°.
3. Calculate the freezing point depression caused by the prescribed concentration of drug in solution.

$$\frac{1\%}{0.07°} = \frac{2\%}{x}; x = 0.14°$$

4. Subtract this from the desired freezing point depression of 0.52°.

$$0.52° - 0.14° = 0.38°$$

5. Decide on an appropriate solute for adjusting the tonicity of the solution: boric acid.

   Note: In this case, the medication order specified boric acid. This chemical is a common ophthalmic additive because it serves the dual purpose of mild buffering and isotonicity adjustment.

6. Using the table, determine the freezing point depression caused by a 1% concentration of this solute in solution: 0.29°.

7. Calculate the concentration of this solute needed to give the remaining freezing point depression.

$$\frac{1\%}{0.29°} = \frac{x\%}{0.38°}; x = 1.3\%$$

8. Calculate the weight of solute in grams needed for the desired quantity of solution.

$$1.3\% \times 15 \text{ mL} = 0.195 \text{ g boric acid}$$

III.   SODIUM CHLORIDE EQUIVALENT METHOD

A. Pharmaceutical scientists decided it would be convenient to have an easier way of calculating the amount of solute to add in adjusting the tonicity of solutions. In 1936 Mellen and Seltzer devised a system to compare the freezing point depression caused by sodium chloride to that of common drugs (2). Sodium chloride was chosen because it is the most common solute used for tonicity adjustment.

B. Mellen and Seltzer developed a factor, called the *Sodium Chloride Equivalent*, which is the weight in grams of sodium chloride that will give an equivalent osmotic effect to that of 1 gram of the designated drug.

C. Sodium Chloride Equivalents for a large number of drugs have been published. Values for many common drugs and chemicals are shown in Appendix D in the column marked $E_{NaCl}^{1\%}$. Some references use the designation "E" (for Equivalent) to designate the Sodium Chloride Equivalents.

D. Ideally, the Sodium Chloride Equivalent should be the same for a given drug at all concentrations, but it can be observed in the extensive tables published in *Remington* and *The Merck Index*, that these values decrease slightly as the solute concentration is increased. This is a demonstration of the increasing effect on colligative properties of molecular and ionic interactions as the concentration of the solute is increased. Although it is always best to use the most precise value available, for pharmaceutical purposes, the E value at 1% concentration is sufficient.

E. The Sodium Chloride Equivalent method is based on the fact that a 0.9% concentration of sodium chloride in water gives an isotonic solution. This isotonic solution is also known as normal saline, isotonic saline, or isotonic sodium chloride. It is often abbreviated NSS for normal saline solution or NS for normal saline. The Sodium Chloride Equivalent method is illustrated next.

F. Basic steps of the Sodium Chloride Equivalent method
   1. Calculate the number of grams of drug in the solution.
   2. Read from Appendix D the Sodium Chloride Equivalent for the drug (that is, the weight in grams of sodium chloride that is equivalent to one gram of drug).
   3. Calculate the weight in grams of sodium chloride that is equivalent to the weight in grams of the drug in this solution.
   4. Calculate the number of grams of sodium chloride needed to make the desired volume of the drug solution isotonic if no other solute were present.
   5. Subtract the weight in grams of sodium chloride that is equivalent to the weight of the drug from the weight of sodium chloride that would be needed to make the solution isotonic.
   6. Add this amount of sodium chloride to the solution.

Example 11.2   **Rx**   Atropine sulfate   2%

Make isotonic with sodium chloride

Purified Water   qs ad   15 mL

1. Calculate the number of grams of drug in the solution.

$$2\% \times 15 \text{ mL} = 0.3 \text{ g atropine sulfate}$$

2. Read from Appendix D the Sodium Chloride Equivalent for the drug: 0.13 (that is, 0.13 g NaCl is equivalent to 1 g atropine sulfate).

3. Calculate the weight in grams of sodium chloride that is equivalent to the weight in grams of the drug in this solution.

$$\frac{0.13 \text{ g NaCl}}{1 \text{ g atropine sulfate}} = \frac{x \text{ g NaCl}}{0.3 \text{ g atropine sulfate}}; x = 0.039 \text{ g NaCl}$$

4. Calculate the number of grams of sodium chloride needed to make the desired volume of the drug solution isotonic if no other solute were present.

$$0.9\% \times 15 \text{ mL} = 0.135 \text{ g NaCl}$$

5. Subtract the weight in grams of sodium chloride that is equivalent to the weight of the drug from the weight of sodium chloride that would be needed to make the solution isotonic.

$$0.135 \text{ g} - 0.039 \text{ g} = 0.096 \text{ g NaCl needed}$$

6. Add this amount of sodium chloride to the solution.

If the sodium chloride is available as sterile NSS (that is, 0.9% NaCl solution), the amount of this solution needed for isotonicity can be determined easily:

$$\frac{0.9 \text{ g NaCl}}{100 \text{ mL NSS}} = \frac{0.096 \text{ g NaCl}}{x \text{ mL NSS}}; x = 10.7 \text{ mL NSS}$$

In this case, the solution would be made by dissolving the 0.3 g of atropine sulfate in 10.7 mL of NSS and then qs ad 15 mL with Sterile Water.

Example 11.3

As you can see, this method is fairly simple if the tonicity adjustor is sodium chloride. It becomes more difficult if you want to use a different solute to adjust tonicity, such as the boric acid, which was used in the first example. In that case, another set of calculations is necessary to convert the amount of sodium chloride needed to an equivalent amount of the other solute. From Appendix D, the Sodium Chloride Equivalent for boric acid is 0.5. Therefore:

$$\frac{0.5 \text{ g NaCl}}{1 \text{ g boric acid}} = \frac{0.096 \text{ g NaCl}}{x \text{ g boric acid}}; x = 0.192 \text{ g boric acid}$$

Notice that the answer, 0.192 g of boric acid, is very close to the 0.195 g of boric acid that was calculated using the freezing point depression method.

IV. ## USP METHOD (ALSO KNOWN AS THE WHITE–VINCENT METHOD OR THE SPROWLS METHOD)

A. The previous example using boric acid is somewhat common because buffering agents are sometimes desired in isotonic ophthalmic solutions, and they can serve the dual purpose of buffering and tonicity adjustment. When several solutes are being added to a solution, such as when Sorensen's Buffer is used, the mathematics in using the Sodium Chloride Equivalent method become cumbersome.

B. In 1947, White and Vincent developed a simple and easy system to handle these situations (3). They made use of the fact that colligative effects are additive, so when one isotonic solution is added to another isotonic solution, you get an isotonic solution. They reasoned that the easiest way to make an isotonic solution would be to add sufficient water to the desired amount of drug to make an isotonic solution and then qs to the desired volume with an isotonic diluting solution, either normal saline or an isotonic buffer solution.

C. To put this system into practice, the volume of water, which will make an isotonic solution with a given weight of drug, must be determined. For this purpose, White and Vincent developed the following equation:

$$V = w \times E \times 111.1$$

where
V = the volume in milliliters of isotonic solution that will be prepared by mixing the drug with water
w = the weight in grams of the drug
E = the sodium chloride equivalent of the drug
111.1 is the volume in milliliters of the isotonic solution obtained when dissolving 1 g of sodium chloride in water.

Note: The value *111.1* is calculated from the 0.9% w/v concentration of sodium chloride in water, which gives an isotonic solution:

$$\frac{0.9 \text{ g NaCl}}{100 \text{ mL isotonic solution}} = \frac{1 \text{ g NaCl}}{x \text{ mL isotonic solution}}; x = 111.1 \text{ mL isotonic solution}$$

The validity of the White-Vincent equation can be verified using dimensional analysis:

$$\left(\frac{w \text{ g of drug}}{}\right)\left(\frac{E \text{ g NaCl}}{1 \text{ g drug}}\right)\left(\frac{111.1 \text{ mL isotonic soln}}{1 \text{ g NaCl}}\right) = w \times E \times 111.1 \text{ mL isotonic sol'n}$$

D. In 1949, Sprowls published a paper on the use of this type of system for making isotonic solutions in the pharmacy.

    1. The paper, "A Further Simplification in the Use of Isotonic Diluting Systems," appeared in *The Journal of the American Pharmaceutical Association, Practical Pharmacy Edition*, and included a list of calculated V values, the number of milliliters of water that will make given weights of various drugs isotonic (4).

    2. Sprowls's list gave the volume of water to make 0.3 g of drug isotonic. This weight was chosen because 0.3 g is the weight of drug for 1 oz or 30 mL of a 1% solution, a common situation with ophthalmic solutions. Some later tables of V values list the volumes for 1 g of drug. Column V^{1g} in Appendix D uses this later convention.

E. It should be noted that the V values are not experimentally determined; they are derived values calculated from published Sodium Chloride Equivalents. Sodium Chloride Equivalent values, in turn, are also not experimentally determined, but are calculated from freezing point depression values that are measured in the lab.

F. Although the published tables of V values state that these are volumes of **water** needed to make a given weight of drug isotonic, the calculated volumes are really volumes of isotonic **solutions.** Furthermore, the assumption is made that the drug and sodium chloride have the same powder volume. Because isotonic solutions are dilute, the errors introduced by these approximations are small and insignificant for the intended purpose.

G. This method is sometimes called the *USP method* because at one time *USP* Chapter ⟨1151⟩, Pharmaceutical Dosage Forms, published tables with these values and explained this method of making isotonic solutions. This method is illustrated next.

H. Basic steps in the USP method

    1. Calculate the number of grams of drug in the solution.

    2. Read from Appendix D the number of milliliters of water needed to make 1 g of drug isotonic.

    3. Calculate the number of milliliters of water needed to make the desired weight of drug isotonic.

    4. Make this solution.

    5. Qs to the final desired volume with any isotonic solution.

Example 11.4

℞   Atropine sulfate   2%

    Make isotonic

    Purified Water   qs ad   15 mL

1. Calculate the number of grams of drug in the solution.

$$2\% \times 15 \text{ mL} = 0.3 \text{ g}$$

2. Read from Appendix D the number of milliliters of water needed to make 1 g of drug isotonic: 14.3 mL.

3. Calculate the number of milliliters of water needed to make the desired weight of drug isotonic.

$$\frac{1 \text{ g atropine sulfate}}{14.3 \text{ mL water}} = \frac{0.3 \text{ g atropine sulfate}}{x \text{ mL water}} \; ; x = 4.29 \text{ mL water}$$

4. Make this solution.

5. Qs to the final desired volume with any isotonic solution: 0.9% Sodium Chloride, 1.9% Boric Acid solution, Sorensen's Modified Buffer, and so on.

Notice that the 4.3 mL of water calculated in this part plus the 10.7 mL of isotonic saline calculated in the section on Sodium Chloride Equivalents add up to the 15 mL of total solution needed.

I. If you prefer to use a system such as this but do not have V values, you can calculate them easily using published Sodium Chloride Equivalents and the equation by White and Vincent. The sample calculation shown here uses the data from the atropine sulfate examples shown previously.

$$V = w \times E \times 111.1$$

$$V = \left(\frac{0.3 \text{ g atropine}}{1 \text{ g atropine}} \right) \left(\frac{0.13 \text{ g NaCl}}{1 \text{ g atropine}} \right) \left(\frac{111.1 \text{ mL isotonic sol'n}}{1 \text{ g NaCl}} \right) = 4.3 \text{ mL}$$

They may also be calculated from the percent concentration of isotonic sodium chloride solution (0.9%) and the Sodium Chloride Equivalent for the drug.

$$\left(\frac{100 \text{ mL isotonic sol'n}}{0.9 \text{ g NaCl}} \right) \left(\frac{0.13 \text{ g NaCl}}{1 \text{ g atropine}} \right) \left(\frac{0.3 \text{ g atropine}}{} \right) = 4.3 \text{ mL}$$

V. L_{ISO} METHOD

A. As was discussed in the introduction to this chapter, the equation $\Delta T_f = L_{iso} \, c$ can be used to estimate freezing point depressions for solutes in aqueous solution when isotonicity values for freezing point depression or Sodium Chloride Equivalents are not available. It is possible that this will become more common in coming years. For nearly 30 years, two pharmaceutical scientists, Dr. E. R. Hammarlund and Dr. Kaj Pedersen-Bjergaard, were responsible for determining freezing point depression and Sodium Chloride Equivalent values for many drugs and chemicals, and together or individually they published those values in pharmaceutical journals from 1958 until 1989. As new drugs become available, the needed values may not be available for pharmacists to use in making the above calculations, and it will be necessary to rely on estimates based on the general L_{iso} equation.

B. Basic steps of the L_{iso} method
   1. Determine the molar concentration of the drug in solution. (If the prescribed drug concentration is given in percent or weight per volume, locate the molecular weight of the drug and use this to calculate the molar concentration. See the next example and examples in Chapter 8 for molar concentration sample calculations.)
   2. From the chemical structure of the drug, determine its ionic type.
   3. Using Table 11.1, determine the L_{iso} for the ionic type of the drug.
   4. Using the L_{iso} equation, calculate the freezing point depression (ΔT_f) that results from the calculated molar concentration of drug in solution.
   5. Subtract this from the desired freezing point depression of 0.52°.
   6. Decide on an appropriate solute for adjusting the tonicity of the solution.
   7. Using the table in Appendix D, determine the freezing point depression caused by a 1% concentration of this solute in solution.
   8. Calculate the concentration of solute needed to give the remaining freezing point depression.
   9. Calculate the weight of solute in grams needed for the desired quantity of solution.

Example 11.5

For ease of comparison with results obtained from published freezing point depression values, we use the same prescription order as was given in Example 11.1.

℞ Atropine sulfate   2%

   Make isotonic with boric acid

   Purified Water   qs ad   15 mL

1. Determine the molar concentration of drug in solution.

Atropine sulfate is available as the monohydrate with a MW = 695.

$$\left(\frac{\text{mol atropine}}{695 \text{ g atropine}} \right) \left(\frac{2 \text{ g atropine}}{100 \text{ mL solution}} \right) \left(\frac{1{,}000 \text{ mL}}{\text{L}} \right) = 0.0288 \text{ mol/L}$$

2. From the chemical structure of the drug, determine its ionic type: Atropine sulfate is a univalent-divalent electrolyte.
3. Using Table 11.1, determine the L_{iso} for the ionic type of the drug: 4.3.

4. Using the L_{iso} equation, calculate the freezing point depression caused by the calculated molar concentration of drug in solution.

$$\Delta T_f = L_{iso}\ c = 4.3\ (0.0288) = 0.12°$$

5. Subtract this from the desired freezing point depression of 0.52°.

$$0.52° - 0.12° = 0.40°$$

6. Decide on an appropriate solute for adjusting the tonicity of the solution: boric acid.
7. Using the table in Appendix D, determine the freezing point depression caused by a 1% concentration of this solute in solution: 0.29°.
8. Calculate the concentration of solute needed to give the remaining freezing point depression.

$$\frac{1\%\ \text{boric acid}}{0.29°} = \frac{x\%\ \text{boric acid}}{0.40°}; x = 1.38\%\ \text{boric acid}$$

9. Calculate the weight of solute in grams needed for the desired quantity of solution.

$$1.38\% \times 15\ \text{mL} = 0.207\ \text{g boric acid}$$

As is apparent from the results in this example, the estimate of the freezing point depression value from the L_{iso} method (0.40°) is very close to the experimentally determined freezing point depression values (0.38°) as given in Example 11.1, and the amount of boric acid calculated to add in the L_{iso} method (0.207 g) is close to that calculated using a measured freezing point depression (0.195 g). The answer is well within the range that is considered useful for the purpose of making isotonic solutions.

REFERENCES

1. Wells JM. Rapid method for calculating isotonic solutions. J Am Pharm Assoc Pract Ed 1944; 5: 99–106.
2. Mellen M, Seltzer LA. A ready method for the extemporaneous preparation of isotonic collyria. J Am Pharm Assoc Sci Ed 1936; 25: 759–763.
3. White AI, Vincent HC. Diluting solutions in preparation of adjusted solutions. J Am Pharm Assoc Pract Ed 1947; 8: 406–411.
4. Sprowls JB. A further simplification in the use of isotonic diluting solutions. J Am Pharm Assoc Pract Ed 1949; 10: 348–351.

Part 3

Compounding Drug

Preparations

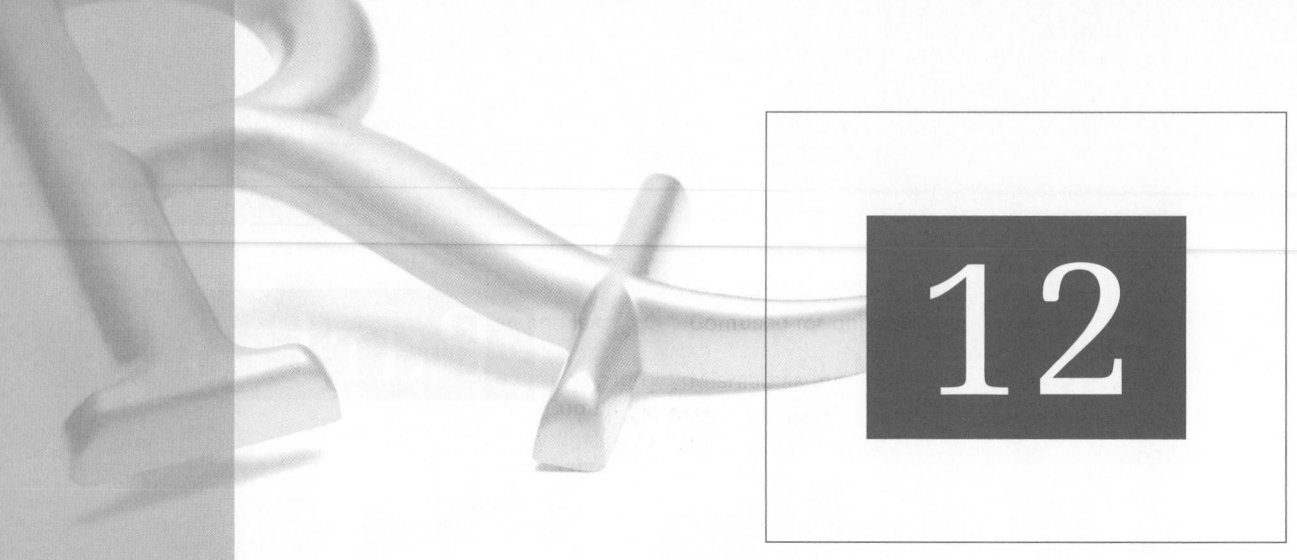

General Guidelines for Preparing Compounded Drug Preparations

I. DEFINITIONS

It is very important to define and distinguish between pharmacy compounding and pharmaceutical manufacturing because compounding is a part of professional practice, a function regulated primarily by state laws with enforcement by state government agencies, whereas manufacturing is regulated by the Food and Drug Administration (FDA) through the Federal Food, Drug, and Cosmetic Act (FDCA). Though differentiating between compounding and manufacturing would appear to be simple, in recent years it has been the subject of much controversy and even court cases, including one that was argued before the U.S. Supreme Court. In the United States, with multiple layers of regulation and enforcement (federal, state, and local), plus a long and strong legacy of individual rights, it is understandable that positioning of jurisdictional lines has the potential for dispute.

A. The following are definitions of compounding and manufacturing from the 2007 *National Association of Boards of Pharmacy* (NABP) *Model State Pharmacy Act*. They are also included in the NABP *Good Compounding Practices Applicable to State Licensed Pharmacies*. (The complete text of the current version of these documents can be accessed on the NABP Internet Web site at http://www.nabp.net, accessed December 2007.)

1. Compounding:

the preparation of Components into a drug product (i) as the result of a Practitioner's Prescription Drug Order or initiative based on the Practitioner/patient/Pharmacist relationship in the course of professional practice, or (ii) for the purpose of, or as an incident to, research, teaching, or chemical analysis and not for sale or Dispensing. Compounding includes the preparation of Drugs or Devices in anticipation of receiving Prescription Drug Orders based on routine, regularly observed prescribing patterns (1).

2. Manufacturing:

the production, preparation, propagation, conversion, or processing of a Drug or Device, either directly or indirectly, by extraction from substances of natural origin or independently by means of chemical or biological synthesis. Manufacturing includes the packaging or repackaging of a Drug or Device or the Labeling or relabeling of the container of a Drug or Device for resale by pharmacies, Practitioners, or other Persons (1).

B. Both *USP* Chapter ⟨795⟩ Pharmaceutical Compounding—Nonsterile Preparations, and Chapter ⟨1075⟩, Good Compounding Practices, have sections that describe and define compounding and differentiate it from manufacturing.

  1. Chapter ⟨1075⟩ states:

  > Compounding involves the preparation, mixing, assembling, packaging, and labeling of a drug or device in accordance with a licensed practitioner's prescription or medication order under an initiative based on the practitioner/patient/pharmacist/compounder relationship in the course of professional practice. Compounding includes the following:
  >
  >   **a)** Preparation of drugs or devices in anticipation of prescription drug orders based on routine, regularly observed prescribing patterns.
  >
  >   **b)** Reconstitution or manipulation of commercial products that may require the addition of one or more ingredients as a result of a licensed practitioner's prescription drug order.
  >
  >   **c)** Preparation of drugs or devices for the purposes of, or as an incident to, research, teaching, or chemical analysis (2).

  2. Chapter ⟨795⟩ lists three characteristics that differentiate compounding from manufacturing: "the existence of specific practitioner-patient-compounder relationships; the quantity of medication prepared in anticipation of receiving a prescription or prescription order; and the conditions of sale, which are limited to specific prescription orders" (3).

C. The Pharmacy Compounding Accreditation Board (PCAB) Standards contain a definition of compounding that includes the elements given in Chapter ⟨1075⟩ and adds compounding for practitioner administration (e.g., medical office use), for non-food animal patients (veterinary practice), and non-legend compounded preparations, in all cases as federal and state regulations allow (4).

D. The FDA gave its definition of compounding in the background information of a 2002 FDA study, "Survey of Drug Products Compounded by a Group of Community Pharmacies: Findings from a Food and Drug Administration Study":

  > Combining, mixing, or altering of ingredients by a licensed pharmacist to create a customized drug (e.g. removal of a dye due to patient allergy, conversion to a different dosage form for ease of administration) for a patient based on the receipt of a valid prescription or in anticipation of prescriptions based on an order history from pharmacist-physician-patient relationship. Excludes: mixing, reconstituting, or other acts in accordance with directions in FDA approved labeling (5).

  (Notice that though the *USP* and PCAB definitions include reconstitution of commercial products as part of compounding, the FDA specifically excludes this act when it is performed according to FDA-approved labeling.)

E. Finally, in a 2002 U.S. Supreme Court decision that dealt with the application of federal law to pharmacy compounding, Justice O'Connor, in the opinion of the Court, described compounding. In a concise statement, Justice O'Connor communicated the essence of drug compounding.

  > Drug compounding is a process by which a pharmacist or doctor combines, mixes, or alters ingredients to create a medication tailored to the needs of an individual patient. (6)

II.   EVOLUTION AND CURRENT STATUS OF COMPOUNDING IN PHARMACY PRACTICE

A. Though compounding drug dosage forms has been an integral part of the profession of pharmacy since antiquity, over the last 100 years, with the birth and growth of the pharmaceutical industry, there has been a significant decline in compounding by pharmacists. In the more recent past, starting in the mid-1980s, compounding customized drug preparations by pharmacists has increased and, in fact, has emerged as a specialty practice for some pharmacists. Estimates vary widely on the number of compounded prescriptions that are dispensed by pharmacies: A 2002 FDA estimate placed that number at approximately 250 million compounded prescriptions per year, between 1% and 8% of total prescriptions dispensed (5); a 2007 PCAB press release put the number at 30 million to 40 million compounded prescriptions per year. Even with the large variability in estimates, the number of compounded prescriptions is significant.

B. The reasons for the recent reemergence of compounding are varied.

  1. This increase has been due partly to a shift of interest on the part of the pharmacy profession from merely "dispensing" drugs to an intensified concern for patients and their individual drug therapy needs—the pharmaceutical care movement. The commonly used definition of pharmaceutical care promulgated by Hepler and Strand, "the responsible provision of drug therapy for the purpose of achieving definite outcomes that improve a patient's quality of life" (7), carries with it the tacit requirement for considering individualized dosage and drug delivery systems. Some examples include the following:

   a. Some drugs are available only as tablets or capsules, and some patients, (e.g., pediatric, geriatric, unconscious, very ill) cannot swallow these dosage forms. These patients need the drug formulated in a liquid, suppository, topical, or other specialized dosage form.

   b. Some patients, especially infants, children, and the elderly, need dosage strengths that are not commercially available.

   c. Some patients are allergic to an excipient (e.g., preservative, dye, diluent, binder) in the manufactured dosage form.

   d. Some patients, particularly children and animals, need special flavoring to make the drug more palatable and acceptable.

2. There is a renewed awareness that individual patient therapy needs cannot always be met by drug products from the pharmaceutical industry, which has constraints imposed upon it by mass production and market-share requirements.

   a. This is manifested in several ways: specialty and projected low-profit items are never introduced by a manufacturer, low-volume products are discontinued, and there are periodic shortages (sometimes for considerable lengths of time) for some products.

   b. The latter has become such a difficult and common problem that in the year 2001, the American Society of Health-System Pharmacists (ASHP) published the document, *ASHP Guidelines on Managing Drug Product Shortages*, which is available on the ASHP Internet site (http://www.ashp.org). Both ASHP and FDA (http://www.fda.gov/cder/drug/shortages, accessed February 2008) maintain Internet sites with current lists of drugs in short supply and discontinued products, information on handling drug product shortages, and links for reporting drug shortages.

   c. One obvious alternative for dealing with these problems is for the pharmacist to compound needed drug preparations when they are either temporarily or permanently not available from commercial sources.

3. Another factor that has contributed to an increase in drug compounding has been the trend toward home health care. For various reasons, including cost containment and patient comfort, patients who previously would have been concentrated for treatment in hospitals and medical centers are being treated at home. These patients often require individualized infusion therapy and other treatment modalities. This has created the need for an entire new type of pharmacy practice in which pharmacists in retail settings are required to prepare custom sterile and nonsterile dosage forms.

4. The expansion of custom-compounded drug preparations has been made possible in recent years partly because of the availability of new and useful items of equipment, packaging and labeling materials, excipients, and drugs and chemicals. New companies have been established, and older existing companies have expanded and specialize in marketing these needed compounding supplies.

5. Needed information on compatibility and stability of compounded drug preparations has become available and more widely disseminated.

   a. New books, journals, and technical support from pharmacy organizations and from the vendors of pharmacy supplies have played an important role in enabling compounding to modernize and flourish.

   b. The United States Pharmacopeia (USP), which has for many years provided standards for purity and stability of manufactured drug products, has taken the initiative to develop and publish general information chapters and monographs for compounded drug preparations with tested formulations and stability information.

C. The present status of compounding in pharmacy practice can be judged in part by its inclusion in current written standards of practice, in published national competencies for pharmacist licensure and pharmacy technician certification, and in laws, court decisions, and FDA compliance guidelines on compounding. It is the responsibility of pharmacists and pharmacy technicians to be knowledgeable about these standards.

1. NABP has several Model Rules that address compounding. As indicated at the beginning of this chapter, the complete texts of the documents can be accessed on the NABP Internet site.

    a. *Model Rules for the Practice of Pharmacy*

       (1) In the minimum requirements for a pharmacy: "Each pharmacy shall be of sufficient size to allow for the safe and proper storage of Prescription Drugs and for the safe and proper Compounding and/or preparation of Prescription Drug Orders" (8).

       (2) Included as an act of unprofessional conduct: "Unreasonably refusing to Compound or Dispense Prescription Drug Orders that may be expected to be Compounded or Dispensed by Pharmacies or Pharmacists" (8).

    b. *Good Compounding Practices Applicable to State Licensed Pharmacies*

    c. *Model Rules for Sterile Pharmaceuticals*

2. The competency statements for NAPLEX, the national pharmacist licensing exam, and for PTCE, the certification exam for pharmacy technicians, both include sections on compounding. For the complete NAPLEX competency statements, access the NAPLEX Blueprint through the NABP Internet site; the examination content outline and the knowledge base statements for the PTCE are available on the Pharmacy Technician Certification Board (PTCB) Internet site (https://www.ptcb.org, Accessed February 2008).

3. USP has developed and published standards and informational chapters on compounding, and monographs for compounded drug preparations.

    a. In November 1996, Chapter ⟨1161⟩ Pharmacy Compounding Practices was introduced in the fifth Supplement to *USP 23–NF 18*. This chapter was subsequently renamed as Pharmaceutical Compounding—Nonsterile Preparations and was renumbered as Chapter ⟨795⟩, which places it in that section of the *USP* that has traditionally been used for potentially legally enforceable standards. This chapter has become the basic standard of compounding practice for nonsterile dosage forms.

    b. Chapter ⟨1206⟩ Sterile Drug Products for Home Use was originally introduced as a general information chapter in *USP* for compounding sterile preparations for home health care. In the years between 2002 and 2007, a huge amount of work was done on this chapter in revising and expanding the content, and it has been renumbered and renamed as Chapter ⟨797⟩ Pharmaceutical Compounding—Sterile Preparations. It is now considered the standard of practice for sterile compounding in all health care settings.

    c. *USP* Chapter ⟨1191⟩, Stability Consideration in Dispensing Practice, has been updated, and three additional compounding chapters have been added to *USP* including ⟨1075⟩, Good Compounding Practices, ⟨1160⟩ Pharmaceutical Calculations, and ⟨1163⟩, Quality Assurance in Pharmaceutical Compounding.

    d. The first four modern compounding monographs became official with the ninth Supplement to *USP 23–NF 18* in 2002; 15 were included in *USP 24–NF 19*, and by the 2008 *USP 31–NF 26*, there were 129 official compounding monographs. The USP Pharmacy Compounding Expert Committee is very active in this area of development, and the number of these monographs continues to grow.

    e. In 2005, the first *USP Pharmacists' Pharmacopeia* was published. Though both *USP* and *NF* were originally books of recognized formulas for physicians and pharmacists to use in practice, the *USP–NF* (the "big red book" that is now published yearly in a three-volume set) has become a book that primarily addresses standards for the pharmaceutical industry. It was recognized that a similar book was needed to focus on standards for pharmacists. The *Pharmacists' Pharmacopeia* contains the General Notices, pertinent chapters from *USP–NF*, compounding monographs, abbreviated drug and excipient substance monographs with chemical structures, therapeutic categories, descriptions, solubilities, and packaging and storage information and a wealth of informational articles, and reference tables. The second printed edition of the *Pharmacists' Pharmacopeia* was published in 2008.

4. Federal law and FDA guidances

    a. In November 1997, Congress passed Public Law 105-115. Section 127. Application of Federal Law to Practice of Pharmacy Compounding. This law was part of the FDA Modernization Act of 1997 (FDAMA). It added a section, Sec. 503 A. Pharmacy Compounding, to the FDCA. This provision supported the right of licensed pharmacists and physicians to compound drug preparations, but with certain restrictions. Though the Supreme Court later held that a section of this law is an unconstitutional restriction of commercial free speech, the Court opinion supported the general concept of extemporaneous compounding of drug preparations by pharmacists and physicians (6). (For a discussion of the provisions of this law, applicable court cases, and current status, see the following section on historical perspective.)

  b. FDA's compliance policy guidance on pharmacy compounding states that it recognizes that pharmacists traditionally have extemporaneously compounded and manipulated drug products upon receipt of a valid prescription (9).

5. ASHP has been very active in the area of standards of practice for both sterile and nonsterile compounding. Their members developed some of the first written guidelines and technical assistance bulletins in these areas. They continue to offer a wide array of services, publications, seminars, and written guidelines on compounding. In addition, their general guidelines that set minimum standards for pharmacies and pharmaceutical services (*ASHP Guidelines: Minimum Standard for Pharmacies in Hospitals* and *ASHP Guidelines: Minimum Standard for Pharmaceutical Services in Ambulatory Care*) have requirements for providing extemporaneous compounding and sterile products for patients who need these services. Several ASHP guidelines that address specific areas of compounding are listed below; the complete documents can be accessed on the ASHP Web site.

 a. *ASHP Technical Assistance Bulletin on Compounding Nonsterile Products in Pharmacies*

 b. *ASHP Guidelines on Quality Assurance for Pharmacy-Prepared Sterile Products*

 c. *ASHP Guidelines on Handling Hazardous Drugs*

 d. *ASHP Guidelines on Pharmacy-Prepared Ophthalmic Products*

 e. *Safe Use of Automated Compounding Devices for the Preparation of Parenteral Nutrition Admixtures*

6. The International Academy of Compounding Pharmacists (IACP) was founded in 1991 as a not-for-profit association of compounding pharmacists. By 2008, with a membership of nearly 2,000 pharmacists, the organization works to promote the practice of pharmacy compounding by lobbying efforts at the state and national levels. It provides timely print and electronic newsletters, position papers, and documents from national legislative and regulatory government agencies. It serves its members by providing a network of pharmacists with a common interest in compounding and a referral service for patients or health care providers needing a pharmacy compounding service. Information about IACP is available at its Internet site at www.iacprx.org.

7. Various national and state pharmacy organizations sponsor and support special interest groups for compounding pharmacists. In addition, in 2004, eight national organizations, including the American College of Apothecaries, the American Pharmacists Association, the IACP, the NABP, the National Community Pharmacists Association, the National Council of State Pharmacy Association Executives, the National Home Infusion Association, and the USP, collaborated to establish the Pharmacy Compounding Accreditation Board (PCAB). The purpose of the PCAB is to improve the quality of compounded medications through the medium of a voluntary accreditation program for pharmacies that do compounding. The first accreditation of a pharmacy was granted in 2006. More information on this organization and the process of accreditation is available on the PCAB Internet site (http://www.pcab.org, accessed February 2008).

D. Historical perspective

From the point of view of compounding, a historical perspective on the regulation of drug quality is more than just interesting, because laws and decisions from 70 and 100 years ago continue to impact our current practice. For example, notice in Table 12.1 the definition of "new drug" from the 1938 Federal Food, Drug and Cosmetic Act. Also notice the two partial lists of drugs that were available before 1938 (e.g., aspirin, phenobarbital, codeine); these are "grandfathered" drugs that were never required to obtain FDA approval. Now, as you read the following brief history, notice how often the terms *new drug* and *non-FDA approved drug* come up in current proposed FDA regulations and court cases that affect pharmacy compounding.

1. Over the first half of the twentieth century, as the pharmaceutical industry became established and grew, there were problems with quality control issues, unsubstantiated therapeutic claims, and questions of safety for industry-prepared drug products. In response, the federal government passed legislation and established administrative bodies aimed at assuring the public of a safe and reliable drug supply. Table 12.1 gives a brief chronologic outline of the federal regulations enacted since 1900. It is important to note the even with robust regulations and oversight by the FDA and rigorous processing controls by much of the pharmaceutical industry, problems with manufactured products still do occur; the FDA, USP, and other agencies and organizations publish and post on their Internet sites current lists of recalled drug products.

2. Some of the same problems that have plagued the pharmaceutical industry are shared by pharmacists in professional practice, and compounded drug preparations have not been free from quality control problems. Several serious compounding incidents occurred in 1990 that alerted pharmacists, the FDA, and the public to some of these problems. These accidents illustrated

Table 12.1	HISTORICAL PERSPECTIVE ON REGULATION OF DRUG QUALITY AND COMPOUNDING

1906—PURE FOOD AND DRUG ACT OF 1906

1. The Act prohibited adulteration and misbranding of foods and drugs in interstate commerce.
2. It was originally administered by the Chemistry Bureau in the U.S. Department of Agriculture; the Food and Drug Administration (FDA) evolved from this Bureau and by 1930 it was known by its present name. In 1940, it was transferred from the Department of Agriculture to the Federal Security Agency, the forerunner to the current Department of Health and Human Services (10).
3. When the Act was amended in 1912 to prohibit false or fraudulent efficacy claims, drug companies were able to circumvent prosecution by omitting all directions for use and so on (10).
4. The *USP* and *NF* were already being published and were the official standards.
5. Drugs available at this time: many of the natural plant alkaloids such as codeine, morphine, cocaine, atropine, scopolamine, caffeine, colchicine, strychnine, etc; aspirin and salicylic acid; acetaminophen; digitalis compounds; phenol; epinephrine; benzocaine; arsenic compounds and many other inorganic compounds such as Epsom salts (magnesium sulfate) and Glauber's salts (sodium sulfate).

1938—FEDERAL FOOD, DRUG AND COSMETIC ACT (FDCA)

1. This Act required premarket documentation of **safety** of *new drugs*, that is, drugs not commonly used before 1938. All those listed above plus phenobarbital and digoxin were exempted by a "grandfather clause." As any of these *old drugs* came off patent, other firms could market them without FDA approval (10).
2. This Act was passed in response to the sulfanilamide elixir tragedy in which more than 100 people died as the result of taking an elixir that was made with a toxic solvent, diethylene glycol (antifreeze).
3. New Drug Applications, or NDAs, were used as the screening and approval mechanism for new drug safety, but the 1938 Act did not require proof of efficacy or therapeutic effectiveness (10).
4. Examples of drugs marketed after 1938 but before 1962, which were governed solely by the safety requirement, include hydrocortisone, prednisone, many antibiotics, such as penicillin and tetracycline, and many antihistamines, such as chlorpheniramine and diphenhydramine, warfarin, chlorpromazine, chlorthiazide, and isoniazid.

1962—FEDERAL FOOD, DRUG AND COSMETIC ACT (FDCA), AS AMENDED

1. The Amended Act requires premarket proof of **safety and efficacy** of new drugs (10). The efficacy requirement brings with it the necessity of bioavailability testing.
2. The grandfather clause for drugs marketed prior to 1938 was left intact.
3. Congressional mandate required that drugs approved between 1938 and 1962 solely on safety be reevaluated on efficacy. Any drug not recognized as effective would be considered a *new drug* subject to all regulations and requiring an NDA.

1967—DRUG EFFICACY STUDY IMPLEMENTATION (DESI)

1. The FDA contracted with the National Academy of Science/National Research Council to do evaluations of the 1938–1962 drugs.
2. Thirty panels basically completed their work by mid-1969, but some products were still in study and litigation in the 1990s. During the interim, these were classified as "less than effective."

1970—ABBREVIATED NEW DRUG APPLICATIONS (ANDA) FOR DESI DRUGS

1. The FDA introduced ANDAs for new products of 1938–1962 drugs that had cleared a DESI panel as efficacious. These required bioequivalence testing but no clinical testing for efficacy.
2. Manufacturers of new generic products for drugs that were introduced after 1962 had to complete a "paper NDA" that gave literature citations on efficacy plus bioequivalence testing. Manufacturers of innovator drugs found that they could prevent or delay the release of a generic equivalent to their product by not publicly publishing the efficacy studies on their post-1962 drugs.

1974—CONGRESS SET UP PANELS TO STUDY PROBLEMS OF CHEMICAL-THERAPEUTIC EQUIVALENCE

1. The Office of Technology Assessment (OTA) of the U.S. Congress set up a panel of nine experts to review the relationship between chemical and therapeutic equivalence and the ability of current technology to determine this.

(continued)

Table 12.1	HISTORICAL PERSPECTIVE ON REGULATION OF DRUG QUALITY AND COMPOUNDING (*continued*)

1977—FIRST PUBLISHED LIST "THERAPEUTICALLY EQUIVALENT DRUGS"

1. This list gave currently marketed drug products with their manufacturers that have complied with NDA or ANDA requirements.
2. Drugs not expected to have bioequivalence problems were given the designation "A," and those with documented or potential problems were given a "B" rating.

1978—CURRENT GOOD MANUFACTURING PRACTICE IN MANUFACTURE, PROCESSING OR HOLDING OF HUMAN AND VETERINARY DRUGS (CGMP OR GMP)

1. The FDA issued these regulations to aid them in assuring the public of safe, pure, and high-quality drug products that have the appropriate identity, strength, quality and purity at the time of use (11).
2. They give the FDA the authority to inspect manufacturing facilities, and they require manufacturers to have written quality control procedures and stability testing programs.

1980—FIRST ANNUAL *APPROVED DRUG PRODUCTS WITH THERAPEUTIC EQUIVALENCE EVALUATIONS* ("ORANGE BOOK") PUBLISHED

1. This update of the FDA's "Therapeutically Equivalent Drugs" includes definitions of terms such as *pharmaceutical and therapeutic equivalents, bioavailability, and bioequivalent drug products.*
2. Published annually, this book of bioequivalence ratings of drug products becomes the basis for generic product evaluation and selection by pharmacists.

1984—DRUG PRICE COMPETITION AND PATENT TERM RESTORATION ACT

1. Eliminated "paper NDAs" and allowed generic equivalents of post-1962 drug products coming off patent to be marketed using ANDAs. This made it easier to market generic products.
2. Innovator drug firms are compensated by being assured of a certain length of time to market new products under patent.

1992—FDA ISSUES COMPLIANCE POLICY GUIDE 7132.16 ON PHARMACY COMPOUNDING (14)

1. Recognizes that pharmacists traditionally have compounded drugs on a prescription from a practitioner for an individual patient.
2. States its intent to enforce FDCA with pharmacies the FDA considers to be manufacturing under the guise of compounding.
3. Does not consider pharmacies exempt from the "new drug" approval provisions of the FDCA.

1997—FOOD AND DRUG ADMINISTRATION MODERNIZATION ACT (FDAMA) OF 1997 (16)

1. Sec. 503 A. Pharmacy Compounding is added to the FDCA.
2. Codifies the right of pharmacists (and physicians) to compound drug preparations but with certain restrictions and exempts these compounded drugs from the FDCA "new drug" approval process.

2002—U.S. SUPREME COURT RULES ON FDAMA SEC. 503A. (6)

1. Court holds that the prohibition of advertising and solicitation in Sec. 503 A. is an unconstitutional restriction of commercial free speech; does not rule on other sections of the FDAMA.
2. Court affirms that the FDCA new-drug approval process is important and should be preserved.
3. Court also affirms the importance of compounding in meeting patient needs; finds that requiring compounded drugs to comply with the FDCA "new-drug" approval process would be too costly and onerous and therefore rejects this.

2002—FDA ISSUES COMPLIANCE POLICY GUIDE (CPG) 460.200 PHARMACY COMPOUNDING (9)

1. Published in response to the Supreme Court ruling.
2. Contains most of the features of the 1992 CPG except the provision on advertising and solicitation.

2008—MEDICAL CENTER PHARMACY, ET AL. V. GONZALES, ET AL. U.S. DISTRICT COURT (15)

1. Holds that compounded drugs, when created for an individual patient on a prescription from a licensed practitioner, are exempt from the "new-drug" definitions of the FDCA and states that the FDA may not enforce this portion of CPG 460.200.

what can happen when proper compounding procedures and controls are not used. In one case, a pharmacist prepared indomethacin ophthalmic drops that were not properly sterilized and preserved; the result was 12 patients who had eye infections and 2 patients who had to have an eye surgically removed (12,13). In the second case, a hospital pharmacy prepared drug solutions that were intended to be sterile for use in a surgical unit; they were contaminated, and two patients died (12,13).

3. These incidents caused the FDA, with its role in protecting public health, to consider ways of addressing these problems, but in each of the foregoing cases, the drug preparations were made by compounding in a hospital or retail pharmacy, and as indicated at the beginning of this chapter, pharmacy compounding is a part of professional practice, a function regulated primarily by state laws with enforcement by state government agencies. The FDA regulates pharmaceutical manufacturing through the FDCA and has lacked jurisdiction over professional practice unless misbranding or adulteration is involved. Therefore, starting in 1992, the FDA has attempted to expand its authority to include compounded preparations as "new drugs" under the FDCA. It issued a Compliance Policy Guide (CPG) that claimed that compounded drugs are subject to certain provisions of the FDCA (14). This expanded interpretation of a *new drug* has not been upheld (6,15), largely for practical reasons—there is an obvious need for unique dosage forms for patients, and the pharmaceutical industry does not and cannot make doses or dosage forms uniquely.

4. To clarify the issue of jurisdiction over compounded drugs, Public Law 105-115. Section 127. Application of Federal Law to Practice of Pharmacy Compounding, was enacted by the U.S. Congress on November 9, 1997.

   a. This law was part of the FDAMA and added a section, Sec. 503 A. Pharmacy Compounding, to the FDCA.

   b. Though the new law supported the right of licensed pharmacists and physicians to compound drug products, it did establish certain restrictions. Some of the provisions of the FDAMA, as they apply to pharmacists (and physicians) who compound drug products, are briefly summarized here (16).

   (1) There must be a valid prescription based on an established relationship between the patient, an authorized prescribing practitioner, and the pharmacist.

   (2) Compounded quantities are limited to those for a patient on an individual prescription and based on a history of such valid prescriptions (i.e., limited anticipatory compounding is allowed).

   (3) The substances used in compounding must either (i) comply with standards for *USP–NF* monographs and the *USP* chapter on pharmacy compounding, (ii) be a component of an FDA-approved product, or (iii) be on a list of substances approved by a committee of the FDA.

   (4) Substances used in compounding cannot be on a list published in the *Federal Register* by the FDA after having been removed from the market because they have been found to be unsafe or not effective.

   (5) Drug products that are copies of commercially available products may not be compounded regularly or in inordinate amounts.

   (6) Drug preparations may not be compounded if they have been identified by the FDA as too difficult to compound so that they may not be safe or may be ineffective when compounded.

   (7) The drug product must be compounded either (i) in a state that has a memorandum of understanding with the FDA concerning inordinate amounts of compounded drug products distributed outside the state, or (ii) the amount sent outside of state by the compounder may not exceed 5% of the total prescriptions dispensed by that pharmacy.

   (8) The compounding pharmacist may not advertise or promote the compounding of a particular drug or class of drugs (16).

   c. Western States Medical Center *v.* Shalala

   (1) In 1998, a group of pharmacists challenged that section of the new law that restricted their right to advertise, asserting that this violated their First Amendment right to free speech. The case was originally heard in the U.S. District Court in Nevada, which found for the plaintiffs, but the decision was appealed by the federal government to the Ninth U.S. Circuit Court of Appeals.

   (2) Though both courts held that the advertising restriction of the law violated the plaintiffs' right to commercial free speech, the Court of Appeals also held that the restriction on advertising and solicitation in Section 127 could not be separated from the main part of the law, and therefore found the entire compounding provisions of Section 127 of FDAMA invalid.

  d. Thompson, Secretary of Health and Human Services, et al. *v.* Western States Medical Center et al.

    (1) On February 26, 2002, the federal government appealed the Circuit Court decision to the U.S. Supreme Court. On April 29, 2002, in a 5 to 4 decision, the Supreme Court held that FDAMA's advertising and solicitation prohibitions are an unconstitutional restriction of commercial free speech (6). In the opinion of the court, written by Justice O'Connor, it was found that the restrictions on speech were more extensive than necessary and that the government could rather use other restrictions, such as prohibiting compounding pharmacists from using commercial-scale manufacturing or testing equipment or limiting the amount that can be compounded to that for prescriptions already received or banning compounded drugs products from being sold at wholesale to other state licensed entities (6).

    (2) Because the Supreme Court did not rule on the separability issue, the status of Section 503a has remained in limbo; on January 10, 2008, the Fifth Circuit Federal Court of Appeals heard a case that considered this issue, and at the time of this writing, a decision has not been rendered. (The entire Supreme Court decision, including the dissenting opinion, can be accessed on the CD that accompanies this book.)

5. In May 2002, in response to the Supreme Court decision, the FDA issued a new Compliance Policy Guides Manual, Sec. 460.200 Pharmacy Compounding (CPG 460.220). This guidance, while it does not have the force of law, is intended to inform both FDA staff and the individuals involved with compounding about FDA's current views on the topic of pharmacy compounding and the sort of practices that FDA will consider to be violations of the FDCA.

  a. The introductory paragraph in the discussion begins as follows:

> FDA recognizes that pharmacists traditionally have extemporaneously compounded and manipulated reasonable quantities of human drugs upon receipt of a valid prescription for an individually identified patient from a licensed practitioner. This traditional activity is not the subject of this guidance. (9)

  b. If the FDA considers that the range of compounding activities of a pharmacy place it more in the category of a manufacturer, and that there are significant violations of the new drug, adulteration, or misbranding regulation of the FDCA, the FDA will consider federal enforcement of that pharmacy practice. The Guidance lists nine items that it will consider in making this determination (9):

    (1) Compounding drug preparations in anticipation of receiving prescription orders, except in limited amounts

    (2) Compounding drug preparations using drugs that have been removed from the market for safety reasons. The FDA provided a list of these drugs in Appendix A of the Compliance Guide.

    (3) Compounding from bulk active ingredients that are not components of FDA-approved drugs products without an investigational new drug application

    (4) Purchasing and using drugs without a written assurance from the supplier that the drug was made in an FDA-registered facility

    (5) Receiving, storing, or using drug components that are not in compliance with official compendia (i.e., *USP* or *NF*) requirements

    (6) Using commercial-scale manufacturing or testing equipment for compounding

    (7) Compounding drug preparations for third parties for resale

    (8) Compounding drug preparations that are essentially copies of FDA-approved manufactured products. If a preparation varies slightly from the FDA approved product, there should be documented medical need for this preparation for the particular patient.

    (9) Failure to operate in accordance with applicable state pharmacy practice laws (9)

  (The full text of this document is available at the FDA Internet Web site, http://www.fda.gov.)

6. In August 2006, in Medical Center Pharmacy, et al. *v.* Gonzales, et al., the U.S. District Court reiterated that a compounded drug preparation that is made for individual patient on the basis of a prescription from a licensed practitioner is not a new drug under federal law and that the FDA may not enforce provisions of its CPG 460.000 that conflict with the court decision [e.g., this court order contradicts aforementioned item (3) in the FDA CPG] (15). The court stated:

Public policy supports exempting compounded drugs from the new drug definitions. If compounded drugs were required to undergo the new drug approval process, the result would be that patients needing individually tailored prescriptions would not be able to receive the necessary medication due to the cost and time associated with obtaining approval... It is in the best interest of public health to recognize an exemption for compounded drugs that are created based on a prescription written for an individual patient by a licensed practitioner (15).

7. The FDA continually states that it is not against the compounding of drugs and that it only brings enforcement actions against those pharmacies that the FDA contends are manufacturing drug products under the pretext of pharmacy compounding (17). Some pharmacies and pharmacy organizations take exception to that characterization, especially when the FDA contends that all compounded drug preparations are "new drugs" under the FDCA and that drugs that are not in FDA-approved products cannot be used in compounding.

III. GUIDELINES FOR PROVIDING SAFE AND EFFECTIVE COMPOUNDED DRUG PREPARATIONS

A. As is apparent from this historical perspective, the exact line between compounding and manufacturing continues to be controversial. Fortunately, all parties agree that compounding drug preparations for patients on the written order of a practitioner is a necessary and important function in modern drug therapy. Therefore, the task of pharmacists and pharmacy technicians is to perform this function in a manner that assures patients of safe and effective compounded medications. Unfortunately, problems with unacceptable compounded preparations continue to be reported. Several examples are useful to note and analyze.

1. In a June 23, 2002, feature story in the *San Francisco Chronicle*, the investigative reporters related a list of recent compounding accidents: 4,200 cancer patients in the Kansas City, Missouri, area who received diluted chemotherapy agents; 4 patients in Atlanta who were hospitalized after taking a compounded thyroid preparation that was 1,000 times its intended potency; and 8 patients in Memphis who had neurologic damage due to a drug error in an implanted pump. In addition, two separate incidents were reported with *serratia* contamination in drug solutions that were intended to be sterile: In one of the incidents, 38 patients received contaminated spinal injections, and 3 of these patients died (18).

2. In December 2002, the Centers for Disease Control and Prevention reported that a compounding pharmacy in South Carolina had made and dispensed injectable methylprednisolone acetate suspensions that were contaminated with the fungal agent *Exophiala dermatitidis*. The report described five cases of infection caused by these injections; one patient had died. An inspection of the pharmacy showed an autoclave that did not perform properly and a series of practices that did not meet guidelines for pharmacy-prepared sterile products, including lack of sterility testing and inadequate clean-room procedures (19).

3. In March 2007, at least two people died after receiving intravenous (IV) colchicine in an alternative-medicine pain clinic. Colchicine is a drug with a known narrow therapeutic window. The IV solution was prepared in a compounding pharmacy, and it contained 4 mg/mL of colchicine but was labeled to contain 0.5 mg/mL (20).

B. Though we all know that accidents do happen (e.g., the U.S. Institute of Medicine's *To Err Is Human*), the foregoing pattern of incidents is clearly unacceptable. In analyzing compounding medication accident cases, they occur for a variety of reasons. Though most incidents are truly accidents, the Kansas City case described earlier was an exception in that increased profit was the motive behind the pharmacist intentionally dispensing subpotent antineoplastic preparations. For other cases, the causes, though unintentional, have the similar result of unsafe or ineffective medications being provided to patients. Some of the identified causes include the following:

1. Lack of knowledge of accepted standards, especially in making sterile preparations
2. Inadequate training
3. Disregard of published guidelines for environmental controls or compounding procedures
4. Mathematical errors in calculating doses or quantities of formulation ingredients or dosage form amounts
5. Weighing or measuring errors
6. Improper ingredient selection
7. Compounding procedural errors

C. Minimizing compounding errors involves both general common-sense principles and specific recommended practices.

1. It is obvious that pharmacists and pharmacy technicians need to be both knowledgeable and careful.
   a. They need good education and training in their respective fields followed by life-long learning.
   b. If embarking on a new or specialty area of practice, they should read and study available literature, guidelines, and standards; get training from well-respected sources; network with a diverse set colleagues; obtain information from a variety of professional organizations and governmental agencies; and use both basic science knowledge and critical thinking skills to make good judgments. The recent addition of the PCAB Standards and accreditation procedure provides a great opportunity for pharmacists to learn the latest accepted standards of practice for compounding and a mechanism to measure their own practice against these standards.
   c. Both pharmacists and pharmacy technicians need to recognize their limitations and never engage in activities for which they lack the needed level of expertise.

2. There are also specific techniques and practices that have been found to reduce the likelihood of errors, especially those that reach the patient.
   a. When doing mathematical calculations:
      (1) **Write** down each step **with units.**
      (2) Be especially careful with decimal points.
      (3) Use independent colleague verification when possible. The essential feature of this technique is the word *independent*. It means that rather than show your calculation to a colleague and ask for verification, you should present the problem and ask for an independent calculation. Then compare your answers.
   b. For weighing and measuring functions and ingredient selection, at minimum use the self "triple-check" system, which has been advocated for many years, and whenever possible, use colleague verification.
   c. Use extreme caution when using potent drugs, those with narrow therapeutic limits, antineoplastic agents, and electrolytes. Be especially careful when compounding for vulnerable patients, such as pediatric and geriatric individuals. Check and recheck and recheck!
   d. Be actively conscious of every step in the compounding process. If you find that you are using an unusual quantity of an ingredient, get independent verification that you are using the correct amount.
   e. Label items for intermediate steps and have a label prepared in advance for the final preparation. Use the 5-second rule—nothing sits for longer than 5 seconds without a label.
   f. Be organized.
   g. Use quality control procedures, and when feasible, have compounded preparations analyzed by an independent laboratory.

3. Use well-documented procedures, which includes master compounding formula sheets and compounding record sheets, and when applicable, written standard operating procedures. These are recommended and discussed in *USP* Chapters ⟨795⟩, ⟨1075⟩, and ⟨1163⟩.
   a. Chapter ⟨795⟩ states that the master compounding record sheet should include the name, strength, and dosage form of the preparation, the quantity or number of doses, all ingredients and their quantities, any special equipment needed, explicit compounding instructions, dispensing container and storage instructions, beyond-use date, and quality control tests. A sample master compounding record sheet is shown in Figure 12.1, and the use of these sheets is illustrated in each of the sample prescriptions given in the dosage form chapters of this book.
   b. The compounding record sheet should contain the name and strength of the preparation, a number to link this record to the appropriate master formula sheet, the quantity or number of doses made, the date prepared and the beyond-use date, the prescription or control number, a list of all ingredients used with the quantity, manufacturer, lot number, and expiration date of each, results of quality control tests (such as weights of capsules, pH of aqueous liquids, etc.), and identification of the person who prepared and the person who checked or approved the compounding steps. A sample compounding record sheet is shown in Figure 12.2, and the use of these sheets is illustrated in each of the sample prescriptions given in the dosage form chapters of this book.
   c. Standard operating procedures (SOPs) are recommended for all significant procedures performed in the pharmacy. They are used both as documents for training personnel and to ensure that procedures are performed in a timely, uniform, and consistent manner. A sample SOP is shown in Figure 12.3 for testing a Class III torsion balance. Often SOPs are used in conjunction with a log or check-off sheet. In the sample case, the main SOP document

is used with the balance-testing sheet given in Figure 14.1 in Chapter 14 of this book. Pharmacy personnel can write their own SOPs, but samples are also readily available through sources such as the *International Journal of Pharmaceutical Compounding*.

IV. STEPS TO FOLLOW IN THE COMPOUNDING PROCESS

The following are basic steps to use when compounding any drug preparation for the first time. This assumes that both a master formulation record (Fig. 12.1) and a record of compounding (Fig. 12.2) are made at this time. Each time a refill is made, the master formulation record should be followed and a record of compounding completed. The recommendations given here are a composite of information given in (i) *Good Compounding Practices Applicable to State Licensed Pharmacies*, (ii) *ASHP Technical Assistance Bulletin on Compounding Nonsterile Products in Pharmacies*, and (iii) *USP* Chapters ⟨795⟩, ⟨1075⟩, and ⟨1163⟩.

1. Carefully read and interpret the prescription or medication order. It may be necessary or helpful to consult with the prescriber and the patient about the intent of the drug preparation and preferences or limitations of the patient.
2. Note any missing or confusing information; clarify, gather, and add this information to the drug order.
3. Perform the following steps and record the information on the master compounding formulation record and/or the compounding record sheet.
   a. Check the dose, dosage regimen, dosage form, and route of administration for appropriateness.
   b. Determine all preparation ingredients based on availability and considerations of the prescribed dosage form (e.g., bulk drug or chemical versus manufactured dosage form, salt/base form of the drug).
   c. Check compatibility and stability information for the individual ingredients and the ingredient combination in the formulation, and determine the dispensing container, storage conditions and a beyond-use date. If there are any problems in this regard, consult with the prescriber to resolve the issues.
   d. Perform the necessary calculations. Include quantities of ingredients weighed or measured for intermediate steps when making aliquots or dilutions.
   e. List the names and quantities of all ingredients on the master formulation record sheet. This includes active ingredients and excipients (e.g., vehicles, solvents, ointment and suppository bases, emulsifying and viscosity-inducing agents, levigating agents, flavors, colors, buffers, preservatives).
   f. Retrieve and consult Material Safety Data Sheets for all bulk ingredients and determine whether any special personal protective equipment is needed.
   g. Choose and inspect appropriate compounding equipment. All equipment and apparatus must be clean and functioning properly.
   h. Determine and write the compounding procedure based on the available ingredients, equipment, and the prescribed dosage form.
   i. Determine appropriate quality control procedures that will be used for this preparation.
   j. If possible, have a colleague verify all calculations and procedures for appropriateness and accuracy. The master compounding record should identify both the person who prepared the master formulation record and the person who checked it.
4. Wash hands and don a clean lab coat or other protective apparel and disposable gloves.
5. Assemble the required ingredients, equipment, apparatus, and the dispensing container. Record the names, quantities, manufacturers, lot numbers, and expiration dates for all ingredients on the compounding record (first check of the ingredient identity for the triple check system).
6. Using recommended techniques and the written compounding procedure on the master formulation record, compound the preparation. If any procedural changes are needed, document these on the formulation record (second check of ingredient identity).
7. Inspect the finished preparation and perform the quality control procedures. Record the results on the compounding record.
   a. Visual inspection of the preparation should always be done.
   b. Make measurements when this is possible and appropriate (e.g., capsule weights, pH measurements, final weight or volume compared to the theoretical values).
8. Package the preparation in the dispensing container.
9. Label the container, including recommended auxiliary labels.
10. Recheck all work. Clean all equipment and return ingredients to stock (third check of ingredient identity).

MASTER COMPOUNDING FORMULATION RECORD

NAME, STRENGTH AND DOSAGE FORM OF PREPARATION:

QUANTITY: **FORMULATION RECORD ID:**

THERAPEUTIC USE/CATEGORY: **ROUTE OF ADMINISTRATION:**

INGREDIENTS:

Ingredient	Quantity	Physical Description	Solubility	Function

COMPATIBILITY, STABILITY, AND SPECIAL PROCESSING PROCEDURES:
(with references when available)

RECOMMENDED PACKAGING AND STORAGE CONDITIONS:

BEYOND-USE DATE:
(with references when available)

CALCULATIONS:

MSDS AND RECOMMENDED PERSONAL PROTECTIVE EQUIPMENT:

SPECIALIZED EQUIPMENT (IF NEEDED):

COMPOUNDING PROCEDURE:

DESCRIPTION OF FINISHED PRODUCT:

QUALITY CONTROL TESTS:

LABELING INFORMATION:
(Product content and auxiliary labels)

PATIENT/CAREGIVER/STAFF INSTRUCTIONS:

MASTER FORMULA SHEET PREPARED BY: **CHECKED BY:**

DATE: **VERSION:**   **PAGE _____ OF _____**

FIGURE 12.1. SAMPLE MASTER COMPOUNDING FORMULATION RECORD.

COMPOUNDING RECORD

NAME, STRENGTH AND DOSAGE FORM OF PREPARATION:

QUANTITY: **DATE PREPARED:** mm/dd/yy   **BEYOND-USE DATE:** mm/dd/yy

FORMULATION RECORD ID: **CONTROL/RX NUMBER:**

INGREDIENTS USED:

Ingredient	Quantity	Manufacturer Lot Number	Expiration Date	Weighed/ Measured by	Checked by

QUALITY CONTROL DATA:

FIGURE 12.2. SAMPLE COMPOUNDING RECORD

11. Document any additional information on the compounding record sheet and sign or initial the prescription document and the compounding records.
12. Deliver the product to the patient or caregiver with appropriate consultation, and check for understanding of use of the preparation.
13. In all cases, the user-patient should be instructed to watch for any change in the preparation that may indicate that physical instability, chemical degradation, or microbial growth has occurred; the patient should be told to contact the pharmacist if there are questions or concerns. If there is any problem with a compounded preparation, corrective steps should be taken: Recall the preparation, investigate the reason for the failure and, after finding a solution to the problem, reformulate the preparation. Inform the prescriber of the problem and the corrective action taken. If the formulation was prepared according to a *USP* monograph, the pharmacist should submit a USP Monograph Experience Reporting Form (3). Document all these activities.

NAME OF PHARMACY

Page 1 of ___
SOP 001.1

Title: (e.g., Balance Testing for a Torsion Balance)

Number/Revision: (e.g., 001.1, which would be SOP number 1, version 1)

Purpose: (e.g., To ensure that the balance used in compounding meets or exceeds the tolerances for a Class III torsion balance as specified in *USP* Chapter ⟨1176⟩ Prescription Balances and Volumetric Apparatus. This is necessary to make certain that ingredients weighed for compounded prescriptions are within a range of ± 5% of the desired weight.)

Responsibility: (e.g., Who will perform the procedure, and who will approve a passable procedure or take corrective action in the event of a failed procedure or test)

Equipment/Supplies Needed: (e.g., Balance brand and model number and test weights brand and class)

Frequency: (e.g., The first Monday of each month)

Procedure: (e.g., Use attached procedure log sheet; in this case, see Figure 14.1 in Chapter 14)

References: (if applicable)

Written by: **Date:**

Checked/Approved by: **Date:**

FIGURE 12.3. SAMPLE STANDARD OPERATING PROCEDURE.

REFERENCES

1. National Association of Boards of Pharmacy. Model State Pharmacy Act and Model Rules of the National Association of Boards of Pharmacy. Mount Prospect, IL: Author, 2007; 207.

2. The United States Pharmacopeial Convention, Inc. Chapter ⟨1075⟩ 2008 USP 31/NF 26. Rockville, MD: Author, 2007; 500–503.

3. The United States Pharmacopeial Convention, Inc. Chapter ⟨795⟩ 2008 USP 31/NF 26. Rockville, MD: Author, 2007; 315–319.

4. Pharmacy Compounding Accreditation Board. PCAB Standards with compliance indicators. Washington, DC: Author, 2006; 26–27.

5. Subramaniam V, Sokol G, Zenger V, et al. Survey of drug products compounded by a group of community pharmacies: Findings from a Food and Drug Administration study. Rockville, MD: Food and Drug Administration, 2002.

6. Thompson, Secretary of Health and Human Services, et al. *v.* Western States Medical Center et al. 535 U.S. 2 (2002).

7. Hepler CD, Strand LM. Opportunities and responsibilities in pharmaceutical care. Am J Hosp Pharm 1990; 47: 533–543.

8. National Association of Boards of Pharmacy. Model rules for the practice of pharmacy. Mount Prospect, IL: Author, 2007.

9. Food and Drug Administration. Compliance policy guide, Chapter 4, Sec. 460.200. Pharmacy compounding. Rockville, MD: Author, May 2002.

10. Fink JL, Marquardt KW, Simonsmeier LM, eds. Pharmacy law digest, 26th rev. St. Louis: Facts and Comparisons, Inc., 1995; DC-3–DC-4.

11. Vadas EB. Stability of pharmaceutical products. In: Gennaro AR, ed. Remington: The science and practice of pharmacy, 19th ed. Easton, PA: Mack Publishing Co., 1995; 639.

12. Bloom MZ. Compounding in today's practice. Am Pharm 1991; 31: 31–37.

13. Conlan MF. Compounding versus manufacturing. Where is the line? Drug Topics 1992; 136: 46–51.

14. Food and Drug Administration. Compliance policy guide, Chapter 32—Drugs general (7132.16). Rockville, MD: Author, March 16, 1992; 1.

15. Medical Center Pharmacy, et al. *v.* Gonzales, et al. U.S. Western District of Texas Court (August 30, 2006).

16. Public Law 105-115. Section 127. Application of Federal Law to Practice of Pharmacy Compounding.

17. Foxhall K. FDA says it's not against compounding. Drug Topics 2007; http://www.drugtopics.com/drugtopics/content/printContentPopup.jsp?id=461195. Accessed October 2007.

18. Hallissy E, Russell S. Who's mixing your drugs? Bad medicine: Pharmacy mix-ups a recipe for misery; some drugstores operate with very little oversight. *San Francisco Chronicle*, June 23, 2002; A-1.

19. Centers for Disease Control and Prevention. *Exophiala* infection from contaminated injectable steroids prepared by a compounding pharmacy—United States, July–November 2002. MMWR Morb Mortal Wkly Rep 2002; 51: 1109–1112.

20. Centers for Disease Control and Prevention. Deaths form intravenous colchicine resulting from a compounding pharmacy error—Oregon and Washington, 2007. MMWR Morb Mortal Wkly Rep 2007; 56(40): 1050–1052.

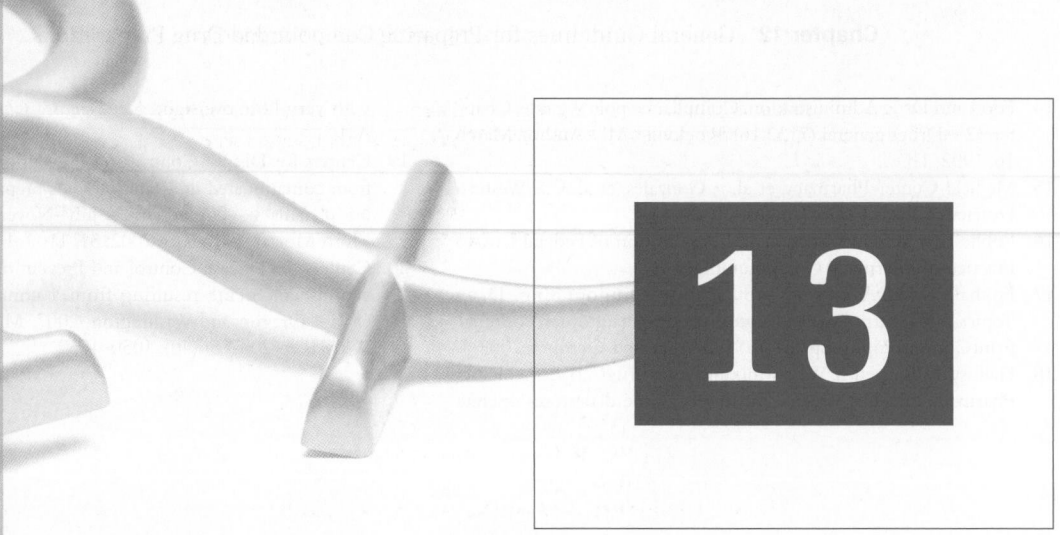

13

Selection, Storage, and Handling of Compounding Equipment and Ingredients

I. COMPOUNDING FACILITIES AND EQUIPMENT

A. Legal requirements

The minimum requirements for equipment and facilities for pharmacies are usually set by state pharmacy practice acts. At one time, these acts had very specific requirements, such as minimum number of square feet in the pharmacy; number and types of mixing, measuring, and weighing equipment; types and even titles of mandated reference books; and so on. Now most state laws follow the guidelines of the NABP *Model Rules for the Practice of Pharmacy* with more general statements, such as a compounding area of "sufficient size" to allow for safe and proper compounding, and "The Pharmacy shall carry and utilize the equipment and supplies necessary to conduct a Pharmacy in a manner that is in the best interest of the patients served" (1). Consult your state statutes for applicable information for your practice site.

B. Professional standards for nonsterile compounding equipment and facilities

USP Chapter ⟨795⟩ Pharmaceutical Compounding—Nonsterile Preparations and Chapter ⟨1075⟩ Good Compounding Practices have sections on compounding equipment and facilities for nonsterile compounding. These chapters do not distinguish between compounding done in pharmacies and that done in medical offices, clinics, or hospitals. Though they do not give lists of specific required equipment (e.g., balances, mortars, graduated cylinders), they address both facilities and equipment in more general ways (2,3). The *ASHP Technical Assistance Bulletin on Compounding Nonsterile Products in Pharmacies* has a similar section devoted to facilities and equipment for nonsterile compounding (4).

1. Compounding facility (2–4)
   a. The compounding area should be of adequate size and design for the type of compounding done in the facility. If possible, the area should be separated from other activities of the pharmacy or professional practice. Both of the *USP* chapters and the *ASHP Technical Assistance Bulletin* place special emphasis on ensuring that the location and amount of space is sufficient for storage, compounding, packaging, and labeling so as to minimize dust and particulate matter and prevent cross-contamination and mix-ups of ingredients or preparations during compounding.
   b. The facility, including the storage area, is to be kept in a clean, sanitary, and orderly condition with regular and proper disposal of waste and trash.
   c. It should have appropriate lighting, ventilation, and temperature control so that the area meets storage conditions as set forth in *USP* monographs and FDA and manufacturer recommendations for drugs and chemicals stored and used in the facility.
   d. The facility should have a sink with hot and cold tap (potable) water, hand-soap and dish detergent, and air dryer or single-use towels to be used for washing hands and for washing glassware and other compounding equipment.
      (1) The potable water should meet the requirements of the Environmental Protection Agency's (EPA) National Primary Drinking Water Regulations, as given in 40 CFR Part 141.
      (2) Potable water is acceptable for washing hands, glassware, and compounding equipment, but it is not to be used as an ingredient in making drug preparations. Purified water USP is to be used as the water ingredient for nonsterile preparations and for rinsing compounding equipment. For water requirements for sterile products, see Chapter 15 in this book and *USP* water monographs.

2. Compounding equipment (2–4)
   a. Compounding equipment is to be of the appropriate type, design, and size for the intended use.
   b. Equipment surfaces that come in contact with ingredients or compounded preparations should not be reactive, additive, or sorptive so that the purity of preparations is not compromised during compounding and packaging.
   c. All equipment used in compounding (including analytical devices used to verify the strength and properties of ingredients and finished preparations) should be routinely inspected, cleaned, maintained, and checked for expected performance. All equipment should be used in conformance with manufacturer's recommendations. Devices that are used for measurement or analysis should be calibrated on a regularly scheduled basis, and records should be kept of these activities. It is highly recommended that standard operating procedures (SOPs) be written and used for all compounding and analytical equipment.
   d. Equipment should be stored appropriately so as to maintain it in a clean condition, free from contamination. Just before use, it should be inspected, and immediately after use it should be carefully cleaned.

C. **Recommendations and requirements for sterile compounding**
   Standards for equipment and facilities for compounding sterile products are much more specific. For information on this subject, see Chapter 32 of this book and *USP* Chapter ⟨797⟩.

D. The following is a modest list of equipment that will serve most nonsterile compounding needs. Where appropriate, descriptions, uses, and limitations are given. The CD that accompanies this book has an excellent audio-visual slideshow on the use of balances and much of the compounding equipment described here.

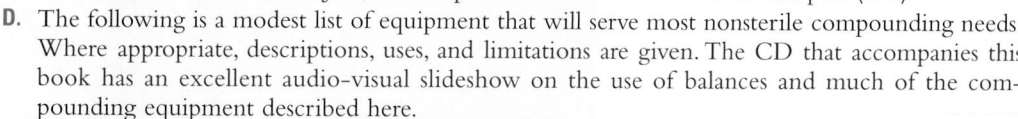

   1. Balances
      For detailed descriptions of balances, their specifications, and proper care and use, see Chapter 14, Selection and Use of Weighing and Measuring Equipment, and the CD with this book.
   2. Volumetric apparatus
      For specifications and descriptions of graduated cylinders and other volumetric apparatus, see Chapter 14 and the CD with this book.
   3. Mortars and pestles
      a. Wedgwood mortars are heavy-duty, durable mortars available in various sizes: 2 oz, 4 oz, 8 oz, 16 oz, and 32 oz. They are made with abradant interior surfaces, making them ideal for particle size reduction and for making emulsions, where efficient shear is desirable. Because of their porous interiors, Wedgwood mortars should not be used for drugs that stain, for drugs present in small quantities, or for very potent or hazardous drugs; and particular care must be taken with cleaning Wedgwood mortars so as to avoid cross-contamination of future preparations. The rough surfaces of Wedgwood mortars do become smooth with

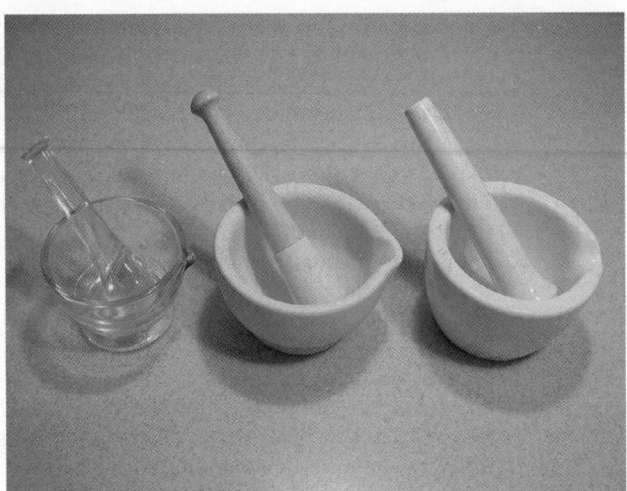

MORTARS AND PESTLES (GLASS, WEDGWOOD, AND CERAMIC).

continued use. When this occurs, some pharmacists triturate washed sand or emery in the mortar in an effort to re-roughen the surfaces, but this procedure has limited success.

b. Porcelain mortars are available in the same sizes as Wedgwood mortars. They have a more attractive white, glazed surface but provide less shearing efficiency than Wedgwood mortars and are somewhat less durable.

c. Ceramic mortars are similar to Wedgwood mortars; they have abradant interior working surfaces and therefore have similar uses and precautions. They are available in sizes ranging from 2 oz to 32 oz. Like porcelain mortars, they are less durable than Wedgwood mortars.

d. Clear glass mortars have smooth, nonporous interior surfaces, making them useful for triturating drugs that stain. Because of their smooth sides, glass mortars are not as efficient as Wedgwood or ceramic mortars in reducing particle size of powders and especially hard crystals, but they are useful for making solutions and suspensions and for diluting creams to lotions. They are not efficient for making emulsions because adequate shear is difficult to achieve with a glass mortar and pestle. They are preferred for triturating highly potent drugs and should always be used if it is necessary to triturate a hazardous drug. Like Wedgwood mortars, they are available in sizes ranging from 2 oz to 32 oz.

e. For maximum efficiency, use pestles that are matched with respect to size and type with the corresponding mortar.

4. Spatulas

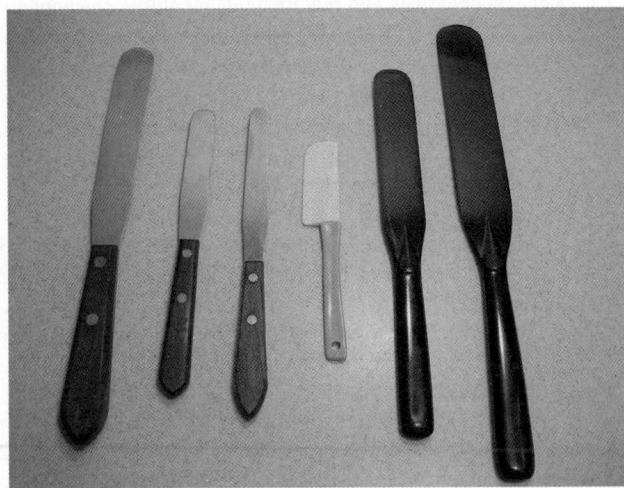

SPATULAS.

a. Stainless steel spatulas with wooden or hard plastic handles are available in various sizes, with blades from 3 to 12 inches in length. It is important to use the appropriate size and type for the task.

(1) The small sizes are used for handling dry chemicals, for scraping materials from other spatulas and from the sides of small mortars and pestles, and for levigating small quantities of drugs and chemicals on ointment pads or slabs.

(2) The larger sizes are used for handling larger quantities of materials. Spatulas with 8- to 12-inch blades are preferred for levigating moderate-to-large quantities of drugs and for mixing or spatulating ointments.

(3) Special spatulas of this type with angled blades are also available.

b. Small, double-bladed, nickel–stainless steel spatulas, sometimes called *micro spatulas*, are useful for withdrawing small amounts of chemicals and drugs from their containers. They are not used for levigation.

c. Hard rubber or Teflon-coated stainless steel spatulas, 4 and 6 inches, are **special purpose only:** They are used in handling drugs and chemicals, such as iodine, that react with metal. In general, they lack the flexibility needed for levigating and spatulating ointments.

d. Flexible, rubber spatulas, sometimes called *rubber policemen* or *rubber scrapers*, have broad, rectangular, flexible rubber, silicone, or plastic scrapers with wooden or plastic handles. These spatulas are very useful for scraping material from the inside surface of mortars when transferring a preparation from the mortar to a packaging container.

5. Funnels are available in both glass and plastic and come in a wide range of capacities and with different stem lengths and diameters.

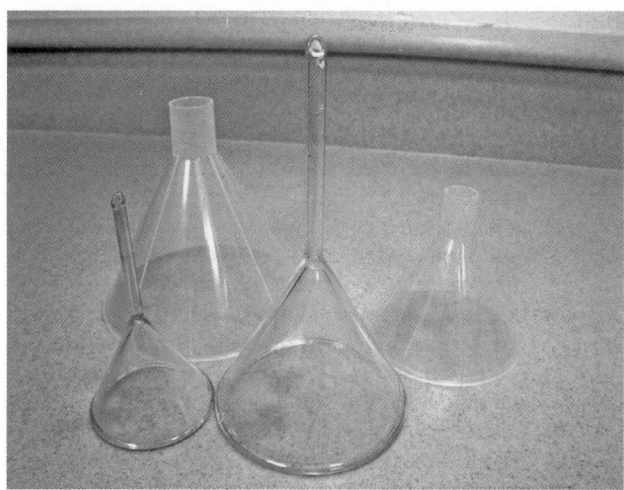

GLASS AND PLASTIC FUNNELS.

a. Funnels with narrow stem diameters are used for transferring solutions from one vessel or bottle to another. These are also used with filter papers in filtering solutions. **Do not try to use them for transferring thick suspensions or emulsions from a mixing vessel to a prescription bottle**—the bore on the glass stem will generally get clogged, and you will have a mess!

b. Powder funnels have short, larger diameter stems. These are useful for transferring powders from mortars and other mixing vessels to dispensing and stock bottles. Depending on the viscosity of the liquid, these may also be used to transfer suspensions and emulsions from mixing vessel to dispensing container.

c. When transferring large quantities of powders or liquids, so-called canning funnels can be useful.

6. Ointment slabs and pads

a. Ointment slabs

(1) Though ointment slabs are called *ointment* slabs because of their use as a surface for levigation and spatulation in compounding ointments, an ointment slab may also be used as a clean, hard surface for holding powders when punching capsules and as a surface for rolling semi-solid materials when marking hand-rolled suppositories or lozenges.

(2) Some ointment slabs have a rough surface on one side to facilitate particle size reduction when levigating powders for ointments. Care must be exercised to avoid getting water-insoluble materials (dyes, tars, etc.) in the pores on this rough side because this surface is difficult to clean and residues may contaminate future preparations.

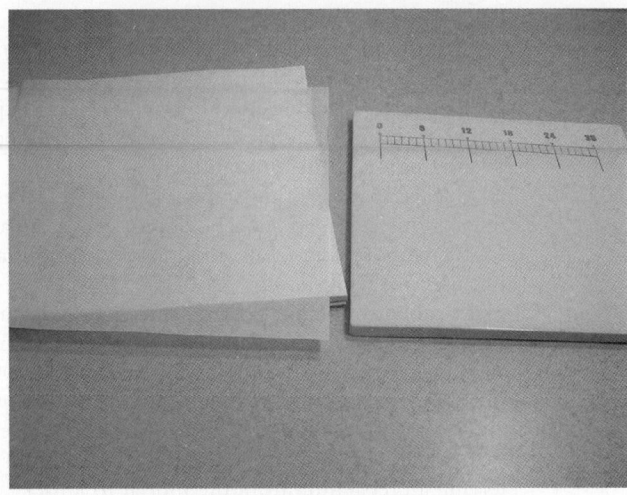

OINTMENT PAD AND OINTMENT SLAB.

   b. Ointment pads
   (1) Ointment pads are convenient because the top sheet is used and then torn off and discarded when the job is completed—a great time-saver.
   (2) They do have some limitations. They soak up liquids, including the water phase of creams, aqueous solutions to be incorporated into ointment bases, and even thick tar-like ingredients; ointment slabs are preferred over pads in these situations.
7. Glass stirring rods are useful for stirring liquid preparations. Spatulas are not to be used as stirring rods.
8. Pyrex or other heat-resistant beakers come in many sizes, from 10 mL to 4 L. The most common sizes used in compounding are 50 mL, 100 mL, 150 mL, 250 mL, 400 mL, 600 mL, and 1,000 mL. These are described in Chapter 14.
9. Pyrex or other heat-resistant Erlenmeyer flasks also come in various sizes, from 25 mL to 6 L. These are useful when making solutions because the contents of the flask can easily be mixed by swirling and there is less danger of spillage than when using a beaker. On the other hand, it is more difficult to add ingredients to an Erlenmeyer flask because of the small flask orifice.
10. Crucibles and evaporating dishes are handy for heating suppository and ointment bases. They can also be used as the water vessel for a simple, improvised hot-water bath.
11. Suppository and troche molds
   a. Aluminum and plastic disposable suppository molds are needed for making suppositories by fusion. These are described and pictured in Chapter 31, Suppositories.
   b. Plastic disposable troche molds are described and pictured in Chapter 26, Capsules, Lozenges, and Other Solid Oral Dosage Forms.
12. Personnel protective equipment (PPE), including lab coats or gowns, safety glasses, and disposable gloves, should be available and used as needed when compounding. When handling some drugs and chemicals, the use of particulate respirators is recommended. These are facemasks that protect personnel from inhalation exposure. They are available in a variety of models, which provide varying degrees of protection and user comfort; some provide protection from aerosols. Select a model or models that are approved by the National Institute for Occupational Safety and Health (NIOSH); a surgical mask does not afford the necessary protection (5).
13. Paper or test strips for measuring pH: These are available in various pH ranges at a nominal price; they are essential for quality control monitoring of preparations containing water.
14. Filter papers, various sizes
15. Cutting devices, such as scissor and single-edge razor blades
16. Wax or other marking pen
17. Brushes of various sizes and shapes for cleaning graduates and funnels
18. Thermometers
   a. A laboratory thermometer is needed for monitoring and adjusting the temperatures of water baths and of liquids and molten semisolids when this is required during compounding.
   b. Ambient temperature thermometers are required for monitoring the temperature in dispensing, compounding, and drug storage areas, including refrigerators and freezers. Models that are available also measure relative humidity, and some have memory features that store

minimum and maximum temperatures during specified periods. Some models have chart recorders that make a hardcopy tracing of the temperature on an ongoing basis.

19. Heating devices

   a. Microwave oven

     (1) As a heating device, a microwave oven is convenient, safe, and fast.

     (2) Because microwave ovens work on the principle of alternating polarity, they do not heat non-polar substances, such as white petrolatum and some waxes and oils. This disadvantage can be overcome by using the microwave oven to heat water in a crucible or beaker; this may then be used as a hot water bath for heating or melting nonpolar items.

     (3) Microwave ovens can develop "hot spots" that may cause overheating and degradation of ingredients.

   b. Hot plate

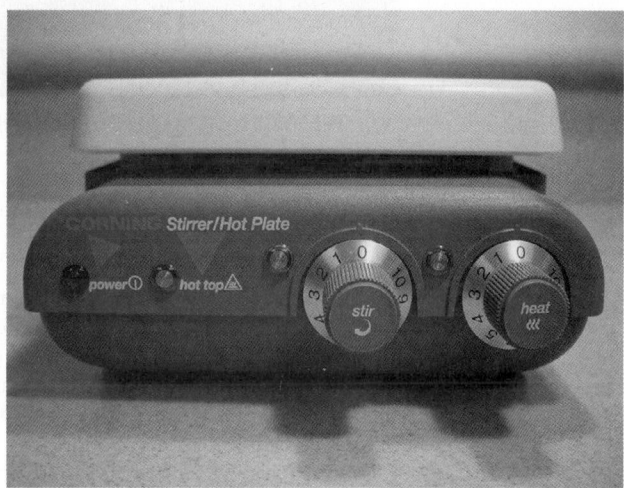

HOT PLATE WITH MAGNETIC STIRRER.

     (1) Hot plates offer fast and direct sources of heat, but they require careful monitoring to avoid overheating or scorching of ingredients. When heating a preparation that must have a carefully controlled temperature and the desired temperature is 100°C or less, a hot-water bath may be the preferred heating device.

     (2) Some hot plates are available with magnetic stirring devices, which can be very handy.

   c. Hot-water bath

     A hot-water bath can be improvised by using two heat-resistant beakers or similar vessels of different sizes. Water is added to the larger vessel, and this is heated either on a hot plate or in a microwave oven. The material to be melted or heated is placed in the smaller vessel and this is then floated in the hot water contained in the larger vessel.

20. Refrigerator (including a freezing compartment) that will maintain temperatures as specified in the *USP*.

21. If sterile products are compounded, special equipment (such as a laminar airflow hood) is required. The equipment and the specialized environment needed for this sort of practice are discussed in Chapter 32, General Principles of Sterile Dosage Form Preparation and in *USP* Chapter ⟨797⟩.

22. A wide variety of other useful pieces of equipment are available. Decisions on the purchase and use of particular equipment depend on the amount and type of compounding performed and economic circumstances of the professional practice. Examples of other types of equipment are listed here.

   a. Sieves, both individual and as sets with various mesh sizes, which are available at a modest cost. These are useful when powders of a particular size are needed for product uniformity or comfort.

   b. A magnetic stirring device. A combination hot plate–magnetic stirrer is more versatile but also more expensive.

   c. Thermostatically controlled hot-water baths, which offer great convenience, especially if formulations that are made require carefully controlled constant temperatures.

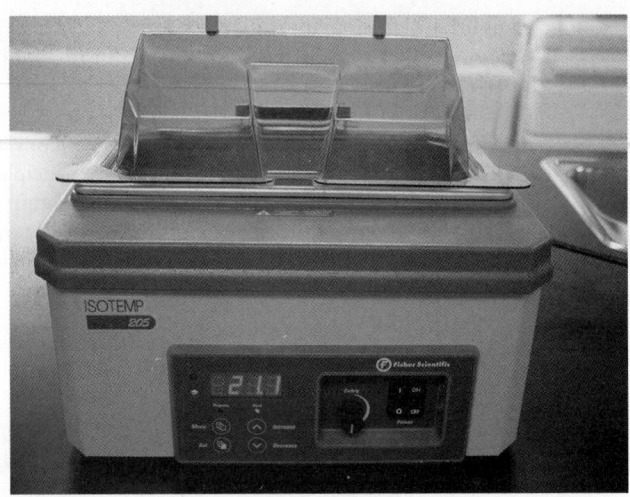

THERMOSTATICALLY CONTROLLED HOT-WATER BATH.

   d. A source of homogenization, such as a hand-homogenizer or a blender.
   e. Electric mixer.
   f. Electronic mortar and pestles systems, such as the Topitec Electric Ointment Mixer and the Unguator Mixing System. These systems are designed to mix suspensions, ointments, and gels directly in special dispensing jars. Because these are closed systems, the compounder is protected from exposure to the ingredients during the mixing process.
   g. A pH meter. This offers both convenience and accuracy but is considerably more expensive than pH paper or strips. Meters are available in both stationary and portable models; some also measure temperature in degrees Celsius.
   h. Ductless containment hoods, glove boxes, and laboratory fume hoods. These provide protection from exposure to compounding ingredients, including powders and particulates, fumes, and vapors. Depending on the amount and type of compounding done, equipment of this type may be required for a compounding facility. Biological safety cabinets are used for protection from hazardous drugs when compounding sterile products. These are discussed in Chapter 32.
   i. Capsule-filling machines, ranging from very simple devices at approximately $20 to motorized machines for more than $5,000. These can be purchased from pharmacy supply vendors.
   j. Ointment mills, which make very fine ointments. This piece of equipment is quite expensive, usually several thousand dollars, so you need to make a lot of ointments for this sort of equipment to make economic sense.
   k. For pharmacies that want to do in-house analysis of their bulk chemicals or drugs or of finished preparations, various kinds of analytical equipment, from melting-point instruments to spectrophotometers.

II. COMPOUNDING INGREDIENTS

A. Definitions and ingredient grade abbreviations

   1. The definitions given next are quoted from the NABP *Model State Pharmacy Act* (6). USP Chapter ⟨795⟩ and federal law 21 CFR 210.3(b)(7)–(8) have similar definitions.
   a. "'Active Ingredients' refer to chemicals, substances, or other Components of articles intended for use in the diagnosis, cure, mitigation, treatment, or prevention of diseases in humans or other animals or for use as nutritional supplements" (6).
   b. "'Added Substances' mean the ingredients necessary to prepare the Drug product but are not intended or expected to cause a human pharmacological response if administered alone in the amount or concentration contained in a single dose of the Compounded Drug product. The term 'added substances' is usually used synonymously with the terms 'inactive ingredients,' 'excipients,' and 'pharmaceutic ingredients'" (6).
   c. "'Component' means any Active Ingredient or Added Substance intended for use in the Compounding of a Drug product, including those that may not appear in such product" (6).
   d. The aforementioned federal law defines an inactive ingredient as any component of a drug product other than the active ingredient. The FDA Center for Drug Evaluation and

Research maintains an Inactive Ingredients Database that gives information (name, concentration or amount, dosage form, etc.) on all the inactive ingredients present in FDA-approved drug products. It is available on their Internet site at www.fda.gov/cder. This information can be used as a guide in determining appropriate inactive ingredients and amounts for compounded preparations.

2. Grade designations for ingredients
    a. USP: The ingredient is certified to meet or exceed the specifications prescribed in the current edition of the *USP*.
    b. NF: The ingredient is certified to meet or exceed the specifications prescribed in the current edition of the *NF*.
    c. FCC: The ingredient is certified to meet or exceed the specifications listed in the current edition of the *Food Chemical Codex*.
    d. ACS: The ingredient is certified to meet or exceed the specifications listed in the current edition of *Reagent Chemicals*, which is published by the American Chemical Society.
    e. AR: Also known as *analytical reagent grade*, this is the grade assigned to chemicals of high purity that are suitable for analytic laboratory work.
    f. Purified: A designation given to chemicals of superior quality for which there is no official standard.
    g. CP: Also known as *chemically pure*, this designation is applied to chemicals that are more refined than technical grade but for which only partial analytic information is available.
    h. Technical: Also called *commercial grade*, this grade is assigned to chemicals of commercial or industrial quality.
    i. Food Grade: This grade is assigned to chemicals that have clearance for use in foods.
    j. Cosmetic Grade: This designation can be given to chemicals approved for use in cosmetics.

B. Selecting bulk components for compounding

It is the responsibility of the pharmacist to choose appropriate, quality ingredients for compounded drug preparations. Several resources give guidance for this task.

1. *USP* Chapters ⟨795⟩ and ⟨1075⟩, *ASHP Technical Assistance Bulletin on Compounding Nonsterile Products in Pharmacies*, and NAPB *Good Compounding Practices Applicable to State Licensed Pharmacies* all give similar guidance on ingredient selection (2–4,7).
    a. The preferred grade for compounding is USP or NF.
    b. If an official USP or NF ingredient is not available, the pharmacist should use professional judgment in the selection of an alternative source so that the safety and purity of the ingredient is ensured. Recommended grades include AR, ACS, and FCC.
    c. When possible, drug substances used for compounding should be made in an FDA-registered facility.
        (1) Many vendors of drugs and chemicals for compounding now state in their catalogs that their products conform to the requirements of cGMPs (current Good Manufacturing Practices) and that their facilities are inspected by and registered with the FDA.
        (2) *USP* Chapter ⟨795⟩ states, "For any substance used in compounding not purchased from a registered drug manufacturer, the pharmacist should establish purity and safety by reasonable means, which may include lot analysis, manufacturer reputation, or reliability of source" (2). This includes requesting a certificate of analysis from the supplier.
    d. Compounding ingredients may not be on the FDA list of components withdrawn or removed from the market for safety reasons.

2. The FDA has expressed its views on the issue of acceptable compounding ingredients with a Compliance Policy Guide for Pharmacy Compounding. In this document, the FDA states that it "recognizes that pharmacists traditionally have extemporaneously compounded and manipulated reasonable quantities of human drugs upon receipt of a valid prescription for an individually identified patient from a licensed practitioner. This traditional activity is not the subject of this guidance" (8). The document then discusses the FDA's concern about pharmacies that practice outside this traditional mode by using large quantities of bulk drugs to produce large quantities of drug preparations and providing these to patients and physicians with only a "remote" professional relationship. The FDA considers this kind of activity to be manufacturing (FDA's realm of enforcement) rather than compounding and has warned that it will consider enforcement action against pharmacies that engage in this type of practice; it gives nine factors that it will consider in making this determination. Four of these factors deal with compounding ingredients:
    a. Using drugs that were withdrawn or removed from the market because of safety issues. [The list of these drugs is included as Appendix A of the Compliance Policy Guide. Because this list

may be updated from time to time, the most current list should be consulted. It is available on the FDA Internet site at www.fda.gov/cder/pharmcomp/default.htm (accessed August 2007).]

  b. Using bulk active ingredients that are not components of FDA-approved products.

  c. Using drug substances without the assurance that they were manufactured in an FDA-registered facility.

  d. Using drug components that do not meet official compendia requirements (8).

C. Manufactured drug products as compounding ingredients

Manufactured drug products, such as tablets, capsules, or injections, are often used as sources of ingredients for compounded preparations. This is illustrated with sample prescriptions in Chapter 25, Powders (sample prescriptions 25.5 and 25.6); Chapter 26, Capsules, Lozenges, and Other Solid Oral Dosage Forms (sample prescriptions 26.2, 26.3, 26.5, and 26.7); and Chapter 28, Suspensions (sample prescriptions 28.5 and 28.6).

  1. To be used as an ingredient in compounding, the manufactured drug product must come from a container that has a batch control number, and the product must be within its stated expiratory date (2).

  2. Certain solid dosage forms should not be crushed and used as ingredients for compounding.

  a. Controlled-release and enteric-coated products are specially formulated or coated to give certain desired or required release characteristics. Crushing the product may destroy these features.

  b. Some drugs are put into capsules or are formulated into tablets that are sugar- or film-coated to mask their unpleasant taste, to protect the mouth or throat from irritation, or to protect the teeth from staining. Crushing the tablets or emptying the contents of the capsules to use them as compounding ingredients destroys this protection.

  c. Sublingual or buccal tablets may contain drugs that require this special route of administration for therapeutic activity.

  d. There are several sources of information on oral drug products that should not be crushed; consult one of the sources given next before using a manufactured oral dosage form as a compounding ingredient.

  (1) The journal *Hospital Pharmacy* periodically publishes a chart with oral solid dosage forms that should not be crushed. These charts can be purchased through their Internet Web site at http://www.factsandcomparisons.com/Products (accessed May 2007).

  (2) The appendix section of Lexicomp's *Pediatric Dosage Handbook* contains a list of tablets and capsules that cannot be crushed or altered.

  (3) Often, prescribing information (i.e., the product package insert) for the particular product also contains this information.

  3. Special care must be exercised when manipulating hazardous drug products (such as anticancer agents, antivirals, and hormonal drugs) as ingredients for compounding. Disposable gloves should be worn, and precautions should be employed, such as using a particulate respirator mask, a glove box, a powder containment hood, or a biological safety cabinet. This sort of powder containment is illustrated with sample prescription 25.6 in Chapter 25: In this example, the tablets are placed in a sealable plastic bag and carefully crushed with a pestle, taking care not to puncture the bag.

  4. Care must be exercised when selecting injectable products as ingredients for other routes of administration.

  a. Some injectable products use prodrugs to enhance solubility of the active ingredient. These prodrugs may or may not be therapeutically active when used by other routes of administration. For example, if the prodrug is an ester, esterases must be present at the site of administration for the drug to be active.

  b. Some drugs that are efficacious when given parenterally may not be therapeutically active orally or topically. This can be caused by such factors as loss by first-pass effect, degradation in the gastrointestinal tract or lack of absorption in the gut when the drug product is given orally, or lack of absorption through the skin or mucous membranes when given topically.

  5. The pharmacist should consider all these factors when deciding to use a manufactured drug product as an ingredient for a compounded drug preparation. The prescribing information should always be consulted for helpful information from the product's manufacturer.

III.   STORAGE CONDITIONS FOR DRUG PRODUCTS AND INGREDIENTS

A. All drugs, chemicals, drug products, and preparations should be stored and distributed under conditions that meet or exceed *USP–NF* or manufacturer's specifications. This includes shipment of these articles to the consumer (9).

Note: *USP* Chapters ⟨795⟩ and ⟨1075⟩ use the term *drug preparation* for compounded dosage forms to distinguish them from drug products, which are manufactured dosage forms (2,3).

B. Definitions of storage temperatures

Storage temperatures as defined in the General Notices of the *USP* are given here (9). The Celsius temperatures are given first with the Fahrenheit temperatures following in parenthesis.

1. Freezer: between −25° and −10° (−13° and 14°)
2. Cold: Not exceeding 8° (46°)
3. Refrigerator: thermostatically controlled between 2° and 8° (36° and 46°) (see 5 Controlled Cold Temperature)
4. Cool: between 8° and 15° (46° and 59°)
   An article that is to be stored in a cool place may be stored and distributed in a refrigerator unless otherwise specified.
5. Controlled Cold Temperature: thermostatically controlled between 2° and 8° (36° and 46°) with allowed excursions between 0° and 15° (32° and 59°) as long as the mean kinetic temperature (MKT, defined in 12.) does not exceed 8° (46°). If the manufacturer labeling allows, transient spikes up to 25° (77°) are permitted as long as they do not exceed 24 hours or manufacturer instructions.
6. Room Temperature: the ambient temperature in the room
7. Controlled Room Temperature: thermostatically controlled between 20° and 25° (68°–77°) with allowed excursions between 15° and 30° (59° and 86°) and transient spikes up to 40° (104°) as long as the MKT does not exceed 25° (77°) and spikes do not exceed 24 hours. Spikes above 40° are permitted if the manufacturer instructs that this is allowed. An article that is to be stored at controlled room temperature may be stored and distributed in a cool place unless otherwise specified.
8. Warm: 30° to 40° (86° to 104°)
9. Excessive Heat: above 40° (104°)
10. Protection from Freezing: protect from temperatures below 0° (32°)
11. Dry place: a place where, at controlled room temperature, the average relative humidity (RH) does not exceed 40% or equivalent humidity at other temperatures. The determination of temperature–relative humidity can be based on actual measurement in the storage place or reported climatic conditions. It is based on not less than 12 equally spaced measurements during a season, a year, or the length of storage of the article. RH values can be up to 45% RH as long as the average RH is 40% or less (9).
12. Mean kinetic temperature: The MKT is a single calculated temperature that gives approximately the same drug product degradation as would occur if the product were subjected to various temperatures. It is calculated using an equation that is derived from the Arrhenius equation and gives a value that is slightly higher than a simple arithmetic mean (10). The definition and equation for MKT are given in *USP* Chapter ⟨1150⟩ Pharmaceutical Stability and the equation with a sample calculation is given in *USP* Chapter ⟨1160⟩ Pharmaceutical Calculations and in Chapter 7 in this book. The calculated MKT is used to any necessary adjustments in the temperature-controlling equipment for the pharmacy or storage space, including refrigerators used to store drugs. If the temperatures in these areas are consistently maintained within the specified ranges, the MKT need not be calculated.
13. Nonspecific storage conditions: When no storage conditions are given in an official monograph or manufacturer's labeling, the item should be stored at controlled room temperature and protected from moisture, freezing, excessive heat, and, when necessary, from light (9).

IV.   CONTAINERS AND CLOSURES

A. The General Notices of the *USP* give the definitions of container types used for packaging and storing drugs, chemicals, pharmaceutic ingredients, and drug products and preparations. (By *USP* definition, the closure is considered to be part of the container.) Additional information that is specific to compounding can be found in the section Packaging and Drug Preparation Containers in *USP* Chapter ⟨1075⟩; various *USP* chapters, described later, also have container requirements and specifications.

B. Some container standards and recommendations are general in nature

1. The container should be clean, and it should not interact physically or chemically with the article placed in it (3,9).
2. The material of the container should be such that it does not change the quantity, strength, or purity of the product or preparation (3,9).

3. Containers should not be stored directly on the floor but rather should be stored and handled in a manner that avoids contamination of the containers and that facilitates inspection of the stock and cleaning of the area. Container stock should be rotated to use the oldest containers first (3).

C. When container specifications are given in official monographs, these apply not only to those products produced by manufacturers but to these same drug products dispensed by the pharmacist (9).

D. **Descriptions of official types of containers**
   1. Well-closed Container: A well-closed container merely provides protection from extraneous solids getting in or the contents of the container getting out under normal conditions (9).
   2. Tight Container: Most drugs, chemicals, and drug products and preparations are stored in tight containers. The General Notices of the *USP* define a tight container as one that provides protection from "contamination by extraneous liquids, solids, or vapors; from loss of the article; and from efflorescence, deliquescence, or evaporation under ordinary or customary conditions of handling, shipment, storage, and distribution, and is capable of tight re-closure" (9). The moisture permeation standards for both tight and well-closed containers are given in *USP* Chapter ⟨671⟩ Containers—Performance Testing (11).
   3. Light-resistant Container: These containers protect the article or product from the effects of light (9). The specifications for maximum percentage of light transmission and details of testing for light-resistant containers are given in *USP* Chapter ⟨671⟩ (11). When an opaque outer wrapper or carton is used by the manufacturer as part of the container for protecting the product from light, this wrapper must not be removed prior to dispensing (9).
   4. Hermetic Container: This is the most secure container type. It is impervious to air or any other gas under normal conditions (9).

E. **Information provided in the USP on containers for dispensing**
   1. *USP* Chapter ⟨660⟩ Containers—Glass and Chapter ⟨661⟩ Containers—Plastic have information on the various materials used to make drug containers and on chemical and physical tests used to determine their suitability for this purpose.
   2. *USP* Chapter ⟨671⟩ describes the light transmission test and specifications for light-resistant containers and has the moisture permeation specifications for well-closed and tight containers. It also sets the moisture permeation standards for multiple-unit prescription containers and single-unit and unit-dose containers. For normal dispensing in multiple-unit containers, the pharmacist does not need to be an expert on the details of light transmission and moisture permeation specifications because the companies that sell these containers specify their type. It is important to purchase dispensing containers and packaging materials from reliable sources.
   3. Repackaging guidelines and requirements
      a. The *USP* has several chapters that address the subject of repackaging by pharmacies. If a pharmacy is repackaging drug products or contracting for repackaging, it is essential that the pharmacist be knowledgeable about the packaging standards for the types of materials and containers used.
      b. *USP* Chapter ⟨681⟩ Repackaging into Single-unit Containers and Unit-Dose Containers for Nonsterile Solid and Liquid Dosage Forms (new in *USP 31*) and Chapters ⟨1136⟩ Packaging—Unit-of Use and ⟨1146⟩ Packaging Practice—Repackaging a Single Solid Oral Drug Product into a Unit-dose Container were written specifically for dispensing practice. They contain requirements and practical recommendations on selecting packaging materials, labeling, equipment, setting beyond-use dates, and record keeping for pharmacies that repackage in single-unit and unit-dose containers (such as blister packs) and customized patient medication packages (mnemonic packaging). Though the details of repackaging standards are beyond the scope of this text, any pharmacy engaged in this type of practice should be knowledgeable about and follow these important guidelines.
   4. Though most pharmacists need not be experts on all the technical aspects of packaging materials and containers, they must be knowledgeable about those standards and requirements that impact their specific practices. They have a responsibility to carefully select suppliers of dispensing and storage containers and should be watchful of container specifications and know the required storage conditions for all drugs, chemicals, preparations, and products stored in their practice site and dispensed to their patients.
   5. Packaging, storage and containers for sterile products are discussed in Chapter 32, General Principles of Sterile Product Preparation and in *USP* Chapter ⟨797⟩.

| | **V.** | **SAFE HANDLING OF DRUGS AND CHEMICALS IN THE PHARMACY** |

A. In 1970, the U.S. Congress enacted the Occupational Safety and Health Act (Title 29 of the U.S. Code). This law created a rule-making and enforcement agency, the Occupational Safety and Health Administration (OSHA), which is part of the U.S. Department of Labor, and a research, information, education, and training arm, the National Institute for Occupational Safety and Health (NIOSH), which is in the Center for Disease Control and Prevention (CDC) in the U.S. Department of Health and Human Services. Though these two agencies work by different means (i.e., enforcement versus education), the aim of both is to promote and ensure the health and safety of employees in the workplace (12,13).

B. Though many people think of OSHA in terms of its industrial and construction safety regulations (e.g., safety guards on machines in factories and hard hats at constructions sites), OSHA is charged with protecting the health and safety of all workers. One way in which it does this for employees of pharmacies, hospitals, health care work environments, laboratories in colleges of pharmacy, and so on is by setting and enforcing the Hazard Communication Standard (HCS). In its Guidelines for Employer Compliance, OSHA says this about the HCS:

> The Hazard Communication Standard (HCS) is based on a simple concept—that employees have both the need and a right to know the hazards and identities of the chemicals they are exposed to when working. They also need to know what protective measures are available to prevent adverse effects from occurring. The HCS is designed to provide employees with the information they need (14).

C. The HCS assigns to manufacturers and importers the responsibility for evaluating the hazards of the chemicals that they produce and distribute. These manufacturers, importers, and distributors are then required to disseminate this hazard information and appropriate protective measures to users of the chemicals. This is to be done through labels on the chemical containers and through more-explicit written information in the form of material safety data sheets (MSDSs) that must be provided with the first shipment of any chemical to a user. OSHA is very clear that evaluation of chemical hazards is technical and complex and, therefore, employers and workers who simply use the chemicals are not required to make hazard evaluations. Both physical hazards (such as flammability or explosive potential) and health hazards (such as tissue irritation or damage, carcinogenic and teratogenic effects, and so on) must be assessed by manufacturers and must be communicated by them to users (14,15).

D. Employers (and pharmacists-in charge) also have responsibilities under the HCS. They are charged with designing, establishing, documenting, and monitoring a workplace program that will provide their employees and the people they supervise with both the information and protections needed for safely working with the chemicals used in their particular work site. OSHA Guidelines for Employer Compliance, which is available through the OSHA Internet site, is an excellent resource for establishing such a program. Though a complete discussion of this subject is beyond the scope of this book, it is useful to be familiar with the broad topics covered in these OSHA guidelines.
  1. Be familiar with the HCS rule. (OSHA publishes a pamphlet, "Chemical Hazard Communication," that is available from its office.)
  2. Identify responsible staff for initial and ongoing activities.
  3. Identify and maintain a list of the hazardous chemicals that are in the workplace.
  4. Prepare and implement a written hazard communication program for the work site. It must include how the facility will meet the requirements for the following:
    a. Hazard labels on all chemical containers
    b. Material safety data sheets
    c. Employee information and training (Additional information on training is available in OSHA Publication No. 2254 that was prepared by OHSA's Training Institute.)
    d. Other requirements (14)

E. What users need to know about safe handling of drugs and chemicals
Users (in this case, primarily pharmacists and pharmacy technicians) and other staff who may be exposed to chemicals (e.g., cleaning and custodial workers) are also responsible for the safe handling and disposal of chemicals in the workplace. To perform this function, all users should be knowledgeable about routes of body exposure, types of health hazards from chemicals, special precautions with hazardous drugs, information given on labels of containers and MSDSs, and protective measures.
  1. Routes of exposure

    a. Inhalation: A very common way in which a chemical substance can enter the body is by inhaling a chemical that is mixed in the surrounding air. To avoid this type of exposure, personnel must use great care when triturating, mixing, and transferring powdered drugs and chemicals; volatile solvents should be contained in tightly closed containers whenever this is possible, even during a compounding process. Chemicals that can become airborne should be used only in well-ventilated areas or, when circumstances dictate, while using proper respiratory protection, such as mask respirators, glove boxes, ductless containment hoods, and fume hoods.

    b. Ingestion: The second way in which chemicals enter the body is through the mouth. Ingestion of chemicals is usually done unknowingly and unintentionally. Occasionally, a person ingests a chemical mistaken for a food or beverage. More likely, however, chemical ingestion occurs when an individual eats or drinks contaminated food or beverages. Therefore, eating and/or drinking should not be permitted in the laboratory or pharmacy. Lab coats or other protective clothing should be worn, and hands should be washed frequently when handling drugs and chemicals, and hands should be washed thoroughly before leaving the lab or pharmacy.

    c. Absorption: The third way in which environmental chemicals enter the body is through the skin. Organic solvents and some other chemicals can be absorbed directly through the skin. Some chemicals cause irritation or tissue damage through direct contact with the skin, eyes, nasal passages, and other accessible body membranes. To protect yourself from accidental absorption or surface contact, wear appropriate personal protective clothing, such as gloves and lab coats or protective gowns; use safety goggles to protect your eyes.

2. General types of health hazards from chemicals

Though OSHA states that it is difficult to completely identify and define the wide range of health hazards, their regulation Health Hazard Definitions (Mandatory) – 1910.1200 App A defines the following terms. Briefly,

    a. Acute effects: rapid effects from short-term exposure

    b. Chronic effects: effects that result from long-term exposure and that are of long duration

    c. Carcinogen: a chemical that has been judged by one of the designated agencies or reports to be a carcinogen or a potential carcinogen

    d. Corrosive: a chemical that causes visible destruction or irreversible alteration in living tissue

    e. Irritant: a chemical that, while not corrosive, causes a reversible inflammatory reaction on living tissue

    f. Sensitizer: a chemical that causes a substantial proportion of exposed individuals to develop an allergic reaction to the chemical on repeated exposures

    g. Highly toxic: chemicals classified in terms of their LD_{50} in mice or rabbits by the various routes of exposure (e.g., an LD_{50} of 50 mg/kg or less when administered orally)

    h. Toxic: chemicals also classified in terms of their LD_{50} in mice or rabbits by the various routes of exposure (e.g., LD_{50} of greater than 50 mg but less than 500 mg/kg, when administered orally) (16)

3. Hazardous drugs

    a. The class of hazardous drugs forms a separate category of chemicals that require special handling. The term *hazardous drugs* was first used and defined in the 1990 ASHP Technical Assistance Bulletin on Handling Cytotoxic and Hazardous Drugs (17). Previously the terms *cytotoxics*, *antineoplastics*, and *chemotherapeutic agents* were used to describe cancer treatment drugs, which were the main source of hazardous drugs in health care settings. At that time, it was decided that a broader term was needed to describe these drugs and others that presented similar handling hazards.

    b. In September 2004, NIOSH published the NIOSH Alert: Preventing Occupational Exposures to Antineoplastic and Other Hazardous Drugs in Health Care Settings; this comprehensive document defines and gives a sample list of hazardous drugs, describes the health hazards associated with acute and chronic exposure to hazardous drugs, and gives recommendations for safely handling these agents in health care facilities (5).

    c. A hazardous drug is defined by the NIOSH Alert as a drug that has one or more of the characteristics listed here.

        (1) Carcinogenicity

        (2) Teratogencity or other developmental toxicity

        (3) Reproductive toxicity

        (4) Organ toxicity at low doses

        (5) Genotoxicity

Table 13.1	NIOSH ALERT SAMPLE LIST OF DRUGS THAT SHOULD BE HANDLED AS HAZARDOUS

Aldesleukin	Dinoprostone	Interferon alfa-2a	Podophyllum resin
Alemtuzumab	Docetaxel	Interferon alfa-2b	Prednimustine
Alitretinoin	Doxorubicin	Interferon alfa-n1	Procarbazine
Altretamine	Dutasteride	Interferon alfa-n3	Progesterone
Amsacrine	Epirubicin	Irinotecan HCl	Progestins
Anastrozole	Ergonovine/	Leflunomide	Raloxifene
Arsenic Trioxide	methyl-ergonovine	Letrozole	Raltitrexed
Asparaginase	Estradiol	Leuprolide acetate	Ribavirin
Azacitidine	Estramustine phosphate Na	Lomustine	Streptozocin
Azathioprine	Estrogen-progestin	Mechlorethamine	Tacrolimus
Bacillus Calmette-Guerin	combinations	Megestrol	Tamoxifen
Bexarotene	Estrogens, conjugated	Melphalan	Temozolomide
Bicalutamide	Estrogens, esterified	Menotropins	Teniposide
Bleomycin	Estrone	Mercaptopurine	Testolactone
Busulfan	Estropipate	Methotrexate	Testosterone
Capecitabine	Etoposide	Methyltestosterone	Thalidomide
Carboplatin	Exemestane	Mifepristone	Thioguanine
Cetrorelix acetate	Finasteride	Mitomycin	Thiotepa
Chlorambucil	Floxuridine	Mitotane	Topotecan
Chloramphenicol	Fludarabine	Mitoxantrone HCl	Toremifene citrate
Choriogonadotropin alfa	Fluorouracil	Mycophenolate mofetil	Tositumomab
Cidofovir	Fluoxymesterone	Nafarelin	Tretinoin
Cisplatin	Flutamide	Nilutamide	Trifluridine
Cladribine	Fulvestrant	Oxiliplatin	Trimetrexate glucuronate
Colchicine	Ganciclovir	Oxytocin	Triptorelin
Cyclophosphamide	Ganirelix acetate	Paclitaxel	Uracil mustard
Cytarabine	Gemtuzumab ozogamicin	Pegaspargase	Valganciclovir
Cyclosporin	Gonadotropin, chorionic	Pentamidine isethionate	Valrubicin
Dacarbazine	Goserelin	Pentostatin	Vidarabine
Dactinomycin	Hydroxyurea	Perphosphamide	Vinblastine sulfate
Daunorubicin HCl	Ibritumomab tiuxetan	Pipobroman	Vincristine sulfate
Denileukin	Idarubicin	Piritrexim isethionate	Vindesine
Dienestrol	Ifosfamide	Plicamycin	Vinorelbine tartrate
Diethylstilbestrol	Imatinib mesylate	Podofilox	Zidovudine

Adapted from National Institute for Occupational Safety and Health. NIOSH alert: Preventing occupational exposures to antineoplastic and other hazardous drug in health care settings. http://www.cdc.gov/niosh/docs/2004-165/. Accessed August 2007.

(6) Structure and toxicity profiles of new drugs that mimic existing drugs determined hazardous by the above criteria. (5)

(See the NIOSH Alert for more details on these categories.)

d. Table 13.1 gives the NIOSH Alert sample list of drugs that should be handled as hazardous. Many of the drugs are antineoplastic agents, but there are also antivirals, immunosuppressants, hormones, and others from miscellaneous categories. For example, podophyllum resin and colchicine are listed as unclassified or miscellaneous hazardous drugs. Though NIOSH stresses that this is not a complete list of hazardous drugs, it is a useful guide to the types of therapeutic agents that should be handled with special precautions (5).

e. Handling hazardous drugs in the pharmacy and health care facilities is extremely important. Though this subject is beyond the scope of this book, pharmacists and pharmacy technicians who handle hazardous drugs should be well informed about this area of practice. Fortunately there are good resources available on this subject including the following:

(1) *NIOSH Alert Preventing Occupational Exposures to Antineoplastic and Other Hazardous Drug in Health Care Settings.* National Institute for Occupational Safety and Health, DHHS (NIOSH) Publication No. 2004-165, available through the NIOSH Internet site: http://www.cdc.gov/niosh/docs/2004-165/ (accessed August 2007)

(2) *OSHA Technical Manual Section VI: Chapter 2 Controlling Occupational Exposure to Hazardous Drugs*, available through OSHA's Internet site at: www.osha.gov/dts/osta/otm/otm_vi/otm_vi_2.html (accessed August 2007)

(3) *OSHA Technical Information Bulletin: Potential Health Hazards Associated with the Process of Compounding Medications from Pharmaceutical Grade Ingredients*, available through OSHA's Internet site at: www.osha.gov/dts/tib/tib_data/tib20011221.html (accessed August 2007)

(4) The American Society of Health-System Pharmacists' *ASHP Guideline on Handling Hazardous Drugs*. As with all of ASHP's practice guidelines, this is available on their Internet site at www.ashp.org.

(5) International Academy of Compounding Pharmacists' *Hazard Alert: Compounding with Hazardous and/or Potent Pharmaceuticals*

4. OSHA-required labels for chemicals

   a. As discussed at the beginning of this section, all containers of chemicals must be labeled with appropriate warning information, including the potential hazards of the substance.

   b. OSHA studied communication theory as it was establishing labeling standards, and it found that the more information that appears on a label, the less likely it is to be read (18). For this reason and to provide as much information as possible in a small space, labels use numbers and symbols to represent types and levels of hazard for labeled chemicals. This means that those who handle chemicals must be trained to accurately interpret key words and label information, including the OSHA definitions of chemical health hazards that are described earlier.

   c. Though OSHA has specific labeling requirements, there is no required format or code system for labels. Two visual code systems commonly seen on bulk chemicals are proprietary; therefore, OSHA does not endorse either system. The National Fire Protection Association (NFPA) uses four colored diamonds grouped together in the shape of a large diamond. The National Paint and Coating Association developed the Hazardous Materials Identification System (HMIS), which is a stacked bar of four colored rectangles.

   (1) Both systems use some of the same color codes (blue for health hazards and red for flammability) and a similar numbering system (0 is the least hazardous, 4 the most dangerous).

   (2) There are some differences: HMIS has an orange section for physical hazards and a white section for personal protective equipment, whereas NFPA has a yellow section for instability and a white section for special hazards, such as unusual reactivity to water. The differences are understandable because the NFPA label was designed primarily for fire fighters and emergency responders and the HMIS label was created to convey health hazard information to people who work with chemicals.

   d. If a bulk drug or chemical is transferred from one container to another, the responsible person must properly label the new container with the identity of the chemical and the appropriate hazard warning information.

   e. The HCS provides exemptions for several types of chemicals found in pharmacies:

   (1) Drugs in a retail setting that are packaged for sale to consumers

   (2) Drugs intended for personal consumption by employees in the workplace

   (3) Any drug, when it is in solid final form, for direct administration to a patient

5. Material safety data sheets

   a. As stated at the beginning of this section, the HCS requires that manufacturers and distributors of chemical products provide hazard information in the form of MSDSs with the first shipment of any chemical to their customers.

   b. Facilities at which chemicals are used are required to have MSDSs accessible to all employees who have contact with the chemicals. In the past, these sheets were kept physically in a file or binder, but the HCS now allows access through electronic files on a computer, as long as the computer is immediately accessible in the area wherein the drug or chemical is used (14). Many vendors of pharmacy supplies offer access to MSDS in several ways: printed copies available on request either by mail or by fax or computer access through their Internet site.

   c. MSDSs are reference documents. They are intended to give brief but complete information about the chemical. As with labels, they use designated technical terms (see foregoing definitions) that should be understood by workers, especially supervisors, who use them. Pharmacists, pharmacy technicians, laboratory students, and any others who use chemicals are encouraged to review these sheets, especially before handling a particular drug or chemical.

d. Information on MSDSs has evolved over time. Though there has been pressure for standardization of format and terminology, this is a complex process; and OSHA currently does not mandate a set format as long as critical information is included on the MSDS. To deal with this problem, a committee of the Chemical Manufacturers Association (now the American Chemistry Council) developed a standardized 16-section MSDS, American National Standards Institute (ANSI) standard Z400.1. Though this format is not required, it is now commonly used, and it has the advantage for workers that the most vital information, such as hazards identification and first aid measures, is located at the beginning of the MSDS (18).

e. For pharmacists and pharmacy technicians, one of the most important sections of an MSDS is the information on exposure control/personal protection (e.g., personal protective equipment, such as gloves, safety goggles, lab coats, and mask respirators, and engineering controls, such as appropriate ventilation and containment hoods). This information should be used in determining what protective measures to use in safely handling the chemical. Most often this information gives several options, each with a different level of protection, and using this information requires judgment in evaluating potential exposure levels (18).

6. Globally Harmonized System (GHS) of Classification and Labeling of Chemicals

In 1992, the United Nations Conference on Environment and Development proposed an international harmonized chemical classification and labeling system. Since that time, much effort has gone into the development of the Globally Harmonized System (GHS) of Classification and Labeling of Chemicals. The GHS has standardized requirements for labels and MSDSs, and it is now available for worldwide implementation. At the time of this writing, the United States was still in the process of deciding whether to adopt the GHS, but International Chemical Safety Cards (similar to the MSDS) covering more than 1,300 substances in 14 languages are available on OSHA's Internet site (18).

VI. SOURCES OF SUPPLY FOR DRUGS AND CHEMICALS, COMPOUNDING EQUIPMENT, PACKAGING MATERIALS, AND TECHNICAL SUPPORT

Compounding of custom drug preparations has been able to expand in recent years partly because of the availability of new and useful items of equipment, packaging and labeling materials, pharmaceutic ingredients, and drugs and chemicals. Most companies that sell drugs and supplies also maintain Internet sites with catalogs and useful compounding information (e.g., Paddock Labs' *Secundum Artem* articles), and some companies also provide personal technical support for compounding questions and problems. Available information on compounding has also greatly expanded in recent years with excellent articles in professional journals, such as the *International Journal of Pharmaceutical Compounding, American Journal of Health-System Pharmacists,* and the *Journal of the American Pharmacists Association.* The International Academy of Compounding Pharmacists (www.iacprx.org) is an excellent source of information on compounding supplies and technical assistance and standards.

REFERENCES

1. National Association of Boards of Pharmacy. Model State Pharmacy Act and Model Rules of the National Association of Boards of Pharmacy. Mount Prospect, IL: Author, 2006; 66–67.

2. The United States Pharmacopeial Convention, Inc. Chapter ⟨795⟩. 2008 USP 31/NF 26. Rockville, MD: Author, 2007; 315–319.

3. The United States Pharmacopeial Convention, Inc. Chapter ⟨1075⟩. 2008 USP 31/NF 26. Rockville, MD: Author, 2007; 500–503.

4. American Society of Health-System Pharmacists. ASHP technical assistance bulletin on compounding nonsterile products in pharmacies. http://www.ashp.org/. Accessed March 2007.

5. National Institute for Occupational Safety and Health. NIOSH alert: Preventing occupational exposures to antineoplastic and other hazardous drug in health care settings. http://www.cdc.gov/niosh/docs/2004-165/. Accessed August 2007.

6. National Association of Boards of Pharmacy. Model State Pharmacy Act and Model Rules of the National Association of Boards of Pharmacy. Mount Prospect, IL: Author, 2006; 3.

7. National Association of Boards of Pharmacy. Model State Pharmacy Act and Model Rules of the National Association of Boards of Pharmacy. Mount Prospect, IL: Author, 2006; 195–196.

8. U.S. Department of Health and Human Services, Food and Drug Administration, Office of Regulatory Affairs, Center for Drug Evaluation and Research. Compliance policy guidance for FDA staff and industry, chapter 4, subchapter 460, section 460.200. Pharmacy Compounding. Washington, DC: Author, May 2002. www.fda.gov/ora/complicance_ref/cpg/cpgdrg/cpg460-200.htm.

9. The United States Pharmacopeial Convention, Inc. General notices. 2008 USP 31/NF 26. Rockville, MD: Author, 2007; 9–11.

10. The United States Pharmacopeial Convention, Inc. Chapter ⟨1150⟩. 2008 USP 31/NF 26. Rockville, MD: Author, 2007; 613.

11. The United States Pharmacopeial Convention, Inc. Chapter ⟨671⟩. 2008 USP 31/NF 26. Rockville, MD: Author, 2007; 255–258.

12. Occupational Safety and Health Administration. OSHA facts: August 2007. http://www.osha.gov/as/opa/oshafacts.html. Accessed August 2007.

13. National Institute for Occupational Safety and Health. About NIOSH. http://www.cdc.gov/niosh/about.html. Accessed August 2007.

14. Occupational Safety and Health Administration. Guidelines for employer compliance (Advisory) 1910.1200 App E. http://www.osha.gov/pls/oshaweb/owadisp.show_document?p_table=STANDARDS&p_id=10104. Accessed August 2007.

15. Occupational Safety and Health Administration. Guidance for hazard determination. http://www.osha.gov/dsg/hazcom/ghd053107.html. Accessed August 2007.

16. Occupational Safety and Health Administration. Health hazard definitions (Mandatory) 1910.1200 App A. http://www.osha.gov/pls/pshaweb/owadisp.show_document?p_table=STANDARDS&P_ID=10100. Accessed August 2007.

17. American Society of Health-System Pharmacists. ASHP technical assistance bulletin on handling cytotoxic and hazardous drugs. Am J Health-Syst Pharm 1990; 47: 1033–1049.

18. Occupational Safety and Health Administration. Hazard communication in the 21st century workplace. http://www.osha.gov/dsg/hazcom/finalmsdsreport.html. Accessed August 2007.

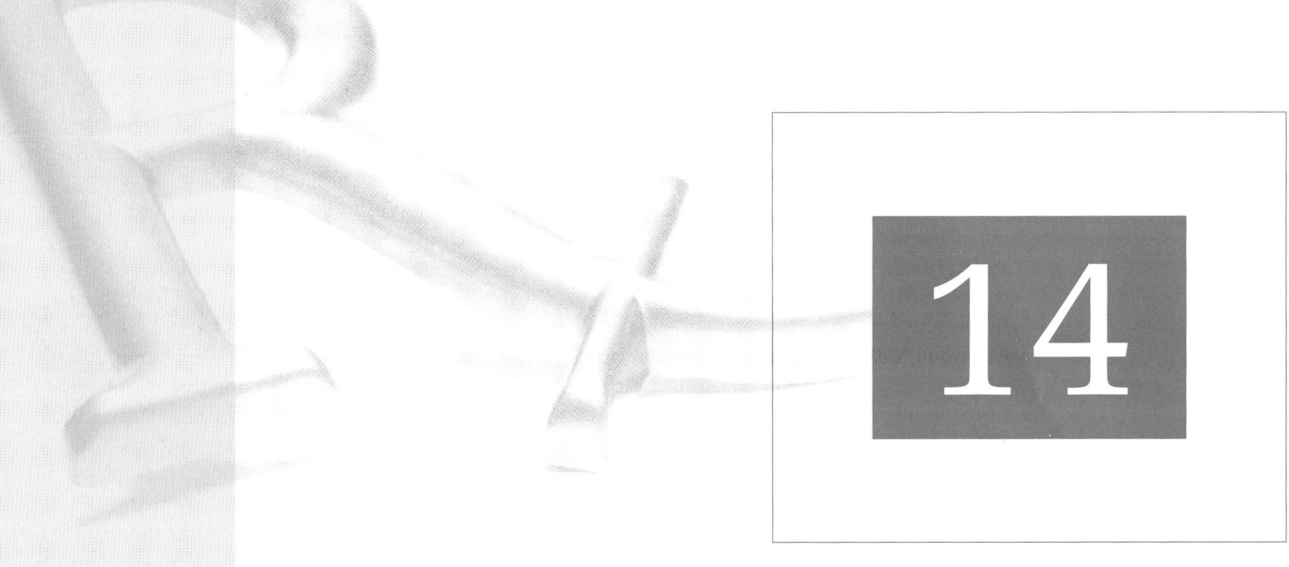

Selection and Use of Weighing and Measuring Equipment

I. STANDARDS AND STANDARD-SETTING AGENCIES

A. Because balances, weights, and volumetric measuring devices are essential tools in the practice of pharmacy, pharmacists need to know how to select and properly use this equipment. In order to access, understand, and use the accepted standards for this equipment, it is necessary to know the organizations and agencies that have responsibility for these areas. In the United States, this is a complex affair. Unlike many other countries, in which authority for weights and measures is centralized in their federal governments, in the United States, this function is decentralized in a patchwork of state and federal agencies and not-for-profit organizations.

 1. **National Institute for Standards and Technology (NIST):** This agency, which was formerly called the National Bureau of Standards (NBS), is a nonregulatory agency in the Department of Commerce. It was established by Congress in 1901 to "serve as a national scientific laboratory in the physical sciences, and to provide fundamental measurement standards for science and industry" (1). It is charged with working with the states to develop laws, codes, and procedures to secure uniformity of weights and measures and methods of inspection. Since 1949, NIST has published the guidebook known as *Handbook 44*. This book contains specifications, tolerances, and other technical requirements for weighing and measuring devices for everything from livestock scales to taximeters to jewelry scales, and it includes standards for prescription balances and volumetric devices used in pharmacies (1). Internet site: www.nist.gov.

 2. **National Conference on Weights and Measures (NCWM):** Though it is not a government agency, the NCWM works with the Office of Weights and Measures of NIST in creating weights and measures standards. The standards in *Handbook 44* are reviewed, revised, amended, and adopted each year at the Annual Meeting of the NCWM (1). Also, in cooperation with the NIST, state

173

government weights and measures officials, and private sector individuals, the NCWM operates the National Type Evaluation Program (NTEP) to evaluate and certify weighing and measuring devices such as electronic balances (2). Internet site: www.ncwm.net.

3. **American Society for Testing and Materials (ASTM):** Now called ASTM International, this not-for-profit organization develops and publishes voluntary standards for materials, products, systems, and services. The "Standard Specifications for Laboratory Weights and Precision Mass Standards" (E 617 – 97), which specifies our classes of weights, is a publication of ASTM. Internet site: www.astm.org.

4. **American National Standards Institute (ANSI):** This is also a not-for-profit, nongovernmental organization. It does not develop standards, but it serves as the U.S. representative to international standard-setting organizations, such as the International Organization for Standardization (ISO). ANSI also accredits national organizations, such as ASTM, that develop standards. Internet site: www.ansi.org.

5. **United States Pharmacopeial Convention (USP):** Since 1820, USP, another not-for-profit, nongovernmental organization, has been setting standards for drugs and medications in the United States. USP publishes the *United States Pharmacopeia* (*USP*) and the *National Formulary* (*NF*), two separate compendia that are now published in a combined volume that is commonly referred to simply as the *USP*. This book of standards contains drug and dosage form monographs that specify the standards for strength, quality, and purity for each monograph entity. *USP* also contains general chapters that describe tests, assays, and practice standards for drug manufacturing and compounding. *USP* Chapter ⟨1176⟩ Prescription Balances and Volumetric Apparatus sets standards for weighing and measuring equipment used in pharmacies (3). Internet site: www.usp.org.

B. With this information in mind, it is important to remember the following:

1. Standards, such as those in *Handbook 44*, ASTM E 617–97, or *USP*, have been developed by government or private agencies for use by the state and federal governments in regulating commerce and protecting public health and safety. Though they are written as voluntary standards, they become legally enforceable if they are written into federal laws (such as the Federal Food, Drug, and Cosmetic Act) or state statutes or administrative codes.

2. Because requirements for weighing and measuring equipment in pharmacies are primarily regulated by state statutes, it is important for pharmacists to be informed about the applicable state codes for pharmacy equipment for their practice sites. For example, if a state statute states that pharmacies must use graduates that conform to the standards in *Handbook 44*, the graduate specifications in that document would be legally enforceable in the pharmacies of that state.

3. Even when nationally recognized standards are not codified in state statutes and federal laws, these standards provide invaluable guidance to pharmacists in selecting and using appropriate weighing and measuring equipment and apparatus.

II. GENERAL PRINCIPLES FOR WEIGHING AND MEASURING

To prepare accurate dosage forms, the pharmacist and pharmacy technician must use weighing and measuring apparatus with care and understanding and must be conscious of the following general principles:

A. **Select** weighing equipment and measuring devices appropriate for the intended purpose.

B. **Use** the devices and operate the equipment with recommended techniques that ensure accuracy of measurement.

C. **Maintain** the equipment so that it is clean and free of chemical contamination and retains the prescribed tolerances.

III. BALANCES AND WEIGHTS

A. **Definitions:** In selecting a balance for purchase or for use in compounding, the pharmacist and pharmacy technician need to be familiar with the following terms:

1. **Capacity:** the maximum weight, including containers and tares, that can be placed on a balance pan

2. **Sensitivity:** also referred to as *Sensitivity Requirement* or *Sensitivity Reciprocal*, the smallest weight that gives a perceptible change in the indicating element (e.g., one subdivision deflection of the indicator pointer on the index plate of a double-pan balance; one number change on the digital display of an electronic balance)

3. **Readability:** for electronic balances, the smallest weight increment that can be read on the digital display of the balance (e.g., 0.001 g). On a double-pan balance, the smallest weight incre-

ment is determined by the value of a hash-mark on the graduated dial or weighbeam (e.g., on the metric scale of the dial, each mark stands for 0.01 g, and on the apothecaries' scale of the dial, each mark stands for 0.2 grains).

4. **Precision:** the reproducibility of the weighing measurement as expressed by a standard deviation. A similar term, *repeatability*, is sometimes used in specifications for electronic balances.

5. **Accuracy:** the closeness of the displayed weight, as measured by the balance, to the true weight, as known by the use of a calibration weight or weights

B. **Prescription balances**

There are two types of balances used for prescription compounding: double-pan torsion balances and single-pan electronic balances.

1. **Double-pan torsion balances**

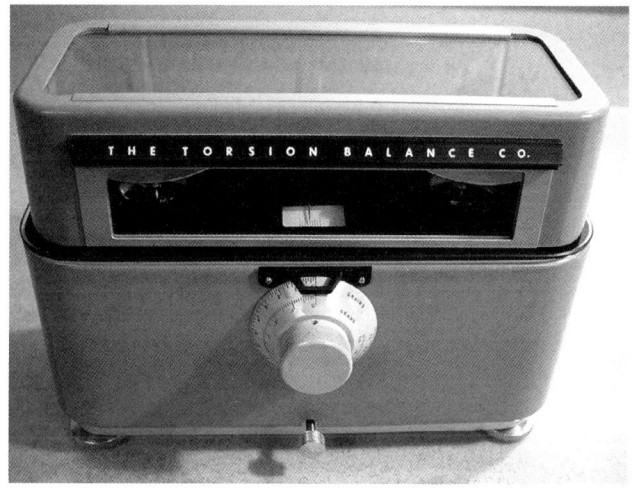

DOUBLE-PAN TORSION BALANCE

a. Specifications for prescription balances are given in Section 2.20 Scales in *Handbook 44*. In general, these balances meet the specifications for NIST Class III scales (formerly designated Class A); however, *Handbook 44* gives some design elements and tolerance specifications that are specific for prescription balances (1).

b. *USP* Chapter ⟨1176⟩ specifies that a Class A (that is, Class III) prescription balance be used for all weighing operations required in prescription compounding (3). (However, see 2.a., which follows, concerning allowance for balances giving equivalent or better accuracy.)

c. Sensitivity: These balances meet or exceed a sensitivity requirement of 6 mg with no load and with a load of 10 g on each pan (1,3).

d. Capacity: The maximum load capacity should be stated in the manufacturer's specifications for that particular balance. Though a balance may have a capacity such as 60 or 120 g, it is usually impractical to weigh amounts >15 to 30 g on a double-pan balance because the volume occupied by larger weights of most powders and dry ingredients is difficult to contain on weighing papers, boats, or dishes without spilling.

e. Because *Handbook 44* is written to describe nearly all types of weighing devices, it is a rather extensive document and is written in technical language. Therefore, for the pharmacist selecting a torsion prescription balance, the most practical procedure is to buy a balance that is certified to meet or exceed the specifications for a NIST Class III prescription balance.

2. **Electronic single-pan balances**

a. Though the *USP* Chapter ⟨1176⟩ specifies that Class A (now Class III) prescription balances be used for all weighing operations required in prescription compounding, a note at the beginning of that chapter states that other balances may be used, provided they give equivalent or better accuracy (3).

b. Sensitivity: It is important to pick an electronic balance that has a sensitivity that is at least equivalent to the 6-mg standard for Class III prescription balances. Electronic, single-pan balances with readability and repeatability of 1 mg are available, and these would exceed this Class III balance sensitivity specification.

c. Capacity: Capacities vary with the brand, model, and price. Often as the capacity goes up, the sensitivity or readability goes down. Some electronic balances come with dual modes:

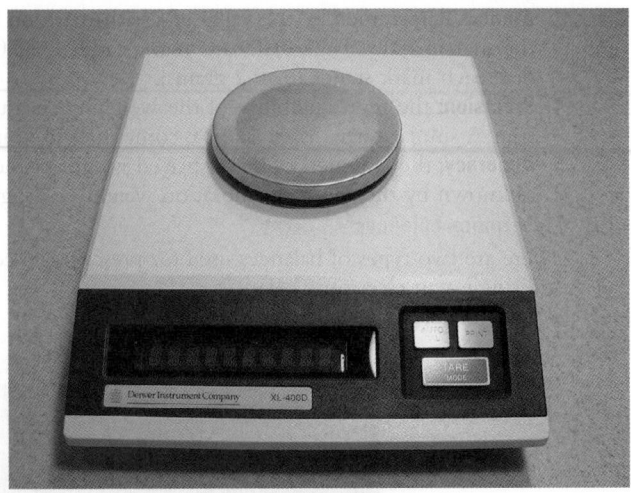

ELECTRONIC BALANCE

one mode for low capacity and high sensitivity and a second mode with larger capacity but lower sensitivity. When using such a balance, it is important to be operating in the proper mode for the weighing task.

d. Electronic balances with an official NTEP rating have been tested and evaluated by the NCWM and are certified to meet applicable U.S. weight and measure standards (2).

e. Most individuals who have used electronic balances find them easier to use and more accurate than a traditional double-pan torsion balance. Though appropriately selected electronic balances meet or exceed the requirements for prescription balances as stated in *Handbook 44* and the *USP*, before purchasing an electronic balance, the pharmacist should consult with his or her state board of pharmacy to determine whether a given balance meets the applicable state statutes or codes for pharmacy equipment.

3. Minimum or least weighable quantity.

It is extremely important to distinguish between the minimum quantity that is possible to detect or weigh on a balance (i.e., the balance's sensitivity) and the minimum quantity that may be weighed if you wish to ensure a desired level of accuracy. The least or minimum weighable quantity (MWQ) allowed for prescription compounding is 20 times the sensitivity or sensitivity requirement as illustrated here.

a. A maximum 5% error is the generally accepted standard for weighing operations used in compounding (3).

b. To avoid errors of 5% or more when weighing on a balance, calculate the MWQ by equating 5% × MWQ with the sensitivity requirement (SR) of the balance. This is because that balance cannot detect differences in weight smaller than the SR; therefore, any smaller amounts could be in error. The general equation is:

$$5\% \times MWQ = SR$$

For example, on a Class III balance with a measured sensitivity requirement of 6 mg, the MWQ is calculated to be 120 mg:

$$5\% \times MWQ = 6 \text{ mg}$$
$$MWQ = \frac{6 \text{ mg}}{0.05} = 120 \text{ mg}$$

c. A more sensitive balance could obviously use a smaller MWQ. For example, a balance with a sensitivity requirement of 1 mg would have a MWQ of 20 mg (checking by percent: 5% × 20 mg = 1 mg).

d. If an amount of drug or chemical is needed that is less than the MWQ determined for that balance, an aliquot method of measurement should be used. Methods of calculating aliquot amounts are presented in Chapter 10, Aliquot Calculations.

4. Balance testing

a. *USP* general guidelines

(1) Chapter ⟨1176⟩ states, "All balances should be calibrated and tested frequently using appropriate test weights, both singly and in combination" (3).

(2) Chapter ⟨795⟩ Pharmaceutical Compounding—Nonsterile states, "Equipment and accessories used in compounding are to be inspected, maintained, cleaned, and validated at appropriate intervals to ensure the accuracy and reliability of their performance" (4).

b. Frequency of testing: As can be seen from the foregoing statements, the frequency of balance testing is not explicitly stated and is therefore a matter of professional judgment and experience with a particular balance and practice patterns with that instrument. It is important to have a written plan for scheduled frequency of testing.

c. Records of testing: A balance-testing record should be maintained by the pharmacy; the record should include the date, the type of testing and calibration procedures performed, the results, and the name or initials of the person who performed the procedures. A sample standard operating procedure (SOP) for testing a Class III torsion balance is given in Chapter 12 Figure 12.3, and a sample testing record sheet used in conjunction with the SOP is shown in Figure 14.1.

d. Testing procedures for electronic balances

(1) Testing and calibration procedures for electronic balances are given in the use and maintenance manual provided by the balance manufacturer.

(2) The usual procedure involves the use of special test calibration weights that may be provided with the balance or purchased separately. Usually ASTM Class 1 (NBS Class S) weights are required.

e. Testing procedures for Class III torsion balances

(1) Test weights: ASTM Class 4 (NBS Class P) or better weights are recommended for testing Class III prescription balances. This weight set should be reserved for testing the balance and for checking weights that are routinely used for compounding (3). **The graduated dial or rider on a double–pan torsion balance may not be used to calibrate the balance** because an internal mechanism does not constitute a valid standard for testing an instrument.

(2) *USP* Chapter ⟨1176⟩ specifies the following tests to be performed on torsion prescription balances. As stated earlier, a sample testing procedure with the details of these tests is shown in Figure 14.1.

(a) Sensitivity requirement

(b) Arm ratio test

(c) Shift tests

(d) Rider and graduated beam tests (3)

(3) The test for sensitivity requirement deserves some additional comment. The *USP* gives the following instructions regarding this test: "Level the balance, determine the rest point, and place a 6-mg weight on one of the empty pans. Repeat the operation with a 10-g weight in the center of each pan. The rest point is shifted not less than one division on the index plate each time the 6-mg weight is added" (3). Unfortunately, many weight sets available to pharmacies do not contain the 6-mg weight required for this test; the smallest weight in a set may be a 10-mg weight. A modified sensitivity requirement test may still be performed using other weights of comparable size, provided a linear relationship is established for the range of measurement. The procedure is as follows:

(a) Put weighing papers or weighing dishes on each balance pan.

(b) Bring the balance into equilibrium using the leveling feet at the front of the balance.

(c) Place one 10-mg weight on the right-hand balance pan.

(d) Release the pan arrest and read the number of divisions the balance indicator is deflected on the index plate: _____

(e) Repeat steps (c) and (d) using a 20-mg weight. How many units is the balance indicator shifted on the index plate now? _____

A linear relationship exists if the number found in (e) is two times that in (d); that is, double the weight gives double the deflections. If a linear relationship exists, the sensitivity requirement can be calculated as shown next. For this example, a 10-mg weight was found to give 1.5 deflections, and a 20-mg weight gave 3 deflections (a linear relationship was established).

$$\frac{10 \text{ mg weight}}{1.5 \text{ deflections}} = \frac{x \text{ mg weight}}{1 \text{ deflections}}; x = 6.7 \text{ mg}$$

In this example, the balance does not meet the Class III balance requirement. Remember, for a Class III balance, the sensitivity requirement must be 6 mg or less. In this example, a weight greater than 6 mg (6.7 mg) was needed to give one deflection.

Test	Results	Pass/Fail
Sensitivity Requirement		
1. Place a 6-mg weight on one of the empty balance pans. Release the balance pans. How many divisions is the indicator deflected on the index plate? To pass, the indicator must deflect 1 or more divisions.		
2. Place a 10-g weight in the center of each pan and place the 6-mg weight on one of the empty pans. How many divisions is the indicator deflected on the index plate? To pass, indicator must deflect 1 or more divisions		
Arm Ratio Test		
1. Place a 30-g weight in the center of each balance pan. Release the balance pans. Is the indicator deflected on the index plate? If no deflection, pass. If indicator deflected, perform 2.		
2. Place a 20-mg weight on the balance pan for the lighter side. Is the indicator back to the rest point or farther? If yes, pass; if no, fail.		
Shift Test		
1. Place a 10-g weight in the center of the left pan. Place a second 10-g weight on the right pan and successively move that weight toward the right, left, front, and back of the pan. In each case, is the indicator deflected? If no, pass. If indicator deflected, perform 2.		
2. If indicator deflected with any of the above shifts, add a 10-mg weight to the balance pan of the lighter side. Is the indicator back to the rest point or farther? If yes, pass; if no, fail.		
3. Place a 10-g weight in the center of the right pan. Place another 10-g weight on the left pan and successively move that weight toward the right, left, front, and back of the pan. If each case, is the indicator deflected? If no, pass. If indicator deflected, perform 4.		
4. If indicator deflected with any of the above shifts, add a 10-mg weight to the balance pan of the lighter side. Is the indicator back to the rest point or farther? If yes, pass; if no, fail.		
5. Move the 10-g weights to all different positions on both balance pans, e.g., both left, both right, one left and one right, both back, both front, one back and one front, etc. Is the indicator deflected on the index plate? If no, pass. If indicator deflected, perform 6.		
6. If indicator deflected with any of the above shifts, add a 10-mg weight to the balance pan of the lighter side. Is the indicator back to the rest point or farther? If yes, pass; if no, fail.		
Rider and Graduated Beam Tests		
1. Place a 500-mg weight on the left balance pan. Move the rider or the graduated dial weight to the 500-mg position. Is the indicator deflected on the index plate? If no, pass. If the indicator is deflected, perform 2.		
2. If the indicator is deflected, place a 6-mg weight on the balance pan for the lighter side. Is the indicator back to the rest point or farther? If yes, pass; if no, fail		
3. Place a 1-g weight on the left balance pan. Move the rider or the graduated dial weight to the 1-g position. Is the indicator deflected on the index plate? If no, pass. If the indicator is deflected, perform 4.		
4. If the indicator is deflected, place a 6-mg weight on the balance pan for the lighter side. Is the indicator back to the rest point or farther? If yes, pass; if no, fail.		

Date_____

Balance Brand and Model Number_____

Test Weight Brand and Class_____

Pharmacist/Technician_____

Before proceeding with the balance tests, do the following:

1. Position the balance on flat, level surface away from drafts and air currents.
2. Check that the weighbeam rider or dial-in weights are at zero.
3. Using balance leveling feet, bring balance into equilibrium with the indicator at the zero position on index plate. Check this before each of the following tests.

This balance passes the above performance tests.   Signed:_____

FIGURE 14.1. BALANCE TESTING FOR A TORSION BALANCE.

f. Repair and reconditioning of balances: For balances that need to be repaired or reconditioned, contact the service department of the balance manufacturer. There are also companies that have the equipment and expertise to test, calibrate, recondition, and repair torsion and electronic balances. One such company is Pharmaceutical Balance Systems; information is available at their Internet site at www.PharmacyBalances.com or Email: info@pharmacy-balances.com.

C. Weights

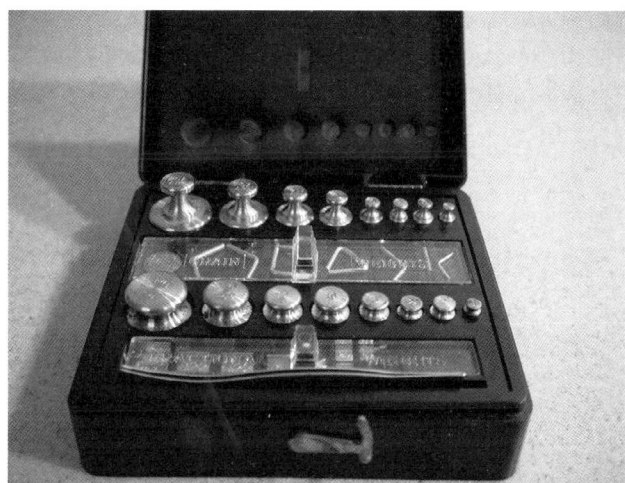

WEIGHT SET

1. Metric weights are the preferred weights to use in compounding. Some weight sets contain both metric and apothecary weights in the same box. These sets should be used with extreme caution because it is easy to select a weight from the wrong system. This is especially true when people who are not familiar with both systems use these weights.

2. All weights must have cylindrical construction, and coin-type weights should not be used (3).

3. Weights are to be stored in a rigid, compartmentalized box and should be handled with special forceps or tweezers to prevent contamination (3).

4. Recommended classes for prescription weights

   a. The situation with classes of weights is a bit confusing because as the class designations have changed over the years, and many older documents and standards still contain the former class designations.

      (1) Prior to 1978, weight classifications and specifications were contained in NBS Circular 547, which used letter designations such as *P* and *Q* to specify weight classes (5).

      (2) In 1978, NBS Circular 547 was superseded by ASTM E 617 (Standard Specification for Laboratory Weights and Precision Mass Standards), which uses number designations 0 through 7 (5).

      [The ASTM standard has a fixed designation of E 617 with a number immediately following that indicates the year of latest revision and sometimes followed by a number in parenthesis with the year of latest reapproval. For example, in the year 2007, the document designation was E 617-97 (2003), which means 1997 was the year of last revision, and 2003 was the year the standard was most recently reapproved (6).]

      (3) The international standard, International Recommendation R 111, from Organisation Internationale de Metrologie Legale (OIML), uses classes E1, E2, F1, F2, M1, M2, and M3 (6).

      (4) Table 14.1 gives a comparison of the various class designations (5); this is especially useful when using documents or catalogs written with either NBS letter weight classes or R111 classes. From this table, it is easy to see that NBS Class P is approximately equivalent to ASTM Class 4. Table 14.2 has the more detailed specifications for the various weight classes (7).

   b. For prescription compounding with a torsion balance, *USP* Chapter ⟨1176⟩ recommends the use of Class P (ASTM Class 4) or better weights but states that Class Q (ASTM Class 5) weights may be used because they do have tolerances within the limits of accuracy for Class III prescription balances (3).

Table 14.1	ACCURACY CLASSES FOR WEIGHTS

OIML R 111 1994	ASTM E 617-1997	NBS CIRCULAR 547 SUPERSEDED 1978	NIST 105-1 1990
Extra-fine accuracy			
E1	—	—	—
E2	0	—	—
	1	M, S	—
Fine accuracy			
F1	2	—	—
	3	S-1	—
F2	—	—	—
Medium accuracy			
—	4	P	—
M1	5	Q	—
M2	6	T	F
M3	7	—	—

Adapted from Weights and Measures Division, NIST. Commonly asked questions about mass standards. http://ts.nist.gov/WeightsAndMeasures/caqmass.cfm. Accessed September 2007.

Table 14.2	METRIC WEIGHT TOLERANCES

	INTERNATIONAL ORGANIZATION R111				ANSI/ASTM E 617						NBS CIRCULAR 547 SECTION 1					NIST
Size	F1	F2	M1	M2[a]	Class 1[b]	Class 2[b]	Class 3	Class 4	Class 5	Class 6	M[b]	S	S-1	P	Q	105-1 F
100 g	0.5	1.5	5	15	0.25	0.50	1.0	2.0	9	10	0.50	0.25	1.0	2.0	9.0	20
50 g	0.30	1.0	3.0	10	0.12	0.25	0.6	1.2	5.6	7	0.25	0.12	0.60	1.2	5.6	10
30 g	—	—	—	—	0.074	0.15	0.45	0.90	4.0	5	0.15	0.074	0.45	0.90	4.0	6.0
20 g	0.25	0.8	2.5	8	0.074	0.10	0.35	0.70	3.0	3	0.10	0.074	0.35	0.70	3.0	4.0
10 g	0.20	0.6	2.0	6	0.05	0.074	0.25	0.50	2.0	2	0.050	0.074	0.25	0.50	2.0	2.0
5 g	0.15	0.5	1.5	5	0.034	0.054	0.18	0.36	1.3	2	0.034	0.054	0.18	0.36	1.3	1.5
3 g	—	—	—	—	0.034	0.054	0.15	0.30	0.95	2	0.034	0.054	0.15	0.30	0.95	1.3
2 g	0.12	0.4	1.2	4	0.034	0.054	0.13	0.26	0.75	2	0.034	0.054	0.13	0.26	0.75	1.1
1 g	0.10	0.3	1.0	3	0.034	0.054	0.10	0.20	0.50	2	0.034	0.054	0.10	0.20	0.50	0.9
500 mg	0.08	0.25	0.8	2.5	0.010	0.025	0.080	0.16	0.38	1	0.010	0.025	0.080	0.16	0.38	0.72
300 mg	—	—	—	2.0	0.010	0.025	0.070	0.14	0.30	1	0.010	0.025	0.070	0.14	0.30	0.61
200 mg	0.06	0.20	0.6	1.5	0.010	0.025	0.060	0.12	0.26	1	0.010	0.025	0.060	0.12	0.26	0.54
100 mg	0.05	0.15	0.5	—	0.010	0.025	0.050	0.10	0.20	1	0.010	0.025	0.050	0.10	0.20	0.43
50 mg	0.04	0.12	0.4	—	0.010	0.014	0.042	0.085	0.16	—	0.010	0.014	0.042	0.085	0.16	0.35
30 mg	—	—	—	—	0.010	0.014	0.038	0.075	0.14	—	0.010	0.014	0.038	0.075	0.14	0.30
20 mg	0.03	0.10	0.3	—	0.010	0.014	0.035	0.070	0.12	—	0.010	0.014	0.035	0.070	0.12	0.26
10 mg	0.025	0.08	0.25	—	0.010	0.014	0.030	0.060	0.10	—	0.010	0.014	0.030	0.060	0.10	0.21
5 mg	0.020	0.06	0.20	—	0.010	0.014	0.028	0.055	0.080	—	0.010	0.014	0.028	0.055	0.080	0.17
2 mg	0.020	0.06	0.20	—	0.010	0.014	0.025	0.050	0.060	—	0.010	0.014	0.025	0.050	0.060	0.12
1 mg	0.020	0.06	0.20	—	0.010	0.014	0.025	0.050	0.050	—	0.010	0.014	0.025	0.050	0.050	0.10

Note: All tolerances for these class and ranges are in milligrams.
[a]Maintenance tolerances.
[b]Individual.
Source: Troemner Mass Standards Handbook. Philadelphia, PA: Troemner, Inc., 2000; 6–7.

   c. As indicated in the section on balance testing, ASTM Class 1 weights are usually required for testing and calibration of electronic balances, and ASTM Class 4 or better weights are recommended for testing Class III torsion prescription balances (3).

   d. Sometimes there is confusion over the standards for weights given in *USP* Chapter ⟨1176⟩ Prescription Balances and Volumetric Apparatus and Chapter ⟨41⟩ Weights and Balances. Chapter ⟨1176⟩ was written specifically for prescription compounding. The standards for weights given in section ⟨41⟩ of the *USP* were written for "accurate weighing" in *USP* assays and not for general prescription compounding by pharmacists. The recommendation that a weight class be chosen so that the tolerance of the weights does not exceed 0.1% of the amount weighed as given in Chapter ⟨41⟩ is not a requirement for weighing done in prescription compounding (8).

   e. When purchasing a weight set for use in compounding or balance testing, the pharmacist should require information from the vendor on the class of the weight or weight set because catalog descriptions such as "precision metric weight set" and "accurate weights" do not give sufficient information.

D. Weighing papers and dishes

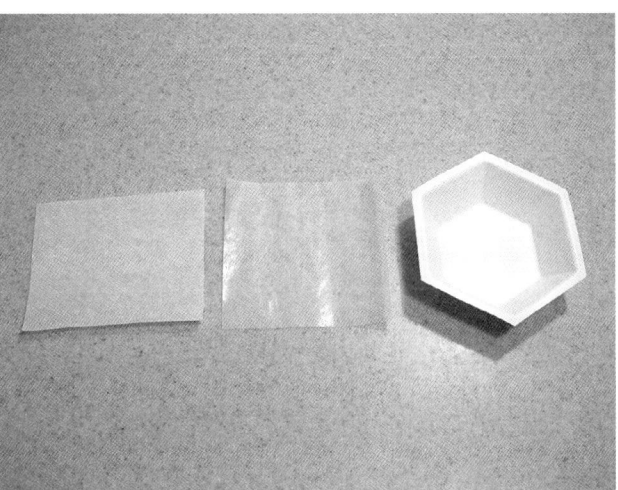

WEIGHING PAPERS AND DISHES

1. When weighing drugs or chemicals, these substances are never placed directly on the balance pan; a disposable weighing paper, boat, or dish is placed on the balance pan, and drug or chemical is placed on the paper or in the boat or dish. A fresh weighing paper or dish is used for each drug or chemical weighed. There are several reasons for using these devices: (i) they protect the balance pan from harmful or corrosive chemicals, (ii) they prevent cross-contamination of drugs and chemicals, and (iii) they eliminate the necessity of washing the balance pan between weighing different drugs or chemicals.

2. Weighing paper

   a. Glassine papers are preferred for weighing. They have a smooth, shiny surface that does not absorb materials placed on them, and drugs and chemicals are easily slipped off for complete transfers. Glassine papers come in various sizes, from 3″ × 3″ to 6″ × 6″.

   b. Some pharmacists use powder papers as weighing papers because they prefer the rectangular shape or sizes available. These papers are available in vegetable parchment paper and come in various sizes. They are acceptable for most purposes, but they are more absorbent than glassine and should not be used for weighing thick liquids, such as coal tar and ichthammol.

   c. Weighing papers should be creased to create a depression or "boat," which helps to contain the substance being weighed and prevents spilling on the balance pans or balance platform. The easiest way to make a weighing boat is to separately pinch together each of the four corners of the paper. A depression can also be made by folding the paper in quarters and then opening the sheet or making 1/4- to 1/2-inch lengthwise folds along each side of the paper.

3. Weighing dishes

   a. Weighing dishes are available in a variety of sizes, shapes, and materials. Most vendors of compounding supplies have dishes made of aluminum and polystyrene plastic. They come in capacity sizes ranging from approximately 5 to 250 mL and shaped as round pans, rectangles, boats, canoes, and hexagons.

b. Though weighing dishes are very handy and they more securely contain substances being weighed, they are also more expensive than weighing papers. They have the added advantage of being useful for weighing liquids because they have rigid sides that contain more securely the liquid being weighed.

IV.   RECOMMENDED WEIGHING PROCEDURES

The following section gives general information and procedures for weighing on a torsion double-pan balance and on an electronic digital balance. These procedures are also demonstrated on the CD that accompanies this book, and abbreviated checklist procedures are given in Figures 14.2 and 14.3.

A. Weighing on a torsion balance

1. Position the balance on a flat, level surface in an area that is away, as much as is possible, from drafts or air currents.

2. Check to be sure that the weighbeam rider or the graduated dial are at the zero position.

3. Using the leveling feet at the front of the balance, bring the balance into equilibrium. Equilibrium is reached when the index pointer, called the *balance indicator*, either comes to rest at the center on the index plate or when it travels an equal number of divisions to the right and left of the center. If air currents in the room affect the movement of the balance pans, the balance lid should be closed. This is also true when determining balance during the weighing procedure.

4. Place a weighing paper or dish on each balance pan. These should be positioned on the balance pans so that they do not interfere with the free movement of the pans.

---

1. Position the balance on a flat, level surface in an area that is away from drafts or air currents

2. Check to be sure that the weighbeam rider or the graduated dial are at the zero position.

3. Using the leveling feet at the front of the balance, bring the balance into equilibrium. If air currents in the room affect the movement of the balance pans, the balance lid should be closed. This is also true when determining balance during the weighing procedure.

4. Place a weighing paper or dish on each balance pan. These should be positioned on the balance pans so that they do not interfere with the free movement of the pans.

5. With the weighing papers or dishes in place, repeat the process of using the leveling feet to bring the balance pans into equilibrium.

6. During the entire weighing procedure, keep the balance pans arrested when adding anything to the balance pans.

7. Add the appropriate external and dial weights to the balance. Handle external weights with tweezers or forceps. **External weights are added to the right-hand balance pan.** This is important because the dial and rider weights are added to that side.

8. Using a spatula, add **material to be weighed** to the weighing paper or dish **on the left-hand balance pan.**

9. Release the arresting mechanisms and observe the balance pointer to determine if you have transferred the desired amount of material, or if too much or too little material was added.

10. If the pans are not in balance, arrest the pans before adding or removing material. Repeat steps 8 and 9 until the index pointer indicates that equilibrium has been reached. As you approach the required weight of material, you may release the balance arrest as you slowly and carefully add very small amounts of material until the exact weight is reached.

11. Arrest the balance pans and remove the weights, both external and dial or rider. As you do this, recheck the weights to be sure you have selected the desired weights. Return the external weights to their appropriate compartments in the weight box.

12. If any powder or liquid was inadvertently spilled on the balance pan or platform, clean the balance.

FIGURE 14.2. PROCEDURE FOR WEIGHING ON A TORSION BALANCE.

1. Position the balance on a flat, level surface in an area that is away from drafts or air currents.

2. Turn the balance on and press the tare button; the digital display should show 0.000 g. If air currents in the room are affecting the balance (the numbers on the digital display will drift up and down), the balance lid should be closed or an air current shield should be put in place. This is also true when determining balance during the weighing procedure.

3. Place a weighing paper or dish on the balance pan. If a weighing paper is being used, it should be positioned so that it does not interfere with the balance lid if it needs to be closed during the weighing procedure.

4. Press the tare button again to tare out the weight of the weighing paper or dish; the digital display should show 0.000 g.

5. Using a spatula, add material to be weighed to the weighing paper or dish on the balance pan until the desired weight appears on the digital display.

6. If any powder or liquid was inadvertently spilled on the balance pan or platform, clean the balance.

FIGURE 14.3. PROCEDURE FOR WEIGHING ON AN ELECTRONIC BALANCE.

5. With the weighing papers or dishes in place, repeat the process of using the leveling feet to bring the balance pans into equilibrium. This is necessary because there may be minor differences in the weights of weighing papers or dishes even with the same type and size.

6. During the entire weighing procedure, keep the balance pans arrested when adding anything to the balance pans. This protects the balance mechanism. Some newer torsion balances allow for the dial weights to be adjusted without arresting the balance pans.

7. Add the appropriate external and dial or rider weights to the balance. Some double-pan prescription balances have two scales on the same graduated dial, one in the metric (0.01-g) system and one in the apothecaries' (0.2-gr) system. **Great care must be exercised when using these dials to ensure that the intended scale is being read.**

8. Handle external weights with tweezers or forceps, never with your fingers. External weights are added to the right-hand balance pan. This is important because the dial or rider weights are added to that side. If you were to use a combination of external and dial weights for a given weight, putting the external weights on the wrong side would result in a weight that is the difference of the two rather than the desired sum of the two. If you have not done weighing recently and have forgotten which is the proper side for the external weights, dial in some weight and observe which balance pan goes down; that is the side for the weights.

9. Using a spatula, add material to be weighed to the weighing paper or dish on the left-hand balance pan. When using a spatula for this purpose, you may find it helpful to hold the spatula between your thumb and middle finger so that the index finger is free to tap the blade of the spatula. This is a good way to tap off small, controlled amounts of drug from the spatula blade.

10. Release the arresting mechanism and observe the balance indicator to determine whether you have transferred the desired amount of material or whether too much or too little material was added.

11. If the pans are not in balance, arrest the pans before adding or removing material. Repeat steps 9 and 10 until the position of the balance indicator on the index plate shows that equilibrium has been reached. As you approach the required weight of material, you may release the balance arrest as you slowly and carefully add very small amounts of material until the exact weight is reached.

12. Arrest the balance pans and remove the weights, both external and rider or dial. As you do this, recheck the weights to be sure you have selected the desired weights. Return the external weights to their appropriate compartments in the weight box.

13. If any powder or liquid was inadvertently spilled on the balance pan or platform, clean the balance.

B. Weighing on an electronic balance

Refer to the operator's manual for weighing instructions specific to that balance. Some balances have several modes for different weighing systems and dual capacity weighing ranges; be sure the balance is in the proper mode for weighing in the metric system and in the appropriate range for the weighing being done. The following steps give general procedures for most electronic balances. A brief stepwise version is given in Figure 14.3.

1. Position the balance on a flat, level surface in an area that is away, as much as is possible, from drafts or air currents.
2. Turn the balance on and press the tare button; the digital display should show 0.000 g. If air currents in the room are affecting the balance (the numbers on the digital display will drift up and down), the balance lid should be closed, its draft shield put in place, or the balance repositioned in a less drafty area. This is also true when determining balance during the weighing procedure.
3. Place a weighing paper or dish on the balance pan. Be sure it is positioned so that it does not interfere with the balance lid or draft shield if either needs to be used during the weighing procedure.
4. Press the tare button again to tare out the weight of the weighing paper or dish; the digital display should show 0.000 g.
5. Using a spatula, add material to be weighed to the weighing paper or dish on the balance pan. When using a spatula for this purpose, you may find it helpful to hold the spatula between your thumb and middle finger so that the index finger is free to tap the blade of the spatula. This is a good way to tap off small, controlled amounts of drug from the spatula blade. As you approach the required weight of material, carefully add very small amounts of material until the exact weight is reached. If you overshoot the target weight, simply remove any excess powder or material with the spatula.
6. If any powder or liquid was inadvertently spilled on the balance pan or platform, clean the balance.

V. VOLUMETRIC DEVICES

A. Definitions
1. **Capacity:** the designated volume, at the maximum graduation, that the vessel will contain (labeled as "TC," meaning "to contain") or deliver (labeled as "TD," meaning "to deliver") at the temperature indicated on the vessel. Generally, graduates, pipettes, and burettes are calibrated TD, whereas volumetric flasks are calibrated TC.
2. **Cylindrical graduate:** a measuring vessel that is a right circular cylinder, that is, with sides parallel to each other and perpendicular to the base.

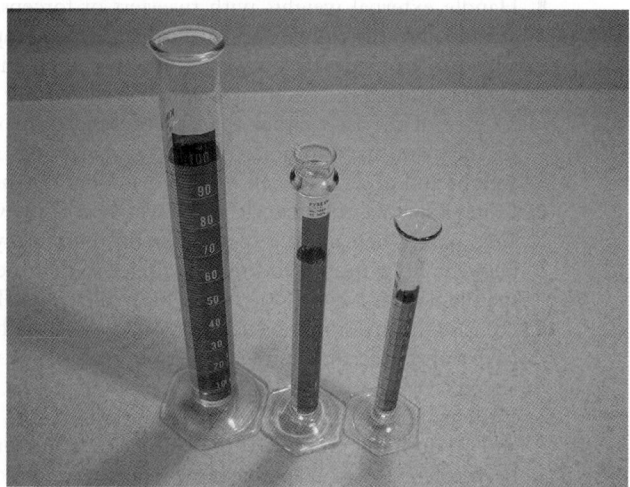

CYLINDRICAL GRADUATES

3. **Conical graduate:** a measuring vessel whose cross-section is circular but whose sides flare outward from its base. The circumference of the vessel is larger at the top graduation than at the lowest graduation marking.
B. Volumetric apparatus recommended in *USP* Chapter ⟨1176⟩
1. *USP* has two chapters on volumetric devices. Chapter ⟨31⟩ Volumetric Devices is written for precise volume measurements used in *USP* assays. Chapter ⟨1176⟩ was written for prescription practice; it lists the following pharmaceutical devices for measuring volumes of liquids when compounding and dispensing.
    a. Burettes
    b. Pipettes

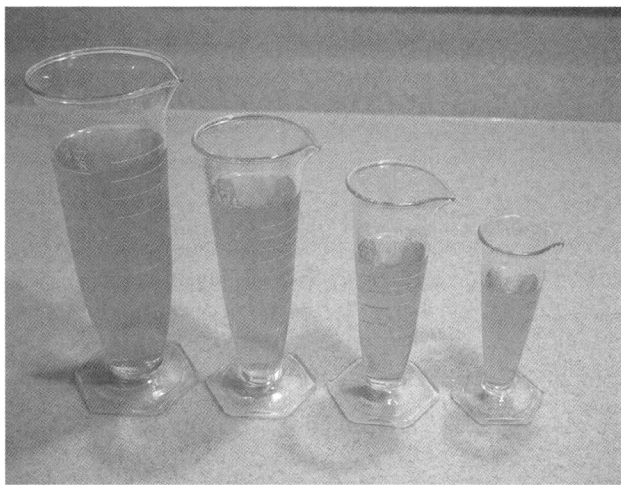

CONICAL GRADUATES

    c. Cylindrical graduates
    d. Conical graduates
    e. Medicine droppers
2. Burettes, pipettes, and cylindrical graduates (metric or apothecaries')
    a. Chapter ⟨1176⟩ states that for pharmaceutical uses, these devices should meet standards set down in NTIS★ COM-73-10504 (3). This document is NBS Circular 602 Testing Glass Volumetric Apparatus. It was issued by the NBS (now the NIST) in 1959, and though it is now out of print and therefore cannot be ordered from NTIS, it is available in pdf format through the NIST Internet site (9).
    b. NBS Circular 602 is a 14-page document with technical information and specifications for many types of glass volumetric apparatus; however, standards for conical graduates are not included in this document (10).
    c. Following is a summary from Circular 602 of specifications for burettes, pipettes, and graduated cylinders used in the pharmacy. This information should be helpful to you in making informed decisions on the purchase of these devices. Many brands of volumetric devices that are available and marketed to pharmacies do not meet these particular standards. (Remember that conformity with standards such as these is not legally required unless mandated by state or federal law. Consult applicable pharmacy codes and statutes to find out what is required for your practice site.)
        (1) Made of good-quality glass, transparent and free from defects
        (2) Circular cross-section that allows complete emptying and draining and thorough cleaning
        (3) Graduation marks that are fine, clear, permanent, and of uniform width and with clear space between adjacent lines
        (4) Graduation marks in only one scale, either metric or apothecaries', but not both
        (5) Graduated either "to contain" or "to deliver" (In other words, graduated cylinders that have a numbered scale running up and also an inverse scale running down the side of the cylinder do not meet this standard.)
        (6) No subdivision lines between the base and the first numbered graduation line
        [NBS Circular 602 has no stated requirement for the initial interval (e.g., one-fifth the capacity of the graduate) as there is for cylindrical and conical graduates in *Handbook 44.*]
        (7) A permanent inscription with the capacity, the temperature (either 20° or 25°C) at which the graduate is to be used, and whether it is calibrated TC (to contain) or TD (to deliver) (10).
3. Conical graduates
    a. Chapter ⟨1176⟩ also lists conical graduates as acceptable measuring devices for prescription compounding, and it requires these graduates to meet the standards described in *Handbook*

★NTIS (National Technical Information Service) is not to be confused with NIST; NTIS is an agency in the U.S. Commerce Department that serves as the repository and disseminator of government documents and information.

44, 4th ed. (3). (As is described at the beginning of this chapter, *Handbook 44* was first published in 1949, and it is issued each year following the Annual Meeting of NCWM, so it is now well past the 4th ed. The complete document, current and several previous editions, is available on the NIST Internet site.)

b. Though Chapter ⟨1176⟩ only specifies that conical graduates meet the standards of *Handbook 44*, the section on graduates in *Handbook 44* does address both cylindrical and conical graduates (1,3).

c. Next is a summary of specifications from the Graduates section of *Handbook 44*. To comply with Chapter ⟨1176⟩ standards, conical graduates for use in compounding should have these characteristics. In states where statutes require that graduates comply with *Handbook 44*, all graduates used in compounding should follow these standards.

(1) Made of good-quality glass, clear, transparent, free of defects, of uniform thickness, and not excessively thick

(2) Graduation marks that are continuous, uniform, clear, and permanent

(3) An initial interval that is not subdivided and that is not less than one-fifth or more than one-fourth of the graduate capacity (e.g., for a graduate with a capacity of 100 mL, the first graduation mark cannot be less than 20 mL or more than 25 mL)

(4) Graduated "to deliver" at 20°C and permanently and conspicuously marked with this information

(5) Graduates with capacity greater than 15 mL (4 fluid drams) may be either cylindrical or conical, but graduates with capacity less than 15 mL must be cylindrical.

(6) Graduates may have a dual scale (milliliters and ounces); for single-scale graduates, the main graduations should completely encircle the graduate, and the subordinate graduations should extend at least half way around; for double-scale graduates, there must be a clear space between the ends of the main graduations on the two scales (1).
(Recall that NBS Circular 602 does not allow dual scales; this is probably one reason why cylindrical graduates have single scales, but conical graduates, which need only comply with *Handbook 44*, are available with dual scales.)

d. Capacities, graduation ranges and intervals, and number of graduations for the various sizes are given in a table of values in *Handbook 44* (1). See that document for details.

4. Medicine droppers

a. Standards are described for medicine droppers in *USP* Chapter ⟨1176⟩ and Chapter ⟨1101⟩ Medicine Dropper.

b. Graduated medicine droppers are described in Chapter ⟨1101⟩; when held vertically, they deliver drops of water each of which weighs between 45 mg and 55 mg. Chapter ⟨1101⟩ states that the volume error for these droppers should not exceed 15% (11).

c. Nongraduated medicine droppers are described in Chapter ⟨1176⟩; the dropper tip external dimension is the same as for a graduated medicine dropper (3 mm), and the drop size is essentially the same, but the standard is written in terms of 20 drops of water weighing 1 g at a temperature of 15°C with a tolerance of 10% (3).

d. Notice that for both types of droppers, the calibration is given in terms of water. Other liquids have different surface tensions and viscosities, which give different drop volumes. Therefore, if a dropper is to be used for measuring a liquid, it should be calibrated with the liquid to be measured. This is done by holding the dropper vertically and delivering a given number of drops into a small graduated cylinder and accurately measuring the volume.

e. Because of the general availability and greater accuracy offered by syringes and pipettes, medicine droppers now have limited usefulness as measuring devices for compounding.

C. Other volumetric apparatus

Though the following are not listed as volumetric devices in *Handbook 44*, NBS Circular 602, or the *USP*, pharmacists and pharmacy technicians often use these for measuring volumes when compounding prescriptions. Each has advantages and limitations that should be carefully considered.

1. Syringes

a. Plastic disposable syringes are available in sizes ranging from 0.5 mL to 60 mL.

b. Small syringes of 1- and 3-mL capacities are useful for measuring volumes less than the 2-mL minimum recommended for a 10-mL graduated cylinder. Micropipettes are also handy for this purpose.

c. Syringes of the appropriate size may be preferred over graduated cylinders for measuring viscous liquids, such as glycerin or mineral oil, because these thick liquids drain slowly and sometimes incompletely from graduated cylinders.

2. Graduated beakers

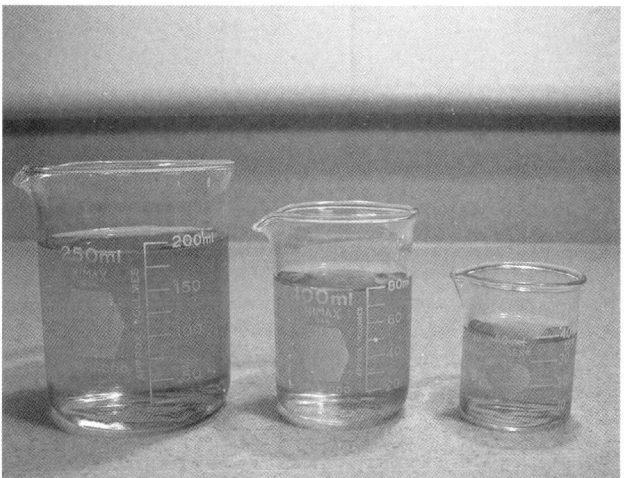

GRADUATED BEAKERS

a. Beakers are used in the pharmacy as vessels for compounding liquids and for many other purposes. They are commonly available in sizes ranging from 50 to 1,000 mL, and larger-capacity beakers are available from some suppliers.

b. Most glass beakers have painted graduation marks. Usually these markings do not give precise volume measurements and are not intended for accurate measuring. Unless these beakers are calibrated and marked using water measured in a graduated cylinder, they should not be used when accurate measuring is required, such as when "q.s.'ing" a preparation to a desired volume.

3. Graduated prescription bottles

a. Amber plastic prescription bottles, called *prescription ovals*, are used for dispensing liquid drug products and preparations. They are commonly available in the following sizes: 2, 3, 4, 6, 8, and 16 oz, which correspond to metric capacities of 60, 90, 120, 180, 240, and 480 mL. They have graduation marks that are embossed in the plastic and run up the side of the bottle.

b. Like graduated beakers, the volume markings on graduated prescription bottles are approximate.

(1) The capacity markings are sufficiently accurate for measuring and dispensing a manufactured liquid product where the strength of the product is not dependent on the accuracy of the capacity markings.

(2) Though graduated prescription bottles are not intended for the accurate measuring needed in compounding, in recent years the quality of some brands of prescription ovals has improved to the point where the graduation markings are quite accurate and well within the usual standard of $\pm$ 10%. Pharmacists often prefer to "q.s." compounded liquid preparations in the final prescription bottles, especially when compounding viscous liquid preparations, because there is no loss of material in transferring from a measuring cylinder. If prescription ovals are being used in this manner, the calibration markings on the bottles should be checked. To do this, accurately measure water or other compatible mobile liquid in a graduated cylinder and use this to check the graduation and capacities markings on the bottle.

VI. RECOMMENDTIONS FOR USING VOLUMETRIC DEVICES

A. For maximum accuracy in measuring, select a graduate or other volumetric device with a capacity equal to or slightly larger than the volume to be measured (3). For graduates, the smaller the volume to be measured as a percentage of the graduate capacity, the larger the potential percentage error from a given deviation in reading the meniscus. **The general rule is to measure volumes no less than 20% of the capacity of the graduate.**

B. Cylindrical graduates are preferred for measurement over conical graduates. Because of the constant diameter of a cylindrical graduate, a given deviation in reading (e.g., $\pm$ 1 mm) gives a constant error in a measured volume throughout the entire length of the graduate. This is not true for conical graduates, where the diameter continually increases from the base to the top graduation mark. Therefore, an error in reading the meniscus of ± 1 mm can cause a volume error of 0.5 mL at any point on a 100-mL cylindrical graduate, but this same ± 1-mm deviation can cause a much greater volume error (~1.8 mL) at the 100-mL mark of a 4-oz conical graduate (3).

C. According to the *USP* Chapter ⟨1176⟩, conical graduates having a capacity of less than 25 mL should not be used in prescription compounding (3). *Handbook 44* puts this limitation at 15 mL (1).

D. When reading the volume of liquid in a graduate or other volumetric measuring device, the graduation mark, the meniscus of the liquid, and the line of sight should all be in alignment. This minimizes errors caused by the parallax effect.

E. As indicated in the discussion of specifications for volumetric devices, they are to be permanent inscribed with the temperature at which they calibrated; most often this temperature is 20°C. While ideally any measurements using the device should be done at the calibration temperature, in most compounding situations, a modest deviations from this temperature does not cause an unacceptable error in measured volume. If a very precise volume is needed (e.g., for analytical purposes), either the liquid and ambient temperature should be the same as the device calibration temperature, or a volume-temperature correction should be made. NBS Circular 602 has a table of these correction values for water (10).

REFERENCES

1. Weights and Measures Division, NIST. NIST Handbook 44—2006 Edition, Specifications, tolerances, and other technical requirements for weighing and measuring devices. Gaithersburg, MD: Author, 2006.

2. National Conference on Weights and Measures. National type evaluation program (NTEP). http://www.ncwm.net/ntep/. Accessed September 2007.

3. The United States Pharmacopeial Convention, Inc. Chapter ⟨1176⟩. 2008 USP 31/NF 26. Rockville, MD: Author, 2007: 642–643.

4. The United States Pharmacopeial Convention, Inc. Chapter ⟨795⟩. 2008 USP 31/NF 26. Rockville, MD: Author, 2007: 316.

5. Weights and Measures Division, NIST. Commonly asked questions about mass standards. http://ts.nist.gov/WeightsAndMeasures/caqmass.cfm. Accessed September 2007.

6. American Society for Testing and Materials. E 617–97 (2003) Standard specifications for laboratory weights and precision mass standards. West Conshohocken, PA: Author, 2003.

7. Troemner Mass Standards Handbook. Philadelphia: Troemner, Inc., 2000; 6–7.

8. The United States Pharmacopeial Convention, Inc. Chapter ⟨41⟩. 2008 USP 31/NF 26. Rockville, MD: Author, 2007; 67.

9. National Institute of Standards and Technology. Technical notes and publications. http://www.cstl.nist.gov/div836/836.01/Publications.html. Accessed September 2007.

10. Hughes JC. Testing glass volumetric apparatus. National Bureau of Standards Circular 602. Springfield, VA: The National Technical Information Service, 1959; 1–14.

11. The United States Pharmacopeial Convention, Inc. Chapter ⟨1101⟩. 2007 USP 30/NF 25. Rockville, MD: Author, 2006; 578.

Part 4

Pharmaceutical

Excipients

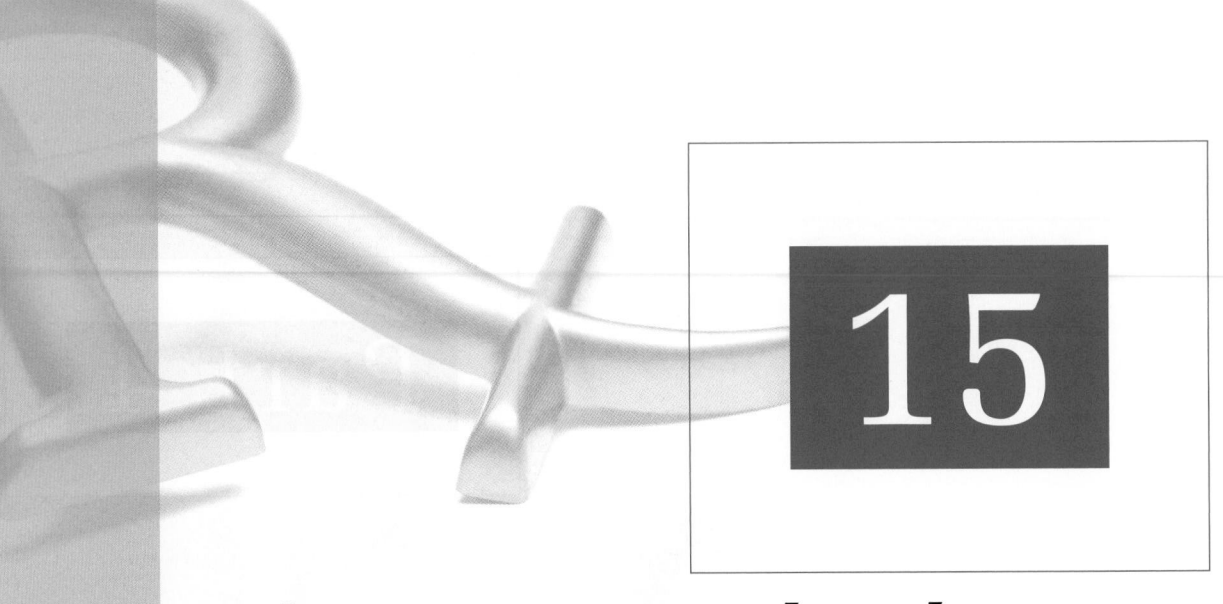

15

Pharmaceutical Solvents and Solubilizing Agents

Melgardt de Villiers, PhD

I. GENERAL INFORMATION

A. Water is the most commonly used and most desirable solvent-vehicle for liquid drug products and preparations for all uses.

B. Other solvent-vehicles frequently used as ingredients in drug products and compounded preparations include alcohol, isopropyl alcohol, glycerin, propylene glycol, and polyethylene glycol 400.

C. Some other solvents are used pharmaceutically in processing drug products, for assays and tests, or for making specialty products and preparations such as Flexible Collodion. Examples include acetone, ether, and chloroform.

D. Oils used as pharmaceutical solvents-vehicles include a variety of vegetable oils and mineral oil. Examples include corn oil, cottonseed oil, and almond oil. Some special vegetable and essential oils are used primarily as flavors and scents. The *National Formulary* section of the *USP–NF* (1) has monographs for various oils of this type, such as anise oil, lemon oil, and rose oil. These are discussed in Chapter 21, Colors, Flavors, Sweeteners, and Scents.

E. The *USP–NF* lists official articles classified as solvents and vehicles by categories in a table of excipients in the Front Matter of the *NF* section (2). These are given in Table 15.1. Notice that some articles are listed in both categories and some, such as Sterile Water for Inhalation and Dehydrated Alcohol, are not listed at all. The following chapter describes those articles most frequently encountered in pharmacy compounding and practice.

F. In reading and interpreting the current chapter, note that this text employs the usual convention of using upper-case first letters for words designating official *USP–NF* articles (e.g., Alcohol,

Table 15.1	USP AND NF EXCIPIENTS CATEGORIZED AS SOLVENTS AND VEHICLES

SOLVENT	VEHICLE
Acetone	FLAVORED AND/OR SWEETENED
Alcohol	Aromatic Elixir
Alcohol, Diluted	Benzaldehyde Elixir, Compound
Amylene Hydrate	Dextrose
Benzyl Benzoate	Peppermint Water
Butyl Alcohol	Sorbitol Solution
Canola Oil	Syrup
Caprylocaproyl Polyoxylglycerides	OLEAGINOUS
Corn Oil	Alkyl (C12-15) Benzoate
Cottonseed Oil	Almond Oil
Diethylene Glycol Monoethyl Ether	Canola Oil
Ethyl Acetate	Corn Oil
Glycerin	Cottonseed Oil
Hexylene Glycol	Ethyl Oleate
Isopropyl Alcohol	Isopropyl Myristate
Lauroyl Polyoxylglycerides	Isopropyl Palmitate
Linoleoyl Polyoxylglycerides	Mineral Oil
Methyl Alcohol	Mineral Oil, Light
Methylene Chloride	Octyldodecanol
Methyl Isobutyl Ketone	Olive Oil
Mineral Oil	Peanut Oil
Oleoyl Polyoxylglycerides	Safflower Oil
Peanut Oil	Sesame Oil
Polyethylene Glycol	Soybean Oil
Polyethylene Glycol Monomethyl Ether	Squalane
Propylene Glycol	STERILE
Sesame Oil	Sodium Chloride Injection, Bacteriostatic
Stearoyl Polyoxylglycerides	Water for Injection, Bacteriostatic
Water for Injection	SOLID CARRIER
Water for Injection, Sterile	Sugar Spheres
Water for Irrigation, Sterile	
Water, Purified	

From the United States Pharmacopeial Convention Inc. USP 30/ NF 25. 2006: Front Matter—NF: Excipients. Rockville, MD: Author, 2007, with permission.
Source: 2007 USP 30/ NF 25. Rockville, MD: The United States Pharmacopeial Convention Inc., 2006: Front Matter—NF: Excipients.

Purified Water) and lower-case first letters for words designating the chemical substances (e.g., ethanol, water).

G. Recently, the *USP* also started listing some cyclodextrins that are used as solubilizing agents.

II. WATER

A. General information

  1. Water is such an important substance and component of pharmaceutical dosage forms that the *USP* describes and sets standards for various types of water in the General Notices official monograph, and Chapter ⟨1231⟩ Water for Pharmaceutical Purposes.

  2. There are eight official types of water. These are USP Purified Water; USP Water for Injection; USP Water for Hemodialysis; USP Sterile Water for Injection; USP Sterile Water for Inhalation; USP Bacteriostatic Water for Injection; USP Sterile Water for Irrigation; and USP Sterile Purified Water. (3). The *USP* designation means that the water is the subject of an official monograph in the current *USP* with various specifications for each type. The latter four waters are "finished" products that are packaged and labeled as such. The USP Purified Water, USP Water for Injection, and USP Water for Hemodialysis conversely, are components or "ingredient materials" as they are termed by the *USP*, intended to be used in the production of drug products.

3. When water is used in making official *USP* preparations, it must meet the criteria specified in the *USP* for the type of preparation being made. For example, the water used for making parenteral products must meet the requirements for injections found in Chapter ⟨1⟩ Injections of the *USP* (4).

4. The basic starting ingredient for all *USP* water items is potable (drinking) water as defined in the General Notices of the *USP*: "Potable water meeting the requirements for drinking water as set forth in the regulations of the federal Environmental Protection Agency may be used in the preparation of official substances" (1). This means that drinking water may be used in the manufacturing and preparation of USP drug substances, including water articles. Drinking or tap water does not, however, meet the standards as an ingredient in dosage forms. Water for making dosage forms must be one of the official *USP* monograph water articles as described further.

5. In addition to Water for Injection and Purified Water USP, in Europe there is a third class of water called *highly purified water*, like a super grade of Purified Water USP. Unlike Water for Injection, which is traditionally produced with a still, highly purified water is not boiled. Instead, it goes through various pretreatment steps, one or two reverse osmosis passes, a deionization step, and sometimes ultraviolet radiation and a final filtration step. The end result is highly purified water that is equivalent to Water for Injection but produced at a lower cost.

B. ***USP–NF* water articles**
1. Purified Water USP (3,5)

$$H_2O \quad MW = 18.02$$

   a. Preparation
      (1) Made from water complying with the U.S. Environmental Protection Agency (EPA) National Primary Drinking Water Regulations or comparable regulations of the European Union or Japan
      (2) Processed by distillation, ion-exchange treatment, reverse osmosis, or other suitable method
      (3) No added substances (such as preservatives)
   b. Description: clear, colorless, odorless liquid
   c. Standards
      (1) Meets USP requirements for Total Organic Carbon ⟨643⟩ and Water Conductivity ⟨645⟩
      (2) Bacterial endotoxins (pyrogens): no standard
      (3) Bacteriologic purity: complies with EPA regulations for drinking water
   d. Packaging and storage: When packaged, use tight containers.
   e. Labeling: When packaged, label method of preparation.
   f. Uses
      (1) *USP* Chapter ⟨795⟩ states that for nonsterile compounding, pharmacists must use USP-grade purified water (6), which must meet criteria (e.g., for dissolved solids, pH) that ensure the stability of preparations.
      (2) It is used as a solvent-vehicle for the preparation of pharmaceutical dosage forms for internal or external use.
      (3) It is not for use when sterility is required unless it meets the requirements under *USP* Sterility Tests ⟨71⟩ or is first sterilized by filtration or autoclaving. It must then be protected from microbial contamination.
      (4) It is not for use in making parenteral products unless it can be assured that it meets the requirements for sterility and bacterial endotoxins for parenteral administration.

2. Sterile Purified Water USP (3,5)
   a. Preparation
      (1) Made from Purified Water that has been sterilized and suitably packaged
      (2) No added substances (such as preservatives)
   b. Description: clear, colorless, odorless liquid
   c. Standards
      (1) Meets USP requirements for Total organic carbon ⟨642⟩ and Water conductivity ⟨645⟩. Total organic carbon (TOC) is an indirect measure of organic molecules present in pharmaceutical waters measured as carbon. Electrical conductivity in water is a measure of the ion-facilitated electron flow through it and Water conductivity is therefore a measure of the presence of extraneous ions
      (2) Bacterial endotoxins (pyrogens): no standard

(3) Bacteriologic purity: meets requirements in Chapter ⟨71⟩ for Sterility. Portions of this general chapter in the USP have been harmonized with the corresponding texts of the European Pharmacopeia and/or the Japanese Pharmacopeia

(4) pH: between 5.0 and 7.0

(5) Other standards as given in the *USP* for ammonia, calcium, chloride, sulfate, and oxidizable substances

  d. Packaging and storage: suitable tight containers

  e. Labeling: Label with method of preparation and that this is not for parenteral use.

  f. Uses

    (1) It is used as a solvent-vehicle for the preparation of pharmaceutical dosage forms for internal or external use.

    (2) It is not for parenteral administration.

3. Water for Injection USP (3,5)

  a. Preparation

    (1) Purified by distillation or reverse osmosis not by deionization because bacterial endotoxins can grow in a deionizing chamber to a level exceeding USP requirements

    (2) No added substances (such as preservatives)

  b. Description: clear, colorless, odorless liquid

  c. Standards

    (1) Bacterial endotoxins (pyrogens, *USP* Chapter ⟨151⟩ Pyrogen Test): not more than 0.25 USP Endotoxin Units per mL (*USP* Chapter ⟨85⟩ Bacterial Endotoxins Test)

    (2) All requirements for Purified Water

  d. Uses: Water for Injection is a starting material for making parenteral products. It must be processed further either before use or during product preparation. The *USP* monograph has the following note on its use:

> NOTE—Water for Injection is intended for use as a solvent for the preparation of parenteral solutions. Where used for the preparation of parenteral solutions subject to final sterilization, use suitable means to minimize microbial growth, or first render the Water for Injection sterile and thereafter protect it from microbial contamination. For parenteral solutions that are prepared under aseptic conditions and are not sterilized by appropriate filtration or in the final container, first render the Water for Injection sterile and thereafter, protect it from microbial contamination (5).

4. Sterile Water for Injection USP (3,5)

  a. Preparation

    (1) Made from Water for Injection that is sterilized and suitably packaged

    (2) No added substances (such as preservatives)

  b. Description: clear, colorless, odorless liquid

  c. Standards

    (1) All requirements given for Sterile Purified Water

    (2) Particulate matter: Meets requirements in *USP* Chapter ⟨788⟩ Particulate Matter in Injections. In this context, particulate matter is defined as mobile, randomly sourced, extraneous substances, other than gas bubbles, that cannot be quantitated by chemical analysis because of the small amount of material present (7). Injectable solutions, including solutions constituted from sterile solids intended for parenteral use, must be free from particulate matter that can be observed on visual inspection (4,7).

    (3) Bacterial endotoxins (pyrogens): not more than 0.25 USP Endotoxin Units per mL

    (4) Bacteriologic purity: meets requirements given for Sterile Purified Water (Chapter ⟨71⟩ Sterility Tests)

  d. Packaging and storage: single-dose glass or plastic containers not larger than 1 liter. Glass containers of Type I or Type II glass are preferred.

  e. Labeling: Label to indicate that no preservative or other substance has been added. Also label that it is not suitable for intravascular injection unless it is first made approximately isotonic by the addition of a suitable solute.

  f. Uses

    (1) Base vehicle for large-volume parenteral fluids

    (2) Solvent for drugs intended for parenteral use

5. Sterile Water for Inhalation USP (3,5)

  a. Preparation

    (1) Made using Water for Injection that is sterilized and suitably packaged

(2) No added substances, except that antimicrobial agents may be added when the water is to be used in humidifiers or other devices in which it may become contaminated

b. Description: clear, colorless solution

c. Standards

   (1) All requirements given for Sterile Purified Water except pH
   (2) Bacterial endotoxins (pyrogens): not more than 0.5 USP Endotoxin Units per mL
   (3) Bacteriologic purity: meets USP sterility requirements
   (4) pH: 4.5 to 7.5

d. Packaging and storage: Glass or plastic containers; Type I and II glass preferred for glass containers

e. Labeling: Label that it is for inhalation therapy only and not for parenteral use.

f. Uses

   (1) In humidifiers to add moisture to the environment
   (2) As a solvent for drugs to be administered by inhalation
   (3) The following is a note on use in the *USP* monograph:
       NOTE—"Do not use Sterile Water for Inhalation for parenteral administration or for other sterile compendial dosage forms" (5).

6. Sterile Water for Irrigation USP (3,5)

a. Preparation

   (1) Made from Water for Injection that is sterilized and suitably packaged
   (2) No added substances (such as preservatives)

b. Description: clear, colorless, odorless liquid

c. Standards

   (1) All requirements given for Sterile Purified Water
   (2) Bacterial endotoxins (pyrogens): meets the endotoxin test under Water for Injection
   (3) Bacteriologic purity: meets requirements given for Sterile Purified Water

d. Packaging and storage: single-dose glass or plastic containers. Glass containers of Type I or Type II glass are preferred. Containers may have volumes in excess of 1 liter and may be designed with a closure to facilitate easy, rapid emptying.

e. Labeling: Label to indicate that no preservative or other substance has been added. Also, the labels "For irrigation only" and "Not for injection" must be conspicuous.

f. Uses

   (1) Irrigation fluid
   (2) Solvent for drugs to be administered by irrigation, usually for local effect

7. Bacteriostatic Water for Injection USP (3,5)

a. Preparation

   (1) Made from Sterile Water for Injection that has been sterilized and suitably packaged
   (2) Added substances: one or more suitable antimicrobial agents are added

b. Description: clear, colorless liquid, odorless, or possibly having the odor of the added antimicrobial agent(s)

c. Standards

   (1) Particulate matter: meets requirements for Sterile Water for Injection
   (2) Bacterial endotoxins (pyrogens): not more than 0.5 USP Endotoxin Units per mL
   (3) Bacteriologic purity: meets USP sterility requirements
   (4) pH: 4.5 to 7.0
   (5) Meets the effectiveness requirements of Chapter ⟨51⟩ Antimicrobial Effectiveness Testing and label claim for content of the antimicrobial agent(s) in Chapter ⟨341⟩ Antimicrobial Agents–Contain
   (6) Meets all requirements for Sterile Purified Water except pH, ammonia, chloride, and oxidizable substances

d. Packaging and storage: single-dose or multiple-dose glass or plastic containers not larger than 30 mL. Glass containers of Type I or Type II glass are preferred.

e. Labeling: Label with name and quantity of preservative(s). Also label in boldface capital letters with contrasting color (preferably red): **NOT FOR USE IN NEWBORNS.**

f. Uses

   (1) As a solvent for drugs to be given parenterally when a preserved solution is desired and when the antimicrobial agent(s) do not cause compatibility problems with the chosen drug or drugs
   (2) Is not to be used when large volumes are needed for parenteral administration. If large volumes are needed (>30 mL), Sterile Water for Injection should be used. Even with moderate volumes (>5 mL), Sterile Water for Injection is preferred.

| III. | **ALCOHOLS** |

A. General information

1. In organic chemistry, alcohols have the general formula R–OH, where R represents a general hydrocarbon group. In pharmacy, when the term *alcohol* is used, it has a more restricted meaning. The General Notices section of the *USP* states (1):

> **Alcohol**—All statements of percentages of alcohol, such as under the heading *Alcohol content*, refer to percentage, by volume of C_2H_5OH at 15.56°. Where reference is made to C_2H_5OH, the chemical entity possessing absolute (100%) strength is intended.
>
> *Alcohol*—Where "alcohol" is called for in formulas, tests, and assays, the monograph article *Alcohol* is to be used (1).

Therefore, when a prescription order or pharmaceutical formula calls for alcohol, the monograph product Alcohol USP is to be used. Another alcohol, such as isopropyl alcohol, should not be used when the term *alcohol*, without modifier, is written.

2. If a prescription order calls for a specific alcohol, such as isopropyl alcohol, that specified alcohol must be used. Different alcohols may not be substituted in prescription or medications orders without the consent of the prescriber, any more than, for example, aspirin may be substituted for acetaminophen. Alcohols vary greatly in their relative toxicities; a single carbon atom separates the pharmaceutically useful ethanol from the toxic methanol. Be sure to use only alcohols that are approved for the intended purpose, either external or internal use, or as a solvent for processing. Methanol is very toxic and is never used in the preparation of dosage forms.

3. Calculations involving content and labeling of alcohol have been the subject of some confusion. Explanations and multiple examples can be found in Chapter 8, Quantity and Concentration Expressions and Calculations.

B. *USP–NF* Alcohol (R-OH) articles

1. Alcohol (Ethanol, Ethyl Alcohol) (5)

$$CH_3CH_2OH \qquad C_2H_6O \qquad MW = 46.07$$

a. Alcohol USP (1,5,8)
   (1) Content: not less than 92.3% and not more than 93.8%, by weight (w/w), corresponding to not less than 94.9% and not more than 96.0%, by volume (v/v), of C_2H_5OH
   (2) Description: clear, colorless, mobile, volatile liquid; flammable; boils at 78°; has a characteristic odor
   (3) Specific gravity: between 0.812 and 0.816
   (4) Labeling: "The content of alcohol in a liquid preparation shall be stated on the label as a percentage (v/v) of C_2H_5OH" (1).
   (5) Solubility: miscible with water, isopropyl alcohol, glycerin, acetone, propylene glycol, polyethylene glycol 400, ether, and chloroform; will mix with castor oil, but not other fixed oils and not with mineral oil
   (6) It is used as a solvent-vehicle for the preparation of pharmaceutical dosage forms for internal or external use. It is an effective antiseptic-disinfectant, being germicidal in concentrations above 60%. Its usual concentration as an antiseptic-disinfectant is 70%.
   (7) Packaging and storage: tight containers, remote from fire

b. Dehydrated Alcohol USP (5,8)
   (1) Content: not less than 99.2%, by weight (w/w), corresponding to not less than 99.5%, by volume (v/v), of C_2H_5OH
   (2) Description: clear, colorless, mobile, volatile liquid; flammable; boils at 78°; has a characteristic odor
   (3) Specific gravity: not more than 0.7964
   (4) Use this preparation when "dehydrated" or "absolute" alcohol is written in a formula (1).
   (5) Packaging and storage: tight containers, remote from fire

c. Dehydrated Alcohol for Injection USP (5,8)
   (1) The injection is dehydrated alcohol that is suitable for parenteral use.
   (2) Description: clear, colorless, mobile, volatile liquid; flammable; boils at 78°; has a characteristic odor
   (3) Specific gravity: not more than 0.8035

(4) It meets the requirements for Dehydrated Alcohol plus the requirements for parenteral products found in *USP* Chapter ⟨1⟩ Injections. These include specifications for sterility, pyrogenicity, particulate matter, and other contaminants.

(5) Packaging and storage: single-dose containers with Type I glass preferred. Container headspace may have inert gas.

d. Diluted Alcohol NF (8,9)

(1) Content: a mixture of Alcohol and water with not less than 41.0% and not more than 42.0%, by weight (w/w), corresponding to not less than 48.4% and not more than 49.5%, by volume (v/v), of C_2H_5OH

Diluted Alcohol may be prepared as follows:

Alcohol 500 mL

Purified Water 500 mL

Measure the Alcohol and the Purified Water separately at the same temperature, and mix. If the water and the Alcohol and the resulting mixture are measured at 25°C, the volume of the mixture will be about 970 mL.

(2) Description: clear, colorless, mobile liquid with a characteristic odor

(3) Specific gravity: between 0.935 and 0.937

(4) Packaging and storage: tight containers, remote from fire

e. Rubbing Alcohol USP (5,8)

RUBBING ALCOHOL SHOULD NEVER BE CONFUSED WITH ISOPROPYL RUBBING ALCOHOL, WHICH IS DISCUSSED LATER.

(1) Alcohol content: 68.5% to 71.5% by volume of dehydrated alcohol

(2) Other content: It is made in accordance with the specifications of Formula 23-H (U.S. Treasury Department, Bureau of Alcohol, Tobacco, and Firearms): 8 parts by volume of acetone, 1.5 parts by volume of methyl isobutyl ketone, and 100 parts by volume of ethanol. In addition to containing water, ethanol, and denaturants, Rubbing Alcohol may also contain stabilizers, perfumes, or dyes that are FDA-approved for use in drugs. In each 100 mL, it has not less than 355 mg sucrose octaacetate or not less than 1.4 mg of denatonium benzoate.

(3) Description: like Alcohol, except it may be colored because of addition of dye; odor depends on presence of other additives such as perfumes.

(4) Specific gravity: between 0.869 and 0.877

(5) Rubbing Alcohol is for external use only. It may be used as a solvent-vehicle for drugs that are being formulated into topical products. It is an effective antiseptic-disinfectant.

(6) Labeling: Label that it is flammable.

(7) Packaging and storage: tight containers, remote from fire

2. Isopropyl alcohol (2-Propanol) (5)

$$CH_3CHOHCH_3 \qquad C_3H_8O \qquad MW = 60.10$$

a. Isopropyl Alcohol USP (5,8)

(1) Content: not less than 99.0% of C_3H_8O

(2) Description: transparent, colorless, mobile, volatile, flammable liquid with a characteristic odor

(3) Specific gravity: between 0.783 and 0.787

(4) Solubility: miscible with water, alcohol, glycerin, propylene glycol, polyethylene glycol 400, acetone, ether, and chloroform. It is immiscible with fixed oils and mineral oil.

(5) Isopropyl Alcohol is for external use only. It may be used as a solvent-vehicle for drugs that are being formulated into topical products. In concentrations ≥70%, it is an effective disinfectant. It is somewhat superior to ethanol as an antiseptic.

(6) Packaging and storage: tight containers, remote from heat

b. Isopropyl Rubbing Alcohol USP (5,8)

(1) Content: not less than 68.0% and not more than 72.0% by volume (v/v) of isopropyl alcohol, the remainder consisting of water, with or without stabilizers, perfume oils, and color additives that are certified by the FDA for use in drugs

(2) Description: like Isopropyl Alcohol, except it may be colored because of addition of dye. Odor depends on the presence of other additives, such as perfumes.

(3) Specific gravity: between 0.872 and 0.883

(4) Isopropyl Rubbing Alcohol is for external use only. It may be used as a solvent-vehicle for drugs that are being formulated into topical products. It is an effective antiseptic-disinfectant.

(5) Packaging and storage: tight containers, remote from heat

c. Azeotropic Isopropyl Alcohol USP (5,8)

(1) Content: not less than 91.0% and not more than 93.0% of isopropyl alcohol, by volume (v/v), the remainder consisting of water

(2) Description: like Isopropyl Alcohol

(3) Specific gravity: between 0.815 and 0.810

(4) Packaging and storage: tight containers, remote from heat

C. The use of alcohol in drug products for children

1. For a long time the American Academy of Pediatrics has warned about the use of alcohol in oral medications for children (10). This eventually led the FDA to set the following maximum limits on alcohol concentration in over-the-counter (OTC) drug products intended for oral ingestion (11).

a. For products labeled for use by adults and children 12 years of age and over, the amount of alcohol in the product shall not exceed 10%.

b. For products labeled for used by children 6 to younger than 12 years of age, the amount of alcohol in the product shall not exceed 5%.

c. For products labeled for use by children younger than 6 years of age, the amount of alcohol in the product shall not exceed 0.5%.

2. In addition the amount of alcohol present in a product shall be stated in terms of v/v% of absolute alcohol at 60°F (15.56°C) and a statement expressing the percentage of alcohol present in a product shall appear prominently and conspicuously on the "principal display panel." In addition, for any OTC drug product intended for oral ingestion containing >0.5% alcohol and labeled for use by children ages 6 to younger than 12 years of age, the labeling shall contain the following statement in the directions section: "Consult a physician for use in children under 6 years of age."

3. The following drug products are temporarily exempt from these provisions: (i) Aromatic Cascara Fluidextract, (ii) Cascara Sagrada Fluidextract, and (iii) orally ingested homeopathic drug products. Ipecac syrup is exempt from the provisions for children younger than 6 years of age because ipecac syrup is an important OTC product that is used to cause vomiting when poisoning occurs. Alcohol is used in the preparation of the syrup to ensure complete extraction of the alkaloids from the ipecac powder. As a result, ipecac syrups contain between 1.0 and 2.5% alcohol. To comply with this exception ipecac product labels must contain a statement conspicuously boxed and in red letters that states: "For emergency use to cause vomiting in poisoning. Before using, call physician, the poison Control Center, or hospital emergency room immediately for advice." The labeling must also state: "Usual dosage: 1 tablespoon (15 milliliters) in person over 1 year of age."

4. These FDA regulations only affect orally ingested OTC medications; thus, products such as mouthwashes, which contain a high alcohol content, remain exempt. Furthermore, greater flexibility is allowed for prescription products and preparations. See Sample Prescription 31.2 in Chapter 31 for considerations and sample calculations involving alcohol in a prescribed pediatric compounded preparation.

IV.   GLYCOLS

A. General information

1. Glycols are simply dihydroxy alcohols. Because of their chemical structure, they have more than one site for hydrogen bonding and therefore, relative to their molecular weights, they have higher water solubility and higher boiling points (are less volatile) than a comparable single hydroxy alcohol. For example, ethanol boils at 78°C, whereas the structurally comparable dihydroxy ethylene glycol has a boiling point of 197°C. Ethylene glycol owes its usefulness as an antifreeze to its unique glycol properties of low freezing point, high boiling point, and high water solubility. Similarly, polyethylene glycols have high water solubility even though they are high-molecular-weight organic compounds.

2. As with alcohols, glycols vary greatly in their relative toxicities, and a single carbon atom separates the pharmaceutically useful and nontoxic propylene glycol from the very toxic ethylene glycol. Be sure to use only glycols approved for the intended purpose, either external or internal use.

B. *USP–NF* glycol articles

   1. Glycerin USP (glycerol) (5,8)

$$C_3H_8O_3 \qquad MW = 92.01$$

   a. Content: not less than 99.0% and not more than 101.0% of $C_3H_8O_3$
   b. Description: clear, colorless, viscous liquid; practically odorless, hygroscopic, neutral pH
   c. Specific gravity: not less than 1.249
   d. Solubility: miscible with water, ethanol, isopropyl alcohol, propylene glycol, and polyethylene glycol 400; is soluble to the degree of 1 g/15 mL in acetone; insoluble in chloroform, ether, fixed oils, mineral oil, and volatile oils
   e. It is used as a solvent-vehicle for the preparation of pharmaceutical dosage forms for internal or external use. It has humectant and preservative properties.
   f. Packaging and storage: tight container
   Note: In May 2007, the FDA issued a warning to pharmaceutical manufacturers, suppliers, drug repackers, and health professionals who compound medications to be especially vigilant in ensuring that glycerin, a sweetener commonly used worldwide in liquid OTC and prescription drug products, is not contaminated with diethylene glycol (DEG). DEG is a known poison used in antifreeze and as a solvent. The most recent poisoning incident occurred in Panama in September 2006 and involved DEG-contaminated glycerin used in cough syrup, which resulted in dozens of hospitalizations for serious injury and more than 40 deaths. In late 1995 and early 1996, at least 80 children died in Haiti owing to DEG-contaminated glycerin in acetaminophen syrup. Between 1990 and 1998, similar incidents of DEG poisoning reportedly occurred in Argentina, Bangladesh, India, and Nigeria and resulted in hundreds of deaths. In 1937, more than 100 people died in the United States after ingesting DEG-contaminated Elixir Sulfanilamide, a drug used to treat infections. This incident led to the enactment of the Federal Food, Drug, and Cosmetic Act, which is the nation's primary statute on the regulation of drugs (12).

   2. Glycerin Oral Solution USP (5,8)
   a. Content: not less than 95.0% and not more than 105.0% of $C_3H_8O_3$
   b. Description: like Glycerin USP except pH between 5.5 and 7.5
   c. Solubility: like Glycerin USP
   d. It is used as a solvent-vehicle for the preparation of pharmaceutical oral dosage forms.
   e. Packaging and storage: tight containers

   3. Glycerin Ophthalmic Solution USP (5,8)
   a. Content: not less than 98.5% of $C_3H_8O_3$; may contain one or more suitable antimicrobial preservatives
   b. Description: like Glycerin Oral Solution USP except it is sterile
   c. Solubility: like Glycerin USP
   d. For ophthalmic use
   e. Packaging and storage: Tight containers of glass or plastic with volume not greater than 15 mL and protected from light. The container or carton is sealed and tamper-proof so that sterility is ensured at opening.

   4. Propylene Glycol USP (5,8,13)

$$C_3H_8O_2 \qquad MW = 76.09$$

   a. Content: not less than 99.5% of $C_3H_8O_2$
   b. Description: clear, colorless, viscous liquid; practically odorless, hygroscopic
   c. Specific gravity: between 1.035 and 1.037
   d. Solubility: miscible with water, ethyl and isopropyl alcohol, acetone, glycerin, polyethylene glycol 400, chloroform, and ether; dissolves many volatile oils, but is immiscible with fixed oils and mineral oil

     e. It is used as a solvent-vehicle for the preparation of pharmaceutical dosage forms for internal or external use. It is also useful as a humectant and preservative.

  5. Polyethylene Glycol NF (8,9,13)

     a. Polyethylene Glycol, also known as PEG, is an addition polymer of ethylene oxide and water. It has the formula $H(OCH_2CH_2)_nOH$, where n represents the number of oxyethylene groups.

     b. PEG is labeled with a number indicating the average nominal molecular weight of the polyethylene glycol. The numbers range from 200 to 8,000; polyethylene glycols 200, 300, 400, and 600 are liquids at room temperature, and the higher molecular polymers are waxy solids. (See Chapter 24, Table 24.1.)

     c. Polyethylene glycol 400 is the most common liquid PEG used as a solvent-vehicle in making pharmaceutical dosage forms for both internal and external use. It is a clear, colorless, slightly hygroscopic, viscous liquid with a slight odor. It congeals at 6°C and has a specific gravity at 25° of 1.12.

     d. Solubility: All PEGs are soluble in water, and many are organic solvents. PEG 400 is miscible with water, ethyl and isopropyl alcohol, acetone, glycerin, and propylene glycol. It is immiscible with fixed oils and mineral oil.

     e. Recommended packaging: tight containers

V. KETONES

A. General information

  1. There are only two official solvent-vehicles in the ketone group, Acetone and Methyl Isobutyl Ketone. Methyl ethyl ketone is not an official substance, but it is described in the reagent section of the *USP* because it is used as a solvent for assays, tests, and processing.

  2. Official ketones have limited usefulness because of their volatility, flammability, and toxicity. They do have some unique solvent properties that make them useful.

B. Acetone NF (9,13)

$$CH_3COCH_3 \qquad C_3H_6O \qquad MW = 58.08$$

  1. Description: transparent, colorless, mobile, volatile liquid that boils at 56.5°C. Has a distinctive odor. A 1 in 2 solution with water has neutral pH.
CAUTION: *Acetone is very flammable. Do not use where it may be ignited.*

  2. Specific gravity: 0.788 (not >0.789)

  3. Solubility: miscible with water, alcohol, ether, chloroform, and most oils

  4. Packaging and storage: tight containers and stored remote from fire

VI. OILS

A. General information

  1. The solvent-vehicle oils official in the *USP-NF* are listed in Table 15.1.

  2. As stated in the introduction to this chapter, some special vegetable and essential oils are used primarily as flavors and scents. The *National Formulary* section of the *USP–NF* has monographs for various oils of this type such as Anise Oil, Lemon Oil, and Rose Oil. These are discussed in Chapter 21, Colors, Flavors, Sweeteners, and Scents.

B. *USP–NF* oils

  1. Almond Oil NF (8,9)

     a. Description: clear, pale, straw-colored or colorless, oily liquid; clear at −10°C, congeals at −20°C

     b. Specific gravity: 0.910 to 0.915

     c. Solubility: insoluble in water, slightly soluble in alcohol, miscible with mineral oil, other fixed oils, ether, chloroform, and solvent hexane

  2. Castor Oil USP (5,8)

     a. Description: pale, yellowish or nearly colorless, transparent, viscid liquid; has a faint, mild odor

     b. Specific gravity: 0.957 to 0.961

    c. Solubility: insoluble in water and mineral oil, soluble in alcohol, miscible with dehydrated alcohol, other fixed oils, glacial acetic acid, chloroform, and ether

3. Corn Oil NF (8,9)
    a. Description: clear, light yellow, oily liquid with a faint characteristic odor
    b. Specific gravity: 0.914 to 0.921
    c. Solubility: insoluble in water, slightly soluble in alcohol, miscible with mineral oil, other fixed oils, ether, chloroform, and solvent hexane

4. Cottonseed Oil NF (8,9)
    a. Description: pale yellow, oily liquid. Odorless or nearly so. Particles of fat may separate beginning at 10°C, solidifies at 0° to −5°C.
    b. Specific gravity: 0.915 to 0.921
    c. Solubility: insoluble in water, slightly soluble in alcohol, miscible with mineral oil, other fixed oils, ether, chloroform, and solvent hexane

5. Mineral Oil USP (5,8)
    a. Description: colorless, transparent, oily liquid; odorless at room temperature
    b. Specific gravity: 0.845 to 0.905
    c. Solubility: insoluble in water and in alcohol, soluble in volatile oils; miscible with most fixed oils but not with castor oil

6. Light Mineral Oil NF (8,9)
    a. Description: colorless, transparent, oily liquid, odorless at room temperature
    b. Specific gravity: 0.818 to 0.880
    c. Solubility: insoluble in water and in alcohol, soluble in volatile oils; miscible with most fixed oils but not with castor oil

7. Olive Oil NF (8,9)
    a. Description: pale yellow or light greenish-yellow oily liquid; has a characteristic odor
    b. Specific gravity: 0.910 to 0.915
    c. Solubility: insoluble in water, slightly soluble in alcohol, miscible with mineral oil, other fixed oils, ether, and chloroform

8. Peanut Oil NF (8,9)
    a. Description: colorless or pale yellow oily liquid; may have a nutty odor
    b. Specific gravity: 0.912 to 0.920
    c. Solubility: insoluble in water, very slightly soluble in alcohol, miscible with mineral oil, other fixed oils, ether, and chloroform

9. Safflower Oil USP (5,8)
    a. Description: light yellow oil; becomes thick and rancid on prolonged exposure to air
    b. Specific gravity: 0.921
    c. Solubility: insoluble in water, slightly soluble in alcohol, miscible with other fixed oils, ether, and chloroform

10. Sesame Oil NF (8,9)
    a. Description: pale yellow, oily liquid; practically odorless
    b. Specific gravity: 0.916 to 0.921
    c. Solubility: insoluble in water, slightly soluble in alcohol, miscible with mineral oil, other fixed oils, ether, chloroform, and solvent hexane

11. Soybean Oil USP (5,8,14)
    a. Description: clear, pale yellow oily liquid with a characteristic odor
    b. Specific gravity: 0.916 to 0.922
    c. Solubility: insoluble in water, slightly soluble in alcohol, miscible with mineral oil, other fixed oils, ether, and chloroform

VII.   CYCLODEXTRINS

A. General information

1. Cyclodextrins, cyclic oligosaccharides, were discovered more than 100 years ago (15). Cyclodextrins are chemically and physically stable molecules formed by the enzymatic modification of starch. Typical cyclodextrins contain a number of glucose monomers ranging from six to eight units in a ring, creating a cone shape. The most common cyclodextrins are α-cyclodextrin: six-sugar-ring molecule; β-cyclodextrin: seven sugar-ring-molecule; and γ-cyclodextrin: eight-sugar-ring molecule.

2. Being starch derivatives, cyclodextrins are generally regarded as essentially nontoxic materials. Worldwide α, β and γ-cyclodextrin are fully registered in all major chemical inventories (16).

In the United States, both β and γ-cyclodextrin have Generally Regarded As Safe (GRAS) status. However, β-cyclodextrin can form insoluble complexes with cholesterol that disrupt the function of the kidneys, so it should not be used in parenteral applications, and its oral use should be limited to a daily maximum dose of 5 mg/kg.

3. In the presence of water, hydrophobic molecules or functional groups of molecules can be included in the cyclodextrin cavity if their molecular dimensions correspond to those of the cyclodextrin cavity. The formed inclusion complexes are relatively stable. One, two, or three cyclodextrin molecules contain one or more entrapped "guest" molecules; this is the essence of "molecular encapsulation."

4. In pharmaceutical dosage forms, cyclodextrins have mainly been used as complexing agents to increase the aqueous solubility of poorly water-soluble drugs and to increase their bioavailability and stability. See example 27.2 in Chapter 27 solutions for a compounded formulation that uses a cyclodextrin in solubilize a drug.

B. *USP–NF* cyclodextrins

1. α-Cyclodextrin: Alfadex NF (9,16)

$$(C_6H_{10}O_5)_6, MW = 972.84$$

a. Alfadex is composed of six alpha-(1-4) linked D-glucopyranosyl units. It contains not less than 98.0% and not more than 101.0% of $(C_6H_{10}O_5)_6$, calculated on the anhydrous basis.

b. Appearance: white crystalline powder

c. Water content: not more than 11.0%

d. Solubility: soluble in water, slightly soluble in alcohol (17)

2. β-Cyclodextrin: Betadex NF (9,16)

$$(C_6H_{10}O_5)_7, MW = 1,135$$

a. Betadex is a nonreducing cyclic compound composed of seven alpha-(1-4) linked D-glucopyranosyl units. It contains not less than 98.0% and not more than 102.0% of $(C_6H_{10}O_5)_7$, calculated on the anhydrous basis.

b. Appearance: white crystalline powder

c. Water content: not more than 14.0%

d. Solubility: soluble in water, slightly soluble in alcohol (17)

3. β-Cyclodextrin derivatives (13,16)

a. 2-Hydroxylpropyl-beta-cyclodextrin (HP-β-CD) is an alternative to alpha-, beta- and gamma-cyclodextrin; it has improved water solubility and may be more toxicologically benign. It is well tolerated in humans, with the main adverse event being diarrhea, and there has been no adverse event on kidney function documented to date (18). Owing to its unique properties, it is frequently used to solubilize poorly soluble drugs. For example, Sporanox (itraconazole) injection is a sterile, pyrogen-free, clear, colorless-to-slightly-yellow solution for intravenous infusion. Each milliliter contains 10 mg of itraconazole, solubilized by hydroxypropyl-β-cyclodextrin (400 mg) as a molecular inclusion complex.

b. Sulfobutylether-β-cyclodextrin (Captisol) is another chemically modified cyclodextrin rationally designed to increase drug solubility yet, unlike natural cyclodextrins, it is toxicologically acceptable in injectable formulations. Abilify (aripiprazole) Injection is a (7.5 mg/mL) clear, colorless, sterile, aqueous solution for intramuscular use that contains 150 mg/mL of sulfobutylether β-cyclodextrin as a solubilizer.

REFERENCES

1. The United States Pharmacopeial Convention Inc. General notices. 2007 USP 30/NF 25. Rockville, MD: Author, 2006.

2. The United States Pharmacopeial Convention Inc. 2007: Front Matter—NF: Excipients. USP 30/NF 25. Rockville, MD: Author, 2006.

3. The United States Pharmacopeial Convention Inc. Chapter ⟨1231⟩ 2007 USP 30/NF 25. Rockville, MD: Author, 2006; 687–694.

4. The United States Pharmacopeial Convention Inc. Chapter ⟨1⟩ 2007 USP 30/NF 25. Rockville, MD: Author, 2006: 33–36.

5. The United States Pharmacopeial Convention Inc. USP Monographs 2007. USP 30/NF 25. Rockville, MD: Author, 2006.

6. The United States Pharmacopeial Convention Inc. Chapter ⟨795⟩ 2007 USP 30/NF 25. Rockville, MD: Author, 2006; 330.

7. The United States Pharmacopeial Convention Inc. Chapter ⟨788⟩ 2007 USP 30/NF 25. Rockville, MD: Author, 2006; 321.

8. The United States Pharmacopeial Convention Inc. References: Descriptions and Solubilities. 2007 USP 30/NF 25. Rockville, MD: Author, 2006.

9. The United States Pharmacopeial Convention Inc. NF Monographs. 2007 USP 30/NF 25. Rockville, MD: Author, 2006.

10. American Academy of Pediatrics, Committee on Drugs. Ethanol in liquid preparations intended for children. Pediatrics 1984; 73: 405–407.

11. Food and Drug Administration, Department of Health and Human Services. Code of Federal Regulations, Title 21, vol. 5, Revised as of April 1, 2001. Chapter I—Part 328—Over-the-counter drug products intended for oral ingestion that contain alcohol [Original March 13, 1995, as amended at 61 FR 58630, Nov. 18, 1996.] Washington, DC: Author, 1996.

12. U.S. Department of Health and Human Services, Food and Drug Administration, Center for Drug Evaluation and Research. Guidance for industry: Testing of glycerin for diethylene glycol (http://www.fda.gov/cder/guidance/7654fnl.pdf) May 2007.

13. Rowe R, Sheskey P, Weller, P. eds. Handbook of pharmaceutical excipients, 5th ed. Washington, DC: APhA Publications, 2005.

14. Thompson, MICROMEDEX, Inc. USP DI Vol. III, 27th ed. Englewood, CO: Author, 2007.

15. Villiers A. Sur la transformation de la fécule en dextrine par le ferment butyrique. Compt Rend Fr Acad Sci 1891; 435–438.

16. Szejtli J. Cyclodextrin technology, vol 1. New York: Springer, 1988.

17. Sabadini E, Cosgrovea T, do Carmo Egídio F. Solubility of cyclomaltooligosaccharides (cyclodextrins) in H$_2$O and D$_2$O: A comparative study, Carbohydr Res 2006; 341: 270–274.

18. Gould S, Scott RC. 2-Hydroxypropyl-beta-cyclodextrin (HP-beta-CD): A toxicology review. Food Chem Toxicol 2005; 43: 1451–1459.

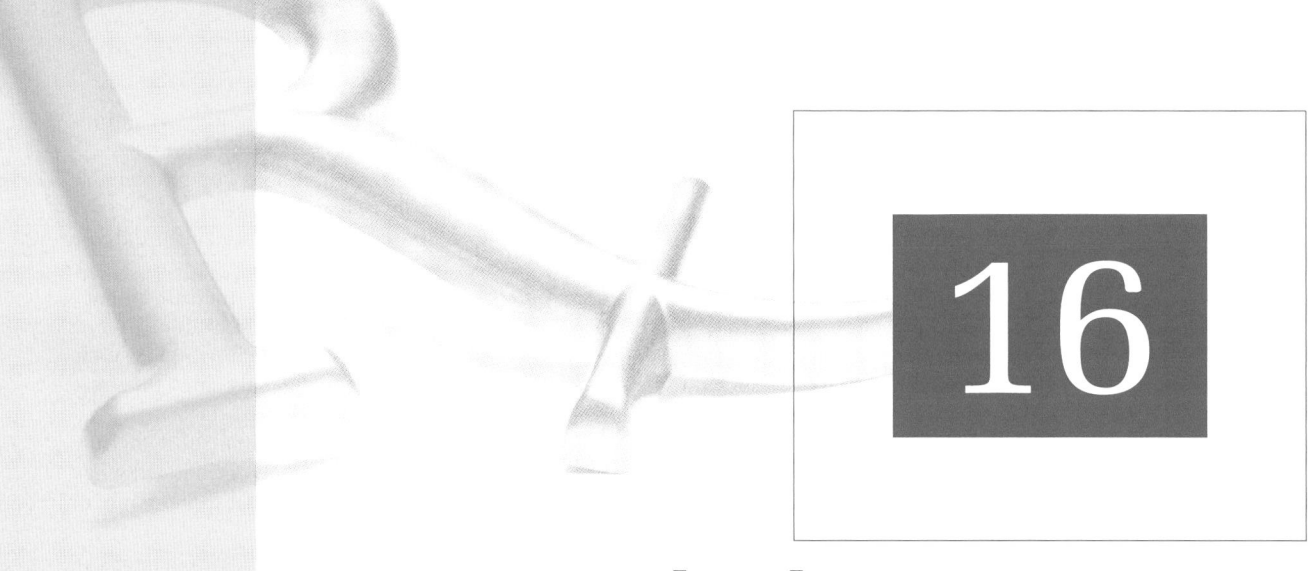

Antimicrobial Preservatives

Melgardt de Villiers, PhD

I. DEFINITION

Antimicrobial preservatives are substances added to nonsterile dosage forms to protect them from microbiological growth or from microorganisms that are introduced inadvertently during or subsequent to the manufacturing process. In the case of sterile articles packaged in multiple-dose containers, antimicrobial preservatives are added to inhibit the growth of microorganisms that may be introduced from repeatedly withdrawing individual doses.

Antimicrobial agents should not be used as a substitute for good manufacturing practices or solely to reduce the viable microbial population of a nonsterile product or to control the presterilization bioburden of multidose formulations during manufacturing (1).—*USP*

II. USES OF PRESERVATIVES

A. Preservatives should be added to extemporaneously compounded preparations when there is a possibility of microbial contamination and growth, either at the time of preparations or during use by the patient or caregiver (1,2).

B. In *USP* Chapter ⟨1151⟩ Pharmaceutical Dosage Forms, antimicrobial agents are explicitly mentioned and required for most dosage forms containing water and for one nonaqueous system, ophthalmic ointments (3).

1. Emulsions (including semisolid or ointment-type emulsions): "All emulsions require an antimicrobial agent because the aqueous phase is favorable to the growth of microorganisms."
2. Suspensions: "Suspensions intended for any route of administration should contain suitable antimicrobial agents to protect against bacteria, yeast, and mold contamination."
3. Oral solutions: "Antimicrobial agents to prevent the growth of bacteria, yeasts, and molds are generally also present."
4. Ophthalmic solutions: "Each solution must contain a suitable substance or mixture of substances to prevent the growth of, or to destroy, microorganisms accidentally introduced when the container is opened during use. Where intended for use in surgical procedures, ophthalmic solutions, although they must be sterile, should not contain antibacterial agents, since they may be irritating to the ocular tissues."
5. Ophthalmic ointments: "Ophthalmic ointments must contain a suitable substance or mixture of substances to prevent growth of, or to destroy, microorganisms accidentally introduced when the container is opened during use, unless otherwise directed in the individual monograph, or unless the formula itself is bacteriostatic."

C. The requirements for antimicrobial agents in parenteral products are treated in *USP* Chapter ⟨1⟩, Injections (4):

> A suitable substance or mixture of substances to prevent the growth of microorganisms must be added to preparations intended for injection that are packaged in multiple-dose containers, regardless of the method of sterilization employed, unless one of the following conditions prevails: (1) there are different directions in the individual monograph; (2) the substance contains a radionuclide with a physical half-life of less than 24 hours; (3) the active ingredients are themselves antimicrobial. Such substances are used in concentrations that will prevent the growth of or kill microorganisms in the preparations for injection (4).

III.   WHEN IS IT NOT NECESSARY TO ADD A PRESERVATIVE?

A. The preparation will be used immediately. This assumes that the preparation is made using appropriate techniques that avoid contamination while it is being made and administered.
B. No water is present. Generally, microorganisms require water for growth, so products that contain no water, such as tablets, powders, and hydrocarbon ointments, are not media for growth. Exceptions to this rule include ophthalmic ointments and nonaqueous injections when the *USP* specifically requires an antimicrobial agent.
C. The pH of the medium is either <3 or >9.
   Note: Though this pH range for inhibition of growth holds true for most microorganisms, certain resistant molds have been shown to grow in media with pH <3 (5).
D. Ingredient(s) that have antimicrobial properties are already present in the formulation.

IV.   WHEN ARE PRESERVATIVES CONTRAINDICATED?

A. Neonates
B. Ophthalmic solutions intended for use in eyes during eye surgery, with non-intact corneas, or for intraocular injection
C. Parenteral products with volumes >30 mL

V.   ALTERNATIVE STRATEGIES WHEN PRESERVATIVES ARE NEEDED BUT ARE CONTRAINDICATED

A. Prepare a single dose and use immediately.
B. Prepare a limited quantity that will be used within a short time period, store under refrigeration, and label with a short expiration period.

VI.   PROPERTIES OF THE IDEAL PRESERVATIVE

A. Effective at a low, nontoxic concentration against a wide variety of organisms
B. Chemically stable under normal conditions of use over a wide pH and temperature range
C. Soluble at the required concentration
D. Compatible with a wide variety of drugs and excipients
E. Free from objectionable odor, taste, color, or stinging
F. Nontoxic and nonsensitizing both internally and externally at the required concentration
G. Reasonable cost
H. Unreactive (does not adsorb, penetrate, or interact) with containers or closures

Table 16.1	ANTIMICROBIAL PRESERVATIVES LISTED IN THE *USP 30-NF 25*

Benzalkonium Chloride	Benzalkonium Chloride Solution	Benzethonium Chloride
Benzoic Acid	Benzyl Alcohol	Butylparaben
Cetrimonium Bromide	Cetylpyridinium Chloride	Chlorobutanol
Chlorocresol	Cresol	Ethylparaben
Methylparaben	Methylparaben Sodium	Phenol
Phenoxyethanol	Phenylethyl Alcohol	Phenylmercuric Acetate
Phenylmercuric Nitrate	Potassium Benzoate	Potassium Sorbate
Propylparaben	Propylparaben Sodium	Sodium Benzoate
Sodium Dehydroacetate	Sodium Propionate	Sorbic Acid
Thimerosal	Thymol	

Source: 2007 USP 30/ NF 25. Rockville, MD: The United States Pharmacopeial Convention Inc. 2006: Front Matter—NF:Excipients.

VII. ANTIMICROBIAL PRESERVATIVES LISTED IN THE *USP 30–NF 25*

A. Table 16.1 gives the articles listed as antimicrobial preservatives in the *USP 30–NF 25* (6). Some chemicals, though not listed by the *USP* as preservatives, have antimicrobial properties and may be useful as preservatives in formulated preparations.

B. The preservatives used most commonly in extemporaneous compounding are described in sections VIII through X of this Chapter.
1. To facilitate selection of an antimicrobial preservative when formulating a preparation, the agents are organized by suitability for route of administration (e.g., oral, topical, and ophthalmic).
2. The descriptions and solubilities presented here give a composite of information from the Chemistry and Compendial Requirements section of the *USP DI Vol. III* (7), *The Merck Index* (8), the *Handbook of Pharmaceutical Excipients* (2), and other references as cited. For additional information on each agent, consult the *Handbook of Pharmaceutical Excipients.*

C. In reading and interpreting the current chapter, note that this text employs the usual convention of using upper-case first letters for words designating official *USP-NF* articles (e.g., Alcohol, Purified Water) and lower-case first letters for words designating the chemical substances (e.g., ethanol, water).

VIII. PRESERVATIVES FOR ORAL DOSAGE FORMS

A. **Alcohols and glycols**
1. Ethyl Alcohol

$$CH_3CH_2OH \qquad MW = 46.07$$

a. Official articles of ethyl alcohol that are suitable for oral use:
(1) Alcohol USP
(2) Dehydrated Alcohol USP
(3) Dehydrated Alcohol Injection USP
(4) Diluted Alcohol NF
Note: Rubbing Alcohol USP is a product containing ethyl alcohol, but it may **not** be used orally. It contains denaturants that are toxic orally.
b. Description and solubility: See Chapter 15, Pharmaceutical Solvents and Solubilizing Agents
c. Effective concentration
(1) Effective concentration depends on the pH of the solution and the amount of "free water."
Note: "Free water" is the water in a preparation that is not bound by interaction with other molecules. Originally, the term was used to represent the amount of water in a preparation that is not tied up by interaction with sucrose in the ratio of 85 g of sucrose to 45 mL of water. This 85:45 ratio of sucrose to water is called the *USP Syrup Equivalent* because it is the proportion of these ingredients in the formula for Syrup NF (Simple Syrup), which is a saturated, self-preserving solution. Obviously, other dissolved molecules can also reduce the activity of water. For example, a salt, such as potassium chloride, or a highly hydrated polymer, such as methylcellulose, also binds water in an

aqueous solution, but the degree of these interactions has not been documented. It is important to realize that these interactions do occur, and when these ingredients are in a liquid preparation, they do effectively reduce the "free water" in that product.

(2) **The alcohol concentration should be 15% (Acid)—17.5% (Neutral or mildly alkaline) of the free water (9).**

(3) Though the 15% to 17.5% range seems high, the percentage actually needed for most preparations is far less because these percentages apply only to the "free water." Consider the following example:

Mineral Oil Emulsion USP (10)

Mineral Oil	500 mL
Acacia	125 g
Syrup	100 mL
Vanillin	40 mg
Alcohol	60 mL
Purified Water, a sufficient quantity to make	1,000 mL

If you add the approximate volumes of all the ingredients (in the case of the solids—acacia and vanillin—you have to estimate the powder volume) and subtract this quantity from 1,000 mL, you get the approximate free water volume: 1,000 mL − [500 + 100 + 60 + ~40 (powder volume estimate)] = 300 mL. This is the amount of water that must be preserved with alcohol. The quantity of ethyl alcohol in this prescription is 95% × 60 mL = 57 mL. This quantity represents only 5.7% of the total product, but it is 19% of the free water (19% × 300 mL = 57 mL).

Some syrups are protected from microbial growth by virtue of their high solute concentrations that create an unfavorable osmotic environment for these organisms. However, more dilute syrups are good media for microbial growth and require the addition of preservatives. This is another example in which alcohol or another preservative should be added to preserve the free water.

(4) One commonly seen guideline of alcohol content for preservation of liquid formulations is **5% to 10%** alcohol. In using this figure, one should be aware of its origins: It comes from a rough estimate of the free water available in the "average" product. Therefore, if you have a prescription order that contains a large proportion of free water, you should add extra alcohol for adequate preservation.

2. Propylene Glycol

$$C_3H_8O_2 \qquad MW = 76.09$$

a. Official article Propylene Glycol USP
b. Description and solubility: See Chapter 15, Pharmaceutical Solvents and Solubilizing Agents.
c. Effective concentration
   (1) In most situations, propylene glycol is effective at a concentration of **10% w/v,** although inhibition of growth of certain molds requires up to 30% w/v (11,12).
   (2) Propylene glycol potentiates several other preservatives. A 2% to 5% concentration of propylene glycol, though ineffective as a sole preservative, potentiates the effect of a methyl and propyl paraben combination. Various combinations tested were found to be effective against bacteria, molds, and yeast but were ineffective against bacterial spores until they entered the vegetative stage (13). This effect on paraben efficacy is especially useful because the concentration at which the parabens exert their antimicrobial effect is so close to their solubility. Though parabens are particularly useful for preserving vulnerable syrups that have a neutral pH, because of their poor water solubility, it is often difficult to dissolve a sufficient concentration of parabens to achieve adequate preservation. In this study, both a 2% and a 5% concentration of propylene glycol allowed the

minimum inhibitory concentration of methylparaben to be reduced from 0.18% to 0.1% when combined with 0.02% propylparaben (13).

3. Glycerin

$$C_3H_8O_3 \quad MW = 92.01$$

HO⌒⌒OH
OH

a. Official article Glycerin USP
b. Description and solubility: See Chapter 15, Pharmaceutical Solvents and Solubilizing Agents.
c. Effective concentration
 (1) Though glycerin **preserves at concentrations ≥50%,** at lower concentrations it may actually act as a nutrient for some microorganisms. This is because glycerin's activity as an antimicrobial agent depends solely on an osmotic effect rather than any innate toxicity to microorganisms (13).
 (2) Though glycerin is not often used as a sole preservative, it is frequently used with alcohol to reduce the volume of alcohol necessary to preserve a preparation.

4. Benzyl Alcohol

$$C_7H_8O \quad MW = 108.14$$

a. Official article Benzyl Alcohol NF
b. Description: colorless liquid; faint, aromatic odor; sharp, burning taste; neutral pH; flammable
c. Solubility: 1 g/30 mL water; freely soluble in 50% alcohol; miscible with alcohol and fixed and volatile oils
d. Effective concentration: bacteriocidal at **1% to 2%** (14)
e. Benzyl alcohol is listed here because it is approved for oral products; however, it is not typically used in these preparations because of its sharp, burning taste. It is used frequently in manufactured parenteral products, in which it is especially useful because of its local anesthetic properties. It may be used in topical preparations and, in fact, has been used therapeutically as a local anesthetic to relieve itching when mixed with equal parts of alcohol and water (15). Though listed as an approved preservative for ophthalmic products (2), it is not commonly found in ophthalmic preparations (16).
f. Benzyl alcohol is most effective at pH less than 5 and has minimal activity at pH 8 and above. It is incompatible with methylcellulose and its activity is reduced by nonionic surfactants, such as polysorbate 80 (2).

B. Organic acids
 1. Benzoic Acid/Sodium Benzoate/Potassium Benzoate
  a. Official articles include the following:
   (1) Benzoic Acid USP

$$C_7H_6O_2 \quad MW = 122.12$$

   (2) Sodium Benzoate NF
   (3) Potassium Benzoate NF
  b. Descriptions
   (1) Benzoic acid: white crystals, scales, or needles; slight aromatic odor; volatile at warm temperatures; $pK_a = 4.19$; pH of a saturated solution = 2.8
   (2) Sodium benzoate: white granular or crystalline powder; practically odorless; slightly hygroscopic but stable in air. Has an unpleasant sweet and salty taste. Sodium benzoate is the most commonly used salt of benzoic acid.

(3) Potassium benzoate: white granular or crystalline powder; practically odorless; stable in air

c. Solubilities

(1) Benzoic acid: 1 g/300 mL of water (0.33%), or 3 mL of alcohol; soluble in fixed oils

(2) Sodium benzoate: 1 g/2 mL of water, or 75 mL of alcohol.

(3) Potassium benzoate: soluble in water and alcohol

d. Effective concentration

(1) Benzoic acid is the active preservative form, and its effective concentration is **0.1% to 0.3%** (17).

(2) Because its effective concentration is so close to its solubility, benzoic acid is often dissolved as the sodium salt (sodium benzoate), which is very water-soluble. The amount present as the active form is then dependent on the pH of the solution. This amount can be estimated using the Henderson–Hasselbalch equation.

(3) Benzoic acid/sodium benzoate is ineffective in solutions with a pH above 5. This means that in deciding the effectiveness of this preservative, you must know the pH of the liquid you wish to preserve. Most fruit-flavored and cola fountain syrups have pHs around 3 and are effectively preserved with benzoic acid/sodium benzoate. Depending on method of preparation, Syrup NF has a pH of 5 to 6.5, so it may or may not be adequately protected. Methylcellulose 1% gel has a pH of approximately 6, and sodium carboxymethylcellulose 1% gel has a pH of about 7, so these would probably not be preserved. The monographs of some official liquid preparations give pH ranges for these liquids. The pH of manufactured liquid drug products is often given in the product package insert. An alternative easy way to determine the approximate pH of a liquid product or preparation is to use pH paper or a pH meter. This is illustrated in the sample prescription quality control section for numerous water-containing preparations in Part 5, Nonsterile Dosage Forms and their Preparation, of this book.

(4) Its effectiveness may be reduced by such nonionic surfactants as polysorbate 80.

(5) Benzoic acid/sodium benzoate is widely used as a preservative, especially in foods. It has most of the properties of an ideal preservative. Its biggest drawback is the pH dependence of its effectiveness.

2. Sorbic Acid/Potassium Sorbate

a. Official articles include the following:

(1) Sorbic Acid NF

$$C_6H_8O_2 \qquad MW = 112.13$$

(2) Potassium Sorbate NF

b. Descriptions

(1) Sorbic acid: white crystalline powder; pK_a 4.76

(2) Potassium sorbate: white crystals or powder

c. Solubilities

(1) Sorbic acid: listed in *Remington: The Science and Practice of Pharmacy* as 1 g/1,000 mL of water (0.1%); *The Merck Index* gives a water solubility of 0.25% (1 g/400 mL) at 30° and 3.8% (1 g/26 mL) at 100°. The solubility in alcohol is 1 g/10 mL and in propylene glycol, 1 g/19 mL.

(2) Potassium sorbate: very soluble in water, 1 g/4.5 mL, and moderately soluble in alcohol, 1 g/35 mL

d. Effective concentration

(1) Sorbic acid is the active form, with an effective concentration of **0.05% to 0.2%** (17).

(2) Sorbic acid has properties and problems that are similar to those of benzoic acid. Like benzoic acid, sorbic acid has an effective concentration that is very close to its solubility. Because of this, the salt form, potassium sorbate, which is very soluble in water, is often used. As with benzoic acid, the amount that is present in the active acid form is dependent on the pH of the solution. Because sorbic acid has a slightly higher pK_a than benzoic acid, it has a higher ratio of active to inactive form at the pH levels common to oral products. It reportedly has little antimicrobial activity above pH 6 (18).

(3) Sorbic acid is widely used as a preservative in foods. It is one of the least toxic preservatives, with a reported oral LD_{50} in rats of 7.36 g/kg (7). Though it has low toxicity orally, irritation of the skin in topical products has been reported.

C. Esters of *p*-Hydroxybenzoic Acid (Parabens)

1. Official articles of parabens include the following:

    a. Methylparaben NF

$$C_8H_8O_3 \qquad MW = 152.15$$

    b. Methylparaben Sodium NF

    c. Propylparaben NF

$$C_{10}H_{12}O_3 \qquad MW = 180.20$$

    d. Propylparaben Sodium NF

2. Descriptions

    a. Methylparaben: small, colorless crystals, or white, crystalline powder; practically odorless; slight burning taste

    b. Methylparaben sodium: white, hygroscopic powder

    c. Propylparaben: small, colorless crystals, or white powder

    d. Propylparaben sodium: white, odorless, hygroscopic powder

3. Solubilities

    a. Methylparaben: 1 g/400 mL of water (0.25%), or 3 mL of alcohol. It is soluble in glycerin (1 g/60 mL) and propylene glycol (1 g/5 mL) but insoluble in mineral oil; solubility in fixed oils varies.

    b. Propylparaben: 1 g/2,500 mL of water (0.04%), or 1.5 mL of alcohol

    c. The sodium salts are more soluble, but they are formed only at a relatively high pH (~9), and at this pH, the molecule is fairly unstable because of hydrolysis of the ester group.

4. Effective concentration

    a. Methylparaben: **0.05% to 0.25%** (The lower part of the range is effective only when used in combination with another preservative, such as propylparaben, benzyl alcohol, or propylene glycol.)

       Methylparaben has a water solubility that is essentially identical to its effective concentration. Because it is a rather hydrophobic powder, it is somewhat difficult to dissolve in aqueous solutions. If the product will tolerate a small amount of alcohol or propylene glycol, the powder can first be dissolved in a minimal amount of alcohol or propylene glycol. Methylparaben has many properties of an ideal preservative, including activity over a wide pH range, 4 to 8 (2,16,17). Its major problem is its poor water solubility. Its effectiveness is enhanced by 2% to 5% propylene glycol (13,19).

    b. Propylparaben: **0.02% to 0.04%** (Most effective when used in combination with another preservative such as methylparaben. A concentration of 0.035% is the maximum acceptable concentration for parenteral products.)

       Propylparaben would be a great preservative if it were more water-soluble. It is rarely used by itself because it is impossible to get enough dissolved for sufficient preservative action. It is most often used in combination with methylparaben. Combinations of paraben esters have a synergistic effect. A combination of 0.18% of methylparaben to 0.02% propylparaben is common and has been approved for use as a preservative for certain parenteral products. Like methylparaben, propylparaben is hydrophobic and is difficult to dissolve in water. Furthermore, propylparaben is used in such a small amount that for the small quantities used in extemporaneous formulation, an aliquot is required. If the product will tolerate a small amount of alcohol or propylene glycol, the powder can first be dissolved in a minimal amount of alcohol or propylene glycol. One possible stock solution has the following formula:

Methylparaben	9 g
Propylparaben	1 g
Propylene Glycol qs ad	100 mL

Two milliliters of this stock solution in each 100 mL or 100 g of preparation will provide 0.18% methylparaben, 0.02% propylparaben, and approximately 2% propylene glycol.

5. Parabens are FDA-approved for use in a wide range of dosage forms, including oral, topical, rectal, vaginal, urethral, ophthalmic, nasal, inhalation, irrigation, and parenteral products (16). Though not common, parabens can cause hypersensitivity reactions, most commonly delayed-contact dermatitis. Irritation has also been reported when parabens are used ophthalmically and parenterally (2).

IX. PRESERVATIVES FOR TOPICAL PREPARATIONS

A. Alcohols and glycols
1. Ethyl alcohol: See earlier description and in Chapter 15, Pharmaceutical Solvents and Solubilizing Agents.
   One official article of ethyl alcohol that is not suitable for oral use but may be used topically is Rubbing Alcohol USP. It is described in Chapter 15.
2. Isopropyl Alcohol $CH_3CHOHCH_3$

$$C_3H_8O \qquad MW = 60.10$$

   a. Though isopropyl alcohol may not be used internally because of its toxicity, it is safe for external use and is an effective preservative for topical products.
   b. Official articles, Descriptions, and Solubility: See Chapter 15, Pharmaceutical Solvents and Solubilizing Agents.
   c. Effective concentration: Same as ethyl alcohol
3. Propylene Glycol: See section VIII.
4. Glycerin: See section VIII.
5. Benzyl Alcohol: See section VIII.

B. Organic acids
1. Benzoic Acid: See section VIII.
2. Sorbic Acid: See section VIII.

C. Esters of *p*-Hydroxybenzoic Acid (Parabens): See foregoing description.

D. Organic mercurial derivatives
1. Official articles
   a. Phenylmercuric Acetate NF

$$C_8H_8HgO_2 \qquad MW = 336.74$$

   b. Phenylmercuric Nitrate NF

Phenylmercuric Nitrate is a mixture of phenylmercuric nitrate and phenylmercuric hydroxide (20).

c. Thimerosal USP

$$C_9H_9HgNaO_2S \qquad MW = 404.81$$

d. Thimerosal Topical Solution USP
e. Thimerosal Tincture USP

2. Descriptions
- **a.** Phenylmercuric acetate: white crystalline powder; odorless; pH of a saturated solution = 4
- **b.** Phenylmercuric nitrate: white crystalline powder with mild aromatic odor; affected by light. Saturated solutions are acid to litmus.
- **c.** Thimerosal: light cream–colored, crystalline powder with a slight odor; affected by light; pH of a 1% solution = 6.7
- **d.** Thimerosal Topical Solution USP: clear liquid; sensitive to some metals; affected by light; pH, 9.6–10.2.
- **e.** Thimerosal Tincture USP: transparent, mobile liquid with the odor of acetone and alcohol; sensitive to some metals; affected by light; alcohol content, 45.0% to 55.0%.

3. Solubilities
- **a.** Phenylmercuric Acetate (PMA): listed in *Remington's Pharmaceutical Sciences,* 18th ed., as 1 g/ 180 mL water, 225 mL alcohol; *The Merck Index* gives 1 g/600 mL water, soluble in alcohol and acetone.
- **b.** Phenylmercuric Nitrate (PMN): listed in *Remington's Pharmaceutical Sciences,* 18th ed., as 1 g/ 600 mL water, slightly soluble in alcohol or glycerin; *The Merck Index* gives 1 g/1,250 mL water, slightly soluble in alcohol, moderately soluble in glycerin; soluble in propylene glycol. **Note:** The *Handbook of Pharmaceutical Excipients* states for both compounds that the compendial values and laboratory values on solubility vary considerably. This can be seen in the foregoing values.
- **c.** Because PMN and PMA are used in very dilute concentrations, stock solutions are useful. Convenient concentrations of aqueous stock solutions are 1:2,000 and 1:10,000.
- **d.** Thimerosal: 1 g/1 mL water, 8 mL (*Merck*) or 12 mL (*Remington*) alcohol

4. Effective concentrations
- **a.** Phenylmercuric Acetate and Nitrate: may be used for **topical** products in a range of **0.002% to 0.01%.** The usual concentration for **ophthalmic** solutions is **0.002% to 0.004%**, with 0.004% the maximum allowed for eye products (21).

  Used primarily to preserve parenterals and eye and nasal products. All mercurial compounds can be sensitizing.
- **b.** Thimerosal: **0.001% to 0.02%.** The maximum acceptable concentration for **ophthalmic** products is **0.01%** (21); the maximum for parenteral products is 0.04%.

5. Incompatibilities
- **a.** Phenylmercuric acetate and nitrate precipitate with halides and anionic emulsifying agents, suspending agents, and drugs such as penicillin and fluorescein. They also are incompatible with tragacanth, starch, talc, silicates, sodium metabisulfite, aluminum and other metals, ammonia and its salts, amino acids, sulfur compounds, rubber, and some plastics. Disodium edetate and sodium thiosulfate may cause inactivation of PMN or PMA. Activity may be lost because of sorption onto polyethylene surfaces of containers, closures, or droppers (2,7).
- **b.** Thimerosal is a sodium salt that precipitates in acidic solutions. It also is incompatible with aluminum and other metals, silver nitrate, sodium chloride solutions, lecithin, phenylmercuric compounds, large cations such as quaternary ammonium compounds, thioglycolate, and proteins. Sodium metabisulfite and the EDTA compounds can reduce its antimicrobial effectiveness. In solution, it may sorb to some plastics and rubber closures (2,7).

E. Salts of quaternary ammonium bases

Note: Though the quaternary ammonium preservatives may be used in oral dosage forms, they are listed here because they are used primarily in topical and ophthalmic drug products and preparations.

1. Official articles

   a. Benzalkonium Chloride NF

$$R = C_8H_{17} \text{ to } C_{18}H_{37}$$

Benzalkonium Chloride is a mixture of alkyl-benzyldimethylammonium chlorides with the general formula $[C_6H_5CH_2N(CH_3)_2R]Cl$, in which R represents a mixture of alkyls, including groups beginning with n-C_8H_{17} and extending through higher homologs, with n-$C_{12}H_{25}$, n-$C_{14}H_{29}$, and n-$C_{16}H_{33}$ providing the majority of R groups (20).

   b. Benzalkonium Chloride Solution NF

Benzalkonium Chloride Solution contains benzalkonium chloride in solution. The solution may also contain a suitable coloring agent and may contain not more than 10% alcohol. This solution should not be mixed with ordinary soaps or with anionic detergents as they may decrease or destroy its bacteriostatic activity (20).

   c. Benzethonium Chloride USP

$$C_{27}H_{42}ClNO_2 \qquad MW = 448.08$$

   d. Benzethonium Chloride Concentrate USP

Benzethonium Chloride Concentrate contains not less than 94.0% and not more than 106.0% of the labeled amount of benzethonium chloride ($C_{27}H_{42}ClNO_2$).

   e. Benzethonium Chloride Topical Solution USP

Benzethonium Chloride Topical Solution is an aqueous solution of the chemical (10).

   f. Benzethonium Chloride Tincture USP has the formula shown here (10):

Benzethonium Chloride	2 g
Alcohol	685 mL
Acetone	100 mL
Purified Water, a sufficient quantity to make	1,000 mL

   g. Cetylpyridium Chloride USP

$$C_{21}H_{38}ClN \cdot H_2O \qquad MW = 358.00$$

   h. Cetylpyridinium Chloride Topical Solution USP

Cetylpyridinium Chloride Topical Solution is a solution of the chemical (10).

2. Descriptions

   a. Benzalkonium Chloride (BAC): white or yellowish-white amorphous powder, thick gel or gel-like pieces; hygroscopic; mild odor with a very bitter taste; slightly alkaline (pH = 5–8 for a 10% w/v solution). Solutions foam when shaken.

   b. Benzethonium Chloride: white crystals; mild odor with a bitter taste. The pH of a 1% solution = 4.8–5.5.

    c. Cetylpyridinium Chloride: white powder; mild odor with a bitter taste

    d. Cetylpyridinium Chloride Topical Solution USP: clear, colorless solution with an aromatic odor and bitter taste; may be colored if dye is added

3. Solubilities

    a. Benzalkonium Chloride: very soluble in water, alcohol, and acetone

    b. Benzethonium Chloride: 1 g/mL of water, alcohol, or acetone

    c. Cetylpyridinium Chloride: very soluble in water and alcohol

4. Effective concentrations

    a. Benzalkonium Chloride: **0.004% to 0.02%** (22). The **usual concentration for preservation is 0.01%, with 0.013% the maximum allowed for ophthalmics** (21). The preservative action of Benzalkonium Chloride is somewhat unpredictable at the 0.01% concentration used for ophthalmic solutions. Its bacteriocidal properties are improved by the addition of 0.1% Edetate (EDTA). It can be irritating to the eye, and its solutions may be sensitizing. Benzalkonium chloride is available as 1:750, 10%, 17%, and 50% w/v aqueous solutions and as a 1:750 tincture.

    b. Benzethonium Chloride: **0.01% to 0.02%** (22). The usual preservative concentration and the **maximum allowed for ophthalmics is 0.01%** (21). Benzethonium Chloride is available as the powder.

    c. Cetylpyridinium Chloride: **0.01% to 0.02%** (22). Cetylpyridinium Chloride is available as the powder.

5. Incompatibilities: The salts of quaternary ammonium bases have many incompatibilities. For example, *Martindale: The Extra Pharmacopeia* lists the following incompatibilities for benzalkonium chloride: soaps, anionic drugs and detergents, nonionic surfactants in high concentrations, citrates, iodides, nitrates, permanganates, salicylates, silver salts, tartrates, fluorescein sodium, hydrogen peroxide, kaolin, lanolin, some sulfonamides, some components of commercial rubber mixes, and boric acid 5% (but not less than or equal to 2%) (23). The *Handbook of Pharmaceutical Excipients* also lists zinc oxide and zinc sulfate (2). Cetylpyridinium Chloride, but not Benzalkonium Chloride, is reported to be inactivated by methylcellulose (24).

X. PRESERVATIVES FOR OPHTHALMIC PREPARATIONS

A. All ophthalmic products must be sterile. Preparations in multi-dose containers must contain a suitable preservative to prevent the growth of microorganisms that may be introduced inadvertently into the product during use.

B. Preservatives commonly used in commercial ophthalmic products are given in Table 16.2 (25). Chlorobutanol, which is not used for oral or topical preparations, is described here. Preservatives that are frequently used in extemporaneous compounding of ophthalmic preparations but that are also used in oral and topical preparations have been described previously.

C. Chlorobutanol

$$C_4H_7Cl_3O \text{ (anhydrous)} \qquad MW = 177.46$$

and/or (hemihydrate) 186.46

1. Official article Chlorobutanol NF (20)

2. Description: colorless to white crystals with a camphor-like odor and taste

Table 16.2	PRESERVATIVES COMMONLY USED IN OPHTHALMIC PRODUCTS	
Benzalkonium Chloride	Benzethonium Chloride	Cetylpyridium Chloride
Chlorhexidine	Chlorobutanol	Disodium ETDA
Methylparaben	Phenylethyl Alcohol	Phenylmercuric Acetate
Phenylmercuric Nitrate	Propylparaben	Sodium Benzoate
Sodium Propionate	Sorbic acid	Thimerosal

Source: Handbook of Nonprescription Drugs, 13th ed. American Pharmaceutical Association, Washington DC, 2002.

   3. Solubility: 1 g/125 mL water, although it is somewhat difficult to dissolve. Also, 1 g/0.6 mL alcohol and 10 mL glycerin. It is freely soluble in volatile oils.
   4. Effective concentration: **0.5%** (21)
   5. Incompatibilities
      a. Is incompatible with silver nitrate and the sodium salts of sulfonamides
      b. Hydrolyzes to hydrochloric acid in solutions with pH's at or above neutrality; should be used in solutions buffered at 5.0–5.5
      c. Activity may be lost because of sorption onto polyethylene or rubber surfaces of ophthalmic containers or droppers.
      d. Is inactivated by the macromolecules polysorbate 80 and polyvinylpyrrolidone, but not by methylcellulose (24). Also interacts with carboxymethylcellulose, with resulting reduced antimicrobial activity (2)
   6. Chlorobutanol is used for ophthalmic and parenteral products. It is not used for oral preparations because of its camphor-like odor and taste. Its use as an ophthalmic preservative is limited because of its instability except at acid pH and because it acts slowly in killing organisms.

XI.   NEED FOR PRESERVATIVE-FREE FORMULATIONS

A. It is well known that traditional preservatives are effective in preventing microbial growth. However, there have been reports of irritation from some preserved products (26,27).

B. Disodium edetate (EDTA) and benzalkonium chloride (BAC) are often present as preservatives or stabilizing agents in nebulizer solutions used to treat asthma and chronic obstructive pulmonary disease (28). However, benzalkonium chloride is a potent bronchoconstrictor when inhaled in concentrations similar to those in which it is present in these solutions. Inclusion of BAC (together with EDTA) in the ipratropium bromide (Atrovent) nebulizer solution resulted in paradoxic bronchoconstriction in some asthmatic patients and an overall reduction in bronchodilator efficacy. The use of preservative-free bronchodilator nebulizer solutions does not result in clinically significant bacterial contamination if they are dispensed in sterile unit-dose vials in volumes and concentrations that do not require modification by the user (28).

C. In the case of nasal spray delivery, preservatives can be irritating to the patient mucosa, causing some unpleasant itching, but more seriously can also slow down or even stop the mucociliary clearance that is an essential natural mechanism for the protection of the upper airways (26,27).

D. Parabens are used as preservatives in many thousands of cosmetic, food, and pharmaceutical products to which the human population is exposed. Though recent reports of the estrogenic properties of parabens have challenged current concepts of their toxicity in these consumer products, the question remains as to whether any of the parabens can accumulate intact in the body from the long-term, low-dose levels to which humans are exposed. Initial reported studies showed that parabens can be extracted from human breast tissue and detected by thin-layer chromatography (29).

E. Thimerosal is a preservative that has been used in some vaccines since the 1930s, when it was first introduced by the Eli Lilly Company. At concentrations found in vaccines, it met the requirements for a preservative as set forth by the United States Pharmacopeia; that is, it kills the specified challenge organisms and is able to prevent the growth of the challenge fungi. However, owing to public perceptions of mercury and its toxicity, the use of mercury-containing preservatives in vaccines has declined markedly since 1999, and the FDA is continuing its efforts toward reducing or removing thimerosal from all existing vaccines. In this regard, all vaccines routinely recommended for children 6 years of age or younger and marketed in the United States contain no thimerosal or only trace amounts (1 μg or less mercury per dose), with the exception of inactivated influenza vaccine, which was first recommended by the Advisory Committee on Immunization Practices in 2004 for routine use in children 6 to 23 months of age.

REFERENCES

1. The United States Pharmacopeial Convention Inc. Chapter ⟨51⟩ 2007 USP 30/NF 25. Rockville, MD: Author, 2006; 79.
2. Rowe R, Sheskey P, Weller P, eds. Handbook of pharmaceutical excipients, 5th ed. Washington, DC: APhA Publications, 2005.
3. The United States Pharmacopeial Convention Inc. Chapter ⟨1151⟩ 2007 USP 30/NF 25. Rockville, MD: Author, 2006; 620–631.
4. The United States Pharmacopeial Convention Inc. Chapter ⟨1⟩ 2007 USP 30/NF 25. Rockville, MD: Author, 2006; 34.
5. Barr M, Tice LF. The preservation of aqueous sorbitol solutions. JAPhA Sci Ed 1957; 46: 221–223.
6. The United States Pharmacopeial Convention Inc. 2007 USP 30/NF 25. Front Matter—NF: Excipients. Rockville, MD: Author, 2006.
7. USP DI vol. III, 27th ed. Englewood, CO: Thompson, MICROMEDEX, Inc. 2007.
8. O'Neil MJ, ed. The Merck Index, 13th ed. Rahway, NJ: Merck & Co., Inc., 2001.

9. Gabel LF. The relative action of preservatives in pharmaceutical preparations. JAPhA 1921; 10: 767–768.

10. The United States Pharmacopeial Convention Inc. 2007 USP 30/ NF 25. USP Monographs. Rockville, MD: Author, 2006.

11. Rae J. The preservative properties of ethylene and propylene glycol. Pharm J 1938; 140: 517.

12. Barr M, Tice LF. A study of the inhibitory concentrations of glycerin-sorbitol and propylene glycol-sorbitol combinations on the growth of microorganisms. JAPhA Sci Ed 1957; 46: 217–218.

13. Prickett PS, Murray HL, Mercer NH. Potentiation of preservatives (parabens) in pharmaceutical formulations by low concentrations of propylene glycol. J Pharm Sci 1961; 50: 316–320.

14. Leszczynska-Bakal H, Smmazynski T. Preservation of pharmaceutical preparations by chemical compounds with antibacterial activity. Paper presented at Symposium on Preservatives used in Cosmetics, Bointe Pollena, May 30, 1974.

15. Swinyard EA, Harvey SC. In: Hoover JE, ed. Remington's pharmaceutical sciences, 14th ed. Easton, PA: Mack Publishing Co., 1970; 1066.

16. Inactive Ingredient Guide (redacted) January 1996. http://www.fda.gov/cder/drug/iig/default.htm . Accessed January 2008.

17. Entrekin DN. Relation of pH to preservative effectiveness: I. Acid media. J Pharm Sci 1961; 50: 743–746.

18. Eklund T. The antimicrobial effect of dissociated and undissociated sorbic acid at different pH levels. J Appl Bacteriol 1983; 54: 383–389.

19. Aalto TR, Firman MS, Rigler NE. p-Hydroxybenzoic acid esters as preservatives. JAPhA Sci Ed 1953; 42: 449–457.

20. The United States Pharmacopeial Convention Inc. NF Monographs. 2007 USP 30/NF 25. Rockville, MD: Author, 2006.

21. FDA Advisory Review Panel on OTC Ophthalmic Drug Products. Final Report, December 1979.

22. Allen LV. Preservatives and compounding. US Pharmacist 1994; 19: 84.

23. Reynolds JEF, ed. Martindale: The extra pharmacopoeia, 30th ed. London: The Pharmaceutical Press, 1993; 785.

24. Cadwallader DE. EENT preparations In: King RE, ed. Dispensing of medication, 9th ed. Easton, PA: Mack Publishing Co., 1984; 148.

25. American Pharmaceutical Association. Handbook of nonprescription drugs, 13th ed. Washington DC: Author, 2002.

26. Furrer P, Mayer JM, Gurny R. Ocular tolerance of preservatives and alternatives. Eur J Pharm Biopharm 2002; 53: 263–280.

27. Tripathi BJ. New generation of polymer-based preservatives for contact lens solutions less toxic. Ophthalmology Times, December 15, 1992; 24.

28. Beasley R, Fishwick DM, Jon F, Hendeles L. Preservatives in nebulizer solutions: Risks without benefit. Pharmacotherapy 1998; 18(1): 130–139.

29. Darbre PD, Aljarrah A, Miller WR, et al. Concentrations of parabens in human breast tumours. J Appl Toxicol 2004; 24(1): 5–13.

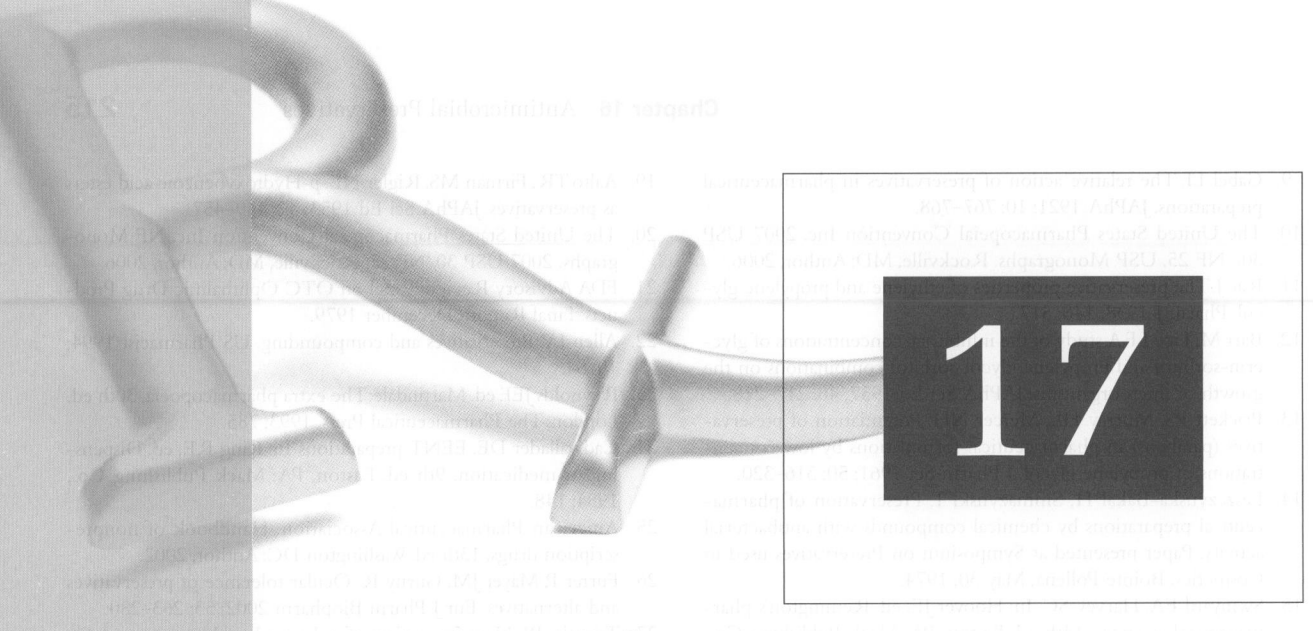

17

Antioxidants

Melgardt de Villiers, PhD

I. DEFINITIONS

A. **Oxidation/reduction** (redox) reactions involve the transfer of one or more oxygen or hydrogen atoms or the transfer of electrons (1). (See Table 17.1 for examples.) Writing an electron transfer in equation form, where e^- represents an electron and n the number of electrons:

$$\text{reduced form} \leftrightarrow \text{oxidized form} + ne^-$$

The section on oxidation in *USP* Chapter ⟨1191⟩, Stability Considerations in Dispensing Practice, describes and relates oxidation to pharmaceutical preparations as follows:

> The molecular structures most likely to oxidize are those with a hydroxyl group directly bonded to an aromatic ring (e.g., phenol derivatives such as catecholamines and morphine), conjugated dienes (e.g., vitamin A and unsaturated free fatty acids), heterocyclic aromatic rings, nitroso and nitrite derivatives, and aldehydes (e.g., flavorings). Products of oxidation usually lack therapeutic activity. Visual identification of oxidation, for example, the change from colorless epinephrine to its amber colored products, may not be visible in some dilutions or to some eyes.
>
> Oxidation is catalyzed by pH values that are higher than optimum, polyvalent heavy metal ions (e.g., copper and iron), and exposure to oxygen and UV illumination. The latter two causes of oxidation justify the use of antioxidant chemicals, nitrogen atmospheres during ampul and vial filling, opaque external packaging, and transparent amber glass or plastic containers (2).

Table 17.1	EXAMPLES OF OXIDATION TYPES	
PROCESS	**REDUCED FORM**	**OXIDIZED FORM**
Electron transfer	Fe^{+2}	Fe^{+3}
	H_2	$2 H^+$
	$2 I^-$	I_2
	H_2O_2	$O_2 + 2H^+$
Addition of oxygen (or loss of hydrogen)	CH_4	CH_3OH
	CH_3OH	$H_2C{=}O$
	$H_2C{=}O$	HCOOH
	HCOOH	CO_2
Loss of hydrogen	RCH_2CH_2R	$RCH{=}CHR + H_2$
	$2 RSH$	$RSSR + H_2$

B. **Auto-oxidations** are oxidations that occur spontaneously under normal conditions of preparation, packaging, and storage.

C. **A free radical** is a chemical species that has an unshared electron in its outer shell. [Oxygen (O_2) has an electronic configuration with two unshared electrons in its outer shell.]

D. **Antioxidants** are substances that prevent or inhibit oxidation. They are added to dosage forms to protect components of the dosage form that are subject to chemical degradation by oxidation.

E. **Chelating agents** are organic compounds that can form complexes with metal ions and, in so doing, inactivate the catalytic activity of the metal ions in the oxidation process.

II. PREVENTING OXIDATION

The pharmacist can try the following to prevent or minimize oxidation during compounding (3):

A. Use deaerated water. Boil Purified Water for 5 minutes and immediately cover it so that it does not come into contact with air that may redissolve in it. Although deaerated water is not an official USP article, the *USP* recognizes this type of water in Chapter ⟨1231⟩, Water for Pharmaceutical Purposes, and in the Reagents section of *USP*, where it states that deaerated water is produced by boiling vigorously for 5 minutes and cooling or by applying ultrasonic vibration (4,5).

B. Incorporate the antioxidants in the preparation as early in the process as possible. If a system with multiple phases is made, such as an emulsion, place an antioxidant in each phase as early in the process as possible.

C. Do not use a mixing method or device that incorporates air into the system.

D. Use a mixing container that has minimal headspace and/or replace the air in the headspace with nitrogen.

E. Add a buffer system to maintain a desired pH.

F. Use ingredients with low heavy-metal content.

G. Decrease the temperature during preparation, if possible.

III. USES OF ANTIOXIDANTS

A. Antioxidants and/or chelating agents may be added to manufactured pharmaceutical products and to extemporaneously compounded preparations when the product or preparation contains an ingredient or ingredients—either an active ingredient or a dosage form component—that is subject to chemical degradation by oxidation.

B. For compounded preparations, the decision by the pharmacist whether or not to add an antioxidant or chelating agent is made by taking into consideration the susceptibility of the ingredient(s) to degradation, the dosage form, the targeted site of drug delivery (e.g., topical, oral, ophthalmic, parenteral), the packaging for the preparation, the anticipated conditions of storage and use of the preparation, and the beyond-use date desired or needed.

| **IV.** | **MECHANISM FOR AUTO-OXIDATION OF PHARMACEUTICAL COMPOUNDS** |

To appreciate how antioxidants and chelating agents function in preventing or retarding oxidation, it is help-ful to have a basic understanding of the oxidation process. Oxidation is complex, and the following is just a brief outline of that process. For an excellent review on the subject of oxidation in pharmaceutical prod-ucts and preparations, see the chapter on oxidation and photolysis in *Chemical Stability of Pharmaceuticals* (6).

A. Oxidation reactions

Auto-oxidation of pharmaceutical ingredients occurs by a series of free radical chain reactions, including initiation, propagation, and termination.

1. Initiation

$$\text{Initiator} \rightarrow R\cdot + H\cdot$$

Note: This reaction may be catalyzed by heat, light, and metal ions.

2. Propagation

$$R\cdot + O_2 \rightarrow RO_2\cdot \text{(peroxy radical)}$$
$$RO_2\cdot + RH \rightarrow ROOH + R\cdot$$

3. Termination

$$RO_2\cdot + RO_2\cdot \rightarrow \text{stable products}$$
$$RO_2\cdot + R\cdot \rightarrow \text{stable products}$$
$$R\cdot + R\cdot \rightarrow \text{stable products}$$

B. To prevent or inhibit oxidation, the stabilizing compound must prevent or interfere with initia-tion or propagation or it must participate in a termination step.

1. Chelating agents inhibit oxidation by complexing metal ions that act as catalysts for some oxi-dation reactions.

a. Metal ions, such as Fe^{+3}, Cu^{+2}, Co^{+3}, Ni^{+2}, and Mn^{+2}, can act as initiators of oxidation because they each have an unshared electron in their outer shell.

b. Drug products and preparations may easily be contaminated by trace amounts of metals because these contaminants may be present in minute amounts, even in high-quality compounding ingredients and on the surfaces of compounding equipment and packaging materials.

c. Chelating agents, such as ethylenediaminetetraacetic acid (also known as *EDTA* or *edetic acid*), citric acid, and tartaric acid, act by binding the metal ions through complexation. Their bind-ing capacity is pH dependent because it depends on the degree of ionization of these organic acids; they are most effective when fully ionized so they lose their ability to complex at low pH.

2. Antioxidants may function by one of the following mechanisms:

a. Some are compounds that are easily oxidized; they have lower oxidation potentials than the drugs they are intended to protect and are preferentially oxidized. These agents act as so-called oxygen scavengers. Examples include the sulfites, ascorbic acid, monothioglycerol, and sodium formaldehyde sulfoxylate.

b. Some antioxidants act as chain terminators. They provide a readily available hydrogen atom or an electron and, in the process, are converted to free radicals that are not sufficiently reac-tive to sustain the chain reaction. Their free radicals either are intrinsically stable or they will combine with other radicals in a termination step. All of the oil system antioxidants listed in section IX of this Chapter act as chain terminators. The water-soluble antioxidant monothi-oglycerol may also act as a chain terminator.

c. Some antioxidants are reducing agents; they reduce a drug or component that has been oxi-dized. Ascorbic acid and sodium thiosulfate may act as reducing agents.

C. Environmental factors that affect oxidation, such as temperature, light, and pH, are discussed in Chapter 37.

| **V.** | **PROPERTIES OF THE IDEAL ANTIOXIDANT/CHELATING AGENT** |

A. Effective at a low, nontoxic concentration
B. Stable and effective under normal conditions of use, over a wide pH and temperature range
C. Soluble at the required concentration
D. Compatible with a wide variety of drugs and pharmaceutical excipients
E. Free from objectionable odor, objectionable taste, or stinging

Table 17.2	**ANTIOXIDANTS LISTED IN THE *USP 30/NF 25* CLASSIFIED ACCORDING TO SOLUBILITY AND LISTING USUAL CONCENTRATION RANGE**

ANTIOXIDANT	SOLUBILITY			CONCENTRATION RANGE (%)
	WATER	ALCOHOL	OIL	
Ascorbic Acid	Yes	Yes	No	0.02–0.1
Ascorbyl Palmitate	Yes	Yes	Yes	0.01–0.2
Butylated Hydroxyanisole	No	Yes	Yes	0.005–0.02
Butylated Hydroxytoluene	No	Yes	Yes	0.005–0.02
Hypophosphorous Acid	Yes	—	—	—
Monothioglycerol	Yes	Yes	—	0.1–1.0
Potassium Metabisulfite	Yes	No	No	0.01–1.0
Propyl Gallate	Slightly	Yes	Slightly	0.001–0.15
Sodium Bisulfite	Yes	Slightly	No	0.05–1.0
Sodium Formaldehyde Sulfoxylate	Yes	Slightly	—	0.005–0.15
Sodium Metabisulfite	Yes	Slightly	—	0.01–1.0
Sodium Sulfite	Yes	No	No	0.01–0.2
Sodium Thiosulfate	Yes	No	—	0.05
Sulfur Dioxide	Yes	Yes	Yes	—
Tocopherol	No	Yes	Yes	0.01–0.1
Tocopherols Excipient	No	Yes	Yes	0.01–0.1

Source: 2007 USP 30/NF 25. Rockville, MD: The United States Pharmacopeial Convention, Inc., 2006: Front Matter—NF: Excipients. Allen LV. Featured excipient: antioxidants. International Journal of Pharmaceutical Compounding, 1999; Vol. 3 No. 1 Jan/Feb.

F. Colorless in both the original and oxidized form

G. Nontoxic and nonsensitizing both internally and externally at the required concentration

H. Reasonable cost

I. Unreactive (does not adsorb, penetrate, or interact) with containers or closures

VI.   ANTIOXIDANTS LISTED IN THE *USP 30/NF 25*

Table 17.2 shows the chemicals listed as antioxidants in the *USP 30/NF 25* (7). This table has classified the antioxidants according to their solubility in water, alcohol, and oil (3).

VII.   CHELATING AGENTS LISTED IN THE *USP 30/NF 25*

A. Edetate calcium disodium, edetate disodium, and EDTA are the three compounds listed by the *USP/NF* as chelating agents (7).

B. Although not listed as chelating agents, Citric Acid USP and Tartaric Acid NF are official compounds that may act as chelating agents.

VIII.   ANTIOXIDANTS FOR AQUEOUS SYSTEMS

The descriptions and solubilities presented here give a composite of information from the *Handbook of Pharmaceutical Excipients* (8), the Chemistry and Compendial Requirements section of the *USP DI Vol. III* (9), and *The Merck Index* (10). For additional information on each agent, consult the *Handbook of Pharmaceutical Excipients*. As noted in the previous Chapters of Part 4, this text employs the usual convention of using upper-case first letters for words designating official *USP-NF* articles (e.g., Alcohol, Purified Water) and lower-case first letters for words designating the chemical substances (e.g., ethanol, water).

A. Ascorbic Acid USP

1. Description: white or slightly yellow crystals or powder; odorless; gradually darkens on exposure to light; reasonably stable in dry state but oxidizes in solution. Solutions have a sour, acid taste, with a pH of 2 to 3. $pK_{a1} = 4.17$, $pK_{a2} = 11.57$.
2. Solubilities: 1 g/3 mL water, 30 mL alcohol, 20 mL propylene glycol, 100 mL glycerin; practically insoluble in vegetable oils
3. Effective concentration: 0.05% to 3.0% (11)

B. **Sodium Bisulfite ($NaHSO_3$), Sodium Metabisulfite ($Na_2S_2O_5$), and Sodium Sulfite (Na_2SO_3)**
   1. Descriptions
      a. Sodium bisulfite: white or yellowish white crystals or powder with the odor of sulfur dioxide; disagreeable taste; unstable in air, losing some SO_2 and gradually oxidizing to the sulfate. Aqueous solutions are acid to litmus. Although sodium bisulfite is not an official article in *USP* or *NF*, it is listed in the Excipient section of *NF* and the Reagents section of *USP*, where it directs use of reagent grade sodium metabisulfite for sodium bisulfite (5,7).
      b. Sodium Metabisulfite NF: colorless crystals or white powder with a sulfurous odor; acid and saline taste; slowly oxidizes to sulfate on exposure to air and moisture; aqueous solutions are acid to litmus with pH of 5% solution = 3.5 to 5.0. The metabisulfite is less hygroscopic and more stable than the bisulfite.
      c. Sodium Sulfite NF: colorless crystals or powder. Aqueous solutions have a pH of approximately 9.
   2. Solubilities
      a. Sodium bisulfite: 1 g/4 mL water, 70 mL alcohol
      b. Sodium metabisulfite: 1 g/2 mL water; soluble in glycerin; slightly soluble in alcohol
      c. Sodium sulfite: 1 g/3.2 mL water; soluble in glycerin; nearly insoluble in alcohol
   3. Effective concentrations
      a. Sodium bisulfite: 0.1% (12)
      b. Sodium metabisulfite: 0.02% to 1.0% (11)
      c. Sodium sulfite: 0.01% to 0.2% (3)
   4. Sulfite warnings: Sulfites are known to cause allergic-type reactions in certain susceptible individuals. Although the number of affected individuals is small, in 1986, a section (§ 201.22) was added to the Food, Drug and Cosmetic Act to require a warning on all prescription drug products that contain sulfite. The warning statement is: "Contains (*insert the name of the sulfite, e.g., sodium metabisulfite*), a sulfite that may cause allergic-type reactions including anaphylactic symptoms and life-threatening or less severe asthmatic episodes in certain susceptible people. The overall prevalence of sulfite sensitivity in the general population is unknown and probably low. Sulfite sensitivity is seen more frequently in asthmatic than in nonasthmatic people" (13). Although this warning is not required on prescription labels, it is prudent to discuss with a patient the addition of a sulfite to any compounded preparation. It also is wise to include on the prescription label the name and quantity of any sulfite added to a drug preparation.

C. **Sodium Thiosulfate USP** $Na_2S_2O_3 \cdot 5H_2O$
   1. Description: large colorless crystals or coarse crystalline powder. It effloresces in dry air at temperatures above 33° and slightly deliquesces in moist air. Aqueous solutions are neutral or slightly alkaline (pH 6.5 to 8).
   2. Solubility: 1 g/0.5 mL water; insoluble in alcohol
   3. Effective concentration: 0.05% (3)

D. **Sodium Formaldehyde Sulfoxylate NF** $HOCH_2SOONa$
   1. Description: white crystals or hard white masses with an odor of garlic; aqueous solutions practically neutral
   2. Solubility: freely soluble in water; slightly soluble in alcohol
   3. Effective concentration: 0.005% to 0.5% (11)

IX. ANTIOXIDANTS FOR OIL SYSTEMS

The descriptions and solubilities presented here give a composite of information from the *Handbook of Pharmaceutical Excipients* (8), the Chemistry and Compendial Requirements section of the *USP DI Vol. III* (9), and *The Merck Index* (10). For additional information on each agent, consult the *Handbook of Pharmaceutical Excipients*.

A. Ascorbyl Palmitate NF

1. Description: white to yellowish white powder with a characteristic odor
2. Solubility: very slightly soluble in water and in vegetable oils; 1 g in 9.3 mL alcohol
3. Effective concentration: 0.01% to 0.2% (11)

B. Butylated Hydroxyanisole (BHA) and Butylated Hydroxytoluene (BHT)

Butylated Hydroxyanisole

Butylated Hydroxytoluene

1. Descriptions
   a. Butylated Hydroxyanisole NF (BHA): white or slightly yellow powder or waxy solid with a faint odor
   b. Butylated Hydroxytoluene NF (BHT): white or pale yellow crystalline solid with a faint odor
2. Solubilities
   a. Butylated hydroxyanisole (BHA): insoluble in water; freely soluble in alcohol (95%) and propylene glycol; soluble in 50% or higher alcohol, isopropyl alcohol, fats, and oils
   b. Butylated hydroxytoluene (BHT): insoluble in water, glycerin, and propylene glycol; soluble in alcohol, isopropyl alcohol, and acetone. It is more soluble in vegetable oils and fats than is BHA.
3. Effective concentrations
   a. Butylated hydroxyanisole (BHA): 0.005% to 0.01% (14)
   b. Butylated hydroxytoluene (BHT): 0.01% (14)

C. Propyl Gallate NF

1. Description: white, crystalline powder with a very slight odor; pH of a 0.1% solution = 5.9; has some antimicrobial activity in addition to its antioxidant properties; unstable at high temperatures.

2. Solubility: slightly soluble in water (1 g/1,000 mL at 20°); freely soluble in alcohol (1 g/3 mL at 20°); 1 g/2.5 mL propylene glycol. Solubility in fixed and mineral oils varies with the oil.
3. Effective concentration: 0.005% to 0.15% (14)

D. Vitamin E USP (α-Tocopherol)

Vitamin E is a form of α-tocopherol ($C_{29}H_{50}O_2$). It includes the following: d- or dl-α-tocopherol ($C_{29}H_{50}O_2$); d- or dl-α-tocopheryl acetate ($C_{31}H_{52}O_3$); d- or dl-α-tocopheryl acid succinate ($C_{33}H_{54}O_5$) (15).

1. Description: clear, yellow, or greenish yellow viscous oil; practically odorless; unstable to light and air, so store in airtight container under inert gas, protected from light.
2. Solubility: insoluble in water; soluble in alcohol; miscible with acetone and vegetable oils
3. Effective concentration: 0.01% to 0.1% (14)

X.　CHELATING AGENTS

The descriptions and solubilities presented here give a composite of information from the *Handbook of Pharmaceutical Excipients* (8), the Chemistry and Compendial Requirements section of the *USP DI Vol. III* (9), and *The Merck Index* (10). For additional information on each agent, consult the *Handbook of Pharmaceutical Excipients*.

A. Edetic Acid NF

1. Description: white, crystalline powder. The pH of a 0.2% solution is 2.2, with the four pK_a values = 2.00, 2.67, 6.26, and 10.26. Edetic Acid NF has some reported independent antimicrobial activity and has synergistic effect with some antimicrobial agents, such as benzalkonium chloride and parabens.
2. Solubility: very slightly soluble in water (1 g/2,000 mL given in *The Merck Index*; 1 g/500 mL given in *Handbook of Pharmaceutical Excipients*)
3. Effective concentration: 0.1% (11)

B. Edetate Disodium USP

1. Description: white, crystalline powder, slightly acid taste. pH of solutions reported as 4.3 to 4.7 and as 5.3. The disodium salt of edetate is reported to reduce the antimicrobial activity of the mercurial antimicrobial agents phenylmercuric nitrate and thimerosal.
2. Solubility: soluble in water (1 g/11 mL); slightly soluble in alcohol
3. Effective concentration: 0.1% (14)

C. Edetate Calcium Disodium USP

1. Description: white crystalline granules or powder; odorless; tasteless; slightly hygroscopic but stable in air. pH of solutions reported as approximately 7 and as 4 to 5. The synergistic effect on antimicrobial activity is reported to be lost in the presence of calcium ions.
2. Solubility: soluble in water (1 g/2 mL), very slightly soluble in alcohol
3. Because the calcium in edetate calcium disodium is preferentially exchanged for lead and other toxic heavy metals, this compound is used primarily as a therapeutic agent for lead poisoning and for removing other heavy metals from the circulation while not removing calcium from the circulation, cells, and bones. It is available as Edetate Calcium Disodium Injection USP, Calcium Disodium Versenate, which is 200 mg/mL (20%).
4. Effective concentration: 0.1% (14)

D. Citric Acid USP

1. Description: colorless or translucent crystals or white granular or crystalline powder. Is available as both the monohydrate and anhydrous solid, and these powders will take up water or effloresce, depending on the form and the relative humidity. The pH of a 1% solution is 2.2, with the three pK_a values = 3.13, 4.76, and 6.40.
2. Solubility: 1 g/mL in water and alcohol
3. Effective concentration: 0.3% to 2.0% (8)
4. Citric acid is used primarily to adjust pH and as a buffering agent, but it is used as an antioxidant synergistically with other agents because of its chelating properties.

E. Tartaric Acid USP

1. Description: Colorless or translucent crystals or white crystalline powder; odorless; tart; stable in air. The pH of a 1.5% solution is 2.2, with its two pK_a values = 2.93 and 4.23.
2. Solubility: 1 g/0.75 mL water and 2.5 mL alcohol; soluble in glycerin
3. Effective concentration: varies
4. Tartaric acid is used primarily to adjust pH and as a buffering agent, but it is used as an antioxidant synergistically with other agents because of its chelating properties.

REFERENCES

1. Connors KA, Amidon GL, Stella VJ. Chemical stability of pharmaceuticals, 2nd ed. New York: John Wiley & Sons, 1986; 83.
2. The United States Pharmacopeial Convention Inc. Chapter ⟨1191⟩. 2007 USP 30/NF 25. Rockville, MD: Author, 2006; 655.
3. Allen LV. Featured excipient: antioxidants. Int J Pharm Compound 1999; 3 (1).
4. The United States Pharmacopeial Convention Inc. Chapter ⟨1231⟩. 2007 USP 30/NF 25. Rockville, MD: Author, 2006; 693.
5. The United States Pharmacopeial Convention Inc. Reagents, indicators, and solutions. 2007 USP 30/NF 25. Rockville, MD: Author, 2006.
6. Connors KA, Amidon GL, Stella VJ. Chemical stability of pharmaceuticals, 2nd ed. New York: John Wiley & Sons, 1986; 82-114.
7. The United States Pharmacopeial Convention Inc. Front matter—NF: Excipients. 2007 USP 30/NF 25. Rockville, MD: Author, 2006.
8. Rowe R, Sheskey P, Weller P, eds. Handbook of pharmaceutical excipients, 5th ed. Washington, DC: APhA Publications, 2005.
9. Thompson, MICROMEDEX, Inc. USP DI Vol. III, 27th ed. Englewood, CO: Author, 2007.
10. O'Neil MJ, ed. The Merck index, 13th ed. Rahway, NJ: Merck & Co., 2001.
11. Swarbrick J, Boylan JC, eds. Encyclopedia of pharmaceutical technology, vol. 1. New York: Marcel Dekker Inc., 1988; 441.
12. FDA Advisory Review Panel on OTC Ophthalmic Drug Products. Final report, Dec. 1979.
13. 21CFR 8 201.22 (b).
14. Lachman L. Antioxidants and chelating agents as stabilizers in liquid dosage forms. Drug Cosm Ind Jan–Feb 1968.
15. The United States Pharmacopeial Convention Inc. USP monographs. 2007 USP 30/NF 25. Rockville, MD: Author, 2006.

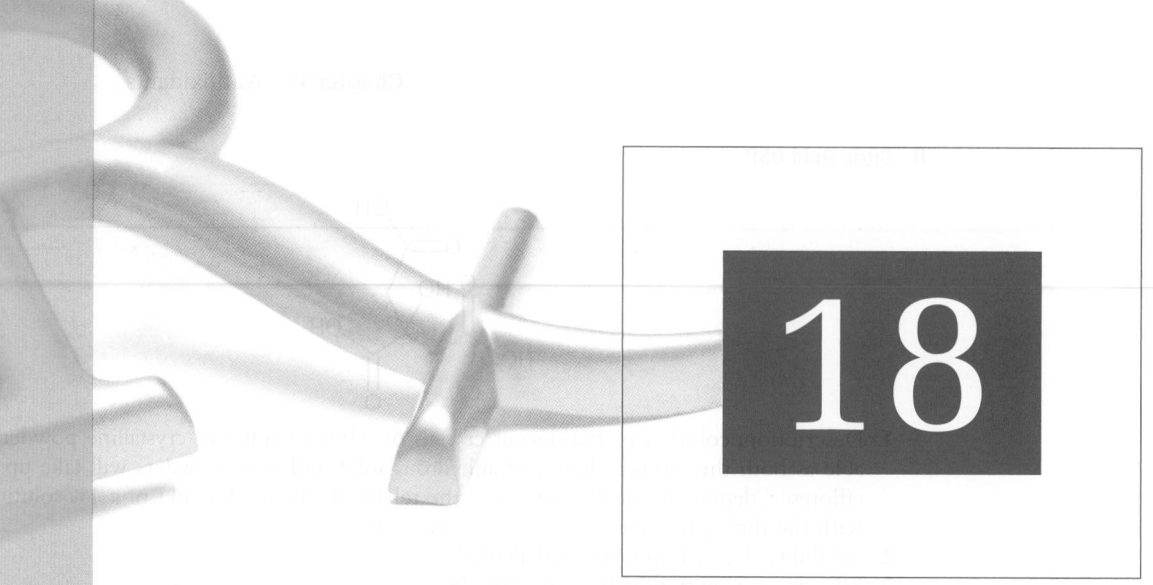

18

Buffers and pH Adjusting Agents

Melgardt de Villiers, PhD

I. DEFINITIONS

A. An **acid** may be defined as
   1. A substance that, when dissolved in water, yields hydrogen ions, H^+ (Arrhenius theory).
   2. A species that yields protons, H^+ (Bronsted-Lowry theory).
   3. An electron pair acceptor (Lewis theory).
B. A **base** may be defined as
   1. A substance that, when dissolved in water, gives hydroxide ions, OH^- (Arrhenius theory).
   2. A species that can accept a proton (Bronsted-Lowry theory).
   3. An electron pair donor (Lewis theory).
   In pharmaceutical systems, we usually are dealing with solutions that contain water; therefore, the Arrhenius and Bronsted-Lowry definitions are most suitable for our purposes.
C. A **buffer** is a compound or a mixture of compounds that, when present in a solution, resists changes in the pH of the solution when small quantities of acid or base are added to the solution.
D. **Buffer capacity** is a measure of the resistance to change in the pH of a solution when acids or bases are added to the solution.
E. Many useful equations have been derived to deal with the subject of acid-base chemistry. A list of those equations most useful in pharmaceutical systems is given in Table 18.1. Example calculations using these equations are also given.

II. USES OF BUFFERS AND pH ADJUSTING AGENTS

Buffers or agents to adjust the pH of solutions may be added to manufactured pharmaceutical products or to extemporaneously compounded preparations for any of the following reasons:

A. For preparations that are intended to be applied to the sensitive membranes of the eye or nasal passages or that may be injected into muscles, blood vessels, organs, tissue, or lesions, it is desirable to adjust the pH of the preparation to a level that is close to the physiologic pH of the tissue. This is done to minimize tissue damage and pain or discomfort experienced by the patient.

B. The absorption, and therefore the therapeutic effectiveness, of certain drugs may be improved when they are present either in an ionized or nonionized state. This state may be manipulated and maintained by adjusting the pH of the medium.

C. The chemical stability of many drugs in solution may be improved by maintaining the pH of the solution in a particular range.

D. The aqueous solubility of many organic drugs depends on the degree to which these weak electrolytes are present in ionic form. This, in turn, may depend on the pH of the solution.

III. BUFFER CAPACITY

A. Buffer capacity, β, is defined by the formula:

$$\beta = \frac{\Delta B}{\Delta pH}$$

where ΔB is the gram equivalents per liter of strong acid or strong base added to the buffer solution and ΔpH is the resulting pH change. The larger β is, the greater the buffer capacity of the system (that is, its ability to resist a pH change).

B. While buffer capacity can be determined for a system by using the formula just given, it is not often calculated in compounding situations. Because of the limited beyond-use datings needed for compounded drug preparations, exact buffer capacities are not required. For a detailed treatment of the subject of buffer capacity, refer to a book on physical pharmacy (1).

C. Even though we rarely calculate buffer capacity, it is helpful to understand the concept in principle and to understand the circumstances under which buffer capacity is maximized.
   1. Solutions of strong acids such as HCl will resist a change in pH at or below pH 3. In fact, the standard buffer solution identified by the *USP* for the pH range 1.2 to 2.2 is a 0.2 M solution of HCl to which KCl has been added as a neutral salt for proper electrolyte concentration (2).
   2. Similarly, strong bases such as NaOH give good buffer capacity at pH 11 or higher.
   3. The most common buffer systems consist of a combination of a weak acid and its salt (i.e., its conjugate base) or a weak base and its salt (i.e., its conjugate acid).
      a. The Henderson-Hasselbalch equation, also known as the *buffer equation*, relates the pH of a solution, which contains an acid-base conjugate pair, to the pair's dissociation constant and the concentrations of the species in the solution. This equation and sample problems are shown in Table 18.1.
      b. Acid-base conjugate pairs have their greatest buffer capacity when the pH of the solution is equal to their pK_a, and buffer capacity of an acid-base pair is effective in the range pH = $pK_a \pm 1$.
   4. Buffer capacity is related to the concentration of the buffer; the greater the concentration of the buffer, the greater the resistance to a change in pH.
   5. High buffer capacity is sometimes undesirable. For example, when a drug is most stable at a pH that differs considerably from the physiologic pH at the site of administration, a compromise must be found. One possible solution is to use a buffer that maintains the pH at the desirable level for stability but has a relatively low buffer capacity, so that on administration, the body's natural buffering systems will rapidly alter the pH of the solution to a more comfortable level.

IV. SELECTING A BUFFER SYSTEM OR A COMPOUND TO ADJUST pH

A. **First, consider the route of administration for the dosage form.**
   1. Ingredients to buffer or adjust pH must be nontoxic for the intended route of administration. This is an important factor to consider. For example, boric acid and sodium borate are common ingredients for ophthalmic solutions; these would not be satisfactory for systemic drug preparations because borate is toxic systemically.
   2. Agents for any route of administration should be nonirritating at the needed concentration.
   3. For oral liquid preparations, buffer compounds should not have a disagreeable odor or taste.
   4. Agents used for parenteral preparations must be in sterile form or must be rendered sterile.

GENERAL EQUATIONS DEFINING pH AND pK

$pH = -\log [H_3O^+]$

$pOH = -\log [OH^-]$

$pH + pOH = pK_w = 14$

$pK_a = -\log K_a$

$pK_b = -\log K_b$

$pK_a + pK_b = pK_w = 14$

K_a is the dissociation constant for a weak acid.

For: $HA + H_2O \rightleftharpoons H_3O^+ + A^-$

$$K_a = \frac{[H_3O^+][A^-]}{[HA]}$$

K_b is the dissociation constant for a weak base

For: $B + H_2O \rightleftharpoons BH^+ + OH^-$

$$K_b = \frac{[BH^+][OH^-]}{[B]}$$

Generally K values for all drugs, both acids and bases, are now reported as K_as.

SPECIFIC EQUATIONS	EXAMPLES
For a strong acid: $pH = -\log [C_a] = -\log [H^+]$	0.1 N HCl $pH = -\log [C_a] = -\log [0.1] = 1$
For a strong base: $pOH = -\log [OH^-] = -\log [C_b]$ or $pH = pK_w + \log [C_b]$	0.1 N NaOH $pH = pK_w + \log [C_b] = 14 + \log [0.1]$ $= 14 - 1 = 13$
For a weak acid: $pH = \frac{1}{2} pK_a - \frac{1}{2} \log [C_a]$	0.1 N acetic acid HOAc; $pK_a = 4.76$ $pH = \frac{1}{2}(4.76) - \frac{1}{2}\log [0.1]$ $= 2.38 - (-0.5) = 2.88$
For a weak base: $pOH = \frac{1}{2} pK_b - \frac{1}{2} \log [C_b]$ or $pH = \frac{1}{2} pK_w + \frac{1}{2} pK_a + \frac{1}{2} \log [C_b]$	0.1 N sodium acetate (the conjugate base of acetic acid) NaOAc $pH = 7 + 2.38 + \frac{1}{2} \log [0.1] = 8.88$
For a diprotic (H_2A) acid: Solution with only the acid $pH = \frac{1}{2} pK_{a1} - \frac{1}{2} \log [C_a]$ Notice that this is the same equation as for a weak acid.	0.1 M carbonic acid H_2CO_3; $pK_{a1} = 6.37$; $pK_{a2} = 10.33$ $pH = \frac{1}{2}(6.37) - \frac{1}{2}\log [0.1]$ $= 3.185 - (-0.5) = 3.685$
For a diprotic (H_2A) acid: Solution with only the ampholyte HA^- $pH = \frac{1}{2} pK_{a1} + \frac{1}{2} pK_{a2}$	0.1 M sodium bicarbonate $NaHCO_3$ $pH = \frac{1}{2}(6.37) + \frac{1}{2}(10.33)$ $= 3.185 + 5.165 = 8.35$
For a diprotic (H_2A) acid: Solution with only the diacidic base, A^{-2} $pH = \frac{1}{2} pK_w + \frac{1}{2} pK_{a2} + \frac{1}{2} \log [C_b]$	0.1 M sodium carbonate Na_2CO_3 $pH = \frac{1}{2}(14) + \frac{1}{2}10.33 + \frac{1}{2}\log(0.1)$ $= 7 + 5.165 + (-0.5) = 11.67$
For conjugate acid-base pairs: $pH = pK_a + \log \frac{[conjugate\ base]}{[conjugate\ acid]}$	Ex. #1: 0.1 M HOAc and 0.1 M NaOAc $pH = 4.76 + \log \frac{[0.1]}{[0.1]} = 4.76 + \log 1$ $= 4.76 + 0 = 4.76$
For acids this is often written: $pH = pK_a + \log \frac{[salt]}{[acid]}$	Ex. #2: 0.1 M HOAc and 0.2 M NaOAc $pH = 4.76 + \log \frac{[0.2]}{[0.1]} = 4.76 + 0.30$ $= 5.06$
For bases this is often written: $pH = pK_a + \log \frac{[base]}{[salt]}$	Ex. #3: 0.1 M ammonia NH_4OH and 0.1 M ammonium chloride NH_4Cl $pK_b = 4.76$ pK_a (for conjugate acid) $= 9.24$ $pH = 9.24 + \log \frac{[0.1]}{[0.1]} = 9.24$
These are all equivalent forms of the Henderson. Hasselbalch equation.	Ex. #4: 0.1 M NH_4OH and 0.2 M NH_4Cl $pH = 9.24 + \log \frac{[0.1]}{[0.2]} = 9.24 - 0.30 = 8.94$

Note: You may recall from previous coursework that the equations presented in this table are simplified versions of more complex (and more accurate) equations. They are based on assumptions that do not hold in all cases. (For example, $pK_w = 14$ only at 25°C.) They do give the sort of approximations that are helpful in the practical situations encountered in compounding. For a detailed treatment of this subject, the reader may wish to review chapters on ionic equilibria and buffered and isotonic solutions in a book on physical pharmacy (1) or an equivalent text.

Table 18.2	MODIFIED WALPOLE ACETATE BUFFER		
pH	ACETIC ACID 99% (mL/100 mL)	SODIUM ACETATE ANHYDROUS (g/100 mL)	SODIUM CHLORIDE TO MAKE ISOTONIC (g/100 mL)
3.6	1.11	0.123	0.28
3.8	1.06	0.197	0.28
4.0	0.98	0.295	0.27
4.2	0.88	0.435	0.26
4.4	0.76	0.607	0.24
4.6	0.61	0.804	0.22
4.8	0.48	0.984	0.21
5.0	0.35	1.156	0.19
5.2	0.25	1.296	0.18
5.4	0.17	1.402	0.17
5.6	0.11	1.484	0.16

Note: This buffer is suitable for internal, external, or ophthalmic use.
Source: Reprinted with permission from Schumacher GE. Buffer formulations. Am J Hosp Pharm 1966; 23: 629.

5. Ophthalmic solutions are ordinarily buffered at the pH of maximum stability for the drugs they contain, but if this pH is more than 1 pH unit from neutrality (i.e., outside the range of 6.5 to 8.5), a system with a low buffer capacity should be used (3) so that when the ophthalmic solution is dropped into the eye, the buffer system of the tears will quickly bring the pH of the solution back to that of the tears. Generally, a buffer capacity less than 0.05 is desired with a pH in the range of 4 to 8 (4,5). See Chapter 33 for more details on pH and buffering considerations for ophthalmic solutions.

B. **Consider the easiest systems first.**
   1. If a formula merely calls for the adjustment of pH to a given level, usually a dilute solution (0.1 to 0.2 N) of HCl or NaOH may be used. Be aware of possible compatibility considerations with the chloride ion in HCl. For example, if a drug is available as a salt with an uncommon anion, such as mesylate, the chloride may cause precipitation because the hydrochloride salt of that drug is less soluble; the preservatives phenylmercuric acetate and nitrate precipitate with halides, etc.
   2. Sodium Bicarbonate Injection is often used to raise the pH of some parenteral preparations. It is sterile and nontoxic, but it too may have compatibility issues. Always check for compatibility with all formulation components.
   3. For oral or topical liquids, consider using a preformulated vehicle. Many of the available flavored syrups and liquid vehicles contain buffers or ingredients that function as buffers. See Chapter 22, Vehicles for Liquid Preparations, for descriptions and specifications, and examples in Sample Prescriptions 28.5 and 28.6 in Chapter 28 and 30.7 in Chapter 30 of this book.
   4. For an easily made buffer in the low- to mid-pH range (3.6 to 5.6), the Acetate Buffer given in Table 18.2 is useful (6). It may be used for systemic, topical, or ophthalmic drug preparations. If isotonicity is needed, the appropriate quantities of sodium chloride are also given; if any of the preparation ingredients are incompatible with halides, sodium nitrate or dextrose in equal osmolar quantities (see Chapter 11) can be substituted for the sodium chloride.
   5. For preparations to be buffered between pH 6 and 8, Sorensen's Phosphate Buffer is a useful system. It can be used for systemic, topical, or ophthalmic preparations. Its formula is shown in Table 18.3 (7,8). It has a relatively high buffer capacity. If an isotonic solution is needed, sodium chloride in the amounts given in the table can be added; if any of the preparation ingredients are incompatible with halides, sodium nitrate or dextrose in equal osmolar quantities (see Chapter 11) can be substituted for the sodium chloride. The use of this buffer in an ophthalmic solution is illustrated in Sample Prescription 33.2 in Chapter 33.
   6. If a **concentrated** multi-purpose buffer solution is desired in the low- to mid-pH range (2.5 to 6.5), the Citrate Buffer in Table 18.4 can be used. When combined in the ratios given, the resulting solution has a molarity of 0.33 M. This buffer can be diluted 10-fold and still have adequate buffer capacity (6).
   7. For ophthalmic solutions that require buffering in the mid–acid range (~5), an aqueous solution of Boric Acid 1.9% is isotonic, easy to make, and has an appropriately low buffer capacity

Table 18.3	SORENSEN'S MODIFIED PHOSPHATE BUFFER

ACID STOCK SOLUTION, M/15 SODIUM BIPHOSPHATE		ALKALINE STOCK SOLUTION, M/15 SODIUM PHOSPHATE	
*Sodium Biphosphate, Anhydrous	8.006 g	Sodium Phosphate, Anhydrous	9.473 g
Purified Water, qs ad	1,000 mL	Purified Water, qs ad	1,000 mL

mL OF M/15 SODIUM BIPHOSPHATE SOLUTION	mL OF M/15 SODIUM PHOSPHATE SOLUTION	pH	SODIUM CHLORIDE REQUIRED FOR ISOTONICITY (g/100 mL)
90	10	5.9	0.52
80	20	6.2	0.51
70	30	6.5	0.50
60	40	6.6	0.49
50	50	6.8	0.48
40	60	7.0	0.46
30	70	7.2	0.45
20	80	7.4	0.44
10	90	7.7	0.43
5	95	8.0	0.42

*Sodium biphosphate, monohydrated 9.208 g may be used.
This buffer is suitable for internal, external, or ophthalmic use.
Source: Deardorff DL. Ophthalmic solutions. In: Hoover JE, ed. Remington's pharmaceutical sciences, 14th ed. Easton, PA: Mack Publishing Co., 1970; 1553–1555. Sörensen SL. Enzyme studies. II. The measurement and importance of the hydrogen ion concentration in enzyme reactions. Biochem Z 1909; 21: 131 and 22: 352.

Table 18.4	CONCENTRATED MULTI-PURPOSE BUFFER SOLUTION (CITRATE BUFFER)

ACID STOCK SOLUTION, M/3 CITRIC ACID		ALKALINE STOCK SOLUTION, M/3 SODIUM CITRATE	
*Citric Acid Monohyrate	70 g	Sodium Citrate Dihydrate	98 g
Purified Water, qs ad *Citric Acid Anhydrous 64 g may be substituted	1,000 mL	Purified Water, qs ad	1,000 mL

mL OF M/3 CITRIC ACID SOLUTION	mL OF M/3 SODIUM CITRATE SOLUTION	pH
92	8	2.5
82	18	3.0
68	32	3.5
58	42	4.0
44	56	4.5
28	72	5.0
14	86	5.5
6	94	6.0
2	98	6.5

Both compounds combined yield a concentration of 0.33 M.
This buffer is suitable for internal, external, or ophthalmic use.

Table 18.5	PALITZSCH OPHTHALMIC BUFFER		

ACID STOCK SOLUTION		ALKALINE STOCK SOLUTION	
Boric Acid	12.404 g	Sodium Borate Decahydrate	19.108 g
Purified Water, q.s. ad	1,000 mL	Purified Water, q.s. ad	1,000 mL

mL OF 0.2 M BORIC ACID SOLUTION	mL OF 0.05 M SODIUM BORATE SOLUTION	pH
97	3	6.8
94	6	7.1
90	10	7.4
85	15	7.6
80	20	7.8
75	25	7.9
70	30	8.1
65	35	8.2
55	45	8.4
45	55	8.6
40	60	8.7
30	70	8.8
20	80	9.0
10	90	9.1

Source: Palitzsch S. Use of borax and boric acid solutions in the colorimetric measurement of the hydrogen ion concentration of sea water. Biochem Z 1915; 70: 333.

for this situation. Its use is illustrated in Sample Prescription 33.1 in Chapter 33. An example of a borate buffer system at higher pH, the Palitzsch buffer, is given in Table 18.5 (9). Numerous other borate buffers are reported in the literature (7,10–12).

C. **If a customized buffer solution must be made, follow these steps:**

   1. Select a compound or combination of compounds that can give you a pH in the range you desire.

      a. As discussed earlier, this may be a strong acid, a strong base, or a conjugate pair. If using a conjugate pair, the pK_a of the conjugate acid should be within one pH unit of the desired pH.

      b. For possible conjugate pairs, you may want to consult the table in the appendix section of the CD that accompanies this book. This table gives the pK_as of a large number of drugs and reference compounds.

      c. Be sure that your choice is chemically stable, is sufficiently soluble, is compatible with the other ingredients in the formulation, is free from odor and color, and is nonsensitizing and nontoxic by the route of administration being used.

      d. Examples of some possible choices are given in Table 18.6.

Table 18.6	BUFFER CHOICES FOR SPECIFIC pH RANGES

pH RANGE	BUFFER
pH 1–3	HCl
pH 2.5–6.5	Citrate Buffer
pH 3.6–5.6	Acetate Buffer
pH 6–8	Sorenson's Phosphate Buffer
pH 8–9	Sodium Bicarbonate
pH 9–11	Sodium Bicarbonate/Sodium Carbonate
pH 11–13	NaOH

Table 18.7	USP 30/NF 25 ARTICLES CATEGORIZED AS ACIDIFYING, ALKALIZING, OR BUFFERING AGENTS

ACIDIFYING AGENT	ALKALIZING AGENT	BUFFERING AGENT
Acetic Acid	Ammonia Solution, Strong	Acetic Acid
Acetic Acid, Glacial	Ammonium Carbonate	Adipic Acid
Citric Acid, Anhydrous	Diethanolamine	Ammonium Carbonate
Citric Acid Monohydrate	Potassium Hydroxide	Ammonium Phosphate
Fumaric Acid	Sodium Bicarbonate	Boric Acid
Hydrochloric Acid	Sodium Borate	Citric Acid, Anhydrous
Hydrochloric Acid, Diluted	Sodium Carbonate	Citric Acid Monohydrate
Malic Acid	Sodium Hydroxide	Lactic Acid
Nitric Acid	Trolamine	Phosphoric Acid
Phosphoric Acid		Potassium Citrate
Phosphoric Acid, Diluted		Potassium Metaphosphate
Propionic Acid		Potassium Phosphate, Dibasic
Sulfuric Acid		Potassium Phosphate, Monobasic
Tartaric Acid		Sodium Acetate
		Sodium Citrate
		Sodium Lactate Solution
		Sodium Phosphate, Dibasic
		Sodium Phosphate, Monobasic
		Succinic Acid

Source: The United States Pharmacopeial Convention Inc. 2007 USP 30/NF 25. Front matter—NF: excipients. Rockville, MD: Author, 2006.

2. Calculate the concentration of each compound needed.
    a. You may use the appropriate equation from Table 18.1 (remembering that these equations can only give approximations) or one of the buffer formulas from Tables 18.2 through 18.5.
    b. If an acid-base conjugate pair is selected, recall that the Henderson-Hasselbalch equation gives you just the ratio of concentrations. From the calculated ratio, select the specific concentrations for the ingredients based on the fact that adequate buffer capacity can be had with final concentrations of 0.05 to 0.5 M (1).

3. After the solution is made, use pH paper or a pH meter to measure the pH of the solution and make adjustments as needed.

V. ACIDIFYING, ALKALIZING, AND BUFFERING AGENTS

Table 18.7 shows compounds that are official articles in the USP30/NF25 and that are categorized by USP–NF as excipients used as acidifying, alkalizing, and buffering agents (13).

REFERENCES

1. Sinko PJ. Martin's physical pharmacy and pharmaceutical sciences, 5th ed. Baltimore, MD: Lippincott Williams & Wilkins, 2006.
2. The United States Pharmacopeial Convention Inc. Reagents: buffer solutions. 2007 USP 30/NF 25. Rockville, MD: Author, 2006.
3. Gonnering R, et al. The pH tolerance of rabbit and human corneal epithelium. Invest Ophthalmol Vis Sci 1979; 18: 3373–3390.
4. Allen LV. Compounding ophthalmic liquids. Secundum Artem, volume 6, number 4 (http://www.paddocklabs.com/images/PadSec_v6n4.pdf).
5. Anonymous. Buffer solutions for ophthalmic preparations. Int J Pharm Compound 1998; 2(3): 190–191.
6. Schumacher GE. Buffer formulations. Am J Hosp Pharm 1966; 23: 629.
7. Deardorff DL. Ophthalmic solutions. In: Hoover JE, ed. Remington's pharmaceutical sciences, 14th ed. Easton, PA: Mack Publishing Co., 1970; 1553–1555.
8. Sörensen SL. Enzyme studies. II. The measurement and importance of the hydrogen ion concentration in enzyme reactions. Biochem Z 1909; 21: 131 and 22: 352.
9. Palitzsch S. Use of borax and boric acid solutions in the colorimetric measurement of the hydrogen ion concentration of sea water. Biochem Z 1915; 70: 333.
10. Gifford SR. Reaction of buffer solution and of ophthalmic drugs. Arch Ophthalmol 1935; 13: 78.
11. Neuwald F, et al. Galenical and pharmacological research on the composition of aqueous ophthalmic pharmaceuticals. I. Stability of some compounds used as ophthalmic pharmaceuticals. II. A generally useful buffer. Pharm ZtgVer Apotheker-Ztg 1957; 102: 40, 51–52 and 1958; 103: 12.
12. Atkins WR, Pantin GF. Buffer mixture for the alkaline range of hydrogen-ion concentration determinations. Biochem J 1926; 20: 102.
13. The United States Pharmacopeial Convention Inc. Front matter-NF: excipients. 2007 USP 30/NF 25. Rockville, MD: Author, 2006.

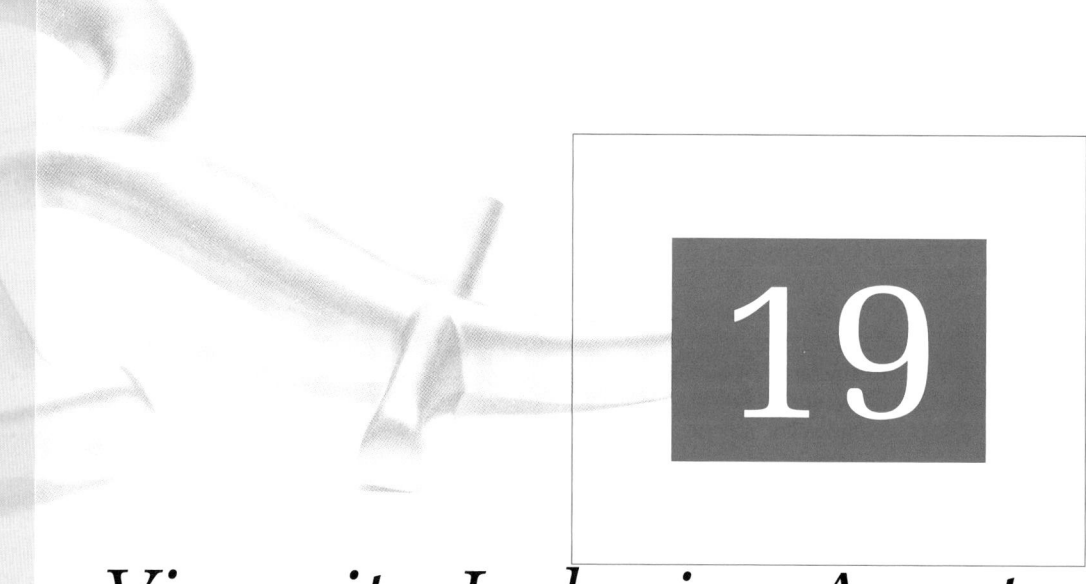

Viscosity-Inducing Agents

Melgardt de Villiers, PhD

I. DEFINITIONS

A. **Viscosity** is a measure of the resistance to flow of a system under an applied stress. The more viscous a liquid, the greater the applied force required to make it flow at a particular rate. This is expressed mathematically by Newton's Law of Flow (1):

$$\frac{F}{A} = \eta \frac{dv}{dr}$$

where F/A is shearing stress, the force per unit area required to bring about flow; dv/dr is the rate of shear; and η is the coefficient of viscosity, usually referred to as just *viscosity*.

B. The traditional unit of viscosity is the **poise,** which is defined as the shearing force in dynes required to produce a velocity of 1 cm/s between two parallel planes of a liquid each 1 cm^2 in area and separated by a distance of 1 cm.

C. The unit of viscosity commonly used in pharmacy is the **centipoise** (cp; plural, cps), which is equal to 0.01 poise.

D. In the more recently adopted International System of Units (SI), the basic unit of viscosity is **Pascal sec** (Pa s) or Newton/m^2–sec^{-1}, which equals 10 poise. The SI unit of viscosity commonly used to report viscosities of pharmaceutical liquids is the **milliPascal sec** (mPa s), which conveniently is numerically equal to the viscosity value in centipoise. The various units of viscosity can be illustrated with the viscosity of water, which is approximately 1 cps at 20°C.

$$1 \text{ cps} = 0.01 \text{ poise} = 0.001 \text{ Pa s} = 1 \text{ mPa s}$$

The SI System's mPa s viscosity units are now used for reporting viscosity values in books such as the *Handbook of Pharmaceutical Excipients* (2).

E. While "thick" liquids are generally more viscous than "thin" liquids, there is not a direct relationship between perceived thickness and viscosity. The viscosity values for some common substances are given in Table 19.1; these give some feeling for relative centipoise (or mPa s) values.

Table 19.1	ABSOLUTE VISCOSITY OF SOME NEWTONIAN LIQUIDS AT 20°C	
LIQUID	**VISCOSITY (CPS)**	
Castor oil	1,000	
Chloroform	0.563	
Ethyl alcohol	1.19	
Glycerin 93%	400	
Olive oil	100	
Water	1.0019	

Reprinted with permission from Sinko PJ. Martin's Physical Pharmacy and Pharmaceutical Sciences, 5th ed. Baltimore, MD: Lippincott Williams & Wilkins, 2006. Copyright Lippincott, Williams & Wilkins Co., Baltimore.

F. **Viscosity-inducing agents** are molecules that interact with water molecules to form a structured system that interrupts the flow of the molecules past one another. They are hydrophilic colloids that are classified either as soluble macromolecules or particulate association colloids (3).

1. The soluble macromolecules are linear or branched-chain polymers that dissolve molecularly in water. The resulting preparations are classified as colloidal dispersions because the individual molecules are in the colloidal particle size range, exceeding 50 to 100 Å. The macromolecules are further classified into one of three groups: natural polymers, semisynthetic cellulose derivatives, and synthetic polymers.

2. The particulate association colloids are water-insoluble particles that hydrate strongly. They include inorganic silicates, colloidal silicon dioxide, and microcrystalline cellulose.

3. When in liquid form colloidal dispersions are sometimes referred to as *sols*, when these systems are semisolids or solids they are called *gels*.

G. Newtonian and non-Newtonian flow (1)

1. Pure liquids and dilute solutions (such as those in Table 19.1) exhibit **Newtonian flow,** which means that their viscosity, η, is characterized by a single value. The relationship between shearing stress (F'/A) and rate of shear (dv/dr) is linear: a plot of shearing stress versus rate of shear gives a straight line; the slope of the line, η, is constant and the line passes through the origin (Fig. 19.1A).

2. Many pharmaceutical systems exhibit non-Newtonian flow patterns. The viscosity of these systems is not constant; rather, it depends on the shearing stress or force applied. Liquid and solid heterogeneous dispersions, such as suspensions, emulsions, colloidal dispersions, and ointments and creams, are non-Newtonian systems. These are further classified into three different groups, based on their flow characteristics: plastic, pseudoplastic, and dilatant. It is helpful for pharmacists who compound drug preparations to have some understanding of these systems. A brief description follows; for a more detailed treatment, refer to a book on physical pharmacy (1) or the chapter on rheology in *Remington's The Science and Practice of Pharmacy* (4).

   a. **Pseudoplastic systems** are sometimes called *shear thinning systems* because their viscosity decreases with increasing shear stress. In this case, a plot of shearing stress versus rate of shear initially starts at the origin and appears Newtonian, but the slope begins to decrease, giving a curved line (Fig. 19.1B). Pharmaceutical systems that exhibit pseudoplastic behavior are the colloidal dispersions of the natural gums, such as acacia and tragacanth, and the synthetic and semisynthetic hydrophilic polymers, such as methylcellulose and carboxymethylcellulose.

   b. **Plastic systems** exhibit Newtonian flow patterns, but only after a certain shearing stress, called the *yield value*, is reached. In this case, the plot of shearing stress versus rate of shear does not go through the origin. In other words, a plastic system exhibits infinite viscosity (the slope, $\eta = \infty$) and does not flow at all until the yield value is reached; once flow is established, the system behaves like a Newtonian system (Fig. 19.1C). Plastic flow is a desirable property in disperse systems in which the force of gravity on small particles is not enough to overcome the yield value; that is, suspension particles do not settle and emulsion droplets do not cream but, under the larger stresses of shaking, pouring, rubbing, or syringing, the system flows. Plastic flow is produced by structured systems of flocculated particles in concentrated suspensions or emulsions.

   c. **Thixotropy** is a property of many plastic and pseudoplastic systems in which the consistency lost when shear is applied (e.g., shaking) takes some finite amount of time for recovery (Fig. 19.1D). This is a desirable property of liquid pharmaceutical dispersions: The dispersion becomes fluid when the product is shaken; the product remains fluid long enough for a dose

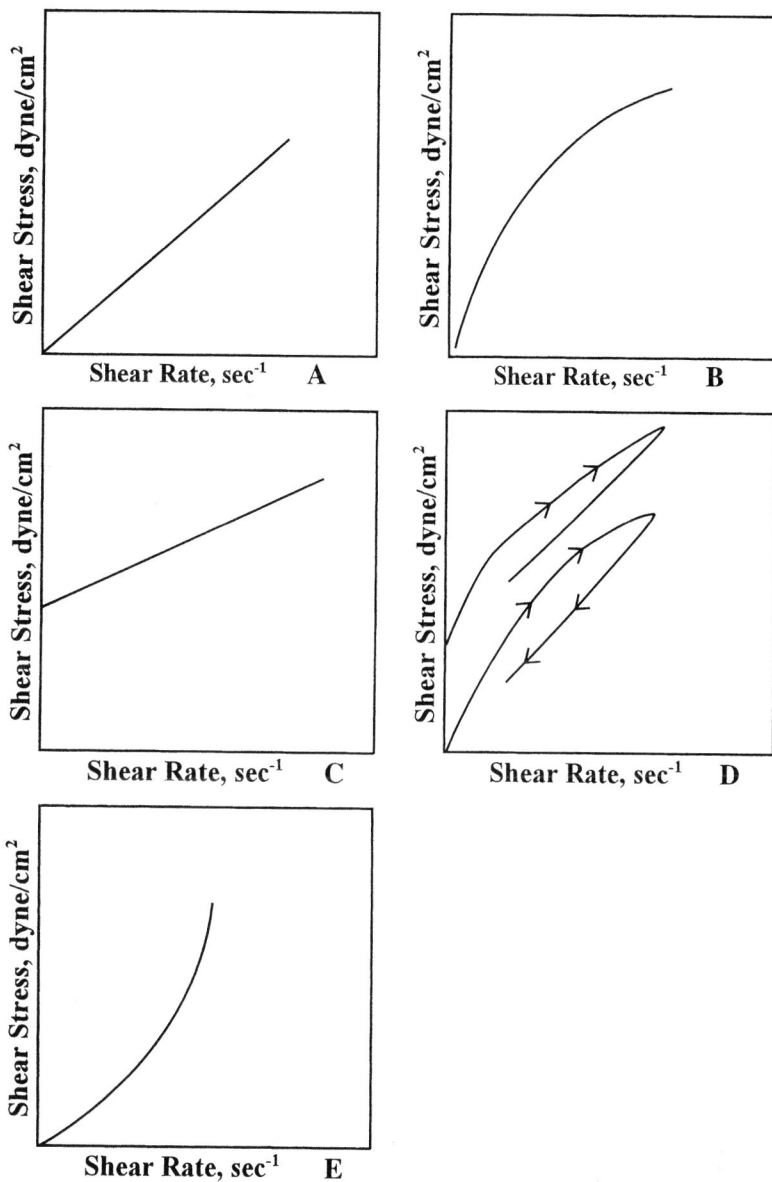

FIGURE 19.1. A: FLOW CURVE FOR A NEWTONIAN SYSTEM. B: FLOW CURVE FOR A PSEUDOPLASTIC SYSTEM. C: FLOW CURVE FOR A PLASTIC SYSTEM. D: FLOW CURVE OF A SYSTEM EXHIBITING THIXOTROPY. E: FLOW CURVE FOR A DILATANT SYSTEM.

to be poured or a topical product to be applied; the system then regains its consistency rapidly enough on standing so that the suspended particles do not settle. Catsup is a nonpharmaceutical example of a thixotropic system. Bentonite Magma, consisting of flocculated colloidal clay particles, and several of the structured liquids marketed as suspending vehicles for compounding, are examples of pharmaceutical thixotropic systems.

d. Dilatant systems act in a manner opposite that of pseudoplastic systems. They are called *shear-thickening systems* because their viscosity increases with increasing shear stress (Fig. 19.1E). Suspensions that have high concentrations of deflocculated particles may exhibit dilatant behavior. One common example of a dilatant system is a starch-in-water slurry. This system flows when left at rest but firms up when pressure is applied. Dilatant systems may cause problems with high-speed mixing equipment used in formulation; these materials may solidify under conditions of high shear and damage the equipment. Dilatancy must also be avoided in injectable suspensions because the high shear stress that results when pushing a liquid through a small needle bore may cause the syringe to lock—not a pleasant experience for the patient.

II.   THE ROLE OF VISCOSITY IN FORMULATION

A. Increased viscosity can offer both advantages and disadvantages with respect to formulating liquid and semisolid preparations. Understanding the meaning of viscosity and the various types of flow behavior is useful to the pharmacist in selecting appropriate formulation ingredients.

B. For topical preparations, appropriate viscosity is essential in achieving desirable smoothness and consistency so that the preparation will be easy to apply, will remain in contact with the affected area, and will feel good to the patient.

C. Palatability of oral liquid preparations is often enhanced by formulating the preparation with appropriate viscosity. This provides what is sometimes referred to as desirable *mouth feel.* Viscous vehicles also may improve the perceived flavor of oral liquids by reducing the contact of bad-tasting drugs with the taste buds on the tongue.

D. High viscosity is a disadvantage when dissolving drugs to make solutions because diffusion, and therefore rate of dissolution, decreases as viscosity increases. This is why compounders do not dissolve drugs directly in viscous vehicles but rather first dissolve them in a minimum quantity of water or other low-viscosity solvent and then combine the resulting solution with the desired viscous vehicle.

E. If increased viscosity is the only formulation goal, a high-viscosity liquid, such as glycerin, or a concentrated aqueous solution of a soluble micromolecule, such as sucrose or sorbitol, may be used.

F. If a structured system is needed to retard the settling or creaming rate of the particles or oil droplets in dispersed systems, the selection and addition of a viscosity-inducing agent that gives pseudoplastic, plastic, or thixotropic flow is required.

III.   SUSPENDING AND/OR VISCOSITY-INDUCING AGENTS LISTED IN *USP 30/NF 25*

A. Table 19.2 gives the articles listed as suspending and/or viscosity-increasing agents in the *USP 30/NF 25* (5). This is not a complete list of all agents used in this way; some compounds, although not on this list, are used for these purposes in manufactured products and compounded preparations.

Table 19.2	*USP* AND *NF* EXCIPIENTS CATEGORIZED AS SUSPENDING AND/OR VISCOSITY-INCREASING AGENTS

Acacia	Gelatin
Agar	Gellan Gum
Alamic Acid	Guar Gum
Alginic Acid	Hydroxyethyl Cellulose
Aluminum Monostearate	Hydroxypropyl Cellulose
Attapulgite, Activated	Hypromellose (formerly Hydroxypropyl
Attapulgite, Colloidal Activated	Methylcellulose)
Bentonite	Magnesium Aluminum Silicate
Bentonite, Purified	Maltodextrin
Bentonite Magma	Methylcellulose
Carbomer 910	Microcrystalline Cellulose
Carbomer 934	Pectin
Carbomer 934P	Polyethylene Oxide
Carbomer 940	Polyvinyl Alcohol
Carbomer 941	Povidone
Carbomer 1342	Propylene Glycol Alginate
Carbomer Copolymer	Silicon Dioxide
Carbomer Homopolymer	Silicon Dioxide, Colloidal
Carbomer Interpolymer	Sodium Alginate
Carboxymethylcellulose Calcium	Starch, Corn
Carboxymethylcellulose Sodium	Starch, Potato
Carboxymethylcellulose Sodium 12	Starch, Tapioca
Carrageenan	Starch, Wheat
Cellulose	Tragacanth
Dextrin	Xanthan Gum

Source: The United States Pharmacopeial Convention, Inc. Front matter—NF: Excipients. 2007 USP 30/NF 25. Rockville, MD: Author, 2006.

B. The agents used most commonly as suspending or viscosity-increasing agents in extemporaneous compounding are described in the following section. This text employs the usual convention of using upper-case first letters for words designating official *USP/NF* articles (e.g., Alcohol, Purified Water) and lower-case first letters for words designating the chemical substances (e.g., ethanol, water). For each agent, the text gives the information needed for selection and use of a suitable compound: a description of each compound, including the pH of its dispersions, its solubility, incompatibilities, suggestions for preparing and preserving its dispersions, possible uses for the compound, and some advantages and disadvantages of its use.

IV.   VISCOSITY-INDUCING AGENTS

The descriptions and solubilities presented here give a composite of information from *Remington's The Science and Practice of Pharmacy* (6), the *Handbook of Pharmaceutical Excipients* (2), *The Merck Index* (7), official monographs in the *USP 30/NF 25* (8,9), the Chemistry and Compendial Requirements section of the *USP DI Vol. III* (10), and other references as cited. Additional information on each agent, including references to original research journal articles, can be found in the *Handbook of Pharmaceutical Excipients* (2).

A. Semisynthetic cellulose derivatives

Cellulose is a polymer of β-D-Glucose, with –CH$_2$OH groups alternating above and below the plane of the cellulose molecule, thus producing long, unbranched chains. The absence of side chains allows cellulose molecules to lie close together and form rigid structures. Cellulose is the major structural material of plants. Cellulose may be modified to produce many semisynthetic cellulose derivatives.

General chemical structure of cellulose

1. Methylcellulose USP
   a. Description
      (1) Methylcellulose is a polymer formed by the methylation of cellulose to form methyl ether linkages. In other words, some of the hydrogens on the –OH groups are replaced with methyl (–CH$_3$) groups. The degree of methylation is regulated to yield polymers with a controlled number of sites for hydrogen bonding. This, together with polymer chain length, determines the degree to which the polymer increases the viscosity of its water solutions or gels. These solutions or gels exhibit pseudoplastic flow characteristics.
      (2) Methylcellulose is a white, fibrous powder or granules. The pH of a 1% dispersion is 5.5 to 8.0.
      (3) Methylcellulose is available in various viscosity grades: 15, 25, 100, 400, 1,500, and 4,000 cps are the most commonly available grades. The grade number refers to the viscosity of a 2% aqueous solution at 20°C.
   b. Solubility: Methylcellulose is insoluble or practically insoluble in acetone, alcohols, glycols, hot water, and saturated salt solutions, but it is soluble in glacial acetic acid. It swells in water and produces a clear to opalescent, viscous colloidal solution that is neutral to litmus.
   c. Incompatibilities
      (1) Methylcellulose is stable to alkalies and dilute acids but coagulates from solution with high concentrations of salts of mineral acids, with moderate to high concentrations of salts of polybasic acids, and with phenols and tannins. This is reported to be prevented by the addition of alcohol or glycol diacetate (6).
      (2) It is also incompatible with aminacrine hydrochloride, chlorocresol, mercuric chloride, silver nitrate, cetylpyridium chloride (but not benzalkonium chloride), *p*-hydroxybenzoic acid, *p*-aminobenzoic acid, and the parabens (2). Benzyl alcohol is also stated to be incompatible with methylcellulose.
   d. Preparation of dispersions
      While the hydrogen bonding sites make possible the formation of clear viscous gels of methylcellulose, they are also responsible for the difficulty with which its solutions are made.

If you were to add water at room temperature to methylcellulose powder, a clumpy mess would result. This is because water forms hydrogen bonds rapidly with the methylcellulose on the outside of the powder bed, forming a very viscous layer and preventing water penetration to the rest of the powder. Hydration of the powder and clear gel formation would eventually occur, but this takes a long time. Listed below are three methods for successful dispersion of methylcellulose in water:

(1) Heat to boiling a portion (approximately one third) of the total water needed for the dispersion. Add the methylcellulose powder and stir to completely wet the powder. Add the remaining water as cold water or ice chips and stir. This method is useful when you need to make a relatively clear solution quickly.

(2) Heat to boiling the total amount of water needed for the solution. Disperse the methylcellulose in the water. Put the cloudy dispersion in a refrigerator and gently stir or agitate frequently until a clear viscous solution results. This method is not useful when you need the solution immediately because it takes a minimum of 4 hours to convert the nonviscous, cloudy dispersion to a clear, viscous gel.

(3) Place the methylcellulose powder in a glass mortar and wet the powder completely with a minimum amount of alcohol or glycerin; then, with trituration, gradually add cold water to the final desired volume. This method is useful when boiling water is not readily available; however, the gels that result may not be crystal clear. Furthermore, there may be cases when you want to avoid alcohol or glycerin in a formulation. This method is particularly handy when the formulation contains an alcohol or glycol as an ingredient and the end product is a suspension or emulsion in which clarity is not essential.

e. Preservation of aqueous dispersions

(1) Although pure solutions or gels of methylcellulose do not support bacterial or mold growth as readily as comparable preparations of the natural polymers (e.g., acacia and tragacanth), preservatives are recommended for methylcellulose solutions because they are liable to microbial spoilage.

(2) Because the pH of methylcellulose solutions is between 5.5 and 8.0, the organic acid preservatives benzoic acid/sodium benzoate and sorbic acid/potassium sorbate would not be effective unless the pH of the solution is adjusted to a level of 5.0 or lower.

(3) As stated earlier, methylcellulose is incompatible with the parabens, benzyl alcohol, and cetylpyridium chloride. For methylcellulose solutions with pH exceeding 5.0, this leaves the following possibilities for preservatives: alcohol, propylene glycol, and benzalkonium or benzethonium chloride.

f. Uses

(1) Methylcellulose is used extensively by the pharmaceutical industry in both oral and topical products. It is used both in solid dosage forms and in emulsions, suspensions, and solutions.

(2) These polymers are also used therapeutically as bulk laxatives, as diet aids, and in artificial tears products. These manufactured products are sometimes used as vehicles or excipients for compounding. For example, artificial tears are useful vehicles for compounding sterile ophthalmic solutions (11). The use of the methylcellulose bulk laxative powder Citrucel is illustrated with Sample Prescription 28.5 in Chapter 28, Suspensions.

(3) In compounding, methylcellulose is useful for making sugar-free vehicles to use in formulating oral solutions and suspensions. It can also be used as a viscosity–inducing agent for topical liquid and gel preparations when a film is acceptable.

(4) A 1% gel of methylcellulose 1,500 cps dispersed in Purified Water or Water for Irrigation gives a liquid vehicle that is useful for many purposes. Although there are published formulas like this that are preserved with 0.2% sodium benzoate, the pH of methylcellulose solutions is not favorable to preservation with this agent.

(5) A 5% gel of methylcellulose 1,500 cps dispersed in Purified Water or Water for Irrigation gives a soft semisolid gel that can be used for topical or vaginal preparations.

g. Advantages of methylcellulose

(1) It produces aesthetically pleasing, clear, colorless, odorless gels.

(2) Its gels have a neutral pH and are stable over a wide pH range, approximately 3 to 12.

(3) It is a nonelectrolyte with no ionizable groups, so it is compatible with many other ingredients and drugs; it is not reactive with quaternary nitrogen compounds (such as benzalkonium chloride), weak acids, or the salts of weak bases.

(4) It is relatively unaffected by moderate concentrations of univalent ions.

(5) Although not soluble in alcohol or most other organic solvents, its solutions tolerate relatively high alcohol concentrations.

(6) It is not a sugar, so it is useful when a sugar-free vehicle is needed.

(7) It is effective as a viscosity-inducing agent at low concentrations, so vehicles made with methylcellulose are not hypertonic. If necessary, its solutions can be made isotonic by adding compatible solutes.

(8) Methylcellulose solutions and gels are less susceptible to bacterial and mold growth than are the natural polymer dispersions.

h. Disadvantages

(1) Flavoring and sweetening are required for palatability when the solutions are used as vehicles for oral drug preparations.

(2) Because methylcellulose depends on hydrogen bonding for its solubility in water, drugs or chemicals that strongly associate with water can dehydrate methylcellulose molecules and cause their separation from solution. Compatibility problems occur with high concentrations of univalent ions and moderate concentrations of polyvalent ions. (See Sample Prescription 27.2 in Chapter 27, Solutions.) Methylcellulose is also dehydrated by phenolic substances, including phenol and resorcinol. (See Sample Prescription 28.3 in Chapter 28, Suspensions.)

(3) Methylcellulose is not soluble in alcohol or most other organic solvents, although its aqueous solutions do tolerate fairly high concentrations of alcohol.

(4) The solutions support bacterial or mold growth, especially when nutrients such as organic drugs, sweeteners, or flavors are added.

(5) The solutions are somewhat difficult to prepare.

2. Carboxymethylcellulose Sodium USP (Sodium CMC)

a. Description

(1) Sodium CMC is structurally similar to methylcellulose except that the methyl groups are replaced with $—CH_2COO^-Na^+$ moieties. Although sodium CMC has properties similar to methylcellulose, there are some differences, due mainly to the ionic centers in sodium CMC molecules.

(2) It is a white to cream-colored powder or granules. The powder is hygroscopic and, in conditions of high humidity, it can absorb large amounts of water. It has a pK_a of 4.3, and a 1% w/v aqueous solution has a pH of approximately 7.5.

(3) Sodium CMC comes in three basic viscosity grades: low, medium, and high. These are sometimes designated LF (1% aqueous solution = 25 to 50 cps), MF (1% aqueous solution = 400 to 800 cps), and HF (1% aqueous solution = 1,500 to 3,000 cps).

(4) Table 19.3 gives the percent concentrations in water of various viscosity-inducing agents needed to give a viscosity of 800 cps. Notice that a 1.7% methylcellulose 1,500 cps solution gives approximately the same viscosity as a 1.9% solution of medium-viscosity sodium CMC. Based on this observation, you can conclude that methylcellulose 1,500 cps is approximately equal to medium-viscosity sodium CMC in its ability to induce viscosity. Table 19.3 gives useful information when it is necessary to substitute one viscosity-increasing agent for another in a formulation.

Table 19.3	COMPARATIVE VISCOSITIES OF VARIOUS SUSPENDING AGENTS
SUSPENDING AGENT	**% CONCENTRATION TO GIVE 800 cps**
Acacia	35 (for 600 cps)
Tragacanth	2.8
Methylcellulose 100 cps	3.5
Methylcellulose 400 cps	2.4
Methylcellulose 1,500 cps	1.7
Carboxymethylcellulose, low	4.1
Carboxymethylcellulose, medium	1.9
Carboxymethylcellulose, high	0.7
Bentonite	6.3
Veegum	6.0

Reprinted with permission from Gerding PW, Sperandio GJ. JAPhA Prac Ed 1954;15:356.

    b. Solubility: Sodium CMC is insoluble or practically insoluble in acetone, alcohol, glycols, and most other organic solvents. Its solubility in water varies with the degree of substitution on the polymer. It disperses in both hot and cold water to form clear, colloidal solutions.

    c. Incompatibilities

      (1) Because sodium CMC molecules interact with water using both hydrogen bonding and ion-dipole interactions, they are less susceptible to dehydration than methylcellulose but are subject to the normal incompatibilities of its weak electrolyte group.

      (2) Because it is the salt of a weak carboxylic acid, it is more sensitive to pH than methylcellulose. Although they will tolerate a fairly wide pH range (2 to 10), its solutions are most stable in the range of pH 5 to 10 and exhibit maximum viscosity at pH 7 to 9 (2).

      (3) Its solutions tolerate a fairly high concentration of alcohol or glycols.

      (4) Sodium CMC, as a large anionic molecule, has potential incompatibilities with quaternary nitrogen compounds such as benzethonium and benzalkonium chloride and with acids and the salts of some weak bases.

      (5) It is also incompatible with soluble iron salts and some other metals such as aluminum, mercury, and zinc (2).

    d. Preparation of dispersions

      (1) *Remington*'s statement that it is easily dispersed in water to form colloidal solutions is somewhat of an overstatement: When water is added to the powder or granules, clumps of partially hydrated powder result; fortunately, the powder hydrates fully and disperses to form a clear solution in 1 to 2 hours.

      (2) Although sodium CMC gels are made more easily than are methylcellulose solutions, CMC powder clumps initially when either hot or cold water is added. As stated previously, these solutions clear in 1 to 2 hours, irrespective of the temperature of the water added.

      (3) Carboxymethylcellulose Sodium Paste USP is a thick semisolid with a concentration of 16.5% sodium CMC in water (8).

      (4) Gels of sodium CMC can be made from sols by the addition of controlled amounts of polyvalent cations, such as aluminum. If too much electrolyte is added or if it is added too rapidly, precipitation of the polymer results (12).

    e. Preservation of aqueous dispersions

      (1) It is recommended that aqueous solutions of sodium CMC be preserved if stored for an extended period (2).

      (2) Selection of a preservative for sodium CMC sols poses a dilemma. The pH of its solutions is too high for effective use of the organic acids, and sodium CMC is incompatible with the quaternary ammonium preservatives. Methylparaben by itself does not preserve these solutions adequately, but the combination with propylparaben in propylene glycol, which is described in Chapter 16, can be used. Alcohol and/or propylene glycol are possibilities, depending on the circumstances.

    f. Uses: Its uses are similar to those of methylcellulose.

    g. Advantages of sodium carboxymethylcellulose

      (1) Because of its ionic centers, sodium CMC interacts with water through ion-dipole interactions and is therefore less easily dehydrated than is methylcellulose, which depends solely on hydrogen bonding with water. As a result, sodium CMC gels are less affected by high concentrations of electrolytes. Sample Prescription 27.2 in Chapter 27, Solutions, illustrates this effect. As stated previously, controlled amounts of polyvalent cations cause gelation of CMC solutions.

      (2) Although it is not soluble in alcohol or most other organic solvents, its solutions tolerate high alcohol concentrations.

      (3) It is more stable than methylcellulose to phenolic-type compounds. This is illustrated in Sample Prescription 28.3 in Chapter 28, Suspensions.

    h. Disadvantages

      (1) Because of its ionic centers, which are salt forms of weak carboxylic acids, it has the potential for interactions and incompatibilities characteristic of these groups.

      (2) Its gels have a pH of approximately 7.5; therefore, preservatives such as benzoic acid/Na benzoate and sorbic acid/K sorbate, which require a pH of 5 or less for activity, are not effective in solutions of sodium CMC.

3. Hypromellose (formerly Hydroxypropyl Methylcellulose) USP

    a. Description

      (1) Hypromellose is a propylene glycol ether of methylcellulose. It is official in the *USP* (8) with varying degrees of substitution, which confer several levels of viscosity induction.

(2) It is a white or slightly off-white, fibrous or granular powder. It is odorless and tasteless.

(3) Its solutions have a pH similar to that of methylcellulose, with a 1% solution having a pH range of 5.5 to 8.0.

b. Solubility: It swells in water to produce a clear or opalescent, viscous colloidal dispersion. On heating, it is converted from a sol to a gel. This can be reversed with cooling. It is practically insoluble in alcohol but is soluble in mixtures of water and alcohol or water and isopropyl alcohol as long as the alcohol content does not exceed 50%.

c. Incompatibilities

(1) Like methylcellulose, hypromellose does not have any ionic groups, so it does not have incompatibilities associated with these groups.

(2) It solutions are most stable between pH 3 and 11 (2).

d. Preparation of liquid dispersions

Solutions of hypromellose are prepared in a manner similar to those of methylcellulose.

(1) One method is to add the hypromellose powder to hot water (80° to 90°C) with agitation to ensure complete wetting of the powder; cold water or ice chips are then added to form a clear, gel-like solution (2,13).

(2) An alternative method may be used when the formulation contains alcohol or glycol as an ingredient. With this method, the hypromellose is added to the organic solvent in a ratio of 5 to 8 parts of solvent to 1 part of the powder. Cold water is then used to qs the preparation to desired volume (2).

(3) A manufactured gel vehicle of hypromellose is Liqua-Gel. In addition to Purified Water and the polymer, Liqua-Gel contains propylene glycol and glycerin plus preservatives and pH-adjusting and buffering agents. It is described in Chapter 22, Vehicles for Liquid Preparations.

e. Preservation of aqueous dispersions

(1) As with methylcellulose, the pH of hypromellose solutions is between 5.5 and 8.0, so the organic acid preservative benzoic acid/sodium benzoate would not be effective unless the pH of the solution is adjusted to a level of 5.0 or lower. Sorbic acid/potassium sorbate would also be ineffective unless the pH is 6.0 or lower.

(2) Manufactured ophthalmic solutions of hypromellose are preserved with benzalkonium chloride, so this would be a good choice as a preservative. Alcohol and propylene glycol are also possible preservatives, depending on the dosage form and route of administration.

(3) The following incompatibilities have been documented only with methylcellulose but, because hypromellose is structurally similar to methylcellulose, the following preservatives should be avoided: parabens, benzyl alcohol, and cetylpyridium chloride.

4. Hydroxypropyl Cellulose NF

a. Description

(1) Hydroxypropyl cellulose, also known as Klucel, is a partially substituted poly(hydroxypropyl) ether of cellulose. It is official in the *National Formulary* (*NF*), which states that it contains not more than 80.5% of hydroxypropyl groups. It may contain not more than 0.6% of silica or other anticaking agent (9).

(2) It is an off-white, odorless, and tasteless powder.

(3) Its solutions have a pH similar to that of methylcellulose, with a 1% solution having a pH range of 5.0 to 8.5.

b. Solubility: It is freely soluble in water below 38°C but is insoluble in hot water and precipitates as flocs between 40° and 45°C; it is soluble in many polar solvents such as short-chain alcohols (alcohol, isopropyl alcohol, etc.) and glycols such as propylene glycol but is insoluble in glycerin. It is also insoluble in aliphatic hydrocarbons such as oils and aromatic hydrocarbons. For a thorough description of the solubility characteristics of this interesting compound, refer to the *Handbook of Pharmaceutical Excipients* (2).

c. Incompatibilities

(1) Like methylcellulose, hydroxypropyl cellulose does not have any ionic groups, so it does not have incompatibilities associated with these groups.

(2) It is incompatible with methylparaben and propylparaben (2).

(3) Solutions of hydroxypropyl cellulose are stable at pH 6 to 8; at low pH, hydroxypropyl cellulose is subject to acid hydrolysis and at high pH it may undergo oxidative degradation (2).

(4) As with methylcellulose, hydroxypropyl cellulose can be dehydrated by moderate to high concentrations of electrolytes. For a rather complete table of compatibility with inorganic salts at a range of concentrations, see the hydroxypropyl cellulose monograph in the *Handbook of Pharmaceutical Excipients* (2).

d. Preparation of liquid dispersions

Preparing colloidal dispersions of hydroxypropyl cellulose requires some patience.

(1) The powder is sprinkled, in portions, on Purified Water or a hydroalcoholic solution; a water or water-alcohol mixture is required for gel formation because a gel may not form if alcohol alone is used (14).

(2) Allow each portion to become thoroughly wetted without stirring. (Do not stir or agitate the preparation until **all** the powder is thoroughly wetted.)

(3) The preparation is then agitated (stirred or shaken), and it is allowed to stand with occasional agitation for 24 hours. It may be placed in a refrigerator.

(4) If needed, Purified Water is added to bring the preparation to the desired final volume, and the preparation is agitated to obtain a uniform, clear dispersion.

e. Preservation of aqueous dispersions

(1) Because of its high degree of substitution, hydroxypropyl cellulose is relatively resistant to growth of bacteria and molds. When in aqueous solution, a preservative is recommended if prolonged storage is required (2).

(2) Alcohol, isopropyl alcohol, or propylene glycol would be acceptable preservatives, depending on the use of the preparation (e.g., no isopropyl alcohol for internal use).

f. Uses: The substitution of hydroxypropyl groups reduces the water solubility of this compound but promotes its solubility in alcohols and glycols. This makes it a useful viscosity-inducing agent for elixirs and topical alcoholic gels. Sample Prescription 30.6 in Chapter 30 illustrates the use of hydroxypropyl cellulose for making a gel preparation.

B. Natural polymers

1. Acacia NF

a. Description

(1) Also known as *gum arabic*, acacia is a natural gum harvested from the stems and branches of various species of the acacia tree. As a natural product, it is a mixture of components, the main constituents being calcium, magnesium, and potassium salts of arabic acid, a polysaccharide. As such, acacia contains large anions and its solutions are acid to litmus. The pH of a 5% w/v solution is 4.5 to 5.0.

(2) Acacia is available as flakes, spheroidal tears, granules, or powder. It is ivory or yellowish white, has a bland taste, and is odorless.

b. Solubility: Acacia forms light-beige colloidal dispersions in twice its weight of water. It is soluble in glycerin (1 g/20 mL), propylene glycol (1 g/20 mL), and water (1 g/2.7 mL). It is practically insoluble in alcohol.

c. Incompatibilities

(1) Acacia is similar to sodium CMC in that it interacts with water using both hydrogen bonding and ion-dipole interactions. This makes it less susceptible to dehydration than methylcellulose but, like sodium CMC, it is subject to the normal incompatibilities of its weak electrolyte groups.

(2) Acacia powder contains peroxidase, which acts as an oxidizing agent for drugs or other ingredients that are susceptible to oxidation. Examples of labile drugs include phenolic and catechol compounds, tannins, and alkaloids such as atropine, morphine, cocaine, physostigmine, and related compounds. The peroxidase can be destroyed by heating acacia solutions at 100°C for a few minutes (6).

(3) It is precipitated from solution by heavy metals and borax. The borax precipitation can be prevented by the addition of glycerin (6).

(4) It is incompatible with large cations, such as quaternary ammonium compounds.

(5) It contains the polyvalent ions calcium and magnesium and has incompatibilities associated with these ions.

(6) More complete lists of incompatibilities can be found in older editions of *Remington's Pharmaceutical Sciences* and *Martindale: The Extra Pharmacopoeia* (now *Martindale: The Complete Drug Reference*).

d. Preparation of liquid dispersions

(1) Although acacia is almost completely soluble in twice its weight of water, like methylcellulose and CMC it tends to clump up when mixed directly with water. This clumping can be prevented by first wetting the acacia powder with glycerin or by first diluting the acacia powder with other powdered ingredient(s) present in the formulation. This latter method is used in preparing Acacia Syrup NF (9), which is described in Chapter 22, Vehicles for Liquid Preparations.

(2) Acacia Mucilage, which was formerly official in the *NF*, is a solution of 35% w/v acacia in water with 0.2% benzoic acid as a preservative.

  e. Preservation of aqueous dispersions

    (1) Because acacia is a natural product, its raw material could contain microbial contamination. The *NF* monograph for acacia states that it must meet the requirements of the tests for absence of *Salmonella* (9). Appropriate precautions should be taken with the purchase of acacia and with making aqueous preparations, including the use of preservatives, conservative beyond-use dates, and, when possible, refrigeration.

    (2) With the pH of its solutions in the 4.5 to 5.0 range, aqueous liquid preparations of acacia are ideal for using the organic acid preservatives benzoic acid/sodium benzoate and sorbic acid/potassium sorbate. Alcohol and propylene glycol may also be used.

    (3) Because acacia is incompatible with large cations, the quaternary ammonium preservatives benzalkonium chloride, benzethonium chloride, and cetylpyridium chloride should not be used.

  f. Uses

    (1) Acacia Syrup was at one time a very commonly used vehicle for extemporaneous compounding of oral solutions and suspensions. It has, in recent years, been largely replaced by gels of the semisynthetic gums, such as methylcellulose and sodium CMC, and by specialty manufactured vehicles such as Ora Sweet, Ora Plus, and Suspendol.

    (2) Acacia powder is unique in that it forms stable oil-in-water emulsions using simple compounding equipment such as a mortar and pestle.

  g. Advantages of acacia

    (1) It is stable over a wide pH range of 2 to 10.

    (2) Although it is not soluble in alcohol, its solutions tolerate alcohol concentrations up to 35% (6).

    (3) Its mucilages contain no sucrose, so they are useful when a sugar-free vehicle is needed. (Acacia does contain polysaccharides.) Note that Acacia Syrup contains a large amount of sucrose, so this preparation may not be used when a sugar-free vehicle is required.

  h. Disadvantages

    (1) Flavoring and sweetening are required for palatability. (Acacia Syrup is flavored and sweetened; Acacia solutions are often mixed with flavored syrups such as Syrup NF, or artificially flavored cherry or orange syrup.)

    (2) Acacia has numerous compatibility problems, as just described.

    (3) Unless preserved with an antimicrobial agent, acacia solutions and emulsions are excellent media for bacterial or mold growth. Fortunately, acacia is compatible with several preservatives, as described earlier. Usually refrigeration is also recommended for acacia preparations that contain water.

    (4) Like the semisynthetic cellulose polymers, acacia dispersions are somewhat difficult to prepare.

    (5) Because they do not have that colorless, crystal-clear appearance, acacia solutions are not as aesthetically appealing as the solutions made with synthetic and semisynthetic polymers.

2. Tragacanth NF

  a. Description

    (1) Like acacia, tragacanth is a natural gum. It comes from various species of the plant *Astragalus*.

    (2) Tragacanth contains bassorin, which is a complex mixture of methoxylated acids that absorb water to form a gel. It also contains tragacanthin, which is a polysaccharide of glucuronic acid and arabinose. This fraction forms a colloidal solution when mixed with water. The pH of a 1% w/v aqueous dispersion is 5 to 6.

  b. Solubility: Although tragacanth is practically insoluble in water, alcohol, and other organic solvents, it swells in ten times its weight of either hot or cold water to give beige-colored colloidal dispersions, which are sols or semi-gels depending on the concentration and conditions.

  c. Incompatibilities

    (1) Tragacanth contains anionic species that have the same types of incompatibilities as sodium CMC and acacia.

    (2) It is compatible with moderate to relatively high salt concentrations (2).

    (3) It has some reported compatibility problems with various preservatives, and some of these are pH dependent. For example, at pH 7, it reportedly reduces the antimicrobial effectiveness of methylparaben and chlorobutanol, but it does not have this adverse effect at pH 5 and lower. As expected, it reduces the effectiveness of the quaternary ammonium compound benzalkonium chloride and also has some effect on phenylmercuric acetate and phenol (2).

d. Preparation of liquid dispersions

(1) Pure tragacanth dispersions are very difficult to make. The following description from the 21st edition of *Remington* illustrates this point:

Introduced into water, tragacanth absorbs a certain proportion of that liquid, swells very much, and forms a soft adhesive paste, but does not dissolve. If agitated with an excess of water, this paste forms a uniform mixture; but in the course of one or two days the greater part separates, and is deposited, leaving a portion dissolved in the supernatant fluid. The finest mucilage is obtained from the whole gum or flake form. Several days should be allowed for obtaining a uniform mucilage of the maximum gel strength (6).

(2) When other ingredients are permitted in a formulation, the preparation of liquid dispersions of tragacanth is easier.

(a) The tragacanth powder can be wetted first with glycerin or propylene glycol using trituration in a mortar. An aqueous solution may then be added gradually with trituration until a smooth, thick liquid or gel is obtained.

(b) If the formulation contains powdered ingredients such as sucrose, the dry tragacanth should be mixed with the powder first and then the liquid ingredients added with trituration.

(3) Tragacanth mucilage was last official in *NF XII*. This preparation is an aqueous solution that contains benzoic acid 0.2% w/w and glycerin 18% w/w in addition to tragacanth 6% w/w (6).

e. Preservation of aqueous dispersions

(1) Because tragacanth is a natural product, its raw material could contain bacterial contamination, and reports of contamination have been published (2). The *NF* monograph for tragacanth states that it must meet the requirements of the tests for absence of *Salmonella* and *Escherichia coli* (9). Appropriate precautions should be taken with the purchase of tragacanth and with making aqueous preparations of this natural product, including the use of preservatives, conservative beyond-use dates and, when possible, refrigeration.

(2) With the normal pH of its solutions in the 5 to 6 range, aqueous preparations of tragacanth may be preserved by the organic acid preservative sorbic acid/potassium sorbate. If the pH is controlled at pH 5 or lower, benzoic acid/sodium benzoate or methylparaben may be used (2). Alcohol and propylene glycol are also possible preservatives.

(3) Because tragacanth is incompatible with large cations, the quaternary ammonium preservatives benzalkonium chloride, benzethonium chloride, and cetylpyridium chloride may not be used.

f. Uses

(1) Tragacanth is rarely used by itself but is useful as an auxiliary emulsifier and viscosity-increasing agent.

(2) Gels of tragacanth can be made by adding glycerin or propylene glycol. These elements decrease the solubility of the tragacanth and produce a semisolid gel. Ephedrine Sulfate Jelly NF XII contains 1% ephedrine sulfate, 1% tragacanth, and 15% glycerin in Purified Water. The formula and method of preparation are given in Table 23.2 in Chapter 23, Ointment Bases.

g. Advantages of tragacanth: As can be observed from Table 19.3, tragacanth is a better viscosity-inducing agent than acacia.

h. Disadvantages

(1) Tragacanth dispersions are very difficult to make.

(2) Tragacanth contains anionic species that have the same types of incompatibilities as sodium CMC and acacia.

(3) As with acacia, solutions of tragacanth are prone to mold and microbial growth.

(4) In most cases, tragacanth solutions and gels require the use of additional viscosity-inducing agents or flavored syrups for quality preparations.

(5) Because they lack that colorless, crystal-clear appearance of the synthetic and semisynthetic polymers, tragacanth solutions are not as aesthetically appealing.

3. Xanthan Gum NF

a. Description

(1) Xanthan gum is a high-molecular-weight polysaccharide gum that is made by fermentation of a carbohydrate, then purified by recovery with isopropyl alcohol. It contains three different monosaccharides: glucose, mannose, and glucuronic acid as the sodium, potassium, or calcium salt.

(2) It is a cream-colored fine powder, is tasteless, and has a slight odor. The pH of a 1% solution is in the range 6 to 8.

b. Solubility: It is soluble in hot and cold water to give viscous dispersions. Information on its solubility in alcohol is conflicting. *Remington* states that 1 g dissolves in 3 mL of alcohol and *Dispensing of Medication* says that it is freely soluble in alcohol (15); however, the *Handbook of Pharmaceutical Excipients* (2) says that it is practically insoluble in alcohol.

c. Incompatibilities
   (1) Solutions of xanthan gum are compatible with nearly all univalent and divalent cations, with polyols, alcohol, and chelating agents, and with most preservatives (13).
   (2) Aqueous solutions are stable over a wide pH range, reported as 1 to 10 (13) or 3 to 12 (2), and over a temperature range of 10°C to 60°C (2).
   (3) Because of the anionic nature of the glucuronic acid groups, xanthan gum shows incompatibilities that are similar to sodium CMC and acacia: it is incompatible with large cationic drugs, surfactants, polymers, and preservatives.
   (4) Solutions of xanthan gum are stable to the addition of up to 60% of water-miscible solvents such as acetone, alcohol, and isopropyl alcohol (2).
   (5) Xanthan gum has reported incompatibility with sodium CMC and some drugs such as amitriptyline, tamoxifen, verapamil, and aluminum hydroxide gel (2). For additional information on compatibility and stability, refer to the xanthan gum monograph in the *Handbook of Pharmaceutical Excipients* (2).

d. Preparation of liquid dispersions
   (1) If a pure dispersion in water is needed, place the water in a beaker and, using a high-speed stirrer (such as a magnetic stirring device), stir the water to form a vortex. Slowly sprinkle the xanthan gum onto the water to obtain a uniform dispersion. Dispersion may be aided by the use of moderate heat (45°C or less).
   (2) When other ingredients are permitted in the formulation, the preparation of a liquid dispersion of xanthan gum can be made by first wetting the powder with glycerin or propylene glycol using trituration in a mortar. An aqueous solution may then be added gradually with trituration until a smooth, thick liquid or gel is obtained.

e. Preservation of aqueous dispersions
   (1) Because xanthan gum is made by a fermentation process, microbiologic contamination would be possible. The *NF* monograph for xanthan gum states that it must meet the requirements of the tests for absence of *Salmonella* and *Escherichia coli* (9). Appropriate precautions should be taken with the purchase of xanthan gum and with making aqueous preparations, including the use of preservatives.
   (2) With the normal pH of its solutions in the 6 to 8 range, aqueous liquid preparations of xanthan gum may be preserved with a combination of methylparaben and propylparaben. If the pH is controlled at 5 or lower, benzoic acid/sodium benzoate or sorbic acid/potassium sorbate may be used. Alcohol and propylene glycol are also possible preservatives.
   (3) Because xanthan gum is incompatible with large cations, the quaternary ammonium preservatives benzalkonium chloride, benzethonium chloride, and cetylpyridium chloride may not be used.

f. Uses
   (1) Xanthan gum is used as a suspending and emulsifying agent in concentrations of 0.2% to 0.5%. At concentrations of 1% and higher, it gives viscous, soft-gel solutions (12).
   (2) There are five official liquid vehicle preparations of xanthan gum in the *NF 25*, including Xanthan Gum Solution, Suspension Structured Vehicle, Sugar-Free Suspension Structured Vehicle, Vehicle for Oral Suspension, and Vehicle for Oral Solution Sugar-Free (9). Furthermore, there are several manufactured liquid vehicles that contain xanthan gum, including Ora Plus, Ora-Sweet SF, and Suspendol-S. All of these are discussed in Chapter 22, Vehicles for Liquid Preparations.

4. Sodium Alginate NF
   a. Description
      (1) Sodium alginate is a polysaccharide product extracted from brown seaweeds using dilute alkali. It consists mainly of the sodium salt of Alginic Acid, which is a polyuronic acid (12).
      (2) It is a yellowish-white coarse or fine powder that is practically odorless and tasteless. The pH of a 1% w/v solution is 7.2.

   b. Solubility

     (1) It is slowly soluble in water, forming viscous colloidal solutions that may be converted into a gel by the addition of divalent cations, particularly calcium, or by the reduction of pH (12).

     (2) It is insoluble in alcohol and in hydroalcoholic solutions that contain greater than 30% alcohol. It is also insoluble in aqueous solutions when the pH is below 3. This is because of the conversion of its carboxylate ions to un-ionized carboxylic acids groups.

   c. Incompatibilities

     (1) Sodium alginate solutions are most stable between pH 4 and 10 (2). As stated earlier, below pH 3, the free acid precipitates.

     (2) Sodium alginate is reported to be incompatible with acridine derivatives, crystal violet, phenylmercuric acetate and nitrate, and heavy metals. Alcohol concentrations of greater than 5% are also reported to be incompatible (2).

     (3) As mentioned previously, the addition of calcium salts and other divalent cations causes gelation; depending on the situation, this can be considered either a desired outcome or an incompatibility. Other electrolytes also affect the viscosity of sodium alginate solutions, with low concentrations causing an increase in viscosity and high concentrations a precipitation of the polymer. For example, a sodium chloride concentration of 4% or greater causes precipitation of sodium alginate from solution (2).

   d. Preparation of liquid dispersions

     (1) Preparation of sodium alginate solutions is similar to that for xanthan gum. If a pure dispersion in water is needed, place the water in a beaker and, using a high-speed stirrer (such as a magnetic stirring device), stir the water to form a vortex. Slowly sprinkle the sodium alginate onto the water to obtain a uniform dispersion. Dispersion may be aided by the use of moderate heat (45°C or less).

     (2) When other ingredients are permitted in the formulation, the preparation of a liquid dispersion of sodium alginate can be made by first wetting the powder with glycerin or propylene glycol using trituration in a mortar. An aqueous solution may then be added gradually with trituration until a smooth, thick liquid or gel is obtained.

   e. Preservation of aqueous dispersions

     (1) Because sodium alginate is extracted from seaweed, microbiologic contamination is possible. The *NF* monograph for sodium alginate states that the total bacterial count may not exceed 200 per gram, and tests for *Salmonella* and *Escherichia coli* must be negative (9). Appropriate precautions should be taken with the purchase of sodium alginate and with making aqueous preparations, including the use of preservatives, conservative beyond-use dates and, when possible, refrigeration.

     (2) With the normal pH of its solutions at 7.2, aqueous liquid preparations of sodium alginate may be preserved with a combination of methylparaben and propylparaben or, for external use preparations, either 0.1% chlorocresol or 0.1% chloroxylenol (2). If the pH of the preparation is controlled at pH 5 or lower, benzoic acid/sodium benzoate or sorbic acid/potassium sorbate may be used. Alcohol has limited usefulness because, as stated previously, sodium alginate is incompatible with an alcohol content of 5% or greater.

     (3) Because sodium alginate is the salt of a polycarboxylic acid compound, it is probably incompatible with large cations such as the quaternary ammonium preservatives benzalkonium chloride, benzethonium chloride, and cetylpyridium chloride. These should not be used as preservatives.

   f. Uses: Sodium alginate is used as a suspending agent in concentrations of 1% to 5% and as a stabilizer for emulsions at 1% to 3%. At concentrations of 5% to 10%, it gives creams and pastes (2). It is used in the food and pharmaceutical industries for multiple purposes.

  5. Carrageenan NF

   a. Description

     (1) Carrageenan is a hydrocolloid extracted from red seaweeds using water or dilute alkali. It consists mainly of potassium, sodium, calcium, magnesium, and ammonium sulfate esters of galactose and 3,6-anhydrogalactose copolymers (9). There are three types of carrageenan—kappa and iota, which are gelling polymers, and lambda, which is a non-gelling polymer (2).

     (2) It is a yellowish brown to white, coarse or fine powder and is odorless and tasteless.

   b. Solubility

     (1) All three types hydrate rapidly in cold water, but only lambda-carrageenan (all salts) and sodium carrageenan (all types) dissolve completely at 20°C. Aqueous solutions of the gelling types, kappa–carrageenan and iota–carrageenan, must be heated to 80°C for dissolution when potassium and calcium ions are present.

(2) Carrageenan mixtures are generally insoluble in organic solvents and in oils.

c. Incompatibilities

(1) Carrageenan solutions are most stable at pH 9. In acid solution, carrageenan reportedly depolymerizes (7).

(2) Carrageenan reacts with cationic compounds (2). It precipitates proteins if the pH of the solution is below the isoelectric point for the protein (7).

d. Preparation of liquid dispersions

(1) The *NF* monograph states that not more than 30 mL of water is required to dissolve 1 g at 80°C (9).

(2) When other ingredients are permitted in the formulation, the preparation of a liquid dispersion of carrageenan can be made by first wetting the powder with glycerin or propylene glycol using trituration in a mortar. An aqueous solution may then be added gradually with trituration until a smooth, thick liquid or gel is obtained.

e. Preservation of aqueous dispersions

(1) Because carrageenan is extracted from seaweed, microbiologic contamination is possible. The *NF* monograph for carrageenan states that the total bacterial count may not exceed 200 per gram, and tests for *Salmonella* and *Escherichia coli* must be negative (9).

(2) With the normal pH of its solutions in the basic range, carrageenan may be preserved with a combination of methylparaben and propylparaben. If the pH of the preparation is controlled at pH 5 or lower, benzoic acid/sodium benzoate or sorbic acid/potassium sorbate may be used.

(3) As stated earlier, carrageenan reacts with cations and therefore is probably incompatible with the quaternary ammonium preservatives benzalkonium chloride, benzethonium chloride, and cetylpyridium chloride. These would not be good choices as preservatives.

f. Uses

(1) Carrageenan is used as a suspending agent, as a viscosity-inducing agent, and as an excipient in tablet, capsule, and suppository formulations. It is used in the food and pharmaceutical industries for multiple purposes.

(2) Carrageenan is an ingredient in Vehicle for Oral Suspension NF (9). The formula is given in Chapter 22, Vehicles for Liquid Preparations.

C. Synthetic polymers

1. Carbomer NF

a. Description

(1) Also known as *Carbopol*, carbomer is a high-molecular-weight copolymer of acrylic acid. As can be seen in Table 19.2, various types and grades are official in the *NF*. Several of these are available from vendors of compounding drugs and chemicals. The "P" suffix identifies a highly purified product that is suitable for oral use. The *NF* monographs for carbomers without a "P" specify that these compounds be labeled to indicate that they are not for internal use (9).

(2) Carbomers are white, fluffy powders furnished as the free acid. They are hygroscopic and have a slight characteristic odor. The pH of a 1% aqueous dispersion is 2.5 to 3.0.

(3) Carbomers 934 and 940 are two readily available carbomers. Their *NF* monographs state that after January 1, 2011, those compounds that are manufactured without the use of benzene will be titled as Carbomer Homopolymers (9).

(a) In Carbomer 934, the acrylic acid is cross-linked with allyl ethers of sucrose. Carbomer 934 forms clear **gels with water**. The viscosity of a neutralized 0.5% aqueous dispersion of this copolymer is between 30,500 and 39,400 cps (9).

(b) In Carbomer 940, the acrylic acid is cross-linked with allyl ethers of pentaerythritol. Carbomer 940 forms similar clear **gels with hydroalcoholic systems**. The viscosity of a neutralized 0.5% aqueous dispersion of this copolymer is between 40,000 and 60,000 cps (9).

b. Solubility: Carbomers are soluble in water. After dispersion in aqueous media, the acid groups of these polymers are neutralized with an alkali hydroxide or amine base to give very-high-viscosity gelled systems. After neutralization, they are soluble in alcohol and glycerin.

c. Incompatibilities

(1) Carbomers are incompatible with phenol and resorcinol, cationic polymers, strong acids, and high concentrations of electrolytes (2).

(2) The viscosity of carbomer gels may be decreased by the addition of electrolytes (12). Some grades are more tolerant than others to ion content.

(3) As indicated later in the section on preparation, the viscosity and quality of a carbomer dispersion depend on the pH of the solution. The viscosity of the system is greatly reduced if the pH is adjusted above 12 or below 3 (2).

(4) Carbomer dispersions are photosensitive and should be protected from light (16). Stability to light is reportedly improved by the addition of benzophenone with 0.05% to 0.1% Edetic Acid (EDTA) (2,16).

d. Preparation of liquid dispersions

(1) Liquid dispersions of carbomers are made by carefully dusting the powder onto the desired liquid vehicle with vigorous stirring or use of a high-speed mixer. When the dispersion is in this fluid form, other ingredients can easily be added and dispersed. The preparation is then allowed to stand until entrapped air bubbles can escape.

(2) The dispersions are gelled by adding an inorganic base, such as sodium, potassium, or ammonium hydroxide, borax, or sodium carbonate or bicarbonate. An amount of base approximately equivalent to 0.4 g of sodium hydroxide is needed to neutralize 1 g of carbomer (2,16). Organic amine bases such as triethanolamine may also be used (7,16,17). The formulas and methods of preparation of several carbomer gels are given in Table 23.2 in Chapter 23, Ointment Bases.

(3) The final pH of the preparation is an important factor in gel viscosity and quality. Some sources recommend that it be adjusted to neutrality (12), while others state that a range of 6 to 11 is satisfactory (2,16).

(4) The viscosity of these systems can be increased by the addition of polyols, such as propylene glycol and glycerin, because they hydrogen-bond with the polymer (12).

e. Preservation of aqueous dispersions

(1) Aqueous dispersions of carbomer are susceptible to microbial growth and should be preserved. Recommended preservatives include 0.1% chlorocresol, 0.18% methylparaben with 0.02% propylparaben, or 0.1% thimerosal (2).

(2) Benzalkonium chloride and sodium benzoate at a concentration of 0.1% or greater give cloudy dispersions with reduced viscosity (2).

f. Uses

(1) Although Carbomer 934P is approved for oral use, carbomers are used most frequently in topical products.

(2) Carbomers may be used as emulsifying agents (0.1% to 0.5% concentration), suspending agents (0.5% to 1% concentration), and gelling agents (0.5% to 2% concentration) (2).

2. Poloxamer NF

a. Description

(1) Also know as *Pluronic*, poloxamer is a block copolymer of ethylene oxide and propylene oxide. It is available in several types; the properties of a particular type depend on the average molecular weight of the type and on the relative proportions of polyoxyethylene and polyoxypropylene present in the copolymer.

(2) The physical state of the polymer type is designated by a letter attached to the name, "L" for liquid, "P" for paste, and "F" for flake. The *NF* lists five poloxamers in the Poloxamer monograph: four that are solids—188 (commercial grade F-68), 237 (commercial grade F-87), 338 (commercial grade F-108), and 407 (commercial grade F-127)—and one that is liquid—124 (commercial grade L-44) (2,9).

(3) The type of poloxamer most often seen in formulas for compounded preparations is poloxamer 407, brand name Pluronic F-127. This compound is a white, practically odorless, tasteless solid with an average molecular weight of 9,840 to 14,600. It melts at 56°C. The pH of a 2.5% solution is 5.0 to 7.4 (2,9,18).

(4) Poloxamers have the unique property of forming micelles at low concentrations and clear, thermoreversible gels at concentrations at or above 20%. Thermoreversibility means that they are liquids at cool (e.g., refrigerated) temperatures but are gels when warmed to body temperature (18).

b. Solubility: Solubility varies with the type and grade; poloxamer 407 is freely soluble in water, alcohol, and isopropyl alcohol (2,18).

c. Incompatibilities

(1) Although poloxamers are relatively stable solids, they are subject to oxidation. The official monograph states that they may contain a suitable antioxidant, but the product must be labeled with the name and quantity of the antioxidant added (9).

(2) Aqueous solutions of poloxamers are also quite stable and are reported to tolerate the presence of acids, alkalis, and metal ions (2).

(3) Inorganic salts can cause compatibility problems with poloxamer gels if the concentration of the salt in solution is too high. It is important to be aware of this property, because formulas for poloxamer gels often contain buffer solutions; if the concentration of the buffer is too high, the desired gel will not form. The critical molal concentrations of the salts vary with the salt but are in the range of 0.1 to 0.3 molal (19).

(4) Poloxamer 188 is reported to be incompatible with phenols and parabens at some concentrations (2).

d. Preparation

(1) Poloxamer gels are not difficult to make, but they do take time. They can be prepared by adding the granules or flakes to water and stirring to dissolve. At the 20% concentration, a "snowball" is often the result, so stirring to dissolve is not possible. Amazingly, when this preparation is placed in a refrigerator for several hours or overnight, a clear, viscous liquid solution results. A sample formula and procedure for making a poloxamer gel is given in Table 23.2 in Chapter 23, Ointment Bases.

(2) Prepared poloxamer 20% gels, which are buffered and preserved, may be purchased from pharmaceutical vendors. A typical formulation includes a citrate/phosphate buffer with sorbic acid and methyl- and propylparaben as preservatives.

(3) Often poloxamer gels are combined with a lecithin-isopropyl palmitate solution (LIPS), which acts as an emollient, emulsifier, and penetration enhancer. The LIPS may be prepared by adding 10 g of soya lecithin to 10 g of isopropyl palmitate and allowing the mixture to set overnight. Prepared LIPS is also available from several pharmaceutical vendors. The manufactured solution comes already preserved but, if the solution is made in the pharmacy, a preservative must be added. Typically, 20 g of LIPS is included for each 100 mL of finished poloxamer gel. This mixture is also known as *poloxamer lecithin organogel*. Sample Prescription 30.7 in Chapter 30 illustrates the use of this poloxamer-lecithin organogel in a compounded preparation.

e. Preservation of aqueous dispersions

(1) Poloxamer aqueous solutions are subject to microbial growth and must be preserved.

(2) Depending on the pH of the solution, the organic acid preservatives benzoic acid/sodium benzoate or sorbic acid/potassium sorbate may or may not be effective. Some formulas include citrate and/or phosphate buffers or other pH–adjusting agents to control the pH at 5 or lower and then use sorbic acid or potassium sorbate as the preservative.

(3) Because poloxamer is soluble in either alcohol or isopropyl alcohol, these may also be considered, depending on the concentration and use. (Isopropyl alcohol may not be used for internal use preparations.) Propylene glycol is also a possible preservative, as are the parabens.

f. Uses

(1) Depending on the type, poloxamer polymers have a wide variety of uses in pharmaceutical products. They are used as emulsifiers, suspending agents, solubilizing agents, wetting agents, and binders or coating ingredients in tablets (2).

(2) For compounding, poloxamers are used most often as viscosity-inducing agents for topical gels.

3. Polyvinyl alcohol and povidone or polyvinylpyrrolidone are two other examples of synthetic polymers used as viscosity-inducing agents. They are available from vendors of compounding products and supplies. For information on these agents, consult the *Handbook of Pharmaceutical Excipients*.

D. Particulate association colloids

1. Bentonite NF

a. Description

(1) Bentonite is a natural clay product that consists mainly of colloidal, hydrated aluminum silicate ($Al_2O_3 \cdot 4SiO_2 \cdot H_2O$). It may also contain calcium, magnesium, and iron. The *NF 25* lists two solid bentonite articles, Bentonite and Purified Bentonite, and the aqueous suspension Bentonite Magma (9). Purified Bentonite is bentonite that has been processed to remove grit and nonswellable ore components (9). Veegum is a silicate with similar properties; it is the purified product of magnesium aluminum silicate.

(2) Bentonite has the disadvantage of having a rather unappealing, gray appearance and an "earthy" taste. Veegum is white or cream-colored and odorless and has a somewhat better appearance.

(3) Both are anionic, and their dispersions have pHs in the range of 9 to 10.5.

b. Solubility: Bentonite is insoluble in water but instead absorbs water and swells to approximately 12 times its original volume to form suspensions or gels. It is practically insoluble in alcohol, isopropyl alcohol, glycerin, and fixed oils.

c. Incompatibilities

(1) Although bentonite is insoluble in water-miscible solvents, its aqueous suspensions will tolerate these in fairly high concentrations: 30% alcohol, isopropyl alcohol, propylene glycol, or polyethylene glycol, and 50% glycerin (2).

(2) The ability of bentonite to absorb water is decreased by acids and acid salts, which cause its suspensions and gels to break down. In contrast, small amounts of alkaline compounds such as magnesium oxide will enhance its gelling properties. It is most stable at pH 7 and higher (6).

(3) Bentonite particles are anionic, and either flocculation or breakdown of the suspension is possible with the addition of electrolytes or positively charged suspensions; the outcome depends on the concentrations (2).

d. Preparation of dispersions

(1) Bentonite Magma NF is a 5% w/w suspension of bentonite in water. Its formula and method of preparation are given in the *NF* (9):

Bentonite	50 g
Purified Water, a sufficient quantity to make	1,000 g

Sprinkle the Bentonite, in portions, upon 800 g of hot purified water, allowing each portion to become thoroughly wetted without stirring. Allow it to stand with occasional stirring for 24 hours. Stir until a uniform magma is obtained, add Purified Water to make 1,000 g, and mix (9).

Making Bentonite Magma is a very finicky process, so follow these instructions to the letter. The *NF* also gives a method using a high-speed blender, but this method is not as reliable and can be very messy.

(2) When bentonite is included as an ingredient in an aqueous formulation, it should first be triturated with a nonaqueous liquid such as glycerin or with the formulation powdered ingredients before adding the water or aqueous portion (2).

(3) Bentonite Magma has a tendency to get thicker and more gel-like with aging; this factor should be considered in determining quantities to prepare for stock suspensions and when setting beyond-use dates on formulated preparations.

e. Preservation of aqueous dispersions

(1) The monographs of all three *NF* articles Bentonite, Purified Bentonite, and Bentonite Magma contain microbial limits that state that these articles must meet the test for absence of *Escherichia coli* (9).

(2) Bentonite and Veegum both absorb cationic preservatives, therefore probably reducing their effectiveness. Nonionic and anionic preservatives are reported to be unaffected by the clay itself (2), but since bentonite and Veegum lose their viscosity below pH 6, preservatives, such as the organic acids, that are effective only below pH 5 or 6 would not be useful in aqueous preparations of bentonite or Veegum. Possible effective preservatives include the parabens, alcohol, isopropyl alcohol (for external-use products), and propylene glycol.

(3) The official Bentonite Magma NF does not contain a preservative.

f. Uses

(1) Bentonite and Veegum are approved for both oral and topical use. In suspensions, they offer the advantage of producing plastic, thixotropic systems, so they are very good at suspending solid ingredients. They are most useful in preparations that have sufficient quantities of opaque solids because these solid powders mask the somewhat unappealing appearance of bentonite and veegum. An example of this is Calamine Topical Suspension USP, which contains calamine and zinc oxide and uses Bentonite Magma as the suspending medium.

(2) Bentonite and Veegum can be made in concentrations ranging from 2% to 10%: the 2% concentration gives a rather thin lotion, the 5% magma has a nice thixotropic structure that is easily pourable when shaken, the 7% suspension is just pourable, and the 10% concentration produces a semisolid preparation.

2. Colloidal Silicon Dioxide NF and Silicon Dioxide NF

a. Description

(1) Colloidal Silicon Dioxide NF (9), also known as *colloidal silica* or *Cab-O-Sil*, is SiO_2. It is a submicroscopic silica prepared by high-temperature vapor hydrolysis of a silicon compound.

(2) Colloidal Silicon Dioxide is distinguished in the *NF* from plain silicon dioxide. Silicon Dioxide NF, SiO_2xH_2O, is obtained by precipitating dissolved silica in a solution of sodium silicate. The *NF* further distinguishes two types of plain silicon dioxide, depending on the method of preparation, and instructs that the type be appropriately labeled (9). One type, silica gel, is prepared by adding a mineral acid to the sodium silicate solution; the second type, precipitated silica, is very fine particles produced by destabilization of a sodium silicate solution.

(3) Colloidal silicon dioxide is a light, white, very fine (approximately 15 nm) powder; it is odorless, tasteless, hygroscopic, and nongritty. The pH of 4% dispersions is in the range 3.5 to 4.4.

b. Solubility: Both regular and colloidal silicon dioxide are insoluble in water and practically insoluble in organic solvents and acids (except hydrofluoric acid) but are soluble in hot solutions of alkali hydroxides. Colloidal silicon dioxide forms colloidal dispersions with water.

c. Incompatibilities

(1) Both forms are quite inert and do not have significant compatibility problems.

(2) Colloidal silicon dioxide is an effective viscosity-inducing agent when in aqueous dispersions at pH of 7.5 and lower. Above pH 7.5, the viscosity-inducing property decreases up to pH 10.7, when the compound dissolves to form soluble silicates (2).

d. Method of preparation of liquid dispersions

Although insoluble in water, silicon dioxide and colloidal silicon dioxide are easily wet by water. Colloidal silicon dioxide forms aqueous dispersions at pH 7.5 and lower.

e. Preservation of aqueous dispersions

(1) Aqueous dispersions of colloidal silicon dioxide have a pH in the acid range (3.5 to 4.4), where the organic acid preservatives are effective.

(2) Because silicon dioxide is unreactive, most other preservatives should be effective antimicrobial agents in its aqueous dispersions.

f. Uses

(1) The silica gel type of silicon dioxide is used in compounding as a filtering aid and as a suspending agent. For example, it is a suspending ingredient in the official compounded formulation for Morphine Sulfate Suppositories USP (8).

(2) Colloidal silicon dioxide is widely used in the pharmaceutical industry as a glidant in tablets and capsules and as a suspending and thickening agent in emulsions, suspensions, suppositories, and aerosols. It confers structure and thixotropy on suspensions, gels, and semisolid systems (2).

3. Microcrystalline Cellulose NF and Microcrystalline Cellulose and Carboxymethylcellulose Sodium NF

a. Description

(1) Microcrystalline cellulose, also known as *Avicel*, is cellulose that has been partially depolymerized by treatment with mineral acids, and the resulting material is purified (9). Although it is a derivative of cellulose, it is classified as a particulate association colloid because it does not dissolve molecularly in water.

(2) Microcrystalline cellulose is also available combined with the semisynthetic cellulose derivative sodium CMC in an official *NF* product that is a colloid-forming mixture (9).

(3) Microcrystalline cellulose is a fine, white, free-flowing, crystalline powder that is odorless and tasteless. It is available in a variety of grades with varying particle sizes and moisture contents, which confer different properties and uses.

(4) The combination product Microcrystalline Cellulose and Carboxymethylcellulose Sodium NF is a whitish powder that is tasteless and odorless. Particle size varies from fine to coarse. The pH of its dispersions is in the range of 6 to 8. The sodium CMC portion makes up between 8.3% and 18.8%, depending on the grade.

b. Solubility

(1) Microcrystalline cellulose is insoluble in water, dilute acids, and most organic solvents. It is slightly soluble in dilute alkali (e.g., 5% NaOH).

(2) The combination product is also insoluble in organic solvents and dilute acids, but the powder will swell in water and gives a white, opaque dispersion or gel with nice structure for suspending solid particles.

c. Incompatibilities: Microcrystalline cellulose is a very stable compound, but it is incompatible with strong oxidizing agents (2). The combination product has the incompatibilities of sodium CMC (see that description earlier in section IV.A.2).

d. Preparation of liquid dispersions

(1) Microcrystalline cellulose is generally not used by itself as a viscosity-increasing agent for liquid preparations.

(2) The combination product is used to produce dispersions or gels with nice structure for suspending solid particles. The method of preparing a liquid dispersion of this combination is essentially the same as for sodium CMC.

e. Preservation of aqueous dispersions

(1) When in solid state, microcrystalline cellulose does not require a preservative.

(2) As stated previously, for liquid dispersions the combination product of microcrystalline cellulose with sodium CMC (or a similar combination) is used. In this case, the acceptable preservatives are limited to those useful for dispersions of the soluble polymer, such as for sodium CMC (see previous section IV.A.2).

f. Uses

(1) Microcrystalline cellulose is a useful ingredient in making tablets and capsules; it is used as a binder, diluent, lubricant, and disintegrant (2).

(2) Because it has good flow properties, microcrystalline cellulose is useful as a diluent in compounding capsules using small-scale "capsule machines." For this purpose, it has the advantage over soluble polymers in that it does not hydrate rapidly to form viscous gels surrounding the capsule powder when it comes into contact with the aqueous solutions in the stomach. Such viscous layers can retard the release of active ingredient from the capsule material.

(3) The combination product microcrystalline cellulose and sodium CMC produces thixotropic dispersions that are useful as suspending vehicles (2).

REFERENCES

1. Sinko PJ. Martin's physical pharmacy and pharmaceutical sciences, 5th ed. Baltimore, MD: Lippincott Williams & Wilkins, 2006; 562–569.
2. Rowe R, Sheskey P, Weller P, eds. Handbook of pharmaceutical excipients, 5th ed. Washington, DC: APhA Publications, 2005.
3. Bowman BJ, Ofner CM, Schott H. Colloidal dispersions. In: University of the Sciences in Philadelphia, ed. Remington: The science and practice of pharmacy, 21st ed. Baltimore MD: Lippincott Williams & Wilkins, 2005; 293–318.
4. Schaare RL, Block LH, Rohan LC. Rheology. In: University of the Sciences in Philadelphia, ed. Remington: The science and practice of pharmacy, 21st ed. Baltimore, MD: Lippincott Williams & Wilkins, 2005; 338–357.
5. The United States Pharmacopeial Convention, Inc. Front matter—NF: Excipients. 2007 USP 30/NF 25. Rockville, MD: Author, 2006.
6. Reilly WJ. Pharmaceutical necessities. In: University of the Sciences in Philadelphia, ed. Remington: The science and practice of pharmacy, 21st ed. Baltimore, MD: Lippincott Williams & Wilkins, 2005; 1058–1092.
7. O'Neil MJ, ed. The Merck index, 13th ed. Rahway, NJ: Merck & Co., 2001.
8. The United States Pharmacopeial Convention, Inc. USP monographs. 2007 USP 30/NF 25. Rockville, MD: Author, 2006.
9. The United States Pharmacopeial Convention, Inc. NF monographs. 2007 USP 30/NF 25. Rockville, MD: Author, 2006.
10. MICROMEDEX, Inc. Chemistry and compendial requirements. USP DI Vol. III, 22nd ed. Englewood, CO: Author, 2002.
11. Reynolds LA, Closson RG, eds. Extemporaneous ophthalmic preparations. Vancouver, WA: Applied Therapeutics, 1993; 6–7.
12. Lieberman HA, Rieger MM, Banker GS, eds. Pharmaceutical dosage forms: Disperse systems, vol 2, 2nd ed. New York: Marcel Dekker, Inc., 1996; 407–409.
13. Lieberman HA, Rieger MM, Banker GS, ed. Pharmaceutical dosage forms: Disperse systems, vol 2, 2nd ed. New York: Marcel Dekker, Inc., 1996; 204–205.
14. Allen LV, ed. Piroxicam 0.5% in an alcoholic gel. IJPC 1997; 1: 181.
15. Booth RE, Dale JK. Compounding and dispensing information. In: King RE, ed. Dispensing of medication, 9th ed. Easton, PA: Mack Publishing Co., 1984; 517.
16. Allen LV, ed. Featured excipient carbopols (carbomers). IJPC 1997; 1: 265–266.
17. Siegel FP, Ecanow B. Dermatologicals. In: King RE, ed. Dispensing of medications, 9th ed. Easton, PA: Mack Publishing Co., 1984; 80.
18. Allen LV, ed. Featured excipient: poloxamer. IJPC 1997; 1:190–191.
19. Pandit NK, Kisaka J. Loss of gelation ability of Pluronic® F127 in the presence of some salts. Int J Pharmaceut 1996; 145: 129–136.

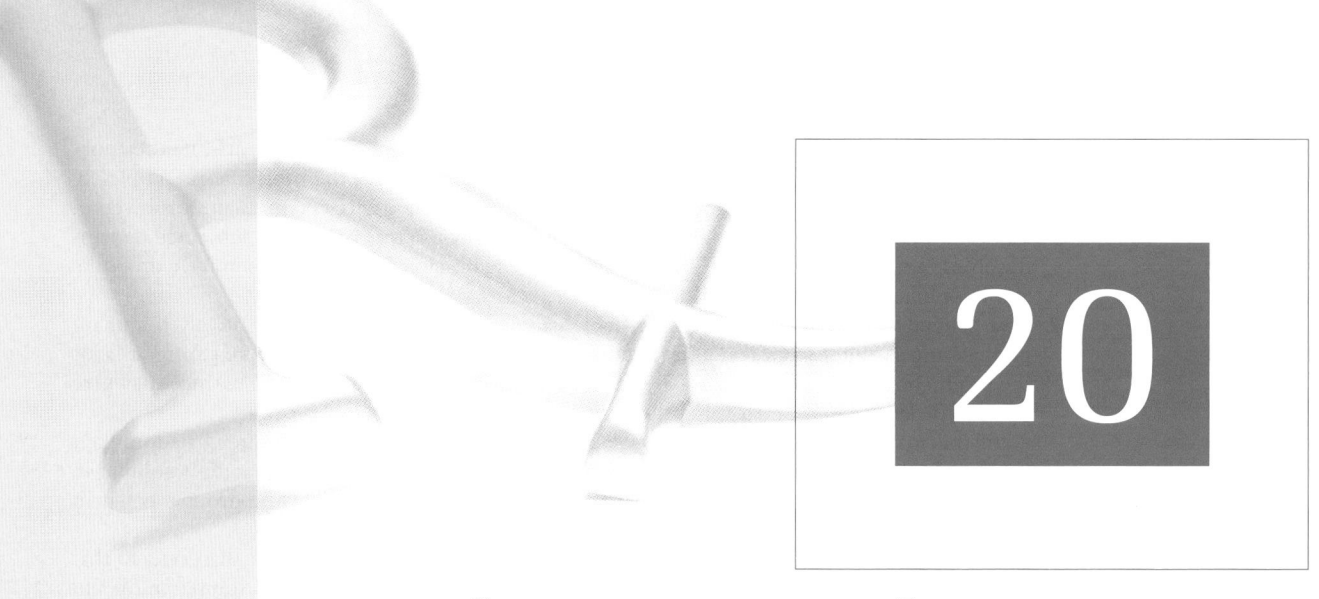

Surfactants and Emulsifying Agents

Melgardt de Villiers, PhD

I. DEFINITIONS

A. **Surface-active agents,** also called **surfactants**, are molecules or ions that are adsorbed at interfaces (1,2).

1. The molecular structure of these substances is composed of two parts: a hydrophilic (water-loving) portion, which orients itself toward water or other relatively polar liquids or solids, and a hydrophobic (water-hating) or lipophilic (oil-loving) part, which orients itself toward oil or other nonpolar solids, liquids, or gas (e.g., air).

2. Surfactants orient themselves at interfaces so as to reduce the interfacial free energy produced by the presence of the interface (2). They lower the surface tension between a liquid and a gas (e.g., air) or the interfacial tension between two liquids.

3. Surfactants can function as wetting agents, detergents, foaming agents, dispersing agents, solubilizers, and emulsifying agents.

   Note: A detailed discussion of interfacial phenomena is beyond the scope of this text. For more information on this subject refer to a book on physical pharmacy (1) or the chapters on interfacial phenomena, colloidal dispersions, and coarse dispersions in *Remington's The Science and Practice of Pharmacy* (2–4).

B. An **emulsifying agent** is a compound that concentrates at the interface of two immiscible phases, usually an oil and water. It lowers the interfacial free energy, reduces the interfacial tension between the phases, and forms a film or barrier around the droplets of the immiscible, discontinuous phase as they are formed, preventing the coalescence of the droplets.

   A discussion of the emulsification process and of liquid emulsions can be found in Chapter 29, Liquid Emulsions. Semisolid emulsions, also known as *creams,* are described in Chapters 23, Ointment Bases, and Chapter 30, Semisolids: Ointments, Creams, Gels, Pastes, and Collodions.

II. DESIRABLE PROPERTIES OF EMULSIFYING AGENTS

A. Molecular structure

1. Although emulsifying agents must contain both hydrophilic and lipophilic parts, neither portion may be too strongly dominant (2,5). If the hydrophilic part of the molecule is completely dominant, the substance does not concentrate at the water–oil interface; it remains dissolved in the water phase. By the same token, if the lipophilic portion is too strong, the substance remains dissolved in the oil. A good emulsifier should have a reasonable balance between its hydrophilic and lipophilic groups.

2. As a general rule, emulsifying agents in which the hydrophilic groups are relatively dominant produce oil-in-water (o/w) emulsions; those in which the lipophilic groups are strongest favor the production of water-in-oil (w/o) emulsions; and those with nearly equal balance may give either type, depending on the circumstances (5). The examples below illustrate.

   a. In the soap sodium stearate, the hydrophilic group —COO^-Na^+ is somewhat dominant over the lipophilic hydrocarbon chain $C_{17}H_{35}$—. As a result, sodium stearate is soluble in water and insoluble in oil. It does possess sufficient balance between the groups so that it concentrates at the oil–water interface and it produces o/w emulsions (6).

   b. In contrast, calcium stearate contains two long hydrocarbon chains, rather than one, so that the lipophilic groups dominate. Calcium stearate is insoluble in water and soluble in oil and promotes the formation of w/o emulsions (5).

   c. In both cases, the ionic portion is required. If a substance such as an acid is added to an emulsion stabilized by one of these emulsifiers, the equilibrium for the reaction R-COO$^-$ $\rightleftharpoons$ R-COOH shifts to the right. The un-ionized form now predominates; the required hydrophilic-lipophilic balance is destroyed and the emulsifier leaves the water–oil interface and dissolves in the oil.

B. The emulsifier must produce a stable film at the interface.

   1. Some surface-active agents are capable of producing emulsions, but the emulsions separate on standing or storage because the surfactant is incapable of producing stable, strong barriers to prevent the coalescence of the dispersed droplets (5).

   2. Agents such as these may be useful if combined with a second substance that acts as a stabilizer. The surfactant is then referred to as the *primary* emulsifying agent and the stabilizer as the *secondary* or *auxiliary* emulsifier (5). An example of such a system is the use of the primary emulsifier sodium lauryl sulfate with the auxiliary emulsifier stearyl alcohol in Hydrophilic Ointment USP (6).

C. The emulsifying agent should be stable to chemical degradation.

D. The emulsifying agent should be reasonably inert and should not interact chemically with any of the other ingredients in the formulation.

E. If the emulsifier is liable to microbiologic attack, adequate precautions must be taken.

   1. In the emulsion section of *USP* Chapter ⟨1151⟩ Pharmaceutical Dosage Forms, it is stated that all emulsions require the addition of a suitable preservative because the water phase is vulnerable to the growth of microorganisms (7).

   2. Other possible precautions when emulsifiers favor the growth of microorganisms include the use of refrigeration and short beyond-use datings.

F. The substance should be nontoxic and nonirritating to skin or mucous membranes.

G. Depending on its use, it should be relatively odorless, tasteless, and colorless.

H. It should have a reasonable cost.

III. CLASSIFICATION AND CHARACTERISTICS OF SURFACTANTS AND EMULSIFYING AGENTS

A. Table 20.1 lists the *USP 30/NF 25* articles categorized as surfactants and emulsifying agents (8).

B. **Water-soluble polymers**

   The water-soluble or hydrophilic polymers may be grouped either by their origin or on the basis of their electrical charge (4).

   1. Based on their origin, there are three classes of water-soluble polymers: natural polymers, derivatives of cellulose, and synthetic hydrophilic polymers.

      a. The natural polymers include polysaccharides, such as acacia, agar, pectin, sodium alginate, xanthan gum, and tragacanth, and polypeptides, such as casein and gelatin.

      b. The cellulose derivatives are semisynthetic products, made by chemical modification of cellulose to yield soluble polymers. Examples include methylcellulose, sodium carboxymethylcellulose, hypromellose, and hydroxyethyl and hydroxypropyl cellulose.

      c. The synthetic water-soluble polymers include vinyl polymers such as polyvinyl alcohol and povidone (polyvinylpyrrolidone), carbomer (which is a copolymer of acrylic acid), and polyethylene glycols.

Table 20.1	*USP* AND *NF* EXCIPIENTS CATEGORIZED AS EMULSIFYING AND/OR SOLUBILIZING AGENTS

Acacia	Carbomer Copolymer
Carbomer Interpolymer	Cholesterol
Coconut Oil	Diethylene Glycol Stearates
Ethylene Glycol Stearates	Glyceryl Distearate
Glyceryl Monolinoleate	Glyceryl Monooleate
Glyceryl Monostearate	Lanolin Alcohols
Lecithin	Mono- and Di-glycerides
Poloxamer	Polyoxyethylene 50 Stearate
Polyoxyl 10 Oleyl Ether	Polyoxyl 20 Cetostearyl Ether
Polyoxyl 35 Castor Oil	Polyoxyl 40 Hydrogenated Castor Oil
Polyoxyl 40 Stearate	Polyoxyl Lauryl Ether
Polyoxyl Stearyl Ether	Polysorbate 20
Polysorbate 40	Polysorbate 60
Polysorbate 80	Propylene Glycol Monostearate
Sodium Cetostearyl Sulfate	Sodium Lauryl Sulfate
Sodium Stearate	Sorbitan Monolaurate
Sorbitan Monooleate	Sorbitan Monopalmitate
Sorbitan Monostearate	Sorbitan Sesquioleate
Sorbitan Trioleate	Stearic Acid
Wax, Emulsifying	

Source: The United States Pharmacopeial Convention, Inc. Front matter—NF: Excipients. 2007 USP 30/NF 25. Rockville, MD: Author, 2006.

2. Based on electrical charge, the hydrophilic polymers are either uncharged or anionic; cationic polymers are uncommon.
   a. Examples of the nonionic or uncharged polymers include methylcellulose and ethylcellulose, hypromellose, hydroxyethyl and hydroxypropyl cellulose, pyroxylin, polyethylene oxide, polyvinyl alcohol, and povidone (polyvinylpyrrolidone),
   b. Examples of anionic polymers include acacia, alginic acid, pectin, tragacanth, xanthan gum, and carbomer at a pH favoring the ionic form of the acid group, and sodium alginate and sodium carboxymethylcellulose.
3. Water-soluble polymers have the following characteristics in common:
   a. They favor o/w emulsions.
   b. They have the advantage of being viscosity-building agents in addition to having surface activity.
   c. With the exception of some of the natural gums, most of the water-soluble polymers are used as auxiliary emulsifying agents.
4. Other properties of the water-soluble polymers depend on the particular chemical structure of the polymer. These agents are discussed in detail in Chapter 19, Viscosity-Inducing Agents. Information is given on their individual properties, solubilities, incompatibilities, formulation methods, and uses.

C. **Anionic soaps and detergents**
   1. Soft soaps
      a. These are salts of fatty acids in which the positive ion is univalent, such as Na^+, K^+, and NH_4^+. The most common fatty acids are stearic (C-18), oleic (C-18, consisting mainly of (Z)-9-octadecenoic acid), palmitic (C-16), and lauric (C-12).
      b. Often the emulsifier is formed at the time of emulsification by adding an alkali base (e.g., NaOH, KOH, NH_4OH, sodium borate) or an organic amine base (e.g., triethanolamine) to a fixed oil that contains a sufficient amount of fatty acid. For this reason, these are often called *nascent* (which means "having recently come into exisitence") soap emulsifiers.
         (1) Soaps with an organic amine as the cation are more balanced and less hydrophilic and form more stable emulsions than the alkali soap emulsifiers (5).
         (2) Emulsions made with alkali soap emulsifying agents sometimes require the addition of auxiliary emulsifiers for stable emulsions.

   c. Soft soaps are water-soluble and/or water-dispersible.

   d. They usually form o/w emulsions.

     (1) The classic vanishing creams and other water-washable creams of this type are **o/w** emulsions that use soft-soap emulsifiers.

     (2) Two exceptions are Rose Water Ointment and Cold Cream. These are **w/o** emulsions formed when a solution of sodium borate (borax) is added to melted white and cetyl ester waxes, which contain sufficient fatty acids for the formation of a soap emulsifier.

   e. Soft soaps give emulsions with a pH in the basic range.

     (1) The alkali soap emulsions have a pH in the range of 8 to 10 (9) and are most stable above pH 10 (5).

     (2) The organic bases give soaps that have a lower neutrality point (about pH 8), with the pH of the emulsions nearer to neutrality and more stable to changes in pH (5).

   f. Soap emulsifiers are weak electrolytes (salts of a carboxylic acid [$R\text{-}COO^-$], a weak acid) and require this ionic center for their surface activity. This means that any drug or other ingredient that neutralizes that ionic center will destroy an emulsion stabilized by these emulsifiers. Problematic ingredients include drugs or additives that are acids or that produce an acid pH (e.g., phenol, salicylic acid), because lowering the pH shifts the equilibrium in favor of the weakly dissociated, oil-soluble $R\text{-}COOH$ form.

   g. Soft soaps are incompatible with multivalent cations (Mg^{++}, Ca^{++}) because these replace the univalent ion, forming the multiple hydrocarbon chain soap of the multivalent ion. This shifts the hydrophilic-lipophilic balance of the molecule in favor of the lipophilic type. This new emulsifier favors the opposite type of emulsion (w/o) and may cause the emulsion to "crack" or coalesce.

   h. Soaps are also incompatible with high concentrations of electrolytes and with high-molecular-weight cations such as the preservatives benzalkonium chloride and benzethonium chloride (9). The anionic portion of the soap binds these preservatives and renders them inactive.

   i. Soft soaps are unsuitable emulsifiers for internal-use emulsions because of their soapy taste and laxative action (5).

  2. Hard soaps

   a. These are salts of fatty acids in which the positive ion is divalent or trivalent (Ca^{+2}, Mg^{+2}, Zn^{+2}, Al^{+3}). The most common hard soap is calcium oleate. This is formed by reacting calcium hydroxide in Calcium Hydroxide Topical Solution (also known as *lime water*) with oleic acid found in olive oil and certain other fixed oils.

   b. Hard soaps are oil-soluble and water-insoluble.

   c. They form w/o emulsions.

   d. Like soft soaps, these are salts of a carboxylic acid ($R\text{-}COO^-$), a weak acid, which gives the weakly dissociated $R\text{-}COOH$ form on addition of drugs or other ingredients that are acids or that produce an acid pH. Hard soaps are particularly sensitive to acid ingredients (5).

   e. The $R\text{-}COO^-$ groups of hard soaps may interact with and bind high-molecular-weight cations like benzalkonium chloride.

   f. Hard soaps are unsuitable for internal-use emulsions.

  3. Detergents

   a. These are salts of alkyl sulfates, sulfonates, phosphates, and sulfosuccinates. Two examples of detergents from this group that are commonly used in pharmaceuticals are sodium lauryl sulfate and dioctyl sodium sulfosuccinate (docusate sodium).

   b. Detergents are very hydrophilic and are soluble in water.

   c. They always form o/w emulsions.

   d. As strong electrolytes, they are more stable to acids, such as phenolic compounds and salicylic acid, and are not sensitive to high concentrations of electrolytes.

   e. Because their ionic centers strongly repel each other, detergents do not form firm, intact barriers. These surfactants are most often used in conjunction with secondary non-ionic emulsifiers such as cetyl or stearyl alcohol.

   f. Like soaps, detergents are unsuitable for internal-use emulsions because of their soapy taste and laxative action.

D. Cationic surfactants

  1. The cationic surfactants are quaternary ammonium compounds such as benzalkonium chloride, benzethonium chloride, and cetylpyridinium chloride.

  2. They are very hydrophilic and are very soluble in water.

  3. Cationic surfactants do not make good emulsifiers but are useful as antimicrobial agents. Their properties and uses as antimicrobial agents are discussed in Chapter 16 Antimicrobial Preservatives.

E. Finely divided solids

1. These are usually finely divided hydrophilic inorganic solids. When these solids are in a very fine state of subdivision, they tend not to be easily wetted by liquids, and they orient at interfaces, forming a barrier to coalescence. The most common examples of this type include the colloidal clays bentonite and Veegum and metallic hydroxides, such as magnesium oxide and zinc oxide.

2. Large quantities of finely divided solids, which are in a product formulation for therapeutic purposes, may function as emulsifiers if an appropriate order of mixing is used. An example is the emulsification of 25% mineral oil with 75% magnesia magma (Haley's M-O).

3. The finely divided solids are not usually used by themselves but are useful as auxiliary emulsifiers. An exception is the magnesia magma–mineral oil emulsion mentioned previously. Here, the finely divided magnesium oxide of magnesia magma serves as the sole emulsifier agent for the mineral oil (9).

4. Hydrophilic solids favor o/w emulsions and are used most often as auxiliary emulsifier for this emulsion type. There are, however, examples of hydrophilic solids present in w/o formulations. An example is the presence of the hydrophilic solids calamine and zinc oxide in Calamine Liniment NF IX, a w/o emulsion that has calcium oleate as the primary emulsifying agent.

5. Finely divided hydrophobic solids favor the formation of w/o emulsions. If a large quantity of a hydrophobic solid is added to a system with the primary emulsifier favoring an o/w emulsion, the final emulsion type is difficult to predict. An example is the formulation of an oral o/w emulsion of the water-insoluble hydrophobic drug sulfadiazine, with a non-ionic emulsifying system that favors an o/w emulsion. Depending on the exact conditions, the result may be either a w/o or an o/w emulsion. Because o/w emulsions are preferred for oral products, the formation of a w/o emulsion in this case may create a compounding problem.

F. Natural non-ionic surfactants

1. These include fatty acid alcohols, such as stearyl alcohol and cetyl alcohol, wool fat or wool wax and its derivatives, wool alcohols and cholesterol, and derivatives of other natural waxes, such as spermaceti and cetyl esters wax (synthetic spermaceti). These are available as fractions of the natural products or their synthetic versions.

2. Some of the natural waxes, such as wool wax, Lanolin USP (wool fat, the waxlike substance from the wool of sheep, that has been cleaned, decolorized, and deodorized), Modified Lanolin USP (wool fat that has been processed to reduce the contents of free lanolin alcohols and detergent and pesticide residues), and hydrous lanolin (hydrous wool fat) and its synthetic version Hydrophilic Petrolatum USP are complex mixtures of oils, waxes, and emulsifiers (6). The purified emulsifying agents in Hydrophilic Petrolatum are the non-ionic emulsifiers stearyl alcohol and cholesterol. Lanolin and hydrous lanolin contain mixtures of similar natural emulsifiers. All are capable of absorbing water to form w/o emulsions. These are discussed in more detail in Chapter 23, Ointment Bases.

3. Although the purified fractions and their synthetic counterparts may be used to produce w/o emulsions, they are also commonly used as auxiliary emulsifiers to stabilize o/w emulsions when a powerful o/w emulsifying agent, such as a detergent, is present as the primary emulsifier. An example of such a system is the o/w cream Hydrophilic Ointment USP (6). In this product, sodium lauryl sulfate is the primary emulsifier, with stearyl alcohol as the auxiliary emulsifying agent.

G. Synthetic non-ionic surfactants

1. These are complex esters and ester-ethers, derived from polyols, alkylene oxides, fatty acids, and fatty alcohols. The hydrophilic portion of these molecules consists of free hydroxyl and oxyethylene groups. The lipophilic part has long-chain hydrocarbons of fatty acids and fatty alcohols. Although they are given a chemical designation based on the primary component, these are actually complex mixtures of closely related derivatives. For example, sorbitan monooleate, also known as *Span 80*, is a mixture, but the primary component is sorbitan monooleate. Polysorbate 80 (Tween 80) is polyoxyethylene 20 sorbitan monooleate; the 20 indicates that there are approximately 20 moles of ethylene oxide for each mole of sorbitol and sorbitol anhydride. Commonly used non-ionic surfactants include various Spans, Tweens, Arlacels, and Myrjs.

2. Non-ionic surfactants have the following characteristics in common:
   a. They are neutral compounds that are stable over a wide pH range.
   b. They are relatively insensitive to the presence of high concentrations of electrolytes.
   c. They are heat stable.
   d. Because these compounds do not possess significant innate ability as viscosity-inducing agents, depending on the water–oil phase ratio and the melting point of the oil phase,

emulsions made with these agents may require auxiliary viscosity-inducing agents or a viscous vehicle for the external phase.

   e. Non-ionic surfactants are mixed in various proportions to give either w/o or o/w emulsions. The appropriate amounts of individual emulsifiers needed to form a specific emulsion type can be determined using a mathematic system called the *HLB system*. This system assigns numeric values to fats and oils and to emulsifiers based on the relative amounts of hydrophilic and lipophilic portions present in these molecules. Examples of the calculation and use of the HLB system can be found in Chapter 29, Liquid Emulsions.

H. Amphoteric or zwitterionic surfactants

   1. These surfactants can be anionic, cationic, or non-ionic in solution, depending on the acidity or pH of the water. They are usually mild, making some of them particularly suited for use in pharmaceutical products and preparations.

   2. An amphoteric surfactant frequently used in pharmaceutical dosage forms is Lecithin NF, a complex mixture of phosphatides, mainly phosphatidyl choline (8). Two major sources of the phosphatides are egg yolks and soya beans. Lecithins are mainly used as dispersing, elmulsifying, and stabilizing agents (10). Lecithin is often included in injectable products, especially parenteral nutrition solutions. Therapeutically, lecithin and derivatives have been used as pulmonary surfactants. Lecithin also forms a component of the bilayers of liposomes (3).

   3. Lecithin is a major component of Pluronic (poloxamer) lecithin organogel (PLO gel). This transdermal vehicle is used by compounding pharmacists to administer medications through the skin when the medication is to be absorbed through the skin for almost immediate effect. This use is illustrated with Sample Prescription 30.7 in Chapter 30.

REFERENCES

1. Sinko PJ. Martin's physical pharmacy and pharmaceutical sciences, 5th ed. Baltimore, MD: Lippincott Williams & Wilkins, 2006; 446–447.
2. Bummer PM. Interfacial phenomena. In: University of the Sciences in Philadelphia, ed. Remington: The science and practice of pharmacy, 21st ed. Baltimore, MD: Lippincott Williams & Wilkins, 2005; 280–292.
3. Bowman BJ, Ofner CM, Schott H. Colloidal dispersions. In: University of the Sciences in Philadelphia, ed. Remington: The science and practice of pharmacy, 21st ed. Baltimore, MD: Lippincott Williams & Wilkins, 2005; 293–318.
4. Swarbrick J, Rubino JT, Rubino OP. Coarse dispersion. In: University of the Sciences in Philadelphia, ed. Remington: The science and practice of pharmacy, 21st ed. Baltimore, MD: Lippincott Williams & Wilkins, 2005; 319–337.
5. Spalton LM. Pharmaceutical emulsions and emulsifying agents. Brooklyn, NY: Chemical Publishing, Inc., 1950; 4–6.
6. The United States Pharmacopeial Convention, Inc. USP monographs. 2007 USP 30/NF 25. Rockville, MD: Author, 2006.
7. The United States Pharmacopeial Convention, Inc. Chapter ⟨1151⟩. 2007 USP 30/NF 25. Rockville, MD: Author, 2006; 623.
8. The United States Pharmacopeial Convention, Inc. Front matter—NF: Excipients. 2007 USP 30/NF 25. Rockville, MD: Author, 2006.
9. Ecanow B. Liquid medications. In: King RE, ed. Dispensing of medications, 9th ed. Easton, PA: Mack Publishing Co., 1984; 112–113.
10. Rowe R, Sheskey P, Weller P, eds. Handbook of pharmaceutical excipients, 5th ed. Washington, DC: APhA Publications, 2005.

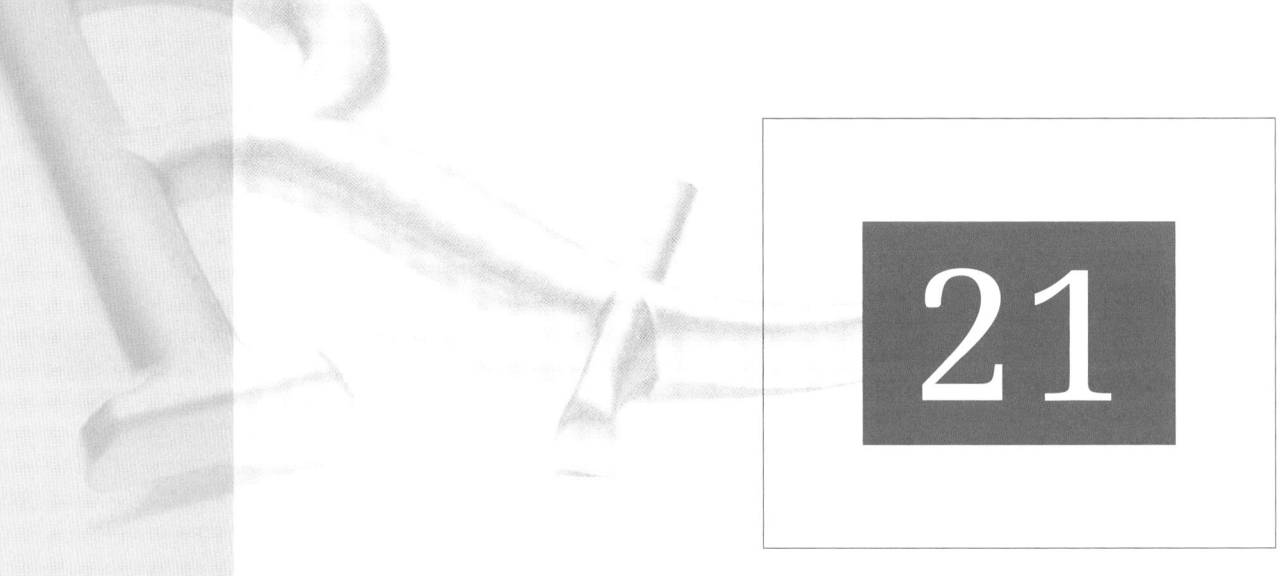

21

Colors, Flavors, Sweeteners, and Scents

Melgardt de Villiers, PhD

I. COLORS

A. Technically, a color additive is any dye, pigment, or substance that can impart color when added or applied to a food, drug, or cosmetic or to the human body.

B. Colors are substances added to drug products and preparations solely for imparting color.
1. They must be nontoxic and inactive pharmacologically.
2. Color additives that are permitted for general use may not be used in the area of the eye or in injections unless such use is specified in the color additive listing regulation. (1,2).
3. The use of colors must follow FDA regulations (1).
4. They should not be employed to disguise poor product quality.

C. Colors are added to improve patient acceptance of a product or preparation.
1. The color added to an oral dosage form is usually selected to coincide with or complement the flavor given to the preparation. For example, cherry-flavored preparations are usually colored red, orange-flavored preparations are colored orange, and mint-flavored preparations may be green or white.
2. Flesh-toned colors may be added to topical preparations so that the preparation blends with the color of the skin and is less visible.
3. Color matters because it is functional and subliminally and overtly communicates information and provides many other operational benefits. Viagra, a diamond-shaped blue pill, was introduced in 1997 and immediately became an overnight sensation. In 2002, the marketing groups of a rival product, Levitra, brainstormed the issue of color for their brand. Extensive market research found that consumers thought that the blue color was too cool and was equated with being sick. For this reason, Levitra's manufacturers made Levitra's color orange, an extremely vibrant and energetic color.

D. The colors used in pharmaceutical dosage forms are either natural colors or synthetic dyes.
1. Two main categories make up the FDA's list of permitted color additives (2). Certifiable color additives are human-made, derived primarily from petroleum and coal sources. Examples are

Table 21.1	COLOR ADDITIVES APPROVED FOR USE IN DRUG PRODUCTS BUT SUBJECT TO BATCH CERTIFICATION

COLOR	USES AND RESTRICTIONS
FD&C Blue No. 1	Ingested and externally applied drugs, including around the eye
FD&C Blue No. 2	Ingested drugs
D&C Blue No. 4	Externally applied drugs
FD&C Green No. 3	Drugs generally
D&C Green No. 5	Drugs generally, including area around eye
D&C Green No. 6	Externally applied drugs
D&C Green No. 8	Externally applied drugs [NTE 0.01% (by weight)]
D&C Orange No. 4	Externally applied drugs
D&C Orange No. 5	Externally applied drugs, including mouthwashes (NTE 5 mg/daily dose of drug)
D&C Orange No. 10 and 11	Externally applied drugs
FD&C Red No. 3	Ingested drugs
FD&C Red No. 4	Externally applied drugs
D&C Red No. 17	Externally applied drugs
D&C Red No. 21 to 30	Drugs generally
D&C Red No. 31	Externally applied drugs
D&C Red No. 33	Ingested drugs (NTE 0.75 mg/daily dose of drug); externally applied drugs, including mouthwashes and dentifrices
D&C Red No. 34	Externally applied drugs
D&C Red No. 36	Ingested drugs (NTE 1.7 mg/daily dose for drugs taken less than 1 yr; NTE 1.0 mg/daily dose for drugs taken more than 1 yr); externally applied drugs
D&C Red No. 39	Quaternary ammonium type germicidal solutions for external application (NTE 0.1% w/w of finished drug product)
FD&C Red No. 40	Drugs generally, including area around eye
D&C Violet No. 2	Externally applied drugs
FD&C Yellow No. 5	Ingested drugs generally; externally applied drugs, including around eye
FD&C Yellow No. 6	Drugs generally
D&C Yellow No. 7 and 8	Externally applied drugs
D&C Yellow No. 10	Drugs generally with some modification of uses and restrictions
D&C Yellow No. 11	Externally applied drugs

NTE, not to exceed.
Source: U.S. Department of Health & Human Services, U.S. Food & Drug Administration, Center for Food Safety & Applied Nutrition. Food Ingredients and Packaging. Summary of Color Additives Listed for Use in the United States in Food, Drugs, Cosmetics, and Medical Devices. http://www.cfsan.fda.gov/~dms/opa-col2.html#table2A; FDA Consumer Health Information/U.S. Food and Drug Administration. December 10, 2007. How Safe Are Color Additives? www.fda.gov/consumer/updates/coloradditives121007.html.

listed in Table 21.1. Other color additives are "exempt" from batch certification. These are obtained largely from plant, animal, or mineral sources. Examples such as caramel color and grape color extract are listed in Table 21.2.

2. Approval of a color additive for one intended use does not mean approval for other uses. For example, no color additives have been approved for injection (2).

3. Natural colors that are used in drug products and preparations fall into two classes: mineral pigments and plant pigments.
   a. Examples of mineral pigments include red ferric oxide, titanium oxide, and carbon black. Red ferric oxide is the red component that, when added to white zinc oxide powder, gives the pink-colored powder calamine. Titanium oxide is a white pigment that is often added to oral or topical preparations and cosmetics. It is also used in tablet coatings and in capsule shells to render them opaque.
   b. Plant pigments include colors such as indigo, saffron, and beta-carotene.

4. Synthetic dyes
   a. As their name indicates, synthetic dyes are chemically synthesized. The first dyes of this sort were synthesized from aniline; because aniline was extracted from coal tar, this whole class of colors is often referred to either as aniline dyes or coal tar dyes.
   b. Synthetic dyes owe their colors to the presence of certain unsaturated groups called *chromophores*. Often conjugation of unsaturated systems is a requirement for color. The color of

Table 21.2	COLOR ADDITIVES APPROVED FOR USE IN DRUG PRODUCTS AND EXEMPT FROM BATCH CERTIFICATION
COLOR	**USES AND RESTRICTIONS**
Alumina [dried Al(OH)$_3$]	Drugs generally
Annatto extract	Ingested drugs generally; external drugs, including eye area use
Calcium carbonate	Drugs generally
Canthaxanthin	Ingested drugs generally
Caramel	Ingested and topically applied drugs generally
β-Carotene	Ingested drugs generally; external drugs, including eye area use
Cochineal extract	Ingested and externally applied drugs
Chlorophyllin-copper complex	Dentifrices that are drugs; NTE 0.1%
Dihydroxyacetone	Externaxternally applied drugs intended solely or in part to impart a color to the human body
Bismuth oxychloride	Externally applied drugs, including eye area use
Synthetic iron oxide	Ingested or topically applied drugs; ingested dosage by humans NTE 5 mg/day (as Fe)
Ferric ammonium ferrocyanide	Externally applied drugs, including eye area use
Ferric ferrocyanide	Externally applied drugs, including eye area use
Chromium hydroxide green	Externally applied drugs, including eye area use
Chromium oxide greens	Externally applied drugs, including eye area use
Guanine	Externally applied drugs, including eye area use
Mica-based pearlescent pigments	Ingested drugs NTE 3%; iron NTE 55 wt %
Pyrophyllite	Externally applied drugs
Mica	Externally applied drugs, including eye area use
Talc	Drugs generally
Titanium dioxide	Drugs generally, including eye area use
Aluminum powder	Externally applied drugs, including eye area use
Bronze powder	Externally applied drugs, including eye area use
Copper powder	Externally applied drugs, including eye area use
Zinc oxide	Externally applied drugs, including eye area use

NTE, not to exceed.
Source: U.S. Department of Health & Human Services, U.S. Food & Drug Administration, Center for Food Safety & Applied Nutrition. Food Ingredients and Packaging. Summary of Color Additives Listed for Use in the United States in Food, Drugs, Cosmetics, and Medical Devices. http://www.cfsan.fda.gov/~dms/opa-col2.html#table2A; FDA Consumer Health Information/U.S. Food and Drug Administration. December 10, 2007. How Safe Are Color Additives? www.fda.gov/consumer/updates/coloradditives121007.html.

the dye or its intensity can be altered by the presence of other groups called *auxochromes* (3).

c. Dyes used in foods, drugs, and cosmetics must be certified by the FDA for such use, because the Federal Food, Drug, & Cosmetic (FD&C) Act of 1938 made food color additive certification mandatory and transferred the authority for its testing from the USDA to the FDA. To avoid confusing color additives used in food with those manufactured for other uses, three categories of certifiable color additives were created:

  (1) Food, Drug, and Cosmetic (FD&C)—color additives with application in foods, drugs, or cosmetics;

  (2) Drug and Cosmetic (D&C)—color additives with applications in drugs or cosmetics;

  (3) External Drug and Cosmetic (External D&C)—color additives with applications in externally applied pharmaceutical dosage forms (e.g., ointments) and in externally applied cosmetics.

d. It is important to keep abreast of the current legal status of dyes used in drug products and preparations, because changes do occur. This is illustrated with the following examples.

  (1) Amaranth, formerly certified FD&C Red #2, was at one time used extensively in processed food products and was the most frequently used dye in compounding pharmaceutical preparations. In 1976, it was banned from use in foods, drugs, and cosmetics.

  (2) For prescription drugs for human use containing FD&C Yellow No. 5 that are administered orally, nasally, vaginally, or rectally, or for use in the area of the eye, the labeling shall bear the warning statement, "This product contains FD&C Yellow No. 5 (tartrazine),

Table 21.3	STABILITY OF SOME FD&C CERTIFIED DYES TO VARIOUS FACTORS THAT MAY INFLUENCE THEIR COLOR STABILITY IN PHARMACEUTICAL PREPARATIONS					
FD&C CERTIFIED DYES	**ACID**	**ALKALI**	**LIGHT**	**REDUCING AGENTS**	**OXIDIZING AGENTS**	**pH VALUE**[a]
FD&C Blue #1 (Brilliant Blue)	Moderate	Moderate	Good	Good	Poor	4.9–5.6
FD&C Blue #2 (Indigo Carmine)	Good	Moderate	Poor	Moderate	Poor	8.5
FD&C Green #3 (Fast Green FCF)	Good	Poor	Good	Good	Poor	4.2–5.8
FD&C Red #3 (Erythrosine)	Poor	Good	Fair	Moderate	Fair	7.7
FD&C Yellow #5 (Tartrazine)	Good	Good	Good	Poor	Fair	6.8
FD&C Yellow #6 (Sunset Yellow FCF)	Good	Good	Good	Poor	Fair	6.6
FD&C Red #40	Good	Good	Good	Poor	Fair	7.3

[a]pH values of 1% aqueous solutions (or suspensions).
Source: Adapted from Booth RE, Dale JK. Compounding and dispensing information. In: King RE, ed. Dispensing of medications, 9th ed. Easton, PA: Mack Publishing Co., 1984; 397.

which may cause allergic-type reactions (including bronchial asthma) in certain susceptible persons. Although the overall incidence of FD&C Yellow No. 5 (tartrazine) sensitivity in the general population is low, it is frequently seen in patients who also have aspirin hypersensitivity" (4). This warning statement must appear in the precautions section of the labeling.

(3) The labeling for over-the-counter and prescription drug products intended for human use administered orally, nasally, rectally, or vaginally containing FD&C Yellow No. 6 shall specifically declare the presence of FD&C Yellow No. 6 by listing it using the name FD&C Yellow No. 6 (4).

e. Dyes may be affected by changes in pH, and most are labile to either oxidation or reduction reactions. These changes may affect the dye's solubility and its color or hue or may destroy its color all together. Table 21.3 lists several water-soluble FD&C certified dyes that are currently available from vendors of compounding drugs and chemicals. The table shows factors that affect the stability of each of these dyes (5). This information is helpful in selecting a particular dye for a dosage form being prepared.

5. Recommended dye concentrations for drug preparation
   a. Appropriate concentrations of dye can best be determined by trial. The following general guidelines may be helpful.
   b. Liquids
      (1) The concentration of dye needed to impart a satisfactory color to a liquid drug preparation is so small that it is usually most convenient to make a stock solution of the dye and use a dropper or 1-mL syringe to measure the desired quantity.
      (2) Color may develop with a concentration of 0.001% to 0.0005%; a tint may result with a concentration as low as 0.0001% (3).
      (3) Rather than purchasing powdered dyes, some pharmacists find it more convenient to buy food coloring from the grocery store. These colors are FD&C approved and may be used for drug preparations. Their stability in the preparation, however, cannot be predicted unless the exact dye is specified on the label. Some labels do give this information.
   c. Powders
      A concentration of approximately 0.1% would give a pastel color to white powders (3). The dye should be incorporated using geometric dilution and trituration. Certifiable powder color additives are available as either "dyes" or "lakes." Dyes dissolve in water and are manufactured as powders, granules, liquids, or other special-purpose forms. Lakes are the water-insoluble form of the dye. Lakes are more stable than dyes and are ideal for coloring preparations containing fats and oils or items lacking sufficient moisture to dissolve dyes.

II.   FLAVORS AND SWEETENERS

A. Although intuitively we all know what flavor is, this characteristic is difficult to adequately define and quantify in precise terms. This is because flavor embodies a group of sensations including taste, smell, touch, sight, and even sound.

B. The human tongue has 10,000 taste buds. This means that even a single sensation such as taste is difficult to describe: Although the four primary tastes are sweet, sour, salty, and bitter, even a combination of these taste types could never be expected to describe the taste of a ripe strawberry or a frosty glass of root beer.

C. Flavors and sweeteners are added to oral dosage forms to improve patient acceptance of the preparation. Selecting a desirable flavor for a compounded drug preparation is important because patient compliance with a medication regimen may depend on the flavor of the drug preparation. This is especially true with children.

1. Flavors may be added to improve the palatability of a bland preparation or to mask the unpleasant taste of an active ingredient. Bitter is the most objectionable taste to patients and is, unfortunately, the most common taste for drugs.

2. As with coloring, determining the type and amount of flavor and sweetener is best done by trial.

3. When possible, selection of flavoring for a drug preparation should be done in consultation with the patient.

    a. Flavor preference is somewhat age-related. Children tend to prefer sweet, fruity, and bubblegum-type flavors, whereas adults often favor such flavors as chocolate, coffee, licorice, maple, or butterscotch.

    b. Flavors are also a matter of personal preference; for example, some patients love the taste of chocolate, whereas others dislike it. Although a certain flavor may do the best job of masking a particular drug taste, it is not useful if the intended patient dislikes that flavor.

    c. Be aware that some patients associate bitter taste with drug potency and effectiveness.

    d. Always check with patients for possible allergy to specific flavors.

4. Flavors are also often used to make medicines tasty for animals. For example, for birds, grape, molasses, orange, pina colada, and tutti-frutti are considered the best. For cats, beef, butterscotch, cheese, chicken, liver, molasses, peanut butter, salmon, sardine, and tuna seem most appropriate. Dogs prefer beef, cheese, chicken, liver, marshmallow, molasses, peanut butter, raspberry, and strawberry. Horses like alfalfa-, apple-, blue grass-, caramel-, cherry-, molasses-, and clover-flavored medications. Many exotic pets also prefer specific flavors. Ferrets like foods that taste like fish, fruits, and molasses, while gerbils, iguanas, and rabbits prefer fruit- or vegetable-flavored items (6).

D. It is useful to recognize that there are some correlations between certain chemical types and the four primary tastes.

1. Sour taste is the result of H+ ions and is proportional to the hydrogen ion concentration and the compound's lipid solubility (3). Therefore, obviously, acids and phenols would generally exhibit sour tastes, but tannins, alum, and lactones are also reported to have this characteristic (3).

2. Salty tastes are associated with inorganic or low-molecular-weight ionic compounds, such as sodium chloride (thus the name "salt"), ammonium chloride, potassium gluconate, and sodium salicylate.

3. When one of the ions in a salt is a high-molecular-weight compound, such as diphenhydramine HCl, the taste is usually bitter. Free bases and amides such as caffeine, amphetamine, and codeine are also bitter.

4. Sweetness is most often associated with the low-molecular-weight polyhydroxy compounds, such as sucrose, sorbitol, and mannitol, but various other groups may give intensely sweet compounds. Imides such as saccharin, amino acid combinations such as those in aspartame, and some chlorinated sugars such as sucralose are very sweet; these structure-activity relationships are unpredictable and, in fact, these compounds, widely used as sweeteners, were discovered by accident.

5. Unsaturation in organic compounds may give sharp, burning tastes (3).

E. Methods of improving the palatability of oral preparations (3,7)

1. Blending

    a. Blended flavors often give improved taste. For example, Compound Orange Spirit, which is illustrated later, is a blend that has been found to give a pleasant flavor.

    b. Try to select a flavor that either blends with or is associated with the drug taste or type. Further improvement may be achieved by then adding a sweetener or blending in another complementary flavor.

    (1) A sour drug tastes best when flavored with a citrus or fruity flavor plus an added sweetener.

(2) Antacids are most often associated with mint flavor, so this would be a good choice for this type of preparation. The flavor will be improved further by adding a sweetener.

(3) Bitter taste can often be improved by adding a salty, sweet, or sour flavor.

2. Masking or overshadowing

a. To cover up the taste of the drug, add a flavor and/or sweetener that has an intense, long-lasting taste. Peppermint, wintergreen (methyl salicylate), and licorice (glycyrrhiza) are examples of compounds of this type.

b. Up to a point, increasing the concentration of a flavor or sweetener increases the intensity of its flavor.

3. Physical

a. Because solubility is a requirement for taste, a bad-tasting drug can be rendered tasteless by using an insoluble form of the drug or by precipitating the drug from solution by altering the pH or the solvent system of the drug preparation.

b. Oils can be emulsified; for example, castor oil emulsions are much more palatable than is liquid castor oil.

c. A viscous vehicle can be used to reduce the contact of the drug with the taste buds on the tongue.

4. Chemical

Chemical methods are used most frequently in drug product manufacturing. In this case, the drug may be complexed, a pro-drug can be made, and so on.

5. Physiologic

a. The addition of an extremely small quantity of an anesthetizing agent can be used. Examples include menthol, peppermint oil, and sodium phenolate.

b. Effervescence can be added to the preparation or the patient may be instructed to take the medication with a carbonated beverage. Carbon dioxide anesthetizes the taste buds.

c. The preparation can be stored in the refrigerator. Cold both reduces the intensity of disagreeable tastes and anesthetizes the taste buds.

6. Certain flavors are also suggested for specific drugs classes (7): for antibiotics, cherry, maple, pineapple, orange; for antihistamines, apricot, cherry, cinnamon, grape, and honey; for decongestants and expectorants, anise, apricot, butterscotch, and cherry; and for electrolyte and geriatric solutions, cherry, grape, and lemon-lime (8). Mint and marshmallow are the best flavors for metallic-tasting drugs such as ibuprofen.

F. Sweeteners

1. Table 21.4 gives the articles listed as sweetening agents in the *USP 30/NF 25* (9). Although this list is representative of the most commonly used agents, it is not a complete list of all agents used as sweeteners in foods and in drug products and preparations. The *Handbook of Pharmaceutical Excipients* lists and describes a number of other compounds used by manufacturers and pharmacists (10). The *Food Chemicals Codex* (FCC) is also a good source of information. In 2007, it was acquired by USP from the Institute of Medicine; starting in 2008, a new edition will be published every 2 years. Some very nice natural sweeteners, such as stevia powder, are available from some pharmaceutical vendors and health food stores.

2. Desirable properties of sweeteners include being colorless, odorless, and soluble in water at the concentration needed for sweetness; having a pleasant taste with no bitter aftertaste; and being chemically stable at normal temperatures of use and storage, stable over a broad pH range, noncarcinogenic, and nontoxic. The sweetness of selected sweeteners relative to sugar is listed in Table 21.5.

3. Polyhydroxy compounds

Note: The solubilities and descriptions given in this section are abstracted from Remington's *The Science and Practice of Pharmacy* (3), *The Merck Index* (11), and other references as cited. As noted in previous Chapters of Part 4, this text uses the convention of upper-case first letters for official USP-NF article and lower-case first letters for words designating the chemical substances.

a. Sucrose NF

(1) Description: colorless or white crystals or powder; odorless; sweet taste; neutral to litmus

(2) Solubility: 1 g/0.5 mL water, 170 mL alcohol, less than 0.2 mL boiling water

(3) Available as pure crystals or powder, as Syrup NF (described in Chapter 22, Vehicles for Liquid Preparations), and as Confectioner's Sugar NF, which is 96% sucrose mixed with cornstarch in a fine, white powder (12).

b. Sorbitol NF

(1) Description: white powder, granules, or flakes; hygroscopic; odorless; neutral to litmus

(2) Solubility: 1 g/0.45 mL water; slightly soluble in alcohol

(3) Sweetness: approximately 0.5 to 0.7 times as sweet as sucrose (13)

Table 21.4	*USP* AND *NF* EXCIPIENTS CATEGORIZED AS FLAVORS, PERFUMES, AND SWEETENING AGENTS

FLAVORS AND PERFUMES	SWEETENING AGENTS
Almond Oil	Acesulfame Potassium
Anethole	Aspartame
Benzaldehyde	Aspartame Acesulfame
Ethyl Acetate	Dextrates
Ethyl Vanillin	Dextrose
Lactitol	Dextrose Excipient
Maltol	Erythritol
Menthol	Fructose
Methyl Salicylate	Galactose
Monosodium Glutamate	Maltitol
Peppermint	Maltose
Peppermint Oil	Mannitol
Peppermint Spirit	Saccharin
Rose Oil	Saccharin Calcium
Rose Water, Stronger	Saccharin Sodium
Thymol	Sorbitol
Vanillin	Sorbitol Solution
	Sucralose
	Sucrose
	Sugar, Compressible
	Sugar, Confectioner's
	Syrup
	Tagatose

Source: The United States Pharmacopeial Convention, Inc. Front matter—NF: Excipients. 2007 USP 30/NF 25. Rockville, MD: Author, 2006.

(4) Available as powder or as the 70% Sorbitol Solution USP (described in Chapter 22, Vehicles for Liquid Preparations)

(5) When vigorously mixed with liquid Polyethylene Glycol (e.g., PEG 300 or 400), a waxy, water-soluble gel with a melting point of 35° to 40°C may result (10).

   c. Mannitol USP

(1) Description: white, crystalline powder or granules; odorless; neutral to litmus

(2) Solubility: 1 g/5.5 mL water, 83 mL alcohol, 18 mL glycerin

(3) Sweetness: approximately 0.7 times as sweet as sucrose; very smooth "mouth feel" (13)

(4) For nonsterile products and preparations, mannitol is available as powder and as granules. It is also available as a sterile injection in concentrations ranging from 5% to 25%,

Table 21.5	SWEETNESS LEVELS OF SELECTED SWEETENERS

SWEETENER	SWEETNESS LEVEL RELATIVE TO SUGAR
Sorbitol	0.5%–0.7%
Mannitol	0.7%
Saccharin	60 mg equivalent to 30 g
Sodium Saccharin	300%
Aspartame	180%
Stevia	200%
Sucralose	600%
Maltitol	90%

Source: Reilly WJ. Pharmaceutical necessities. In: University of the Sciences in Philadelphia, ed. Remington: The science and practice of pharmacy, 21st ed. Baltimore, MD: Lippincott Williams & Wilkins, 2005; 1060–1069; Murphy DH. A practical compendium on sweetening agents. Am Pharm 1983; 23: 32–37; Cardello HMAB, Da Silva MAPA, Damasio MH. Measurement of the relative sweetness of stevia extract, aspartame and cyclamate/saccharin blend as compared to sucrose at different concentrations. Plant Foods Hum Nutr 1999; 54(2): 119–130.

which are used parenterally for the treatment of oliguria and to treat elevated intracranial and intraocular pressures. Incompatibilities of these solutions can be found in a current edition of *The Handbook of Injectable Drugs.*

(5) Mannitol is an isomer of sorbitol and, whereas sorbitol is hygroscopic, mannitol does not sorb water even at high relative humidity (10).

4. Saccharin compounds
    a. Saccharin NF
        (1) Description: white, odorless crystals or powder; solutions acid to litmus (pH = 2.0)
        (2) Solubility: 1 g/290 mL water, 31 mL alcohol, 25 mL boiling water, 50 mL glycerin
        (3) Sweetness: approximately 500 times as sweet as sucrose in dilute solution, with sweetness detectable at 1:100,000 concentration (11). Sixty milligrams is equivalent in sweetening power to 30 g of sucrose (3).
        (4) Available as powder, saccharin is used in a concentration of 0.02% to 0.5% (10).
    b. Saccharin Sodium USP (also known as *soluble saccharin*)
        (1) Description: white, odorless crystals or powder. The dihydrate effloresces; the pH of a 10% solution is reported to be 6.6 (10).
        (2) Solubility: 1 g/1.5 mL water, 50 mL alcohol, 3.5 mL propylene glycol
        (3) Sweetness: approximately 300 to 500 times as sweet as sucrose in dilute solution (11,13). A bitter aftertaste is noticeable at moderate to high concentration (13); approximately 25% of people using sodium saccharin at normal concentrations notice a metallic aftertaste (10).
        (4) Available as pure powder and the manufactured product Sweet 'N Low, which contains dextrose, cream of tartar, and calcium silicate for anticaking and to improve handling and flow properties. Sweet 'N Low is available in boxes of single-use packets as well as in bulk containers and 8-oz liquid bottles. It also comes in tablets, each weighing ¼ grain. The tablets come in a handy one-click dispenser containing 200 tablets. An official USP article, Saccharin Sodium Oral Solution, has a pH range of 3.0 to 5.0 (14).
        (5) Sodium saccharin has the advantage of high water solubility. In oral solutions and syrups, it is used in a concentration range of 0.04% to 0.6%. It is stable under normal conditions of compounding, storage, and use. It works synergistically with other sweeteners such as aspartame and cyclamates (10).
    c. Saccharin Calcium USP
        (1) Description: white, odorless crystals or powder
        (2) Solubility: 1 g/2.6 mL water, 4.7 mL alcohol
        (3) Sweetness: approximately 300 times as sweet as sucrose in dilute solution (3)
        (4) Available as powder
        (5) Calcium saccharin has the advantage of good solubility in both water and alcohol, so it is easy to use in both syrups and elixirs.
    d. Since 1974, when studies released by the Canadian Health Protection Branch linked saccharin to induction of bladder tumors in rats, there has been controversy about the safety of saccharin. Manufactured products or processed foods that contain saccharin must bear a warning about the possible carcinogenicity of this compound. It is generally thought that in moderate amounts, saccharin is safe for consumption. The Joint Food and Agriculture Organization/World Health Organization (FAO/WHO) Expert Committee on Food Additives recommends 2.5 mg/kg as an acceptable daily intake for saccharin or one of its salts (8).

5. Aspartame NF
    a. Aspartame is a chemical combination of two amino acids, L-aspartic acid and L-phenylalanine in its methyl ester form. Both amino acids are found in regular protein foods. Neither is sweet by itself (13).
    b. Description: white, odorless powder. The pH of a 0.8% solution is 4.5 to 6.0 (10). Aspartame is available as the pure powder and as the manufactured product Equal, which contains dextrose and maltodextrin as diluents for improved handling and flow properties.
    c. Solubility: slightly soluble in water, 1 g/100 mL, with increased solubility in acidic solutions (13); slightly soluble in alcohol (10). Diluents or other excipients in commercial products may have more limited water solubility.
    d. Sweetness: Aspartame is approximately 180 times as sweet as sucrose (13, 15). It works synergistically with other sweeteners such as saccharin (10).
    e. Aspartame is not stable to heat (e.g., heat sterilization, baking in an oven).
    f. Because aspartame contains phenylalanine, it should not be used by phenylketonurics (people with an inherited inability to metabolize phenylalanine).

6. Acesulfame Potassium NF
   a. Description: colorless, odorless crystalline powder with good stability both in solid state and aqueous solution; pH = 3 to 3.5 (10). It is available as the pure powder and as a manufactured product, brand names Sunette/Sweet One, which contains dextrose, cream of tartar, and calcium silicate for anticaking and to improve handling and flow properties.
   b. Solubility: soluble in water, 1 g/ 3.7 mL, but only 1 g/1,000 mL alcohol (10)
   c. Sweetness: an intense sweetening agent 180 to 200 times sweeter than sugar (10)
   d. Critics of the use of acesulfame potassium say the chemical may be carcinogenic, although these claims have been dismissed by the U.S. FDA (16).

7. Sucralose NF
   a. Sucralose is a nonnutritive, high-intensity sweetener made from the chlorination of sucrose with the resulting replacement of 3 hydroxyl (−OH) groups with chlorine (−Cl) atoms on the sucrose molecule (11).
   b. Description: a free-flowing, white crystalline powder. The manufactured product Splenda contains maltodextrin and dextrose as diluents to give the powder improved flow properties and a volume for measurement approximately that of table sugar.
   c. Solubility: water-soluble (17)
   d. Sweetness: on average, about 600 times sweeter than sugar (17)
   e. In determining the safety of sucralose, the FDA reviewed data from more than 110 studies in humans and animals. No toxic effects were found, and the FDA's approval is based on its finding that sucralose is safe for human consumption (18).

8. Maltitol NF
   a. Maltitol is a sugar alcohol (a polyol) used as a sugar substitute (19,20).
   b. It is used to replace table sugar because it has fewer calories (maltitol = 2.1 calories per gram; sugar = 4.0 calories per gram), does not promote tooth decay, and has a somewhat lesser effect on blood glucose.
   c. Maltitol is unique because it not only tastes like sugar but also acts like sugar and provides bulk or volume like sugar. Hence, it is used as a direct cup-for-cup replacement for sugar.

G. **Flavors**
   1. Table 21.4 gives the articles listed as flavors and perfumes in the *USP 30/NF 25* (9).
      a. Although this list is representative of some commonly used agents, it is not a very complete list of flavors used in foods and in drug products and preparations.
      b. *Remington's The Science and Practice of Pharmacy* has a more complete list of flavoring agents and has monograph descriptions for a number of compounds used by manufacturers and pharmacists (3). The *Food Chemicals Codex* also has extensive information on flavors.
   2. A wide variety of flavor concentrates are available from numerous sources.
      a. Vendors of compounding drugs and chemicals are a good source of flavors. Catalogs from some of these companies have long lists of available flavor concentrates; some companies even offer special flavors, such as beef, liver, and fish, which are intended for compounding for animals. Some of the concentrates indicate that they can be used at concentrations of 0.2% to 0.5%.
      b. Food stores, including grocery stores and stores that specialize in supplies for baking and candy making, are another source of flavors.
      c. Some pharmaceutical suppliers also specialize in marketing flavors and scents for compounding. One such company is LorAnn Oil (http://www.lorannoils.com/).
   3. Most flavors are available either as oils (e.g., lemon oil, orange oil) or as alcoholic concentrates. If an oil is to be added to an aqueous solution, it must be solubilized first by adding it to alcohol, glycerin, propylene glycol, or a similar solvent that is approved for oral use.
   4. Often blended flavors give improved taste. Two examples of blended flavors are Compound Orange Spirit NF and Compound Cardamom Tincture NF. The formula given here for Compound Orange Spirit (12) illustrates this type of flavoring agent.

Orange Oil	200 mL
Lemon Oil	50 mL
Coriander Oil	20 mL
Anise Oil	5 mL
Alcohol, a sufficient quantity to make	1,000 mL

III.   SCENTS

A. Scents may be added to topical preparations to improve their aesthetic appeal.

B. As stated earlier, Table 21.4 gives the articles listed as flavors and perfumes in the *USP 30/NF 25* (9).

C. Two readily available scents are

    1. Methyl Salicylate NF, which is synthetic oil of wintergreen.

    2. Rose scent, which is available in a variety of forms.

        a. The official forms are Rose Oil NF, which is a colorless or light yellow oil, and Stronger Rose Water NF, which is a saturated solution of Rose Oil in water. Stronger Rose Water can be diluted with an equal volume of Purified Water to make Rose Water (12).

        b. Vendors of compounding supplies may also have rose scent available as artificial rose oil and/or soluble rose fluid.

D. As stated previously, some pharmaceutical suppliers specialize in marketing flavors and scents for compounding.

REFERENCES

1. U.S. Department of Health & Human Services, U.S. Food & Drug Administration, Center for Food Safety & Applied Nutrition. Food ingredients and packaging. Summary of color additives listed for use in the United States in food, drugs, cosmetics, and medical devices. http://www.cfsan.fda.gov/~dms/opa-col2.html#table2A.

2. FDA Consumer Health Information/U.S. Food and Drug Administration. December 10, 2007. How Safe Are Color Additives? www.fda.gov/consumer/updates/coloradditives121007.html.

3. Reilly WJ. Pharmaceutical necessities. In: University of the Sciences in Philadelphia, ed. Remington: the science and practice of pharmacy, 21st ed. Baltimore, MD: Lippincott Williams & Wilkins, 2005; 1060–1069.

4. 21CFR201.20. Title 21, Volume 4. Revised as of April 1, 2002. Declaration of presence of FD&C Yellow No. 5 and/or FD&C Yellow No. 6 in certain drugs for human use.

5. Booth RE, Dale JK. Compounding and dispensing information. In: King RE, ed. Dispensing of medications, 9th ed. Easton, PA: Mack Publishing Co., 1984; 397.

6. Allen LV, Jr. Veterinary compounding. Secundum Artem. 7(2): http://www.paddocklabs.com/forms/secundum/volume_7_2.pdf.

7. Roy GM. Taste masking in oral pharmaceuticals. Pharm Technol 1994; 18: 84–99.

8. Ecanow B. Liquid medications. In: King RE, ed. Dispensing of medications, 9th ed. Easton, PA: Mack Publishing Co., 1984; 126–127

9. The United States Pharmacopeial Convention, Inc. Front matter-NF: Excipients. 2007 USP 30/NF 25. Rockville, MD: Author, 2006.

10. Rowe R, Sheskey P, Weller P, eds. Handbook of pharmaceutical excipients, 5th ed. Washington, DC: APhA Publications, 2005.

11. O'Neil MJ, ed. The Merck index, 13th ed. Rahway, NJ: Merck & Co., Inc., 2001.

12. The United States Pharmacopeial Convention, Inc. NF monographs. 2007 USP 30/NF 25. Rockville, MD: Author, 2006.

13. Murphy DH. A practical compendium on sweetening agents. Am Pharm 1983; 23: 32–37.

14. The United States Pharmacopeial Convention, Inc. USP monographs. 2007 USP 30/NF 25. Rockville, MD: Author, 2006:

15. Cardello HMAB, Da Silva MAPA, Damasio MH. Measurement of the relative sweetness of stevia extract, aspartame and cyclamate/saccharin blend as compared to sucrose at different concentrations. Plant Foods Hum Nutr 1999; 54(2): 119–130.

16. Kroger M, Meister K, Kava R. Low-calorie sweeteners and other sugar substitutes: A review of the safety issues. Compr Rev Food Sci Food Safety 2006; 5(2): 35–47.

17. Grice HC, Goldsmith LA. Sucralose-an overview of the toxicity data. Food Chem Tox 2000; 238: S1–6.

18. Whitmore A. FDA talk paper. FDA approves new high-intensity sweetener sucralose. http://www.fda.gov/bbs/topics/ANSWERS/ANS00859.html.

19. Heume M, Rapaille A. Versatility of maltitol in different forms as a sugar substitute. In: Grenby TH, ed. Advances in sweeteners. New York: Springer Publshing Co, 1996; 85–108.

20. Kato K, Moskowitz AH. Maltitol. Food Sci Technol 2001; 112(Alternative Sweeteners): 283–295.

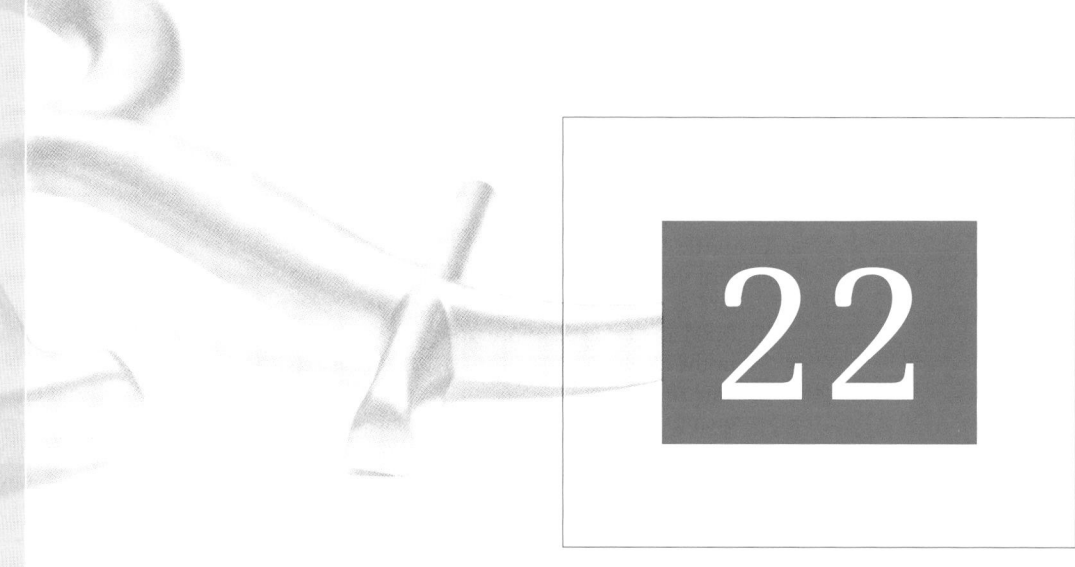

Vehicles for Liquid Preparations

Melgardt de Villiers, PhD

CHAPTER OUTLINE

Introduction

Vehicles for Oral Liquid Preparations

Vehicles for Topical Liquid Preparations

I. INTRODUCTION

A. A vehicle for a liquid dosage form may be a pharmaceutical solvent, a solution, an emulsion, or a suspension.

B. The desired or required properties of the vehicle depend on the route of administration for the preparation and the type of solvent system needed or desired. The definitions and descriptions of pharmaceutical solvents are given in Chapter 15. The various types of liquid systems, such as syrup, elixir, spirit, suspension, and emulsion, are given in Chapters 27 through 29, which discuss each individual liquid dosage form type. The ingredients used in liquid vehicles are described in Chapters 15 through 21.

C. This chapter discusses the general properties of liquid vehicles for oral and topical products and gives examples and descriptions of potential vehicles. For ease of use, the information in this chapter is divided into two sections: vehicles for oral use and vehicles for topical use.

D. As noted in previous chapters of Part 4, this text uses the convention of upper-case first letters for official *USP-NF* articles and lower-case first letters for words designating chemical substances or generic preparation.

II. VEHICLES FOR ORAL LIQUID PREPARATIONS

A. Restrictions

  1. Neonates (birth to 1 month): Add only the essentials.

    a. Alcohol and preservatives should not be added. The organ and enzyme systems of these tiny infants are not fully mature and do not metabolize alcohol and preservatives efficiently (1–5).

    b. Because colors, flavors, and sweeteners are not needed, they also should be avoided.

    c. Hypertonic solutions should not be used—that is, no concentrated sugar syrups, 70% sorbitol, and so on. The gastrointestinal (GI) tracts of neonates are delicate; there are reports of injury to the GI tracts of neonates caused by administration of hypertonic solutions (6–8).

    d. A 1% methylcellulose gel that is preservative-free is a suitable liquid vehicle for this age group.

2. Children: Use judgment based on the child's age; young infants are obviously more sensitive than are 6-year-olds.

    a. Use little to no alcohol (1,2). In practical terms, this means use the minimum amount of alcohol that is absolutely necessary for solubility purposes if a solution is needed. Do not use alcohol as a preservative when there are alternatives.

        (1) Food and Drug Administration recommendations for alcohol use in children are discussed in the alcohol section of Chapter 15, Pharmaceutical Solvents and Solubilizing Agents.

        (2) The American Academy of Pediatrics Committee on Drugs has recommended that the quantity of ethanol contained in a single dose of a drug product or preparation should not be able to cause a blood concentration greater than 25 mg/100 mL. The Academy's published article, "Ethanol in Liquid Preparations Intended for Children," gives equations and tables of values that allow prescribers and pharmacists to calculate the volumes and concentrations of preparations containing alcohol that will result in safe blood concentrations in children (1). An example of the use of this equation is given with Sample Prescription 31.2 in Chapter 31.

        (3) Alcohol content can be minimized even for solubility purposes by the addition of a less toxic solvent such as glycerin. For example, a recommended formula for phenobarbital elixir cuts down on the alcohol content by the addition of glycerin. This is illustrated with Example 37.5 and Table 37.7 in Chapter 37, Compatibility and Stability of Drug Products and Preparations.

    b. Preservatives are not contraindicated but, especially for infants, should be used only when necessary. In some cases, you may substitute refrigeration and a short beyond-use date for the preservative. If this is done, be certain that the caregiver understands the importance of proper storage conditions and the hazards associated with administering a preparation that has passed its beyond-use date.

3. Patients with restrictions based on allergies or medical or physiologic conditions

    a. Diabetics: no sugar; alcohol only if necessary and never with oral antidiabetic agents, such as chlorpropamide, which may give a disulfiram reaction

    b. Patients on a ketogenic diet: no carbohydrates, including maltodextrin (9), which is a filler in many nonsugar sweeteners

    c. Patients with nasogastric tubes: no restrictions, but there is no need to add auxiliary agents such as flavors, sweeteners, or colors

    d. Patients who are alcoholics or patients on a drug that gives a disulfiram reaction: no alcohol

B. Liquid vehicles prepared in the pharmacy

1. At one time, many pharmacies, particularly those in hospitals, made their own vehicles for compounding oral liquid dosage forms. Over the last few decades, many excellent liquid vehicles have become available commercially. These manufactured vehicles should be used when possible because they have well-tested formulations with generally longer expiration dates, and they are made with quality control processes that are difficult to duplicate in most pharmacies. Many of these commercial vehicles are described later in section II.C.

2. In some situations, a pharmacy-prepared liquid vehicle is needed. Examples include the following:

    a. Special formulation requirements exist. These might include vehicles that are preservative-free or carbohydrate-free, vehicles requiring a very low osmolarity or a particularly low or high pH, and vehicles that meet patient preferences for flavor, components, or vehicle consistency.

    b. A vehicle is needed immediately and the pharmacy does not have in stock the needed commercial product.

    c. A needed vehicle is temporarily not supplied by the manufacturer.

3. The following are some vehicles that can be made in the pharmacy when this is necessary. Some may be customized and made with or without preservatives, alcohol, flavors, and sweeteners. The first group of vehicles contain sucrose, the second group includes sugar-free vehicles and components, and the final section gives an anhydrous oral liquid vehicle. When the vehicle has a *USP* or *NF* monograph, a compounding procedure may be found in the official compendia, including the *USP Pharmacists' Pharmacopeia*.

4. Sucrose-containing oral vehicles

    a. Syrup NF (Simple Syrup) (10)

        (1) This saturated solution of sucrose in water is highly hypertonic. It is an 85% w/v or 65% w/w solution of sucrose in water. Its specific gravity is 1.3.

(2) It has the following formula (10):

Sucrose	85 g
Purified Water, a sufficient quantity to make	100 mL

This solution is most easily made by adding sucrose to boiling water, but the *NF* monograph describes a percolation method that does not use heat. If heat is used, care must be exercised to prevent caramelization of the sucrose.

(3) When made correctly, Syrup NF is fully saturated and self-preserving. However, if it is diluted in any way, it will support mold or other microbial growth. When Syrup is diluted in compounding, use precautions such as storage under refrigeration or addition of a preservative. The *NF* monograph states that it should contain a preservative unless it is used immediately after preparation (10). Syrup has a pH in the range of 5 to 7.

(4) It is available from pharmaceutical vendors, in which case it is preserved, usually with sodium benzoate or potassium sorbate. The paraben-propylene glycol preservative described in Chapter 16 is also an acceptable preservative.

(5) Syrup can be diluted to give liquid vehicles of various concentrations, and other ingredients, such as flavors may be added. It is more useful for compounding oral solutions than suspensions because it does not contain ingredients that provide the structure helpful for suspending particles in a suspension.

b. Citric Acid Syrup

(1) This syrup, also known as *Syrup of Lemon*, was formerly official in the *USP*. It contains 1 g of citric acid dissolved in 1 mL of Purified Water, 1 mL of Lemon Tincture, and Syrup sufficient to make 100 mL of preparation (11). Other artificial fruit flavors may be used in place of the Lemon Tincture.

(2) This syrup is useful when a vehicle with an acidic pH is needed, such as for drugs that need an acid vehicle for stability or solubility purposes. It has a pH of approximately 2.5.

(3) Like Syrup NF, Citric Acid Syrup is a saturated sucrose solution which is hypertonic and self-preserving unless diluted. Sodium benzoate and potassium sorbate are useful preservatives for this preparation.

c. Vehicle for Oral Solution NF (10)

(1) This is a sugar-based vehicle that is intended for making oral solutions. Like Syrup, it is not as well suited for making suspensions because it does not contain ingredients to provide the structure helpful for suspending particles in a suspension. It does contain both an antimicrobial preservative system and a buffer to maintain the pH at 4 to 5, a range favorable to the stability of many drugs. It has a content that is similar to that of the commercial vehicle Ora-Sweet.

(2) The official formula contains (10):

Sucrose	80 g
Glycerin	5 g
Sorbitol	5 g
Sodium Phosphate, Dibasic	120 mg
Citric Acid, Monohydrate	200 mg
Potassium Sorbate	100 mg
Methylparaben	100 mg
Purified Water, a sufficient quantity to make	100 mL

The vehicle can be prepared as follows: Place about 30 mL of Purified Water in a beaker that has been precalibrated at 100 mL. Heat the water to 70° to 75°C. Add the glycerin and methylparaben and stir well until the methylparaben is dissolved. Add the dibasic sodium phosphate, citric acid, potassium sorbate, and sorbitol to the beaker and mix thoroughly. Gradually add the sucrose with mixing until it is completely dissolved. Remove the beaker from the heat and allow the solution to cool. Add Purified Water to the calibration mark and mix well. Check the pH of the solution and adjust if necessary to within the range of 4 to 5 (10).

(3) The *NF* monograph instructs packaging this preparation in a tight, light-resistant container and storing at controlled room temperature; under these conditions, a beyond-use date of 6 months is recommended (10).

(4) Vehicle for Oral Solution, sometimes in combination with Vehicle for Oral Suspension NF (see section B. 5. C. (4) of this chapter) is a formulation component in many *USP* compounded oral liquid preparations.

d. Suspension Structured Vehicle NF (10)

(1) This vehicle has the advantage of including a preservative–buffer system and xanthan gum, an ingredient that confers some structure and makes this useful as a suspending vehicle for making suspensions. Its disadvantage is that it is more difficult to make than the simpler sucrose-based vehicles.

(2) The formula below is official in *NF 25* (10).

Potassium Sorbate	150 mg
Xanthan Gum	150 mg
Citric Acid, Anhydrous	150 mg
Sucrose	20 g
Purified Water, a sufficient quantity to make	100 mL

To prepare this vehicle, a temperature-controlled hot plate with a magnetic stirring device is very useful, although not essential. Place the potassium sorbate in a beaker pre-calibrated at 100 mL and add 50 mL of Purified Water to dissolve the potassium sorbate. Use the magnetic stirring device or manual stirring to create a vortex in the solution; then slowly sift the xanthan gum into the solution vortex. Using minimal heat (about 45°C), add the citric acid and the sucrose and stir to dissolve these and obtain a homogeneous mixture. Add Purified Water to the calibration mark and mix well.

(3) The *NF* monograph instructs packaging this preparation in a tight, light-resistant container, storing at controlled room temperature, and avoiding freezing; under these conditions, a beyond-use date of 30 days is recommended. Because this is a suspension, it should be labeled for the user to shake well before using (10).

e. Natural product flavored syrups

(1) Several other sucrose-containing syrup-type vehicles are official in the *NF*. These include Acacia Syrup, Cherry Syrup, Chocolate Syrup, Orange Syrup, and Tolu Balsam Syrup. Because these syrups contain natural juices and flavors as ingredients, they are best when freshly made. For example, the Orange Syrup monograph warns that it should not be used if it has a terebinthine odor or taste (10).

(2) These natural product syrups are very time-consuming to make; they require special procedures for crushing and expressing fruit and macerating natural plant materials. These procedures are well described in their *NF* monographs.

(3) Most patients, especially children, find these natural product vehicles to be less tasty than the manufactured artificially flavored fountain-type syrups. Furthermore, some of the natural components in these vehicles are subject to oxidative degradation and also have been known to cause some compatibility problems with some drugs. Still, "natural" syrups may be preferred and requested by some patients.

f. Vehicles containing alcohol

(1) Aromatic Elixir NF is useful when a sweetened, flavored, hydroalcoholic vehicle is needed. Also known as *Simple Elixir*, it contains approximately equal quantities of Syrup NF, Alcohol USP, and Purified Water. The original formula contained Compound Orange Spirit NF 1.2% for the flavoring agent. (The formula for this flavor is given in Chapter 21, Colors, Flavors, Sweeteners, and Scents.) The formula for Aromatic Elixir in more recent editions of *NF* simply lists "suitable essential oil(s)" (10). The final alcohol content of Aromatic Elixir is 21% to 23%. The ingredient list and procedure for making this elixir are in the *NF*.

(2) Iso-Alcoholic Elixir, also known as Iso-Elixir, was formerly official in the *NF*. It actually consists of two elixirs: Low-Alcoholic Elixir, which contains sucrose, glycerin, compound orange spirit, and 8% to 10% alcohol; and High-Alcoholic Elixir, which has saccharin in place of the sucrose and contains 73% to 78% alcohol. These elixirs are mixed in established ratios to give vehicles of desired alcohol concentrations. The formulas for Low and High Alcoholic Elixirs and the Volume-Percent Alcohol table can be found in older editions (18th and prior) of *Remington's The Science and Practice of Pharmacy*.

(3) An easier way to make an alcohol-containing vehicle is to add alcohol in the needed quantity to an appropriate oral liquid vehicle. This is illustrated with example 8.27 in Chapter 8, Quantity and Concentration Expressions and Calculations, and with example 37.5 in Chapter 37, Compatibility and Stability of Drug Products and Preparations, and on the CD that accompanies this book.

5. Sugar-free liquid vehicles

a. Sorbitol-based vehicle

(1) Sorbitol is the monosaccharide D-glucitol. It has a pleasant, nonartificial, sweet taste with about one-half the sweetness of sucrose. It is added as a sweetener to sugar-free products. It has the added advantage in liquid preparations of preventing sugar crystallization or "cap lock." Its properties are described in Chapter 21, Colors, Flavors, Sweeteners, and Scents.

(2) The official Sorbitol Solution USP is an aqueous solution containing in each 100 g of solution 70 g of total solids consisting mostly of D-sorbitol with small amounts of mannitol and other isomer polyhydric alcohols (12). Sorbitol Solution can be made from Sorbitol NF by dissolving 70 g in 30 g (mL) of Purified Water. This is a saturated solution (sorbitol has a water solubility of 1 g in 0.45 mL of water). It is a clear, colorless, odorless liquid with the consistency of syrup. It has a sweet taste and is neutral to litmus. Its specific gravity is 1.285 (13).

(3) Sorbitol Solution can be diluted to give liquid vehicles of various concentrations. Such other ingredients as flavors may be added. Saturated solutions are self-preserving, but lesser concentrations require the same precautions as sucrose syrups. The official 70% w/w solution is also available from pharmaceutical vendors.

(4) Although not a sugar, sorbitol is a carbohydrate and should not be used in preparations made for patients on ketogenic diets (9). If large quantities of sorbitol solution are consumed, the syrup can have a laxative effect.

b. Vehicles made with natural and synthetic polymers

(1) The polymers most commonly used are the semisynthetic cellulose derivatives methylcellulose (MC) and sodium carboxymethylcellulose (Sodium CMC). Details about these compounds, including their properties, solubilities, incompatibilities, and methods for preparing and preserving their solutions, are given in Chapter 19, Viscosity-Inducing Agents.

(a) MC and Sodium CMC can be purchased as pure powders from various vendors of compounding supplies. Solutions and gels of these agents can be made in a wide range of viscosities by selecting an appropriate grade and concentration. As indicated previously, methods of preparing solutions of these agents and suitable preservatives are discussed in Chapter 19.

(b) Solutions of MC and sodium CMC are clear, odorless, and tasteless. A 1% solution of either MC 1,500 cps or sodium CMC medium viscosity (sometimes labeled 7MF) has appropriate viscosity and is a sugar-free, nonhypertonic liquid vehicle that is suitable for making oral liquid preparations for neonates or other patients requiring this type of vehicle. Because MC and sodium CMC are not digestible carbohydrates, they can also be used for making oral liquid preparations for patients on ketogenic diets.

(c) If used for older children or adults, solutions of MC or Sodium CMC may be customized by adding flavors or sweeteners to improve palatability. Sample Prescription 27.2 in Chapter 27, Solutions, illustrates this technique.

(d) Solutions of MC and sodium CMC are often mixed with Syrup or a flavored syrup to give a vehicle that has appropriate viscosity and good "mouth feel" but that is not as sweet or as highly hypertonic as a saturated sucrose or sorbitol syrup.

(e) Methylcellulose is also available as the over-the-counter bulk laxatives Citrucel (orange-flavored with sucrose for sweetening) and Citrucel SF (orange-flavored with aspartame for sweetening). These powders contain no preservatives and give vehicles of moderate osmolarity, so they are especially useful when preparing oral liquid products for infants and children. A proportion of 1 g Citrucel for each 30 mL of water gives a vehicle with good consistency. The resulting liquid has a pH of approximately 4, so either sodium benzoate or potassium sorbate may be used as a preservative if desired. The use of Citrucel in making a compounding oral vehicle is illustrated in Sample Prescription 28.5 in Chapter 28, Suspensions.

(2) Unsweetened, nonflavored mucilages of the natural polymers acacia and tragacanth were formerly official preparations. The concentrations of these mucilages were 35% for acacia and 6% for tragacanth. Each contained benzoic acid 0.2% as a preservative.

(a) Details about acacia and tragacanth, including their properties, solubilities, incompatibilities, and methods for preparing and preserving their solutions, are given in Chapter 19, Viscosity-Inducing Agents.

(b) If used for oral preparations, sweeteners and flavors may be added to improve palatability. The official preparation Acacia Syrup NF contains 10 g acacia, 80 g sucrose,

100 mg sodium benzoate, 0.5 mL of vanilla tincture, and sufficient Purified Water for 100 mL of syrup (10). (The secret to making this syrup is to combine and mix the dry solid ingredients first before adding a portion of the water, and then using mild heat with patient mixing until the solids are dissolved before qs'ing to final volume.)

(c) Although these natural polymers were once primary ingredients in liquid vehicles, they are used much less frequently now because they offer no real advantages over solutions of the synthetic polymers, and they have the disadvantage of being difficult to make and are especially good media for growth of molds and other microorganisms. Furthermore, they do not offer the aesthetically pleasing clear, colorless solutions of the synthetic polymers.

c. Structured vehicles

The following official preparations all contain xanthan gum, which gives vehicles with good consistency and some structure for suspending insoluble ingredients. Incorporating the xanthan gum does require some technique and patience. Details about xanthan gum, including its properties, solubilities, incompatibilities, and methods for preparing and preserving its dispersions, are given in Chapter 19, Viscosity-Inducing Agents. See the description of the method of preparation for Suspension Structured Vehicle NF, which was given earlier (section II.B.4.d), for a recommended procedure when making formulations with xanthan gum. The *NF* monographs for each preparation listed here give complete compounding procedures.

(1) Xanthan Gum Solution NF (10)

This is a simple unflavored and unsweetened vehicle that can be used as a base for oral or topical preparations. The formula ingredients include (10):

Xanthan Gum	
for 0.1% Solution	100 mg
for 1.0% Solution	1.0 g
Methylparaben	100 mg
Propylparaben	20 mg
Purified Water, a sufficient quantity to make	100 mL

(2) Vehicle for Oral Solution, Sugar Free NF (10)

This is the sugar-free counterpart to Vehicle for Oral Solution NF, which is described in the preceding section on sucrose-containing vehicles (section II.B.4.c). Like Vehicle for Oral Solution, it contains both an antimicrobial preservative system and a buffer to maintain the pH at 4 to 5. Because of the inclusion of xanthan gum, it does have some structure. It has a content that is similar to that of the commercial vehicle Ora-Sweet SF, and it contains the following ingredients (10):

Xanthan Gum	50 mg
Glycerin	10 mL
Sorbitol Solution	25 mL
Saccharin Sodium	100 mg
Citric Acid, Monohydrate	1.5 g
Sodium Citrate	2.0 g
Potassium Sorbate	100 mg
Methylparaben	100 mg
Purified Water, a sufficient quantity to make	100 mL

The monograph states that it should be packaged in a tight, light-resistant container and stored at controlled room temperature; under those conditions, it has a recommended beyond-use date of 6 months. It should be labeled to indicate that it is for use in compounding sugar-free oral solutions and suspensions (10).

(3) Sugar-Free Suspension Structured Vehicle NF (10)

This is the sugar-free counterpart to Suspension Structured Vehicle NF, which is described in the section on sucrose-containing vehicles (section II.B.4.d). It has the same pH-adjusting agent and preservative but contains the nonsucrose sweeteners sodium saccharin, sorbitol, and mannitol instead of sucrose. Because of the sorbitol and mannitol content, this vehicle is not appropriate for preparations made for patients on ketogenic diets.

Xanthan Gum	200 mg
Saccharin Sodium	200 mg
Potassium Sorbate	150 mg
Citric Acid	100 mg
Sorbitol	2 g
Mannitol	2 g
Glycerin	2 mL
Purified Water, a sufficient quantity to make	100 mL

The vehicle should be packaged in a tight, light-resistant container and stored at controlled room temperature; under those conditions, the beyond-use date is 30 days from the day of compounding. It should be labeled for the user to shake well before using (10).

(4) Vehicle for Oral Suspension NF (10)

This is an unflavored and unsweetened vehicle with some structure for suspending insoluble ingredients. Although intended for oral preparations, it contains no flavors or sweeteners so it could also be used for topical preparations. It contains ingredients similar to those in the commercial product Ora-Plus. It has the following formula (10):

Cellulose Microcrystalline	800 mg
Xanthan Gum	200 mg
Carrageenan	150 mg
Carboxymethylcellulose Sodium, High Viscosity	25 mg
Sodium Phosphate, Dibasic	120 mg
Citric Acid, Monohydrate	250 mg
Simethicone	0.1 mL
Potassium Sorbate	100 mg
Methylparaben	100 mg
Purified Water, a sufficient quantity to make	100 mL

The monograph states that it should be packaged in a tight, light-resistant container and stored at controlled room temperature; under these conditions, it has a recommended beyond-use date of 6 months. It has a pH of 4 to 5 and should be labeled to indicate that it is for use in compounding oral solutions and suspensions (10).

6. Anhydrous oral liquid vehicle (14)

This anhydrous oral liquid vehicle can be used when a drug needs to be prepared in the absence of water.

Saccharin	100 mg
Butylated hydroxytoluene (BHT)	100 mg
Flavor	qs
Almond oil, a sufficient quantity to make	100 mL

The flavor selected must be oil-soluble. This product must be stored in tight, light-resistant containers. A beyond-use date of 6 months can be assigned to this product (14).

C. Manufactured liquid vehicles

   1. A wide variety of liquid vehicles for oral preparations is currently available.

   a. These products offer the obvious advantage of convenience.

   b. All of these vehicles contain preservatives, which is beneficial from the viewpoint of microbiologic stability but which may limit their usefulness in certain populations such as neonates.

   c. For certain standard vehicles such as Syrup NF and cherry syrup (fountain-type syrup, not NF), and some popular commercial vehicles such as Ora-Sweet, Ora-Sweet SF, and Ora-Plus, peer-reviewed stability studies for numerous drugs have been published. This is helpful to the pharmacist in assigning beyond-use dates.

   2. Sugar-based vehicles

   a. Syrup NF (Simple Syrup), artificially fruit-flavored syrups such as cherry, strawberry, and orange syrup, chocolate syrup, and cola syrup are available from vendors of pharmacy compounding supplies and from some food stores and candy and soda fountain supply wholesalers. These syrups have pHs in the acid range and usually contain either sodium benzoate or potassium sorbate as a preservative. Most of these vehicles are hypertonic.

    b. Ora-Sweet is a citrus-berry flavored vehicle especially made for compounding oral liquid preparations. It contains sucrose, glycerin, and sorbitol to prevent "cap-lock," methyl-paraben and potassium sorbate as preservatives, flavors, and citric acid and sodium phosphate as a buffer and antioxidant system. It has a pH of 4.2. Although the vehicle itself is hypertonic with an osmolality of 3,240 mOsm/kg, it may be diluted up to 50% without losing its taste and texture properties (15–17). Paddock Labs now makes a product called Ora-Blend that is a 50–50 mixture of Ora-Sweet and Ora-Plus (see the description of Ora-Plus given later). The blend is less sweet and has a lower osmolality than Ora-Plus, and it has the advantage of some structure for retarding sedimentation of suspended particles. Sample Prescription 28.6 in Chapter 28 uses a 50–50 blend of Ora-Sweet and Ora-Plus.

    c. Aromatic Elixir NF is available from several vendors of compounding ingredients and supplies. It contains 21% to 23% alcohol and is described in the previous section as a useful vehicle when a flavored and sweetened hydroalcoholic system is needed.

  3. Sugar-free, artificially sweetened vehicles

    a. Sorbitol Solution USP is available as the 70% w/w solution from several vendors of compounding ingredients and supplies. Its formula and description are given in the previous section on pharmacy-prepared vehicles. This is a hypertonic solution.

    b. Ora-Sweet SF is a citrus-berry flavored, sugar-free, alcohol-free vehicle made for compounding oral liquid preparations when a specialized vehicle of this type is needed. It contains xanthan gum, glycerin, and sorbitol to give it body and texture, sodium saccharin for sweetness, methyl- and propylparaben and potassium sorbate as preservatives, citric acid and sodium citrate as a buffering and antioxidant system, and flavors. It has a pH of 4.2. Although the vehicle itself is hypertonic with an osmolality of 2,150 mOsm/kg, it may be diluted up to 50% without losing its taste and texture properties (15–17). Paddock Labs now makes a product called Ora-Blend SF that is a 50–50 mixture of Ora-Sweet SF and Ora-Plus (see description of Ora-Plus given later). It is less sweet and has a lower osmolality than Ora-Sweet SF, and it has the advantage of some structure for retarding sedimentation of suspended particles.

    c. Various other sugar-free vehicles are available from compounding supply companies such as Gallipot, Hawkins, and Humco. Check their supply catalogs and Internet sites for the specific formulas and properties.

  4. Structured vehicles

    a. These vehicles provide structured systems especially useful for suspending insoluble ingredients in liquid preparations. They may be used as vehicles for either oral or topical preparations but must be sweetened and/or flavored if a palatable preparation for oral use is needed.

    b. Ora-Plus is a thixotropic vehicle containing microcrystalline cellulose, sodium CMC, xanthan gum, and carrageenan as suspending agents, preservatives, buffers, and an antifoaming agent. It contains no sugar, sweeteners, flavors, or alcohol. It has a pH of 4.2 and a more nearly isotonic osmolality of 230 mOsm/kg. It may be diluted up to 50% without losing its suspending properties. It is marketed specifically for compounding oral suspensions (15–17). As noted earlier, Paddock Labs now makes 50–50 blends of Ora-Plus with Ora-Sweet and Ora-Sweet SF.

    c. Suspendol-S is marketed for compounding suspensions for vaginal and rectal use but may also be used for compounding oral suspensions (15,16). It is described below in the section on vehicles for topical administration (section III.C.1.a).

    d. Various other excellent suspension vehicles are available from compounding supply companies such as Gallipot, Hawkins, Humco, and others. Check their supply catalogs and Internet sites for the specific formulas and properties.

III.   VEHICLES FOR TOPICAL LIQUID PREPARATIONS

A. Restrictions

Restrictions on vehicles for preparations intended for topical administration are not as numerous as those on vehicles for oral preparations.

  1. The pharmacist must be sure that the patient is not allergic to any of the ingredients in the preparation.

2. Ingredients that may be sensitizing or irritating should be avoided.
3. If the product is to be used on denuded areas, osmolarity should be considered.

B. **Pharmacy-prepared liquid vehicles for topical administration**

1. Various natural and synthetic polymers can be used by the pharmacist to make liquid vehicles for topical preparations. The semisynthetic cellulose derivatives MC and sodium CMC, and the natural gums acacia, tragacanth, and xanthan gum were described earlier in this chapter and in Chapter 19, Viscosity-Inducing Agents. Sample Prescription 28.3 in Chapter 28 illustrates the use of sodium CMC in a topical suspension. Other semisynthetic polymers such as hypromellose and hydroxypropyl cellulose, which are used for topical preparations, are also described and discussed in Chapter 19. Sample Prescription 30.6 in Chapter 30 illustrates the use of hydroxypropyl cellulose in making a topical gel preparation.

2. Synthetic polymers, such as carbomer and poloxamer, are described in Chapter 19, Viscosity-Inducing Agents. Sample Prescription 30.7 in Chapter 30 illustrates the use of poloxamer in making a compounded topical gel preparation.

3. Hydrophilic particulate colloids, such as bentonite, Veegum, colloidal silicon dioxide, and microcrystalline cellulose, are described in Chapter 19, Viscosity-Inducing Agents. Sample Prescription 28.1 in Chapter 28 illustrates the use of Bentonite Magma.

C. **Manufactured liquid vehicles**

1. Some liquid vehicles that are made specifically for compounding topical preparations are available from pharmaceutical suppliers. Several examples are given here to illustrate useful ingredients and formulations. This list is just a sampling; other products of this type can be found in the ointment and lotion base sections of drug information references such as *Drug Facts and Comparisons* (18) or *The Handbook of Nonprescription Drugs* (19).

   a. Suspendol-S is especially marketed as vaginal and rectal preparations, but it is also a general suspending vehicle. It contains an acrylic polymer resin, a silicone defoaming agent, methylparaben, polysorbate 80, and buffers for a pH of 5.5 (15).

   b. Liquiderm–A is a hydroalcoholic solution that was formulated as a vehicle for topical preparations with active ingredients that require a high concentration of alcohol/glycol solvents for dissolution. It contains 68% isopropyl alcohol, 20% propylene glycol, 3% glycerin, and the emulsifying-wetting agent laureth-4 (polyoxyethylene 4 lauryl ether). It has a pH of 5.5 and is sold in a special 2-oz bottle with an applicator filter top (18,19).

   c. Liqua–Gel is a water-soluble liquid lubricating gel with a viscosity of approximately 80,000 cps. It contains Purified Water, propylene glycol, glycerin, hydroxypropyl methylcellulose (now called *hypromellose*), sodium phosphate and boric acid as pH adjusting agents, and potassium sorbate, diazolidinyl urea, methylparaben, and propylparaben as preservatives. It has a pH of approximately 5.0 (15). Other similar vehicles include K-Y Jelly and Lubricating Jelly (18,19).

   d. Vehicle/N Solutions were recently discontinued, but a recent paper in the *International Journal of Pharmaceutical Compounding* describes formulas for these vehicles. Vehicle/N contained 45% SD alcohol 40, laureth-4, propylene glycol, and 4% isopropyl alcohol; Vehicle/N Mild Solution contained 37.5% SD alcohol 40, laureth-4, and 5% isopropyl alcohol (20).

   e. Solvent-G Liquid contains 55% SD alcohol 40B, laureth-4, propylene glycol, and isopropyl alcohol (18).
   Note: The letters *SD* with alcohol stand for "specially denatured"; the numbers, such as 40 and 40B, signify the particular denaturants used (21). For more detailed information on this topic, consult the Code of Federal Regulations, Title 27, Volume 1, Parts 1 to 199, which is available on the Internet at http://www.atf.treas.gov/regulations/27cfr21.htm, accessed February 2008.

2. Many commercial topical liquids marketed for other purposes (e.g., cleansers, lubricants, and emollients) are suitable suspending media for topical products. Three examples are given here.

   a. Cetaphil Lotion contains cetyl alcohol, stearyl alcohol, sodium lauryl sulfate, propylene glycol, and parabens (18). Its use as a compounding aid is illustrated in Sample Prescription 28.2 in Chapter 28.

   b. Spectro-Jel contains iodo-methylcellulose, carboxypolymethylene, cetyl alcohol, sorbitan monooleate, fumed silica, triethanolamine stearate, glycol polysiloxane, propylene glycol, glycerin, and 5% isopropyl alcohol (18,22).

   c. Nutraderm Lotion contains mineral oil, sorbitan stearate, stearyl alcohol, sodium lauryl sulfate, cetyl alcohol, carbomer-940, parabens, and triethanolamine (18).

REFERENCES

1. American Academy of Pediatrics, Committee on Drugs. Ethanol in liquid preparations intended for children. Pediatrics 1984; 73: 405–407.
2. Code of Federal Regulations, Title 21, Volume 5, Revised as of April 1, 2001. Chapter I—Food and Drug Administration, Department of Health and Human Services. Part 328—Over-the-Counter Drug Products Intended for Oral Ingestion that Contain Alcohol. (Original Mar. 13, 1995, as amended at 61 FR 58630, Nov. 18, 1996.)
3. Gershanik J, Boecler B, Ensley H, et al. The gasping syndrome and benzyl alcohol poisoning. N Engl J Med 1982; 307: 1384–1388.
4. Martin G, Finberg L. Propylene glycol: A potentially toxic vehicle in liquid dosage form. J Pediatr 1970; 77: 877–878.
5. Arulanantham K, Genel M. Central nervous system toxicity associated with ingestion of propylene glycol. J Pediatr 1978; 93: 515–516.
6. White KC, Harkavy KL. Hypertonic formulas resulting from added oral medications. Am J Dis Child 1982; 136: 931–933.
7. Charney EB, Bodurtha JN. Intractable diarrhea associated with the use of sorbitol. J Pediatr 1981; 98: 157–158.
8. Ernst JA, Williams JM, Glick M, et al. Osmolality of substances used in the intensive care nursery. Pediatrics 1983; 72: 347–352.
9. McElhiney LF. Challenges of compounding for patients on the ketogenic diet. IJPC 2007; 11(2): 114–117.
10. The United States Pharmacopeial Convention, Inc. NF monographs. 2007 USP 30/NF 25. Rockville, MD: Author, 2006.
11. Swinyard EA, Lowenthal W. Pharmaceutical necessities. In: Gennaro AR, ed. Remington's pharmaceutical sciences, 17th ed. Easton, PA: Mack Publishing Co., 1985; 1294.
12. The United States Pharmacopeial Convention, Inc. USP monographs. 2007 USP 30/NF 25. Rockville, MD: Author, 2006.
13. Reilly WJ. Pharmaceutical necessities. In: University of the Sciences in Philadelphia, ed. Remington: The science and practice of pharmacy, 21st ed. Baltimore, MD: Lippincott Williams & Wilkins, 2005; 1060–1069.
14. Anonymous. Oral liquid vehicle, anhydrous. IJPC 2007; 11(2): 157.
15. Paddock Laboratories Product Information. Minneapolis, MN: Paddock Laboratories, Inc. (http://www.paddocklabs.com/).
16. Personal correspondence with Paddock Laboratories Customer Service Department. Minneapolis, MN: Paddock Laboratories, Inc.
17. Allen LV, Jr. Featured excipient: Oral liquid vehicles. IJPC 2001; 5(1): 65.
18. Drug Facts and Comparisons, 60th ed. St. Louis, MO: Facts and Comparisons, Wolter Kluwers Health, 2006.
19. Berardi RR, ed. Handbook of nonprescription drugs, 13th ed. Washington, DC: American Pharmaceutical Association, 2002.
20. Anonymous. Vehicle N formulas. IJPC 2007; 11(4): 337.
21. Allen LV, Jr. Featured excipient: Specially denatured alcohols. IJPC 2002; 6(5): 380–383.
22. Spectro Skincare. GlaxoSmithKline, Consumer Healthcare Inc. Oakville, Ontario, Canada, http://www.spectroskincare.com/.

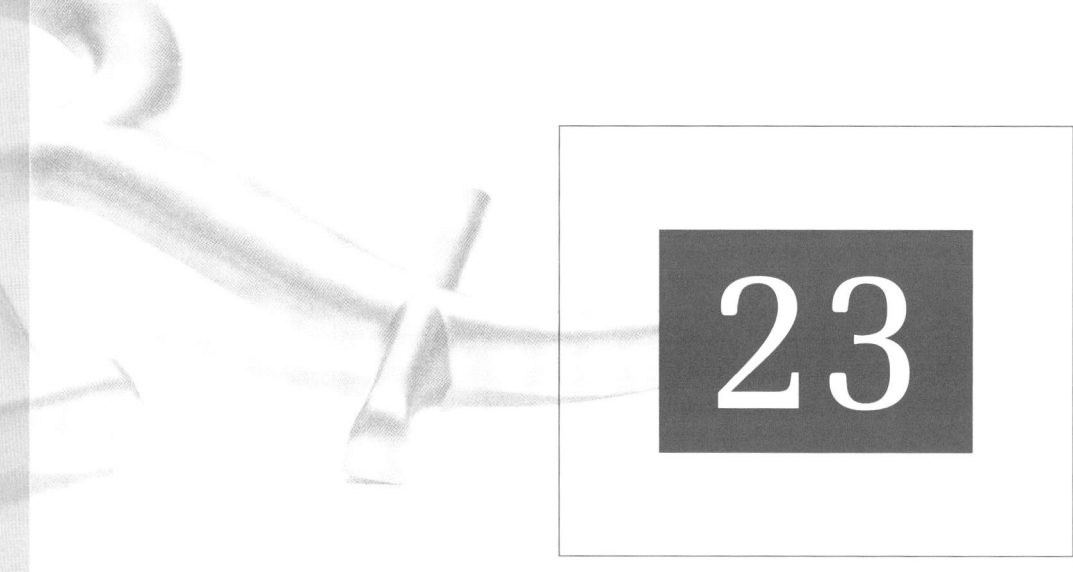

Ointment Bases

Melgardt de Villiers, PhD

I. INTRODUCTION

The purpose of this chapter is to give you basic knowledge about ointment bases and their ingredients. This information is important for two reasons: First, it will help you in guiding prescribers and patients in selecting topical products (e.g., answering the question, which is better for this purpose, an ointment or a cream?). Second, knowledge of the properties of ointment base classes and their ingredients is essential to working successfully with these ingredients when compounding with them and when developing formulations with specific properties.

In learning about ointment bases, you first need to know some definitions and terminology. Second, ointment bases have conveniently been grouped into classes that generally define their properties; knowledge about these class traits helps greatly in selecting an appropriate base for a particular use. Finally, it is useful to know something about the specific properties of ointment base ingredients; it will help you in understanding the labels of ointment products, and specific information such as solubility, melting point, and other properties will aid in selecting and using these ingredients. The ingredient section is meant as a resource for this purpose.

II. DEFINITIONS

Definitions and nomenclature for pharmaceutical dosage forms are currently in transition between use of traditional terms and definitions and a more systematic approach that has been proposed to more accurately and consistently describe drug products and preparations. During this time, it is important that pharmacists and pharmacy technicians know the traditional terms but also understand proposed definitions and nomenclature. The rationale for the changes and the development of the proposed system are discussed at the beginning of Chapter 27, Solutions, and the comparison of nomenclature and definitions specific to semisolids such as ointments, creams, gels, and pastes is presented at the beginning of Chapter 30, Semisolids: Ointments, Creams, Gels, Pastes, and Collodions. Those definitions needed for understanding the information in this chapter follow. For additional information on this subject, consult Chapters 27 and 30.

A. Ointment

1. Traditionally the term *ointment* has been used for (i) the general class name for all external-use semisolids and (ii) the subclass, oleaginous semisolids. For example, *USP 31* Chapter ⟨1151⟩ defines ointments very generally as "semisolid preparations intended for external application to the skin or mucous membranes" (1). However, pharmaceutical manufacturers use the word *ointment* more specifically to indicate that a drug is incorporated into an oleaginous ointment base; for example, the name Hydrocortisone Ointment means that hydrocortisone is incorporated into an oil-type semisolid base.

2. Under the proposed nomenclature, this situation would be clarified; the term *semisolid* would be used for naming the general class, and the term *ointment* would be redefined more narrowly as "a viscous oleaginous or polymeric semisolid dosage form" (2), which is consistent with current usage by the pharmaceutical industry.

3. According to the *USP* Chapter ⟨1151⟩, there are four general classes of ointment (i.e., semisolid) bases (1). These are listed here and are described in more detail in Chapter ⟨1151⟩ and in section III of this chapter.
   - **a.** Hydrocarbon
   - **b.** Absorption
   - **c.** Water-removable
   - **d.** Water-soluble

4. Within these classes, the following ointment bases are listed in the excipient table at the front of the *NF* (3):

   Caprylocaproyl Polyoxylglycerides; Diethylene Glycol Monoethyl Ether; Lanolin, Lauroyl Polyoxylglycerides; Linoleoyl Polyoxylglycerides; Hydrophilic Ointment; White Ointment; Yellow Ointment; Oleoyl Polyoxylglycerides; Polyethylene Glycol Monomethyl Ether; Petrolatum; Hydrophilic Petrolatum; White Petrolatum; Rose Water Ointment; Squalane; Stearoyl Polyoxylglycerides; Type II Vegetable Oil

B. Cream

1. Although creams meet the general definition of an ointment, they have been given a separate section in *USP 31* Chapter ⟨1151⟩. This section has more of a historical description of this term than a specific definition. Although it states that creams are "semisolid dosage forms containing one or more drug substances dissolved or dispersed in a suitable base" (1), it then discusses the evolution of this term to include or exclude certain types of semisolid emulsions and aqueous microcrystalline dispersions.

2. The proposed new nomenclature both simplifies and clarifies the situation by defining a cream as "a dosage form comprising a viscous semisolid emulsion" (2). Under this definition, creams would fall into two of the four general ointment base classes listed earlier: both water-containing absorption bases and water-removable bases.

C. Paste

1. As with creams, pastes meet the general definition of an ointment, but they have been given a separate section in *USP 31* Chapter ⟨1151⟩. They are defined as "semisolid dosage forms that contain one or more drug substances intended for topical application" (1). Then, to more clearly distinguish a paste from other topical semisolids, Chapter ⟨1151⟩ lists two classes of pastes and gives an example of each. One group consists of very stiff ointments with a high concentration of solid particles in an oleaginous base: Zinc Oxide Paste USP is an example of this group. The other subclass is also very thick but has a single aqueous phase with a high polymer content: Carboxymethylcellulose Sodium Paste is an example of this group (2).

2. The proposed new nomenclature defines a paste as "a semisolid preparation with a stiff consistency containing a relatively high concentration of solids" (2).

D. Gel

1. Many, but not all, gels fit within the Chapter ⟨1151⟩ general definition of an ointment; some would be considered thick suspensions rather than semisolids, and some are for oral rather than topical administration. As with creams and pastes, gels are classified separately in Chapter ⟨1151⟩ and are defined there as "semisolid systems consisting of either suspensions made up of small inorganic particles or large organic molecules interpenetrated by liquid" (1). The proposed definition is quite similar: "a dispersion of small inorganic particles or a solution of large organic molecules rendered jellylike in consistency" (2).

2. The gels that are thick suspensions of small inorganic particles are systems such as Aluminum Hydroxide Gel USP. Some are called *magmas* if the size of the dispersed phase is large (e.g., Bentonite Magma) (1). These gels must be labeled "Shake before use." Some are thixotropic, forming semisolids on standing but becoming a liquid when shaken.

3. The gels that have a more jelly-like consistency have large organic polymer molecules like carbomer, methylcellulose, and poloxamer dispersed in a liquid, usually water or a hydroalcoholic solution. An example of this type of gel is Hydrocortisone Gel USP, which is hydrocortisone in a hydroalcoholic gel base (4).

E. Emollient: An agent that softens the skin or soothes irritation in skin or mucous membrane.

F. Protective: A substance that protects injured or exposed skin surfaces from harmful or annoying stimuli.

G. Occlusive: A substance that promotes retention of water in the skin by forming a hydrophobic barrier that prevents evaporation of moisture from within the skin.

H. Humectant: A substance that causes water to be retained because of its hygroscopic properties.

III. DESIRABLE PROPERTIES OF OINTMENT BASES

Certain properties are desired for all ointment bases, no matter what their particular use. These include the following:

A. Chemically and physically stable under normal conditions of use and storage

B. Nonreactive and compatible with a wide variety of drugs and auxiliary agents

C. Free from objectionable odor

D. Nontoxic, nonsensitizing, and nonirritating

E. Aesthetically appealing, easy to apply, and nongreasy

F. Remains in contact with the skin until removal is desired, then is removed easily

IV. CLASSIFICATION AND CHARACTERISTICS OF OINTMENT BASES

A. Many factors determine the choice of an ointment base. These include the action desired, the nature of the medication to be incorporated and its bioavailability and stability, and the desired shelf life of the finished product (1). The choice of a particular base matches these factors with the properties of an ointment base class.

B. Ointment Bases

As stated previously, the *USP* recognizes four general classes of ointment bases to be used therapeutically or as vehicles for active ingredients (1). Each has very specific and unique characteristics (5,6). As noted in the previous chapters of Part 4, this text employs the usual convention of using upper-case first letters for words designating offical *USP-NF* articles (e.g., Alcohol, Purified Water) and lower-case first letters for words designating the chemical substance (e.g., ethanol, water).

1. Hydrocarbon or oleaginous bases

   a. See Table 23.1 for characteristics and examples of these bases; see Table 23.2 for some sample formulas.

   b. Advantages

     (1) Inexpensive

     (2) Nonreactive

     (3) Nonirritating

     (4) Good emollient, protective, and occlusive properties

     (5) Not water-washable so they stay on the skin and keep incorporated medications in contact with the skin

   c. Disadvantages

     (1) These bases have poor patient acceptance because of their greasy nature.

     (2) They are not removed easily with washing when this is desired (**Note:** may be removed using mineral oil, which is then washed off with soap and warm water).

     (3) They cannot absorb water and can absorb only limited amounts of alcoholic solutions, so most liquid ingredients are difficult to incorporate into hydrocarbon bases. Possible strategies for dealing with this difficulty are discussed in Chapter 30, Semisolids: Ointments, Creams, Gels, Pastes, and Collodions, and are illustrated with Sample Prescriptions 30.4 and 30.5.

     (4) Because these bases do not absorb or mix with aqueous solutions, aqueous skin secretions do not readily dissipate.

2. Absorption bases

   a. See Table 23.1 for characteristics and examples of these bases; see Table 23.2 for some sample formulas.

   b. Absorption bases have two subgroups:

     (1) Anhydrous absorption bases

     These are hydrocarbon bases that contain an emulsifier or emulsifiers that form water-in-oil emulsions when water or an aqueous solution is added.

(text continued on page 283)

Table 23.1	CHARACTERISTICS OF OINTMENT BASES AND GELS		
BASE TYPE	**CHARACTERISTICS**	**USES**	**EXAMPLES**
Hydrocarbon (oleaginous) oils and fats	Insoluble in water Not water-washable Anhydrous Will not absorb water Emollient Occlusive Greasy Drug release poor	Protectant Emollient Vehicle for drugs prone to hydrolysis	White Petrolatum White Ointment Vaseline
Anhydrous absorption hydrocarbon base + w/o surfactant	Insoluble in water Not water-washable Anhydrous Can absorb water Emollient Occlusive Greasy Drug release poor but better for hydrophobic drugs	Protectant Emollient Vehicle for aqueous solutions Vehicle for solids and drugs	Hydrophilic Petrolatum Lanolin Aquaphor Aquabase Polysorb
Water-in-oil emulsion absorption hydrocarbon base + <45% w/w water + w/o surfactant with HLB ≤ 8	Insoluble in water Not water-washable Contain water Can absorb water (limited) Emollient Occlusive Greasy Drug release fair to good	Emollient Cleansing cream Vehicle for liquids Vehicle for solids and drugs	Hydrous Lanolin Cold Cream Eucerin Hydrocream Rose Water Ointment Nivea
Water-removable (oil-in-water emulsion) hydrocarbon base + >45% w/w water + o/w surfactant with HLB ≥ 9	Insoluble in water Water-washable Contain water Can absorb water Nonocclusive Nongreasy Drug release fair to good	Emollient Vehicle liquids Vehicle for solids and drugs	Hydrophilic Ointment Vanishing Cream Dermabase Velvachol
Water-soluble	Water-soluble Water-washable May contain water Can absorb water (limited) Nonocclusive Nongreasy Lipid-free Mix well with skin secretions Drug release good	Emollient Vehicle for liquids Vehicle for solids and drugs Local anesthetic	Polyethylene Glycol Ointment Polybase
Gels: single-phase systems	Water-soluble Water-washable Contain water May contain alcohol Can absorb additional water Nonocclusive Nongreasy Lipid-free Drug release good	Vehicle for liquids Vehicle for solids and drugs Ideal for applying drugs to mucous membranes Lubricant gels Spermicidal gels Anesthetic gels	Methylcellulose Gel Sodium Carboxymethyl-cellulose Gel Hydroxypropyl Methyl-cellulose Gel (Liqua-Gel) Hydroxypropyl Cellulose Gel Carbomer Gel Poloxamer Gel

Table 23.2	OINTMENT BASE FORMULAS

HYDROCARBON (OLEAGINOUS) BASES

White Ointment USP (4)

White Wax	50 g
White Petrolatum	950 g
To make	1,000 g

Melt the white wax in a suitable dish on a warm-water bath (65° to 70°C). Add the white petrolatum and continue heating until liquefied. Remove from the heat and stir the mixture until it begins to congeal.

Other Names: Simple Ointment

ANHYDROUS ABSORPTION BASES

Hydrophilic Petrolatum USP (4)

Cholesterol	30 g
Stearyl Alcohol	30 g
White Wax	80 g
White Petrolatum	860 g
To make	1,000 g

Melt the stearyl alcohol and white wax together on a warm-water bath (65° to 70°C), then add the cholesterol and stir until completely dissolved. Add the white petrolatum and stir to mix. Remove from the bath and stir until the mixture congeals.

Polysorb

Petrolatum
Wax
Sorbitan Sesquioleate

Aquaphor

Petrolatum
Mineral Oil
Mineral Wax
Wool-wax Alcohol

Aquabase

Petrolatum
Mineral Oil
Mineral Wax
Wool-wax Alcohol
Sorbitan Sesquioleate

These bases will absorb significant amounts of water.

WATER-IN-OIL EMULSION ABSORPTION BASES

Rose Water Ointment USP (4)

Cetyl Esters Wax	125 g
White Wax	120 g
Almond Oil	560 g
Sodium Borate	5 g
Stronger Rose Water	25 mL
Purified Water	165 mL
Rose Oil	200 μL
To make about	1,000 g

Cut the cetyl esters wax and the white wax into small pieces and melt them on a warm-water bath (65° to 70°C). Add the almond oil with stirring and continue heating until the temperature of the mixture reaches 70°C. Dissolve the sodium borate in the Stronger Rose Water and Purified Water that has been warmed to 70°C. Remove the oil phase from the heat and gradually, with stirring, add the warm-water solution to the melted oil phase and stir rapidly and continuously until the mixture has congealed (about 45°C). Stir in the Rose Oil.

Note: The formula for Cold Cream (formerly USP) is the same as for Rose Water Ointment except mineral oil replaces the almond oil and 190 mL of Purified Water is used since no fragrance is added (13). Neither Cold Cream nor Rose Water Ointment will absorb significant amounts of water.

Hydrocream

Petrolatum	Mineral Oil
Mineral Wax	Cholesterol
Wool-wax Alcohol	Parabens
Imidazolidinyl urea	Water

Eucerin

Petrolatum	Mineral Oil
Wool-wax Alcohol	Preservative
Mineral Wax	Water

Although they each contain water, Eucerin and Hydrocream will absorb a moderate amount of extra water.

(continued)

Table 23.2	**OINTMENT BASE FORMULAS** (*continued*)

WATER-REMOVABLE (OIL-IN-WATER EMULSION) BASES

Hydrophilic Ointment USP (4)

Methylparaben	0.25 g
Propylparaben	0.15 g
Sodium Lauryl Sulfate	10 g
Propylene Glycol	120 g
Stearyl Alcohol	250 g
White Petrolatum	250 g
Purified Water	370 g
To make about	1,000 g

Melt the stearyl alcohol and the white petrolatum on a warm-water bath (65° to 70°C). Continue heating until the temperature of the mixture is about 75°C. Add the other ingredients to the water and heat to 75°C. Add the aqueous portion to the wax mixture with stirring. Remove from the heat and stir continuously until the mixture has congealed.

Soft Water-Washable Base (10)

Stearic Acid	7 g
Cetyl Alcohol	2 g
Glycerin	10 g
Mineral Oil (Light)	20 g
Triethanolamine	2 g
Purified Water to make about	100 g

Combine the cetyl alcohol, stearic acid, and the mineral oil and melt on a water bath. Continue heating until the temperature of the mixture is about 70°C. Add the other ingredients to the water and heat to 70°C. Add the aqueous portion to the wax mixture with stirring. Stir continuously until the mixture has congealed.

Dermabase

Parabens
Sodium Lauryl Sulfate
Propylene Glycol
Cetyl and Stearyl Alcohols
Mineral Oil
Isopalmitate
Imidazolidinyl urea
White Petrolatum
Water

Hydrophilic Ointment and its brand counterparts such as Dermabase will absorb about 30% water without thinning.

Vanishing Cream Base (10)

Stearic Acid	18 g
Light Mineral Oil	2 g
Lanolin	0.5 g
Arlacel 83	2 g
Potassium Hydroxide	0.2 g
Sorbitol Solution 70%	3.7 g
Purified Water to make about	100 g

Combine the stearic acid, the lanolin, the Arlacel, and the mineral oil and melt on a water bath. Continue heating until the temperature of the mixture is about 70°C. Add the other ingredients to the water and heat to 70°C. Add the aqueous portion to the oil mixture with stirring. Stir continuously until the mixture has congealed.

WATER-SOLUBLE BASE

Polyethylene Glycol Ointment NF (11)

Polyethylene Glycol 3350	400 g
Polyethylene Glycol 400	600 g
To make	1,000 g

Combine the two PEG ingredients and heat on a warm-water bath until the mixture is about 65°C. Remove and stir until congealed. If a firmer ointment is desired, 100 g of PEG 400 may be replaced with an equal weight of PEG 3350. To make an ointment that will absorb 6%–25% of an aqueous solution, replace 50 g of PEG 3350 with an equal weight of stearyl alcohol.

PASTE

Zinc Oxide Paste USP (4)

Zinc Oxide	250 g
Starch	250 g
White Petrolatum	500 g
To make	1,000 g

Incorporate the zinc oxide and starch in the white petrolatum and levigate until a smooth paste is obtained. To achieve a smooth paste, the powders should be added in small portions to portions of white petrolatum and then combined.

Table 23.2	OINTMENT BASE FORMULAS (*continued*)

GELS

Carbomer 934 Aqueous Jelly (16)

Carbomer 934	2 g
Triethanolamine	1.65 mL
Methylparaben	0.2 g
Propylparaben	0.05 g
Purified Water, to make	100 mL

Dissolve the parabens in 95 mL of warm water and allow to cool. Add the carbomer in small amounts to the solution while stirring vigorously (or use a high-speed stirrer) until a uniform dispersion is obtained. Allow to stand until entrapped air can escape. Add the triethanolamine dropwise, stirring carefully to avoid entrapping air. Add Purified Water to make 100 mL.

Carbomer 934 Hydroalcoholic Jelly

Carbomer 934	0.625 g
Alcohol USP	50 mL
10% NaOH	dropwise to pH 6–7
Purified Water	49 mL

Disperse the Carbomer 934 in the Purified Water slowly with continuous stirring until a uniform dispersion is obtained. Dropwise add the NaOH solution to form the gel and obtain a pH in the range of 6–7. Very gradually add the Alcohol in small amounts with constant stirring. If the Alcohol is added too quickly, the gel will fall apart. Also, this formula will not work with Carbomer 940.

Carbomer 940 Alcoholic Gel

Carbomer 940	0.5 g
Isopropyl Alcohol 70%	71 mL
Triethanolamine	0.67 g
Purified Water	28 mL

Slowly add the Carbomer 940 to the isopropyl alcohol with constant stirring. Add the triethanolamine to the Purified Water, then add this solution to the carbomer–IPA solution while stirring slowly. Mix thoroughly until the gel forms.

Poloxamer Gel

Poloxamer 407	20 g
Parabens	0.2 g
Purified Water, to make	100 mL

Dissolve the parabens in 95 mL of warm water and allow to cool. Add the Poloxamer to the solution. (Do not be surprised if you get a "snowball.") Cover the container, put in the refrigerator, and allow to hydrate overnight. A clear gel will result. Add Purified Water to make 100 mL.

Note: A manufactured 20% Poloxamer Gel that is preserved with sorbic acid and parabens and buffered with a citrate–phosphate buffer is available. Often poloxamer gels are combined with a lecithin-isopropyl palmitate solution (LIPS), which adds emollient, emulsifier, and penetration enhancement properties. The lecithin–palmitate solution may be purchased or may be prepared by adding 10 g of soya lecithin to 10 g of isopropyl palmitate and allowing the mixture to set overnight. Usually 20 g of the LIPS is added for each 100 mL of finished poloxamer gel. The manufactured lecithin solution comes already preserved but, if the solution is made in the pharmacy, a preservative must be added. Sample Prescription 30.7 in Chapter 30 shows an example of a preparation of this type.

Ephedrine Sulfate Jelly NF XII (17)

Ephedrine Sulfate	10 g
Tragacanth	10 mL
Methyl Salicylate	0.1 g
Eucalyptol	1.0 mL
Pine Needle Oil	0.1 mL
Glycerin	150 g
Purified Water	830 mL

Dissolve the ephedrine sulfate in the Purified Water and add the glycerin, tragacanth, and the essential oils. Mix well and store in a closed container for 1 week, stirring or agitating occasionally.

---

(2) Water-in-oil emulsions

These are absorption bases that contain water, the amount depending on the base. As semi-solid emulsions, they are classified as creams under the proposed nomenclature scheme.

c. Advantages

(1) Absorption bases have moderately good protective, occlusive, and emollient properties.

(2) They do not wash off easily so they hold incorporated medications in contact with the skin.

(3) They can absorb liquids.

(a) Anhydrous absorption bases can absorb significant amounts of water and moderate amounts of alcoholic solutions. This is illustrated with Sample Prescription 30.4 in Chapter 30.

    (b) Because they already contain water, emulsion absorption bases absorb variable amounts of water and/or alcohol.

  (4) Some lanolin-types have compositions somewhat like the sebaceous secretions of the skin. These are thought to have superior emollient properties. *Martindale: The Extra Pharmacopoeia* states that wool-fat preparations mixed with suitable vegetable oils or with petrolatum give emollient ointments that penetrate the skin and enhance absorption (7,8).

  d. Disadvantages

    (1) Some bases in this group have poor patient acceptance.

      (a) The anhydrous absorption bases have a greasy nature similar to that of hydrocarbon bases.

      (b) Some lanolin-type bases are somewhat sticky and have a mildly unpleasant odor.

    (2) They are not easily removed with washing.

    (Note: As with hydrocarbon bases, they may be removed using mineral oil.)

    (3) Those bases containing wool wax or wool-wax alcohols may be sensitizing. Efforts have been made to remove offending principles, including detergents and natural free fatty alcohols, which is reported to reduce the incidence of hypersensitivity to almost zero (9).

    (4) Those bases with soap-type emulsifiers (e.g., Cold Cream, Rose Water Ointment) can have the compatibility problems associated with this type of emulsifying agent. This is discussed in the section on soft soaps in Chapter 20, Surfactants and Emulsifying Agents.

    (5) Those that contain water may have chemical stability problems with ingredients that are sensitive to hydrolysis.

    (6) Those containing water are also subject to microbial growth, and the *USP* requires that these contain a preservative (1).

  3. Water-removable bases

    a. See Table 23.1 for characteristics and examples of these bases; see Table 23.2 for some sample formulas.

    b. These are oil-in-water emulsions and are classified as creams under both traditional and the proposed nomenclature schemes.

    c. Advantages

      (1) Water-removable bases are nongreasy and therefore aesthetically pleasing.

      (2) They can be removed from the skin by washing.

      (3) They can absorb some water or alcohol. If the amount of liquid added reaches a critical amount, the base will thin out to a lotion. This property can be used to advantage, as is illustrated in the use of a cream in making a lotion for Sample Prescription 28.4 in Chapter 28, Suspensions.

      (4) They will allow the dissipation of fluids from injured skin.

    d. Disadvantages

      (1) These bases are less protective, less emollient, and less occlusive than hydrocarbon or absorption bases.

      (2) Those with soap-type emulsifiers can have compatibility problems. As stated previously, this is discussed in the section on soft soaps in Chapter 20, Surfactants and Emulsifying Agents.

      (3) Because these bases contain water, there may be chemical stability problems with ingredients that are sensitive to hydrolysis.

      (4) The water phase is also subject to microbial growth, and the *USP* requires that preparations of this type contain a preservative (1).

      (5) Because water is the external phase, these bases may "dry out" due to evaporation of the water. This can be minimized by storage in tight containers. Humectants may be added to retard dehydration; glycerin and propylene glycol in concentrations of 2% to 5% are commonly used for this purpose (10).

  4. Water-soluble bases

    a. See Table 23.1 for characteristics and examples of these bases; see Table 23.2 for a sample formula.

    b. These are greaseless ointment bases that are water-soluble. Most are polyethylene glycol–type ointment bases, and Polyethylene Glycol Ointment NF is an official preparation in this class (11).

    c. Advantages

      (1) Water-soluble bases are soluble in water and so are easily removed by washing.

      (2) They leave no oil residue.

      (3) They can absorb some water or alcohol; as the amount of liquid added increases, the base begins to thin out and eventually dissolves. The water-absorbing potential of Polyethylene

Glycol Ointment can be improved by adding stearyl alcohol; the formula for this is shown in Table 23.2.

    d. Disadvantages

        (1) These bases can be irritating, especially on denuded or abraded skin or mucous membranes.

        (2) They have little to no emollient properties.

        (3) PEG-type bases may have compatibility problems with incorporated drugs that are subject to oxidation.

        (4) Those that contain water may have the compatibility and stability problems associated with water, and a preservative is required.

C. Pastes

    1. Fatty pastes

        a. Fatty pastes have properties similar to those of ointments, but they are usually thicker and seem less greasy and more absorptive than ointments. This is because they contain high concentrations of solid ingredients that absorb water and aqueous solutions.

        b. Because they are better at absorbing skin secretions, they are useful when treating lesions that are weeping or oozing. They are less penetrating and stay in place on the skin better than ointments.

        c. Zinc Oxide Paste USP is an official product of this type.

    2. Single-phase aqueous gel: An example of this type of paste is Carboxymethylcellulose Sodium Paste USP, which contains 16% to 17% Sodium Carboxymethylcellulose (4).

    3. For animal patients, pastes are an oral rather than a topical dosage form and are described as concentrated, viscous oral dosage forms usually delivered by syringes and not intended for topical application. (See Table 36.3 in Chapter 36, Veterinary Pharmacy Practice.)

D. Gels

As indicated in the definitions given at the beginning of this chapter, gels are semisolids that may be either single-phase or two-phase systems. Gels may be used topically, may be introduced into body cavities (nasal, vaginal, etc.), or may be used internally (e.g., Aluminum Hydroxide Gel).

    1. Single-phase systems

        a. The single-phase systems contain soluble macromolecules, which are linear or branched-chain polymers, dissolved molecularly in water. They are classified as colloidal dispersions because the individual molecules are in the colloidal particle size range, exceeding 50 to 100 Å.

        b. The polymers are classified into one of three groups: natural polymers (e.g., tragacanth), semisynthetic cellulose derivatives (e.g., methylcellulose), and synthetic polymers (e.g., carbomer). These groups are discussed in detail in Chapter 19, Viscosity-Inducing Agents. Sample Prescriptions 30.6 and 30.7 in Chapter 30 illustrate the use of polymers in making topical gels.

        c. The continuous phase for these gels is usually aqueous, but alcohols, polyols, and oils may also be used.

    2. Two-phase systems

        a. The two-phase systems consist of a concentrated network of particulate association colloids. These are water-insoluble particles that hydrate strongly. Examples include the official preparations Aluminum Hydroxide Gel and Bentonite Magma.

        b. These are thixotropic suspensions that are semisolids on standing but become fluid when agitated. The term *gel* is used when the dispersed particles are very small, and the term *magma* is used for gels with larger-sized particles.

        c. Several compounds that form association colloidal gels, including bentonite, microcrystalline cellulose, and colloidal silicon dioxide, are discussed in Chapter 19, Viscosity-Inducing Agents.

V.   INGREDIENTS FOR OINTMENT BASES

A. The ingredients, formulas, methods of preparation, and/or descriptions of some ointment bases are given in Table 23.2.

B. Descriptions of ointment base ingredients, such as solvents, preservatives, viscosity-inducing agents and surfactants, which are contained in numerous types of dosage forms, can be found in the chapters covering those specific ingredient types (Chapters 15 through 21).

C. Ingredients specific to ointment bases are described here. These include waxes, fatty alcohols, acids, and esters, and miscellaneous ointment bases and ingredients. The descriptions and solubilities presented here give a composite of information from *Remington's The Science and Practice of*

Pharmacy (12,13), the *Handbook of Pharmaceutical Excipients* (14), official monographs in the *USP–NF* (4,11), and other references as cited. A melting point is given for each ingredient; this information is especially useful when using the ingredient for making a semisolid dosage form by fusion. Additional information on each agent, including references to original research journal articles, can be found in the *Handbook of Pharmaceutical Excipients*.

1. Petrolatum USP and White Petrolatum USP
   a. Description
      (1) Petrolatum and white petrolatum are mixtures of purified semisolid saturated hydrocarbons extracted from petroleum. White petrolatum has undergone additional treatment so that it is nearly decolorized, and it is preferred for pharmaceutical preparations because it is reported to cause fewer hypersensitivity reactions. The *USP* monographs for both compounds state that they may contain suitable stabilizers (4).
      (2) Petrolatum is a yellowish, translucent, soft unctuous mass. White petrolatum is similar but, as its name indicates, it is white in color. Both are tasteless, odorless, and greasy to touch. They have a melting point range of 38° to 60°C, and the specific gravity of the melt is 0.815 to 0.880.
   b. Solubility: Petrolatum and white petrolatum are practically insoluble in water, hot or cold alcohol, acetone, and glycerin; they are soluble in most volatile and fixed oils.
   c. Incompatibilities: The petrolatum bases are quite stable, and there are few problems with incompatibilities. Because the purified forms are more labile to oxidation, the *USP* allows addition of small amounts of antioxidants (14). Petrolatum does not mix with aqueous or hydroalcoholic solutions.
   d. Uses
      (1) White petrolatum is an, all-purpose, soft ointment base. It has a smooth texture, incorporates powders easily, and spreads evenly on the skin. It is used both by itself and as a major component of combination ointment bases.
      (2) If a stiffer base is desired, a portion of White Wax may be added. (See the formula for White Ointment in Table 23.2.)
   e. Other names
      (1) Petroleum: mineral jelly, petroleum jelly
      (2) White petrolatum: white mineral jelly, white petroleum jelly, white soft paraffin, Vaseline

2. Lanolin USP and Modified Lanolin USP
   a. Description
      (1) Lanolin and modified lanolin are the purified, fatty, waxlike substances obtained from the wool of sheep. These substances are purified, cleaned, decolorized, and deodorized. Modified lanolin has undergone additional treatment to reduce the contents of free lanolin alcohols and detergent and pesticide residues. This modified product is intended to reduce hypersensitivity reactions. The *USP* monographs for both compounds state that they contain not more than 0.25% water and they may contain not more than 0.02% of a suitable antioxidant (4).
      (2) Lanolin is a yellow, tenacious, unctuous mass with a slight characteristic odor. It melts at between 38° and 44°C to give a clear or nearly clear yellow liquid. At 15°C it has a specific gravity of 0.932 to 0.945.
      (3) There is often confusion between Lanolin and hydrous lanolin. Hydrous lanolin, also known as *Hydrous Wool Fat*, contains 25% to 30% water. It is a yellowish white ointment with a mild characteristic odor. Prior to *USP 23*, hydrous lanolin was officially known as *Lanolin*, and the product now known as Lanolin was officially known as *Anhydrous Lanolin*. With *USP 23*, hydrous lanolin was deleted from the *USP* and the monograph for Anhydrous Lanolin was renamed *Lanolin*. You will still find references that use the older nomenclature.
   b. Solubility: Lanolin is practically insoluble in water but will take up twice its weight of water without separation. It is sparingly soluble in cold alcohol but more soluble in boiling alcohol.
   c. Incompatibilities: Lanolin is a natural product that may contain components that can act as oxidizing agents to sensitive ingredients.
   d. Uses
      (1) Lanolin may be used by itself, but it will also mix with vegetable oils or petrolatum to give an emollient base that is reported to penetrate the skin and give improved absorption of active ingredients (14).
      (2) As stated earlier, it will take up to twice its weight of water to form a water-in-oil emulsion.
   e. Other names: wool fat, anhydrous lanolin, refined wool fat

3. Paraffin NF
   a. Description

- **(1)** Paraffin is a purified mixture of solid hydrocarbons from petroleum (11).
- **(2)** It is a colorless or white translucent solid, is tasteless and odorless, and is slightly greasy to the touch. It has a congealing range of 47° to 65°C, depending on the grade, and the specific gravity of the melt is in the range of 0.84 to 0.89.
- **b.** Solubility: Paraffin is practically insoluble in water, alcohol, and acetone but freely soluble in volatile oils and most warm fixed oils.
- **c.** Incompatibilities: Paraffin is a stable, nonreactive compound.
- **d.** Uses: Paraffin is used as a stiffening ingredient in ointment bases.
- **e.** Other names: paraffin wax, hard paraffin, mineral wax

4. White Wax NF
- **a.** Description
    - **(1)** White wax is the bleached, purified wax of honeybees (11). It consists mainly of esters of long-chain hydrocarbons, with myricyl palmitate the principle ester. It also contains free fatty acids and carbohydrates with a small amount of free wax alcohols.
    - **(2)** It is a yellowish white translucent solid, nearly tasteless but having a faint odor. The melting point is 62° to 65°C; the specific gravity of the melted wax is approximately 0.95.
- **b.** Solubility: White wax is insoluble in water and sparingly soluble in alcohol. It is soluble in fixed and volatile oils.
- **c.** Incompatibilities: White wax is a fairly unreactive compound. The free fatty acids portion can react with bases such as sodium hydroxide to form soaps. This can be used to advantage in making an emulsion-type ointment base.
- **d.** Uses: White wax is used as a stiffening ingredient in ointment bases.
- **e.** Other names: bleached wax, white beeswax

5. Cetyl Esters Wax NF
- **a.** Description
    - **(1)** Cetyl esters wax is a mixture primarily of esters of saturated fatty alcohols and fatty acids (C_{14} to C_{18}) (11). Cetyl esters wax is a synthetic substitute for the natural product spermaceti, which was formerly extracted from the head of sperm whales.
    - **(2)** It is white to off-white translucent flakes with a faint odor and bland, mild flavor. Its melting point is 43°C to 47°C. When melted at 50°C, the specific gravity is 0.82 to 0.84.
- **b.** Solubility: Cetyl esters wax is insoluble in water, practically insoluble in cold alcohol, but soluble in boiling alcohol. It is soluble also in volatile and fixed oils. Its solubility in mineral oil is 14 to 22 mg/mL.
- **c.** Incompatibilities: Cetyl esters wax is quite stable and nonreactive, but it is incompatible with strong acids or bases (14).
- **d.** Uses: Cetyl esters wax is a stiffening ingredient and emollient in ointment bases.
- **e.** Other names: synthetic spermaceti

6. Cetyl Alcohol NF
- **a.** Description
    - **(1)** Cetyl alcohol is at least 90% cetyl alcohol, $CH_3(CH_2)_{14}CH_2OH$, with the remainder related alcohols (11), chiefly stearyl alcohol.
    - **(2)** It is white, waxy flakes or granules with a faint odor and a bland, mild flavor. Its melting point is 45°C to 50°C, the specific gravity of the melt being 0.908.
- **b.** Solubility: Cetyl alcohol is insoluble in water but soluble in alcohol and in vegetable oils. When melted, it is miscible with fats, mineral oils, and paraffins.
- **c.** Incompatibilities: Cetyl alcohol is quite stable and nonreactive, but it is incompatible with strong oxidizing agents (14).
- **d.** Uses (14)
    - **(1)** Cetyl alcohol is used as a stiffening ingredient and emollient not only in ointment bases but also in liquid emulsions and lotions, suppositories, and controlled-release solid dosage forms.
    - **(2)** It is widely used in manufactured topical products because of its favorable properties for such formulations: emollient, water absorptive, and emulsifying. It also gives these dosage forms a fine texture and good consistency.
    - **(3)** When applied to the skin, it is absorbed and retained in the epidermis. This accounts for its emollient, lubricating property. It leaves the skin feeling soft and smooth.
    - **(4)** When added to oleaginous bases such as petrolatum, it increases their ability to absorb water. In fact, when 5% is added to petrolatum, the combination will absorb 40% to 50% of its weight in water (14).

(5) It is used as an auxiliary emulsifier for both water-in-oil and oil-in-water emulsions. It is frequently used with detergent surfactants such as sodium lauryl sulfate to form improved barriers to coalescence in emulsion systems.

7. Stearyl Alcohol NF
   a. Description
      (1) Content: Stearyl Alcohol NF is at least 90% stearyl alcohol, $CH_3(CH_2)_{16}CH_2OH$, the remainder being related alcohols (11), chiefly cetyl alcohol.
      (2) It is hard, white, waxy flakes or granules with a faint odor and bland, mild flavor. Its melting point is 55°C to 60°C, and the specific gravity of the melt is 0.88 to 0.91.
   b. Solubility: Stearyl alcohol is insoluble in water but soluble in alcohol, propylene glycol, and vegetable oils.
   c. Incompatibilities: Stearyl alcohol is quite stable and nonreactive, but it is incompatible with strong oxidizing agents (14).
   d. Uses (14)
      (1) Stearyl alcohol is used mainly as a stiffening ingredient, but it does have some emollient, water-absorptive, and emulsifying properties. It is used in ointment bases, liquid emulsions and lotions, suppositories, and controlled-release solid dosage forms.
      (2) As with cetyl alcohol, when added to oleaginous bases such as petrolatum, it increases their ability to absorb water.
      (3) In a concentration of 6% to 25%, it is used in Polyethylene Glycol Ointment NF to increase the water-absorbing ability of that water-soluble base. (See the Polyethylene Glycol Ointment formula in Table 23.2.)

8. Lanolin Alcohols NF
   a. Description
      (1) Lanolin alcohol is a mixture of aliphatic alcohols, triterpenoid alcohols, and sterols that are obtained by the hydrolysis of lanolin. It contains not less than 30% of sterol, calculated as cholesterol. It may contain an antioxidant (11).
      (2) It is a hard, waxy, amber solid with a characteristic odor. Its melting point is not below 56°C.
      (3) This product is a purified version of wool alcohols, which consist of a separated fraction containing cholesterol and other alcohols prepared by the saponification of grease from the wool of sheep (12).
   b. Solubility: Lanolin alcohol is insoluble in water, slightly soluble in alcohol, and soluble 1 part in 25 parts of boiling alcohol.
   c. Incompatibilities: Lanolin alcohol is incompatible with coal tar, ichthammol, phenol, and resorcinol (14).
   d. Uses (14)
      (1) Lanolin alcohol is used mainly as an auxiliary emulsifying agent in ointments and other topical preparations, but it does have some emollient and water-absorptive properties.
      (2) As with cetyl and stearyl alcohol, when lanolin alcohol is added to oleaginous bases such as petrolatum, it increases their ability to absorb water; 5% lanolin alcohol added to petrolatum increases threefold its ability to absorb water .
   e. Other names: wool alcohols, wool-wax alcohol

9. Cholesterol NF

$C_{27}H_{46}O$ MW = 386.65

   a. Description: Cholesterol is white to light yellow leaflets, needles, powder, or granules. It is almost odorless, has a melting point of 147° to 150°C, and is affected by light.
   b. Solubility: Cholesterol is insoluble in water, sparingly soluble in alcohol (1g/100 mL) and dehydrated alcohol (slowly, 1g/50 mL), and soluble in acetone, hot alcohol, and vegetable oils.
   c. Incompatibilities: Cholesterol is a stable and nonreactive compound.

  d. Uses (14)

  (1) Cholesterol is used as an emulsifying agent in ointments and other topical preparations in concentrations of 0.3% to 5%.

  (2) It also has emollient and water-absorptive properties.

10. Glyceryl Monostearate NF

  a. Description

  (1) Glyceryl monostearate is a mixture primarily of the monoesters of glycerin with stearic acid, $CH_3(CH_2)_{16}COOH$, and palmitic acid, $CH_3(CH_2)_{14}COOH$. It may contain an antioxidant (11).

  (2) It is a whitish, waxlike solid with a slight agreeable fatty odor and taste. It does not melt below 55°C, and the specific gravity of the melt is 0.92. Glyceryl monostearate is affected by light.

  b. Solubility: Glyceryl monostearate is insoluble in water but soluble in hot alcohol, acetone, mineral, or fixed oils.

  c. Incompatibilities: The grades of glyceryl monostearate that are self-emulsifying (e.g., Arlacel 165, Hodag CMS-D) are incompatible with acidic compounds.

  d. Uses (14)

  (1) Glyceryl monostearate is used as a nonionic emulsifier for both oil-in-water and water-in-oil emulsions, both liquids and semisolids. It also has emollient properties and imparts texture and viscosity to topical preparations of various types.

  (2) It is also used in solid dosage forms for multiple purposes, including as a lubricant in tablet and capsule making and as a release modifier for controlled-release oral dosage forms, suppositories, and implants. Self-emulsifying glyceryl monostearate is an ingredient in the commercial fatty acid suppository base Fattibase.

  (3) Although glyceryl monostearate is the most commonly used ingredient of this type, there are numerous other glyceryl fatty acid esters such as glyceryl monooleate. For information on the uses and unique properties of these materials, consult *The Handbook of Pharmaceutical Excipients*.

11. Stearic Acid NF

  a. Description

  (1) Stearic Acid NF is a mixture primarily of stearic acid, $CH_3(CH_2)_{16}COOH$, and palmitic acid, $CH_3(CH_2)_{14}COOH$. The content of stearic acid is not less than 40%, and the content of the both stearic and palmitic acids is not less than 90% (11). The *NF* also has a monograph article Purified Stearic Acid in which the stearic acid content is not less than 90% and the combined acids is not less than 96% of the total (11).

  (2) Stearic acid is a hard, white to faintly yellowish, glossy, crystalline solid or powder with a slight odor and taste of tallow; it melts at approximately 55°C, with the purified acid melting at 69° to 70°C.

  (3) Both Stearic Acid and Purified Stearic Acid must be labeled for external use only, unless they are made entirely from edible sources (11).

  b. Solubility: Stearic acid is practically insoluble in water. It is soluble as 1 g/20 mL alcohol or 25 mL acetone and in propylene glycol.

  c. Incompatibilities

  (1) As discussed in d.(2), stearic acid reacts with alkali and organic bases to form stearate soaps. In most cases, this is an intended reaction, as with nascent soap emulsifying agents and with the in situ formation of sodium stearate in Glycerin Suppositories USP.

  (2) It also reacts with metal hydroxides to form water-insoluble stearates, and salts of zinc and calcium are reported to react with stearic acid in ointment bases to give lumpy preparations (14).

  d. Uses

  (1) Stearic acid is widely used as an emulsifying and solubilizing agent in topical preparations. It is also used as a lubricant in tablet and capsule making.

  (2) Stearic acid is the fatty acid part of a soap emulsifier used for water-removable o/w emulsion bases. The base part may be sodium or potassium hydroxide, sodium carbonate, or triethanolamine. When excess stearic acid is added, the unneutralized stearic acid is emulsified as part of the oil phase. This free stearic acid gives these creams a pearlescent luster; they are known as *vanishing creams*. Because of the inherent compatibility problems of soap emulsifiers, some newer vanishing cream formulations use nonionic surfactants, but stearic acid is still added for the desirable pearl luster.

12. Polyethylene Glycol NF (PEG) (11,15)

   a. Description

      (1) PEG has the general formula H—[OCH_2CH_2—]$_n$OH.

      (2) Polyethylene glycols are available as various grades from 200 to 8,000, where the assigned number indicates the average molecular weight (11). Those with numbers 200 through 600 are clear, viscous liquids, PEG 900 and 1,000 are soft solids, and PEGs 1,450 to 8,000 are white, waxy solids or flakes. All are odorless and tasteless, and the pH of a 5% solution is in the range of 4.5 to 7.5. See Table 24.1 in Chapter 24 for more information on the densities and melting points of the individual grades.

   b. Solubility: Although all PEGs are soluble in water and in many organic solvents, their solubilities depend on their molecular weight. See Table 24.1 in Chapter 24 for the solubility of individual grades in water. The liquid PEGs are soluble in acetone, alcohol, glycerin, and glycols; solid PEGs are soluble in acetone and alcohol and slightly soluble in aliphatic hydrocarbons but are insoluble in fats, fixed oils, and mineral oil.

   c. Incompatibilities (14)

      (1) Although these compounds are quite stable, polyethylene glycols may cause problems for compounds subject to oxidation because of the presence of residual peroxide impurities from the manufacturing process.

      (2) Other reported incompatibilities include reduced antibacterial activity of some antibiotics, including penicillin and bacitracin; reduced preservative effectiveness of the parabens owing to binding with PEG; liquification of PEG bases with phenol, tannic acid, and salicylic acid (although the original USP formula for Benzoic and Salicylic Acid Ointment, also known as *Whitfield's Ointment*, used PEG Ointment as the base); discoloration of sulfanilamides; precipitation of sorbitol; and softening or other reactions with some plastics and some membrane filters.

   d. Uses (14)

      (1) Polyethylene glycols are widely used in pharmaceutical products and preparations. They are used as ointment and suppository bases, solvents, viscosity-increasing agents, plasticizers, and lubricants in tablet and capsule making. They are approved for use in oral, topical, rectal, ophthalmic, and parenteral products.

      (2) Their usefulness is limited by the fact that they may be irritating to delicate tissues, mucous membranes, and denuded skin. Although their water-solubility would seem to make them good vehicles to use on burned or denuded skin, they must be used with caution in these situations, both because of their irritating nature and because there have been reports of systemic toxicity due to absorption from these areas. There have also been reports of hypersensitivity reactions.

      (3) The limitation for parenteral products is 30% v/v of PEG 300.

   e. Other names: PEG, Carbowax, Atpeg, Hodag PEG

REFERENCES

1. The United States Pharmacopeial Convention, Inc. Chapter ⟨1151⟩. 2008 USP 31/NF 26. Rockville, MD: Author, 2007; 617–621.

2. Marshall K, Foster TS, Carlin HS, Williams RL. Development of a compendial taxonomy and glossary for pharmaceutical dosage forms. Pharmacopeial Forum. Rockville, MD: The United States Pharmacopeial Convention, Inc., 2003; 29(5).

3. The United States Pharmacopeial Convention, Inc. Front matter—NF: Excipients. 2008 USP 31/NF 26. Rockville, MD: Author, 2007.

4. The United States Pharmacopeial Convention, Inc. USP Monographs. 2008 USP 31/NF 26. Rockville, MD: Author, 2007.

5. Marriot JF, Wilson KA, Langley CA, Belcher D. Pharmaceutical compounding and dispensing. London, UK: Pharmaceutical Press, 2006; 155–171.

6. Shrewsbury R. Applied pharmaceutics in contemporary compounding, 2nd ed. Englewood, CO: Morton Publishing Company, 2008; 117–129.

7. Reynolds JEF, ed. Martindale: The extra pharmacopoeia, 30th ed. London: The Pharmaceutical Press, 1993; 1111.

8. Thompson, MICROMEDEX, Inc. USP DI vol. III, 27th ed. Englewood, CO: Author, 2007.

9. Clark EW, et al. Lanolin with reduced sensitizing potential. Contact Dermatitis 1977; 3: 69–74.

10. Ecanow B, Siegel FP. Dermatology. In: King RE, ed. Dispensing of medications, 9th ed. Easton, PA: Mack Publishing Co., 1984; 78–79.

11. The United States Pharmacopeial Convention, Inc. NF Monographs. 2007 USP 30/NF 25. Rockville, MD: Author, 2006.

12. Swinyard EA, Lowenthal W. Pharmaceutical necessities. In: Gennaro AR, ed. Remington's the science and practice of pharmacy, 18th ed. Easton, PA: Mack Publishing Co., 1990; 1310–1312.

13. Reilly WJ. Pharmaceutical necessities. In: University of the Sciences in Philadelphia, ed. Remington: The science and practice of pharmacy, 21st ed. Baltimore, MD: Lippincott Williams & Wilkins, 2005; 1074–1079.

14. Rowe R, Sheskey P, Weller P, eds. Handbook of pharmaceutical excipients, 5th ed. Washington, DC: APhA Publications, 2005.

15. Plaxco JM. Suppositories. In: King RE, ed. Dispensing of medications, 9th ed. Easton, PA: Mack Publishing Co., 1984; 93.

16. Crowley MM. Solutions, emulsions, suspensions, and extracts. In: University of the Sciences in Philadelphia, ed. Remington: The science and practice of pharmacy, 21st ed. Baltimore, MD: Lippincott Williams & Wilkins, 2005; 772.

17. Harvey, SC, Swinyard EA. Sympathomimetic Drugs. In: Martin EW, ed. Remington's Practice of Pharmacy, 12th ed. Easton, PA: Mack Publishing Co., 1961; 831.

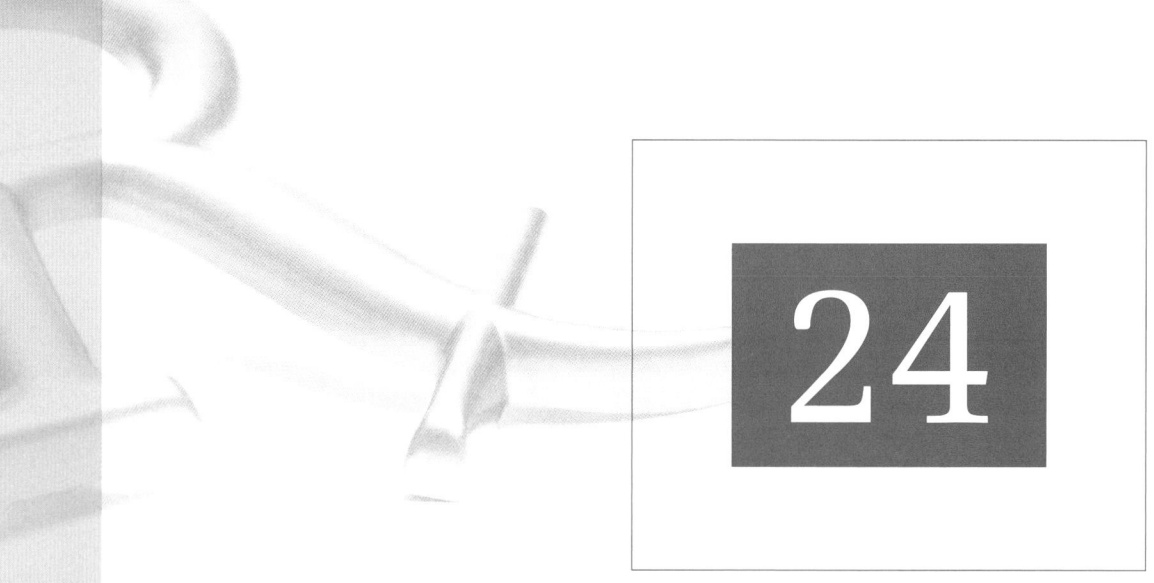

Suppository Bases

Melgardt de Villiers, PhD

I. DEFINITIONS

A. **Suppositories:** "Suppositories are solid bodies of various weights and shapes, adapted for introduction into the rectal, vaginal, or urethral orifice of the human body. They usually melt, soften, or dissolve at body temperature. A suppository may act as a protectant or palliative to the local tissues at the point of introduction or as a carrier of therapeutic agents for systemic or local action" (1). —*USP*

(See the section on definitions and nomenclature in Chapter 31, Suppositories, for a discussion of proposed nomenclature changes for suppository dosage forms.)

B. According to the *USP*, there are six general classes of suppository bases (1):
   1. Cocoa butter
   2. Cocoa butter substitutes
   3. Glycerinated gelatin
   4. Polyethylene glycol base
   5. Surfactant base
   6. Tableted suppositories or inserts

C. According to Allen (2), four classifications of suppository bases are usually described, based on their melting or dissolution properties:
   1. The first is the fat- or oil-type base, which must melt at body temperature to release its medication.
   2. The second is the glycerin-gelatin base suppository, which absorbs water and dissolves to release its medication.
   3. The third is the water-soluble or water-miscible polymers and surface-active agents.
   4. The fourth is a group of bases containing disintegrating agents, natural gums, effervescent agents, collagen, fibrin, hydrogels, etc.

II. DESIRABLE PROPERTIES OF SUPPOSITORY BASES

A. Chemically and physically stable under normal conditions of use and storage
B. Nonreactive and compatible with a wide variety of drugs and auxiliary agents
C. Free from objectionable odor

D. An aesthetically appealing appearance

E. Nontoxic, nonsensitizing, and nonirritating to sensitive tissues

F. Expansion–contraction characteristics such that it shrinks just enough on cooling so that it releases easily from suppository molds

G. Melts or dissolves in the intended body orifice to release the drug

H. Nonbinding of drugs

I. Mixes with or absorbs some water

J. Viscosity low enough when melted to pour easily but high enough to suspend particles of solid drug

K. Some wetting and/or emulsifying properties so that it will spread, disperse in, and release the active ingredient(s) at the administration site

III. CLASSIFICATION AND CHARACTERISTICS OF SUPPOSITORY BASES

The six general classes of suppository bases identified by the *USP* (1) are described here. The descriptions and solubilities for bases or base ingredient are a composite of information from *Remington's The Science and Practice of Pharmacy* (3), the *Handbook of Pharmaceutical Excipients* (4), official monographs in the *USP–NF* (5,6), and other references as cited. Additional information on each agent, including references to original research journal articles, can be found in the *Handbook of Pharmaceutical Excipients*.

A. Cocoa Butter NF

  1. Description

   a. Cocoa butter is the fat from the seeds of *Theobroma cacao* (chocolate beans). It may be obtained either by expressing the oil from the seeds or by solvent extraction. Chemically, it is a mixture of triglycerides of saturated and unsaturated fatty acids, primarily stearic, palmitic, oleic, lauric, and linoleic.

   b. It is a mellow, yellowish solid with a mild odor and bland taste. It is a solid at room temperature but melts at body temperature with a melting point of 31° to 34°C. The specific gravity of the melt is 0.858 to 0.864. It is available as bars or grated.

   c. Cocoa butter does not contain emulsifiers, so it does not absorb significant amounts of water. Tween 61, a tan, waxy, solid, nonionic surfactant, can be added (5% to 10%) to increase the water absorption properties of cocoa butter (7), although addition of nonionic surfactants reportedly gives suppositories with poor stability on storage (8).

  2. Solubility: It is insoluble in water, slightly soluble in alcohol, and soluble in boiling absolute alcohol.

  3. Incompatibilities: The most notable compatibility problem of cocoa butter is the lowering of its melting point with drugs such as chloral hydrate, phenol, and thymol. This can be overcome by the addition of 4% to 6% white wax or 18% to 28% cetyl esters wax, but determining the exact amount that will give an appropriate melting temperature can be difficult and time consuming (9). A group of successful formulas for chloral hydrate suppositories, including some made with cocoa butter, has been published (10).

  4. Advantages

   a. Cocoa butter is bland and nonirritating to sensitive membrane tissues. It is also an excellent emollient and is used alone or in topical skin products for this property.

   b. Because cocoa butter has a variety of uses besides suppository making, it is readily available in many pharmacies. It is also one base that can be used for hand-molding suppositories; no special molds or equipment are needed. These two properties make this base useful when a custom suppository is needed on an emergency basis.

   c. Cocoa butter has a solidification temperature 12° to 13° below its melting point. This makes it easy to pour suppositories before the base solidifies (7).

   d. Cocoa butter is available in grated form. This eliminates one time-consuming aspect of compounding suppositories.

  5. Disadvantages

   a. Because of its relatively low melting point, cocoa butter and its suppositories must be stored either at controlled room temperature or in the refrigerator. It is recommended that storage temperature not exceed 25°C.

   b. Cocoa butter has the further disadvantage of existing in several polymorphic forms that have even lower melting points: 18°, 24°, and 28°C to 31°C (7). Cocoa butter suppositories are therefore somewhat difficult to make by fusion.

    (1) Cocoa butter can very easily be overheated and, when it is, it may solidify as one of the lower melting polymorphs. This means that the suppositories do not set up properly, and they may melt at room temperature, or the suppositories may liquefy when handled by the patient during insertion.

(2) When melting cocoa butter, a warm-water bath should be used and the temperature should be controlled closely. When melted, the base should have a slightly opalescent appearance. Once the molten cocoa butter has completely turned to a clear, straw-colored liquid, the desired melting point has been exceeded; all the stable β-crystals have been destroyed, and the suppositories will melt at a temperature below the desired 34°C to 35°C. A sample procedure with appropriate temperatures for the warm-water bath and the cocoa butter melt is given with example 31.1 in Chapter 31, Suppositories.

c. As with all fatty bases, cocoa butter suppositories may give poor and somewhat erratic release of some drugs. The release of a drug from a fatty suppository base, like cocoa butter, to the aqueous medium in the body cavity depends on the water/base partition coefficient of the drug. Because many organic drug molecules are water-insoluble and lipophilic unless present in an ionized salt form, this can be a problem.

(1) For this reason, from a bioavailability point of view, water-soluble ionized (salt) forms of drugs (these have high water/base partition coefficients) should be used when possible with cocoa butter, particularly when a systemic effect is desired. For example, if a drug such as phenobarbital is being incorporated into a cocoa butter suppository base, the sodium salt of phenobarbital is the preferred form of the drug to use. This principle is illustrated with Sample Prescription 31.2 in Chapter 31.

(2) For drugs, such as acetaminophen, that do not have a water-soluble form, cocoa butter is not a good choice for the suppository base (11).

B. Cocoa butter substitutes

1. Description

a. The *USP* has the following description of cocoa butter substitutes:

> Fat-type suppository bases can be produced from a variety of vegetable oils, such as coconut or palm kernel, which are modified by esterification, hydrogenation, and fractionation to obtain products of varying composition and melting temperatures (e.g., Hydrogenated Vegetable Oil and Hard Fat). These products can be so designed as to reduce rancidity. At the same time, desired characteristics such as narrow intervals between melting and solidification temperatures, and melting ranges to accommodate various formulation and climatic conditions, can be built in (1).

b. Chemically, this type of base is composed primarily of mixtures of triglyceride esters of saturated fatty acids in the C-12 to C-18 range, with lesser amounts of mono- and diglycerides. Other additives include beeswax, lecithin, polysorbates, ethoxylated fatty alcohols, and ethoxylated partial fatty glycerides (4). As can be seen later in the descriptions of some commercially available synthetic fatty bases, some also contain surfactants, self-emulsifying agents, and suspending agents.

c. Substitutes for cocoa butter were first developed in Europe during the Second World War because of the limited availability of natural cocoa butter. In recent years, suppliers of compounding materials in the United States have developed additional products of this type (8). Several of these are described here.

d. Witepsol

(1) Witepsol is a whitish, waxy, brittle solid that melts to a clear to yellowish liquid; it is nearly odorless and has a density of 0.95 to 0.98 at 20°C. It contains emulsifying agents and will absorb a small amount of water (4,8).

(2) Although the *Handbook of Pharmaceutical Excipients* lists 20 different grades of Witepsol, the H15 grade is the most readily available to pharmacists. It has a melting point range of 33.5°C to 35.5°C (4), which is quite close to its congealing range of 32°C to 34°C (8).

(3) Although some pharmacists speak highly of Witepsol bases, others report poor or uneven results. Although suppositories made with this base solidify rapidly and should contract to release easily from the mold, there are reports of problems with suppositories breaking into pieces when being removed from the suppository mold.

e. Fattibase (Paddock Laboratories)

(1) Fattibase is an opaque, white, waxy solid; it is odorless and has a bland taste. Its specific gravity at 37°C is 0.89. It is a mixture of triglycerides from palm, palm kernel, and coconut oils, together with self-emulsifying glyceryl monostearate and polyoxyl stearate, which serve as emulsifiers and suspending agents (12).

(2) It has a melting point range of 32°C to 36.5°C, but instructions from its manufacturer, Paddock Labs, state that the base should be heated slowly and evenly to 49°C to 54°C before adding the active ingredients. The suppositories should be poured when the mixture is 43°C to 49°C. The base should not be heated above 60°C, and use of microwave ovens for heating the base is not recommended (12,13).

(3) Fattibase has the advantages of cocoa butter without the difficulties caused by the sensitive melting point range and polymorphism of cocoa butter. Suppositories made from this base release well from molds; a light spraying of the molds with vegetable oil can be used if needed.

f. Fattyblend (Gallipot Inc.) (14)

(1) The suppository base Fattyblend exhibits the body-temperature melting characteristic inherent in cocoa butter without the polymorphism. It offers uniformity, bland odor, and low irritation characteristics as well as excellent mold release properties as compared with cocoa butter.

(2) It contains triglycerides from palm, palm kernel, and coconut oils, as well as emulsifying and suspending agents.

(3) It has also been used in lip balms and lipsticks because of its bland taste.

g. Supposiblend (Gallipot Inc.) (14)

(1) This is a pellet form of a triglyceride (fatty-acid blend type) suppository base made from vegetable oils, predominantly palm kernel oil that resists oxidation, and does not exhibit the polymorphism of cocoa butter.

(2) It has a melting point range of 34°C to 37°C. It contracts slightly while cooling, which imparts excellent mold release characteristics.

(3) It contains emulsifiers to allow absorption of small amounts of aqueous solutions.

h. Supposibase-F (Hawkins) (15)

(1) Like Supposiblend, Supposibase-F is a pellet-form suppository base that is made from refined, hydrogenated, deodorized vegetable oils, primarily palm kernel oil. It is reported to have good chemical stability, little tendency for oxidation, and physical stability with minimal polymorphism.

(2) It has a melting point range of 34°C to 37°C.

2. Solubility: Cocoa butter substitutes are practically insoluble in water and slightly soluble in warm alcohol.

3. Incompatibilities: The cocoa butter substitutes may have some of the same temperature-lowering difficulties as are seen with cocoa butter.

4. Advantages

a. Fatty bases are favored because they are bland and nonirritating to sensitive membrane tissues.

b. Some of the commercially available synthetic versions of cocoa butter are easier to work with than cocoa butter because they are not as sensitive to minor melting temperature fluctuations and, unlike cocoa butter, they exhibit minimal problems with polymorphic forms.

c. Some of the specially formulated synthetic fatty bases include surfactants and self-emulsifying agents that improve drug release and bioavailability (16).

5. Disadvantages

a. Because of their relatively low melting points, these synthetic cocoa butter bases and their suppositories must be stored either at controlled room temperature or in the refrigerator.

b. As discussed earlier in the section on cocoa butter (see section III.A), fatty bases tend to give poor and somewhat erratic release of water-insoluble drugs, although those bases formulated with surfactants and emulsifiers are reported to be superior in this regard (16). Still, water-soluble ionized (salt) forms of drugs should be used when possible with fatty bases, particularly when a systemic effect is desired. For drugs that do not have water-soluble forms, therapeutic results should be monitored for assurance of adequate drug release from the dosage form. This is illustrated with an indomethacin suppository formulated in Sample Prescription 31.1 in Chapter 31.

C. Glycerinated gelatin bases

1. Description: This base consists of 70 parts of glycerin, 20 parts of gelatin, and 10 parts of water (1). The method of preparation is like that for glycerinated gummy gel base, which is described in Table 26.3 in Chapter 26.

2. These bases are used infrequently because they are more difficult to make and offer few advantages.

3. The base material has a soft, rubbery consistency (rather like the candy, gummy worms), which makes them suitable for vaginal administration but not firm enough for rectal use.

Table 24.1		**PHYSICAL PROPERTIES OF POLYETHYLENE GLYCOLS**					
GRADE (AVG. MW)	MW RANGE	PHYSICAL FORM	DENSITY AT 20°C* OR 60°C**	MELTING RANGE (°C)	SOLUBILITY IN WATER (WT % 20°C)	pH OF 5% SOLUTION
300	285–315	liquid	1.1250*	–15 to –8	Complete	4.5 to 7.5
400	380–420	liquid	1.1254*	4 to 8	Complete	4.5 to 7.5
600	570–630	liquid	1.1257*	20 to 25	Complete	4.5 to 7.5
1,000	950–1,050	soft solid	1.0926**	37 to 40	80	4.5 to 7.5
1,450	1,300–1,600	soft solid or flake	1.0919**	43 to 46	72	4.5 to 7.5
3,350	3,000–3,700	flake or powder	1.0926**	54 to 58	67	4.5 to 7.5
4,600	4,400–4,800	flake or powder	1.0926**	57 to 61	65	4.5 to 7.5
8,000	7,000–9,000	flake or powder	1.0845**	60 to 63	63	4.5 to 7.5

Source: The Dow Chemical Company, Carbowax and Carbowax Sentry Product Data Sheets (http://www.dow.com/polyglycols/carbowax/index.htm).
*Density measurements done at 20° for those grades that are liquid at that temperature (300, 400, 600).
**Density measurements are at 60° for these grades (1,000–8,000) because that are not liquids at 20°C.

4. They do not melt but dissolve slowly in the mucous secretions of the vagina; they have been recommended for sustained release of local antimicrobial agents (7). Glycerinated gelatin suppositories should be moistened before insertion.

5. Glycerinated gelatin suppositories are hygroscopic, so they must be dispensed in tight containers.

6. They are reported to support mold or bacterial growth, so they should be stored in the refrigerator and should contain a preservative (e.g., methylparaben 0.18%, propylparaben 0.02%) (8).

D. **Polyethylene glycol bases**

1. Description: Polyethylene glycol (PEG) suppository bases are composed of blends of polyethylene glycol polymers of various molecular weights. Polyethylene Glycol is described in Chapter 23, Ointment Bases, and properties of some PEG polymers that are used often for pharmaceutical applications are given in Table 24.1. Formulas for some PEG suppository bases are given in Table 24.2.

2. Some commercial polyethylene glycol suppository bases also contain additional components, such as surfactants. Two widely used bases are Polybase (Paddock Labs) and PEGblend (Gallipot Inc.): Both contain a mixture of polyethylene glycols plus the emulsifier polysorbate 80. Polybase is a white solid with an average molecular weight of 3,440 and a specific gravity of 1.177 at 24° C (13,17).

3. PEG suppository bases are formulated so they do not melt at body temperature but rather dissolve in body fluids. Suppositories made from these bases should be moistened with water before insertion.

4. Advantages
   a. PEG suppositories are easily made by fusion.
   b. When formulated with an appropriate PEG blend, they dissolve in body cavity fluids and release the active ingredient(s), both hydrophilic and hydrophobic drugs. Provided there are sufficient aqueous secretions in the body cavity, they provide more reliable release of drug from the dosage form than do fatty bases.
   c. Because their melting points are easily controlled by appropriate blending, these bases and their suppositories do not require carefully monitored storage temperatures.

5. Disadvantages
   a. PEG suppositories are irritating to body cavity tissues, so they have less patient acceptance than do fatty-base suppositories.
   b. They are incompatible with a long list of drugs, especially those prone to oxidation. Specific examples are given in the description of polyethylene glycol in Chapter 23.
   c. They interact with polystyrene, the plastic often used for prescription vials, so they should not be dispensed in these containers unless the suppositories are first wrapped with foil.

E. **Surfactant or water-dispersible bases**

1. Several nonionic surfactants, such as polyoxyethylene sorbitan fatty-acid esters and the polyoxyethylene stearates, are used alone or in combination with other suppository vehicle materials to make suppository bases (1).

Table 24.2	POLYETHYLENE GLYCOL (PEG) BASES	

BASE 1

PEG	8,000	50%
PEG	1,540	30%
PEG	400	20%

Base 1 is a good general-purpose, water-soluble suppository base.

BASE 2

PEG	3,350	60%
PEG	1,000	30%
PEG	400	10%

Base 2 is a good general-purpose base that is slightly softer than base 1 and dissolves more readily.

BASE 3

PEG	8,000	30%
PEG	1,540	70%

Base 3 has a higher melting point, which is usually sufficient to compensate for the melting point lowering of drugs such as chloral hydrate.

BASE 4

PEG	8,000	40%
PEG	400	60%

BASE 5

PEG	8,000	20%
PEG	400	80%

Bases 4 and 5 have been used for progesterone suppositories. Personal communication to the author from practitioners report base 5 to be superior for this purpose.

BASE 6

PEG	8,000	60%
PEG	1,540	25%
Cetyl Alcohol		5%
Water		10%

Base 6 can be used for water-soluble drugs.

Bases 1, 2, 3, 4, and 6 are found in Plaxco JM, Suppositories. In: King RE, ed. Dispensing of medications, 9th ed. Easton, PA: Mack Publishing Co., 1984; 93–94.

2. Bases of this type are not used as frequently for compounding because they are more complicated to formulate.
3. If formulated correctly, these bases have desirable melting points and consistencies. Because they contain surfactants, there are readily dispersed in body cavity fluids.
4. One blend that could be easily made in the pharmacy contains 60% Tween 61 and 40% Tween 60 (7). Both of these compounds are solids at room temperature. They are available through vendors of compounding drugs and chemicals.

F. **Tableted suppositories or inserts**
1. Vaginal suppositories (now usually referred to as *vaginal inserts*) are occasionally prepared by the compression of powdered materials into a suitable shape. They are prepared also by encapsulation in soft gelatin (1).
2. The compression method is suited for suppositories that contain heat-labile drugs or contain a large proportion of insoluble ingredients.

3. This method offers the possibility to make suppositories of many shapes and sizes.

4. The filler used in these suppositories is usually lactose combined with a disintegrating agent, a dispensing agent, and a lubricant.

G. Release of drug from suppository bases is a complicated and unpredictable process. The rate-limiting step in drug release is not only the speed at which fatty bases melt or PEG bases dissolve but also the time required for the drug to partition and diffuse out of the base into the rectal or vaginal lumen. In practice, because bioavailability studies are usually impracticable, it is important to monitor the effectiveness of the drug delivery system by frequent monitoring of therapeutic results.

REFERENCES

1. The United States Pharmacopeial Convention, Inc. Chapter ⟨1151⟩. 2008 USP 31/NF 26. Rockville, MD: Author, 2007; 622–623.

2. Allen LV. Compounding rectal dosage forms. Part II. Secundum Artem, 14(4) (http://www.paddocklabs.com/forms/secundum/volume_14.4.pdf).

3. Block LH. Medicated topicals. In: University of the Sciences in Philadelphia, ed. Remington: The science and practice of pharmacy, 21st ed. Baltimore, MD: Lippincott Williams & Wilkins, 2005; 883–886.

4. Rowe R, Sheskey P, Weller P, eds. Handbook of pharmaceutical excipients, 5th ed. Washington, DC: APhA Publications, 2005.

5. The United States Pharmacopeial Convention, Inc. NF monographs. 2007 USP 30/NF 25. Rockville, MD: Author, 2006.

6. The United States Pharmacopeial Convention, Inc. Front matter—NF: Excipients. 2007 USP 30/NF 25. Rockville, MD: Author, 2006.

7. Coben LJ, Lieberman HA. Suppositories. In: Lieberman HA, Lachman L, Kanig J, eds. The theory and practice of industrial pharmacy, 3rd ed. Philadelphia: Lea & Febiger, 1986; 564–588.

8. Plaxco JM. Suppositories. In: King RE, ed. Dispensing of medication, 9th ed. Easton, PA: Mack Publishing Co., 1984; 93–94.

9. King JC. Suppositories. In: Martin EW, ed. Dispensing of medication, 7th ed. Easton, PA: Mack Publishing Co., 1971; 849.

10. Schumacher GF. Chloral hydrate suppositories. Am J Hosp Pharm 1966; 23: 110.

11. Feldman S. Bioavailability of acetaminophen suppositories. Am J Hosp Pharm 1975; 32: 1173–1174.

12. Fattibase Product Data Sheet, Paddock Laboratories, Minneapolis, MN.

13. Paddock Laboratories Customer Service Department. Personal correspondence. Minneapolis, MN: Paddock Laboratories, Inc.

14. Gallipot Inc. Brochure. 2400 Pilot Knob Road, St. Paul, MN 55120, E-mail: info//www.gallipot.com/).

15. Hawkins Inc. 2008 Hawkins Pharmacy Compounding Catalog. 3000 East Hennepin Avenue, Minneapolis, MN 55413, E-mail: pharmcs//www.hawkinsinc.com/pharmaceutical).

16. Yamazaki M, Soichi I, Sasaki N, et al. Comparison of three test methods for suppositories. Pharmacopeial forum. Rockville, MD: The United States Pharmacopeial Convention, Inc., 1991; Sept–Oct; 2427–2437.

17. The Dow Chemical Company. Carbowax and Carbowax Sentry Product Data Sheets. (http://www.dow.com/polyglycols/carbowax/index.htm).

Part 5

Nonsterile Dosage Forms

and Their Preparation

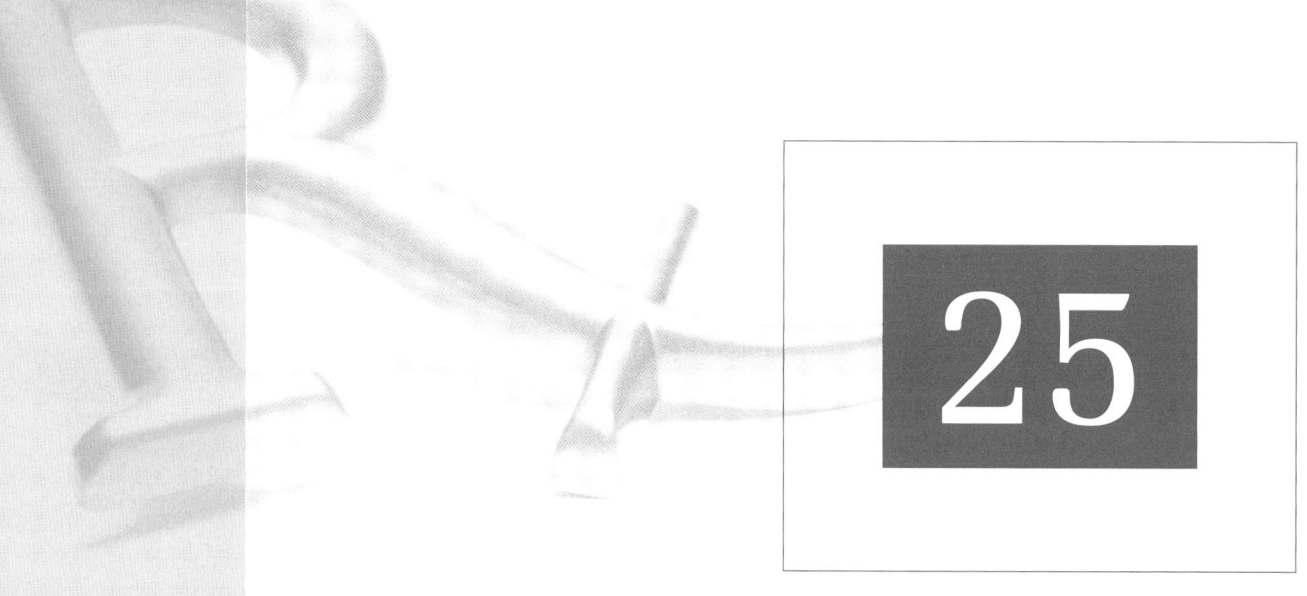

Powders

I. DEFINITIONS

A. **Powders:** Powders are defined in *USP 31* Chapter ⟨1151⟩, Pharmaceutical Dosage Forms, as "intimate mixtures of dry, finely divided drugs and/or chemicals that may be intended for internal (Oral Powders) or external (Topical Powders) use" (1). A similar definition is given in the *CDER Data Standards Manual* published by the FDA Center for Drug Evaluation and Research (CDER), http://www.fda.cder/dsm/DRG/drg00201.htm, accessed March 2008.

B. **Powder:** Proposed new *USP* nomenclature for pharmaceutical dosage forms defines the more general term *powder* as "a solid, or mixture of solids, that has been reduced to a finely divided state" (2). (See the introduction to Chapter 27 for an explanation and discussion of proposed revised *USP* nomenclature.)

C. The following powder types have physical properties that require special handling. In addition to information given in this chapter, compatibility and stability issues for these powders are discussed in Chapter 37.

1. **Efflorescent powders** are drugs or chemicals that contain water of hydration that may be released when the powders are manipulated or are stored under conditions of low relative humidity.

2. **Hygroscopic powders** are solid drugs or chemicals that absorb moisture from the air.

3. **Deliquescent powders** are hygroscopic powders that may absorb sufficient moisture from the air to dissolve and form a solution.

4. **Pharmaceutical eutectic mixture** is a mixture of two or more solid substances that may liquefy when intimately mixed at room temperature.

II. PHARMACEUTICAL USES OF POWDERS

A. Topical bulk powders are applied to the skin for local effect.

B. Bulk powders for internal use offer a convenient method of dispensing nonpotent, powdered drugs that have doses that require moderate to large volumes of powder. Common therapeutic uses for oral bulk powders include antacids, bulk laxatives, antidiarrheal medications, and oral electrolyte mixtures for rehydration. Bulk powders also offer a convenient way for patients to make vaginal douches. Because, at the time of administration, the patient or caregiver measures the dose volumetrically using a household measuring spoon or cup, this dosage form cannot be used for drugs that require precise and accurate dosing.

C. Powders may also be dispensed as divided powders, also known as *chartulae*. In this case, the compounder weighs each dose of powder separately and places it in a small individual packet. At the time of administration, the patient or caregiver mixes the contents of a packet into a liquid or other vehicle. When the medication is for oral use, the powder can be mixed with soft food, such as pudding or applesauce, for ease of administration. This dosage form is useful when a solid dosage form is desired but the medication is not manufactured in the required dose, or when it is supplied as capsules or tablets but the patient cannot swallow these dosage forms.

D. Powders for internal use may also be encapsulated into hard-shell capsules or compressed into tablets. Because the quantity of drug formulated into tablets and capsules can be measured accurately and precisely, these systems are ideal for potent drugs. Compounding of capsules is discussed in Chapter 26.

E. Because nearly all drugs are solids, powders are used as the primary ingredients for most other dosage forms.

III. ADVANTAGES OF SOLID DOSAGE FORMS

A. Drugs and chemicals are most stable as dry solids.

B. Because they are dry and compact, tablets, capsules, and divided powders are packaged, transported, administered, and stored more easily than are drugs formulated in solutions or suspensions.

C. Undesirable taste is less noticeable when substances are in solid form than when in solution. Objectionable taste can be concealed completely by enclosing the solid drug in capsules or coated tablets.

D. Accurate dosing is facilitated with dosage forms furnished as individual units, such as tablets, capsules, and divided powders.

E. Controlled release is much easier to achieve with solid dosage forms than with liquids.

IV. DESIRED PROPERTIES OF POWDERS

A. When intended for topical application, powders should be finely divided and have uniform particle size so as to be smooth to the touch and nonirritating to the skin. They should be free-flowing and should spread easily on the surface of the skin.

B. Powders for internal use should also be finely divided with uniform particle size because the rate of dissolution, and therefore often the bioavailability of the drug, depends on the particle size of the drug.

1. Dissolution rate is expressed mathematically by the Noyes-Whitney equation:

$$\frac{dC}{dt} = KS\,(C_s - C)$$

where

dC/dt = change in concentration with change in time (or rate of dissolution)
K = the dissolution rate constant
S = surface area of the solid
C_s = solubility of the solid
C = concentration of the drug in solution at time = t

2. Because the surface area (S) of a given amount of solid increases as the particle size is decreased for a given weight of solid, the smaller the particle size, the larger the surface area and the faster the rate of dissolution.

C. Even when powder is being used as an ingredient for another dosage form, particle size is important. Not only does it affect the rate of dissolution and bioavailability in these preparations, but it also can affect the rate of settling (in suspensions) and the degree of comfort (in topical suspensions, ointments, and creams).

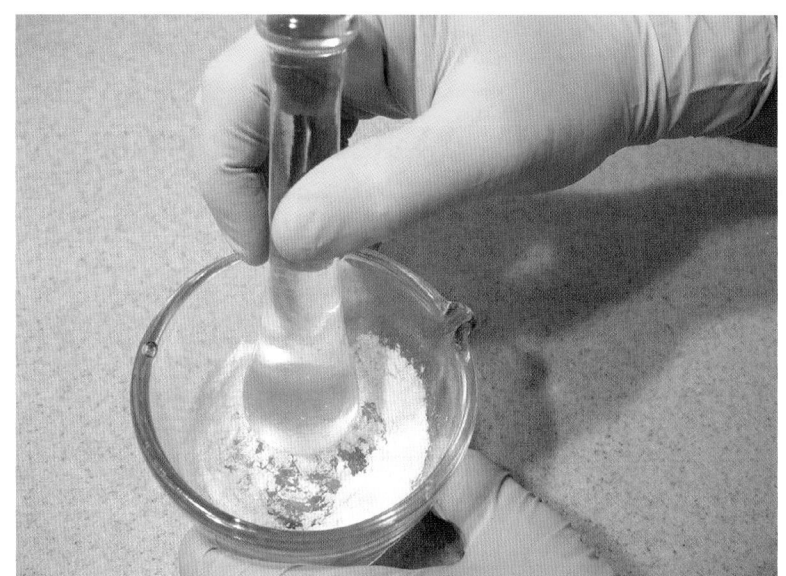

Color Plate 1: Trituration in a glass mortar.

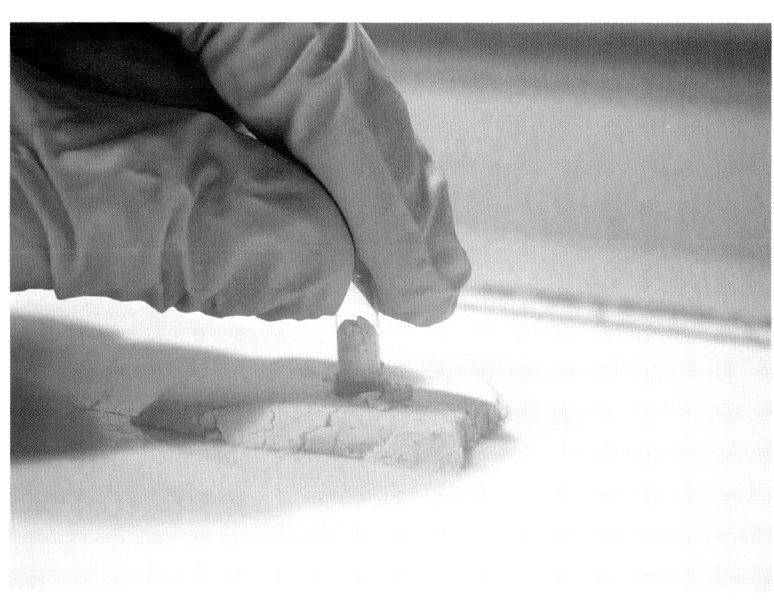

Color Plate 2: Hand-filling a capsule with dry powder.

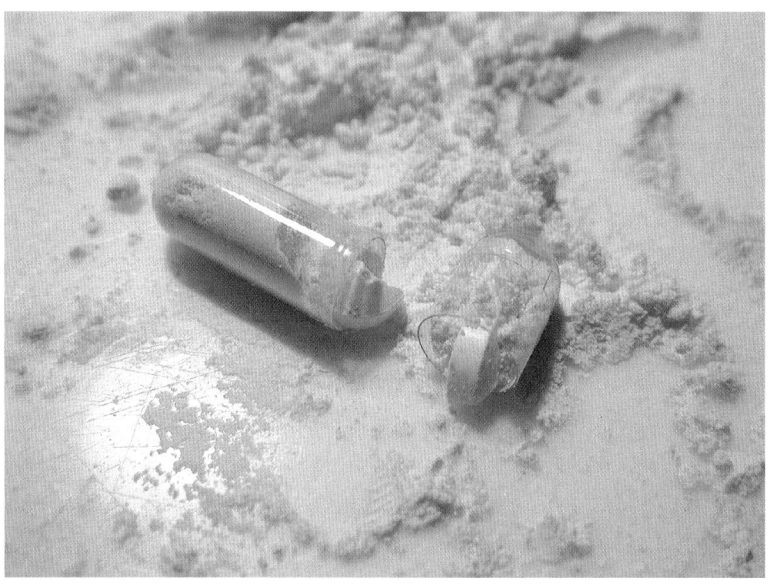

Color Plate 3: Embedding a tablet in capsule powder.

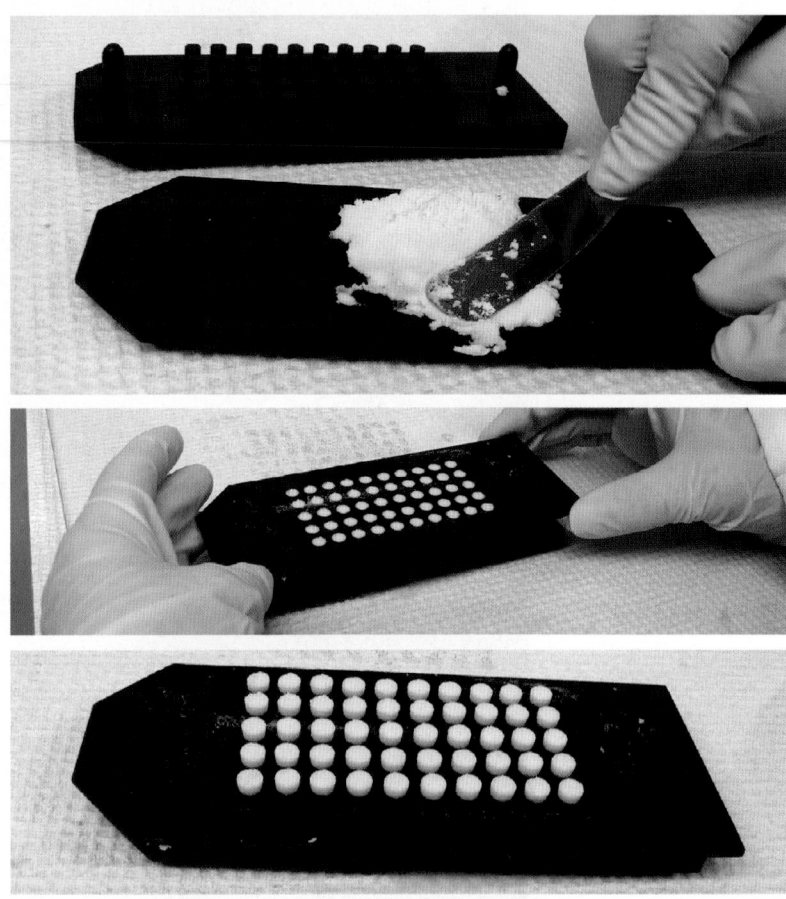

Color Plate 4: Making molded tablets (TTs): pressing the prepared mass into die holes of upper plate **(top)**; centering upper plate over pegs on lower plate and pressing down to push out tablets **(middle)**; and formed tablets drying on lower plate pegs **(bottom)**.

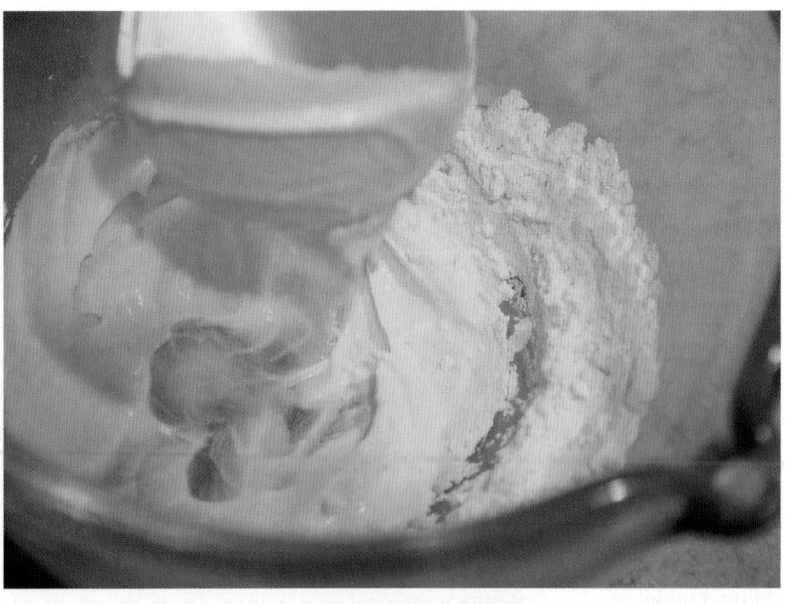

Color Plate 5: Wetting a hydrophobic powder with glycerin.

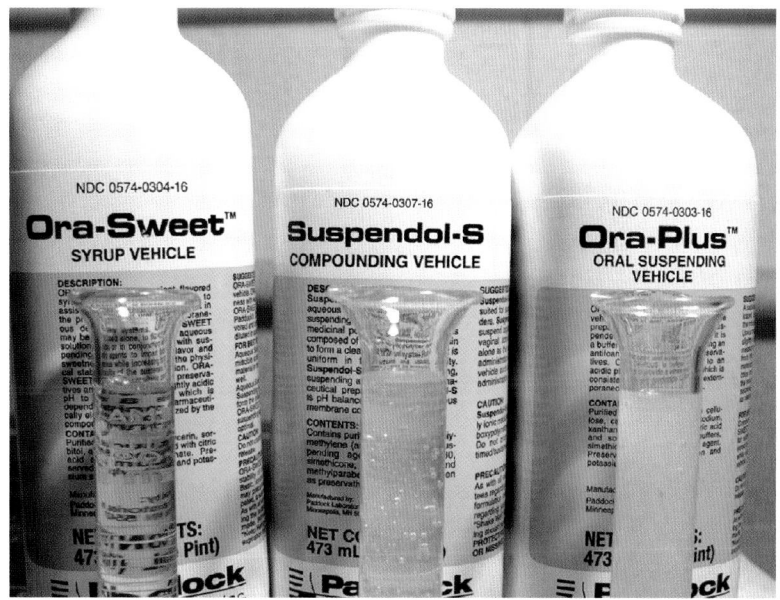

Color Plate 6: A sample of manufactured suspension vehicles for compounding.

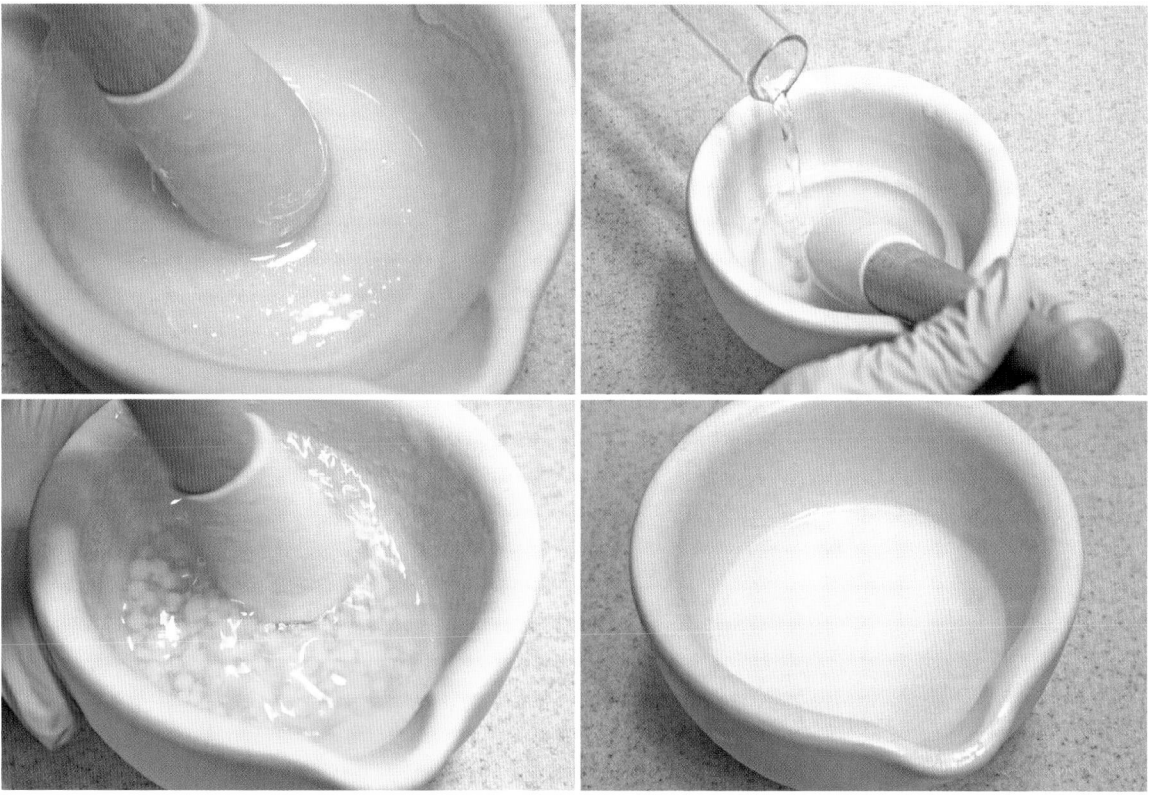

Color Plate 7: Forming an acacia primary emulsion: acacia-oil slurry (**upper left**); adding the water (**upper right**); triturating to form the primary emulsion (**lower left**); formed creamy primary emulsion (**lower right**).

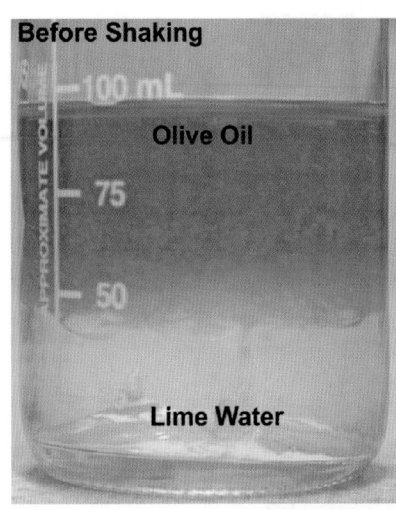
Before Shaking

100 mL

Olive Oil

75

50

Lime Water

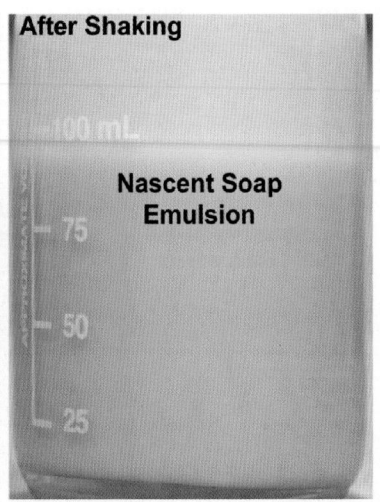
After Shaking

100 mL

Nascent Soap Emulsion

75

50

25

Color Plate 8: Forming a nascent soap emulsion using the bottle method—before **(left)** and after **(right)** emulsification.

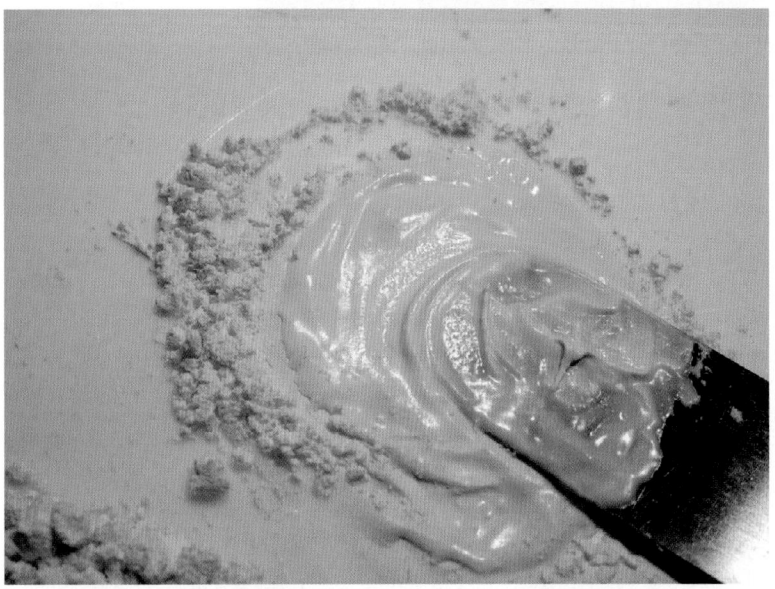

Color Plate 9: Levigation of a powder on an ointment slab.

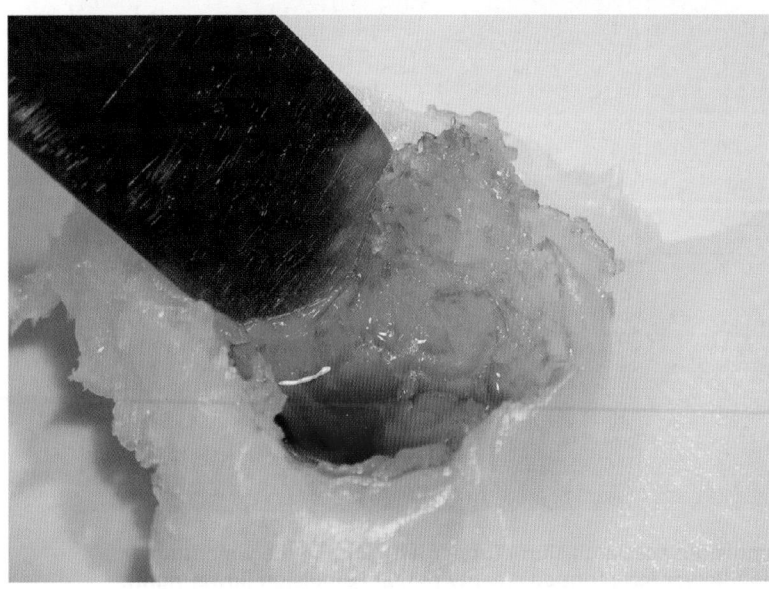

Color Plate 10: Using a depression in hydrophilic petrolatum to incorporate coal tar solution.

D. For bulk powders, it is important for the particle size to be uniform, because particles of different sizes tend to stratify on standing or when a powder is being transported. Stratification can result in inaccurate dosing.

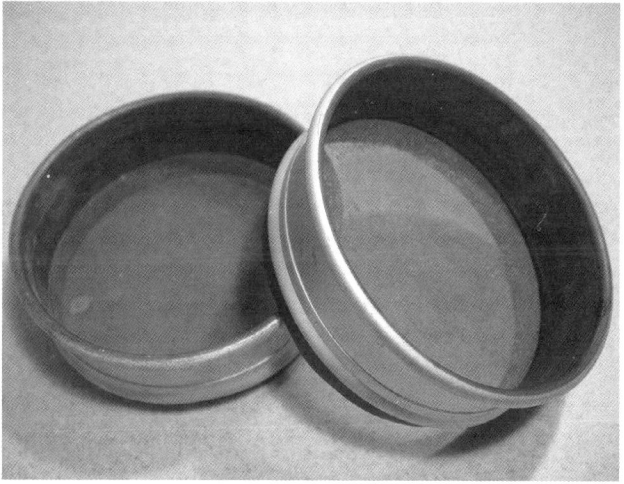

MESH SIEVES

E. Particle size for most pharmaceutical powders is determined by sieving, and the descriptive terms used to classify powders have meaning in terms of percent of the powder sample that will pass through a sieve of a given fineness.

1. Sieve properties are specified in the International Organization for Standardization Specifications ISO 3310-1: Test Sieves—Technical Requirements and Testing, and particle size determination using sieves is described in *USP* Chapter ⟨786⟩, Particle Size Distribution Estimation by Analytical Sieving. Table 25.1 shows the sieve size openings for sieves used to measured particle size for powders of interest in pharmaceuticals. The table column "Sieve U.S. No." gives what is commonly referred to as *mesh size*, a number that comes from the number of openings

Table 25.1	**SIZES OF STANDARD SIEVES**
SIEVE SIZE	**SIEVE U.S. NO.**
4.00 mm	5
2.00 mm	10
1.40 mm	14
1.00 mm	18
850 μm	20
710 μm	25
600 μm	30
500 μm	35
425 μm	40
355 μm	45
300 μm	50
250 μm	60
212 μm	70
180 μm	80
150 μm	100
125 μm	120
106 μm	140
90 μm	170
75 μm	200
63 μm	230

Table 25.2	CLASSIFICATION OF POWDERS BY FINENESS	
CLASSIFICATION OF POWDER		d_{50} **SIEVE OPENING (μm)**
Very coarse		>1,000
Coarse		355–1,000
Moderately fine		180–355
Fine 125–180		
Very fine		90–125

Source: The United States Pharmacopeial Convention, Inc. Chapter ⟨811⟩. 2008 USP 31/NF 26. Rockville, MD: Author, 2007; 339–340.

per linear inch of the sieve mesh. The larger the mesh number, the smaller the sieve openings and the smaller the particles must be to pass through that sieve.

2. Powders almost never have a completely uniform particle size, but rather they have a size distribution. Therefore, even when using sieves to measure particle size, the results are reported as the percent of the sample that passes through a given sieve size plus an upper and lower size boundary, or specifications will state that all the powder must pass through a sieve of a given mesh size. For example, the *USP* compounding monograph for Ketoconazole Oral Suspension states, "If Tablets are used, finely powder the Tablets such that they pass through a 40-mesh or 45-mesh sieve" (3). *USP* also recommends that topical powders, at a minimum, should pass through a size 100-mesh sieve (1).

3. Descriptive terms, such as *fine* or *coarse*, are used to describe powder fineness. The classification used by the *USP* for this purpose is given in Table 25.2, where the designation d_{50} means "the smallest sieve opening through which 50% or more of the material passes" (4).

4. Small (3-inch-diameter) and medium (8-inch-diameter) sieves with mesh sizes useful for compounding are available at a modest price from some vendors of compounding supplies.

V. PRINCIPLES OF COMPOUNDING FOR POWDERS

A. General principles

1. In nearly all compounding situations, solids need to be in a fine state of subdivision. Unless the solid can be purchased as a fine powder, particle size reduction by the compounder is required.

2. The chemical composition and the processing of solids determine their degree of subdivision and physical properties. The properties of a given solid must be understood and considered to properly handle and manipulate the material when fabricating it into a solid dosage form or when incorporating it into another drug delivery system.
    a. Solids that are purchased as fine powders may need no further manipulation.
    b. Some drugs have fine particles, but these may have agglomerated on storage and may need to be broken down into the primary particles originally processed by the manufacturer.
    c. Some drugs and chemicals are available as crystals that can easily be crushed into fine powder using a standard compounding technique, such as trituration, described in B. 2. a.
    d. Some materials are not easy to pulverize. They may be waxy substances or hard crystals that do not crush into fine powder with simple trituration. If a fine state of subdivision is needed, these drugs may require special techniques, such as pulverization by intervention (see B. 2. b.).
    e. Some solids have unique properties, such as deliquescence or intense color, that require special handling.
    f. Some solid drugs and chemicals are cytotoxic or hazardous substances; these, too, require special precautions and handling.

3. When two or more solids are being combined into one mixture, homogeneous blending of the powders is needed.

B. Particle size reduction

1. The process of particle size reduction is called **comminution.** The pharmaceutical industry has elaborate equipment and processes with which to produce finely divided powders with precisely controlled particle size. Although the equipment and methods available in the pharmacy are not nearly as efficient, they work well for the processing done by pharmacists and pharmacy technicians in extemporaneous compounding.

2. Methods of comminution available in the pharmacy

   a. Trituration is the continued rubbing of a solid in a mortar with a pestle to reduce the size of the solid's particles to a desirable degree of fineness. The term is also used to describe the grinding together of two or more substances in a mortar to intimately mix them. Trituration is achieved by firmly holding the pestle and exerting a downward pressure with it while moving it in successively larger concentric circles, starting at the center of the mortar, moving outward to the sides of the mortar, and then back again toward the center. To ensure adequate mixing and uniform particle size reduction, compacted powder is constantly removed from the sides of the mortar and the pestle by scraping with a spatula. Three different types of mortars are available for triturating drugs. Their properties and uses are described in the section on compounding equipment in Chapter 13. The process of trituration is illustrated on Color Plate 1 and is demonstrated in Section 3, Part 3 Compounding Drug Preparations, on the CD that accompanies this book.

   b. Pulverization by intervention

      (1) Some compounds do not lend themselves to direct trituration and must be handled in special ways. For example, some substances have hard crystalline structures that do not crush or triturate easily. The manner in which these drugs are handled depends on their ultimate use. If they are to be added to a liquid or semisolid preparation and if they are soluble in a suitable solvent, they may be dissolved first and incorporated as a solution. If they are to be included in a powdered dosage form, the procedure is more complex. One possible technique is pulverization by intervention. This process is described next.

      (2) Pulverization by intervention uses recrystallization as a method of obtaining fine particles. The word *intervention* refers to the first step of the process, dissolving the drug in a suitable solvent, the solvent being the so-called intervening compound. In this process, the solid is first dissolved in a minimum volume of a volatile solvent such as alcohol.

         (a) If the volume of the liquid is small and the rest of the powder in the preparation is not soluble in the chosen solvent, the solution may be mixed directly with the other powdered ingredients. The powders are then mixed until the solvent has completely evaporated.

         (b) If the other powder ingredients are soluble in the chosen solvent, or if too much solvent is required to dissolve the drug, the solution of the drug in the solvent is spread in a thin layer on the sides of a glass mortar or on the surface of a glass ointment slab. The solvent is allowed to evaporate, and the thin film of fine, solid crystals is then scraped off the glass surface using a metal spatula. The solid can then be blended with the other ingredients in the preparation.

      (3) The most common use of this technique is to obtain fine particles of camphor. Camphor is a hard, chunky solid that does not reduce to a fine powder when triturated in a mortar. When fine crystals of camphor are needed, pulverization by intervention is a useful method.

   c. Levigation is the process of reducing the particle size of a solid by triturating it in a mortar or spatulating it on an ointment slab or pad with a small amount of a liquid in which the solid is not soluble. Optimally, the liquid is somewhat viscous and has a low surface tension to improve the ease of wetting the solid. Mineral oil and glycerin are examples of common levigating agents. Levigation is used most often when incorporating solid ingredients into semisolids (e.g., ointments and creams) and is discussed in more detail in Chapter 30, Semisolids: Ointments Creams, Gels, Pastes, and Collodions. This technique is also illustrated on Color Plate 9 and is demonstrated on the CD that accompanies this book.

C. Blending

  1. The goal in blending powders is to create a homogeneous mixture. This is essential for obtaining uniform doses when mixtures of solid drugs are involved.

  2. Four methods—spatulation, trituration, sifting, and tumbling—are generally described in pharmacy textbooks as methods of blending in extemporaneous compounding. Compounders may also use newer technology, such as electric mixers and blenders.

   a. Spatulation is the mixing of powders on an ointment slab or pad using a spatula. With this method, there is no particle size reduction, so the powders to be mixed must be fine and of uniform size. Because no pressure is used, the resulting powder is usually light and is not compacted. This method should be used when hard trituration is to be avoided, such as when blending powders that have previously been coated to prevent the formation of a liquid eutectic mixture.

b. Trituration is described earlier in this section (see V.B). It is the preferred method of blending under most circumstances because it mixes powders more intimately than other methods. It should always be used when making mixtures that contain small quantities of potent drugs. Because trituration accomplishes two processes at the same time—namely, particle size reduction and blending—this method saves time when powders of unequal particle size are being combined.

c. Clear glass or plastic bottles and zipper-sealed polyethylene bags are useful for mixing powders by **tumbling**. These vessels are especially useful when it is important to carefully contain the powders, such as hazardous or cytotoxic substances or lightweight powders that may get into the air when mixed using trituration or spatulation.

d. Pharmacists and pharmacy technicians who do a lot of compounding use a variety of other equipment for blending. For example, blending moderate to large quantities of powders can be accomplished efficiently with an electric mixer. Special stainless steel sifters, available from vendors of compounding equipment and supplies, can also be used for blending powders.

3. Although visual inspection of the finished powder is an important general quality control measure, visual determination of adequate mixing is usually nearly impossible. This is because most drugs are white powders, so color of the powder mixture is not a good indicator of homogeneity. The following methods are useful for ensuring proper blending of powders.

a. At the beginning of the blending process, a small amount (approximately 0.1%) of a certified dye is added to the mixture; when the dye is evenly dispersed and the color is uniform, the powder is adequately mixed.

b. A more common approach is to use well-tested techniques, such as geometric dilution or alternate addition by portions, and mixing for a length of time found by individual experience to ensure proper blending of the powders.

4. Blending techniques to ensure adequate mixing

a. **Geometric dilution** is used when blending two or more powder ingredients of **unequal quantities**. It is a method designed to help ensure that small quantities of ingredients, usually potent drugs, are uniformly distributed throughout the powder mixture. Trituration usually is the blending method of choice with geometric dilution, because it gives more intimate mixing than other methods. The steps in geometric dilution are given here, and the technique is described in the compounding procedures with Sample Prescriptions 25.2 through 25.5; it is also demonstrated on the CD that accompanies this book.

(1) Weigh all ingredients for the preparation.

(2) Place the ingredient present in the smallest quantity in a mortar.

(3) Select the ingredient present in the next largest quantity and place in the mortar an amount of this ingredient approximately equal in powder volume to that of the first ingredient.

(4) Triturate the powders well until a uniform mixture is achieved.

(5) Add a volume of powder of the second ingredient equal in size to the powder volume of the mixture in the mortar and triturate well.

(6) Continue adding powder to the mortar in this fashion, always adding a volume of powder equal to the volume of powder mixture in the mortar, until all the powder ingredients have been added.

b. When a formulation calls for combining relatively equal amounts of moderate to large quantities of two or more powdered ingredients, a uniform mixture can be obtained most easily by first combining and mixing small portions of each ingredient and then adding additional portions of each alternately, with adequate trituration or mixing with each addition. This process is sometimes referred to as **alternate addition by portions**.

VI. COMPOUNDING BULK POWDERS

A. Topical bulk powders

1. Topical bulk powders often contain one or more active ingredients incorporated in a diluent powder. Powders most often chosen as diluents for external bulk powders are starch and talc.

2. The techniques for preparing and mixing the powders are described in the previous section.

3. Containers for topical powders

a. Although topical powders may be dispensed in a wide-mouth bottle or container, they are much more easily applied by the patient when dispensed in a sifter-topped powder can or shaker canister. Another alternative is a plastic bottle with flip spout, snap cap, or yorker spout.

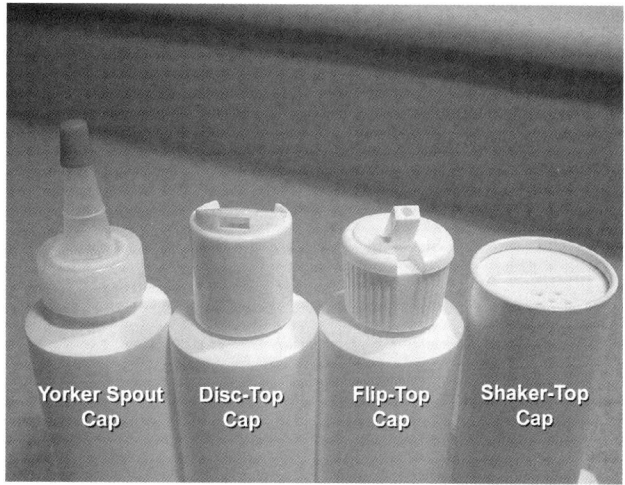

CONTAINERS FOR TOPICAL POWDERS

b. At one time, shaker canisters were made of pasteboard, and therefore these were not tight containers. Bulk powder formulations that contain volatile ingredients can lose these components through evaporation when they are dispensed in nontight containers. Furthermore, moisture from the environment can permeate through these containers and into the contained powder. Shaker containers made from hard plastic are now available, but it is important to check with the container distributor concerning the classification as either a well-closed or tight container. Bulk powders that contain either volatile active ingredients or components that are sensitive to moisture should be dispensed, when possible, in a tight container. If this is not possible or practical, a conservative beyond-use date should be assigned to the preparation. This is illustrated with Sample Prescriptions 25.2 and 25.3.

4. Labeling: The concentrations of active ingredients are expressed as percent weight–weight or as metric weight or units of active ingredient per gram of powder.

B. Bulk powders for internal use

1. Internal-use bulk powders usually do not need added diluent unless required by a particular compounding situation. (One example would be the protection of a potential eutectic mixture, which is discussed in section VIII of this chapter and in section III.B in Chapter 37.) Agents commonly used as diluents or adsorbents for internal products include magnesium carbonate, light or heavy magnesium oxide, calcium carbonate, starch, and lactose.

2. The techniques for preparing and mixing the powders are described in section V of this chapter.

3. Containers for internal-use bulk powders

a. Bulk powders for internal use are dispensed in wide-mouth powder squares, pharmaceutical rounds, or other wide-mouth containers. When the dose to be administered is a teaspoonful or tablespoonful, the container selected should, when possible, allow the patient or caregiver to insert the measuring spoon to withdraw the appropriate dose.

b. As with external bulk powders, the nature of the powder components should be considered when selecting a container, and tight containers should always be used when the situation dictates.

4. Labeling: Internal bulk powders are labeled with the weight of active ingredient per volume to be ingested or administered (e.g., teaspoonful, tablespoonful). To determine the content of active ingredients in this volume, the pharmacist must perform the following procedure:

a. Prepare the formulation as directed in the prescription order.

b. Using the appropriate measuring device (e.g., teaspoon), measure the volume of powder to be taken or administered.

c. Weigh this volume of powder.

d. From the concentration or percent of active ingredient(s) in the prepared powder and the weight of the volume to be administered, calculate the weight(s) of active ingredient(s) in the volume to be administered. An example of this procedure is given in Sample Prescription 25.1.

VII. **COMPOUNDING DIVIDED POWDERS OR CHARTULAE**

A. Divided powders: Also known as *chartulae* or *powder papers*, divided powders have individual doses of powder packaged in folded papers or plastic bags.

B. Preparing the powder

1. Amount of powder

   a. Prepare enough powder for one extra dosage unit, because some powder will be lost in the blending process. If the prescription contains a controlled substance, this loss in compounding must be minimal and should be documented on the prescription order or compounding record sheet.

   b. If the amount of powder for each packet is less than the minimum weighable quantity (MWQ) for the balance being used, an inert diluent powder must be added. This procedure is illustrated in Sample Prescriptions 25.4 and 25.5 in this chapter.

   c. If the amount of powder is above the MWQ but is still small (e.g., less than 300 mg per packet), a diluent such as lactose may be added to bring the quantity of powder per packet to an amount that is convenient for handling and administration. This is illustrated with Sample Prescription 25.6.

      (1) An intermediate amount of powder (200 mg to 500 mg) per packet is desirable.

      (2) Smaller quantities are difficult to handle, and any amount left in the powder paper or bag or spilled by the patient or caregiver significantly affects the dose. In a study, nifedipine divided powders were compounded using crushed nifedipine tablets and lactose as a diluent. Each packet was formulated to contain 1 mg of nifedipine in 500 mg of powder. An analysis showed that the delivered content was 0.92 mg nifedipine per packet and that three-fourths of the loss was found on the powder papers (5). Obviously, the loss of active ingredient would have been greater if the drug had not been diluted with lactose.

      (3) Large quantities of diluent should also be avoided, since larger amounts of powder are more difficult to mix into liquid vehicle or soft food for administration.

2. The techniques for preparing and mixing the powders are described previously in section V of this chapter.

C. Packaging the divided powders

1. Divided powders can be folded into powder papers or packaged in reclosable, so-called zipper-lock polybags or heat-sealed in polyethylene or cellophane bags.

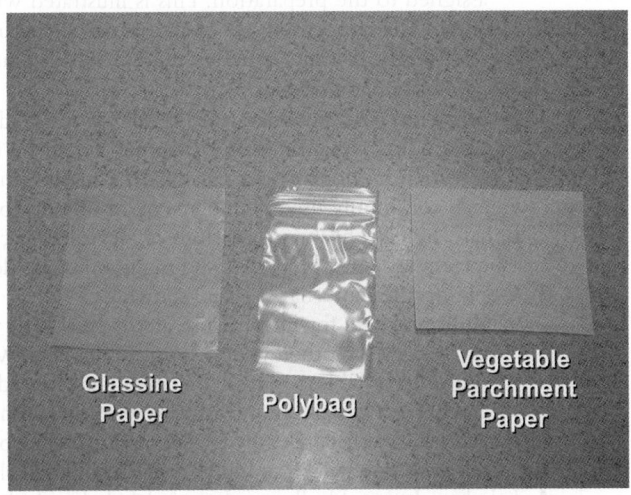

POLYBAGS AND POWDER PAPERS

2. Polybags

   a. Polybags are available in various sizes and can be purchased either with reclosable zipper-type seals or as bags that require a heat-seal or adhesive tape seal. Amber or opaque polybags are also available for drugs that require protection from light.

   b. Preparing divided powders with polybags is quite easy.

      (1) The weighed quantity of prepared powder for one dose is placed in each bag.

      (2) For reclosable bags, the closure is zipped shut. Plain polybags may be sealed by tape or heat-sealed with an impulse sealer.

      (3) The sealed bags may be dispensed in a hinged or telescoping box or may be placed in a powder square or other tight container with a screw top.

3. Folded powder papers

   a. Folded powder papers are used only when other packaging materials for divided powders are not available. Folded powder papers have the following disadvantages over divided powders packaged in polybags: time-consuming preparation, poor moisture barriers, and failure to meet safety-packaging regulations.

b. Types of paper most commonly used for folded powder papers include the following:

   (1) Glassine weighing papers, as described in section III. D. in Chapter 14.

   (2) Powder papers made of vegetable parchment paper, available in a variety of sizes ranging from $2\frac{1}{2}'' \times 3\frac{3}{4}''$ to $4\frac{1}{2}'' \times 6\frac{1}{2}''$.

c. Folding papers for divided powders is demonstrated on the CD that accompanies this book.

D. Use of tablets and capsules in divided powders

One of the main uses of divided powders is for supplying doses for patients who cannot swallow whole tablets or capsules.

1. Always make certain that the manufactured dosage form is one that may be crushed. The topic of oral solid dosage forms that should not be crushed is discussed in section II. C. in Chapter 13.

2. If the dose needed is a **whole unit** of a tablet or capsule, there are some convenient alternatives to making divided powders.

   a. For capsules, the powder can be emptied easily from the capsule shell by the patient or caregiver.

   b. Because tablets need to be crushed, other methods are required. Tablet crushers, intended for use by patients, nurses, or other caregivers, are available at various prices, ranging from less than $10 to deluxe models that cost more than $50. One easy, inexpensive method is for the patient or caregiver to place the tablet in a small plastic bag, such as a sandwich bag, and crush the tablet with the back of a spoon.

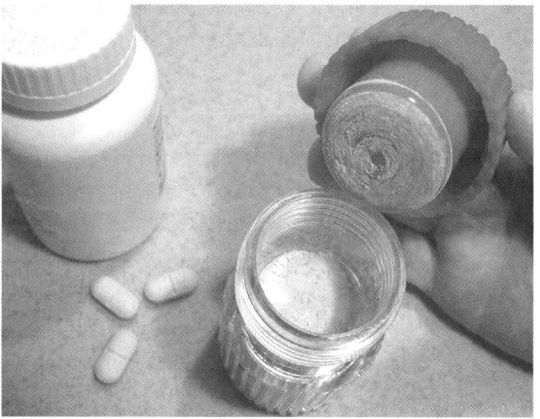

TABLET CRUSHER

3. When the dose needed is either customized with other ingredients or is a fractional part of a manufactured tablet or capsule, divided powders offer a convenient method of administration. Examples of this are shown in Sample Prescriptions 25.5 and 25.6.

4. When crushing tablets that contain cytotoxic or other hazardous drugs, special precautions are necessary. These tablets should be placed in a disposable plastic bag and crushed with a pestle. The bag should be thick enough to avoid being punctured. Sample Prescription 25.6 illustrates this technique.

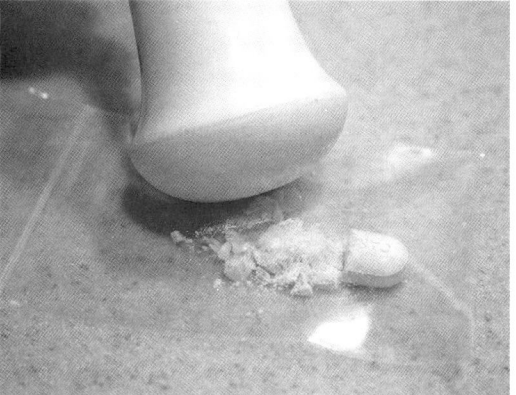

PULVERIZING IN A POLYBAG A TABLET CONTAINING A HAZARDOUS DRUG

E. Labeling: Divided powders are labeled with the metric weight or units of active ingredient(s) per packet.

VIII. COMPATIBIITY, STABILITY, AND BEYOND-USE DATING

A. Physical stability: Although most solids are quite stable physically, a few problems may be encountered with selected drugs and chemicals.

1. The potential physical problems for solids include liquefaction of eutectic mixtures and deliquescent powders, loss of water of hydration for efflorescent powders, and absorption of water by hygroscopic and deliquescent powders. Definitions of these powder types are given at the beginning of this chapter.

2. Methods of handling these incompatibilities of solids are discussed in Chapter 37. Examples are given in the current chapter with Sample Prescriptions 25.2 and 25.5. Some compounding techniques useful for handling drugs with potential problems are demonstrated on the CD that accompanies this book. (See Eutectic in Section 3, Part 3 Compounding Drug Preparations and Rx 25.2 in Part 5 Nonsterile Dosage Forms and Their Preparation.)

3. When a bulk powder contains a drug that requires protection, the compounder should, if possible, use as the protectant an ingredient already in the prescription. Sample Prescription 25.2 illustrates this principle.

4. If the prescription order does not contain an ingredient that is suitable for this purpose, the pharmacist should consult with the prescriber to select a protectant; the agent selected must be suitable for the intended route of administration. Agents commonly used for this purpose are discussed previously and in Chapter 37. Because addition of another ingredient will affect the final weight of the powder and, therefore, the final concentrations of the active ingredients, appropriate adjustments in the amounts of ingredients must be made to keep concentrations at the desired level. Any added ingredients and their quantities must then be recorded, either on the prescription order or in the compounding record kept for that purpose.

B. Chemical stability: Even though most solids are quite stable, it is important to check out ingredients before formulating a preparation.

1. Each sample prescription at the end of this chapter considers the chemical stability of each ingredient in the given dosage form and uses this information in assigning a beyond-use date to the preparation. Examples are given that illustrate the use of various reference resources both to determine stability and to assign beyond-use dates.

2. A few solids are very reactive even in solid state. Most are strong oxidizing (e.g., potassium permanganate, potassium and silver nitrate) or reducing agents that, when mixed together, react; some mixtures are potentially either flammable or explosive. The topic of chemical stability of drugs and chemicals is addressed in Chapter 37.

C. Beyond-use dating: A general discussion on assigning beyond-use dates for solid dosage forms can be found in Chapter 4. *USP* Chapter ⟨795⟩ has the following guidelines for compounded solid dosage forms:

> In the absence of stability information that is applicable to a specific drug and preparation, the following maximum beyond-use dates are recommended for nonsterile compounded drug preparations that are packaged in tight, light-resistant containers and stored at controlled room temperature unless otherwise indicated.
>
> **For Nonaqueous Liquids and Solid Formulations—**
> *Where the Manufactured Drug Product is the Source of Active Ingredient*—The beyond-use date is not later than 25% of the time remaining until the product's expiration date or 6 months, whichever is earlier.
> *Where a USP or NF Substance is the Source of Active Ingredient*—The beyond-use date is not later than 6 months (6).

Sample Prescriptions

SAMPLE PRESCRIPTION 25.1

CASE: Roberta Fifrick is a 135-lb, 5'1"-tall, 63-year-old woman. She is in good general health and her medication profile record shows that she takes estradiol 2 mg daily for postmenopausal vasomotor symptoms ("hot flashes" and "night sweats") and omeprazole 20 mg at bedtime for gastrointestinal reflux disorder (GERD). She usually takes an oral liquid combination antacid product after each meal for gastric symptoms, but she is taking a trip abroad and wants a more "packable" powder that she can mix with water and take as needed while traveling. Dr. Fedder has prescribed the oral bulk antacid powder listed here.

CONTEMPORARY PHYSICIANS GROUP PRACTICE
20 S. PARK STREET, TRITURATE, WI 53706
TEL: (608) 555-1333 FAX: (608) 555-1335

R # *123022*

NAME *Roberta Fifrick*   **DATE** *00/00/00*

ADDRESS *713 Reed Street*

R

Aluminum Hydroxide	3.75 g
Magnesium Hydroxide	3.75 g
Peppermint Oil	qs
Calcium Carbonate	qs ad 15 g

J. Rivera 00/00/00

Sig: One level tsp in water tid pc prn

REFILLS *2*   *H. G. Fedder*   **M.D.**

DEA NO. _____

MASTER COMPOUNDING FORMULATION RECORD

NAME, STRENGTH AND DOSAGE FORM OF PREPARATION: Aluminum and Magnesium Hydroxides 25% and Calcium Carbonate 50% Oral Bulk Powder

QUANTITY: 15 g

THERAPEUTIC USE/CATEGORY: Antacid

FORMULATION RECORD ID: BP001

ROUTE OF ADMINISTRATION: Oral

INGREDIENTS:

Ingredient	Quantity	Physical Description	Solubility	Dose Comparison		Use in the Prescription
				Given	Usual	
Aluminum Hydroxide Dried Gel	3.75 g	white powder	insol in water and alcohol	0.4 g t.i.d.	0.3–0.6 g 4–6 x daily	antacid
Magnesium Hydroxide	3.75 g	white powder	insol in water and alcohol	0.4 g t.i.d.	0.3–0.6 g q.i.d.	antacid
Preppermint Oil	10 drops	pale yellow liqid with peppermint odor	immis w/water mis w/alcohol	—	—	flavor, scent
Calcium Carbonate	7.5 g	white powder	insol in water and alcohol	0.8 g t.i.d	1 g 4–6 × daily	antacid

COMPATIBILITY–STABILITY: All ingredients in this preparation are compatible and very stable when in a solid dosage form.

PACKAGING AND STORAGE: The *USP* monographs recommend storage in well-closed containers for all of these active ingredients when formulated into tablets (3). Dispense this powder in a pharmaceutical round, wide-mouth bottle with a tight cap. Store at controlled room temperature.

BEYOND-USE DATE: Use 6 months as specified in *USP* Chapter ⟨795⟩ for solid formulations made with USP ingredients when the preparation is packaged in a tight container and stored at controlled room temperature (6).

CALCULATIONS

Dose/Concentration

Weight of powder in one level teaspoonful = 1.6 g

Weight of Aluminum Hydroxide and Magnesium Hydroxide per teaspoonful (1.6 g):

$$\frac{3.75 \text{ g Al/Mg hydroxides}}{15 \text{ g powder}} = \frac{x \text{ g Al/Mg hydroxides}}{1.6 \text{ g powder}}; x = 0.4 \text{ g Al/Mg hydroxides}$$

Weight of Calcium Carbonate per teaspoonful (1.6 g):

$$\frac{7.5 \text{ g Ca Carbonate}}{15 \text{ g powder}} = \frac{x \text{ g Ca Carbonate}}{1.6 \text{ g powder}}; x = 0.8 \text{ g Ca Carbonate}$$

Ingredient Amounts

Aluminum Hydroxide and Magnesium Hydroxide: 3.75 g each

Calcium Carbonate: 15 g − (3.75 g + 3.75 g) = 7.5 g

Note: Weight of Peppermint Oil negligible

MSDS AND SAFETY AND PERSONAL PROTECTIVE EQUIPMENT: Review MSDS for all bulk components. Don a clean lab coat and disposable gloves. Avoid inhaling powders.

SPECIALIZED EQUIPMENT: None. All weighing is done on a class III torsion balance.

COMPOUNDING PROCEDURE: Weigh 3.75 g each of magnesium hydroxide and aluminum hydroxide and 7.5 g of calcium carbonate. Place the magnesium and aluminum hydroxides in a 1-gallon zipper-closure plastic bag. Close the bag securely and mix the powders by tumbling until well mixed (approximately 2 minutes). Add the calcium carbonate to the bag and again mix well by tumbling. Add 10 drops of peppermint oil to the powder, distributing the oil droplets as evenly as possible throughout the powder mass. Mix well by tumbling. Calibrate/check the dose by weighing the contents of one level teaspoonful—found to be 1.6 g. Remove the cap from a 2-oz wide-mouth pharmaceutical round bottle, and tare the weight of the bottle. Use a powder funnel to transfer the powder into the bottle; reweigh and record the weight of the powder. Replace the cap and close securely. Label the preparation appropriately and dispense.

DESCRIPTION OF FINISHED PREPARATION: Fine, white powder with a slight odor of peppermint

QUALITY CONTROL: Weigh the powder of one level teaspoonful; it should closely match the 1.6 g noted earlier. It will vary if there is a difference in the bulk density of the final powder, which may result from factors such as a change in manufacturer or lot of ingredients or from processing changes. If there is a substantive change in the weight of powder per teaspoonful, the grams of active ingredient per teaspoonful must be recalculated. Weigh the finished powder; it should closely match the theoretical weight of 15 g.

MASTER FORMULA PREPARED BY: Juanita Rivera, PharmD   **CHECKED BY:** Sue Stein, MS, RPh

COMPOUNDING RECORD

NAME, STRENGTH, AND DOSAGE FORM OF PREPARATION: Aluminum and Magnesium Hydroxides 25% and Calcium Carbonate 50% Oral Bulk Powder

QUANTITY: 15 g   **DATE PREPARED:** mm/dd/yy   **BEYOND-USE DATE:** mm/dd/yy

FORMULATION RECORD ID: BP001   **CONTROL/RX NUMBER:** 123022

INGREDIENTS USED:

Ingredient	Quantity	Manufacturer Lot Number	Expiration Date	Prepared by	Checked by
Aluminum Hydroxide Dried Gel	3.75 g	JET Labs XY1143	mm/yy	bjf	jr
Magnesium Hydroxide	3.75 g	JET Labs XY1144	mm/yy	bjf	jr
Peppermint Oil	10 drops	JET Labs XY1145	mm/yy	bjf	jr
Calcium Carbonate	7.5 g	JET Labs XY1146	mm/yy	bjf	jr

QUALITY CONTROL DATA: Appearance: fine white powder with slight odor of peppermint

Powder weight per teaspoonful:	1.612 g
Weight of powder in bottle (without cap):	52.695 g
Weight of empty bottle (without cap):	37.839 g
Weight of powder:	14.856 g

LABELING

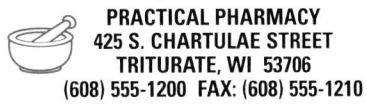

PRACTICAL PHARMACY
425 S. CHARTULAE STREET
TRITURATE, WI 53706
(608) 555-1200 FAX: (608) 555-1210

℞ 123022   Pharmacist: JR   Date: 00/00/00
Roberta Fifrick   Dr. Fedder

Take one level teaspoonful in water three times a day after meals as needed.

Per level teaspoonful of oral powder: Aluminum Hydroxide 0.4 g; Magnesium Hydroxide 0.4 g; Calcium Carbonate 0.8 g

Mfg: Compounded   Quantity: 15 g

Refills: 2   Discard after: Give date

Auxiliary Label: This medicine was compounded in our pharmacy for you at the direction of your prescriber.

PATIENT CONSULTATION: Hello, Ms. Fifrick. I'm Juanita Rivera, your pharmacist. Do you have any drug allergies? Our records show that you take estradiol and omeprazole. Are you taking any other prescription or nonprescription medications? What do you know about this medication? It is my understanding that you are using this antacid powder combination as a substitute for your liquid antacid while you are traveling in Europe. You can use this measuring spoon I am giving you to measure one level teaspoonful of this powder and mix it very well in a glass of water and take it three times a day after meals as needed. This powder contains a combination of antacid ingredients, aluminum and magnesium hydroxide and calcium carbonate; some components can cause constipation, others have a laxative effect, so if you develop any of these symptoms you may want to cut back on the amount you are taking or, if it becomes bothersome, you could stop taking it altogether. This medication should be stored at room temperature, tightly closed, in a cool dry place. Any unused portion should be discarded after 6 months. This prescription has two refills. Do you have any questions?

SAMPLE PRESCRIPTION 25.2

CASE: Max Thompson is a 170-lb, 5'9"-tall, 16-year-old male high school student. A month ago, he joined the swim team at his community pool and soon began to notice intense itching of his feet. His doctor has diagnosed tinea pedis (athlete's foot) and has advised him to purchase over-the-counter (OTC) miconazole cream and to use that with the compounded foot powder prescribed here. Max's medication record shows that he has no recent or current prescription medications but has in the past used antibiotics to treat occasional infections such as strep throat and sinusitis. He reports that the only OTC medicines that he uses are ibuprofen for occasional muscle strains and a daily multivitamin with minerals.

CONTEMPORARY PHYSICIANS GROUP PRACTICE
20 S. PARK STREET, TRITURATE, WI 53706
TEL: (608) 555-1333 FAX: (608) 555-1335

R ℞ #   *123009*

NAME *Max Thompson*   DATE *00/00/00*

ADDRESS *532 Minocqua Court*

℞

Benzocaine		*0.75 g*
Salicylic Acid		*0.75 g*
Benzoic Acid		*1.5 g*
Camphor		*1 g*
Methyl Salicylate qs		
Talc	*qs ad*	*30 g*

J. Johnson 00/00/00

Sig: Apply to feet ut dict q AM and hs

REFILLS *3*   *K. W. Shapiro*   M.D.

DEA NO. _____

MASTER COMPOUNDING FORMULATION RECORD

NAME, STRENGTH, AND DOSAGE FORM OF PREPARATION: Benzoic Acid 5%, Camphor 3.3%, Salicylic Acid and Benzocaine 2.5% Topical Powder

QUANTITY: 30 g

FORMULATION RECORD ID: BP002

THERAPEUTIC USE/CATEGORY: Antifungal/Antipruritic

ROUTE OF ADMINISTRATION: Topical

INGREDIENTS:

Ingredient	Quantity	Physical Description	Solubility	Dose Comparison		Use in the Prescription
				Given	Usual	
Benzocaine	0.75 g	white powder	1 g/2,500 mL water, 5 mL alcohol	2.5%	1–20%	local anesthetic
Salicylic Acid	0.75 g	fine white crystals	1 g/460 mL water, 2.7 mL alcohol	2.5%	1–20%	keratolytic
Benzoic Acid	1.5 g	white needles	1 g/300 mL water, 2.3 mL alcohol	5%	6%	antifungal
Camphor	1.0 g	large chunky crystals	1 g/800 mL water, 1 mL alcohol	3.3%	0.1–10%	antipruritic
Methyl Salicylate	6 drops	clear colorless liquid w/ wintergreen odor	1 g/1,500 mL water, mis w/ alcohol	—	—	scent
Talc	26 g	whitish-gray fine powder	insol in water and alcohol	86.7%	—	vehicle and absorbent

COMPATIBILITY–STABILITY: All ingredients are quite stable; however, the benzocaine, salicylic acid, and camphor have the potential to form a liquefied eutectic mixture if triturated together. In this case, that would be an advantage because camphor is available as hard crystals that do not reduce to a fine powder with direct trituration. Therefore, for this preparation, the preferred treatment is to "force" the eutectic mixture by triturating the benzocaine, salicylic acid, and camphor together in a glass mortar to liquefy these solids. If the mixture does not liquefy adequately to dissolve the camphor, a few drops of alcohol may be added to complete the process. The liquefied eutectic mixture is then adsorbed on the talc powder. The camphor sublimes at room temperature, so there could be some loss if the preparation is not stored in a tight container.

PACKAGING AND STORAGE: To provide ease of use by the patient, a polyethylene bottle with a flip-spout cap will be used as the preparation container. Store at controlled room temperature.

BEYOND-USE DATE: A conservative 3-month beyond-use date is used because it cannot be confirmed that the container/closure system meets the requirements of a tight container. If this preparation is dispensed in a tight, light-resistant container, as recommended in the *USP* monograph for Camphor USP (3), it would be acceptable to use the maximum 6-month beyond-use date as specified in *USP* Chapter ⟨795⟩ for solid formulations packaged in tight containers, stored at controlled room temperature, and made with USP ingredients (6).

CALCULATIONS

Dose/Concentration

$$\% \text{ benzocaine \& salicylic acid: } \frac{0.75 \text{ g benzocaine/s. a.}}{30 \text{ g powder}} = \frac{x}{100}; x = 2.5\%$$

$$\% \text{ camphor: } \frac{1 \text{ g camphor}}{30 \text{ g powder}} = \frac{x}{100}; x = 3.3\%$$

$$\% \text{ benzoic acid: } \frac{1.5 \text{ g benzoic acid}}{30 \text{ g powder}} = \frac{x}{100}; x = 5\%$$

$$\% \text{ talc: } \frac{26 \text{ g talc}}{30 \text{ g powder}} = \frac{x}{100}; x = 86.7\% \text{ (Optional, talc is not an active ingredient)}$$

Ingredient Amounts

All ingredient weights are given on the prescription order except talc.

$$\text{Talc} = 30 \text{ g} - (\text{wt. of other ingredients}) = 30 \text{ g} - (0.75 + 0.75 + 1.5 + 1) \text{ g}$$
$$= 30 \text{ g} - 4 \text{ g} = 26 \text{ g}$$

MSDS AND SAFETY AND PERSONAL PROTECTIVE EQUIPMENT: Review MSDS for all bulk components. Don a clean lab coat and disposable gloves. Avoid inhaling powders.

SPECIALIZED EQUIPMENT: Glass mortar; 3″ 100-mesh sieve; all weighing on an electronic balance

COMPOUNDING PROCEDURE: Weigh 0.75 g of benzocaine and 0.75 g of salicylic acid, 1.5 g of benzoic acid, 1 g of camphor, and 26 g of talc. Transfer the benzocaine, salicylic acid, benzoic acid, and camphor to a glass mortar and triturate these together, "forcing" the eutectic mixture. If the mixture does not liquefy adequately to dissolve the camphor, add a few drops of alcohol. Add the talc to the mortar in portions with trituration, adsorbing the liquid eutectic on the talc. Add 6 drops of methyl salicylate drop-wise to the powder with trituration. Pass the powder through the 100-mesh sieve. Weigh the preparation container. Using a powder funnel, transfer the powder to the container and reweigh to determine the final weight of powder. Label and dispense.

DESCRIPTION OF FINISHED PREPARATION: Fine whitish-gray powder with the scent of camphor and wintergreen.

QUALITY CONTROL: Weigh the finished powder; it should closely match the theoretical weight of 30 g.

MASTER FORMULA PREPARED BY: John Johnson, PharmD   **CHECKED BY:** Sue Stein, MS, RPh

COMPOUNDING RECORD

NAME, STRENGTH, AND DOSAGE FORM OF PREPARATION: Benzoic Acid 5%, Camphor 3.3%, Salicylic Acid and Benzocaine 2.5% Topical Powder

QUANTITY: 30 g   **DATE PREPARED:** mm/dd/yy   **BEYOND-USE DATE:** mm/dd/yy

FORMULATION RECORD ID: BP002   **CONTROL /RX NUMBER:** 123009

INGREDIENTS USED:

Ingredient	Quantity Used	Manufacturer Lot Number	Expiration Date	Weighed by	Checked by
Benzocaine	0.75 g XY1147	JET Labs	mm/yy	bjf	jj
Salicylic Acid	0.75 g XY1148	JET Labs	mm/yy	bjf	jj
Benzoic Acid	1.5 g XY1149	JET Labs	mm/yy	bjf	jj
Camphor1.0 g	JET Labs XY1150	mm/yy	bjf	jj	
Methyl Salicylate	6 drops XY1151	JET Labs	mm/yy	bjf	jj
Talc 26 g	JET Labs XY1152	mm/yy	bjf	jj	

QUALITY CONTROL: Appearance: fine whitish-gray powder with the scent of camphor and wintergreen

Weight of powder in bottle (without cap):   43.830 g

Weight of empty bottle (without cap):   14.082 g

Weight of powder: 29.748 g

LABELING

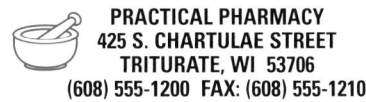

PRACTICAL PHARMACY
425 S. CHARTULAE STREET
TRITURATE, WI 53706
(608) 555-1200 FAX: (608) 555-1210

℞ 123009   Pharmacist: JJ   Date: 00/00/00
Max Thompson   Dr. Shapiro

Apply to feet as directed each morning and at bedtime.

Benzocaine 2.5%; Salicylic Acid 2.5%; Benzoic Acid 5%; Camphor 3.3%; Talc 86.7% (optional) Topical Powder

Mfg: Compounded   Quantity: 30 g

Refills: 3   Discard after: Give date

Auxiliary Labels: For external use only. Keep out of reach of children. This medicine was compounded in our pharmacy for you at the direction of your prescriber.

PATIENT CONSULTATION: Hello, Max. I'm your pharmacist, John Johnson. Do you have any drug allergies? Are you currently taking any prescription or nonprescription drugs? What did Dr. Shapiro tell you about this powder? This foot powder contains a combination of ingredients including camphor, benzoic and salicylic acids, and benzocaine that relieve the itching and treat the fungal infection commonly present with athlete's foot. Apply this powder to your feet as directed each morning and at bedtime. It will help if you use shoes and socks that "breathe"; avoid synthetic materials that don't allow the perspiration to evaporate. Also, carefully dry your feet after you shower. If the condition doesn't improve in a few days, or if it gets worse, contact Dr. Shapiro. Keep this in a cool, dry place, out of the reach of children. This is for external use only. Discard any unused contents after 3 months (give date). This prescription can be refilled three times. Do you have any questions?

SAMPLE PRESCRIPTION 25.3

CASE: Jared Stone is a 15-lb, 4-month-old infant. During the last 3 or 4 days, he has developed severe diaper dermatitis (commonly known as *diaper rash*), with very red and "raw" skin in the diaper area. His previous medication history includes pediatric multivitamins and amoxicillin for otitis media. Dr. Schultz has prescribed the customized topical powder given here to treat Jared's diaper dermatitis. This order has an example of a ratio or ratio strength notation that can be interpreted in two ways, with the colon as a "plus" or as a "qs ad." Pharmacist Barbara Bell called the prescriber, and the intent is one part of Nystatin Powder to (i.e., **plus**) ten parts of the adsorbent powder. This would make sense anecdotally, given the quantity of the bulk powder portion of 20 g, an even multiple of the 1:10 ratio. The other difficulty with interpreting this order concerns the "Nystatin Powder," which could be taken to mean pure Nystatin USP (4,400,000 units/g) or as Nystatin Topical Powder USP (100,000 units/g). Both powders are available. This is addressed in the calculations given next. For this exercise, Pharmacist Bell consulted with Dr. Schultz and determined that the second interpretation, Nystatin Topical Powder, is the desired one.

CONTEMPORARY PHYSICIANS GROUP PRACTICE
20 S. PARK STREET, TRITURATE, WI 53706
TEL: (608) 555-1333 FAX: (608) 555-1335

℞ # *123025*

NAME *Jared Stone*   DATE *00/00/00*

ADDRESS *2530 Lego Lane*

℞

      Mix Nystatin Powder 1:10 with the following:
      Zinc Oxide
      Talc
      Starch
      Calcium Carbonate   *equal quantities to give 20 g*

    Sig: Apply to area with each diaper change

Called Dr. Schultz to confirm ratio interpretation and use of Nystatin
Topical Powder   *B. Bell 00/00/00*

REFILLS *3*   *Aleta Schultz*   M.D.

                         DEA NO.

MASTER COMPOUNDING FORMULATION RECORD

NAME, STRENGTH, AND DOSAGE FORM OF PREPARATION: Nystatin-Adsorbent Topical Powder
QUANTITY: 22 g   **FORMULATION RECORD ID:** BP003
THERAPEUTIC USE/CATEGORY: Antifungal/Adsorbent   **ROUTE OF ADMINISTRATION:** Topical

INGREDIENTS:

Ingredient	Quantity	Physical Description	Solubility	Dose Comparison		Use in the Prescription
				Given	Usual	
Zinc Oxide	5 g	white powder	insol in water and alcohol	22.7%	any	astringent, adsorbent
Talc	5 g	whitish-gray powder	insol in water and alcohol	31.6%*	any	vehicle, adsorbent
Starch	5 g	white powder	insol in water and alcohol	22.7%	any	vehicle, adsorbent
Calcium Carbonate	5 g	white powder	practically insol in water	22.7%	any	astringent, adsorbent
Nystatin Topical Powder 100,000 units/g	2 g	light yellow powder	4 mg/mL water, 1.2 mg/mL alcohol	9,090 units/g	100,000 units/g	antifungal

*This includes 22.7% from the 5 g of added talc plus 8.9% as the diluent in the 2 g of Nystatin Topical Powder.

COMPATIBILITY–STABILITY: The adsorbent powders zinc oxide, talc, starch, and calcium carbonate are compatible and stable in powder form. Nystatin has questionable stability, even in dry powder form. Both *Chemical Stability of Pharmaceuticals* and *Trissel's Stability of Compounded Formulations* report that Nystatin degrades when exposed to heat, light, oxygen, and moisture (7,8).

PACKAGING AND STORAGE: Although the *USP* monograph for Nystatin recommends storage in tight, light-resistant containers, the *USP* monographs for all ingredients used, including Nystatin Topical Powder, allow storage in well-closed containers (3). For convenient use by the caregiver, dispense in a plastic, opaque 2-oz sifter-top powder container, which is not rated as a tight container. Store at controlled room temperature.

BEYOND-USE DATE: When using a manufactured product such as Nystatin Topical Powder, the recommended beyond-use date as specified in *USP* Chapter ⟨795⟩ for solid formulations packaged in tight containers and stored at controlled room temperature is not later than 25% of the time remaining until the product's expiration date or 6 months, whichever is earlier (6). Because the sifter-top container is not rated as a tight container, a more conservative maximum 3-month beyond-use date is used. The beyond-use date will be limited further if 25% times the nystatin product expiration date is less than 3 months.

CALCULATIONS

Dose/Concentration: The 1:10 ratio is to be interpreted as 1 part nystatin powder to 10 parts of bulk adsorbent powder. With 20 g of adsorbent powder, this would mean there should be 2 g of nystatin powder and 22 g of total powder.

Nystatin concentration: If the prescription order is interpreted as Nystatin Topical Powder USP, which is 100,000 units/g:

$$\left(\frac{100{,}000 \text{ units Nys.}}{\text{g Nys. Top. Powder}} \right) \left(\frac{2 \text{ g Nys. Top. Powder}}{22 \text{ g total powder}} \right) = 9{,}090 \text{ units per g}$$

This is approximately one-tenth the usual concentration.

If the prescription order is interpreted as Nystatin USP, apply the units-per-milligram equivalence printed on the bottle of nystatin powder that will be used (a value that varies with the manufacturer and lot number), in this case 6,050 units/mg:

$$\left(\frac{6{,}050 \text{ units Nys.}}{\text{mg Nys. powder}}\right)\left(\frac{2{,}000 \text{ mg Nys. powder}}{22 \text{ g total powder}}\right) = 550{,}000 \text{ units per g}$$

This is approximately 5.5 times the usual concentration.

As indicated in the case information, the pharmacist consulted with the physician and determined that the first interpretation, Nystatin Topical Powder, is the desired one.

Zinc oxide, starch, and calcium carbonate concentrations:

$$\% \text{ Zinc Oxide, Starch, Ca Carb.:} \frac{5 \text{ g Ingred.}}{22 \text{ g powder}} = \frac{x}{100}; x = 22.7\%$$

Talc Concentration: There are two sources of talc in this formulation. In addition to the 5 g of talc in the formula, the Nystatin Topical Powder contains talc. The 2 g of Nystatin Topical Powder contains 200,000 units of nystatin dispersed in talc. The quantity of nystatin and talc in the 2 g can be calculated on a weight basis:

$$\left(\frac{\text{mg nystatin}}{4{,}400 \text{ units nystatin}}\right)\left(\frac{200{,}000 \text{ units nystatin}}{}\right) = 45 \text{ mg nystatin}$$

$$2 \text{ g Nystatin Topical Powder} - 0.045 \text{ g nystatin} = 1.955 \text{ g talc}$$

Therefore, the amount of talc in the formulation is: 5 g + 1.955 g = 6.955 g.

$$\% \text{ Talc:} \frac{6.955 \text{ g Talc}}{22 \text{ g powder}} = \frac{x}{100}; x = 31.6\%$$

Ingredient Amounts

Zinc oxide, talc, starch, calcium carbonate: 20 g/4 = 5 g of each

Nystatin Topical Powder:

$$\frac{1 \text{ part Nys. Top. powder}}{10 \text{ parts other powders}} = \frac{x \text{ g Nys. Top. powder}}{20 \text{ g other powders}}; x = 2 \text{ g Nystatin Top. Powder}$$

MSDS AND SAFETY AND PERSONAL PROTECTIVE EQUIPMENT: Review MSDS for all bulk components. Don a clean lab coat and disposable gloves. Avoid inhaling powders.

SPECIALIZED EQUIPMENT: None. All weighing is done on an electronic balance.

COMPOUNDING PROCEDURE: Weigh 2 g of Nystatin Topical Powder USP 100,000 units/g, and 5 g each of zinc oxide, talc, starch, and calcium carbonate. Mix the adsorbent powders together (for approximately 2 minutes) by tumbling in a 1-gallon zipper-closure bag. Place the Nystatin Topical Powder in a mortar and, using geometric dilution, add the combined adsorbent powders to the Nystatin Topical Powder with trituration to obtain a homogenous powder mix. Weigh the sifter-top preparation container. Using a powder funnel, transfer the powder to the container and reweigh to determine the final weight of powder. Label appropriately and dispense.

DESCRIPTION OF FINISHED PREPARATION: Dosage form is a fine, white, odorless powder.

QUALITY CONTROL: Weigh the finished powder; it should closely match the theoretical weight of 22 g.

MASTER FORMULA PREPARED BY: Barbara Bell, PharmD   **CHECKED BY:** Sue Stein, MS, RPh

COMPOUNDING RECORD

NAME, STRENGTH, AND DOSAGE FORM OF PREPARATION: Nystatin-Adsorbent Topical Powder
QUANTITY: 22 g   **DATE PREPARED:** mm/dd/yy   **BEYOND-USE DATE:** mm/dd/yy
FORMULATION RECORD ID: BP003   **CONTROL/RX NUMBER:** 123025

INGREDIENTS USED:

Ingredient	Quantity	Manufacturer Lot Number	Expiration Date	Weighed by	Checked by
Zinc Oxide	5 g	JET Labs XY1153	mm/yy	bjf	bb
Talc	5 g	JET Labs XY1152	mm/yy	bjf	bb
Starch	5 g	JET Labs XY1155	mm/yy	bjf	bb
Calcium Carbonate	5 g	JET Labs XY1146	mm/yy	bjf	bb
Nystatin Topical Powder 100,000 units/g	2 g	BJF Generics XY1157	mm/yy	bjf	bb

QUALITY CONTROL DATA: Appearance: fine, white, odorless powder

Weight of powder in container (without cap):	32.072 g
Weight of empty container (without cap):	10.215 g
Weight of powder:	21.857 g

LABELING

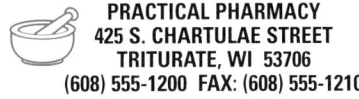

PRACTICAL PHARMACY
425 S. CHARTULAE STREET
TRITURATE, WI 53706
(608) 555-1200 FAX: (608) 555-1210

℞ 123025   Pharmacist: BB   Date: 00/00/00
Jared Stone   Dr. Schultz
Apply to area with each diaper change.
Zinc Oxide, Starch, Calcium Carbonate 22.7% each; Talc 31.6%;
Nystatin 9,090 units/g Topical Powder
Mfg: Compounded   Quantity: 22 g
Refills: 3   Discard after: Give date

Auxiliary Labels: For external use only. This medicine was compounded in
our pharmacy for you at the direction of your prescriber.

PATIENT CONSULTATION: Hello, Mrs. Stone. I'm your pharmacist, Barbara Bell. Does Jared have any
drug allergies? Is he currently using any nonprescription or prescription medications? What did
Dr. Schultz tell you about this powder or how to use it? This is a customized topical powder for

diaper rash; it contains the adsorbent, protective, and healing agents zinc oxide, starch, and calcium carbonate, and the antifungal drug nystatin. It will help keep the area dry and will treat any fungal or yeast infection in the diaper area. You should apply this to the affected area each time you change Jared's diaper, being careful not to get this near Jared's eyes, nose, or mouth. It is also very important to change his diaper frequently—as soon as you notice he is wet and especially when he has had a bowel movement. Carefully cleanse the area first with plain water (baby wipes have a tendency to sting); then gently pat the area dry before applying the powder. If you don't notice any improvement in a few days or if it appears that the area is getting worse, contact Dr. Schultz. This may be stored at room temperature, in an area away from moisture and out of the reach of children. This prescription may be refilled three times. Any unused portion should be discarded after 3 months (give date). Do you have any questions?

SAMPLE PRESCRIPTION 25.4

CASE: Jacob Stone is an 11-year-old boy who weighs 88 pounds and is 58 inches tall. Two years ago he received a multivisceral organ transplant: liver, small bowel, and stomach. He has developed hypertension as a consequence of the physiologic and pharmacologic insults that accompany organ transplantation and subsequent therapy for rejection prophylaxis. For the hypertension, Jacob is being treated with both labetalol and hydralazine (see the prescription here). He is also on a wide array of other medications, and his transplant pharmacist, Brian LaRowe, keeps in close contact with his primary ambulatory pharmacist, Jennie Jackson; Brian provides Jennie with an up-to-date list of Jacob's medications and current medical problems. Some of Jacob's current medications include pantoprazole to suppress gastrointestinal acid production; loperamide, polycarbophil, and pectin for chronic diarrhea; prednisone and tacrolimus for rejection prophylaxis; sodium citrate/citric acid for acidosis; various antibacterial and antifungal agents (e.g., trimethoprim-sulfamethoxazole, acyclovir, and nystatin) for prophylaxis of opportunistic infections; darbepoetin, iron, and folic acid for anemia; and multivitamin and mineral supplements.

CONTEMPORARY PHYSICIANS GROUP PRACTICE
20 S. PARK STREET, TRITURATE, WI 53706
TEL: (608) 555-1333 FAX: (608) 555-1335

R̥ # *123042*

NAME *Jacob Stone* **DATE** *00/00/00*

ADDRESS *521 Lego Circle*

R̥

Hydralazine 0.75 mg/kg/day in four divided doses

M & Ft Chartulae #8

Sig: Take contents of one chart on Cool Whip or pudding qid

J. Jackson 00/00/00

REFILLS *2*   *R. Farrell*   **M.D.**

DEA NO. _____

MASTER COMPOUNDING FORMULATION RECORD

NAME, STRENGTH, AND DOSAGE FORM OF PREPARATION: Hydralazine HCl 7.5-mg Divided Powder Packets

QUANTITY: 9 doses (1 extra for loss on compounding)   **FORMULATION RECORD ID:** DP001

THERAPEUTIC USE/CATEGORY: Antihypertensive   **ROUTE OF ADMINISTRATION:** Oral

INGREDIENTS:

Ingredient	Quantity	Physical Description	Solubility	Dose Comparison		Use in the Prescription
				Given	Usual	
Hydralazine HCl	120 mg weighed/ 67.5 mg used	white powder	1 g/33 mL water, 500 mL alcohol	0.75 mg/kg/day or 7.5 mg q.i.d.	same	antihyper-tensive
Lactose	360 mg weighed for aliquot; 2,430 mg for chartulae diluent	white powder	1 g/5 mL water, v sl sol in alcohol	—	—	diluent

COMPATIBILITY–STABILITY: In a solid dosage form, hydralazine HCl is relatively stable (9).

PACKAGING AND STORAGE: The *USP* monograph for Hydralazine Hydrochloride Tablets recommends storage in tight, light-resistant containers at controlled room temperature (3). Package in individual zipper-lock polyethylene bags and dispense in a 30-dram amber, tight prescription vial with a child-resistant closure. Store at controlled room temperature.

BEYOND-USE DATE: Use the recommended 6-month beyond-use date as specified in *USP* Chapter ⟨795⟩ for solid formulations made with USP ingredients, packaged in tight containers, and stored at controlled room temperature (6).

CALCULATIONS

Dose/Concentration: 0.75 to 1 mg/kg/day in two to four divided doses is the usual initial pediatric dose.

$$\text{Weight of child in kg: } \frac{88 \text{ lb}}{2.2 \text{ lb/kg}} = 40 \text{ kg}$$

$$\text{Dose in mg: } \left(\frac{0.75 \text{ mg}}{\text{kg/day}}\right)\left(40 \text{ kg}\right)\left(\frac{\text{day}}{4 \text{ doses}}\right) = 7.5 \text{ mg/dose}$$

Ingredient Amounts

For nine doses (i.e., eight packets plus one extra dose to compensate for loss of powder in the compounding process):

Hydralazine:

$$\frac{7.5 \text{ mg Hydralazine}}{\text{dose}} \times 9 \text{ doses} = 67.5 \text{ mg Hydralazine}$$

Pure powder will be used, and the amount calculated (67.5 mg) is below the MWQ for the class 3 torsion balance; therefore, an aliquot is needed. If the MWQ of 120 mg of hydralazine is weighed and mixed with 360 mg of lactose to give 480 mg of dilution, the amount of this dilution that will contain the needed 67.5 mg of hydralazine can be calculated:

$$\frac{120 \text{ mg Hydralazine}}{480 \text{ mg dilution}} = \frac{67.5 \text{ mg Hydralazine}}{x \text{ mg dilution}}; x = 270 \text{ mg dilution}$$

Extra lactose diluent to make the final contents of each packet weigh 300 mg:

$$300 \text{ mg} \times 9 = 2{,}700 \text{ mg total powder}$$

$$2{,}700 \text{ mg total powder} - 270 \text{ mg hydralazine aliquot} = 2{,}430 \text{ mg lactose}$$

MSDS AND SAFETY AND PERSONAL PROTECTIVE EQUIPMENT: Review MSDS for hydralazine. Don a clean lab coat and disposable gloves.

SPECIALIZED COMPOUNDING EQUIPMENT: All weighing is done on a class III torsion balance. A glass mortar is used for dilution and mixing of this potent, but finely divided, drug.

COMPOUNDING PROCEDURE: Weigh 120 mg of hydralazine HCl powder and 360 mg lactose. Transfer the hydralazine powder to a glass mortar and add the lactose to the hydralazine powder by geometric dilution, triturating well. Weigh 270 mg of this powder and transfer to a clean glass mortar. Weigh an additional 2,430 mg of lactose and add the lactose to the 270 mg of hydralazine aliquot by geometric dilution, again triturating well. Weigh 300 mg of this powder for each dose and place each dose in a polyethylene zipper-lock bag. Dispense the bags in a 30-dram prescription vial with a tight, child-resistant closure.

DESCRIPTION OF FINISHED PREPARATION: Fine, white powder

QUALITY CONTROL: Each powder packet is weighed to contain 300 mg of powder. A verification check is done as follows: Weigh five empty zipper-lock bags and calculate an average weight per bag; then weigh the finished packets and subtract the average weight of the empty bags from the weight of each packet. The powder in each packet should weigh 300 mg $\pm10\%$.

MASTER FORMULA PREPARED BY: Jennie Jackson, PharmD   **CHECKED BY:** Sue Stein, MS, RPh

---

COMPOUNDING RECORD

NAME, STRENGTH, AND DOSAGE FORM OF PREPARATION: Hydralazine HCl 7.5-mg Divided Powder Packets
QUANTITY: 9 doses (includes 1 extra)   **DATE PREPARED:** mm/dd/yy   **BEYOND-USE DATE:** mm/dd/yy
FORMULATION RECORD ID: DP001   **CONTROL/RX NUMBER:** 123042

INGREDIENTS USED:

Ingredient	Quantity	Manufacturer Lot Number	Expiration Date	Weighed by	Checked by
Hydralazine HCl	120 mg weighed/ 67.5 mg used	JET Labs XY1158	mm/yy	bjf	jj
Lactose	360 mg weighed for aliquot; 2,430 mg used for extra diluent	JET Labs XY1159	mm/yy	bjf	jj

QUALITY CONTROL DATA: Appearance: fine, white powder

Weights (in grams) of five empty zipper-lock packets: 0.517 + 0.519 + 0.525 + 0.510 + 0.515

Average weight (in grams) of empty packet: 0.517 g

Weights (in grams) of eight filled packets: 0.823, 0.818, 0.815, 0.821, 0.812, 0.826, 0.817, 0.820

Approximate weight of powder per packet by subtracting 0.517 g from the weight of each filled packet: 0.306, 0.301, 0.298, 0.304, 0.295, 0.309, 0.3, 0.303

All are within an acceptable range of $\pm10\%$.

LABELING

PRACTICAL PHARMACY
425 S. CHARTULAE STREET
TRITURATE, WI 53706
(608) 555-1200 FAX: (608) 555-1210

R 123042   Pharmacist: JJ   Date: 00/00/00
Jacob Stone   Dr. Farrell

Empty contents of one packet on Cool Whip or pudding and take four
times daily.

Hydralazine 7.5 mg oral divided powder packets

Mfg: Compounded   Quantity: 8 packets

Refills: 2   Discard after: Give date

Auxiliary Labels: Keep out of reach of children. Dizziness warning. This
medicine was compounded in our pharmacy for you at the direction of your
prescriber.

PATIENT CONSULTATION: Hello, Mr. Stone. I'm your pharmacist, Jennie Jackson, and I have Jacob's prescription ready. Does Jacob have any drug allergies? I know that he is taking a large number of other medications, and his transplant pharmacist, Brian LaRowe, has sent me a current list. Is Jacob currently experiencing any problems with his therapies? Did Dr. Farrell or Dr. LaRowe explain what this medication is for? This is hydralazine, and it is used to treat hypertension. You are to empty the contents of one packet onto Cool Whip or some kind of pudding or other soft food and have Jacob eat the total portion prepared. He should do this four times a day. Some side effects that he could possibly experience include headache, dizziness, fast or irregular heartbeat, diarrhea, loss of appetite, nausea, or vomiting. These usually go away after Jacob has taken this for a while. If he notices chest pain, joint pain, sore throat and fever, swelling of his arms or legs, skin rashes, or itching, consult with Dr. Farrell immediately. Store this in a cool, dry place, out of reach of children, and discard any unused portion after the date given on the bottle, which is 6 months from now. Dr. Farrell wrote this order for a small number of doses so that we can try this out to see how well Jacob tolerates this drug and how well he likes taking the drug this way. There are also two refills. If this works well, I can make a larger quantity in the future so you don't have to come into the pharmacy so often. Since these powders must be custom-made, please call in advance when you need more so that I can prepare them and have them ready for you. Do you have any questions?

SAMPLE PRESCRIPTION 25.5

CASE: Larry Bow is a 2-year-old male patient with a history of two febrile seizures at age 1. He has recently experienced several "episodes," and the tentative diagnosis is complex partial seizure disorder. Pharmacist Bill Bailey has received the prescription order given here. On consultation with Mrs. Bow, Pharmacist Bailey is told that Larry weighs 25 lb and that this prescription order is for an initial trial on this drug. Because of Larry's young age, Dr. Bailey checks the dose in two references. For children under 6 years of age, the *Drug Information Handbook* gives an initial carbamazepine dose of 5 mg/kg/day, with increases as necessary every 5 to 7 days up to 20 mg/kg/day; and *Drug Facts and Comparisons* gives an initial dosage range for this age group as 10 to 20 mg/kg/day given in two to three doses. The dose given on the prescription exceeds this recommended dosage range (see calculations next). Based on this information, Dr. Bailey thinks that a recommended initial dosage range for Larry should be: 5 to 10 mg/kg/day × 11.4 kg = 57 to 114 mg per day. Dr. Bailey also thinks that adherence to therapy would be easier if the drug is given just three times a day, with breakfast, lunch, and supper. With three doses per day, a range of 20 to 38 mg per dose is acceptable. Pharmacist Bailey calls Dr. Wurtz; together they decide to change the order from 100 mg per packet to 30 mg per packet and the directions for use are changed from four times a day to three times a day, after breakfast, lunch, and supper.

CONTEMPORARY PHYSICIANS GROUP PRACTICE
20 S. PARK STREET, TRITURATE, WI 53706
TEL: (608) 555-1333 FAX: (608) 555-1335

℞ #   *123045*

NAME *Lawrence Bow*   DATE *00/00/00*

ADDRESS *511 Academy Lane*

℞
                                    30

    Carbamazepine   ~~*400*~~ *mg/powder packet*

            M & Ft Divided Powders #15

                                        Bill Bailey 00/00/00

    Sig: Take contents of one powder packet ~~*tid*~~*, pc* ~~*and hs*~~

                            tid

Changed dose to 30 mg/packet and directions to three times a day
per telephone consult with Dr. Wurtz. BB

REFILLS *5*   *Ozzie Wurtz*   M.D.

                    DEA NO. _____

MASTER COMPOUNDING FORMULATION RECORD

NAME, STRENGTH AND DOSAGE FORM OF PREPARATION: Carbamazepine 30-mg Divided Powder Packets
QUANTITY: 16 units for dispensing 15 packets   **FORMULATION RECORD ID:** DP002
THERAPEUTIC USE/CATEGORY: Anticonvulsant   **ROUTE OF ADMINISTRATION:** Oral

INGREDIENTS:

Ingredient	Quantity	Physical Description	Solubility	Dose Comparison		Use in the Prescription
				Given	Usual	
Carbamazepine 200 mg tablets	480 mg drug from 672 mg crushed tablet powder	pink oblong tablets; pure drug is white powder	practically insoluble in water, sol in alcohol	8 mg/ kg/day	5–20 mg/ kg/day	anticonvulsant
Lactose	4,128 mg	white powder	1 g/5 mL water, v sl sol in alcohol	—	—	diluent

COMPATIBILITY–STABILITY: Even when in a solid dosage form, carbamazepine has some stability concerns, and its solid preparations require special packaging and storage for maximum stability. In two articles reported in the *American Journal of Hospital Pharmacy* and reviewed in the carbamazepine monograph in *Trissel's Stability of Compounded Formulations*, it is reported that the bioavailability of carbamazepine, when in tablet form, can be reduced by one-third if the tablets are exposed to excess moisture. The reduction in bioavailability is reported to be caused by tablet hardening due to the uptake of water by the drug molecule, with the formation of the dihydrate (10–12). This is the reason for the more restrictive packaging and storage conditions recommended by the USP, as given next.

PACKAGING AND STORAGE: The *USP* monograph for Carbamazepine Tablets recommends storage in tight, preferably glass, containers. It also states that the product should be labeled for storage in a dry place, protected from moisture (3). Package in individual zipper-lock polyethylene bags and dispense in an amber, glass, wide-mouth bottle with a tight, child-resistant closure. Store in a dry place at controlled room temperature.

BEYOND-USE DATE: Because of the stability problems with carbamazepine, use a more conservative beyond-use date of 30 days rather than the usual allowable 25% of the time remaining until the product's expiration date or 6 months, whichever is earlier (6).

CALCULATIONS

Dose/Concentration

$$\text{Weight of child in kg: } \frac{25 \text{ lb}}{2.2 \text{ lb/kg}} = 11.4 \text{ kg}$$

$$\text{Original dose (in mg/kg/day): } \left(\frac{100 \text{ mg carbam.}}{\text{dose}} \right) \left(\frac{4 \text{ doses}}{\text{day}} \right) \left(\frac{}{11.4 \text{ kg}} \right) = 35 \text{ mg/kg/day}$$

$$\text{New dose (in mg/kg/day): } \left(\frac{30 \text{ mg carbam.}}{\text{dose}} \right) \left(\frac{3 \text{ doses}}{\text{day}} \right) \left(\frac{}{11.4 \text{ kg}} \right) = 7.9 \text{ mg/kg/day}$$

Ingredient Amounts: For 16 doses, 15 packets plus one extra dose to compensate for loss of powder in the compounding process

Using 30 mg/dose:

$$30 \text{ mg/dose} \times 16 \text{ doses} = 480 \text{ mg of carbamazepine}$$

Carbamazepine is available as 200-mg tablets; three of these are needed, and the weight for three tablets is determined to be 840 mg or 280 mg per tablet. The amount of crushed tablet powder is calculated as follows:

$$\frac{200 \text{ mg carbam.}}{280 \text{ mg tablet powder}} = \frac{480 \text{ mg carbam.}}{x \text{ mg tablet powder}} \text{ ; } x = 672 \text{ mg crushed tablet powder}$$

To make each powder packet weigh 300 mg:

$$300 \text{ mg/packet} \times 16 \text{ packets} = 4{,}800 \text{ mg powder is needed.}$$

The amount of lactose needed:

$$4{,}800 \text{ mg} - 672 \text{ mg} = 4{,}128 \text{ mg lactose}$$

MSDS AND SAFETY AND PERSONAL PROTECTIVE EQUIPMENT: Don a clean lab coat and disposable gloves.

SPECIALIZED EQUIPMENT: All weighing is done on an electronic balance.

COMPOUNDING PROCEDURE: Weigh three carbamazepine 200-mg tablets: 840 mg. The average weight per tablet is 280 mg. Verify the tablet weight if the tablet manufacturer or lot number changes, because weights will vary with different manufacturers and lots. Crush the three tablets and weigh 672 mg of crushed powder, containing 480 mg of active ingredient. Weigh 4,128 mg of lactose and add to the carbamazepine by trituration using geometric dilution. Weigh 300 mg of powder for each dose, and place each dose in an individual polyethylene zipper-lock bag. Dispense the bags in an amber glass, wide-mouth, tight container with a child-resistant closure. Label appropriately.

DESCRIPTION OF FINISHED PREPARATION: White powder with pink flecks of crushed tablet material

QUALITY CONTROL: For each packet, 300 mg of powder is weighed. A verification check is done as follows. Weigh five empty zipper-lock bags and calculate an average weight per bag. Randomly select eight finished packets, weigh each, and subtract the average weight of the empty bags. The powder in each packet should weigh 300 mg ±10 %.

MASTER FORMULA PREPARED BY: Bill Bailey, PharmD   **CHECKED BY:** Sue Stein, MS, RPh

COMPOUNDING RECORD

NAME, STRENGTH, AND DOSAGE FORM OF PREPARATION: Carbamazepine 30-mg Divided Powder Packets

QUANTITY: 16 units for dispensing 15 packets (excess for loss in compounding process)

DATE PREPARED: mm/dd/yy   **BEYOND-USE DATE:** mm/dd/yy

FORMULATION RECORD ID: DP002   **CONTROL/RX NUMBER:** 123045

INGREDIENTS USED:

Ingredient	Quantity	Manufacturer Lot Number	Expiration Date	Weighed by	Checked by
Carbamazepine 200 mg tablets	480 mg drug from 672 mg crushed tablet powder	BJF Generics XY1160	mm/yy	bjf	bb
Lactose	4,128 mg	JET Labs XY1159	mm/yy	bjf	bb

QUALITY CONTROL DATA: Appearance: white powder with pink fleck of crushed tablet material

Weights (in grams) of five empty zipper-lock packets: 0.517 + 0.519 + 0.525 + 0.510 + 0.515

Average weight (in grams) of empty packet: 0.517 g

Weights (in grams) of eight randomly selected filled packets: 0.816, 0.812, 0.823, 0.818, 0.815, 0.821, 0.812, 0.826

Approximate weight of powder per packet by subtracting 0.517 g from the weight of each filled packet: 0.299, 0.295, 0.306, 0.301, 0.298, 0.304, 0.295, 0.309

All are within an acceptable range of ±10 %.

LABELING

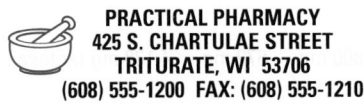

PRACTICAL PHARMACY
425 S. CHARTULAE STREET
TRITURATE, WI 53706
(608) 555-1200 FAX: (608) 555-1210

℞ 123045   Pharmacist: BB   Date: 00/00/00
Lawrence Bow   Dr. Wurtz

Give contents of one packet in soft food three times a day, after breakfast, lunch, and supper.

Carbamazepine 30-mg oral powder packets

Mfg: Compounded   Quantity: 15 packets

Refills: None   Discard after: Give date

Auxiliary Labels: Drowsiness warning. Photosensitivity warning (optional). Store in a dry place. Protect from moisture. Keep out of reach of children. This medicine was compounded in our pharmacy for you at the direction of your prescriber.

PATIENT CONSULTATION: Hi, Mrs. Bow; I have the prescription ready for Larry. Thanks for coming back. I consulted with Dr. Wurtz, and we decided on a dosage adjustment. With this change, Larry will have to take only three doses each day instead of four. This is carbamazepine and it is used to treat seizure disorders. Give him the contents of one packet, mixed with food (e.g., pudding, applesauce), three times a day, after breakfast, lunch, and supper. It is important not to miss any doses but, if you do miss a dose, give it as soon as you remember and then go back to the regular schedule; however, if it's almost time for the next dose, just skip that dose. Does Larry have any drug allergies? Does he take any other medications, either prescription or nonprescription drugs? If he should start on any new medications, be sure to tell the pharmacist that Larry is taking carbamazepine because it does interact with quite a few other drugs. This medication might cause some drowsiness or dizziness, especially initially. Larry should avoid exposure to direct sunlight as much as possible, as it may cause a rash—be sure to apply sunscreen when he will be outdoors in the sunlight. Watch for changes in vision, darkened stool, behavioral changes, or seizures: Contact Dr. Wurtz immediately if you notice any of these changes. Store this medication in a cool, dry place (protect from moisture), out of the reach of children. You have enough medication for 5 days; Dr. Wurtz wants you to call him after 4 days to see how things are going. He will then decide about any needed changes in therapy. Do you have any questions?

SAMPLE PRESCRIPTION 25.6

CASE: John Denali is a 3-year-old boy who was recently diagnosed with acute lymphoblastic leukemia (ALL). He has completed the 4-week induction chemotherapy regimen, which consists of prednisone, vincristine, and asparaginase. He has also received intrathecal therapy (IT) at weeks one and four with methotrexate, hydrocortisone, and cytarabine for central nervous system (CNS) prophylaxis. Nausea and vomiting were adequately controlled by using intravenous (IV) ondansetron prior to and 4 hours after each IT treatment. John has now finished week one of consolidation therapy using IV meds and has been given one dose of intramuscular methotrexate. John's mother has presented Pharmacist Alpine with the prescription given here. She reports that John weighs 30 pounds and is 36 inches tall. She says that she told Dr. Heider that John cannot swallow tablets, so Dr. Heider indicated that the pharmacy could prepare individual packets of powdered medicine for John, and she can give John this medicine by mixing the contents of a packet with a soft food such as pudding, applesauce, or whipped topping. John's medication profile record indicates no known allergies. His previous medications have included amoxicillin/clavulanate for recurrent otitis media and penicillin V for pharyngitis. Before preparing this prescription, Pharmacist Alpine confirmed the appropriateness of the drug and dose for this part of the ALL protocol using information in *Applied Therapeutics*, 7th edition, and *Textbook of Therapeutics*, 8th edition.

CONTEMPORARY PHYSICIANS GROUP PRACTICE
20 S. PARK STREET, TRITURATE, WI 53706
TEL: (608) 555-1333 FAX: (608) 555-1335

℞ # *123047*

NAME *John Denali*   **DATE** *00/00/00*

ADDRESS *296 Mountaineer Rd*

℞

　　　　Mercaptopurine　　　　　　*75 mg/m²/day*

　　M et Ft. Divided Oral Powders # 14

D. Alpine 00/00/00

Sig: Give the contents of one packet with breakfast and one packet with supper.

REFILLS *1*　　　　　　　　*Patsy Heider*　　　　　　**M.D.**

　　　　　　DEA NO.

MASTER COMPOUNDING FORMULATION RECORD

NAME, STRENGTH, AND DOSAGE FORM OF PREPARATION: Mercaptopurine 25-mg Divided Powder Packets

QUANTITY: 15 units for dispensing 14 packets (excess for loss in compounding process)

FORMULATION RECORD ID: DP003

THERAPEUTIC USE/CATEGORY: antineoplastic   **ROUTE OF ADMINISTRATION:** Oral

INGREDIENTS:

Ingredient	Quantity	Physical Description	Solubility	Dose Comparison		Use in the Prescription
				Given	Usual	
Mercaptopurine 50-mg tablets	375 mg drug from 2,123 mg crushed tablet powder	white tablets; pure drug is white powder	insol in water, sol in hot alcohol	75 mg/m^2/day	75 mg/m^2/day	immunosuppressant
Lactose	2.377 g	white powder	1 g/5 mL water, v sl sol in alcohol	—	—	diluent

COMPATIBILITY–STABILITY: In a solid dosage form, mercaptopurine is relatively stable; however, the monograph in *Chemical Stability of Pharmaceuticals* states that degradation of the drug in tablets is minimized by storage in tight, light-resistant containers (13).

PACKAGING AND STORAGE: The *USP* monograph for Mercaptopurine Tablets recommends storage in well-closed containers (3). The National Institute for Occupational Safety and Health (NIOSH) and the FDA recommend proper handling and disposal of this drug as an antineoplastic agent. Package in individual zipper-lock polyethylene bags and dispense in a 30-dram amber, tight prescription vial with a child-resistant closure. Store at controlled room temperature.

BEYOND-USE DATE: Use the recommended beyond-use date as specified in *USP* Chapter ⟨795⟩ for solid formulations made with active ingredients from manufactured drug products when the preparation is stored in a tight container at controlled room temperature: no later than 25% of the time remaining until the product's expiration date or 6 months, whichever is earlier (6).

CALCULATIONS

Dose/Concentration

Dose of 75 mg/m^2/day confirmed as appropriate for patient and condition.

This patient has a body weight of 30 lb and a height of 36″. Based on this weight and height, the body surface area (BSA) from the nomogram in Appendix B is 0.57 m^2.

$$\text{Daily dose: } 75 \text{ mg/m}^2\text{/day} \times 0.57 \text{ m}^2 = 43 \text{ mg/day}$$

The dosage reference states to increase the daily dose to the nearest 25 mg; in this case, increase the 43 mg to 50 mg/day.

$$\text{Dose in mg: } \frac{50 \text{ mg}}{2 \text{ doses/day}} = 25 \text{ mg/dose}$$

Ingredient Amounts:

For 15 doses – 1 extra for loss of powder on compounding

Using 25 mg/dose:

$$25 \text{ mg/dose} \times 15 \text{ doses} = 375 \text{ mg of Mercaptopurine}$$

Mercaptopurine is available as 50-mg tablets, each weighing 283 mg. For 375 mg of mercaptopurine, we will need 7.5 or 8 tablets (225 mg ÷ 50 mg/tablet = 7.5 tablets).

Amount of crushed tablet powder:

$$\frac{50 \text{ mg MP}}{283 \text{ mg tablet powder}} = \frac{375 \text{ mg MP}}{x \text{ mg tablet powder}} \; ; \; x = 2{,}123 \text{ mg tablet powder}$$

Amount of tablet powder to discard:

$$283 \text{ mg} \times 8 \text{ tablets} = 2{,}264 \text{ mg}$$

$$2{,}264 \text{ mg} - 2{,}123 \text{ mg} = 141 \text{ mg to be discarded}$$

To make each powder packet weigh 300 mg:

$$300 \text{ mg/packet} \times 15 \text{ packets} = 4{,}500 \text{ mg powder is needed.}$$

The amount of lactose needed is as follows:

$$4{,}500 \text{ mg} - 2{,}123 \text{ mg} = 2{,}377 \text{ mg lactose}$$

MSDS AND SAFETY AND PERSONAL PROTECTIVE EQUIPMENT: Don a clean lab coat and disposable gloves. Avoid inhaling powders. Mercaptopurine is on the "NIOSH Alert Sample List of Drugs That Should be Handled as Hazardous" (see Table 13.1 in Chapter 13 of this book). This drug requires special handling and disposal as is appropriate for drugs of this type. Therefore, use the following procedure that treats this material as a biohazard.

SPECIALIZED EQUIPMENT: All weighing is done on an electronic balance.

COMPOUNDING PROCEDURE: Tare a zipper-lock bag and then add one or more mercaptopurine 50-mg tablets to the bag and determine the average weight per tablet. This is found to be 283 mg. Verify the tablet weight if the tablet manufacturer or lot number changes, because weights will vary with different manufacturers and lots. Place a total of eight tablets into the bag, close it and, using a pestle on the outside of the bag, crush the tablets to a fine powder. Be careful not to puncture the bag. Withdraw 141 mg of this crushed powder and discard this in another zipper-lock bag that has a BIOHAZARD LABEL on it. Weigh 2.377 g of lactose and add this to the bag containing 2,123 mg of crushed mercaptopurine powder. Close the bag securely and mix the powder well by shaking and manipulating the bag. Reopen the bag and withdraw, transfer, and weigh 300 mg of the powder into a small, dose-sized, tared, zipper-lock bag. Repeat this for a total of fourteen 300-mg portions. Place the filled bags in a tight amber container with a child-resistant closure. Label appropriately. Leave any remaining powder in the zipper-lock bag that was used for mixing, place a biohazard warning label on the bag, and discard it in a biohazard container.

DESCRIPTION OF FINISHED PREPARATION: Fine, white powder

QUALITY CONTROL: Each powder packet is weighed to contain 300 mg of powder. A verification check is done as follows: Weigh five empty zipper-lock bags and calculate an average weight per bag. Weigh each finished packet and subtract the average weight of the empty bags. The powder in each packet should equal 300 mg ±10%.

MASTER FORMULA PREPARED BY: David Alpine, PharmD   **CHECKED BY:** Sue Stein, MS, RPh

COMPOUNDING RECORD

NAME, STRENGTH, AND DOSAGE FORM OF PREPARATION: Mercaptopurine 25-mg Divided Powder Packets

QUANTITY: 15 doses for dispensing 14 packets (excess for loss in compounding process)

DATE PREPARED: mm/dd/yy

FORMULATION RECORD ID: DP003

BEYOND-USE DATE: mm/dd/yy

CONTROL/RX NUMBER: 123047

INGREDIENTS USED:

Ingredient	Quantity	Manufacturer Lot Number	Expiration Date	Weighed by	Checked by
Mercaptopurine 50-mg tablets	375 mg drug from 2123 mg crushed tablet powder	BJF Generics XY1162	mm/yy	bjf	da
Lactose	2.377 g	JET Labs XY1159	mm/yy	bjf	da

QUALITY CONTROL DATA: Appearance: white powder

Weights (in grams) of five empty zipper-lock packets: 0.517 + 0.519 + 0.525 + 0.510 + 0.515

Average weight (in grams) of empty packet: 0.517 g

Weights (in grams) of 14 filled packets: 0.816, 0.812, 0.823, 0.818, 0.815, 0.821, 0.812, 0.826, 0.814, 0.823, 0.818, 0.817, 0.822, and 0.819

Approximate weight of powder per packet by subtracting 0.517 g from the weight of each filled packet: 0.299, 0.295, 0.306, 0.301, 0.298, 0.304, 0.295, 0.309, 0.297, 0.306, 0.301, 0.300, 0.305, and 0.302

All are within an acceptable range of ±10%.

LABELING

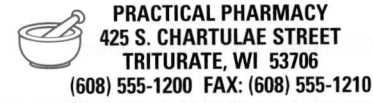

PRACTICAL PHARMACY
425 S. CHARTULAE STREET
TRITURATE, WI 53706
(608) 555-1200 FAX: (608) 555-1210

℞   123047   Pharmacist: DA   Date: 00/00/00
John Denali   Dr. Heider

Give contents of one packet in soft food with breakfast and one packet with supper.

Mercaptopurine 25-mg oral powder packets

Mfg: Compounded   Quantity: 14 packets

Refills: 0   Discard after: Give date

Auxiliary Labels: Keep out of reach of children. Drowsiness warning. This medicine was compounded in our pharmacy for you at the direction of your prescriber.

PATIENT CONSULTATION: So, Mrs. Denali, I have John's prescription ready. Does John have any drug allergies? Is he taking any other prescription or nonprescription medications? Be sure to let me know if he starts other medications, because there are some that interact with this drug. What did Dr. Heider tell you about this medication? These packets contain mercaptopurine, which is an agent used to treat his leukemia. You are to give John the contents of one packet with some pudding or other soft food two times a day, with breakfast and with supper. There are enough packets for 1 week, and I assume that John will be seeing Dr. Heider at that time. Be sure that John drinks plenty of fluids while on this medication. Use caution when handling this medication and be sure to wash your hands after giving John his dose. Possible side effects of this drug include nausea, loss of appetite, diarrhea, and drowsiness or weakness. If John experiences any of these, you can call Dr. Heider or me for suggestions. Because this drug suppresses the immune system, help John with good dental and hygiene habits and protect him, when possible, from sources of infection. Be sure to contact the doctor if John experiences a rash or unusual bruising or bleeding or severe nausea. Store this medication in a dry, cool place, away from sunlight and out of the reach of children. Discard any unused contents after (give date); if you wish, you can return it to our pharmacy for proper disposal. Do you have any questions?

REFERENCES

1. The United States Pharmacopeial Convention, Inc. Chapter ⟨1151⟩. 2008 USP 31/NF 26. Rockville, MD: Author, 2007; 621.

2. Marshall K, Foster TS, Carlin HS, Williams RL. Development of a compendial taxonomy and glossary for pharmaceutical dosage forms. Pharmacopeial forum. Rockville, MD: The United States Pharmacopeial Convention, Inc., 2003; 29(5).

3. The United States Pharmacopeial Convention, Inc. Official monographs. 2008 USP 31/NF 26. Rockville, MD: Author, 2007.

4. The United States Pharmacopeial Convention, Inc. Chapter ⟨811⟩. 2008 USP 31/NF 26. Rockville, MD: Author, 2007; 339–340.

5. Helin MM, Kontra KM, NaaranlahGti TJ, Wallentius KJ. Content uniformity and stability of nifedipine in extemporaneously compounded oral powders. Am J Health-Syst Pharm 1998; 55: 1299–1301.

6. The United States Pharmacopeial Convention, Inc. Chapter ⟨795⟩. 2008 USP 31/NF 26. Rockville, MD: Author, 2007; 317.

7. Connors KA, Amidon GL, Stella VJ. Chemical stability of pharmaceuticals, 2nd ed. New York: John Wiley & Sons, 1986; 631–636.

8. Trissel LA. Trissel's stability of compounded formulations, 3rd ed. Washington, DC: American Pharmacists Association, 2005; 317–319.

9. Trissel LA. Trissel's stability of compounded formulations, 3rd ed. Washington, DC: American Pharmacists Association, 2005; 208–211.

10. Trissel LA. Trissel's stability of compounded formulations, 3rd ed. Washington, DC: American Pharmacists Association, 2005; 71–73.

11. Anon. Moisture hardens carbamazepine tablets, FDA finds. Am J Hosp Pharm 1990; 47: 958.

12. Lowe MMJ. More information on hardening of carbamazepine tablets. Am J Hosp Pharm 1991; 48: 2130–2131.

13. Connors KA, Amidon GL, Stella VJ. Chemical stability of pharmaceuticals, 2nd ed. New York: John Wiley & Sons, 1986; 544–547.

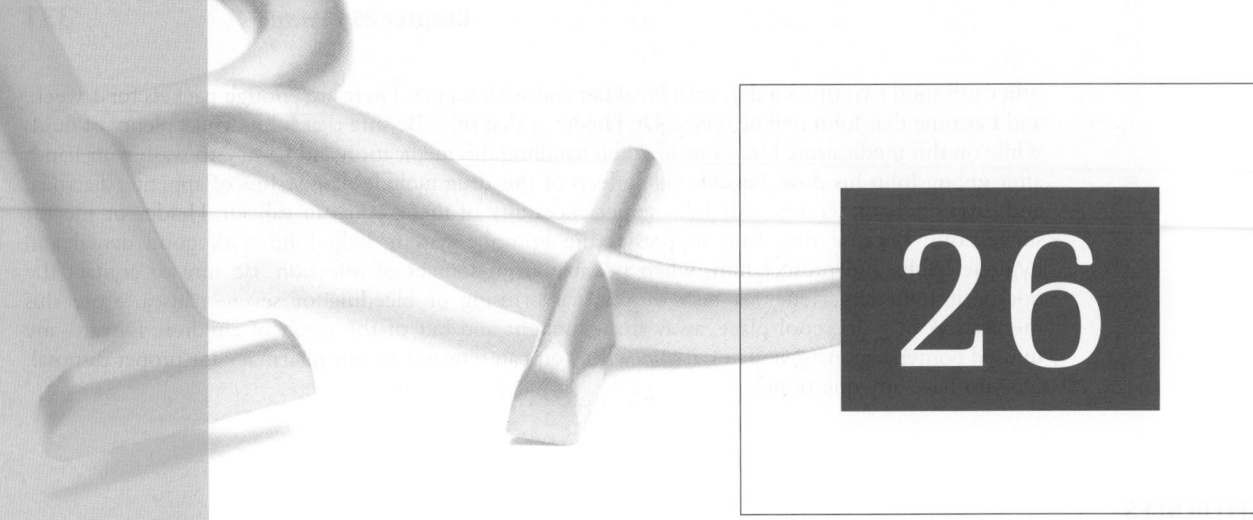

Capsules, Lozenges, and Other Solid Oral Dosage Forms

I. DEFINITIONS

A. Capsules: "Capsules are solid dosage forms in which the drug is enclosed within either a hard or soft soluble container or 'shell.' The shells are usually formed from gelatin; however, they also may be made from starch or other suitable substances" (1).

B. Lozenges: "Lozenges are solid preparations, which are intended to dissolve or disintegrate slowly in the mouth. They contain one or more medicaments, usually in a flavored, sweetened base. They can be prepared by molding (gelatin and/or fused sucrose or sorbitol base) or by compression of sugar based tablets. . . . They are usually intended for treatment of local irritation or infections of the mouth or throat but may contain active ingredients intended for systemic absorption after swallowing" (1).

The definition of lozenge in the FDA *CDER Data Standards Manual* is similar, but it adds, "a lollipop is a lozenge on a stick" (2).

C. Pastilles: *USP 31* states that the term *pastille* is often used for a subclass of lozenges—that is, molded lozenges (1). Although some references make no distinction among lozenges, pastilles, and troches, traditionally pastilles were soft lozenges containing medicament in a transparent glycerinated gelatin base or a base of acacia, sucrose, and water; they usually were flavored and colored to match the flavor (3). Although the proposed new *USP* nomenclature does not include the traditional term *pastille* (4), the 2006 *CDER Data Standards Manual* does list pastille as a dosage form and defines it as "an aromatic preparation, often with a pleasing flavor, usually intended to dissolve in the mouth" (2). (See the introduction to Chapter 27 for a discussion of proposed revised *USP* nomenclature.)

D. Troches: Although some references do not distinguish between lozenges and troches (2,5), *USP 31* states that the term *troches* is often used for the subcategory *compressed lozenges* (1,4), and the *CDER Data Standards Manual* defines a troche as "a discoid-shaped solid containing the medicinal agent in a suitably flavored base" (2).

E. Molded tablets: "Molded tablets are prepared from mixtures of medicinal substances and a diluent usually consisting of lactose and powdered sucrose in varying proportions. The powders are dampened with solutions containing high percentages of alcohol . . . . The dampened powders are pressed into molds, removed, and allowed to dry" (1).

II. CAPSULES

A. Uses: As stated at the beginning of Chapter 25, powders for internal use are often formulated into capsules. Hard-shell capsules offer a customized dosage form that can be made easily and conveniently in the pharmacy. Because the quantity of drug formulated into capsules can be measured accurately, this system is especially ideal for potent drugs and chemicals.

B. Hard-shell capsules

1. Empty hard-shell capsules are available in sizes that range from the largest size, 000, to the smallest size, 5. Larger bolus capsule shells are also available for veterinary use in large animals.

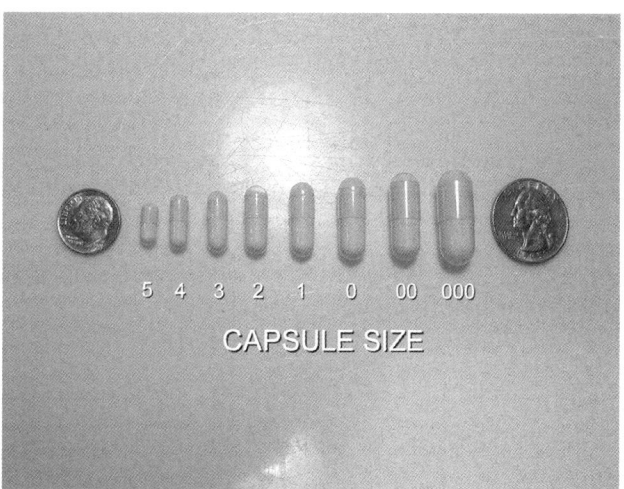

RANGE OF CAPSULE SIZES

   a. Size 00 (double zero) is usually the largest capsule size used orally for humans. For some patients, even size 00 capsules are too large to swallow.

   b. Size 000 (triple zero) capsules are sometimes used to encapsulate medication for rectal or vaginal use. The capsule is then used like a suppository. The capsule should be moistened with lubricating jelly or water before insertion.

2. The approximate capacities, by capsule size, for representative drugs and chemicals are given in Table 26.1. Notice that the weight capacity for a given capsule size is highly dependent on the density of the powder. The approximate volume capacities in milliliters are given in Table 26.2.

3. Empty hard-shell capsules may be purchased from vendors of compounding supplies. They are available as clear, colorless gelatin capsules and in a variety of colors. Some capsule shells are made opaque by the addition of titanium oxide. These are especially useful when it is necessary or desirable to conceal the powder contents, such as when dispensing powders with an unappealing appearance or when making capsules for blind studies.

4. In addition to gelatin, capsule shells may also contain dispersing agents, hardening agents such as sucrose, or preservatives. A certain percentage of water, usually 10% to 15%, must be present in hard-shell capsules (1). Lack of adequate moisture in these shells causes them to be hard and brittle, which makes them difficult to work with and which may affect their dissolution and bioavailability. For this reason, it is advisable to store capsules in tight containers that maintain a constant, adequate relative humidity. Capsules supplied by the manufacturer in paper boxes should be transferred to amber glass powder squares or other tight containers.

Table 26.1	APPROXIMATE CAPACITIES OF GELATIN CAPSULES FOR REPRESENTATIVE DRUGS AND CHEMICALS							
	CAPSULE SIZE							
	5	4	3	2	1	0	00	000
DRUG SUBSTANCE	**CAPACITY (in grams of drug powder)**							
Acetaminophen	0.13	0.18	0.24	0.31	0.42	0.54	0.75	1.10
Aluminum hydroxide	0.18	0.27	0.36	0.47	0.64	0.82	1.14	1.71
Ascorbic acid	0.13	0.22	0.31	0.40	0.53	0.70	0.98	1.42
Aspirin	0.10	0.15	0.20	0.25	0.33	0.55	0.65	1.10
Bismuth subnitrate	0.12	0.25	0.40	0.55	0.65	0.80	1.20	1.75
Calcium carbonate	0.12	0.20	0.28	0.35	0.46	0.60	0.79	1.14
Calcium lactate	0.11	0.16	0.21	0.26	0.33	0.46	0.57	0.80
Corn starch	0.13	0.20	0.27	0.34	0.44	0.58	0.80	1.15
Lactose	0.14	0.21	0.28	0.35	0.46	0.60	0.85	1.25
Quinine sulfate	0.07	0.10	0.12	0.20	0.23	0.33	0.40	0.65
Sodium bicarbonate	0.13	0.26	0.32	0.39	0.52	0.70	0.97	1.43

Source: Adapted from Narducci WA, Newton DW. Extemporaneous formulations. In: King RE, ed. Dispensing of medications, 9th ed. Easton, PA: Mack Publishing Co., 1984; 268, and from data given in Shaw MA. Capsules. In: King RE, ed. Dispensing of medications, 9th ed. Easton, PA: Mack Publishing Co., 1984; 48.

5. Hard-shell capsules consist of two telescoping pieces, a body piece and a cap. In compounding, the two pieces are separated, the body piece is filled with the formulated powder, and then the cap is replaced on the body.

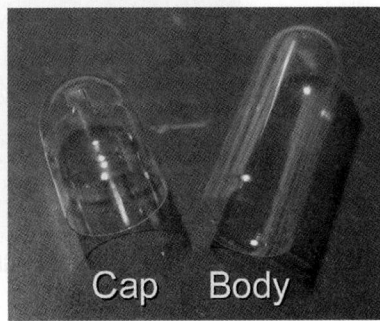

PARTS OF A CAPSULE SHELL

6. Selecting a capsule size for encapsulating a compounded powder
   a. Calculate the weight of the powder to be filled into each capsule. This will include the weight of all active ingredients per capsule plus the weight of any needed diluents.

Table 26.2	APPROXIMATE VOLUME CAPACITY BY CAPSULE SIZE	
	SIZE	**MILLILITERS**
	000	1.36
	00	0.95
	0	0.67
	1	0.48
	2	0.37
	3	0.27
	4	0.20
	5	0.13

b. A diluent may be needed in the following situations.

    (1) If the amount of powder for each capsule is less than the minimum weighable quantity (MWQ) for the balance being used, an inert solid diluent must be added to the active powder ingredients to give a desirable weight per capsule.

    (2) Because the smallest capsule sizes, numbers 4 and 5, are difficult for some compounders to handle, if the quantity of powder is more than the MWQ but is so small that a size 4 or 5 capsule shell is needed, diluent may be added so that a larger capsule size can be used. This is demonstrated with the alternate procedure used for Sample Prescription 26.1 on the CD that accompanies this book.

    (3) Occasionally, the amount of powder per dose does not fit properly in any given capsule size; it is too much powder to fit in one size but gives void space in the next larger size. If this occurs, an inert solid diluent may be added to adjust the powder volume to the larger-size capsule. This is illustrated with Sample Prescription 36.3 in Chapter 36.

    (4) When hand filling capsules, a well-packing diluent may be added to a crystalline or granular powder to improve its ease of packing. Lactose monohydrate (the non-spray-dried variety) and cornstarch are two diluents that work well for this purpose.

    (5) When using a capsule-filling machine, an inert diluent may be needed to improve the flow of the powder so that capsules of uniform weight are obtained. Also, the capsule-filling machine may not have plates for all capsule sizes, so you may be required to add diluent to accommodate the capsules sizes available to you.

c. Consult a capsule capacity table such as Table 26.1.

    (1) If you have a single capsule ingredient and that ingredient is a representative substance in the table, select the capsule size directly from the table.

    (2) Because most formulations are mixtures, selection of a capsule size usually requires judgment and sometimes trial and error. Try to pick a representative substance in the table that has a density similar to that of the ingredient in your formulation that is present in the greatest quantity. If you do not know this information, pick a capsule size that best fits your powder weight for the greatest number of representative drugs and chemicals.

    (3) In selecting a capsule size, you want the smallest size that will produce a filled capsule with no void space. For this reason, if your ingredient weight falls between two weights on the table, try the smaller capsule size first.

d. Selecting a capsule size is something of a compromise. For best bioavailability of the powder, a loosely packed capsule is preferred because the powder disperses easily as the capsule shell dissolves. However, when filling capsules individually by hand, it is easier to fill capsules that are **slightly** packed because, as you fill a number of capsules to a given weight, your fingers will be able to sense the packing pressure that corresponds to the desired weight of capsule ingredients. This makes it easier to achieve the appropriate capsule weight with a minimum number of balance checks. You do not have this sense of pressure with loosely packed capsules.

e. If the amount of powder per unit necessitates a capsule size that is too large for the patient to swallow comfortably, divide the powder per dose in half and put each dose in two capsules. The number of capsules dispensed is then doubled and the directions for use changed to double the number of units administered. The prescriber should be advised of any changes made in the prescription order.

f. The size and color of capsules used for compounding a preparation should be written on the prescription order or included on the compounding record; this will ensure that any refills are prepared with the same capsule size and type. When this information is recorded on the front of the prescription order, the number of the capsule size is usually written inside a triangle, Δ, and the capsule color is recorded beneath the triangle. This is demonstrated for Sample Prescription 26.1 on the CD that accompanies this book.

 7. Procedure for hand filling capsules with dry ingredients

a. Prepare the powder using the techniques and procedures for particle size reduction and blending as described in section V of Chapter 25. Make enough powder for one extra capsule, because there will be some loss in the blending and capsule-filling process. If the prescription contains a controlled substance, this loss in compounding must be minimal and should be documented on the prescription order or compounding record.

b. Place the powder mixture for all the capsules on an ointment slab or pad. Using a spatula, arrange the powder into a compact, flat powder bed of uniform thickness. This is sometimes referred to as "blocking the powder bed." The height of the powder bed should be just slightly shorter than the long dimension of the body piece of the capsule shell. This allows for the most efficient punching of powder into the shell. If the powder bed is even and uniformly packed, it is possible, after punching a few capsules, to get an idea of the number of times to punch powder into each shell body to give the approximate desired weight of powder per capsule.

   c. At one time, it was considered permissible to handle capsules with clean hands, but now it is standard procedure to use disposable gloves. In addition to being more sanitary, the use of gloves protects the compounder from contact exposure to the drugs or chemicals being encapsulated. Furthermore, use of gloves eliminates the problem of fingerprints on capsule shells; any dampness on bare fingers will cause a partial dissolution of the gelatin shell and a smudging of its surface.

   d. Separate the capsule cap from the body of the capsule shell and repeatedly press the open end of the body of the shell downward into the powder bed. This process is called *punching* capsules. It is illustrated on Color Plate 2 and is demonstrated using Sample Prescription 26.1 on the CD that accompanies this book.

   e. Replace the cap on the body loosely and check the weight of the capsule. The weighing procedure for a double-pan torsion balance is given in Figure 26.1 and, for an electronic balance, in Figure 26.2. Add to or empty powder from the capsule shell until the desired weight is achieved. A tolerance in final capsule weight of $\pm 5\%$ usually can be achieved without too much difficulty.

8. Use of capsule-filling machines

   a. Pharmacists who compound capsules routinely or in larger quantities may want to invest in a capsule filler or capsule-filling machine. The nonautomated fillers are available through pharmacy vendors in prices ranging from approximately \$20 to more than \$3,000. There are also motorized capsule-loading machines in the \$5,000 to \$10,000 price range that can fill 300 capsules per batch. These fillers work on a principle of calibrated volume fill rather than weight, and their use requires good quality control procedures to ensure precise and accurate dose per capsule.

   b. When using a capsule-filling machine, the powder must be formulated so that its flow properties give capsules of uniform weight. Because an inert diluent is usually added to the powder when making capsules by volume, this ingredient should be selected carefully with flow properties in mind.

---

1. Place the balance on a smooth, level surface. Be sure the graduated dial or rider are at zero. Release the balance pan arrest and check that the balance is operating properly with balance pans and index pointer moving freely.

2. Using the leveling feet at the front of the balance, bring the balance pans into equilibrium.

3. Put a weighing paper on each balance pan and re-establish equilibrium using the leveling feet. **After this step, do not touch the leveling feet again during this weighing operation.**

4. On the right-hand balance pan, place an empty capsule shell of the appropriate size plus weights to offset the weight of the powder per capsule. Adding weights on the graduated dial at the front of the balance adds weight to the right side of the balance.
Example: If a capsule is to contain 300 mg. of drug, place an empty capsule shell on the right balance pan and add 300 mg in fractional weights to the right balance pan **or** dial 0.3 g on the graduated dial.

5. For each capsule, punch powder into an empty capsule shell and place it on the left balance pan. This will be offset by the weights added or dialed in plus the empty capsule shell placed on the right balance pan. Add or remove powder to the capsule shell until the index pointer is at the center of the index plate or until it moves an equal distance to the right and left of the center.

FIGURE 26.1. PROCEDURE FOR WEIGHING CAPSULES WITH A DOUBLE-PAN TORSION BALANCE

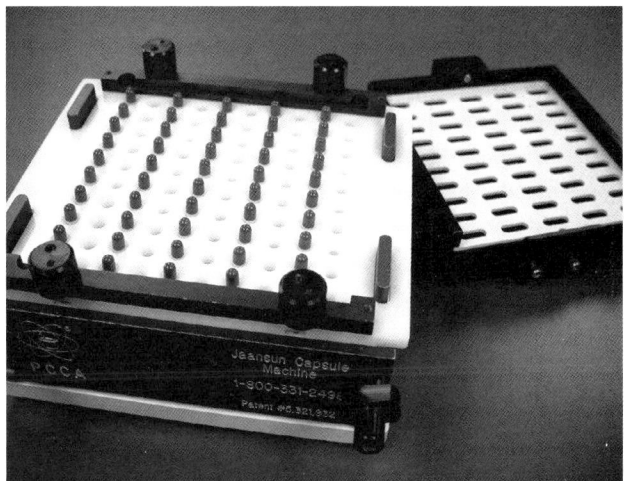

A CAPSULE-FILLING MACHINE

(1) Lactose is a common inert diluent. It is commonly available as the monohydrate, and some suppliers sell the monohydrate in two forms, regular and spray-dried. The regular lactose monohydrate packs well, but it does not have particularly good flow properties. Spray-dried lactose monohydrate has been modified through processing to give a powder with improved flow characteristics. Anhydrous lactose is also available, and it too has good flow properties. Spray-dried lactose monohydrate and anhydrous lactose are good diluents for capsule-filling machines. Check the type carefully when purchasing lactose for use as a diluent in capsule machines.

(2) Microcrystalline cellulose has been used successfully as a diluent for capsule-filling machines. It is a free-flowing powder classified by the NF as a tablet disintegrant and tablet and capsule diluent.

(3) Some granular materials, such as sodium carboxymethylcellulose (CMC), have good flow properties but, depending on the other ingredients in the formulation, they may change the dissolution and absorption characteristics of the drug. Unless specifically called for, natural and synthetic gum powders should be avoided as diluents, because they may form thick viscous barriers around the drug particles when exposed to the aqueous fluid in the stomach and may prevent the drug from being released from the dosage

1. Place the balance on a smooth, level surface. Press the tare button and observe the balance set at 000.0.

2. Place a weighing paper and an empty capsule shell of the appropriate size on the balance pan. Re-zero the balance by pressing the tare button. The digital display should read 000.0 **After this step, do not touch the tare button again during this weighing operation.**

3. Remove the empty capsule shell from the balance pan. The digital display will read a negative value which represents the weight of the capsule shell.

4. For each capsule, punch powder into an empty capsule shell and place it on the balance pan. Add or remove powder to the capsule shell until the digital display shows the desired weight of the capsule powder. The weight of the capsule shell will be offset by the negative value achieved when taring the empty shell at the beginning of the procedure.
   Example: If a capsule is to contain 300 mg of drug, the digital display should read 0.300 g when the completed capsule is on the balance pan.

FIGURE 26.2. PROCEDURE FOR WEIGHING CAPSULES WITH AN ELECTRONIC BALANCE

form. Some sustained-release capsule formulations use synthetic gums to modify drug release, but these formulations should always be thoroughly tested before use.

(4) If flow is a problem, one recommendation is to add a small quantity (less than 1% of the total powder weight) of magnesium stearate, a powdered excipient used as a lubricant in manufacturing tablets (6).

c. As with capsules punched individually, capsules made using a filling machine should always be checked for accuracy and uniformity. A modification of the weight variation test given in Chapter ⟨905⟩ of *USP 23* (7) is useful when evaluating capsules made in this way.

(1) Select 30 capsules and weigh 10 of them individually.

(2) Calculate a mean, a standard deviation, and a relative standard deviation for this sample using these equations:

$$s = \left[\frac{\sum(x_i - \overline{X})^2}{n-1} \right]^{1/2} \qquad RSD = \frac{100s}{\overline{X}}$$

where:

s = sample standard deviation

RSD = relative standard deviation (the sample standard deviation expressed as a percentage of the mean)

$\overline{X}$ = mean of the values obtained from the units tested, expressed as a percentage of labeled amount of drug

n = number of units tested

x_i = individual values of the units tested, expressed as a percentage of the labeled amount of drug

(3) The capsules are satisfactory if all 10 units are within the range of 85% to 115% of the labeled amount of drug per capsule and if the relative standard deviation is less than or equal to 6%.

(4) If this sample of 10 capsules fails to meet these standards, check the 20 additional capsules originally selected; the specifications are met if none of the 30 capsules is outside 75% to 125% and not more than 3 of the 30 is outside 85% to 115% of label claim and the RSD of the 30 capsules does not exceed 7.8% (7).

(5) A quality control record with sample data that utilizes this modified weight variation test is given in Figure 26.3.

d. The modified weight variation test just described checks only for uniformity of fill of the capsules. It assumes that the compounded powder contains the correct amount of active ingredient(s) and that the capsule components are uniformly distributed in the powder mass. To verify that individual capsules contain the labeled amount of drug, pharmacies that routinely compound batches of a given formulation should initially and periodically send batches of the compounded capsules to an analytical lab for testing. If capsules are found to be outside the official *USP* ⟨905⟩ content uniformity standard, corrective action should be taken so that compounded capsules are within acceptable limits.

e. An additional double-check procedure that is useful when doing batch compounding is to weigh the containers of formulation ingredients before and after the compounding procedure. The difference in the weight of each container should coincide with the calculated amount of that ingredient in the batch.

f. Pharmacists who compound batches of capsules routinely should also develop written formula and batch record sheets and written standard operating procedures (SOPs). Sample SOPs for capsule making have been published in the *International Journal of Pharmaceutical Compounding*.

9. Use of manufactured tablets and capsules in compounded hard-shell capsules

a. Manufactured tablets or capsules may be used as ingredients for compounded capsules. Review the discussion on using manufactured dosage forms as compounding ingredients in section II.c. of Chapter 13.

b. Depending on the situation, one of the following techniques may be used:

(1) The tablets may be crushed or the manufactured capsule contents emptied and the resulting powder used as would be any powdered ingredient.

(2) A whole tablet or capsule may be embedded in powder that has been punched into a capsule shell. If the quantity of an ingredient per capsule is the exact quantity in a manufactured tablet or capsule, it may be easier to punch the correct amount of the other ingredients into the shell and then embed the manufactured tablet or capsule in this

1. Date: mm/dd/yy

2. Preparation/Quantity: Estradiol 10 mg Capsules   #100

3. Batch or Prescription Number: XXXX#####

4. Equipment: Handy Dandy Capsule Filling Machine, Model A689X

5. Capsule Size: 0

6. Diluent (Manufacturer/Lot #/Exp. Date):

   Anhydrous lactose, JET Labs, #KYB4856–mm/yy

7. Formulation:

   Calibrated powder weight for anhydrous lactose per capsule: 367 mg

   Capsules were made using the following formula:

Weight of powder for 100 capsules:	36,700 mg
Weight of active ingredient for 100 capsules:	1,000 mg
Weight of diluent for 100 capsules:	35,700 mg

8. Prepare powder and fill 100 capsules.

9. Randomly select 10 filled capsules. Weigh each capsule individually and record the weights in column (2) on the attached table.

10. Select 10 empty capsule shells from the lot used to make the capsules. Determine the combined weight of the 10 shells using an electronic balance and calculate the average weight per shell. Individually weigh 5 capsules to verify that all capsules are within ± 5% of the mean weight of the 10 capsules. Record the mean weight of the capsule shells in column (3) of the attached table.

11. Subtract the average weight of a capsule shell from the weight of each filled capsule to determine the weight of powder in each shell and record this weight in column (4).

12. Using the formulation quantities above, and the true weight of powder in each capsule, calculate the amount of active ingredient in each capsule and record this in column (5). For example, for capsule #1:

$$\frac{10 \text{ mg estradiol}}{367 \text{ mg capsule power}} = \frac{x \text{ mg estradiol}}{343 \text{ mg capsule power}}; x = 9.3 \text{ mg estradiol}$$

13. For each capsule, express the amount of active ingredient as a percentage of label claim (LC) and record this in column (6).

$$\frac{9.3 \text{ mg actual estradiol}}{10 \text{ mg LC estradiol}} \times 100\% = 93\% \text{ of LC}$$

14. Calculate the mean value of the units expressed as a percentage of label claim and record this as $\overline{X}$ in the last row, last column of the table.

15. Calculate the range of 85% to 115% of label claim for this preparation.

    $85\% \times 10 \text{ mg} = 8.5 \text{ mg}$

    $115\% \times 10 \text{ mg} = 11.5 \text{ mg}$

FIGURE 26.3. QUALITY CONTROL RECORD FOR HARD-SHELL CAPSULES (*Continued*)

16. Calculate the range of 75% to 125% of label claim for this preparation.

     75% × 10 mg = 7.5 mg

     125% × 10 mg = 12.5 mg

17. Calculate the standard deviation (*s*) and the relative standard deviation (*RSD*) for this sample. (Note: This may be calculated with a preprogrammed calculator, a computer statistics software program, or using the equations given in this chapter.)

$$ s = \left[\frac{\sum (x_i - \bar{X})^2}{n-1} \right]^{1/2} = 2.18 \qquad RSD = \frac{100\,s}{\bar{X}} = 2.35\% $$

18. Determine if the batch meets the standard of this modified weight variation test:

   a. If any unit is outside the 75% to 125% range, the batch fails. None of our units is outside the range of 7.5 to 12.5 mg.

   b. The batch passes if the amount of active ingredient in not less than 9 of 10 units is within the 85 to 115% range and no unit is outside the 75% to 125% range, and the *RSD* of the 10 units is less than or equal to 6%.

     Our batch passes this test because no capsule is outside the range of 8.5 to 11.5 mg (the range for our sample is 8.9 to 9.7 mg) and the *RSD* of our sample is less than 6% (our *RSD* is 2.35%).

   c. If 2 or 3 units are outside the 85% to 115% range, but none is outside the 75% to 125% range, and/or if the *RSD* is greater than 6%, 20 additional units may be tested. The requirements are met if not more than 3 units of the 30 are outside the 85% to 115% range and none is outside the 75% to 125% range and the *RSD* of the 30 units is not greater than 7.8%.

(1) Capsule Number	(2) Weight of Capsule (mg)	(3) Ave. Weight of Capsule Shell (mg)	(4) Weight of Capsule Contents (mg)	(5) Active Ingredient Weight (mg)	(6) Active Ingredient expressed as a percentage of label claim (x_i)
1	435	92	343	9.3	93
2	419	92	327	8.9	89
3	447	92	355	9.7	97
4	436	92	344	9.4	94
5	431	92	339	9.2	92
6	432	92	340	9.3	93
7	425	92	333	9.1	91
8	439	92	347	9.5	95
9	435	92	343	9.3	93
10	429	92	337	9.2	92
Mean value of the units expressed as a percentage of label claim:				$\bar{X} =$	92.9

FIGURE 26.3. QUALITY CONTROL RECORD FOR HARD-SHELL CAPSULES (*Continued*)

powder. This technique is particularly useful for protecting ingredients from each other when there is a question about compatibility. This method can also be used when encapsulating tablets or capsules for blind studies. In this case, the capsule shell is partially filled with lactose or another inert diluent, and the tablet or capsule containing the active ingredient is concealed by embedding it in the diluent. If a tablet is concealed in this way, it may be split in two so that a smaller capsule shell can be used. This is especially important when making capsules for children and the elderly, who may have difficulty swallowing larger capsules. This technique is illustrated on Color Plate 3 and is used in Sample Prescription 26.2.

10. Procedure for compounding capsules with liquid ingredients

   a. Liquid drugs or solutions or dispersions of drugs may be filled into capsule shells if the shell material is not soluble in the liquid.

   b. Care must be exercised to ensure that the liquid does not leak out of the capsule during storage or use.

   (1) Leakage can be minimized by sealing the capsule cap to the body of the capsule shell by moistening the inside edge of the cap before replacing it on the body. This can be done with a cotton applicator that has been dipped in water or a water/alcohol solution.

   (2) Several brands of capsule shells now are grooved so that the cap snaps in place on the body piece of the capsule. If possible, use capsule shells of this type to prevent leakage of liquid ingredients.

   (3) A third method is to mix the liquid drug with a melted miscible material that is a solid at room temperature but will melt at body temperature or will dissolve in the aqueous fluid in the stomach. The solution of the drug in this melted material is added in liquid form to the capsule shell. Because the material solidifies at room temperature, it will congeal and will not leak out of the capsule shell during storage or use. Examples of such drug vehicles are the fatty bases and appropriate blends of polyethylene glycol polymers.

   c. Capsule shells may be filled with liquids volumetrically using a syringe or a graduated dropper or pipette.

   d. Liquids can also be filled in capsule shells by weight.

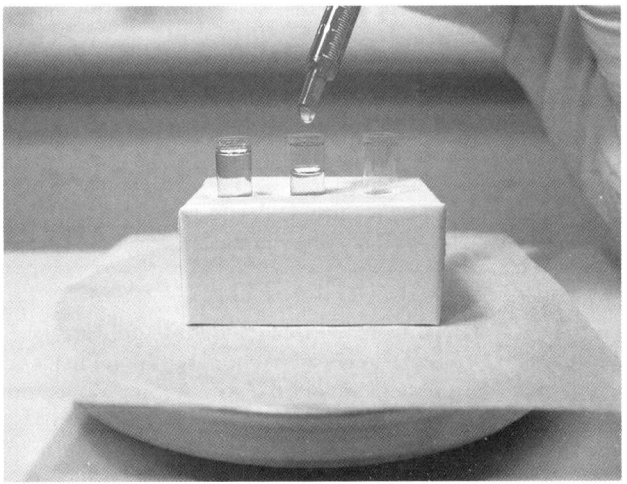

FILLING CAPSULES WITH LIQUID INGREDIENTS

   (1) Insert the bodies of capsule shells in a holder. (The holder may be as simple as the lid of a powder box with holes punched that are the size of the capsule bodies.)

   (2) Place the holder containing the capsule bodies on an electronic balance and tare out the weight.

   (3) Using a syringe, dropper, or pipette, add liquid to each shell body to the predetermined desired weight. This procedure is illustrated with Sample Prescription 26.4.

C. Soft-shell capsules or soft-gels

   1. The principal material for the shells of these capsules is usually gelatin but, as their name implies, the shell is a softer, more pliable material than that used for hard-shell capsules. This is caused by the presence of glycerin and/or sorbitol, each of which acts as a plasticizer. The shells of soft-gels are also thicker than those of hard-shell capsules (1).

2. These capsules are usually filled with liquids; either the physical form of the active ingredient is a liquid, or a solid active ingredient is dissolved or suspended in a liquid vehicle.

3. The liquid vehicle used in soft-shell capsules must be approved for oral use. It is usually a vegetable oil or a nonaqueous, water-miscible liquid glycol, such as polyethylene glycol 400 or one of the other liquid polyethylene glycols (1).

4. The technology and equipment required for making soft-shell capsules is generally not available in pharmacies, so this dosage form is not usually compounded extemporaneously.

5. Manufactured soft-shell capsules are sometimes used as ingredient sources for compounding.

   a. Capsule contents can be extracted either by using a 16- to 20-gauge needle and a syringe to withdraw the liquid contents or by making a slit in the capsule shell and squeezing the contents into the compounding container or measuring device. (See the picture, Extracting surfactant docusate Na from a soft-shell capsule, in Chapter 28.)

   b. If the capsule contents are oleaginous, a compatible oil may be added and the resulting oil solution can be used directly, or an emulsion can be made with the addition of water and an emulsifying agent.

   c. If the capsule contents have a water-miscible base, such as a liquid polyethylene glycol, they may be added directly to an aqueous or water-miscible compounding vehicle.

III.   LOZENGES

A. Uses

1. Lozenges have traditionally been used for local effect—to administer topical anesthetics and demulcents for soothing irritated throat passages experienced with cough and sore throat, and to deliver antibacterial agents intended to promote healing of inflamed or abraded mouth and throat tissues.

2. More recently, lozenges are being used as a way to deliver drugs systemically. As the lozenge slowly dissolves in the mouth, drug is released for absorption in the mouth, either buccally or sublingually, and drug that is swallowed can be absorbed in the gastrointestinal tract.

3. Lozenges are especially useful for patients who have difficulty swallowing oral solid dosage forms. This includes some pediatric and geriatric patients and patients with gastrointestinal blockage.

4. Because lozenges dissolve slowly in the mouth, this dosage form is also useful for medications that give maximum benefit when in prolonged contact with local tissues. Examples include antifungal agents used for the treatment of candidiasis (thrush) and sodium fluoride used for the prevention of dental caries.

5. To enhance patient compliance, especially in children, lozenges are formulated to taste good. Because they may look and taste like candy, lozenges are a potential danger to children; households with children should be warned to keep these preparations out of the reach of children.

B. Types of lozenges

1. Hard lozenges

   a. Hard-candy lozenges are mixtures of sucrose and other sugars and/or carbohydrates in an amorphous state. Although they are made from aqueous syrups, the water, which is initially present, evaporates as the syrup is boiled during processing so that the moisture content in the finished product is 0.5% to 1.5% (5).

   b. Because making hard lozenges is similar to candy making, helpful hints can be found by consulting a comprehensive cookbook or a candy-making reference. Flavorings, colors, and special molds can be purchased from some vendors of compounding supplies and from businesses that specialize in selling supplies for making candies and confectionaries. Hard-candy lollipops have become an especially popular compounded dosage form in recent years, and special molds and sucker sticks and wrappers are available from various vendors.

   c. Successful preparation of smooth hard lozenges depends on careful handling of the syrup and monitoring of temperatures. This is because the crystal-amorphous form of the sugar in the final preparation is temperature and condition dependent. If a formula states that the syrup should not be stirred until a particular temperature is reached, or if it states that the temperature of the syrup must reach 154°C, it is wise to follow these instructions precisely.

   d. The finished hardness of the candy depends partly on its water content. To obtain lozenges that are hard and not tacky, the temperature of the melt must reach 149° to 154°C (300° to 310°F). This is called the *hard crack* stage. This temperature is based on conditions at sea level

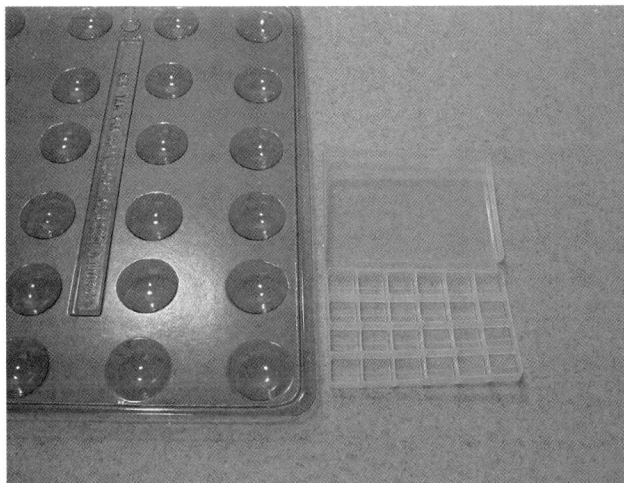

SAMPLE LOZENGE MOLDS

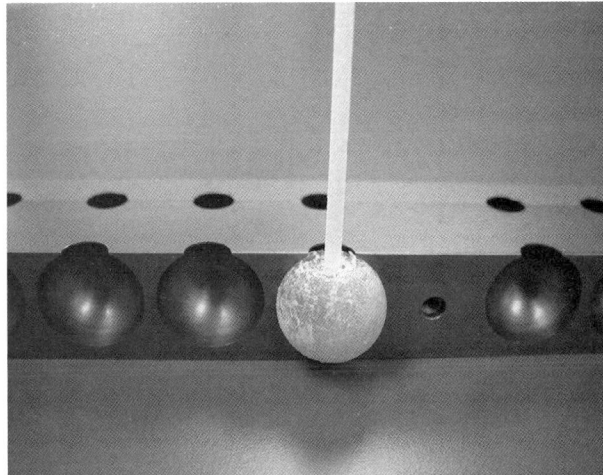

MOLDED HARD-CANDY LOLLIPOP

and average relative humidity. At higher altitudes, these temperatures are lower; on humid days, the syrup should be heated to 1°C higher than usual.

 e. Because of the high temperatures needed to make hard lozenges, drugs or chemicals that are unstable at elevated temperatures should not be incorporated into this dosage form.

 f. Formulas for two hard-lozenge bases are given in Table 26.3.

2. Soft lozenges

Soft lozenges can be made with a flavored fatty base (such as chocolate), a polyethylene glycol (PEG) base, or a sugar–acacia base.

 a. Fatty-base soft lozenges

  (1) The chocolate lozenge base shown in Table 26.3 contains dipping chocolate melted together with a vegetable oil. These lozenges are easy to make and taste good.

   (a) The oil depresses the congealing point of the base to facilitate the homogeneous incorporation of active ingredients and the pouring of accurately measured doses.

   (b) After melting and mixing, this base can be either poured directly or drawn into a syringe and carefully squirted into tared mold cavities, all without congealing. Plastic medication cups work well as extemporaneous molds.

   (c) The finished lozenges should be placed in a freezer to harden for ease of removal from the mold cavities. The removed lozenges should be placed in individual polyethylene bags and stored in the freezer. Because of the presence of oil, these lozenges are too soft to be stored at room temperature. Sample Prescription 26.5 illustrates a compounding procedure for chocolate lozenges.

  (2) Table 26.3 also shows a formula for a fatty-base soft lozenge made with a synthetic cocoa butter base and artificial flavor and sweetener. These have a less appealing taste than the chocolate base. Perhaps the chocolate flavor is a needed complement for the oily feel of such a base.

 b. PEG-base soft lozenges

  (1) These bases are similar to PEG suppository bases except that they are formulated to be less firm. Most commonly, PEG 1,000, with a melting point of 37° to 40°C, or PEG 1,450, with a melting point of 43° to 46°C, is used alone or with added acacia, approximately 0.5 g per 20 g of PEG base. Some formulas are more complex and use a combination of solid and liquid PEGs to give a particular desired consistency. (10–12)

  (2) To make these soft lozenges palatable, flavoring and a heat-stable artificial sweetener, such as sodium saccharin, should be added. Color may be added if desired. A sample compounding procedure is given in Table 26.3. Even with added flavor and sweetener, these lozenges would not be considered tasty. If this sort of base is used, considerable experimentation with flavoring and sweetener must be done to formulate a preparation with a satisfactory taste.

 c. Hand-rolled acacia–sugar lozenges

  (1) The base material for this lozenge is powdered sugar held together by an acacia mucilage.

Table 26.3	**LOZENGE FORMULAS**

CLEAR, HARD-LOZENGE BASE

This formula is modified from a hard-candy formula available from LorAnn Oil, Inc.
70 g Sucrose
40 g Light corn syrup
20 mL Purified Water
0.5 mL Flavoring oil
qs Color (if desired)
qs Active ingredients

Combine the sucrose, corn syrup, and Purified Water in a beaker. Place on a hotplate at medium heat and stir until the sucrose dissolves. Bring to a boil and boil without stirring until the temperature reaches 154°C (310°F). A candy thermometer is useful for monitoring the temperature. Remove from heat. Stir in flavoring oil, active ingredients, and the coloring (if desired). Pour into precalibrated molds that have been lubricated with vegetable spray or dusted with powdered sugar. Alternatively, place mold(s) on an electronic balance and tare out the weight of the mold(s); then pour lozenge material into each mold cavity to the desired weight.

OPAQUE, HARD-LOZENGE BASE (8)

This base has been used to make medicated lollipops.
150 g Sucrose
0.5 g Potassium bitartrate (Cream of Tartar)
50 mL Purified Water
The following should be dissolved in 5 mL of Purified Water:
0.5 mL Flavoring concentrate
qs Color (if desired)
qs Active ingredients

Dissolve the sucrose and potassium bitartrate in the Purified Water in a beaker. Bring to a boil on a hotplate and heat until the temperature reaches 154°C (310°F). Remove from heat. Add the solution containing the active ingredients, but do not stir until the mixture has cooled to 125°C (257°F); then stir until uniform. Pour into a precalibrated mold that has been dusted with powdered sugar. If this is used for lollipops, insert a stick into each lozenge before allowing the preparation to cool.

CHOCOLATE LOZENGE BASE (9)

30 g Dipping chocolate
10 g Vegetable oil (corn, soybean, etc.)
qs Active ingredients

On an electronic balance, tare out the weight of a 150-mL beaker. Add vegetable oil to the beaker to a weight of 10 g. Set the beaker in a warm-water bath. Break the chocolate into pieces and add to the heated oil in portions, melting the chocolate with each addition. Stir until completely melted and well mixed. Weigh the desired amount of chocolate base and active ingredient(s). Add the active ingredient(s) to the base and stir to mix well. Pour into mold cavities to a predetermined weight or volume. The chocolate base material can be stored in the refrigerator. Portions can be weighed and used as needed for preparing chocolate lozenges.

FATTY BASE SOFT LOZENGES (5)

25 g Synthetic cocoa butter base (e.g., Fattibase)
1 g Acacia
qs Flavor
qs Sweetener, e.g. sodium saccharin
qs Active ingredient(s)

Melt the Fattibase on a warm-water bath to approximately 40°C. Gradually add the acacia powder and then the drug, stirring to form a uniform mixture. Add the flavor and the sweetener and stir well. Place a mold(s) on an electronic balance and tare out the weight of the mold(s); then pour lozenge material into each mold cavity to the desired weight.

(continued)

Table 26.3	**LOZENGE FORMULAS** (*Continued*)

POLYETHYLENE GLYCOL BASE SOFT LOZENGES (5,10–12)

Bases of this type contain PEG 1,000 (m.p. 37°–40°C), PEG 1,450 (m.p. 43°–46°C), or a combination of solid and liquid PEGs. In some formulas, acacia is added, approximately 0.5 g per 20 g of PEG.

The PEG is placed in a beaker and melted on a warm-water bath or a hotplate to approximately 70°C. The acacia (if added) and the active ingredient(s) are added and the mixture stirred well. Flavoring and a heat-stable artificial sweetener, such as sodium saccharin, should be added. Color may be added if desired. Either pour the melted material into a precalibrated mold or use the tared mold method described earlier.

HAND-ROLLED SUGAR LOZENGES (5)

10 g Powdered sugar
0.7 g Acacia
qs Purified Water
qs Flavor
qs Color (if desired)
qs Active ingredient(s)

Put the acacia in a mortar and add sufficient Purified Water with trituration to form a mucilage. Using geometric dilution, combine the active ingredient(s) and the powdered sugar and mix thoroughly by spatulation. Put this powder into a sifter and sift together onto an ointment slab. Add the powders to the acacia mucilage in portions to make a mass of a proper consistency for hand rolling. Add the flavor and color (if desired). On the ointment slab, roll the mass into a cylindric pipe. Using a ruler as a gauge, cut the pipe into equal portions. Check the weight of individual pieces; this should be the final weight of the ingredients divided by the number of doses of active ingredient added.

GLYCERINATED GUMMY GEL BASE

This base is similar to a glycerinated gelatin suppository base. Here it is used as a base for oral chewable gummy gels. An easier alternative to making the base is to purchase gummy candy and melt it on a warm-water bath.
18 g Gelatin
70 mL Glycerin
12 mL Purified Water
qs Flavor
qs Color (if desired)
qs Active ingredient(s)

Either weigh 87.5 g or measure 70 mL of glycerin and pour into a 150-mL beaker. Add the Purified Water and stir to mix. Prepare a boiling-water bath using a 600-mL beaker and a stirring hotplate. Heat the glycerin-water together for 4–5 minutes and then slowly and carefully sprinkle the gelatin onto the liquid. Continue stirring until it is a uniform mixture and is free of all lumps. Continue heating for about 40–45 minutes. Remove it from the heat and allow it to cool. Portions of this gel can be weighed and used as a base for preparing gummy gel dosage forms.

(2) These lozenges are among the simplest to make. A sample formula and a procedure are given in Table 26.3 and are illustrated in Sample Prescription 26.7. The general compounding procedure is given later in this section (see III.C.2).

3. Chewable gummy gel lozenges

    a. This lozenge base is similar to the old-fashioned glycerinated gelatin that was used for many years as a base for vaginal suppositories. It made its appearance as a base for chewable oral drug preparations after a candy for children, so-called *gummy worms* or *gummy bears*, was introduced and became popular.

    b. A gummy gel base, such as that shown in Table 26.3, can be made from scratch in the pharmacy. This requires time and patience, because first the material must be heated carefully with stirring for 40 to 45 minutes, and this is only the beginning! To make a palatable product, appropriate flavoring and sweetening must then be added; citric acid is sometimes added to improve the taste—the tartness it provides takes away from the acrid taste of the glycerin. In addition, acacia may be added to provide smoothness. If the active ingredient or ingredients are insoluble in the base, a small amount of a suspending agent, such as bentonite, may also be added (13). In short, making this base is a time-consuming process.

   c. An alternative to making the gummy gel base is to purchase gummy candy. It can be heated in a beaker on a warm-water bath until a fluid is obtained. This gives a flavorful base of a desirable consistency.

C. General compounding methods for lozenges
   1. Lozenges are similar to suppositories in that they can be made either by hand rolling or by fusion. Depending on the compounding method selected, special calculations, compounding techniques, and equipment may be required to give accurate doses of lozenges.
   2. Hand-rolled lozenges
      a. Advantages
         (1) Hand-rolled lozenges do not require special calculations.
         (2) Special equipment is not required for this method. A pill roller is useful, but a broad-bladed spatula or any stiff, flat piece of nonreactive material can be used for this purpose.
      b. Disadvantages
         (1) Preparing and forming hand-rolled lozenges requires experience and good technique.
         (2) Even when well made, hand-rolled lozenges do not have an elegant appearance.
      c. General compounding method (used in Sample Prescription 26.7)
         (1) Check the doses of the active ingredients.
         (2) Using general principles, create a base formula or, if the lozenge base formula is taken from a journal article or book, adapt that formula for your specific use. The desired finished weight per lozenge is usually 1 to 2 g.
         (3) Calculate the quantity of each ingredient needed for compounding the preparation. Make enough material for two extra lozenges.
            (a) Multiply the dose per unit times the number of units to determine the quantity of each active ingredient.
            (b) Multiply the finished weight per unit times the desired number of units.
            (c) Subtract the weight of the active ingredients from the total weight of the lozenges to determine the amount of base material.
         (4) Weigh and prepare the active ingredients and base materials.
         (5) Combine the ingredients to form a cohesive mass.
         (6) Place the mass on an ointment slab and roll into a cylindric pipe of an appropriate length.
         (7) Using a clean razor blade and a ruler for a gauge, cut the pipe into equal pieces of the desired number of dosage units.
         (8) Weigh each piece and shave off extra material if needed to achieve lozenges of the correct weight.
   3. Molded lozenges, fusion method (using heat)
      a. Advantages
         (1) Some of the better-tasting lozenges, such as hard-candy, chocolate, and gummy gel chewable lozenges, can be made only by using heat and molding.
         (2) When well made, the preparations have a finished, professional appearance. Special molds, including those to make lollipops, are available from some vendors of compounding supplies and from confectionaries.
      b. Disadvantages
         (1) Special molds are usually required to make lozenges by molding. It is possible to improvise by using the caps of such items as vials or plastic medication cups for mold forms.
         (2) Handling some types of base materials requires special skill, experience, and care to obtain satisfactory preparations.
         (3) Caution must be used when incorporating drugs sensitive to heat.
         (4) Although the dosage units of molded lozenges may be determined either by weight or by volume, both methods require special equipment, calculations, or procedures.
      c. General compounding methods
         (1) By weight (illustrated with Sample Prescription 26.5)
            (a) When lozenges are compounded to a final weight, an electronic digital balance is nearly a necessity.
            (b) Follow steps (1) through (4) as given previously for hand-rolled lozenges.
            (c) Using heat, prepare the lozenge base material.

(d) Add the active ingredient(s) to the molten base.

(e) Place the lozenge mold(s) on an electronic balance and tare out the weight of the mold(s).

(f) Pour melted lozenge material into each mold cavity to the calculated desired weight per lozenge using the balance digital readout as the gauge. In some cases, it is easier to first draw the lozenge material into a syringe and use this to add the molten material to the mold cavities.

(2) By volume

(a) If volume is used, density calculations, mold calibrations, double-casting, or other procedures are required to give accurate doses.

(b) Because lozenges are solid at room temperature, most of the base components and active ingredients are solids and are measured by weight. The components are then combined, melted, and poured into mold cavities. This means the quantity of the dosage unit is determined by volume—the volume of the mold cavity.

(c) The quantity of active ingredient in each dosage unit therefore depends on two factors: the w/w concentration of active ingredient in the base material and the weight of the mixture contained in each mold cavity. The weight of mixture in the mold cavity depends on the volume of the cavity and the density of the molten mixture.

(d) To determine the quantity of base and active ingredients(s) to weigh when using this method, it is necessary to either calibrate the mold cavities for the desired material or use a double-casting procedure. Descriptions of these procedures are given in examples 31.1 through 31.3 in Chapter 31, Suppositories.

IV. MOLDED TABLETS

A. Molded tablets, sometimes called *tablet triturates* (TTs), are small tablets containing a medicament incorporated in lactose powder that has been formed into a soft mass by addition of a small quantity of a hydroalcoholic solution. A triturate mold is used to produce the tablets from the pliable, soft mass.

B. Molded tablets are small, usually weighing approximately 65 mg (1 grain in the apothecaries' system), and are very soluble in water, so they dissolve quickly and release drug rapidly when used sublingually or buccally. The most common use for molded tablets is as nitroglycerin sublingual tablets, but any potent drug is a candidate for this dosage form. Because the base material is primarily lactose, the resulting tablets are quite fragile, and this somewhat limits their use.

C. In addition to use as a therapeutic dosage form, molded tablets are also useful as dispensing tablets for potent drugs. At one time, potent alkaloids such as atropine sulfate and narcotics such as morphine sulfate were available commercially as molded tablets to use as compounding and dispensing aids. Custom-molded tablets of potent drugs can be compounded to provide a convenient source of small measured quantities of the drug and thereby eliminate the necessity for making serial dilutions. For example, in Sample Prescription 26.3, tablet triturates of atropine sulfate, 0.12 mg each, could be made, and one tablet could be added for each capsule made; this would eliminate the serial dilution required for this formulation.

D. The base material for molded tablets is lactose, but combinations with sucrose, dextrose, and/or mannitol are commonly used. Lactose by itself gives tablets that are too friable, and sucrose produces tablets that are too hard. When mannitol is added, it imparts a smooth, cooling feeling. A recommended mixture uses lactose with 5% to 25% finely powdered sucrose (14). The liquid used for dampening the powder and producing the soft, moldable mass is usually 50% alcohol. The amount of liquid added must be enough to provide adequate cohesion of the mass, but it should be kept as low as possible because excess liquid will require extended drying times and can result in hard, discolored tablets with possible migration of the active ingredient to the surface of the tablets, a condition known as *creep* (15). A typical formula for a triturate mass would be:

Lactose	8 g
Powdered sucrose	2 g
Alcohol 50%	2 mL

E. A triturate mold is used to produce the tablets. Molds are made of hard rubber or metal and consist of two rectangular plates. The upper plate has rows of holes that act as the dies for the tablets, and the lower plate has rows of matching pegs that fit into the holes and punch out the formed tablets when the upper plate is placed on the lower one.

F. To mold the tablets, the upper plate is placed on a smooth surface such as an ointment slab, and the prepared mass is pressed into the holes with a spatula. The upper plate is then centered over the lower plate so the pegs line up with the holes, and the upper plate is carefully pressed down so the formed tablets are pushed out of the holes and rest on top of the pegs of the lower plate. The tablets are allowed to dry and are then gently removed from the tops of the pegs. This procedure is illustrated on Color Plate 4.

G. As with lozenge and suppository molds, triturate molds must be calibrated for the specific triturate base formulation. In this case, the base mass is prepared using a formula such as the one given previously. This material is made into TTs using the method just described. The dried tablets are weighed to determine the weight of base material per tablet, and this information is used in creating individual formulations with active ingredients. In most cases, you subtract an amount of base material equivalent to the amount of active ingredient added; however, it is always best to do a trial batch in case there is a significant unequal displacement of active ingredient for base material.

V. COMPATIBILITY, STABILITY, AND BEYOND-USE DATING

A. **Physical stability:** As was discussed in Chapter 25, most solid dosage forms are quite stable physically.

1. For powders in capsules, the potential physical problems are liquefaction of eutectic mixtures and deliquescent powders, loss of water of hydration for efflorescent powders, and absorption of water by hygroscopic and deliquescent powders. These are discussed in Chapter 25, Powders, and in section III. B of Chapter 37, Compatibility and Stability of Drug Products and Preparations.

2. For lozenges that use melted bases (such as chocolate, cocoa butter, or synthetic fatty acid bases), a potential physical problem is melting during storage. Proper labeling and patient instructions for storage conditions can address this problem.

B. **Chemical stability:** Even though most solids are quite stable, it is important to check out ingredients before formulating a preparation.

1. When water is added during formulation of some lozenges, molded tablets, and popsicles, the potential for hydrolysis of ingredients must be considered.

2. For lozenges made by fusion, degradation of active ingredients can occur during the heating process; ingredients that are labile to this type of instability may not be good candidates for this type of dosage form unless you have definitive stability information for the formulation or a similar preparation.

3. There are a few solids that are very reactive even in solid state. Most are strong oxidizing (e.g., potassium permanganate, potassium and silver nitrate) or reducing agents that, when mixed together, react; some mixtures are potentially either flammable or explosive.

4. Capsules provide a unique method of handling incompatibilities between ingredients. Two mutually incompatible ingredients can be contained in the same capsule shell by first punching one of the ingredients in a smaller shell. The other powder is punched into a larger capsule, and the smaller capsule is then embedded in this powder.

5. Each sample prescription at the end of this chapter considers the chemical stability of each ingredient in the given formulation and dosage form and uses this information in assigning a beyond-use date to the preparation. Examples are given that illustrate the use of various reference resources to determine stability and assign beyond-use dates. The topic of chemical stability of drugs and chemicals is addressed in Chapter 37.

C. **Beyond-use dating:** A general discussion on assigning beyond-use dates for solid dosage forms can be found in Chapter 4. For *USP* compounded formulations, a beyond-use date is given in the monograph (16). As stated in Chapter 25, *USP* Chapter ⟨795⟩ has the following general guidelines for compounded solid dosage forms.

> In the absence of stability information that is applicable to a specific drug and preparation, the following maximum beyond-use dates are recommended for nonsterile compounded drug preparations that are packaged in tight, light-resistant containers and stored at controlled room temperature unless otherwise indicated.
>
> **For Nonaqueous Liquids and Solid Formulations—**
> *Where the Manufactured Drug Product is the Source of Active Ingredient*—The beyond-use date is not later than 25% of the time remaining until the product's expiration date or 6 months, whichever is earlier.
>
> *Where a USP or NF Substance is the Source of Active Ingredient*—The beyond-use date is not later than 6 months (17).

Sample Prescriptions

SAMPLE PRESCRIPTION 26.1

CASE: Jack Heller is a 190-lb, 6'2"-tall, 80-year-old male patient with a long history of asthma. He has had excellent control of his symptoms for more than 40 years by using a commercial combination product containing theophylline, ephedrine sulfate, and phenobarbital. This was a very popular combination product when Mr. Heller was first diagnosed with asthma and, as he has used it successfully all these years, he wants to continue with this combination. Unfortunately, the current manufacturer is not supplying the product, so Dr. Clyde has asked Pharmacist Julia Jacobson to compound an equivalent preparation. Mr. Heller has no known cardiac problems, but he does have mild hypertension that is controlled with hydrochlorothiazide, 25 mg daily, and he has hypercholesterolemia, for which he uses pravastatin, 10 mg at bedtime. He has an albuterol inhaler, but he reports that he rarely uses it. Dr. Jacobson notes that the dose of theophylline on the prescription appears to be high if Mr. Heller were to take the maximum number of daily doses. She has performed the dose calculations shown on the Master Compounding Formulation Record and has called Dr. Clyde to consult with him on this. Dr. Clyde replied that he wrote this prescription in this way to give Mr. Heller some flexibility with timing his doses but has asked Dr. Jacobson to remind Mr. Heller to take no more than 7 capsules in 24 hours and to include this information on the label. This is especially important for this geriatric patient.

CONTEMPORARY PHYSICIANS GROUP PRACTICE
20 S. PARK STREET, TRITURATE, WI 53706
TEL: (608) 555-1333 FAX: (608) 555-1335

R # *123834*

NAME *Jack Heller*   DATE *00/00/00*

ADDRESS *802 Arbor Street*

R

Theophylline	*118 mg*	
Ephedrine Sulfate	*24 mg*	
Phenobarbital	*8 mg*	
Dispense Capsules #6		

J. Jacobson 00/00/00

Sig: 1 – 2 caps q 4 hr prn breathing **Add: Do not take more than**
7 capsules in 24 hours – per Dr. Clyde

1" Red C*

REFILLS *4*   *E. S. Clyde*   **M.D.**

DEA NO. *AC4437922*

---

*Manufacturers of products containing this combination of ingredients usually apply for and are granted exemption as controlled substances but, because this is a compounded preparation, the pharmacy should maintain records of the use of the C-IV phenobarbital.

MASTER COMPOUNDING FORMULATION RECORD

NAME, STRENGTH, AND DOSAGE FORM OF PREPARATION: Theophylline 118 mg, Ephedrine 24 mg, and Phenobarbital 8 mg Oral Capsules

QUANTITY: 6 (plus 1 extra for loss on compounding)

THERAPEUTIC USE/CATEGORY: Asthma

FORMULATION RECORD ID: CP001

ROUTE OF ADMINISTRATION: Oral

INGREDIENTS USED:

Ingredient	Quantity Used	Physical Description	Solubility	Dose Comparison		Use in the Prescription
				Given	Usual	
Theophylline	826 mg	white powder	sl sol water; sp sol in alcohol	118–236 mg q4h prn	max. 900 mg/day	bronchodilator
Ephedrine Sulfate	168 mg	white powder	v sol water; sp sol in alcohol	24–48 mg q4h prn	25–50 mg q3–4h prn	bronchodilator, decongestant
Phenobarbital	120 mg weighed 56 mg used	white powder	v sl sol in water; fr sol in alcohol	8–16 mg q4h prn	10–50 mg 2–3 × daily	sedative
Lactose	240 mg weighed 112 mg used	white powder	fr sl water; v sl sol in alcohol	—	—	diluent

COMPATIBILITY–STABILITY: All ingredients in this preparation are compatible and quite stable when in a solid dosage form. There have been many similar commercial capsules with these components, and expiration dates for these products are a minimum of 2 years.

PACKAGING AND STORAGE: The *USP* monographs for Phenobarbital Tablets and Theophylline Tablets recommend storage in well-closed containers, but the monograph for Ephedrine Sulfate Capsules recommends a tight, light-resistant container (16), so use a tight, amber prescription vial and store at controlled room temperature.

BEYOND-USE DATE: Use the maximum 6-month beyond-use date as specified in *USP* Chapter ⟨795⟩ for solid formulations made with USP ingredients (17).

CALCULATIONS

Dose/Concentration

Ephedrine sulfate: The usual adult dose is 25 to 50 mg every 3 to 4 hours: okay.

Phenobarbital: The sedative dose is 30 to 100 mg daily in two to three divided doses: okay.

Theophylline: The dose of theophylline is 13 mg per kilogram of ideal body weight (IBW) per day or 900 mg/day, whichever is less. The dose is based on IBW because this drug does not distribute into fat tissue.

Mr. Heller, who is 6′2″ tall, has an IBW calculated here:

$$IBW_{kg} = 50 + (2.3 \times 14) = 50 + 32.2 = 82.2 \text{ kg}$$

Daily theophylline dose based on Mr. Heller's IBW: 13 mg/kg × 82.2 kg = 1,068 mg

Therefore, the maximum daily dose for Mr. Heller would be 900 mg; with 118 mg per capsule, the maximum number of capsules per day is 7 capsules (118 × 7 = 826 mg). Since the directions for use in the prescription order would allow for a maximum of 12 capsules per day, the patient should be warned not to exceed 7 capsules per day.

Ingredient Amounts

Calculations are for 7 doses, 1 extra

Theophylline: 118 mg/dose $\times$ 7 doses = 826 mg

Ephedrine Sulfate: 24 mg/dose $\times$ 7 doses = 168 mg

Phenobarbital: 8 mg/dose $\times$ 7 doses = 56 mg

The quantity of phenobarbital is below the MWQ for the class III torsion balance being used to compound this formulation; therefore, an aliquot is needed. If the MWQ of 120 mg of phenobarbital is weighed and mixed with 240 mg of lactose to give 360 mg of dilution, the amount of this dilution that will contain the needed 56 mg of phenobarbital can be calculated as shown here.

$$\frac{120 \text{ mg Pb}}{360 \text{ mg dilution}} = \frac{56 \text{ mg Pb}}{x \text{ mg dilution}}; x = 168 \text{ mg dilution}$$

Because phenobarbital powder is a C-IV substance, we must account for the amount weighed, dispensed, and discarded in making the aliquot and the extra dose to allow for the loss in compounding.

Amount weighed: 120 mg

Amount dispensed: 8 mg/capsule $\times$ 6 capsules dispensed = 48 mg

Amount discarded: 120 mg − 48 mg = 72 mg

Capsule Content Weight

$$\frac{826 \text{ mg Theo.} + 168 \text{ mg Eph.} + 168 \text{ mg Pb aliquot}}{7 \text{ capsules}} = \frac{1{,}162 \text{ mg powder}}{7 \text{ capsules}} = 166 \text{ mg/capsule}$$

With 166 mg of mixed powder per capsule, use a size 4 capsule shell. (See Table 26.1 for approximate capsule shell capacities in grams of various powders.)

An alternative procedure for this prescription is demonstrated on the CD that accompanies this book. With this method, Pharmacist Jacobson wants to use a slightly larger capsule shell (for some people the very small capsules, such as sizes 4 and 5, are difficult to handle), so she adds additional lactose to give a powder weight per unit that will fit in a preferred shell size. View the procedure on the CD for details and calculations for this method.

MSDS AND SAFETY AND PERSONAL PROTECTIVE EQUIPMENT: Review MSDS for all components. Don a clean lab coat and disposable gloves. Avoid inhaling powders.

SPECIALIZED EQUIPMENT: Glass mortar for aliquot; all weighing is done on a class III torsion balance.

COMPOUNDING PROCEDURE: Weigh 120 mg of phenobarbital and 240 mg of lactose; transfer these powders to a glass mortar and triturate well together. Weigh 168 mg of this mixture and place in a mortar. Weigh 168 mg ephedrine SO_4 and add to the Pb aliquot in the mortar with trituration. Weigh 826 mg of theophylline and add to the powder mixture in the mortar with trituration using geometric dilution. For quality control purposes, weigh five no. 4 empty capsule shells, record this weight, and calculate the average weight per capsule shell (should be approximately 38 mg). Punch powder in size 4 clear, colorless capsules so that the powder contents of each capsule weighs 166 mg; balance finished capsules against dial-in weight of 166 mg plus an empty capsule shell on the right balance pan. Place finished capsules in an amber capsule vial with a child-resistant closure and label the vial appropriately.

DESCRIPTION OF FINISHED PREPARATION: The preparation is fine, white powder encapsulated in no. 4 clear, colorless capsule shells.

QUALITY CONTROL: Each capsule is weighed to contain 166 mg of powder. A verification check is done as follows: (1) Weigh five no. 4 empty gelatin capsules and calculate the average weight per capsule shell; (2) weigh each finished capsule; and (3) subtract the average weight per empty capsule shell from the weight of each finished capsule to determine the weight of powder per capsule. The powder in each capsule should weigh 166 mg ±10%. Adjust the content of any capsule that is outside this tolerance.

MASTER FORMULA PREPARED BY: Julia Jacobson, PharmD   **CHECKED BY:** Ted Fifrick, RPh

COMPOUNDING RECORD

NAME, STRENGTH, AND DOSAGE FORM OF PREPARATION: Theophylline 118 mg, Ephedrine 24 mg, and Phenobarbital 8 mg Oral Capsules

QUANTITY: 6 (plus 1 extra)

DATE PREPARED: mm/dd/yy

BEYOND-USE DATE: mm/dd/yy

FORMULATION RECORD ID: CP001

CONTROL/RX NUMBER: 123834

INGREDIENTS USED:

Ingredient	Quantity Used	Manufacturer Lot Number	Expiration Date	Weighed/ Measured by	Checked by
Theophylline	826 mg	JET Labs XY1162	mm/yy	bjf	jj
Ephedrine Sulfate	168 mg	JET Labs XY1163	mm/yy	bjf	jj
Phenobarbital	120 mg weighed/ 56 mg used	JET Labs XY1165	mm/yy	bjf	jj
Lactose	240 mg weighed/ 112 mg used	JET Labs XY1159	mm/yy	bjf	jj

QUALITY CONTROL DATA: The powder in the capsules appears as fine, white powder. The size no. 4 clear, colorless gelatin capsules are full with no dead space. Each capsule has been individually weighed and checked to contain 166 mg $\pm$10% of powder.

Capsule Number	Weight of Capsule (mg)	Capsule Shell Weight (mg)	Weight of Powder (mg)
1	205	38	167
2	204	38	166
3	206	38	168
4	203	38	165
5	204	38	166
6	205	38	167

LABELING

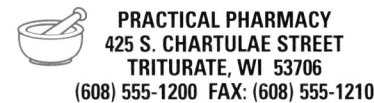

PRACTICAL PHARMACY
425 S. CHARTULAE STREET
TRITURATE, WI 53706
(608) 555-1200 FAX: (608) 555-1210

℞ 123834	Pharmacist: JJ	Date: 00/00/00
Jack Heller		Dr. E. S. Clyde

Take one or two capsules every four hours as needed for breathing.
Do not take more than 7 capsules in 24 hours.

Theophylline 118 mg, Ephedrine Sulfate 24 mg, Phenobarbital 8-mg
Oral Capsules

Mfg: Compounded	Quantity: 6 capsules
Refills: 4	Discard after: Give date

Auxiliary Labels: Drowsiness-alcohol-driving warning. This medicine was
compounded in our pharmacy for you at the direction of your prescriber.
Federal do not transfer label.

PATIENT CONSULTATION: Hello, Mr. Heller. I'm your pharmacist, Julia Jacobson. Do you have any drug allergies? My records show that you are taking hydrochlorothiazide and pravastatin and that you occasionally use an albuterol inhaler for breathing problems associated with your asthma. Are you taking any other prescription or nonprescription medication? I know that you have been taking the commercial equivalent of these capsules for many years. They contain theophylline, ephedrine, and phenobarbital. You are to take 1 or 2 capsules every 4 hours when needed for breathing. Dr. Clyde asked me to remind you that even though this prescription is labeled so that you can take doses every 4 hours, you should not take any more than 7 capsules in a 24-hour period. Do you know the maximum number that you take in a day? Does Dr. Clyde monitor your theophylline levels? As I am sure you know, this medication can cause some excitement, difficulty sleeping, headaches, or a jittery feeling, but it also contains some phenobarbital to help offset these side effects, and phenobarbital can cause drowsiness. Therefore, be sure to monitor how you are feeling before operating a motor vehicle, machinery, and so on. Have you ever had problems with this medication causing you to have an upset stomach? This is usually caused by the theophylline and, if this occurs, it might be helpful to take these with food or milk. If you experience diarrhea or pounding heart, be sure to call Dr. Clyde immediately. Store this bottle in a cool, dry place and discard any unused contents after 6 months (give beyond-use date). I just made a small number of capsules until we see how they work for you; you may refill this four times. Let Dr. Clyde or me know if you want a larger quantity. Do you have any questions?

SAMPLE PRESCRIPTION 26.2

CASE: Shanna Woodruff is a 52-lb, 4′-tall, 7-year-old second grader who has recently undergone a complete neurologic exam and an evaluation by a school psychologist because of problems with poor concentration at school and general impulsivity. The problem with concentration is negatively impacting her ability to learn at school. The psych tests showed that she has an above-average IQ, and the neurologic and electroencephalographic tests ruled out a seizure disorder and other neurologic disorders. She has been tentatively diagnosed with attention deficit disorder (ADD), and her pediatrician, Dr. Runnel, wants to do a blind study with methylphenidate to see if this drug will help her school performance. Shanna has no major health issues, but she is allergic to cats and has seasonal allergies to pollen for which she takes Claritin Reditabs (loratadine), 10 mg daily, when needed.

CONTEMPORARY PHYSICIANS GROUP PRACTICE
20 S. PARK STREET, TRITURATE, WI 53706
TEL: (608) 555-1333 FAX: (608) 555-1335

℞ #   *123822*

NAME *Shanna Woodruff*   DATE *00/00/00*

ADDRESS *863 Wildwood Circle*

℞

For Blind Study:
1) Methylphenidate   5 mg
*   Lactose   qs*
*   Dispense #14 Caps*
Sig: i po at 7 am and 11 am during weeks 1 & 2
Label: Methylphenidate A 5 mg

2) Lactose   qs
*   Dispense #14 Caps*
Sig: i po at 7 am and 11 am during weeks 3 & 4
Label: Methylphenidate B 5 mg

B. Badger 00/00/00

REFILLS *0*   *Adolph Runnel*   M.D.

DEA NO. *AR 3938745*

MASTER COMPOUNDING FORMULATION RECORD

NAME, STRENGTH, AND DOSAGE FORM OF PREPARATION: Methylphenidate 5 mg/Placebo Oral Capsules

QUANTITY: 14 of each   **FORMULATION RECORD ID:** CP002

THERAPEUTIC USE/CATEGORY: ADD blind study   **ROUTE OF ADMINISTRATION:** Oral

INGREDIENTS USED:

Ingredient	Quantity Used	Physical Description	Solubility	Dose Comparison		Use in the Prescription
				Given	Usual	
Methylphenidate 5 mg tabs	14 × 5 mg	light yellow tablets	freely sol in water; sol inalcohol	5 mg bid	5–20 mg 2–3 × daily	hyperactivity, ADD
Lactose	qs	white powder	1 g/5 mL water; v sl sol in alcohol	—	—	diluent/placebo

COMPATIBILITY–STABILITY: In a solid dosage form, methylphenidate is quite stable. In this case, we are merely embedding manufactured tablets in lactose.

PACKAGING AND STORAGE: The *USP* monograph for Methylphenidate Tablets recommends storage in tight containers (16). Use tight, amber prescription vials and store at controlled room temperature.

BEYOND-USE DATE: Use the recommended beyond-use date as specified in *USP* Chapter ⟨795⟩ for solid formulations made with active ingredients from manufactured drug products: no later than 25% of the time remaining until the product's expiration date or 6 months, whichever is earlier (17).

CALCULATIONS

Dose/Concentration: Okay

Ingredient Amounts: No calculations are needed. One 5-mg tablet is put in each capsule for methylphenidate A.

MSDS AND SAFETY AND PERSONAL PROTECTIVE EQUIPMENT: Don a clean lab coat and disposable gloves.

SPECIALIZED EQUIPMENT: Use no. 3 snap-closure, red-cap/red-body gelatin capsules.

COMPOUNDING PROCEDURE: To avoid mixing up the active and placebo capsules, make the vial labels and label the vials first. Punch a small quantity of lactose into the body of a size 3 red capsule. Break a methylphenidate 5-mg tablet in half and embed the two halves into the lactose in the capsule, and then punch more lactose into the capsule, concealing the broken tablet halves. Replace the capsule cap and place this capsule in the capsule vial labeled methylphenidate A 5 mg. Repeat this procedure for 13 more capsules. Then punch 14 no. 3 red capsules with lactose only and be sure that these approximate the size and appearance of "A" capsules. Place these capsules in the capsule vial labeled methylphenidate B 5 mg. Dispense the vials with child-resistant closures.

DESCRIPTION OF FINISHED PREPARATION: The capsules contain a fine, white powder (lactose) encapsulated in no. 3 red capsules. Each of the capsules in the bottle labeled "A" contain two half-tablets embedded in the lactose. All capsules for both vials appear the same.

QUALITY CONTROL: No weighing needed

MASTER FORMULA PREPARED BY: Barry Badger, RPh   **CHECKED BY:** David Albers, RPh, PhD

COMPOUNDING RECORD

NAME, STRENGTH, AND DOSAGE FORM OF PREPARATION: Methylphenidate 5 mg/Placebo Oral Capsules

QUANTITY: 14 of each   **DATE PREPARED:** mm/dd/yy   **BEYOND-USE DATE:** mm/dd/yy

FORMULATION RECORD ID: CP002   **CONTROL/RX NUMBER:** 123822

INGREDIENTS USED:

Ingredient	Quantity Used	Manufacturer Lot Number	Expiration Date	Weighed/ Measured by	Checked by
Methylphenidate 5-mg tabs	14 × 5 mg tablets	BJF Generics XY1166	mm/yy	bjf	bb
Lactose	qs	JET Labs XY1159	mm/yy	bjf	bb

QUALITY CONTROL DATA: The capsules contain a fine, white powder (lactose) encapsulated in no. 3 red capsules. Each of the capsules in the bottle labeled "A" contain two half-tablets embedded in the lactose. Fourteen 5-mg tablets were counted and all were used. Each capsule has been inspected so be sure that in no instance is an edge of a hidden methylphenidate tablet visible. All capsules for both vials appear the same.

LABELING

Vial A

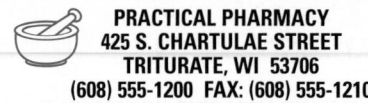

PRACTICAL PHARMACY
425 S. CHARTULAE STREET
TRITURATE, WI 53706
(608) 555-1200 FAX: (608) 555-1210

℞ 123822   Pharmacist: BB   Date: 00/00/00
Shanna Woodruff   Dr. Adolph Runnel

Take one capsule orally twice daily at 7 AM and 11 AM during weeks 1 and 2.

Methylphenidate A 5-mg Oral Capsules

Mfg: Compounded   Quantity: 14 capsules

Refills: 0   Discard after: Give date

Auxiliary Label: Federal do not transfer label. This medicine was compounded in our pharmacy for you at the direction of your prescriber.

Vial B

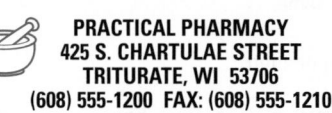

PRACTICAL PHARMACY
425 S. CHARTULAE STREET
TRITURATE, WI 53706
(608) 555-1200 FAX: (608) 555-1210

℞ 123822   Pharmacist: BB   Date: 00/00/00
Shanna Woodruff   Dr. Adolph Runnel

Take one capsule orally twice daily at 7 AM and 11 AM during weeks 3 and 4.

Methylphenidate B 5-mg Oral Capsules

Mfg: Compounded   Quantity: 14 capsules

Refills: 0   Discard after: Give date

Auxiliary Label: Federal do not transfer label. This medicine was compounded in our pharmacy for you at the direction of your prescriber.

PATIENT CONSULTATION: Hello, Mrs. Woodruff. I'm your pharmacist, Barry Badger, and I have Shanna's prescription ready. Does she have any drug allergies? Are you giving her any other medicine, either nonprescription or prescription? I'm sure your doctor has discussed that this is a double-blind study to determine whether Shanna will benefit from this drug, called *methylphenidate*. Neither Shanna, her teacher, Dr. Runnel, nor you should know which of these vials contains capsules with the drug and which has capsules with no drug. I assume that Shanna's teacher will be sending a daily report to you and the school psychologist. If Shanna exhibits any unusual behavior while taking this medication, contact your doctor immediately, because the study might have to be discontinued. Give her one capsule at 7 AM and one at 11 AM every morning for 4 weeks. Notice you give the capsules from vial A on weeks 1 and 2 and switch to giving the capsules from vial B on weeks 3 and 4. Note that the bottles tell you which weeks to give capsules from that bottle. DO NOT MIX UP THE BOTTLES. Store the bottles in a secure, dry place, at room temperature, and away from the reach of children. Discard any unused portion after 6 months (or 25% of expiration date of tablets). This prescription may not be refilled. After the 4-week study, Dr. Runnel will call me to find out the contents of the vials, and you will all be meeting with him to determine how to proceed. Do you have any questions?

SAMPLE PRESCRIPTION 26.3

CASE: Wayne John is a 164-lb, 5′11″-tall, 46-year-old patient with a diagnosis of a "common cold." He has a headache, rhinitis, cough, and mild sore throat but no fever or body aches. He asked Dr. Smitby for an antibiotic to cure his cold, but Dr. Smitby told him that his cold is viral and, in this case, an antibiotic will not help. Mr. John says that he is miserable with his symptoms, he can't get any rest, and he needs something "strong." Dr. Smitby says that he has a custom cold formula that really works well for the symptoms Mr. John describes. Mr. John should take these capsules every 8 hours as needed, and Dr. Smitby has prescribed a guaifenesin-with-codeine cough syrup for Mr. John to take at night so he can get a good night's rest. Mr. John has no chronic health conditions; he is taking no prescription medications but is taking a multivitamin with minerals, vitamin C 500 mg, and vitamin E 400 units. He had his flu shot 2 months ago.

CONTEMPORARY PHYSICIANS GROUP PRACTICE
20 S. PARK STREET, TRITURATE, WI 53706
TEL: (608) 555-1333 FAX: (608) 555-1335

℞ #   *123828*

NAME *Wayne John*   DATE *00/00/00*

ADDRESS *2530 Blackhawk Estates*

℞

Acetaminophen	*325 mg*
Diphenhydramine HCl	*25 mg*
Atropine sulfate	*0.12 mg*
Caffeine	*30 mg*

M et Ft Capsules #6

Sig: 1–2 caps po q 8 hr prn headache, cough, and cold symptoms

B. Boggs 00/00/00

REFILLS *3*   *Lance Smitby* _____ M.D.

DEA NO. _____

MASTER COMPOUNDING FORMULATION RECORD

NAME, STRENGTH, AND DOSAGE FORM OF PREPARATION: Acetaminophen 325 mg, Diphenhydramine 25 mg, Atropine Sulfate 0.12 mg, and Caffeine 30 mg Oral Capsules

QUANTITY: 6 (plus 1 extra for loss on compounding)

THERAPEUTIC USE/CATEGORY: Cold symptoms

FORMULATION RECORD ID: CP003

ROUTE OF ADMINISTRATION: Oral

INGREDIENTS USED:

Ingredient	Quantity Used	Physical Description	Solubility	Dose Comparison		Use in the Prescription
				Given	Usual	
Acetaminophen (APAP)	2,275 mg	white powder	1 g/70 mL water, 10 mL alcohol	325–650 mg q8h	0.3–1 g 3–4 × daily	antipyretic, analgesic
Diphenhydramine (DPH) 50-mg capsules	175 mg in 525 mg powder	white powder	1 g/1 mL water, 2 mL alcohol	25–50 mg q8h	25–50 mg 3–4 × daily	antihistamine
Atropine Sulfate	120 mg weighed/ 0.84 mg used	white powder	1 g/0.5 mL water, 5 mL alcohol	0.12–0.24 mg q8h	0.3–1.2 mg q4–6h	anticholinergic, antispasmodic
Lactose	5,040 mg weighed/ 133 used	white powder	fr sol in water; v sl sol in alcohol	—	—	diluent
Caffeine	210 mg	white powder	1 g/50 mL water, 70 mL alcohol	30–60 mg q8h	100–500 mg prn	counteracts drowsiness of CNS depressants; active for vascular headache

COMPATIBILITY–STABILITY: All ingredients in this preparation are compatible and quite stable when in a solid dosage form.

PACKAGING AND STORAGE: The *USP* monographs for Atropine Sulfate Tablets and Caffeine recommend storage in well-closed containers, but the monographs for Diphenhydramine HCl Capsules and Acetaminophen Tablets are more restrictive and recommend storage in tight containers (16). Package in a tight, amber prescription vial and store at controlled room temperature.

BEYOND-USE DATE: Because the source of one of the active ingredients, diphenhydramine HCl, is a manufactured capsule, use the recommended beyond-use date as specified in *USP* Chapter ⟨795⟩ for solid formulations made with active ingredients from manufactured drug products: no later than 25% of the time remaining until the product's expiration date or 6 months, whichever is earlier (17).

CALCULATIONS

Dose/Concentration: All doses okay

Ingredient Amounts: Calculations are for 7 doses, including 1 extra.

Acetaminophen (APAP): 325 mg/dose × 7 doses = 2,275 mg

Caffeine: 30 mg/dose × 7 doses = 210 mg

Diphenhydramine HCl (DPH): 25 mg/dose × 7 doses = 175 mg

DPH is available as 50-mg capsules with capsule content weight of 150 mg/capsule. For 175 mg of DPH, 4 capsules are needed, and the weight of capsule powder is calculated as:

$$\frac{50 \text{ mg DPH}}{150 \text{ mg capsule powder}} = \frac{175 \text{ mg DPH}}{x \text{ mg capsule powder}}; x = 525 \text{ mg capsule powder}$$

Atropine sulfate: 0.12 mg/dose $\times$ 7 doses = 0.84 mg

This amount is below the MWQ for the class III torsion balance and, because it is such a small amount, a serial dilution is required (see section III in Chapter 10, Aliquot Calculations).

Dilution A: Weigh the MWQ of 120 mg of atropine sulfate and mix with an intermediate amount of lactose, 4,680 mg, to give 4,800 mg of Dilution A. Weigh the MWQ of this dilution. The amount of atropine sulfate in Dilution A is calculated as:

$$\frac{120 \text{ mg Atropine}}{4,800 \text{ mg Dilution A}} = \frac{x \text{ mg Atropine}}{120 \text{ mg Dilution A}}; x = 3 \text{ mg Atropine}$$

To the 120 mg of Dilution A (which contains 3 mg of atropine sulfate), add 360 mg of lactose to give 480 mg of Dilution B. Calculate the amount of Dilution B that will contain 0.84 mg of atropine sulfate:

$$\frac{3 \text{ mg Atropine}}{480 \text{ mg Dilution B}} = \frac{0.84 \text{ mg Atropine}}{x \text{ mg Dilution B}}; x = 134 \text{ mg Dilution B}$$

Capsule Content Weight

$$\frac{2,275 \text{ mg APAP} + 210 \text{ mg Caf} + 134 \text{ mg Atr Alq} + 525 \text{ mg DPH}}{7 \text{ capsules}} = \frac{3,144 \text{ mg powder}}{7 \text{ capsules}} = 449 \text{ mg/capsule}$$

With 449 mg of powder per capsule, size no. 1 capsule shells work well (see Table 26.1).

MSDS AND SAFETY AND PERSONAL PROTECTIVE EQUIPMENT: Review MSDS for all components. Don a clean lab coat, disposable gloves, and safety glasses. Avoid inhaling powders.

SPECIALIZED EQUIPMENT: Glass mortar for aliquot; all weighing is done on a class III torsion balance.

COMPOUNDING PROCEDURE: Weigh 120 mg of atropine sulfate and place in a glass mortar. Weigh 4,680 mg of lactose and mix with the atropine by trituration using geometric dilution. Weigh 120 mg of this first dilution, transfer to a clean glass mortar, and add 360 mg of lactose by geometric dilution and triturate well. Weigh 134 mg of this second dilution and transfer it to a clean mortar. Weigh 210 mg of caffeine and add it to the 134 mg of the second atropine dilution and triturate the powders well. Weigh the contents of a diphenhydramine 50-mg capsule to determine the total powder weight per capsule (150 mg). Weigh 525 mg of powder from 4 capsules and add to the atropine aliquot–caffeine mixture with trituration. Weigh 2,275 mg of acetaminophen and add to above by geometric dilution with trituration. For quality control purposes, weigh five no. 1 empty, clear, colorless capsule shells, record this weight, and calculate the average weight per capsule shell (should be approximately 76 mg). Punch powder in size no. 1 clear, colorless capsules so that the powder contents of each capsule weighs 449 mg; balance finished capsules against dial-in weight of 449 mg plus an empty capsule shell on the right balance pan. Dispense in an amber capsule vial with a child-resistant closure.

DESCRIPTION OF FINISHED PREPARATION: The preparation is fine, white powder encapsulated in no. 1 clear, colorless capsules.

QUALITY CONTROL: Each capsule is weighed to contain 449 mg of powder. A verification check is done as follows: Weigh five no. 1 empty gelatin capsules and calculate the average weight per capsule; then each finished capsule is weighed and the average weight per empty capsule is subtracted. The powder in each capsule should weigh 449 mg $\pm$10%. Adjust the content of any capsule that is outside this tolerance.

MASTER FORMULA PREPARED BY: Brenda Boggs, PharmD   **CHECKED BY:** Ted Fifrick, RPh

COMPOUNDING RECORD

NAME, STRENGTH, AND DOSAGE FORM OF PREPARATION: Acetaminophen 325 mg, Diphenhydramine 25 mg, Atropine Sulfate 0.12 mg, and Caffeine 30 mg Oral Capsules

QUANTITY: 6 (plus 1 extra)   **DATE PREPARED:** mm/dd/yy   **BEYOND-USE DATE:** mm/dd/yy

FORMULATION RECORD ID: CP003   **CONTROL/RX NUMBER:** 123828

INGREDIENTS USED:

Ingredient	Quantity Used	Manufacturer Lot Number	Expiration Date	Weighed/ Measured by	Checked by
Acetaminophen (APAP)	2,275 mg	JET Labs XY1168	mm/yy	bjf	bb
Diphenhydramine (DPH) 50 mg capsules	175 mg in 525 mg powder	BJF Generics XY1168	mm/yy	bjf	bb
Atropine Sulfate	120 mg weighed/ 0.84 mg used	JET Labs XY1170	mm/yy	bjf	bb
Lactose	5,040 mg weighed/ 133 used	JET Labs XY1159	mm/yy	bjf	bb
Caffeine	210 mg	JET Labs XY1172	mm/yy	bjf	bb

QUALITY CONTROL DATA: The powder in the capsules appears as fine, white powder. The size no. 1 clear gelatin capsules are full with no dead space. Each capsule has been individually weighed and checked to contain 449 mg ±10% of powder.

Capsule Number	Weight of Capsule (mg)	Capsule Shell Weight (mg)	Weight of Powder (mg)
1	527	76	451
2	525	76	449
3	526	76	450
4	524	76	448
5	525	76	449
6	528	76	452

LABELING

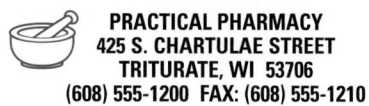

PRACTICAL PHARMACY
425 S. CHARTULAE STREET
TRITURATE, WI 53706
(608) 555-1200 FAX: (608) 555-1210

R 123828   Pharmacist: BB   Date: 00/00/00
Wayne John   Dr. Lance Smitby

Take one to two capsules by mouth every eight hours as needed for
headache, cough, and cold symptoms.

Acetaminophen 325 mg, Diphenhydramine HCL 25 mg, Atropine
Sulfate 0.12 mg, Caffeine 30 mg Oral Capsules

Mfg: Compounded   Quantity: 6 capsules

Refills: 3   Discard after: Give date

Auxiliary Labels: Drowsiness/alcohol-driving warning. This medicine was
compounded in our pharmacy for you at the direction of your prescriber.

PATIENT CONSULTATION: Hello, Mr. John. I'm your pharmacist. Brenda Boggs. Do you have any drug allergies? Are you taking any over-the-counter or prescription medications? What did Dr. Smitby tell you about this medication? He has prescribed this custom cold preparation; it contains acetaminophen for pain, combined with the antihistamine diphenhydramine and atropine sulfate to help dry nasal secretions. The diphenhydramine will also help with your cough. The capsules also contain caffeine to counteract the drowsiness caused by the other ingredients; caffeine also helps with some types of headaches. You may take one or two capsules every 8 hours as needed. Some side effects include drowsiness and dry mouth, but the caffeine may make you a bit jittery. See how you react to this combination therapy before operating a motor vehicle, machinery, and so on. Don't exceed the prescribed dose, and don't take any additional nonprescription medications unless you check with me about their content, because some products contain similar ingredients. This is especially important because large doses of acetaminophen can cause kidney and liver problems. Dr. Smitby has also prescribed a cough medicine for you to take at night. It is okay to take the cough medicine with these capsules. If you don't get relief, if your condition worsens, or if you develop a skin rash, contact Dr. Smitby. It is best not to consume alcoholic beverages or, at least, to be very moderate in their use while taking this medication. Keep this out of the reach of children. This may be refilled three times. Discard any unused portion after 6 months (or 25% of DPH expiration date, whichever is less; give date). Do you have any questions?

SAMPLE PRESCRIPTION 26.4

CASE: Florence Thompson is a 146-lb, 5'5"-tall, 64-year-old patient who has seen her physician for her yearly checkup. She has asked Dr. Shapiro to represcribe estrogen replacement therapy (ERT) for vasomotor symptoms of menopause. Ms. Thompson had a vaginal hysterectomy (ovaries left intact) at age 42, and she reports that she first experienced vasomotor symptoms of menopause at age 53. At that time, she was treated with conjugated equine estrogens, 0.625 mg daily. At various times over the next 9 years, she tried to taper off this product, but the "hot flashes" always returned and were problematic, especially because they disturbed her normal sleep. At age 62, she retired from her full-time job and decided to make a more concerted effort to withdraw from ERT, especially in light of clinical studies recommending only short-term ERT therapy. Shortly after discontinuing estrogen therapy, Ms. Thompson started experiencing significant "hot flashes" and sweating multiple times each day and during the night. She has tried some alternative therapies, such as clonidine, with no improvement. She says that she is miserable and wants to resume estrogen therapy. Dr. Shapiro agrees but says he now prefers to use a compounded bi-estrogen[1] combination. Ms. Thompson has no

---

[1]Although estriol is an official USP article and has been used extensively in compounding, in January 2008 the FDA issued an opinion that pharmacies may not compound drug preparations containing estriol unless they have an FDA-sanctioned investigational new drug application. The reason given is that estriol is not a component of any product approved by FDA for safety and effectiveness. This action has been contested by various compounding organizations, so check on the current legal status of this drug before compounding with this ingredient.

cardiac risk factors: blood pressure 117/75, ideal cholesterol/lipid profile, no history of smoking or diabetes, daily exercise, moderate weight. Dr. Shapiro has told her to take low-dose (80 mg) aspirin daily for blood clot prophylaxis and to be sure to continue her routine breast self-examination and yearly mammogram.

CONTEMPORARY PHYSICIANS GROUP PRACTICE
20 S. PARK STREET, TRITURATE, WI 53706
TEL: (608) 555-1333 FAX: (608) 555-1335

℞ #   *123881*

NAME *Florence Thompson*   DATE   *00/00/00*

ADDRESS *3075 Wausau Court*

℞   *For 50 capsules:*

Estradiol		*0.025 g*
Estriol		*0.1 g*
Peanut Oil	*qs to*	*10 mL*
M. et div.		*Dispense 30 Capsules*

J. Hutter 00/00/00

Sig: 1 cap po q day

REFILLS *2*   *K. W. Shapiro*   M.D.

DEA NO. _____

MASTER COMPOUNDING FORMULATION RECORD

NAME, STRENGTH, AND DOSAGE FORM OF PREPARATION: Estriol 2 mg and Estradiol 500 mcg Oral Capsules
QUANTITY: 30 (plus 20 extra for loss on compounding)   **FORMULATION RECORD ID:** CP004
THERAPEUTIC USE/CATEGORY: Estrogen replacement   **ROUTE OF ADMINISTRATION:** Oral

INGREDIENTS USED:

Ingredient	Quantity Used	Physical Description	Solubility	Dose Comparison		Use in the Prescription
				Given	Usual	
Estradiol	25 mg	white, crystalline powder	pr insol in water; sol in alcohol; sp sol in vegetable oil	500 mcg daily	500 mcg–2 mg daily	estrogen replacement therapy
Estriol	100 mg	white, crystalline powder	insol in water; sp sol in alcohol; sol in vegetable oil	2 mg qd	2 mg qd	estrogen replacement therapy
Peanut Oil	qs to 10 mL	pale yellow oily liquid	immis with water; v sl sol in alcohol	—	—	solvent, vehicle

COMPATIBILITY–STABILITY: All ingredients in this preparation are reported to be compatible and quite stable when in a non-aqueous, oil-based dosage form (19). Commercial products of estradiol are available in various dosage forms with expiration dates of at least 2 years.

PACKAGING AND STORAGE: The *USP* monograph for Estriol recommends storage in a tight container, and the monograph for Estradiol recommends storage in a tight, light-resistant container (16). Package in a tight, amber prescription vial. To minimize possible oil leakage from the capsules and to enhance stability, store in the refrigerator.

BEYOND-USE DATE: A beyond-use date of 6 months is recommended for two similar compounded preparations that are described in the *International Journal of Pharmaceutical Compounding* (18) and *Allen's Compounded Formulations* (19), but no stability data are given. Use a 6-month beyond-use date as specified in *USP* Chapter ⟨795⟩ for nonaqueous liquids made with USP ingredients (17).

CALCULATIONS

Dose/Concentration

Estriol: 100 mg/50 capsules = 2 mg/capsule: okay.

Estradiol: 25 mg/50 capsules = 0.5 mg/capsule = 500 mcg/capsule: okay.

Ingredient Amounts: This example assumes the use of an electronic balance with a MWQ of 20 mg. Because of the small quantities of active ingredients needed and the sensitivity limitations of the balance, the entire quantity for 50 capsules is made. Any excess remaining after the 30 capsules are filled is discarded.

Estradiol: 0.025 g = 25 mg   Estriol: 0.1 g = 100 mg

Peanut Oil:

Volume: Assume a volume of 10 mL with a zero powder volume for the estradiol and estriol because of the very small quantities of powder.

Weight: Peanut Oil has a density of 0.919 g/mL. The weight of Peanut Oil can be calculated:

$$\frac{1 \text{ mL Peanut Oil}}{0.919 \text{ g Peanut Oil}} = \frac{10 \text{ mL Peanut Oil}}{x \text{ g Peanut Oil}}; x = 9.19 \text{ g Peanut Oil}$$

Total weight of capsule contents:

>   9.19 g Peanut Oil
>   0.1 g Estriol
>   <u>0.025 g</u> Estradiol
>   9.315 g

Weight per capsule: 9.315 g/50 capsules = 0.186 g/capsule

MSDS AND SAFETY AND PERSONAL PROTECTIVE EQUIPMENT: Review MSDS for all components. Don a clean lab coat, disposable gloves, and a mask approved by the National Institute for Occupational Safety and Health (NIOSH). Avoid inhaling powders.

SPECIALIZED EQUIPMENT: All weighing is done on an electronic balance.

COMPOUNDING PROCEDURE: Weigh 100 mg of estriol and 25 mg of estradiol. Place the powders in a glass mortar and add approximately 6 mL peanut oil slowly with trituration to form a smooth slurry. Transfer the mixture to a graduated cylinder and add sufficient peanut oil to make 10 mL. Use some of the oil to rinse out the mortar to ensure complete transfer of the estrogen mixture. Stir mixture thoroughly using a glass stirring rod. Place the graduated cylinder containing the compounded mixture in a refrigerator for approximately 1 hour to increase the viscosity of the oil; this will retard settling of the drug particles and ensure a more uniform suspension. Using either an improvised or manufactured capsule holder, place the bodies of size no. 1 green snap-closure capsules on the electronic balance and tare out the weight (see the picture, Filling capsules with liquid ingredients, in this chapter). Remove the compounded suspension from the refrigerator and stir thoroughly using a glass stirring rod. Draw into a 1-mL syringe an amount of the estrogen mixture. Squirt 186 mg of suspension into each capsule body, using the digital readout on the balance to determine the desired weight. Replace the capsule caps and snap in place. Place capsules in an amber prescription vial with a child-resistant closure; label and dispense.

DESCRIPTION OF FINISHED PREPARATION: The oil in the capsules appears as straw-colored liquid with minimal finely divided suspension particles. The size no. 1 green gelatin capsules are approximately one-half full.

QUALITY CONTROL: Weigh each capsule individually to contain 186 mg of oil solution. Each capsule should be inspected to ensure that the cap is snapped securely in place.

MASTER FORMULA PREPARED BY: Julie Hutter, PharmD   **CHECKED BY:** Ted Fifrick, RPh

COMPOUNDING RECORD

NAME, STRENGTH, AND DOSAGE FORM OF PREPARATION: Estriol 2 mg and Estradiol 500 mcg Oral Capsules
QUANTITY: 30 (plus 20 extra)   **DATE PREPARED:** mm/dd/yy   **BEYOND-USE DATE:** mm/dd/yy
FORMULATION RECORD ID: CP004   **CONTROL/RX NUMBER:** 123881

INGREDIENTS USED:

Ingredient	Quantity Used	Manufacturer Lot Number	Expiration Date	Weighed/ Measured by	Checked by
Estradiol	25 mg	JET Labs XY1133	mm/yy	bjf	jh
Estriol	100 mg	JET Labs XY1134	mm/yy	bjf	jh
Peanut Oil	qs to 10 mL	JET Labs XY1135	mm/yy	bjf	jh

QUALITY CONTROL DATA: The oil in the capsules appears as straw-colored. The size no. 1 green gelatin capsules are approximately one-half full. Each capsule has been individually weighed to contain 186 mg of oil solution. Each capsule has been inspected to ensure that the cap is snapped securely in place. (This record sheet could also contain a table similar to those shown for Sample Prescriptions 26.1 and 26.3 with capsule weights/capsule shell weights/liquid fill weights.)

LABELING

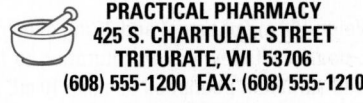

PRACTICAL PHARMACY
425 S. CHARTULAE STREET
TRITURATE, WI 53706
(608) 555-1200 FAX: (608) 555-1210

℞ 123881   Pharmacist: JH   Date: 00/00/00
Florence Thompson   Dr. K. W. Shapiro
Take one capsule by mouth daily.
Estradiol 500 mcg, Estriol 2 mg Oral Capsules
Mfg: Compounded   Quantity: 30 capsules
Refills: 2   Discard after: Give date

Auxiliary Labels: Keep in the refrigerator. This medicine was compounded in our pharmacy for you at the direction of your prescriber.

PATIENT CONSULTATION: Hello, Ms. Thompson. I'm your pharmacist, Julie Hutter. Are you using any other prescription or nonprescription medications? Are you allergic to peanuts, peanut oil, or any other foods or medications? What has Dr. Shapiro told you about this medication? This is an estrogen replacement medication. You are to take one capsule by mouth daily. I know that you formerly took an estrogen tablet, and this medication has similar effects. You will want to report to Dr. Shapiro your response to the medication as well as any adverse effects; sometimes the dosage needs to be adjusted for maximum benefit. Since this is a customized formula, we can easily adjust the dose. The capsules should be stored in the refrigerator. Discard any unused capsules after 6 months (give date). This may be refilled two times. Do you have any questions?

SAMPLE PRESCRIPTION 26.5

CASE: David Brawn is a 42-lb, 44″-tall, 5-year-old kindergartener. His teacher, Mrs. Felz, has noticed that several times each day David has brief episodes of staring. While each spell is very brief (less than 10 seconds), David does not seem to recall anything that has happened during that time period. His pediatrician, Dr. Patsy Heider, has diagnosed simple absence seizures, and this was confirmed by an electroencephalogram. David was initially started with ethosuximide syrup, 125 mg/2.5 mL bid, and the dose was gradually increased to the current 250 mg bid. Serum concentrations are within the normal to high therapeutic range, so Dr. Heider does not want to increase this dose further. Because David's seizures were not adequately controlled, valproic acid was added to the regimen, but David did not tolerate this drug well. Dr. Heider now wants to try clonazepam. The initial dose of clonazepam for children is 0.01 mg to 0.03 mg/kg/day. In consultation with Pharmacist John Dopp, Dr. Heider has prescribed clonazepam 0.1 mg in a chocolate lozenge base; David's starting dose will be 0.1 mg bid. (See dose calculations on the Master Compounding Formulation Record.) Dr. Dopp will dispense enough lozenges for 6 days, and he and Dr. Heider will do a preliminary evaluation of the clinical situation for dosage adjustment after 3 days.

CONTEMPORARY PHYSICIANS GROUP PRACTICE
20 S. PARK STREET, TRITURATE, WI 53706
TEL: (608) 555-1333 FAX: (608) 555-1335

℞ #   *123835*

NAME *David Brawn*   DATE *00/00/00*

ADDRESS *1399 Hyde Park Road*

℞

Clonazepam	*0.1 mg*
Chocolate lozenge base	*q.s.*

Dispense #12 chocolate lozenges   *J. Dopp 00/00/00*

Sig: Take one lozenge bid for absence seizure disorder

1″ Red C

REFILLS *1*   *Patsy Heider*   M.D.

DEA NO. *AH3932464*

MASTER COMPOUNDING FORMULATION RECORD

NAME, STRENGTH, AND DOSAGE FORM OF PREPARATION: Clonazepam 0.1 mg Oral Lozenges

QUANTITY: 12 (plus 2 extra for loss on compounding)

THERAPEUTIC USE/CATEGORY: Absence seizures

FORMULATION RECORD ID: LZ001

ROUTE OF ADMINISTRATION: Oral

INGREDIENTS USED:

Ingredient	Quantity Used	Physical Description	Solubility	Dose Comparison		Use in the Prescription
				Given	Usual	
Clonazepam 1-mg tablets	1.4 mg in 126 mg tablet powder	blue tablets w/ "K" stamped out of center, 1 mg and Klonopin imprinted	v sol in water, fr sol in alcohol	0.1 mg bid	0.1 to 0.3 mg bid	absence seizures
Chocolate lozenge base made from:	27.874 g		immis w/ water and alcohol	—	—	flavored, sweetened base
Dipping Chocolate	30 g	brown semisolid	immis w/ water and alcohol	—	—	flavored, sweetened base
Corn Oil	10 g	yellow oily liquid	immis w/ water and alcohol	—	—	mp and viscosity adjustor

COMPATIBILITY–STABILITY: As a solid dosage form, clonazepam in manufactured tablets is quite stable. Incorporating the crushed tablets in the dipping chocolate should pose no significant compatibility or stability concerns. Crushed clonazepam tablets incorporated in several aqueous suspending vehicles have been studied, and there was no significant loss of drug during various 60-day study periods (20).

PACKAGING AND STORAGE: The *USP* monograph for Clonazepam Tablets recommends packaging in a tight, light-resistant container and storage at room temperature (16); however, this soft chocolate lozenge dosage form should be stored in the freezer. Each lozenge should be individually packaged in a zipper-closure polyethylene bag and then stored in a tight, amber prescription vial.

BEYOND-USE DATE: Because the source of the active ingredient is manufactured tablets, use the recommended beyond-use date as specified in *USP* Chapter ⟨795⟩ for solid formulations made with active ingredients from manufactured drug products: no later than 25% of the time remaining until the product's expiration date or 6 months, whichever is earlier (17).

CALCULATIONS

Dose/Concentration

Initial pediatric dose: 0.01 to 0.03 mg/kg/day

Patient's weight (in kg): $\dfrac{42\ \text{lb}}{2.2\ \text{lb/kg}} = 19.1\ \text{kg}$

Dose (in mg): $\left(\dfrac{0.01\ \text{mg} - 0.03\ \text{mg}}{\text{kg/day}}\right)\left(\dfrac{19.1\ \text{kg}}{}\right) = 0.191\ \text{mg to } 0.573\ \text{mg/day}$

If given in two divided doses, the range is 0.095 to 0.287 mg per dose or 0.1 to 0.3 mg per dose. For this prescription, the dose per lozenge will be 0.1 mg.

Ingredient Amounts: Calculations are for 14 lozenges, including two extra doses.

Clonazepam: 0.1mg/dose $\times$ 14 doses = 1.4 mg

The clonazepam is available as 1-mg tablets, each weighing 90 mg. Two tablets will be needed for 1.4 mg clonazepam. The amount of crushed tablet material is calculated to be:

$$\frac{1 \text{ mg clonazepam}}{90 \text{ mg tablet powder}} = \frac{1.4 \text{ mg clonazepam}}{x \text{ mg tablet powder}}; x = 126 \text{ mg tablet powder}$$

Base: The formula for the base is 30 g of dipping chocolate plus 10 g of corn oil. This is made first, and then the desired amount of base material is weighed for use. The lozenges are made to a weight of 2 g per lozenge.

Total weight of lozenges: 2 g/lozenge $\times$ 14 lozenges = 28 g

Base: 28 g − 0.126 g clonazepam tablet powder = 27.874 g chocolate base

Because clonazepam is a controlled substance in C-IV, we must account for the amount dispensed and discarded or lost when making the 2 extra doses to allow for the loss in compounding.

Quantity used: 2 $\times$ 1 mg/tablet = 2 mg

Quantity dispensed: 0.1 mg/lozenge $\times$ 12 lozenges = 1.2 mg

Quantity discarded: 2 mg − 1.2 mg = 0.8 mg

MSDS AND SAFETY AND PERSONAL PROTECTIVE EQUIPMENT: Don a clean lab coat and disposable gloves.

SPECIALIZED EQUIPMENT: All weighing is done on an electronic balance.

COMPOUNDING PROCEDURE: The weight of clonazepam 1-mg tablets is determined to be 90 mg per tablet. Two tablets are placed in a mortar and the tablets are well triturated to a very fine powder. Weigh 126 mg of this crushed tablet powder. Prepare chocolate lozenge base by melting together 30 g of dipping chocolate and 10 g of corn oil. On the balance, tare out the weight of a 150-mL beaker and add melted chocolate base to a weight of 27.874 g. Transfer the 126 mg of clonazepam crushed tablet powder to the beaker containing the melted chocolate base and stir well to mix. Place a lozenge mold on a piece of weighing paper on the balance and tare out this weight. Pour molten chocolate-drug material into each mold cavity to a weight of 2 g per lozenge. When all 12 lozenges are poured, place the mold in the freezer to cool and solidify the lozenges. When solid, remove lozenges from the mold with a double-ended nickel spatula. Place each lozenge in a small zipper-closure bag and put the bags in an amber prescription vial. Label and dispense. Lozenges are best when stored in the freezer.

DESCRIPTION OF FINISHED PREPARATION: The lozenges are chocolate-brown in color with a smooth surface. The lozenges are round disks with a diameter of 2.5 cm, and each appears uniform in size with a depth of 0.5 cm.

QUALITY CONTROL: To confirm the appropriateness of the lozenge size for this weight of lozenge, the approximate specific gravity of the chocolate base was calculated from the weight fractions of dipping chocolate (0.75) and corn oil (0.25) and their respective specific gravities of 0.861 and 0.915 (= 0.874 g/cm^3), and this was multiplied by the calculated volume of a round lozenge with a diameter of 2.5 cm and height of 0.5 cm: Volume $\times$ density = π r^{2}h $\times$ d = 3.14 $\times$ (1.25 cm)^2 $\times$ 0.5 cm $\times$ 0.874 g/cm^3 = 2.14 g. The theoretical weight of 2.14 g closely matches the actual weight of 2 g. Each lozenge should be individually weighed to contain 2 g $\pm$10%. Reject and repour any lozenge that is outside this tolerance.

MASTER FORMULA PREPARED BY: John Dopp, PharmD   **CHECKED BY:** David Albers, RPh, PhD

COMPOUNDING RECORD

NAME, STRENGTH, AND DOSAGE FORM OF PREPARATION: Clonazepam 0.1 mg Oral Lozenges

QUANTITY: 12 (plus 2 extra)   **DATE PREPARED:** mm/dd/yy   **BEYOND-USE DATE:** mm/dd/yy

CONTROL/RX NUMBER: 123835   **FORMULATION RECORD ID:** LZ001

INGREDIENTS USED:

Ingredient	Quantity Used	Manufacturer Lot Number	Expiration Date	Weighed/ Measured by	Checked by
Clonazepam 1-mg tablets	1.4 mg in 126 mg tablet powder	JET Labs XY1175	mm/yy	bjf	jd
Chocolate lozenge base made from:	27.874 g				
Dipping Chocolate	30 g	Evon T54H	mm/yy	bjf	jd
Corn Oil	10 g	Westle BR72	mm/yy	bjf	jd

QUALITY CONTROL DATA: The lozenges are chocolate-brown in color with a smooth surface. Each lozenge is a round disk with a diameter of 2.5 cm and each appears uniform in size with a depth of 0.5 cm. Each lozenge has been individually weighed to contain 2 g $\pm$10% of total material. Weights of lozenges: 1.975, 2.086, 2.135, 1.947, 1.978, 2.036, 2.106, 2.089, 1.988, 1.964, 2.058, and 1.939.

LABELING

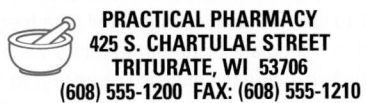

PRACTICAL PHARMACY
425 S. CHARTULAE STREET
TRITURATE, WI 53706
(608) 555-1200 FAX: (608) 555-1210

℞ 123835   Pharmacist: JD   Date: 00/00/00
David Brawn   Dr. Patsy Heider

Suck on one lozenge two times daily for absence seizure disorder.

Clonazepam 0.1 mg Oral Lozenges

Mfg: Compounded   Quantity: 12 lozenges

Refills: 1   Discard after: Give date

Auxiliary Labels: Store in freezer. Keep out of the reach of children. This medicine was compounded in our pharmacy for you at the direction of your prescriber.

PATIENT CONSULTATION: Hello, Mrs. Brawn. I'm your pharmacist, John Dopp, and I have David's prescription ready. Does David have any drug allergies? I know that he takes ethosuximide for his absence seizures, but is he currently taking any other nonprescription or prescription medications? What did Dr. Heider tell you about this medication? These are clonazepam chocolate lozenges that have been specially formulated in our pharmacy. I hope David likes chocolate. Hopefully these will bring more complete control to David's seizures. He should suck on one lozenge twice each day. This medication may make him drowsy, especially at first as his body gets used to this medication. It would probably be best to start this medication on the weekend so it will have a minimal impact at school and you can monitor the effects more easily. If drowsiness continues or if it impairs his performance at school, call Dr. Heider. If David experiences stomach upset with these, give the doses with food or milk and that should help. I understand that Dr. Heider wants you to contact her in 3 days to check on how things are going, and she and I can adjust the dose from there. These are a soft chocolate, so store them in the freezer for ease of handling. Be sure to keep these out of the reach of children; this is especially important because they could be mistaken for candy. Discard any unused contents after 6 months (or 25% rule, whichever is less). You may have one refill. Do you have any questions?

SAMPLE PRESCRIPTION 26.6

CASE: Sarah Davis is a 27-lb, 34″-tall, 2-year-old girl who has recently recovered from acute community-acquired pneumonia. She was treated with Vantin (cefpodoxime proxetil) 100 mg q12h for 14 days. As a result of her therapy with this broad-spectrum antibiotic, she has developed oral *Candidiasis albicans* (thrush). Because of her age and the fact that she has just recovered from a serious illness, Dr. Heider has decided to treat her fungal infection with cherry-flavored nystatin popsicles, which are compounded by Pharmacist Lloyd Thompson at Practical Pharmacy. Sarah has no other medical problems and is not currently using any prescription or nonprescription medications.

CONTEMPORARY PHYSICIANS GROUP PRACTICE
20 S. PARK STREET, TRITURATE, WI 53706
TEL: (608) 555-1333 FAX: (608) 555-1335

R # *123865*

NAME *Sarah Davis*   **DATE** *00/00/00*

ADDRESS *2227 North Rococo Rd.*

R

Nystatin	*2,000,000 units*
Sorbitol 70% Solution USP	*10 mL*
Syrup NF	*30 mL*
Cherry Flavor concentrate	*qs*
Purified Water	*qs ad 100 mL*

M et Div. to make 10 popsicles

L. Thompson 00/00/00

Sig: Eat one popsicle q8h for thrush

REFILLS *2*   *Patsy Heider*   **M.D.**

DEA NO. _____

MASTER COMPOUNDING FORMULATION RECORD

NAME, STRENGTH, AND DOSAGE FORM OF PREPARATION: Nystatin 200,000 unit Oral Popsicles

QUANTITY: 10

THERAPEUTIC USE/CATEGORY: Oral candidiasis infection

FORMULATION RECORD ID: LZ002

ROUTE OF ADMINISTRATION: Oral

INGREDIENTS USED:

Ingredient	Quantity Used	Physical Description	Solubility	Dose Comparison		Use in the Prescription
				Given	Usual	
Nystatin Powder 6,050 units/mg	2,000,000 units 330 mg*	light yellow powder	4 mg/mL in water; 1.2 mg/mL in alcohol	200,000 units q8h	200,000–400,000 units q8h	antifungal
Sorbitol 70% solution	10 mL	clear, colorless viscous liquid	misc with water	—	—	vehicle, sweetener, suspending agent
Syrup NF	30 mL	clear, colorless viscous liquid	misc with water	—	—	sweetened vehicle
Cherry Flavor Concentrate	10 drops	clear, colorless liquid	misc with water	—	—	flavor
Purified Water	qs ad 100 mL	clear, colorless liquid	—	—	—	vehicle

*Check potency on bottle of nystatin powder being used for this preparation because this weight is for a lot that is 6,050 units/mg. Make metric weight adjustments as appropriate.

COMPATIBILITY–STABILITY: Nystatin has some major stability concerns that are described in the nystatin monograph in *Trissel's Stability of Compounded Formulations* (21). Common flavored syrups with low pH (e.g., 2 to 4) should be avoided as compounding vehicles, because low pH is unfavorable to the stability of nystatin; the pH range for official USP Nystatin formulations is 4.5 to 7.0. The measured pH of the prescribed preparation is an acceptable 5. A flavoring concentrate that does not alter the pH may be added to improve the taste. The Nystatin monograph in the 11th edition of *The Merck Index* states that aqueous solutions and suspensions of Nystatin start to lose activity shortly after preparation. Suspensions that were tested at elevated temperature were found to be most stable at pH 7.0 and in moderately alkaline media. They were unstable at pH 2 or less and pH 9 or greater. A formulation similar to the one for this prescription was described in a *Hospital Pharmacy* journal article, in which the drug manufacturer, Squibb, suggested a 2-month beyond-use date for that preparation by (22).

PACKAGING AND STORAGE: *USP* monographs for Nystatin, Nystatin Lozenges, and Nystatin Oral Suspension all recommend packaging in tight, light-resistant containers (16); therefore, place each popsicle in a zipper-closure polyethylene bag and package in a tight, amber or opaque container. The nystatin powder is labeled for storage in the refrigerator but, because this is a popsicle dosage form, store in the freezer.

BEYOND-USE DATE: Based on the preceding information, use a conservative beyond-use date of 30 days.

CALCULATIONS

Dose/Concentration: Nystatin: 2,000,000 units ÷ 10 doses = 200,000 units/dose: okay.

Amounts: Nystatin powder from JET Labs; Lot # XY1178 is 6,050 units/mg, so the needed metric quantity of this powder is calculated:

$$\frac{6,050 \text{ units nystatin}}{\text{mg nystatin}} = \frac{2,000,000 \text{ units nystatin}}{x \text{ mg nystatin}}; x = 330 \text{ mg nystatin}$$

To determine whether this preparation is a solution or suspension, check the solubility of the nystatin in aqueous solution (determined to be 4 mg/mL) and calculate the quantity of water required to dissolve the 330 mg of nystatin:

$$\frac{4 \text{ mg nystatin}}{\text{mL water}} = \frac{330 \text{ mg nystatin}}{x \text{ mL water}}; \ x \ = \ 82.5 \text{ mL water}$$

This preparation will be a solution.

MSDS AND SAFETY AND PERSONAL PROTECTIVE EQUIPMENT: Review MSDS for all components. Don a clean lab coat and disposable gloves. Avoid inhaling nystatin powders.

SPECIALIZED EQUIPMENT: Glass mortar; all weighing is done on a class III torsion balance.

COMPOUNDING PROCEDURE: Weigh 330 mg (2,000,000 units) of nystatin powder. In a 50-mL graduated cylinder, measure 30 mL of Syrup NF and, in a 10-mL graduate, measure 10 mL of sorbitol 70% solution. Put the nystatin in a glass mortar, add the sorbitol 70% solution to the nystatin, and triturate well. Add the Syrup NF in portions while triturating. Using a 100-mL graduated cylinder, measure approximately 55 mL of Purified Water. Slowly add the water to the mortar with trituration. Some of the water may be used, if needed, to first rinse out the graduates used for the Syrup and Sorbitol Solution, with the rinsings added to the mortar. Stir to mix and then pour the solution into a 100-mL graduated cylinder and verify the volume as approximately 95 mL. Using Purified Water, qs ad 100 mL. Using a glass stirring rod, mix well. Measure and record the pH of the solution using a portable pH meter. Using a 10-mL disposable syringe, measure 10-mL portions of the liquid and squirt each portion into one cavity of an ice cube tray. Place in the freezer. When the popsicles are semisolid, insert a popsicle stick into each popsicle. Put the ice cube tray back into the freezer. When the popsicles are completely frozen, remove them from the tray and package in a large zipper-closure bag and place the bag in an opaque or amber tight container; label and dispense.

DESCRIPTION OF FINISHED PREPARATION: The popsicles appear as ice cubes with a slight pale yellow, opaque color.

QUALITY CONTROL: All are uniform in depth at 1.5 cm and each has been individually measured volumetrically to contain 10 mL of liquid. Measure the pH using a portable pH meter: pH = 5.

MASTER FORMULA PREPARED BY: Lloyd Thompson, RPh   **CHECKED BY:** John Albers, PharmD

COMPOUNDING RECORD

NAME, STRENGTH, AND DOSAGE FORM OF PREPARATION: Nystatin 200,000 unit Oral Popsicles

QUANTITY: 10   **DATE PREPARED:** mm/dd/yy   **BEYOND-USE DATE:** mm/dd/yy

FORMULATION RECORD ID: LZ002   **CONTROL/RX NUMBER:** 123865

INGREDIENTS USED:

Ingredient	Quantity Used	Manufacturer Lot Number	Expiration Date	Weighed/ Measured by	Checked by
Nystatin Powder 6,050 units/mg	2,000,000 units 330 mg	JET Labs XY1178	mm/yy	bjf	lt
Sorbitol 70% solution	10 mL	JET Labs XY1179	mm/yy	bjf	lt
Syrup NF	30 mL	JET Labs XY1180	mm/yy	bjf	lt
Cherry Flavor Concentrate	10 drops	JET Labs XZ2096	mm/yy	bjf	lt
Purified Water	qs ad 100 mL	Sweet Springs AL0529	mm/yy	bjf	lt

QUALITY CONTROL DATA: The popsicles appear as ice cubes with a slight pale yellow, opaque color. All are uniform in depth at 1.5 cm and each has been individually measured volumetrically to contain 10 mL of liquid. The pH was measured using a portable pH meter: pH = 5.

LABELING

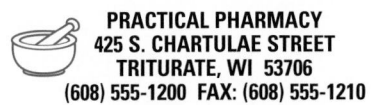

PRACTICAL PHARMACY
425 S. CHARTULAE STREET
TRITURATE, WI 53706
(608) 555-1200 FAX: (608) 555-1210

℞ 123865   Pharmacist: LT   Date: 00/00/00
Sarah Davis   Dr. Patsy Heider

Suck on one popsicle every eight hours for thrush.

Nystatin 200,000 units Oral Popsicles

Mfg: Compounded   Quantity: 10 popsicles

Refills: 2   Discard after: Give date

Auxiliary Labels: Keep out of the reach of children. Store in the freezer. This medicine was compounded in our pharmacy for you at the direction of your prescriber.

PATIENT CONSULTATION: Hello, Mrs. Davis. I'm your pharmacist, Lloyd Thompson. Does Sarah have any drug allergies? Is she currently taking any other medications? What do you know about this medication? What sort of instructions did Dr. Heider give you about using this medication? These are Nystatin popsicles to treat Sarah's oral thrush. You should have her suck on one popsicle every 8 hours. They have been sweetened and flavored with cherry, so hopefully Sarah will like the taste; any objectionable taste is usually helped by the cold popsicle because that tends to numbs her taste buds. If you think she would prefer a different flavor, just let me know because we can make these nearly any flavor that she likes. If these do not help her oral infection, or if the situation worsens, contact Dr. Heider. Store these in the freezer and be sure to keep them out of the reach of children. This is especially important because they look tempting to children. Discard any unused contents after 1 month. You may have two refills. Do you have any questions?

SAMPLE PRESCRIPTION 26.7

CASE: Janet Riemenschneider is a 150-lb, 5′7″-tall 60-year-old female patient with a diagnosis of breast cancer. She is to begin the "classic" CMF (cyclophosphamide, methotrexate, fluorouracil) regimen for breast cancer. Because this chemotherapy regimen causes acute and often late-onset emesis in a majority of patients, Dr. Ashman wants to prevent this adverse reaction to chemotherapy-induced nausea and vomiting (CINV). He has prescribed ondansetron, 24 mg PO, to be taken 30 minutes prior to Ms. Riemenschneider's IV methotrexate and fluorouracil on days 1 and 8 of each cycle, then 8 mg PO bid for 3 days (23). As an adjunct to this antiemetic therapy, Dr. Ashman has prescribed the combination ABH (Ativan, Benadryl, Haldol) antiemetic lozenges. Ms. Riemenschneider is to take one lozenge with the ondansetron 30 minutes prior to the IV therapy and then one lozenge q8h prn for days 1 through 14 of each cycle when Ms. Riemenschneider will be taking oral cyclophosphamide. The combination of ingredients in the lozenge formula works well to prevent anticipatory nausea and vomiting and also offers some antiemetic, antianxiety, and sedative benefits.

CONTEMPORARY PHYSICIANS GROUP PRACTICE
20 S. PARK STREET, TRITURATE, WI 53706
TEL: (608) 555-1333 FAX: (608) 555-1335

℞ #   *123834*

NAME *Janet Riemenschneider*   DATE *00/00/00*

ADDRESS *187 Enurese St.*

℞

Lorazepam	24 mg
Diphenhydramine HCl	600 mg
Haloperidol	96 mg
Acacia	1.65 g
Powdered Sugar	21.63 g
Flavoring	qs
Purified Water	qs

S. White 00/00/00

M et Div. for 24 Lozenges

1″ Red C

Sig: Suck on one lozenge 30 minutes prior to IV chemotherapy; then, one q8h prn N & V for the 14 days of oral cyclophosphamide therapy.

REFILLS *2*   *Linus Ashman*   M.D.

DEA NO. *AA4436677*

MASTER COMPOUNDING FORMULATION RECORD

NAME, STRENGTH, AND DOSAGE FORM OF PREPARATION: Lorazepam 1 mg, Diphenhydramine 25 mg, and Haloperidol 4 mg Oral Lozenges

QUANTITY: 24 (plus 2 extra for loss on compounding)

FORMULATION RECORD ID: LZ003

THERAPEUTIC USE/CATEGORY: Antiemetic

ROUTE OF ADMINISTRATION: Oral

INGREDIENTS USED:

Ingredient	Quantity Used	Physical Description	Solubility	Dose Comparison		Use in the Prescription
				Given	Usual	
Lorazepam 2-mg tablets	26 mg drug, 13 tablets	white tablets Mylan 457	insol in water; sl sol in alcohol	1 mg q8h	2–6 mg/day	antiemetic; amnesiac
Diphenhydramine HCl	650 mg	white powder	1 g/1 mL water, 2 mL alcohol	25 mg q8h	25–50 mg q6h	antiemetic; sedative
Haloperidol 5-mg tablets & 2-mg tablets	104 mg drug: 20 × 5 mg, 2 × 2 mg	5 mg—orange Mylan 327; 2 mg—orange Mylan 214	1 g/78 mL cold water	4 mg q8h	0.5–5 mg q8h	antiemetic, tranquilizer
Acacia	1.788 g	buff powder	sol in water; insol in alcohol	—	—	binder
Powdered Sugar	23.433 g	white powder	sol in water	—	—	sweetener, vehicle
Orange Flavor	5 drops	light yellow liquid	miscible w/ water, alcohol	—	—	flavoring
Purified Water	2.5 mL	clear, colorless liquid	—	—	—	vehicle, wetting agent

COMPATIBILITY–STABILITY: All ingredients in this preparation should be quite stable when in a solid dosage form. The letters ABH stand for Ativan (lorazepam), Benadryl (diphenhydramine HCl), and Haldol (haloperidol). The formula used here is given in the *International Journal of Pharmaceutical Compounding*; unfortunately, the article stated that no stability studies have been reported on this specific formulation (24).

PACKAGING AND STORAGE: The *USP* monograph for Diphenhydramine HCl Capsules recommends packaging in a tight container, but the monographs for both Lorazepam Tablets and Haloperidol Tablets recommend tight, light-resistant containers (16). Place each lozenge in its own small zipper-closure bag and place the bags in a tight, amber prescription vial with a child-resistant closure.

BEYOND-USE DATE: Because water has been added to this preparation, use a conservative 14-day beyond-use date as specified in *USP* Chapter ⟨795⟩ for water-containing formulations (17). If the patient needs extra flexibility, the beyond-use-data may be extended to 30 days; this follows Chapter ⟨795⟩ guidelines for "Other formulations"(17).

CALCULATIONS

Dose/Concentration

Lorazepam: 24 mg/24 doses = 1 mg/dose: okay.

Haloperidol: 96 mg/24 doses = 4 mg/dose: okay.

Diphenhydramine HCl: 600 mg/24 doses = 25 mg/dose: okay.

Ingredient Amounts

Calculations are for 26 lozenges, including 2 extra dosage units.

Lorazepam: 1 mg/dose $\times$ 26 doses = 26 mg needed.

Available as 2-mg tablets; 13 tablets needed; weight of 13 tablets = 1,469 mg

Haloperidol: 4 mg/dose $\times$ 26 doses = 104 mg needed

Generic tablets available as 0.5-, 1-, 2-, and 5-mg tablets. Use twenty 5-mg tablets and two 2-mg tablets for the 104 mg needed; weight of these tablets = 2,560 mg.

Diphenhydramine HCl: 25 mg/dose $\times$ 26 doses = 650 mg needed

Lozenge base materials: The formula for the base material is taken from the *International Journal of Pharmaceutical Compounding* (25).

Powdered Sugar:

$$\frac{21.63 \text{ g powdered sugar}}{24 \text{ lozenges}} = \frac{x \text{ g powdered sugar}}{26 \text{ lozenges}} ; \ x = 23.433 \text{ g powdered sugar}$$

Acacia:

$$\frac{1.65 \text{ g Acacia}}{24 \text{ lozenges}} = \frac{x \text{ g Acacia}}{26 \text{ lozenges}} ; \ x = 1.788 \text{ g Acacia}$$

Total weight of lozenges:

    23.433 g powdered sugar

    1.469 g lorazepam

    2.560 g haloperidol

    1.788 g acacia

    0.650 g diphenhydramine HCl

    <u>2.500 g</u> Purified Water

    32.400 g

Weight per lozenge: 32.4 g/26 lozenges =1.246 g/lozenge

Because lorazepam is a controlled substance in C-IV, we must account for the amount dispensed and discarded when making the 2 extra doses to allow for the loss in compounding.

    Quantity used: 13 $\times$ 2 mg/tablet = 26 mg

    Quantity dispensed: 1 mg/lozenge $\times$ 24 lozenges = 24 mg

    Quantity discarded: 26 mg − 24 mg = 2 mg

MSDS AND SAFETY AND PERSONAL PROTECTIVE EQUIPMENT: Review MSDS for all bulk components. Don a clean lab coat and disposable gloves.

SPECIALIZED EQUIPMENT: All weighing is done on an electronic balance.

COMPOUNDING PROCEDURE: Weigh 650 mg of diphenhydramine HCl powder and place in a mortar. Weigh 13 lorazepam 2-mg tablets (1,469 mg). Crush the 13 lorazepam tablets and add this to the diphenhydramine powder in portions; triturate well after each addition. Take 20 haloperidol 5-mg tablets and 2 haloperidol 2-mg tablets and weigh them (2,560 mg). Transfer them to a mortar, crush and triturate the tablets to a fine powder, and add this powder to the diphenhydramine/lorazepam powder and triturate to mix well. Weigh 1.788 g of acacia and 23.433 g of powdered sugar. Add the acacia to a clean glass mortar and add 2.5 mL of Purified Water and five drops of orange flavoring; then triturate to form a mucilage. Using geometric dilution and spatulation, combine the powdered sugar with the powdered drugs, and then put the powders in a flour sifter and sift the powder onto an ointment pad. Gradually add the mix of drugs and powdered sugar to the acacia mucilage in the mortar. Triturate and mix until a firm but pliable solid forms. Roll the mass into a cylindric shape on a glass ointment slab. Using a clean razor blade and a ruler, cut the cylinder into 24 equal portions. Each lozenge should weigh approximately 1.246 g; adjust the weight of lozenges as needed by shaving or adding material. Place each lozenge in its own small zipper-closure bag, and place the bags in an amber prescription vial with a child-resistant closure. Label and dispense.

DESCRIPTION OF FINISHED PREPARATION: The lozenges are buff in color. They are coin-shaped with a diameter of 1.5 cm and a depth of 0.5 cm.

QUALITY CONTROL: Weigh each lozenge individually; each should be within the range of 1.246 ±10%, or 1.121 g to 1.371 g. Adjust or reject any lozenges that are outside the allowed tolerance.

MASTER FORMULA PREPARED BY: Slappy White, PharmD   **CHECKED BY:** John Albers, PharmD

COMPOUNDING RECORD

NAME, STRENGTH, AND DOSAGE FORM OF PREPARATION: Lorazepam 1 mg, Diphenhydramine 25 mg, and Haloperidol 4 mg Oral Lozenges

QUANTITY: 24 (plus 2 extra)   **DATE PREPARED:** mm/dd/yy   **BEYOND-USE DATE:** mm/dd/yy

FORMULATION RECORD ID: LZ003   **CONTROL/RX NUMBER:** 123856

INGREDIENTS USED:

Ingredient	Quantity Used	Manufacturer Lot Number	Expiration Date	Weighed/ Measured by	Checked by
Lorazepam 2-mg tablets	26 mg drug, 13 tablets	Mylan XY1170	mm/yy	bjf	sw
Diphenhydramine HCl	650 mg	JET Labs XY1183	mm/yy	bjf	sw
Haloperidol 5-mg tablets and 2-mg tablets	104 mg drug: 20 × 5 mg, 2 × 2 mg	Mylan XY1171	mm/yy	bjf	sw
Acacia	1.788 g	JET Labs XY1186	mm/yy	bjf	sw
Powdered Sugar	23.433 g	G & H M86J5	mm/yy	bjf	sw
Orange Flavor	5 drops	JET Labs XY1184	mm/yy	bjf	sw
Purified Water	2.5 mL	Sweet Springs AL0529	mm/yy	bjf	sw

QUALITY CONTROL DATA: The lozenges are buff in color. They are coin-shaped with a diameter of 1.5 mm and a depth of 0.5 cm. The weights (in grams) of the lozenges are: 1.133, 1.285, 1.309, 1.182, 1.240, 1.276. 1.225, 1.296, 1.347, 1.246, 1.168, 1.187, 1.249, 1.310, 1.356, 1.182, 1.193, 1.239. 1.221, 1.235, 1.176, 1.172, 1.242, and 1.252. All are within the range of 1.246 ±10% (1.121 g to 1.371 g).

LABELING

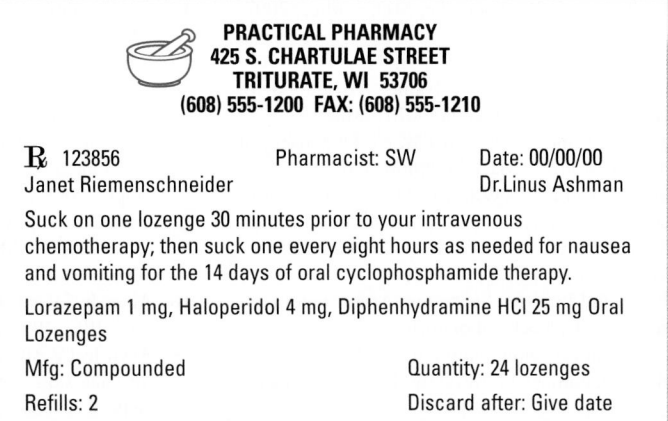

PRACTICAL PHARMACY
425 S. CHARTULAE STREET
TRITURATE, WI 53706
(608) 555-1200 FAX: (608) 555-1210

Ŗ 123856   Pharmacist: SW   Date: 00/00/00
Janet Riemenschneider   Dr.Linus Ashman

Suck on one lozenge 30 minutes prior to your intravenous
chemotherapy; then suck one every eight hours as needed for nausea
and vomiting for the 14 days of oral cyclophosphamide therapy.

Lorazepam 1 mg, Haloperidol 4 mg, Diphenhydramine HCl 25 mg Oral
Lozenges

Mfg: Compounded   Quantity: 24 lozenges

Refills: 2   Discard after: Give date

Auxiliary Labels: Drowsiness/alcohol warning label. Federal transfer label.
Keep out of the reach of children. This medicine was compounded in our
pharmacy for you at the direction of your prescriber.

PATIENT CONSULTATION: Hello, Ms. Riemenschneider. I'm your pharmacist, Slappy White. Do you have any drug allergies? I understand you are about to undergo chemotherapy. Are you currently taking any other medications? What did Dr. Ashman tell you about this medication? These lozenges contain a combination of ingredients—lorazepam, haloperidol, and diphenhydramine—that have been found to be very effective in preventing nausea and vomiting that often accompany chemotherapy. You should suck on one lozenge approximately 30 minutes before your intravenous anticancer therapy at the clinic; then you can suck on one lozenge every 8 hours as needed for the 14 days that you will be using oral therapy. These lozenges will probably make you drowsy, so do not drive or do anything that requires mental alertness if you have taken a lozenge. That means that on the day of your clinic appointment, you should arrange to have someone drive you to and from the clinic. Dr. Ashman has also prescribed another drug, ondansetron, which is also a very effective antinausea drug. I have that prescription ready for you, too. If these medications do not completely control your nausea, call Dr. Ashman or me and we will try some other medications. Also, if you notice any uncontrolled body movements while taking these, contact Dr. Ashman immediately. Do not drink any alcohol while taking this medication, as it will increase your drowsiness, possibly to a hazardous level. Store these in the refrigerator, out of the reach of children. Discard any unused contents after 2 weeks. You may have two refills. Do you have any questions? Good luck with your therapy and call me if I can do anything to help you with your medications.

REFERENCES

1. The United States Pharmacopeial Convention, Inc. Chapter ⟨1151⟩. 2008 USP 31/NF 26. Rockville, MD: Author, 2007; 616–625.

2. CDER Data Standards Manual. Rockville, MD: Food and Drug Administration, 2006: Data Element Name: Dosage Form, http://www.fda.gov/cder/dsm/DRG/drg00201.htm.

3. Miller RH. Tablets and pills. In: Martin EW, ed. Dispensing of medications, 7th ed. Easton, PA: Mack Publishing Co., 1971; 799.

4. Marshall K, Foster TS, Carlin HS, Williams RL. Development of a compendial taxonomy and glossary for pharmaceutical dosage forms. Pharmacopeial forum. Rockville, MD: The United States Pharmacopeial Convention, Inc., 2003; 29(5).

5. Allen Jr. LV. Troches and lozenges. Secundum Artem, volume 4, number 2. Minneapolis: Paddock Laboratories, Inc.

6. Allen Jr. LV. Pharmaceutical compounding tips and hints. Secundum Artem, volume 5, number 12. Minneapolis: Paddock Laboratories, Inc.

7. The United States Pharmacopeial Convention, Inc. Chapter ⟨905⟩. 2002 USP 25/NF 20. Rockville, MD: Author, 2001; 2082–2084.

8. Allen Jr. LV, ed. Tetracaine 20-mg lollipops. IJPC 1997; 1: 112.

9. Allen Jr. LV, ed. Pediatric chocolate troche base. IJPC 1997; 1: 106.

10. Allen Jr. LV, ed. ABH soft troche base. IJPC 1997; 1: 27.

11. Allen Jr. LV, ed. HDDM soft troche base. IJPC 1997; 1: 30.

12. Allen Jr. LV, ed. Tetracycline compound troche. IJPC 1997; 2: 113.

13. Allen Jr. LV, ed. Pediatric chewable gummy gels. IJPC 1997; 1: 107.

14. Sadik F. Tablets. In: King RE, ed. Dispensing of medications, 9th ed. Easton, PA: Mack Publishing Co., 1984; 67.

15. Rudnic E, Schwartz JB. Oral solid dosage forms. In: University of the Sciences in Philadelphia, ed. Remington: The science and practice of pharmacy, 21st ed. Baltimore, MD: Lippincott Williams & Wilkins, 2006; 915.

16. The United States Pharmacopeial Convention, Inc. USP monographs. 2008 USP 31/NF 26. Rockville, MD: Author, 2007.

17. The United States Pharmacopeial Convention, Inc. Chapter ⟨795⟩. 2008 USP 31/NF 26. Rockville, MD: Author, 2007; 316–317.

18. Allen Jr. LV, ed. Progesterone-estradiol-testosterone in oil capsules. IJPC 1998; 2: 54.

19. Allen Jr. LV. Allen's compounded formulations, the *U.S. Pharmacist* collection, 1995–1998. Washington, DC: American Pharmaceutical Association, 1999; 76–77.

20. Trissel LA. Stability of compounded formulations, 3rd ed. Washington, DC: American Pharmacists Association, 2005; 112–113.

21. Trissel LA. Stability of compounded formulations, 3rd ed. Washington, DC: American Pharmacists Association, 2005; 317–319.

22. Dobbins JC. A frozen nystatin preparation. Hosp Pharm 1983; 18: 452–453.

23. Waddell JA, Holder NA, Solimando Jr DA. Cyclophosphamide, methotrexate, and fluorouracil (CMF) regimen. Hosp Pharm 1999; 34: 1268–1277.

24. Allen Jr. LV, ed. ABH sugar troche. IJPC 1997; 1: 27.

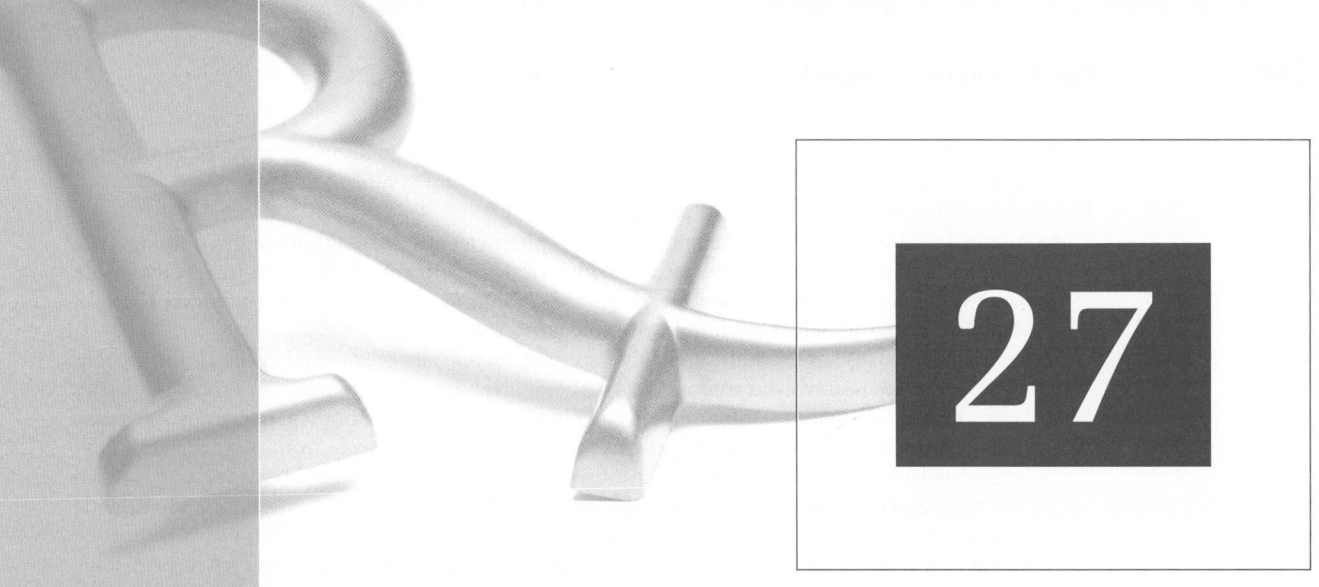

Solutions

I. DEFINITIONS AND SOLUTION NOMENCLATURE

A. **Solutions:** "Solutions are liquid preparations that contain one or more chemical substances dissolved (i.e., molecularly dispersed) in a suitable solvent or mixture of mutually miscible solvents" (1).

B. Traditional pharmaceutical dosage form terms used for solutions are briefly defined and described in the following list. For additional information, see *USP* Chapter ⟨1151⟩, Pharmaceutical Dosage Forms (1), and the FDA *CDER Data Standards Manual* (2).

   1. Spirits: These are alcoholic or hydroalcoholic solutions of volatile substances such as camphor and peppermint. The high alcoholic content of a spirit is usually necessary for solubility of the ingredient(s), so addition of water may cause turbidity or precipitation. These solutions should be stored and dispensed in tight, light-resistant containers to retard evaporation of the volatile ingredients and the alcohol and to minimize oxidation of labile active ingredients (1).

   2. Tinctures: These solutions contain vegetable materials or chemical substances in alcoholic or hydroalcoholic solvents (1,2). Some tinctures, such as Iodine Tincture USP, are made by direct dissolution (3). Other tinctures, such as those containing vegetable materials, are made by special percolation or maceration processes (1). Compound Benzoin Tincture USP, which is an ingredient in Sample Prescription 27.4, is an example of a tincture made using maceration (3).

   3. Aromatic waters: These are clear, saturated aqueous solutions of volatile oils or other aromatic or volatile substances. As with spirits, they should be stored in tight, light-resistant containers (1).

   4. Elixirs: This term is commonly used for oral solutions that use a sweetened hydroalcoholic vehicle (1). *The CDER Data Standards Manual* defines an elixir as, "a clear, pleasantly flavored, sweetened hydroalcoholic liquid containing dissolved medicinal agents" (2).

   5. Syrups: Oral solutions that contain a high concentration of sucrose or other sugars are often called *syrups*, but this term is also used in a more general sense to describe sweet, viscous, oral liquid preparations, including suspensions (1,2).

   6. Lotion: Although this term has been used for a variety of topical dosage forms including suspensions, emulsions, and solutions (1,2), the 2006 *CDER Data Standards Manual* states that the current definition is now limited to liquid emulsions for external application to the skin (2).

7. Otic (ear), ophthalmic (eye), nasal (nose): Words designating the intended route of administration have also been part of the traditional nomenclature for solutions (1).

C. Understanding solution nomenclature

1. As can be seen from the preceding examples, pharmaceutical dosage form terminology is a complex conglomerate; it is the result of historical tradition plus the need to specify in the name of a preparation the physical system (e.g., solution, suspension), the intended route of administration, and, when applicable, the solvent system.

a. Tradition: This has given us such names as *spirit, tincture, elixir, lotion,* and *syrup.* Unfortunately, because they just evolved through usage, these terms are not systematic, and most categories are neither all-inclusive nor mutually exclusive. For example, both peppermint spirit and lemon tincture (i) are solutions, (ii) have similar uses, (iii) are made from plant materials, (iv) have volatile components, and (v) have hydroalcoholic solvent systems; however, one is called a spirit and the other a tincture. On the other hand, the term syrup has been used for a wide array of oral liquids, including two different physical systems—solutions and suspensions.

b. Physical system: Identification of the physical system seems simple but terms such as solid, solution, and semisolid are often in sufficient to adequately describe the dosage form. Terms such as tablet, tincture, and cream are needed, and these terms must be specific and well-defined.

c. Route of administration: Solutions are the most versatile of all dosage forms and may be used for nearly any route of administration. The intended route of administration does impose on the solution certain necessary properties, such as sterility for injections, isotonicity for ophthalmic solutions, and palatability for oral solutions. For example, potassium chloride oral solution and potassium chloride injection both contain the same active ingredient, both are made by simple dissolution, and both are aqueous solutions, but their different intended routes of administration require distinctive components and processing controls that result in very different preparations. Therefore, route of administration is an important part of each preparation's name.

d. Solvent system: The importance of identifying the solvent system can be seen with two official topical solutions: Iodine Topical Solution and Iodine Tincture (3). Pharmaceutically, both are solutions, both are used topically, and both contain 2% iodine, but the fact that one is an aqueous solution and the other has a solvent system containing nearly 50% alcohol makes them very different, and the name of each preparation must reflect this.

2. The numerous dosage form terms and their ambiguity have been sources of confusion among prescribers, pharmacists, and pharmacy technicians, but tradition is a powerful force that often works against needed change. Fortunately, in the relatively recent past, two trends—use of computer technology and globalization—have provided some impetus for the development of a more systematic approach to pharmaceutical dosage form nomenclature.

a. Simple and standard drug dosage form terminology is essential for the efficient (and cost-effective) use of computer technology by government agencies in the drug product approval and monitoring process and by users of patient electronic health information for delivery and monitoring of, and payment for, drug therapy. Impacted organizations and agencies such as USP, the FDA, Health Level Seven (HL7), and the National Committee on Vital and Health Statistics (NCVHS) have been working toward the goal of standardized nomenclature for dosage forms (4).

b. Standardization of terminology is also important for global harmonization of standards. USP and HL7 have been working cooperatively with the International Conference on Harmonization (ICH) on international standards for dosage form nomenclature (4).

c. In 2002, USP formed a group to create a taxonomic scheme that would logically categorize dosage forms and simplify and clarify dosage form nomenclature. Under a system proposed by this group, a dosage form for a drug substance would be identified by the name of the drug, the route of administration (e.g., oral, topical), and the physical system (e.g., tablet, solution, suspension). When appropriate, the release pattern (immediate, extended, etc.) would also be included (4). For example, as of July 2007, Calamine Lotion USP became Calamine Topical Suspension USP (3). The proposed system would eliminate some traditional names such as *elixir* and *spirit.* For more information on this project, see USP's *Pharmacopeial Forum* 29, Sept–Oct 2003 (4).

d. Development and acceptance of and transition to any new nomenclature system will undoubtedly take years, and it will require the understanding and cooperation of all the affected constituencies. Therefore, it is important for health care workers, and particularly pharmacists and pharmacy technicians, to understand proposed dosage form taxonomy and nomenclature but also to recognize the various traditional terms used to describe dosage forms. The definitions and descriptions in this section should help in this regard.

II. ADVANTAGES AND DISADVANTAGES OF SOLUTIONS

A. Advantages

1. Because solutions are molecularly dispersed systems, they offer these advantages:
   a. Completely homogenous doses
   b. Immediate availability for absorption and distribution
2. Solutions also provide a flexible dosage form.
   a. They may be used by any route of administration.
   b. They can be taken by or administered to patients who cannot swallow tablets or capsules.
   c. Doses are easily adjusted.

B. Disadvantages

1. Drugs and chemicals are less stable when in solution than when in dry, solid form.
2. Some drugs are not soluble in solvents that are acceptable for pharmaceutical use.
3. Drugs with objectionable taste require special additives or techniques to mask the taste when in solution.
4. Because solutions are bulkier and heavier than dry, solid dosage forms, they are more difficult to handle, package, transport, and store.
5. Oral solutions in bulk containers require measurement by the patient or caregiver. This is often less accurate than individual solid dosage forms, such as tablets and capsules.

III. USES AND DESIRED PROPERTIES OF SOLUTIONS BY ROUTE OF ADMINISTRATION

A. Oral solutions (1)

1. Oral solutions are liquid preparations intended for oral administration.
2. They contain one or more therapeutically active ingredients dissolved in water or a water-cosolvent system. Solutions are most often made by direct dissolution. Factors that affect this process are described later in this chapter. Sample Prescriptions 27.2 and 27.8 illustrate principles and techniques used in making oral solutions.
3. Oral solutions may contain inactive ingredients to improve their palatability, stability, and/or aesthetic appeal. Examples of such ingredients include flavors, sweetening or coloring agents, viscosity-inducing agents, buffers, antioxidants, and preservatives.
4. As described earlier, syrups are oral solutions containing high concentrations of sugars. Oral solutions may contain other polyols, such as glycerin or sorbitol, which prevent "cap-lock" by inhibiting crystallization of the sugars in the cap and adjacent areas of the container. Depending on the polyol, these additives may also serve as sweetening agents, preservatives, cosolvents, and viscosity-inducing agents to improve "mouth feel."

B. Topical solutions (1,2)

1. Topical solutions are intended for topical application to the skin.
2. They are usually aqueous but may also contain other solvents, such as alcohols and/or polyols or other solvents approved for topical use.
3. They may also contain such additives as preservatives, antioxidants, buffers, humectants, viscosity-inducing agents, colors, or scents. Preparations in Sample Prescriptions 27.1 and 27.4 through 27.6 are examples of topical solutions.

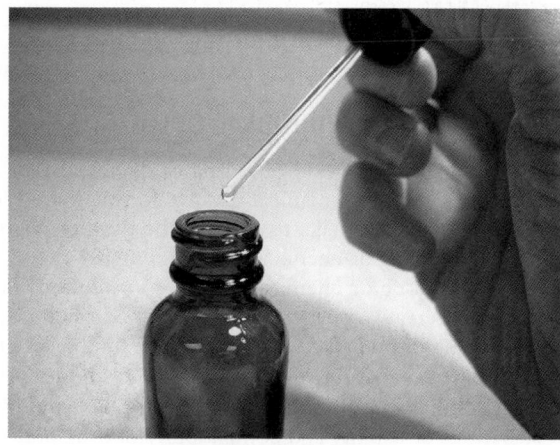

APPLICATOR BOTTLE

4. Specialized containers for topical preparations are available from vendors of compounding supplies. Bottles with glass applicators, with dauber or roller tops, with sprayer assemblies, and with specialized spout or disc caps are convenient administration aids for topical solutions.

C. Otic solutions (1)
1. Otic solutions are intended for instillation in the outer ear.
2. The vehicle may be water or glycerin or a cosolvent system containing water, alcohol, and/or polyols.
3. Otic solutions may also contain such additives as preservatives, antioxidants, buffers, viscosity-inducing agents, or surfactants. Sample Prescription 27.7 illustrates the use of several additive ingredients in an otic preparation.
4. Bottles with dropper closures are available to facilitate administration of otic solutions.

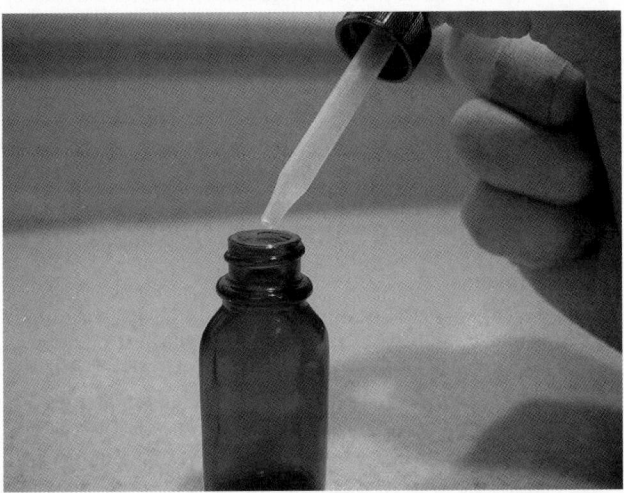

DROPPER BOTTLE

D. The solutions in the following list are sterile preparations and therefore are discussed in the chapters in Part 6, Sterile Dosage Forms and Their Preparation.
1. Ophthalmic solutions are sterile, particle-free solutions formulated for instillation in the eye (1).
2. Nasal solutions are sprayed or instilled into the nasal cavity. Although they are not specifically mentioned as a class in *USP* Chapter ⟨1151⟩ (1), there are official *USP* nasal solutions such as Naphazoline Hydrochloride Nasal Solution (3). Nasal solutions are most often used for local action, but they may also be used for systemic effect (2).
3. Inhalations are drugs, solutions, or suspensions administered either by the nasal or oral route with the respiratory tract as the intended site for local effect or for systemic absorption of an active ingredient (1,2).
4. Irrigations are solutions used to soak, flush, or irrigate open wounds or body cavities, such as the bladder (1,2).
5. Injections are parenteral preparations injected through the skin or a boundary membrane or directly into a blood vessel, muscle, organ, body cavity, or other tissue (1,2).

IV. PRINCIPLES OF COMPOUNDING SOLUTIONS

A. When making a solution of a drug or chemical, consider the following:
1. Will the drug or chemical dissolve in the desired solvent?
2. How long will it take to dissolve the drug or chemical?
3. Will the drug or chemical stay in solution?
4. Will the drug or chemical be stable in solution? For how long?
5. Is a preservative needed to prevent the growth of microorganisms inadvertently introduced at the time of preparation or during use by the patient?

B. Questions 1 and 2 concern the making of solutions (that is, dissolving drug or chemical in a solvent). Methods and factors affecting dissolution are discussed here. Questions 3 through 5 are considerations of stability and compatibility of drug preparations once they are made. These topics are the focus of Chapter 37, Compatibility and Stability of Drug Products and Preparations, and

Chapter 16, Antimicrobial Preservatives, but appropriate consideration of these issues is illustrated in each of the sample prescriptions in this chapter.

C. Will the drug or chemical dissolve in the desired solvent?

   1. Dissolution of solids

   a. To make a solution of a solid in a solvent, the solid must be sufficiently soluble in that solvent. Obviously, a solid will not dissolve above its solubility.

   b. Useful pharmaceutical solvents

   (1) Water is the most commonly used and most desirable solvent.

   (2) Others common solvents include alcohol (i.e., ethanol), isopropyl alcohol, glycerin, propylene glycol, polyethylene glycol 400, and various oils. These and other *USP* solvents are described in Chapter 15, Pharmaceutical Solvents and Solubilizing Agents.

   (3) Some solvents, such as isopropyl alcohol, are approved for topical solutions but may not be used internally because of their systemic toxicity.

   c. When predicting the solubility of a solid in a given solvent, very generally the old saying "Like dissolves like" is a useful guide, where *like* refers to similarity of molecular structure.

   d. Usually more precise information on solubility is required, so the first step in making a drug solution is to check the solubility of the drug. Useful references for this purpose include *The Merck Index* and *Remington: The Science and Practice of Pharmacy*.

Example 27.1

Boric acid   10%

Purified water qs   ad 60 mL

On checking the solubility of boric acid, the compounder finds it to be 1 g/18 mL water, or approximately 5%. This preparation cannot be made because the prescribed concentration, 10%, is above the solubility of boric acid in water.

---

   (1) Remember that solubility is given in grams of solute per milliliter of **solvent,** not per milliliter of solution, so unless you know the density of the saturated solution, you cannot know the precise amount of solution that will result. Therefore, the 5% noted in the preceding example is a rough estimate.

   (2) Useful quantity information on saturated solutions of many chemicals and drugs can be found in the Saturated Solutions table in the Miscellaneous Tables section of older editions (13th and prior) of *The Merck Index*.

   (3) Many times, solubility is given in descriptive terms, such as *soluble, slightly soluble,* and *sparingly soluble.* The numerical equivalents of these terms can be found in the *USP* (5) and other references and are shown in Table 27.1.

   e. If possible, always dissolve the drug in pure solvent. For example, although Syrup NF contains a lot of water, these solvent molecules are tied up through hydrogen bonding with the sucrose and are unavailable for the purposes of interacting with and dissolving additional solute. This principle is illustrated with Sample Prescription 27.2.

   f. Be careful when using hot water to dissolve drugs or chemicals (a useful technique to speed up dissolution), because the drug may precipitate when the preparation cools to room temperature if its concentration is above its solubility at room temperature. In the example with

Table 27.1	**APPROXIMATE SOLUBILITIES—DESCRIPTIVE TERMS**
DESCRIPTIVE TERM	**PARTS OF SOLVENT REQUIRED FOR 1 PART OF SOLUTE**
Very soluble	<1
Freely soluble	1–10
Soluble	10–30
Sparingly soluble	30–100
Slightly soluble	100–1,000
Very slightly soluble	1,000–10,000
Practically insoluble or insoluble	≥10,000

boric acid, the solubility of boric acid is 1 g/4 mL of boiling water, or approximately 25%. The 10% solution could easily be made using hot or boiling water, but some of the boric acid will precipitate out on cooling to room temperature.

g. If the solution is to be stored or used at a temperature other than room temperature (e.g., in the refrigerator), the solubility of the drug at that temperature must be considered.

h. Following are several useful compounding strategies when a drug solution is prescribed but the desired concentration is above the drug's solubility:

(1) Make as a suspension. You may need to add a suspending agent, as described in Chapter 28, Suspensions. Remember to use a "Shake Well" label.

(2) Use a different solvent or a cosolvent system. To calculate an estimate of the volume fraction of each solvent needed in a cosolvent system for the drug, use the equation:

$$log\ S_T = vf_{water}\ log\ S_{water} + vf_{sol}\ log\ S_{sol}$$

where:

$$
\begin{aligned}
S_T &= \text{total concentration of drug in solution} \\
S_{water} &= \text{solubility of the drug in water} \\
S_{sol} &= \text{solubility of the drug in the chosen cosolvent} \\
vf_{water} &= \text{volume fraction of water in the solution} \\
vf_{sol} &= \text{volume fraction of the cosolvent in the solution}
\end{aligned}
$$

Use of this equation is illustrated with Sample Prescription 27.5 and is discussed in the section on cosolvents in Chapter 37.

(3) As described in Chapter 15, Pharmaceutical Solvents and Solubilizing Agents, cyclodextrins are sometimes used to enhance the solubility of poorly water-soluble drugs. Because the "guest" drug molecule is encapsulated in the cavity of one or more cyclodextrin molecules, cyclodextrins are used in **molar ratios** of 1:1, 2:1, 3:1, etc., with the target drug. Therefore, when using cyclodextrin to solubilize a drug for a compounded preparation, start with a molar ratio of 1:1 cyclodextrin to drug. If the drug is not completely dissolved, additional cyclodextrin may be required to satisfy a higher molar ratio.

Example 27.2

A compounding student attempted to make a published formula that contained progesterone (MW = 314) 20 mg, β-cyclodextrin (MW = 1,311) 62 mg, Purified Water qs ad 1 mL. At this concentration of β-cyclodextrin, the progesterone failed to dissolve completely, but complete dissolution was achieved with 84 mg of β-cyclodextrin, consistent with a 1:1 molar ratio as calculated here:

$$\left(\frac{1{,}311\text{ mg }\beta\text{-cyclo.}}{\text{mmol }\beta\text{-cyclo.}}\right)\left(\frac{1\text{ mmol }\beta\text{-cyclo.}}{1\text{ mmol Progest.}}\right)\left(\frac{\text{mmol Progest.}}{314\text{ mg Progest.}}\right)\left(\frac{20\text{ mg Progest.}}{}\right) = 84\text{ mg }\beta\text{-cyclo.}$$

---

(4) Decrease the concentration of the prescribed drug or chemical. Two different examples of this are illustrated in Sample Prescriptions 27.2 and 27.4. For systemic medications, the volume of the dose to be administered must be adjusted to give the prescribed amount of drug per dose.

(5) In all cases where changes are required, consult with the prescriber.

2. Miscibility of liquids

a. Solubility of solids in liquids has a counterpart with the miscibility of liquids with other liquids. When two liquids are completely soluble (i.e., molecularly dispersed) in each other in all proportions, they are said to be *miscible*. Some liquid pairs are partially miscible, which means that they are soluble in each other in definite proportions. Immiscible liquid pairs are imperceptibly soluble in each other in any proportion. Whereas you know that oil and water don't mix (i.e., they are immiscible), consider the miscibility of the following liquid pairs:

- Alcohol and water?   Yes
- Glycerin and water?   Yes
- Glycerin and alcohol?   Yes
- Glycerin and mineral oil?   No
- Alcohol and mineral oil?   No
  (Mineral oil is miscible with chloroform, ether, benzene, and many other oils, but not with alcohol and not with glycerin.)
- Alcohol and cottonseed oil?   No
- Alcohol and castor oil?   Partially

(Castor oil is the only fixed oil that is partially miscible, approximately equal parts, with alcohol.)

- ■ Cottonseed oil and mineral oil?   Yes
- ■ Castor oil and mineral oil?   No

(Castor oil is the only fixed oil not miscible with mineral oil.)

b. Obviously miscibility is not always easily predicted. Therefore, if you do not know the miscibility of two liquids, consult a suitable reference, such as *The Merck Index* or *Remington: The Science and Practice of Pharmacy.*

c. Following are several useful compounding strategies when it is necessary to combine immiscible liquids.

  (1) Make an emulsion by adding an emulsifying agent. Be sure to use a "Shake Well" label. This is described in Chapter 29, Liquid Emulsions.

  (2) Use a different solvent or an appropriate cosolvent system. For example, if you need to make a solution that contains alcohol and an oil, use castor oil rather than cottonseed or another vegetable oil.

  (3) In all cases in which changes are required, consult with the prescriber.

D. How long will it take to dissolve the drug

In other words, what is the rate of dissolution? In practical terms, what we often want to know is, how can we speed up the rate of dissolution? This can be analyzed in terms of the Noyes-Whitney equation, which was given in Chapter 25, Powders, and which is repeated here.

$$\frac{dC}{dt} = KS(C_s = -C)$$

1. From Fick's First Law of Diffusion, it can be shown that the dissolution rate constant, *K,* is equal to D/hV, where D is the diffusion coefficient, h is the thickness of the unstirred layer around the particle, and V is the volume of the solvent into which the drug is dissolved.

2. The diffusion coefficient D is actually composed of several factors expressed in the Stokes-Einstein equation given here. Knowledge of these factors will help the compounder to understand conditions that can be changed or controlled to increase rate of dissolution.

$$D = \frac{kT}{6\pi\eta r}$$

where:

> k is the Boltzmann constant (the gas constant, R, divided by Avogadro's number)
> T is absolute temperature,
> η is viscosity of the medium
> r is the radius of the drug molecule

From the Noyes-Whitney and Stokes-Einstein equations and Fick's First Law of Diffusion, it can be seen that some factors can be controlled or modified to increase the rate of dissolution and some cannot.

$dC/dt,$ the rate of dissolution, is dependent on:

a. T: Temperature is an important factor that can be altered by the compounder. As temperature increases, D increases, so diffusion and the rate of dissolution increase. In practical terms, we can use warm solvents or can heat solutions to increase the rate of dissolution. This is illustrated with Sample Prescription 27.7. Care must be exercised when using heat, because increasing the temperature also increases the rate of degradation of drug molecules.

b. η: Increasing the viscosity of the medium has the opposite effect on diffusion and dissolution rate; increasing viscosity decreases the diffusion coefficient and the rate of dissolution. As a result, drugs dissolve more slowly in viscous vehicles. For this reason, when possible, first dissolve drugs in pure, low-viscosity solvents such as water or alcohol; then add the more viscous necessary liquids, such as glycerin, syrups, or gels. This is illustrated in Sample Prescription 27.2.

c. r: Even though we cannot control the radius of the drug molecule, it is important and helpful to understand how it affects diffusion and the rate of dissolution. The larger the radius (r), the smaller D becomes and the slower the rate of dissolution. This means that, all other things being equal, large drug molecules dissolve more slowly than do smaller molecules. This is especially important when working with macromolecules, such as erythromycin lactobionate and amphotericin B. When making solutions of these drugs, it is necessary to give them sufficient time to dissolve. This is illustrated with Sample Prescription 27.6, a clindamycin topical solution. This factor will have increasing importance as pharmacists and pharmacy technicians handle more peptide and protein drugs, because these are very large molecules.

d. The factor h, which is the thickness of the unstirred layer around the particle, can be affected by stirring. The dissolution rate is faster if the drug-solvent-solution system is agitated or stirred. By stirring, the dissolved drug molecules are moved away from the surface of the solid to the bulk of the solution. This has the effect of decreasing h, which increases K and therefore increases the rate of dissolution.

e. The surface area of the solid, S: As was discussed in Chapter 25, Powders, for a given weight of solid, the surface area of a solid increases as the particle size decreases; therefore, the smaller the particle size, the larger the surface area and the faster the rate of dissolution.

(1) Although important, this principle has limited practical application in modern compounding situations. Most drugs and chemicals are now purchased in a fine state of subdivision. Unless a solid ingredient is in large pieces, any mechanical manipulation, such as trituration, by the pharmacist has only a minor effect on the rate of dissolution. The amount of time saved in speeding the rate of dissolution by decreasing the particle size is usually more than offset by the time lost in the extra steps of weighing, triturating, transferring, and reweighing before dissolving the drug or chemical.

(2) For a few drugs, such as sulfurated potash (used to make White Lotion, as shown in Sample Prescription 28.3), that are available in large chunks or "rocks," particle size reduction is useful for increasing the rate of dissolution.

f. The solubility of the solid, C_s: Although the solubility of the solid is a given property of the drug, it is important to know that poorly soluble drugs may dissolve slowly.

g. C, the concentration of the drug or chemical in solution at time $= t$. As the solution approaches saturation, the quantity $(C_s - C)$ gets smaller and smaller until $C_s = C$. At this point, $(C_s - C) = 0$, saturation is reached and dissolution stops. As saturation is approached, the rate of dissolution may become very slow. This is one reason for making saturated solutions ahead of time, because getting that last little amount to dissolve may take a long time. Some pharmacies maintain stock bottles of saturated solutions with excess drug or chemical on the bottom of the vessel and then decant the saturated solution when it is needed.

V. COMPATIBILITY, STABILITY, AND BEYOND-USE DATING

A. Physical stability of the system: The major concern with regard to physical stability of a solution is precipitation of a soluble component. Change in temperature, evaporation of solvent, or addition of another drug or chemical to a solution may result in precipitation of a drug or chemical from solution. This subject is discussed in section III. D. of Chapter 37, Compatibility and Stability of Drug Products and Preparations.

B. Chemical stability of the ingredients

1. As stated in section II of this chapter, drugs and chemicals are less stable when in solution then when in drug, solid form. For ingredient-specific information, check references such as those listed in Chapter 37. Examples are illustrated with the prescription ingredients in each of the sample prescriptions at the end of this chapter.

2. USP Chapter ⟨795⟩ recommends a **maximum 14-day beyond-use date** for water-containing liquid preparations made with ingredients in solid form when the stability of the ingredients in that specific formulation is not known. This assumes that the preparation will be stored at controlled cold temperature (e.g., under refrigeration) (6). While storage in the refrigerator works well for oral liquids, topical preparations are usually stored at room temperature, and the beyond-use date may need adjustment to compensate for this higher storage temperature. Concerns for chemical stability of labile drugs may necessitate greater limits on beyond-use dates; Sample Prescription 27.1 illustrates this consideration.

3. While technically it is very easy to make solutions, care should always be used in checking and verifying the stability and the beyond-use date of the compounded preparation.

C. Microbiological stability: The USP states that for oral solutions, antimicrobial agents are generally added to protect against bacteria, yeasts, and molds (1). Preservatives should also be considered for topical solutions. If antimicrobial ingredients are prescribed as part of the formulation, extra preservatives are not needed. Antimicrobial agents and their proper use are discussed in Chapter 16, and consideration of preservatives is presented in each of the following sample prescription formulations.

Sample Prescriptions

SAMPLE PRESCRIPTION 27.1

CASE: Ashley Fingerhut is a 110-lb, 5'1"-tall 20-year old female patient who has a painless ulcer on her right hand. She noticed a red papule about 2 months ago and initially self-treated it with various OTC topical creams. When it did not improve and, in fact, ulcerated, she consulted with her pharmacist Jack Jones, who suggested she see her physician. Dr. Attles did a culture of the lesion and has now diagnosed *Sporohiza schenckii*, which Ashley probably got while working with rose bushes at her summer job at a local greenhouse. Dr. Attles has prescribed a potassium permanganate wet dressing and oral itraconazole 100 mg bid for 3 months.

CONTEMPORARY PHYSICIANS GROUP PRACTICE
20 S. PARK STREET, TRITURATE, WI 53706
TEL: (608) 555-1333 FAX: (608) 555-1335

℞ # *123178*

NAME *Ashley Fingerhut*   DATE *00/00/00*

ADDRESS *5487 Social Avenue*

℞

        KMnO₄   *1:6,000*

        Dispense 6 oz.

J. Jones 00/00/00

    Sig: Apply to lesion 2-3 times daily as a wet dressing

REFILLS *0*   *M. Q. Attles*   M.D.

DEA NO.

MASTER COMPOUNDING FORMULATION RECORD

NAME, STRENGTH, AND DOSAGE FORM OF PREPARATION: Potassium Permanganate Topical Solution 0.017%

QUANTITY: 180 mL

THERAPEUTIC USE/CATEGORY: Germicide/antifungal

FORMULATION RECORD ID: SN001

ROUTE OF ADMINISTRATION: Topical

INGREDIENTS:

Ingredient	Quantity Used	Physical Description	Solubility	Dose Comparison		Use in the Prescription
				Given	Usual	
Potassium Permanganate	120 mg weighed, 30 mg used	purple crystals	1 g/4 mL	0.017%	0.004% – 1%	antibacterial, antifungal, germicidal
Purified Water	qs 180 mL	clear, colorless liquid	—	—	—	vehicle

COMPATIBILITY–STABILITY: With regard to physical stability, this solution should be very stable because Potassium permanganate is very water soluble, and this is a very dilute solution. Chemical stability is a very different matter. Potassium permanganate is a very strong oxidizing agent and is not very stable chemically. It can be explosive and flammable if mixed with organic substances such as lactose and glycerin. While it is more stable in aqueous solution, even in this form it has limited stability. This is apparent as solutions turn from purple to brown with the formation of manganese dioxide. With respect to microbiological stability, no added preservative is needed for this solution, because potassium permanganate is an antimicrobial agent.

PACKAGING AND STORAGE: This solution should be dispensed in a tight, light-resistant container. Because this is a topical preparation, controlled room temperature will be the recommended storage condition.

BEYOND-USE DATE: Although it would be possible to use the *USP* Chapter ⟨795⟩ recommended maximum 14-day beyond-use date for compounded water-containing liquid formulations prepared from ingredients in solid form (6), use a more conservative 7-day dating because of the labile nature of potassium permanganate.

CALCULATIONS

Dose/Concentration: Concentration okay for intended use

The 1:6,000 ratio strength may be expressed on the label as a w/v%:

$$\frac{1 \text{ g KMnO}_4}{6{,}000 \text{ mL solution}} = \frac{x \text{ g}}{100 \text{ mL}}; x = 0.017 \text{ g}/100 \text{ mL} = 0.017\%$$

Ingredient Amounts

Potassium permanganate ($KMnO_4$):

$$6 \text{ oz} = 180 \text{ mL}; \frac{1 \text{ g KMnO}_4}{6{,}000 \text{ mL solution}} = \frac{x \text{ g KMnO}_4}{180 \text{ mL solution}}; x = 0.03 \text{ g} = 30 \text{ mg KMnO}_4$$

This amount is below the MWQ for the class III torsion balance used for compounding this preparation; a solid–water aliquot is needed. **Remember:** You may not use any organic diluent (lactose, alcohol, etc.) for potassium permanganate.

Weigh 120 mg $KMnO_4$ and qs ad 12 mL with Purified Water:

$$120 \text{ mg}/12 \text{ mL} = 10 \text{ mg/mL}$$

Because 30 mg is needed, measure 3 mL of this solution: 10 mg/mL $\times$ 3 mL = 30 mg

MSDS AND SAFETY AND PERSONAL PROTECTIVE EQUIPMENT: Review MSDS for potassium permanganate. Don a clean lab coat, disposable gloves, and safety glasses. Use extreme caution in working with the potassium permanganate; it is a strong oxidizing agent and can be explosive and flammable when mixed with organic materials. It is corrosive and causes burns to any area it contacts.

SPECIALIZED EQUIPMENT: All weighing is done on a class III torsion balance; graduated cylinders must be meticulously clean.

COMPOUNDING PROCEDURE: Rinse and precalibrate a 6-oz prescription bottle with Purified Water. Put approximately 5 mL of Purified Water in a 25-mL graduated cylinder. Weigh 120 mg of potassium permanganate, carefully transfer it to the graduated cylinder, and qs to a final volume of 12 mL with Purified Water. Stir to mix. Measure 3 mL of this solution in a 10-mL graduate and transfer this to the precalibrated 6-oz prescription bottle (with a child-resistant closure). Add Purified Water to the 180-mL graduation mark. Replace cap, close tightly, and agitate to mix. Label and dispense.

DESCRIPTION OF FINISHED PREPARATION: The preparation is a clear purple solution with no brown coloration.

QUALITY CONTROL: The actual volume is checked and matches the theoretical volume of 180 mL.

MASTER FORMULA PREPARED BY: Jack Jones, PharmD

CHECKED BY: Mary Ann Kirkpatrick, RPh, PhD

COMPOUNDING RECORD

NAME, STRENGTH, AND DOSAGE FORM OF PREPARATION: Potassium Permanganate Topical Solution 0.017%
QUANTITY: 180 mL **DATE PREPARED:** mm/dd/yy **BEYOND-USE DATE:** mm/dd/yy
FORMULATION RECORD ID: SN001 **CONTROL/RX NUMBER:** 123178

INGREDIENTS USED:

Ingredient	Quantity Used	Manufacturer Lot Number	Expiration Date	Weighed/ Measured by	Checked by
Potassium Permanganate	120 mg weighed, 30 mg used	JET Labs SN2611	mm/yy	bjf	jj
Purified Water	qs 180 mL	Sweet Springs AL0529	mm/yy	bjf	jj

QUALITY CONTROL DATA: The preparation is a clear purple solution with no brown coloration. The actual volume was checked and matches the theoretical volume of 180 mL.

LABELING

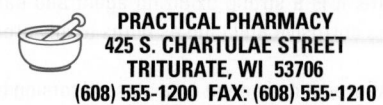

PRACTICAL PHARMACY
425 S. CHARTULAE STREET
TRITURATE, WI 53706
(608) 555-1200 FAX: (608) 555-1210

℞ 123178	Pharmacist: JJ	Date: 00/00/00
Ashley Fingerhut		Dr. Matt Attles

Apply to lesion on your hand as a wet dressing two to three times a day.

Potassium Permanganate 1:6,000 (0.017%) Topical Solution

Mfg: Compounded	Quantity: 180 mL
Refills: None	Discard after: Give date

Auxiliary Labels: For external use only. Keep out of the reach of children. This medicine was compounded in our pharmacy for you at the direction of your prescriber.

PATIENT CONSULTATION: Hello, Ashley, you maybe remember me; I'm your pharmacist, Jack Jones. I see that Dr. Attles has figured out what has caused the sore on your hand. Are you allergic to any drugs? Are you taking or using any prescription or nonprescription medications? What did Dr. Attles tell you about this soaking solution? This is a solution of potassium permanganate that is used to kill fungal organisms. Lay a sterile gauze pad on the lesion on your hand and carefully pour this solution on the gauze and let it soak for about 15 to 30 minutes. The gauze will dry in that time; this procedure is sometimes called "wet to dry." Then carefully pat the area dry with a soft, clean towel; just don't rub the lesion. This preparation will stain clothing, sheets, and so on, so be careful, and keep the bottle tightly closed. This solution should be stored at room temperature, away from light. If you notice that the solution has turned brown, call me and I will make some fresh solution for you. Keep this out of reach of children, and dilute with water and discard any unused portion after 1 week (give date). If your lesion worsens, or doesn't start to improve, I would contact Dr. Attles. He has not authorized refills because he wants to see you in a week. He also has prescribed an oral antifungal agent, which I also have ready for you. Do you have any questions?

SAMPLE PRESCRIPTION 27.2

CASE: Fred Flynn Stone is a 223-lb, 5′10″-tall 62-year old male patient with type 2 diabetes and hypertension. When his diabetes was diagnosed approximately 10 years ago, he quit smoking and drinking of alcoholic beverages and went on a diet and exercise program. He lost 10 pounds, but he realizes that he is still somewhat overweight, and he continually works on this. Both his hypertension and diabetes are currently well controlled with glipizide 10 mg daily, nifedipine XL 30 mg daily, and hydrochlorothiazide 25 mg every morning. A recent lab panel showed a decrease in his serum potassium to 3.3 mEq/L. Dr. Behling has referred Fred to a cardiologist for an evaluation of his condition and medications. In the meantime, he has prescribed sugar-free, alcohol-free potassium gluconate syrup 10 mEq bid. Pharmacist Juanita Juarez has called Dr. Behling to tell him that there is not a commercial product that meets the specifications of his prescription order. She can make a compounded oral liquid that is both sugar-free and alcohol-free, but she will need to change the concentration from 10 mEq per teaspoonful to 10 mEq per tablespoonful because of solvent and solubility constraints. Dr. Behling agrees with this plan.

CONTEMPORARY PHYSICIANS GROUP PRACTICE
20 S. PARK STREET, TRITURATE, WI 53706
TEL: (608) 555-1333 FAX: (608) 555-1335

℞ # *123182*

NAME *Fred Flynn Stone* **DATE** *00/00/00*

ADDRESS *983 Bronto Lane*

℞   *Potassium Gluconate* ~~40 mEq/5 mL~~ **Change to 10 mEq/15 mL**

   M & Ft. Flavored sugar-free, alcohol-free syrup

   Dispense ~~120 mL~~ **Change to 360 mL**

   Change to 15 mL
   Sig: ~~5 mL~~ *bid in juice or water*

Per consult with Dr. Behling, changed concentration,
dose volume, and dispensed volume because of solubility issues.   *J. Juarez 00/00/00*

REFILLS *5*   *F. Behling*   **M.D.**

   DEA NO. _____

MASTER COMPOUNDING FORMULATION RECORD

NAME, STRENGTH, AND DOSAGE FORM OF PREPARATION: Potassium Gluconate Oral Solution 10 mEq/15 mL (2.34 g/15 mL)

QUANTITY: 360 mL

THERAPEUTIC USE/CATEGORY: Potassium supplement

FORMULATION RECORD ID: SN002

ROUTE OF ADMINISTRATION: Oral

INGREDIENTS:

Ingredient	Quantity Used	Physical Description	Solubility	Dose Comparison		Use in the Prescription
				Given	Usual	
Potassium Gluconate	56.16 g	white crystals	1 g/3 mL water prac insol in alcohol	20 mEq per day	20–80 mEq per day	potassium supplement
Grape Flavor	10 drops	clear, colorless liquid	miscible	—	—	flavor
Sodium Saccharin	30 mg	white powder	fr sol in water sp sol in alcohol	—	—	sweetener
Paraben–Propylene Glycol Stock Solution	7.2 mL	clear, colorless, slightly viscous liquid	miscible with water, alcohol	0.18% MP 0.02% PP 2% Pr Gly	0.18% MP 0.02% PP 2% Pr Gly	preservative system
Sodium Carboxymethyl-cellulose (CMC) med. viscosity Solution 1%	qs 360 mL	clear, colorless, viscous liquid	miscible with water, alcohol	—	—	vehicle
Purified Water	170 mL	clear, colorless liquid	—	—	—	solvent, vehicle

Note: MP = methylparaben, PP = propylparaben, Pr Gly = propylene glycol.

COMPATIBILITY–STABILITY: The solubility of the potassium gluconate at the concentration prescribed was checked, and it was determined that it is not sufficiently soluble. It is necessary to change the volumes of the solution (see calculations that follow). This means that both the total volume and dose volume must be changed; the final strength will be 10 mEq per 15 mL, rather than per 5 mL. The dose volume will become 15 mL instead of 5 mL, and the total volume dispensed will be 360 mL so the same number of doses will be dispensed. With regard to chemical stability, potassium gluconate is very stable; there are numerous official *USP* solution monographs for potassium gluconate (3). For the sugar-free syrup, methylcellulose 1,500 cps 1% gel would be a preferred vehicle, but this gum is incompatible with the high electrolyte content of the potassium gluconate solution. Sodium carboxymethylcellulose (CMC) is more stable to concentrated salts solutions, so a 1% gel of medium-viscosity CMC, flavored with grape concentrate and sweetened with sodium saccharin, is the selected vehicle. The usual oral liquid preservatives sodium benzoate and potassium sorbate are not effective preservatives at the basic pH (7.5) of this solution. Use the pharmacy-prepared paraben stock preservative solution described in Chapter 16; it contains 9% methylparaben and 1% propylparaben in propylene glycol. At a concentration of 2 mL of the stock solution per 100 mL of preparation solution, it provides methylparaben 0.18%, propylparaben 0.02%, and propylene glycol 2%.

PACKAGING AND STORAGE: The *USP* monographs for similar preparations recommend packaging in tight containers (3). Recommend storage of this oral solution in the refrigerator.

BEYOND-USE DATE: Although manufactured versions of this formulation are given expiration dates of several years, use a more conservative 30-day beyond-use date, as recommended in *USP* Chapter ⟨795⟩, for other formulations (6).

CALCULATIONS

Dose/Concentration: Dose of 20 mEq/day is within the usual adult prescribing limits, but potassium blood levels should be monitored.

Ingredient Amounts

Grams of potassium gluconate (K gluc) required for this preparation:

$$(\text{K gluc MW} = 234; 1 \text{ mEq K}^+ /\text{mmol K gluc})$$

$$\left(\frac{234 \text{ mg K gluc}}{\text{mmol K gluc}}\right)\left(\frac{\text{mmol K gluc}}{1 \text{ mEq K}^+}\right)\left(\frac{10 \text{ mEq K}^+}{5 \text{ mL}}\right)\left(\frac{120 \text{ mL}}{}\right) = 56,160 \text{ mg} = 56.16 \text{g K gluc}$$

The water solubility of K gluc is 1 g/3 mL. To dissolve the needed 56.16 g of K gluc, the amount of water (or aqueous vehicle) can be calculated:

$$\frac{1 \text{ g K gluc}}{3 \text{ mL water}} = \frac{56.16 \text{ g K gluc}}{x \text{ mL water}}; x = 168 \text{ mL water}$$

The prescribed volume is only 120 mL, so the quantity of salt needed is above its aqueous solubility for this volume. If we multiply all the volumes by three, the drug is sufficiently soluble. In this case, the new dose volume is 15 mL (10 mEq/15 mL), and the dispensing volume is 360 mL. The prescriber was consulted and the patient advised of the change.

The prescription content should be labeled both in terms of milliequivalents per dose and grams or milligrams of the salt per dose (5). It can be observed that with a molecular weight of 234 mg/mmol, a 1 mEq/mmol equivalence, and 10 mEq/dose, that each dose will contain 2,340 mg or 2.34 g per 15-mL dose. This is verified by calculation:

$$\left(\frac{234 \text{ mg K gluc}}{\text{mmol K gluc}}\right)\left(\frac{\text{mmol K gluc}}{1 \text{ m Eq K}^+}\right)\left(\frac{10 \text{ mEq K}^+}{\text{dose}}\right) = 2,340 \text{ mg} = 2.34 \text{ g K gluc}$$

The 1% sodium CMC medium-viscosity gel is available as a stock solution in the pharmacy. For a procedure for making this vehicle, see Chapter 19, Viscosity-Inducing Agents, and Sample Prescription 28.3.

Volume of paraben stock solution:

The paraben–propylene glycol stock solution that is described in Chapter 16 will be used as the preservative system. This solution contains 9 g methylparaben (9%) and 1 g propylparaben (1%) in 100 mL propylene glycol solution. If 2 mL of this stock solution is added per 100 mL of our preparation solution, the final concentrations provided are the recommended amounts: methylparaben 0.18%, propylparaben 0.02%, and propylene glycol 2%. This can be verified by the calculation. For example, for methylparaben:

$$9\% \times 2 \text{ mL} = 0.09 \times 2 \text{ mL} = 0.18 \text{ g per } 100 \text{ mL of preparation or } 0.18\%$$

Calculate the volume of the paraben stock solution needed for this preparation:

$$2 \text{ mL stock solution/100 mL preparation} \times 360 \text{ mL preparation} = 7.2 \text{ mL stock solution}$$

MSDS AND SAFETY AND PERSONAL PROTECTIVE EQUIPMENT: Review MSDS for all components. Don a clean lab coat and disposable gloves.

SPECIALIZED EQUIPMENT: Electronic balance; portable pH meter

COMPOUNDING PROCEDURE: Weigh 56.16 g of Potassium Gluconate and 30 mg of sodium saccharin and transfer them to a clean 400-mL beaker. Add 170 mL Purified Water and stir to dissolve. With stirring, add 120 to 150 mL of sodium CMC 1% solution, 7.2 mL of the paraben stock solution, and 10 drops of grape flavoring concentrate (any water-soluble flavor is acceptable). Using a portable pH meter, check and record the pH of the solution. Transfer the solution from the beaker into a precalibrated 360-mL or 12-oz prescription bottle (or, if not available, use a pint bottle), and qs to the 360-mL mark with additional sodium CMC 1% solution. Tightly cap the bottle and agitate well to mix. Label and dispense.

DESCRIPTION OF FINISHED PREPARATION: The preparation is a clear, colorless, slightly viscous solution.

QUALITY CONTROL: Check the pH of the preparation with a portable pH meter: pH = 7.5. The actual volume is checked and matches the theoretical volume of 360 mL. Store in the refrigerator for 1 hour and inspect for any precipitation. If there is precipitation, reformulate the solution.

MASTER FORMULA PREPARED BY: Juanita Juarez, PharmD

CHECKED BY: Mary Ann Kirkpatrick, RPh, PhD

COMPOUNDING RECORD

NAME, STRENGTH, AND DOSAGE FORM OF PREPARATION: Potassium Gluconate Oral Solution 10 mEq/15 mL (2.34 g/15 mL)

QUANTITY: 360 mL   **DATE PREPARED:** mm/dd/yy   **BEYOND-USE DATE:** mm/dd/yy

FORMULATION RECORD ID: SN002   **CONTROL/RX NUMBER:** 123182

INGREDIENTS USED:

Ingredient	Quantity Used	Manufacturer Lot Number	Expiration Date	Weighed/ Measured by	Checked by
Potassium Gluconate	56.16 g	JET Labs SN2621	mm/yy	bjf	jj
Grape Flavor	10 drops	JET Labs SV2622	mm/yy	bjf	jj
Sodium Saccharin	30 mg	JET Labs SN2623	mm/yy	bjf	jj
Paraben– Propylene Glycol Stock Solution	7.2 mL	Prac. Pharm. JT6814	mm/yy	bjf	jj
Sodium Carboxymethyl- cellulose (CMC) med viscosity Solution 1%	qs 360 mL	Prac. Pharm JT6803	mm/yy	bjf	jj
Purified Water	170 mL	Sweet Springs AL0529	mm/yy	bjf	jj

QUALITY CONTROL DATA: The preparation is a clear, colorless, slightly viscous solution. The pH of the preparation was checked with a portable pH meter: pH = 7.5. The actual volume was checked and matches the theoretical volume of 360 mL. The preparation was stored in the refrigerator for 1 hour and inspected; no precipitation was observed.

LABELING

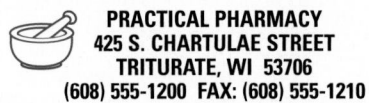

PRACTICAL PHARMACY
425 S. CHARTULAE STREET
TRITURATE, WI 53706
(608) 555-1200 FAX: (608) 555-1210

Rx 123182   Pharmacist: JJ   Date: 00/00/00
Fred Flynn Stone   Dr. F. Behling

Take one tablespoonful (15 mL) two times daily well diluted in water or juice.

Potassium 10 mEq per 15 mL as Potassium Gluconate 2.34 g per15 mL Oral Solution

Mfg: Compounded	Quantity: 360 mL
Refills: 5	Discard after: Give date

Auxiliary Label: Keep in the refrigerator. This medicine was compounded in our pharmacy for you at the direction of your prescriber.

PATIENT CONSULTATION: Hello, Mr. Stone. I'm your pharmacist, Juanita Juarez. Do you have any drug allergies? I notice on your medication record that you are taking nifedipine and hydrochlorothiazide for high blood pressure and glipizide for diabetes. Are you taking any other medications? What did your doctor tell you about this medication? This is a potassium supplement, which is used to increase your body potassium and keep your electrolytes in balance. It has been specially formulated to be sugar-free and alcohol-free. You are to take one tablespoonful (**not 1 teaspoonful** as Dr. Behling may have said; we had to make an adjustment) twice a day in juice or water. It is very important that you dilute this adequately so as to improve its taste and to avoid any stomach problems. To minimize any stomach upset, take it with food or after meals. Other possible side effects include light-headedness, weakness, or irregular heartbeat. If any of these occur, contact Dr. Behling immediately. When did Dr. Behling tell you to have your potassium blood level checked? This is very important. Be sure to store this in a refrigerator, out of the reach of children, and discard any unused portion after 30 days. Check the solution in the bottle when you take a dose; if you notice that any of the drug has formed crystals in the solution, bring the bottle back into the pharmacy so that we can make some adjustments in the formulation; that won't cost you anything extra, so don't hesitate to do that. Dr. Behling has authorized five refills. Do you have any questions?

SAMPLE PRESCRIPTION 27.3

CASE: Dr. Dennis Clomp, DDS, has contacted Pharmacist Bonnie Fingerhut about making a phosphoric acid solution for his orthodontic practice. He has just read an online article in *Angle Orthodontist* about a superior preparation for etching teeth prior to bonding the brackets when applying orthodontic braces (7). The procedure requires a 37% phosphoric acid solution that Dr. Clomp will mix 50:50 with 1.25% acidulated phosphate fluoride (APF) gel. Dr. Clomp has the APF gel and wants Dr. Fingerhut to make the phosphoric acid for him. Dr. Clomp has shared the article with Dr. Fingerhut and, although the article does not state whether the phosphoric acid percent is w/w, w/v, or v/v, they have decided to make it 37% w/w, which follows *USP/NF* precedent for Acetic Acid NF, which is 36% to 37% by weight. It also makes sense because the acid is being mixed with a semisolid gel.

HAPPY SMILE DENTISTRY PRACTICE
20 S. PARK STREET, TRITURATE, WI 53706
TEL: (608) 555-8201 FAX: (608) 555-8205

℞ # *123795*

NAME *Dr. Clomp Orthodontic Office*   **DATE** *00/00/00*

ADDRESS *20 S. Park Street*

℞
　　　　　　　　Phosphoric Acid　　　　*37% w/w*
　　　　　　　　Dispense　　　　　　　　*120 mL*
　　　Sig: Mix with acidulated phosphate fluoride (APF) gel and
　　　　　use for etching teeth prior to applying orthodontic braces.

B. Fingerhut 00/00/00

REFILLS　　　　　　　　　　　*Dennis Clomp*　　　　　　　　**D.D.S.**

DEA NO. _____

MASTER COMPOUNDING FORMULATION RECORD

NAME, STRENGTH, AND DOSAGE FORM OF PREPARATION: Phosphoric Acid Solution 37% w/w
QUANTITY: 120 mL
THERAPEUTIC USE/CATEGORY: Teeth prep for brace application
FORMULATION RECORD ID: SN003
ROUTE OF ADMINISTRATION: Teeth

INGREDIENTS:

Ingredient	Quantity Used	Physical Description	Solubility	Dose Comparison		Use in the Prescription
				Given	Usual	
Phosphoric Acid NF 86% w/w	36.7 mL	colorless, viscous liquid	miscible with water and alcohol	37% w/w	37% w/w	teeth enamel etching
Purified Water	qs ad 120 mL	colorless, clear liquid	—	—	—	diluent

COMPATIBILITY–STABILITY: This preparation is very similar to an official formulation, Diluted Phosphoric Acid NF, which is known to be very stable (3). No additional preservative is needed because this solution has a pH unfavorable to microbial growth.

PACKAGING AND STORAGE: The *NF* monographs for Phosphoric Acid and Diluted Phosphoric Acid recommend packaging in tight containers (3). It should be stored at controlled room temperature.

BEYOND-USE DATE: Although this preparation is known to be very stable, use a conservative 6-month beyond-use date for this compounded preparation.

CALCULATIONS

Dose/Concentration: Okay for intended purpose

Ingredient Amounts

Phosphoric Acid NF is 86.5% w/w H_3PO_4; its specific gravity $= 1.71$.

Number of grams of H_3PO_4 needed for this preparation: To calculate the quantity of Phosphoric Acid NF and Purified Water to make the desired w/w solution, the density or specific gravity of the 37% w/w solution is required. (See section VI, Special Calculations Involving Concentrated Acids, in Chapter 8, Quantity and Concentration Expressions and Calculations.) In the case of phosphoric acid, although we do not have a published value for the density of 37% w/w phosphoric acid in water, *The Merck Index* has values for 100%, 85%, 50%, and 10% w/w aqueous solutions of this acid at 25°C. When these values are plotted using an Excel spreadsheet or similar graph-plotting software, a nice smooth curve results, and the density of the 37% w/w solution can be determined by reading the graph or using the equation fitted to the resulting curve (provided the R^2 is very close to 1, true in this case).

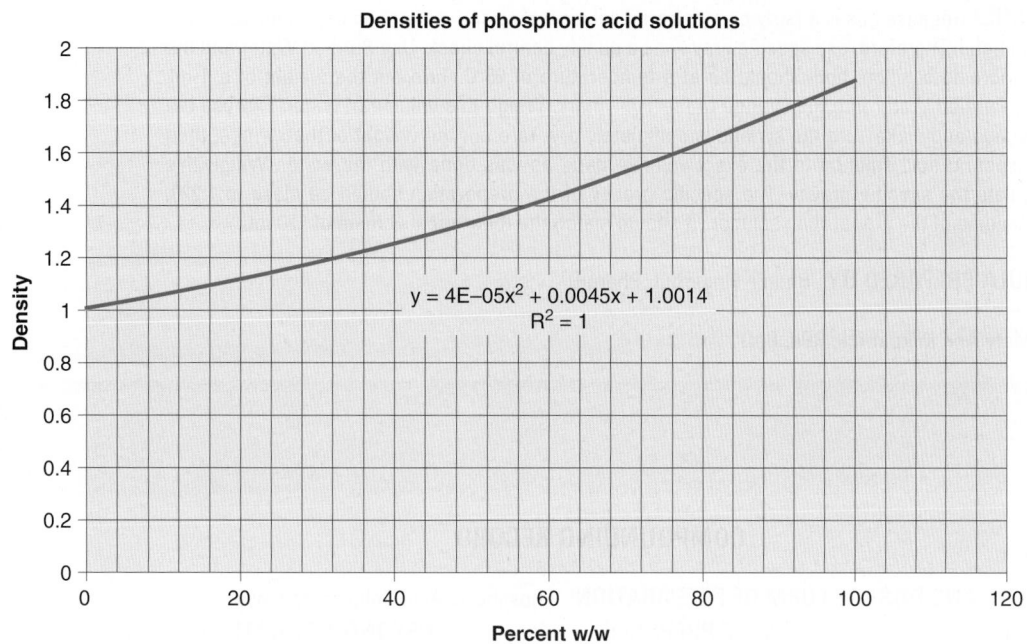

Densities of phosphoric acid solutions

$$y = 4E-05x^2 + 0.0045x + 1.0014$$
$$R^2 = 1$$

Using the equation, the density is calculated to be:

$$y = 4 \times 10^{-5}x^2 + 0.0045 + 1.0014 = 1.223, \text{ where } y = \text{density and } x = \%w/w$$

At 25°C, the density of a 37% w/w solution is 1.223 g/mL. Using this value, the weight of phosphoric acid needed can be calculated:

$$\left(\frac{37 \text{ g H}_3\text{PO}_4}{100 \text{ g 37\% solution}} \right) \left(\frac{1.223 \text{ g 37\% solution}}{\text{mL 37\% solution}} \right) \left(\frac{120 \text{ mL solution}}{} \right) = 54.301 \text{ g H}_3\text{PO}_4$$

Next, the volume of Phosphoric Acid NF that will give this desired quantity of phosphoric acid can be calculated:

$$\left(\frac{\text{mL H}_3\text{PO}_4 \text{ NF}}{1.71 \text{ g H}_3\text{PO}_4 \text{ NF}} \right) \left(\frac{100 \text{ g H}_3\text{PO}_4 \text{ NF}}{86.5 \text{ g H}_3\text{PO}_4} \right) \left(\frac{54.301 \text{ g H}_3\text{PO}_4}{} \right) = 36.7 \text{ mL H}_3\text{PO}_4 \text{ NF}$$

MSDS AND SAFETY AND PERSONAL PROTECTIVE EQUIPMENT: Review MSDS for all components. Don a clean lab coat, disposable gloves, and safety glasses. *NF* states: "Caution—Avoid contact as Phosphoric Acid rapidly destroys tissue" (3).

SPECIALIZED EQUIPMENT: None

COMPOUNDING PROCEDURE: Pour approximately 50 mL of Purified Water into a precalibrated 4-oz prescription bottle with a child-resistant closure. Carefully measure 30 mL of Phosphoric Acid NF (86.5% w/w) in a 50-mL syringe and 6.7 mL in a 10-mL syringe. Carefully transfer the acid to the prescription bottle; then qs to the 120-mL calibration mark with Purified Water. Carefully cap the bottle tightly and agitate to ensure complete mixing of the solution. Check the temperature of the preparation and measure the specific gravity of the solution by comparing the weight of 1 mL of the solution measured in a 1-mL syringe with the weight of an exactly equal quantity of Purified Water. Label the preparation and transfer to the dental office.

DESCRIPTION OF FINISHED PREPARATION: The preparation is a clear, colorless solution with apparent viscosity approximately that of water.

QUALITY CONTROL: Because this is a fairly concentrated solution of strong mineral acid, pH measurement would not be meaningful. Therefore, use specific gravity as a quality control check. Use Purified Water and the prepared phosphoric acid solution; both should be at a temperature of 25°C. Tare out the weight of a 1-mL syringe. Withdraw Purified Water into the syringe to the 1-mL mark. Weigh this volume of water. Express the water from the syringe and make sure the syringe is completely dry. Tare out the weight of the syringe, then withdraw the phosphoric acid solution to the exact volume mark, as was done with the water. Weigh this solution and calculate the specific gravity. The specific gravity of the preparation should be close to 1.223. Check the actual volume of the preparation solution; it should match the theoretical volume of 120 mL.

MASTER FORMULA PREPARED BY: Bonnie Fingerhut, PharmD

CHECKED BY: Mary Ann Kirkpatrick, RPh, PhD

COMPOUNDING RECORD

NAME, STRENGTH, AND DOSAGE FORM OF PREPARATION: Phosphoric Acid Solution 37% w/w
QUANTITY: 120 mL   **DATE PREPARED:** mm/dd/yy   **BEYOND-USE DATE:** mm/dd/yy
FORMULATION RECORD ID: SN003   **CONTROL/RX NUMBER:** 123795

INGREDIENTS USED:

Ingredient	Quantity Used	Manufacturer Lot Number	Expiration Date	Weighed/ Measured by	Checked by
Phosphoric Acid NF 86.5% w/w	36.7 mL	JET Labs SN2631	mm/yy	jet	bf
Purified Water	qs ad 120 mL	Sweet Springs AL0529	mm/yy	jet	bf

QUALITY CONTROL DATA: The preparation is a clear, colorless solution with apparent viscosity approximately that of water. The actual volume was checked and matches the theoretical volume of 120 mL.

Specific gravity data:

$$\text{Weight of 1 mL Purified Water at 25°C} = 0.989 \text{ g}$$

$$\text{Weight of equal volume of prepared phosphoric acid solution at 25°C} = 1.206$$

$$\text{Specific gravity} = \frac{1.206 \text{ g}}{0.989 \text{ g}} = 1.219$$

This is very close to the theoretical value of 1.223, within 0.33%.

LABELING

PRACTICAL PHARMACY
425 S. CHARTULAE STREET
TRITURATE, WI 53706
(608) 555-1200 FAX: (608) 555-1210

℞ 123795   Pharmacist: BF   Date: 00/00/00
Dr. Clomp Dental Office   Dr. Dennis Clomp, DDS

Mix 50:50 with acidulated phosphate fluoride (APF) gel and use for
etching teeth prior to applying orthodontic braces. For Office Use
Only

Phosphoric Acid Solution 37% w/w

Caution: Caustic liquid; wash immediately if in contact with skin.

Mfg: Compounded   Quantity: 120 mL

Refills: None   Discard after: Give date

Auxiliary Label: Keep out of the reach of children.

PATIENT CONSULTATION: Hi, Dennis, this is Bonnie Fingerhut. I have your phosphoric acid solution ready for you. I know that you are aware of the safety precautions with using this solution because you have used similar phosphoric acid preparations in your practice. I did label it with a cautionary statement and a "Keep out of the reach of children" label so that any of your office personnel will be careful with it and will know to keep this safely out of reach of patients. It is quite stable chemically, but you should discard any unused contents after 6 months; just be sure to dilute it first with water before pouring it down a drain or in a toilet bowl; as you well know, it etches porcelain. Store this at controlled room temperature. Do you have any questions?

SAMPLE PRESCRIPTION 27.4

CASE: Pam Perfect is a 145-lb, 5′8″-tall, 25-year-old female patient who has a diagnosis of plantar warts. Pam swims laps every noon hour at Citywide Health Club and has apparently contacted human papillomavirus (HPV) at this facility. She has several warts on the sole of her left foot. Fortunately, she has a desk job, so she is not required to be on her feet continually during the day, but she enjoys hiking and wants to clear up these warts as soon and easily as possible. Dr. Parker has heard from a colleague about good success in treating these plantar warts with a combination podophyllum–salicylic acid in Compound Benzoin Tincture. Dr. Parker checked a reference book for appropriate concentrations of podophyllum and salicylic acid and gave Ms. Perfect the prescription order shown here. Pharmacist Billie Burke checked both the effective therapeutic concentrations and the solubilities of these drugs and contacted Dr. Parker with the suggestion that the salicylic acid concentration be reduced to 15% because this compound is not sufficiently soluble in this combination at 25%. At 15% it would still be effective. Dr. Parker has agreed to this change.

CONTEMPORARY GROUP PRACTICE
20 S. PARK STREET, TRITURATE, WI 53706
TEL: (608) 555-1333 FAX: (608) 555-1335

℞ #   *123780*

NAME   *Pam Perfect*   DATE   *00/00/00*

ADDRESS   *285 Polly Point*

℞

Podophyllum	*12%*
Salicylic Acid	~~*25%*~~ **Changed to 15%**
Compound Benzoin Tincture q s ad 7.5 mL	
Sig: Apply to warts q hs	

Changed concentration of salicylic acid to 15% in consultation with
Dr. Parker because of insufficient solubility of 25%.   *Billie Burke 00/00/00*

REFILLS   *1*   *J. L. Parker*   M.D.

DEA No. _____

MASTER COMPOUNDING FORMULATION RECORD

NAME, STRENGTH, AND DOSAGE FORM OF PREPARATION: Podophyllum 12% and Salicylic Acid 15% in Compound Benzoin Tincture Topical Solution

QUANTITY: 7.5 mL

THERAPEUTIC USE/CATEGORY: Keratolytic/caustic for warts

FORMULATION RECORD ID: SN004

ROUTE OF ADMINISTRATION: Topical

INGREDIENTS:

Ingredient	Quantity Used	Physical Description	Solubility	Dose Comparison		Use in the Prescription
				Given	Usual	
Salicylic Acid	1.125 g	white, crystalline powder	1 g/3 mL alcohol 1 g/460 mL water	15% (changed from 25%)	2%–60%	keratolytic
Podophyllum	900 mg	light brown powder	sol in alcohol insol in water	12%	12%–25%	caustic for warts
Compound Benzoin Tincture	qs ad 7.5 mL	dark brown liquid	miscible with alcohol immis with water	—	—	vehicle, demulcent

COMPATIBILITY–STABILITY: With regard to chemical stability, all ingredients in this preparation are known to be very stable in this alcohol medium. Podophyllum Resin Topical Solution is an official *USP* formulation that contains podophyllum resin in an alcoholic extract of Benzoin. Compound Benzoin Tincture is also an official *USP* preparation, and there are many commercial solutions of salicylic acid. With regard to physical properties, the prescribed concentrations of salicylic acid and podophyllum were checked against their solubility in an alcoholic medium such as Compound Benzoin Tincture, and it was determined that the content of salicylic acid would have to be lowered because of inadequate solubility. The supporting calculations are shown later. No added preservative is needed due to the high alcoholic content of the preparation and the presence of ingredients that are toxic to microbes.

PACKAGING AND STORAGE: The *USP* monographs for similar preparations recommend packaging in tight, light-resistant containers (3). Storage should be at controlled room temperature, and exposure to excessive heat should be avoided. This is a flammable liquid and should be so labeled (3).

BEYOND-USE DATE: Although this formulation is quite stable, it does contain a volatile solvent with concentrations of ingredients near the saturation point. Therefore, use a conservative 1-month beyond-use date for this compounded preparation.

CALCULATIONS

Dose/Concentration: Podophyllum is used in a concentration range of 12% to 25%: okay.

Salicylic acid is used in a range of 2% to 60%: okay.

Ingredient Amounts

Podophyllum: $\qquad$ 12% $\times$ 7.5 mL = 0.12 $\times$ 7.5 mL = 0.9 g = 900 mg

Salicylic acid: 25% $\times$ 7.5 mL = 0.25 $\times$ 7.5 mL = 1.875 g (changed to 1.125 g; see the following calculation)

Solubility:

The solvent here is Compound Benzoin Tincture (Compd. Tr. Benzoin), which is 74% to 80% alcohol. The number of milliliters of alcohol available for dissolving the podophyllum and salicylic acid depends on the final volume of Compd. Tr. Benzoin in the preparation. Because the tincture is used to qs ad 7.5 mL and the powder volume of the podophyllum and salicylic acid is unknown, the volume of Compd. Tr. Benzoin can only be estimated. Some pharmacists use a powder volume estimate of 0.5 mL for 1 g of powder. Using this technique, we calculate a powder volume of:

$$(0.9 \text{ g} + 1.875 \text{ g}) \times 0.5 \text{ mL/g} = 2.775 \text{ g} \times 0.5 \text{ mL/g} = 1.388 \approx 1.4 \text{ mL}$$

The volume of Compd. Tr. Benzoin would be 7.5 mL − 1.4 mL = 6.1 mL. The amount of alcohol available for dissolution would be approximately 77% $\times$ 6.1 mL = 4.7 mL.

Podophyllum: Although podophyllum is listed as soluble in alcohol (1 g/10–30 mL), it should be satisfactory at the 12% concentration because its usual recommended concentration in alcoholic vehicles is 12% to 25%. In this preparation, the high concentration of salicylic acid may tie up solvent and limit the amount of alcohol available for dissolving the podophyllum.

Salicylic Acid: The solubility of salicylic acid in alcohol is given as 1 g/3 mL. In this prescription, we have 1.875 g salicylic acid, so we need 1.875 g $\times$ 3 mL/g = 5.63 mL of alcohol. Because we have only about 4.7 mL of alcohol in this preparation, we have too little to dissolve the salicylic acid. If the salicylic acid concentration is changed to 15%, then the quantity of salicylic acid would be reduced to 0.15 $\times$ 7.5 = 1.125 g, and we would need only 1.125 g $\times$ 3 mL/g = 3.375 mL of alcohol for dissolution. Because this concentration is still in the therapeutically effective range for salicylic acid, it would be acceptable to request a change of concentration of salicylic acid to 15%. Because the preceding is based on estimates, the preparation should be observed for proper dissolution.

MSDS AND SAFETY AND PERSONAL PROTECTIVE EQUIPMENT: Review MSDS for all components. Don a clean lab coat, disposable gloves, and safety glasses. It is advisable to use a facemask when preparing this preparation because both salicylic acid and podophyllum are highly irritant powders that should not be inhaled. The *USP* also warns that podophyllum resin is highly irritating to the eyes and mucous membranes (3).

SPECIALIZED EQUIPMENT: All weighing is done on an electronic balance.

COMPOUNDING PROCEDURE: Weigh 1.125 g salicylic acid and place in a clean 50-mL beaker. Add about 4.5 mL of Compound Benzoin Tincture to dissolve the salicylic acid. Stir to mix and observe for complete dissolution. Weigh 900 mg of podophyllum and dust a portion on top of the solution in the beaker and stir gently. Repeat until all is added and completely dissolved. Precalibrate an applicator bottle at 7.5 mL, using alcohol as the calibration liquid (as water is incompatible with this preparation). Transfer the prepared solution to the bottle. Use additional Compound Benzoin Tincture to rinse the solution from the beaker into the applicator bottle for a complete transfer of active ingredients and qs to the final volume calibration mark. Place the applicator cap on the bottle and close tightly. Agitate the solution to ensure complete mixing. Label and dispense.

DESCRIPTION OF FINISHED PREPARATION: The preparation is a dark brown, viscous solution. There should be no visible precipitate or sediment. It has the characteristic odor of Compound Benzoin Tincture.

QUALITY CONTROL: The actual volume is checked and matches the theoretical volume of 7.5 mL.

MASTER FORMULA PREPARED BY: Billie Burke, PharmD

CHECKED BY: Mary Ann Kirkpatrick, RPh, PhD

COMPOUNDING RECORD

NAME, STRENGTH, AND DOSAGE FORM OF PREPARATION: Podophyllum 12% and Salicylic Acid 15% in Compound Benzoin Tincture Topical Solution

QUANTITY: 7.5 mL **DATE PREPARED:** mm/dd/yy **BEYOND-USE DATE:** mm/dd/yy
FORMULATION RECORD ID: SN004 **CONTROL/RX NUMBER:** 123780

INGREDIENTS USED:

Ingredient	Quantity Used	Manufacturer Lot Number	Expiration Date	Weighed/ Measured by	Checked by
Salicylic Acid	1.125 g	JET Labs SN2641	mm/yy	bjf	bb
Podophyllum	900 mg	JET Labs SN2642	mm/yy	bjf	bb
Compound Benzoin Tincture	qs 7.5 mL	JET Labs SN2643	mm/yy	bjf	bb

QUALITY CONTROL DATA: The preparation is a dark brown, viscous solution. It was observed at 1 hour and showed no visible precipitate or sediment. It has the characteristic odor of Compound Benzoin Tincture. The actual volume was checked and it matches the theoretical volume of 7.5 mL.

LABELING

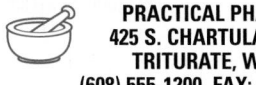

PRACTICAL PHARMACY
425 S. CHARTULAE STREET
TRITURATE, WI 53706
(608) 555-1200 FAX: (608) 555-1210

℞ 123780	Pharmacist: BB	Date: 00/00/00
Pam Perfect		Dr. J. L. Parker

Apply to warts each night at bedtime.

Podophyllum 12%, Salicylic Acid 15% in Compound Benzoin Topical Tincture

Mfg: Compounded	Quantity: 7.5 mL
Refills: 1	Discard after: Give date

Auxiliary Labels: Caution: Flammable. For external use only. Keep out of the reach of children. This medicine was compounded in our pharmacy for you at the direction of your prescriber.

PATIENT CONSULTATION: Hello, Ms. Perfect, I'm your pharmacist, Billie Burke. Do you have any drug allergies? Are you taking or using any prescription or nonprescription medications? This is a specially formulated solution containing podophyllum and salicylic acid in Compound Benzoin Tincture and is used to treat plantar warts. Apply it to your warts each night at bedtime, using the applicator provided in the bottle. You may want to cover the skin surrounding each wart with Vaseline for protection of the healthy skin. Be very careful not to get this near your eyes or mouth and be sure to wash your hands carefully after handling this solution because it is very irritating to healthy skin. If the treated area becomes irritated or the condition worsens, contact Dr. Parker. Keep the bottle tightly closed and store it at room temperature, away from heat, and out of reach of children. It is a flammable liquid that should be kept away from any open flame, lighted smoking materials, or anything else that may ignite it. Discard any unused portion after 1 month. You may get one refill if you need it. Do you have any questions?

SAMPLE PRESCRIPTION 27.5

CASE: Ronnie Snax is a 160-lb, 6′-tall, 50-year old male patient who has just returned from trout fishing. He has a number of small red welts on his legs that itch intensely. He immediately called his primary physician, Roberta Barksen and, fortunately, she was able to see him during her lunch break. She has diagnosed chigger bites and has prescribed a customized hydroalcoholic solution of the local anesthetic benzocaine with the anti-infective benzethonium chloride to prevent any secondary infection of the bite sites. Dr. Barksen also recommended OTC hydrocortisone maximum-strength cream. Ronnie has no other health problems and reports that the only other medications he takes are a multivitamin with minerals and, occasionally, Aleve for muscle strains.

CONTEMPORARY PHYSICIANS GROUP PRACTICE
20 S. PARK STREET, TRITURATE, WI 53706
TEL: (608) 555-1333 FAX: (608) 555-1335

℞ #   *123772*

NAME *Ronnie Snax*   **DATE** *00/00/00*

ADDRESS *425 Instinct Lane*

℞

Benzocaine	*3%*
Benzethonium Chloride	*0.1%*
Alcohol	*qs*
Methyl Salicylate	*qs*
Purified Water	*qs ad 30 mL*

Fernie Bohunting 00/00/00

Sig: Apply to bites 3 to 4 times daily prn for itching

REFILLS *2*   *Roberta Barksen*   **M.D.**

DEA No. _____

MASTER COMPOUNDING FORMULATION RECORD

NAME, STRENGTH, AND DOSAGE FORM OF PREPARATION: Benzocaine 3% and Benzethonium Cl 0.1% Topical Solution
QUANTITY: 30 mL   **FORMULATION RECORD ID:** SN005
THERAPEUTIC USE/CATEGORY: Antiseptic/anesthetic   **ROUTE OF ADMINISTRATION:** Topical

INGREDIENTS:

Ingredient	Quantity Used	Physical Description	Solubility	Dose Comparison		Use in the Prescription
				Given	Usual	
Benzocaine	900 mg	white, crystalline powder	1 g/2,500 mL water or 5 mL alcohol	3%	1%–20%	local anesthetic
Benzethonium Chloride	120 mg weighed, 30 mg used	white crystals	v sol in water sol in alcohol	0.1%	0.1%	antimicrobial, antiseptic
Alcohol	22 mL	clear, colorless mobile liquid	miscible with water	—	—	solvent, preservative
Methyl Salicylate	5 drops	light yellow liquid w/ odor of wintergreen	sl sol in water sol in alcohol	—	—	scent
Purified Water	qs ad 30 mL	clear, colorless liquid	—	—	—	vehicle

COMPATIBILITY–STABILITY: The benzethonium chloride, alcohol, and methyl salicylate in this preparation are compatible and very stable when in a hydroalcoholic solution. In an aqueous solution, the benzocaine presents some concerns for both physical compatibility and chemical stability. With regard to physical compatibility, benzocaine is quite insoluble in water, and a cosolvent system containing alcohol is required for dissolution. Calculations for the relative amounts of water and alcohol are shown later. With regard to chemical stability, benzocaine is an ester that undergoes hydrolysis in aqueous solution. Information on the stability of benzocaine was found in the reference *Chemical Stability of Pharmaceuticals* (8). Benzocaine undergoes both acid and base catalyzed hydrolysis, and it is most stable at neutral pH. The half-life at pH 9 and 30°C is 127 days. This translates to a shelf life under those conditions of about 19 days. This preparation has a neutral pH, so this would provide more stable conditions. No extra preservative is needed because benzethonium Cl is an antimicrobial agent. In addition, the alcohol content is 70%.

PACKAGING AND STORAGE: This preparation should be packaged in a tight container. Controlled room temperature will be the recommended storage conditions.

BEYOND-USE DATE: Using the literature cited earlier as a guide, Pharmacist Bohunting will use a 14-day beyond-use date for this preparation.

CALCULATIONS

Dose/Concentration: Concentrations okay for intended use

Ingredient Amounts

Benzocaine: $3\% \times 30$ mL $= 0.03 \times 30$ mL $= 0.9$ g $= 900$ mg

Benzethonium Cl: $0.1\% \times 30$ mL $= 0.001 \times 30$ mL $= 0.03$ g $= 30$ mg

The 30 mg of benzethonium Cl is below the MWQ for the class III torsion balance, so an aliquot is needed. Benzethonium Cl is very soluble in water, so a solid–liquid aliquot using water would be convenient. If we weigh the MWQ of 120 mg of benzethonium Cl and qs ad 4 mL with water, we get a solution of 120 mg/4 mL $= 30$ mg/mL. One milliliter of this solution measured with a 1-mL syringe will be the amount needed.

Benzocaine has very limited solubility in water (1 g/2,500 mL), but it is very soluble in alcohol (1 g/5 mL). Therefore, a cosolvent system is needed, and the required alcohol content can be estimated using the log solubility equation given in this chapter and shown here:

log solubility equation: $\log S_T = vf_{water} \log S_{water} + vf_{alc} \log S_{alc}$

To use this equation, all concentrations must be expressed using the same units.

Total required solution concentration (S_T) of benzocaine (in mg/mL):

$$3\% = 3 \text{ g}/100 \text{ mL} = 3{,}000 \text{ mg}/100 \text{ mL} = 30 \text{ mg/mL}$$

Water solubility (S_{water}) of benzocaine (in mg/mL):

$$1 \text{ g}/2{,}500 \text{ mL} = 1{,}000 \text{ mg}/2{,}500 \text{ mL} = 0.4 \text{ mg/mL}$$

Alcohol solubility (S_{alc}) of benzocaine (in mg/mL):

$$1 \text{ g}/5 \text{ mL} = 1{,}000 \text{ mg}/5 \text{ mL} = 200 \text{ mg/mL}$$

The sum of the volume fractions is 1: $vf_{water} + vf_{alc} = 1$

Therefore: $vf_{water} = 1 - vf_{alc}$

Substituting: $\log 30 = (1 - vf_{alc}) \log 0.4 + vf_{alc} \log 200$

Solving for the volume fraction of alcohol (vf_{alc}):

$$\log 30 = \log 0.4 - vf_{alc} \log 0.4 + vf_{alc} \log 200$$

$$\log 30 - \log 0.4 = vf_{alc} \log 200 - vf_{alc} \log 0.4 = vf_{alc} (\log 200 - \log 0.4)$$

$$vf_{alc} = \frac{(\log 30 - \log 0.4)}{(\log 200 - \log 0.4)} = \frac{1.87506}{2.69897} \approx 69.5\% \text{ Å } 70\%$$

Based on an alcohol-water cosolvent system with 70% alcohol, we can calculate the volume of ethanol (C_2H_5OH) needed for our preparation: 70% × 30 mL = 21 mL. Using Alcohol USP 95%, we can calculate the number of milliliters of this needed for our cosolvent system:

$$\frac{95 \text{ mL C}_2\text{H}_5\text{OH}}{100 \text{ mL Alcohol USP}} = \frac{21 \text{ mL C}_2\text{H}_5\text{OH}}{x \text{ mL Alcohol USP}}; \; x = 22 \text{ mL Alcohol USP}$$

MSDS AND SAFETY AND PERSONAL PROTECTIVE EQUIPMENT: Review MSDS for all components. Don a clean lab coat and disposable gloves.

SPECIALIZED EQUIPMENT: Class III torsion balance

COMPOUNDING PROCEDURE: Weigh 900 mg of benzocaine and transfer to a clean beaker. Measure 22 mL of Alcohol USP in a 25-mL graduated cylinder and add to the benzocaine to dissolve it. Weigh 120 mg of benzethonium Cl, transfer it to a 10-mL graduated cylinder, and qs ad 4 mL with Purified Water. Stir with a glass stirring rod to completely dissolve and mix. With a 1-mL disposable syringe, measure 1 mL of the benzethonium Cl solution and add this to the benzocaine solution. Add 5 drops of methyl salicylate and transfer the solution to a 50-mL graduated cylinder and qs to the 30-mL mark using Purified Water. Using a pH range 2 to 9 test strip, check and record the pH of the solution. Pour this solution into a 1-oz dauber bottle and tightly cap the bottle. Label and dispense.

DESCRIPTION OF FINISHED PREPARATION: The preparation is a clear, colorless solution with apparent viscosity approximately that of alcohol. It has the characteristic odor of alcohol and wintergreen.

QUALITY CONTROL: The pH of the preparation is checked with a pH range 2 to 9 test strip: pH = 5.5. The actual volume is checked and matches the theoretical volume of 30 mL.

MASTER FORMULA PREPARED BY: Fernie Bohunting, RPh

CHECKED BY: Mary Ann Kirkpatrick, RPh, PhD

COMPOUNDING RECORD

NAME, STRENGTH, AND DOSAGE FORM OF PREPARATION: Benzocaine 3% and Benzethonium Cl 0.1% Topical Solution
QUANTITY: 30 mL   **DATE PREPARED:** mm/dd/yy   **BEYOND-USE DATE:** mm/dd/yy
FORMULATION RECORD ID: SN005   **CONTROL/RX NUMBER:** 123772

INGREDIENTS USED:

Ingredient	Quantity Used	Manufacturer Lot Number	Expiration Date	Weighed/ Measured by	Checked by
Benzocaine	900 mg	JET Labs SN2651	mm/yy	bjf	fb
Benzethonium Chloride	120 mg weighed, 30 mg used	JET Labs SV2652	mm/yy	bjf	fb
Alcohol	22 mL	JET Labs SN2653	mm/yy	bjf	fb
Methyl Salicylate	5 drops	JET Labs SN2654	mm/yy	bjf	fb
Purified Water	qs 30 mL	Sweet Springs AL0529	mm/yy	bjf	fb

QUALITY CONTROL DATA: The preparation is a clear, colorless solution with apparent viscosity approximately that of alcohol. It has the characteristic odor of wintergreen and alcohol. The pH of the preparation was checked with a pH range 2 to 9 test strip: pH = 5.5. The actual volume was checked and matches the theoretical volume of 30 mL.

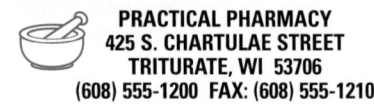

LABELING

PRACTICAL PHARMACY
425 S. CHARTULAE STREET
TRITURATE, WI 53706
(608) 555-1200 FAX: (608) 555-1210

℞ 123772   Pharmacist: FB   Date: 00/00/00
Ronnie Snax   Dr. R. Barksen

Apply to affected bites three to four times a day as needed for itching.

Benzocaine 3%, Benzethonium Cl 0.1% Topical Solution

Contains Alcohol 70%

Mfg: Compounded   Quantity: 30 mL

Refills: 2   Discard after: Give date

Auxiliary Labels: Caution: Flammable. For External Use Only. Keep out of the reach of children. This medicine was compounded in our pharmacy for you at the direction of your prescriber.

PATIENT CONSULTATION: Hello, Mr. Snax, I'm Pharmacist Fernie Bohunting. I have your prescription for your chigger bites. Are you taking or using any other prescription or nonprescription medications currently? Do you have any allergies? What did Dr. Barksen tell you about this medication? This is a custom formula used by Dr. Barksen for chigger and other insect bites. It contains the local anesthetic benzocaine for the itching and also has benzethonium chloride and alcohol to prevent any infection. You are to dab this on the bites three to four times a day as needed for the itching. I have had other patients tell me that it works pretty well, but if your bites don't improve or they worsen, contact Dr. Barksen so we can try something else. Store this at room temperature and away from sunlight. This is for external use only and should be kept out of the reach of children. It does contain a fairly large percentage of alcohol, so be careful not to get it near your eyes, and wash your hands after applying it. It is a flammable liquid that should be kept away from any open flame, lighted smoking materials, or anything else that may ignite it, and the bottle should be kept tightly closed. Discard any unused portion after 2 weeks (give date). If needed, you may have this refilled two times. Because I have helped other patients with these nasty bites, I did go online and found some good information on The Ohio State University Extension Internet site. It gives suggestions on preventing contact with chiggers and other useful hints for dealing with these pests. If you have a computer, I would check it out; otherwise, let me know and I could print something for you. Do you have any questions?

SAMPLE PRESCRIPTION 27.6

CASE: Lilly La Lane is a 110-lb, 5′3″-tall, 16-year-old female patient with acne vulgaris. For the past 4 weeks, she has been using with good success a commercially available 1% clindamycin suspension. Recently, the manufacturer has not been able to supply the product to pharmacies and wholesalers, so Pharmacist Becky Bilder has offered to compound a similar preparation until the manufactured product becomes available again. Miss La Lane's medication profile record shows that she uses sumatriptan for migraine headaches and ibuprofen for menstrual pain. She reports that she uses OTC Dayquil when she gets a cold.

CONTEMPORARY PHYSICIANS GROUP PRACTICE
20 S. PARK STREET, TRITURATE, WI 53706
TEL: (608) 555-1333 FAX: (608) 555-1335

℞ # *123756*

NAME *Lilly La Lane*   DATE *00/00/00*

ADDRESS *592 Pirate Cove Apts.*

℞

Clindamycin		*1%*
Propylene Glycol		*1.5 mL*
Isopropyl Alcohol 50%	*aa qs ad*	
Purified Water		*15 mL*

B. Bilder 00/00/00

Sig: Apply as directed to acne q am and hs

Refills *3*   *Ozzie Wurtz*   M.D.

DEA No. _____

MASTER COMPOUNDING FORMULATION RECORD

NAME, STRENGTH, AND DOSAGE FORM OF PREPARATION: Clindamycin 1% Topical Solution

QUANTITY: 15 mL

THERAPEUTIC USE/CATEGORY: Antiacne

FORMULATION RECORD ID: SN006

ROUTE OF ADMINISTRATION: Topical

INGREDIENTS:

Ingredient	Quantity Used	Physical Description	Solubility	Dose Comparison Given	Dose Comparison Usual	Use in the Prescription
Clindamycin (as HCl)	150 mg (base) (1 capsule)	white powder	freely sol in water and alcohol	1%	1%	antibiotic
Propylene Glycol	1.5 mL	clear, colorless, viscous liquid	miscible with water and alcohol	10%	varies	solvent, humectant, antiseptic
Isopropyl Alcohol (IPA) 70%	7.1 mL to make 10 mL 50% IPA	clear, colorless, mobile liquid	miscible with water	22.5%	varies	solvent, antiseptic
Purified Water	qs 15 mL	clear, colorless liquid	—	—	—	vehicle

COMPATIBILITY–STABILITY: With regard to chemical stability, topical clindamycin solutions in this type of solvent system have been evaluated and reported in the literature. A good review of this subject can be found in the clindamycin monograph in *Trissel's Stability of Compounded Formulations*. At 25°C, these formulations were stable for at least 6 months, but a 6- to 8-week beyond-use date was recommended (9). With regard to solubility and physical stability, Clindamycin HCl is freely soluble (1 g/1–10 mL) in water and soluble (1 g/10–30 mL) in alcohol. This means that the 0.15 g of clindamycin (as the HCl salt) in this preparation should dissolve in 0.15 to 1.5 mL water or 1.5 to 4.5 mL of alcohol. This information is important because capsule contents are being used for this preparation, and there may be insoluble excipients in those contents. If a solution is to be made, the preparation should be filtered. Although we want to filter out the inert ingredients, we don't want to filter any drug. Therefore, we want to be certain to dissolve all of the drug from the capsule contents. To ensure complete dissolution of this large molecule, it is recommended that the capsule contents be put in a sufficient amount of the solvent system (approximately 30 mL for four capsules) and the liquid shaken for 30-second time intervals and repeated several times over a 10- to 15-minute period before filtering out the excipients. Additional solvent is then added to the remaining solids and the process repeated, rinsing this portion through the same filter (9). No additional preservative is needed for this preparation, because the formula contains both the antibacterial clindamycin and 23% isopropyl alcohol.

PACKAGING AND STORAGE: Because the *USP* monographs for clindamycin solutions recommend packaging in tight containers, this is recommended for this preparation (3). Use a dauber bottle for convenient application. Storage should be at controlled room temperature.

BEYOND-USE DATE: Using the literature cited earlier as a guide, use a 1-month beyond-use date for this preparation; however, because this solution uses the contents of a commercial capsule, the beyond-use date for the preparation may not exceed 25% of the time left of the expiration date of the capsules.

CALCULATIONS

Dose/Concentration: Concentrations/strengths/doses for clindamycin are expressed in terms of the base, even though the drug is in the salt form in commercial products. A 1% concentration of clindamycin (base) is appropriate for the intended use.

Propylene glycol (PG): % v/v concentration is calculated to be:

$$\frac{1.5 \text{ mL PG}}{15 \text{ mL solution}} = \frac{x \text{ mL PG}}{100 \text{ mL solution}}; x = 10 \text{ mL PG/100mL solution} = 10\%$$

Isopropyl alcohol (IPA): % v/v concentration is calculated here.

Assuming a zero powder volume for the clindamycin and additive volumes for the liquids, the volume of the 1:1 mixture of Water and 50% IPA in the final solution is:

$$\frac{(15 \text{ mL} - 1.5 \text{ mL})}{2} = \frac{13.5 \text{ mL}}{2} = 6.75 \text{ mL}$$

The amount of pure IPA in 6.75 mL of 50% IPA is: $50\% \times 6.75 \text{ mL} = 3.38 \text{ mL}$.

The % v/v IPA in the finished preparation is:

$$\frac{3.38 \text{ mL IPA}}{15 \text{ mL solution}} = \frac{x \text{ mL IPA}}{100 \text{ mL solution}} \ x = 22.5 \text{ mL IPA/100 mL solution} = 22.5\% \approx 23\%$$

Ingredient Amounts

Clindamycin: $1\% \times 15 \text{ mL} = 0.01 \times 15 \text{ mL} = 0.15 \text{ g}$ clindamycin, which is the quantity in one 150-mg capsule.

50% isopropyl alcohol (IPA): Need to make this from the 70% IPA available in the pharmacy. The amount made may be any reasonable amount equal to or greater than 6.75 mL. It is decided that 10 mL of a 50% solution will be made. The amount of pure IPA needed is:

$$50\% \times 10 \text{ mL} = 0.5 \times 10 \text{ mL} = 5 \text{ mL}$$

The volume of 70% IPA to give 5 mL of IPA is:

$$\frac{70 \text{ mL IPA}}{100 \text{ mL of 70\% solution}} = \frac{5 \text{ mL IPA}}{x \text{ mL of 70\% solution}}; x = 7.1 \text{ mL of 70\% solution}$$

Measure 7.1 mL of 70% IPA and qs to 10 mL with Purified Water.

MSDS AND SAFETY AND PERSONAL PROTECTIVE EQUIPMENT: Review MSDS for all components. Don a clean lab coat and disposable gloves.

SPECIALIZED EQUIPMENT: None

COMPOUNDING PROCEDURE: Make 10 mL of 50% IPA by measuring 7.1 mL of 70% IPA in a 10-mL graduated cylinder and qs ad 10 mL with Purified Water. Transfer this solution to a 25-mL graduated cylinder and add 10 mL of Purified Water to this to make a 50:50 solution of Purified Water and 50% IPA. Stir to mix. Empty the contents of one clindamycin 150-mg capsule into a beaker and add 6 mL of the 50:50 solvent mixture to dissolve the drug. Allow it to dissolve with intermittent stirring over 10 to 15 minutes. Filter this solution into a 25-mL graduated cylinder. Using a 3-mL syringe, measure 1.5 mL of propylene glycol and add this to the drug solution. Using another 6-mL portion of the 50:50 solvent mixture, rinse the beaker and filter into the drug solution to ensure complete dissolution and transfer of the drug. Then qs to 15 mL with the 50:50 solvent mixture. Using a glass stirring rod, mix the solution well. Using a portable pH meter, check and record the pH of the solution. Transfer the solution to a dauber bottle. Label and dispense.

DESCRIPTION OF FINISHED PREPARATION: The preparation is a clear, colorless solution with apparent viscosity approximately that of a water–alcohol solution. It has the characteristic odor of isopropyl alcohol.

QUALITY CONTROL: Check the pH of the preparation using a portable pH meter: pH = 5.5. The actual volume is checked and should match the theoretical volume of 15 mL.

MASTER FORMULA PREPARED BY: Becky Bilder, PharmD

CHECKED BY: Mary Ann Kirkpatrick, RPh, PhD

COMPOUNDING RECORD

NAME, STRENGTH, AND DOSAGE FORM OF PREPARATION: Clindamycin 1% Topical Solution
QUANTITY: 15 mL   **DATE PREPARED:** mm/dd/yy   **BEYOND-USE DATE:** mm/dd/yy
CONTROL/RX NUMBER: 123756   **FORMULATION RECORD ID:** SN006

INGREDIENTS USED:

Ingredient	Quantity Used	Manufacturer Lot Number	Expiration Date	Weighed/ Measured by	Checked by
Clindamycin (as HCl)	150 mg (base) (1 capsule)	Premium Generics SN2661	mm/yy	bjf	bb
Propylene Glycol	1.5 mL	JET Labs SV2662	mm/yy	bjf	bb
Isopropyl Alcohol (IPA) 70%	7.1 mL to make 10 mL 50% IPA used 6.75 mL of the 50% solution	JET Labs SN2663	mm/yy	bjf	bb
Purified Water	q.s. 15 mL	Sweet Springs AL0529	mm/yy	bjf	bb

QUALITY CONTROL DATA: The preparation is a clear, colorless solution with apparent viscosity approximately that of a water–alcohol solution. It has the characteristic odor of isopropyl alcohol. The pH of the preparation was checked using a portable pH meter: pH = 5.5. The actual volume was checked and matches the theoretical volume of 15 mL.

LABELING

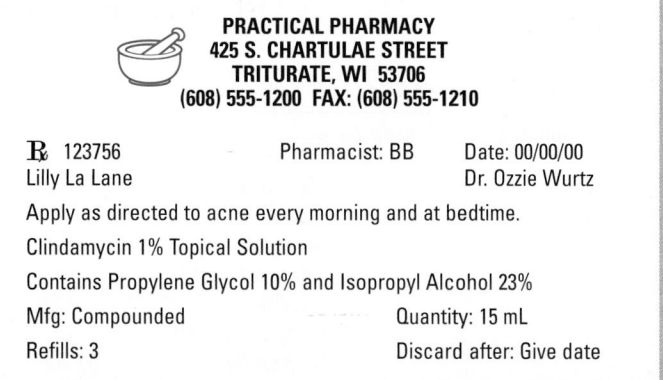

PRACTICAL PHARMACY
425 S. CHARTULAE STREET
TRITURATE, WI 53706
(608) 555-1200 FAX: (608) 555-1210

℞ 123756   Pharmacist: BB   Date: 00/00/00
Lilly La Lane   Dr. Ozzie Wurtz

Apply as directed to acne every morning and at bedtime.

Clindamycin 1% Topical Solution

Contains Propylene Glycol 10% and Isopropyl Alcohol 23%

Mfg: Compounded   Quantity: 15 mL

Refills: 3   Discard after: Give date

Auxiliary Labels: Flammable; keep away from heat and flame. For External Use Only. This medicine was compounded in our pharmacy for you at the direction of your prescriber.

PATIENT CONSULTATION: Hello, Miss La Lane, I'm your pharmacist, Becky Bilder. Do you have any drug allergies? Are you taking any prescription or over-the-counter medications? This is the custom compounded clindamycin solution to treat your acne. You can use it just like the commercial product that you have been using. Apply it to your acne every morning and every evening at bedtime. Wash and rinse the area carefully, then wait about 15 minutes to a half-hour before applying the solution. Apply to entire area, not just to pimples. You have used these dauber bottles before; have they worked well for you? This solution contains alcohol so keep it away from your eyes or other sensitive parts, and wash your hands after applying the solution. Because it is a flammable liquid, it should be kept away from any open flame, lighted smoking materials, or anything else that may ignite it. Have you experienced any adverse effects when using the commercial clindamycin? A rare but serious side effect is signaled by the onset of severe abdominal cramping or diarrhea, so if you experience this, stop using this solution and get in touch with Dr. Wurtz immediately. This preparation is for external use only. The bottle should be kept tightly closed and should be stored at room temperature and out of the reach of children. You may have three refills. Discard any unused portion after 1 month (or 25% rule; give date). Do you have any questions?

SAMPLE PRESCRIPTION 27.7

CASE: Beavus Budhead is a 145-lb, 5′10″-tall, 16-year-old male patient with external otitis (swimmer's ear). He recently started a job at the local YMCA summer camp on Crystal Lake, where he works as a lifeguard and swimming instructor. This morning he awoke with a very painful left ear. He saw Dr. Osgood's physician's assistant, Susette Thompson, who diagnosed inflammation and mild infection of the external ear canal. She and Dr. Osgood want to try topical treatment before going to a systemic antibiotic. Beavus reports no other current medical problems. He has attention deficit disorder (ADD), but he takes medication for this only during the school year. He says that he applies Vaseline Intensive Care Blockout as a sunscreen several times each day when he is outdoors on the waterfront.

CONTEMPORARY PHYSICIANS GROUP PRACTICE
20 S. PARK STREET, TRITURATE, WI 53706
TEL: (608) 555-1333 FAX: (608) 555-1335

℞ # *714*

NAME *Beavus Budhead*   **DATE** *00/00/00*

ADDRESS *931 Dumbdy Lane*

℞

Antipyrine	*5%*
Hydrocortisone	*0.5%*
Neomycin sulfate	*5 mg/mL*
Na metabisulfite	*0.1%*
Glycerin	*25%*
Propylene Glycol	*25%*
Purified Water *qs ad*	*30 mL*

Al Bungy 0/00/00

Sig: Instill 4 drops in left ear 3-4 times daily

REFILLS *0*   *Norace Osgood*   **M.D.**

DEA NO. _____

MASTER COMPOUNDING FORMULATION RECORD

NAME, STRENGTH, AND DOSAGE FORM OF PREPARATION: Antipyrine 5%, Hydrocortisone 0.5%, and Neomycin Sulfate 0.5% Otic Solution

QUANTITY: 30 mL

THERAPEUTIC USE/CATEGORY: External otitis infection

FORMULATION RECORD ID: SN007

ROUTE OF ADMINISTRATION: Otic

INGREDIENTS:

Ingredient	Quantity Used	Physical Description	Solubility	Dose Comparison		Use in the Prescription
				Given	Usual	
Antipyrine	1.5 g	white powder	1 g/mL water or 1.3 mL alcohol	5%	5%	antipyretic, analgesic
Hydrocortisone	150 mg	white powder	v sl sol in water, 1 g/40 mL alcohol	0.5%	0.5%–2.5%	anti-inflammatory
Neomycin Sulfate	150 mg	white powder	1 g/mL water, v sl sol alcohol	5 mg/mL (0.5%)	5 mg/mL	antibiotic
Sodium Metabisulfite	120 mg weighed, 30 mg used	white powder	1 g/2 mL water, v sl sol alcohol	0.1%	0.1%	antioxidant
Glycerin	7.5 mL	clear, colorless viscous liquid	miscible with water or alcohol	25%	varies	humectant, preservative, vehicle
Propylene Glycol	7.5 mL	clear, colorless liquid	miscible with water or alcohol	25%	varies	humectant, preservative, vehicle
Purified Water	qs 30 mL	clear, colorless liquid	—	—	—	vehicle

COMPATIBILITY–STABILITY: No stability data for this specific formulation is available. Because of the multiple ingredients and the cosolvent system in this preparation, it is a difficult formulation to evaluate. From a chemical stability standpoint, the antipyrine in aqueous solution has been evaluated and found to be reasonably stable, although storage in tight, light-resistant containers is recommended (10). Aqueous solutions of neomycin sulfate are reported to be stable over a fairly wide pH range, pH 2 to 9, but the drug is subject to oxidation, and tight, light-resistant containers should be used (11). The hydrocortisone is somewhat more difficult to assess. It undergoes oxidation and other complex degradation reactions. It is most stable at pH 3.5 to 4.5, and its stability is quite dependent on pH, with steep slopes for its pH profile in both the acidic and basic regions (12). The presence of the antioxidant sodium metabisulfite should stabilize both the neomycin and hydrocortisone to oxidative degradation. The physical stability of this solution is also difficult to predict. The antipyrine does not pose a problem, because it is soluble in both water and organic solvents such as glycerin and propylene glycol. In contrast, neomycin sulfate is soluble in water but not very soluble in organic solvents, while hydrocortisone is relatively soluble in organic solvents [e.g., 12.7 mg/mL in propylene glycol (12)] but very slightly soluble in water. Fortunately, both the hydrocortisone and neomycin sulfate are present in low concentrations, and the preparation uses a cosolvent system, but it is difficult to predict with certainty whether a solution will result. Order of mixing is important in making this solution: Begin by adding the water-soluble ingredients to water and the hydrocortisone to the organic solvents; then carefully combine. Finally, it is necessary to observe the finished preparation for complete dissolution of all components. No extra preservative is needed because 50% of the preparation is a glycerin–propylene glycol cosolvent, and both of these ingredients act as preservatives at this concentration.

PACKAGING AND STORAGE: Packaging should be in a tight, light-resistant container, with recommended storage at controlled room temperature.

BEYOND-USE DATE: Use the *USP* recommended maximum 14-day beyond-use date for compounded water-containing liquid formulations prepared from ingredients in solid form when there is no stability information for the formulation (6).

CALCULATIONS

Dose/Concentration: All concentrations are okay.

A % w/v concentration for labeling the neomycin sulfate can be calculated as follows:

$$\frac{0.005 \text{ g neomycin sulfate}}{\text{mL solution}} = \frac{x \text{ g neomycin sulfate}}{100 \text{ mL solution}}; x = 0.5\% \text{ neomycin sulfate}$$

Ingredient Amounts

Antipyrine: $\qquad 5\% \times 30 \text{ mL} = 0.05 \times 30 \text{ mL} = 1.5 \text{ g}$

Hydrocortisone: $\qquad 0.5\% \times 30 \text{ mL} = 0.005 \times 30 \text{ mL} = 0.15 \text{ g} = 150 \text{ mg}$

Neomycin sulfate: $\qquad 5 \text{ mg/mL} \times 30 \text{ mL} = 150 \text{ mg}$

Sodium metabisulfite: $\qquad 0.1\% \times 30 \text{ mL} = 0.001 \times 30 \text{ mL} = 0.03 \text{ g} = 30 \text{ mg}$

Glycerin and propylene glycol: $\qquad 25\% \times 30 \text{ mL} = 0.25 \times 30 \text{ mL} = 7.5 \text{ mL of each}$

Sodium metabisulfite aliquot:

Weigh four times the amount needed, 120 mg, qs ad 8 mL with water, and take $^1/_4$ that volume, 2 mL, to give 30 mg. The validity of this may be checked as follows:

$$120 \text{ mg/8 mL} = 15 \text{ mg/mL}$$

$$15 \text{ mg/mL} \times 2 \text{ mL} = 30 \text{ mg}$$

MSDS AND SAFETY AND PERSONAL PROTECTIVE EQUIPMENT: Review MSDS for all components. Don a clean lab coat and disposable gloves. Avoid inhaling powders.

SPECIALIZED EQUIPMENT: Class III torsion balance

COMPOUNDING PROCEDURE: Weigh 150 mg of neomycin sulfate, transfer to a clean beaker, and dissolve in 4 mL of Purified Water. Weigh 120 mg of sodium metabisulfite, transfer it to a 10-mL graduated cylinder, and qs ad 8 mL with Purified Water. Stir to mix. Measure 2 mL of this solution and add it to the beaker containing the neomycin sulfate. Next weigh 1.5 g of antipyrine and add this to the beaker. It should dissolve in the 6 mL of water present, but a small amount of additional water may be added for complete dissolution. Weigh 150 mg of hydrocortisone and place in a separate clean beaker. The hydrocortisone is soluble in glycerin and propylene glycol, but it is not easily wetted by these viscous liquids, so wet the hydrocortisone with a few drops of Alcohol. Add 7.5 mL each of glycerin and propylene glycol and swirl to mix. Put the beaker in a warm-water bath and heat gently to dissolve the hydrocortisone. (A few seconds in a microwave oven also works, but there may be concern about drug degradation.) Transfer both drug solutions to a 50-mL graduated cylinder. Use Purified Water to rinse the beakers to ensure complete transfers of the solutions and to qs to the 30-mL mark. Using a glass stirring rod, mix well and inspect to verify a clear solution with no precipitates. Using a portable pH meter, check and record the pH of the solution. Transfer the solution to a ½-oz dropper bottle and cap tightly. Label and dispense.

DESCRIPTION OF FINISHED PREPARATION: The preparation is a clear, colorless or slightly yellowish solution with apparent viscosity slightly greater than that of water.

QUALITY CONTROL: Use a portable pH meter to check the pH of the preparation: pH = 6. The actual volume is checked and matches the theoretical volume of 30 mL.

MASTER FORMULA PREPARED BY: Al Bungy, PharmD

CHECKED BY: Mary Ann Kirkpatrick, RPh, PhD

COMPOUNDING RECORD

NAME, STRENGTH, AND DOSAGE FORM OF PREPARATION: Antipyrine 5%, Hydrocortisone 0.5%, and Neomycin Sulfate 0.5% Topical Solution

QUANTITY: 30 mL **DATE PREPARED:** mm/dd/yy **BEYOND-USE DATE:** mm/dd/yy
CONTROL/RX NUMBER: 123714 **FORMULATION RECORD ID:** SN007

INGREDIENTS USED:

Ingredient	Quantity Used	Manufacturer Lot Number	Expiration Date	Weighed/ Measured by	Checked by
Antipyrine	1.5 g	JET Labs SN2691	mm/yy	bjf	ab
Hydrocortisone	150 mg	JET Labs SN2692	mm/yy	bjf	ab
Neomycin Sulfate	150 mg	JET Labs SN2693	mm/yy	bjf	ab
Sodium Metabisulfite	120 mg weighed, 30 mg used	JET Labs SN2694	mm/yy	bjf	ab
Glycerin	7.5 mL	JET Labs SS2813	mm/yy	bjf	ab
Propylene Glycol	7.5 mL	JET Labs SV2662	mm/yy	bjf	ab
Purified Water	qs 30 mL	Sweet Springs AL0529	mm/yy	bjf	ab

QUALITY CONTROL DATA: The preparation is a clear, colorless solution with apparent viscosity slightly greater than that of water. The pH of the preparation was checked using a portable pH meter: pH = 6. The actual volume was checked and matches the theoretical volume of 30 mL.

LABELING

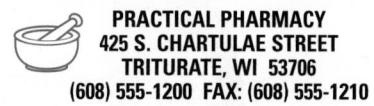

PRACTICAL PHARMACY
425 S. CHARTULAE STREET
TRITURATE, WI 53706
(608) 555-1200 FAX: (608) 555-1210

℞ 123714   Pharmacist: AB   Date: 00/00/00
Beavus Budhead   Dr. Norace Osgood

Put four drops in your left ear three to four times daily.

Antipyrine 5%, Hydrocortisone 0.5%, Neomycin Sulfate 0.5% Otic
Solution

Contains: Sodium Metabisulfite 0.1%, Glycerin 25%, Propylene Glycol
25%

Mfg: Compounded   Quantity: 30 mL

Refills: None   Discard after: Give date

Auxiliary Label: For the Ear. This medicine was compounded in our
pharmacy for you at the direction of your prescriber.

PATIENT CONSULTATION: Hello, Mr. Budhead, I'm your pharmacist, Al Bungy. Are you currently using any prescription or nonprescription medication? Are you allergic to any drugs? What has Ms. Thompson or Dr. Osgood told you about this medication? This is a custom-compounded solution containing a combination of drugs used to treat ear infections. It contains neomycin, which is an antibiotic, plus hydrocortisone and antipyrine, ingredients to treat the pain and inflammation. You are to place four drops into your left ear canal three to four times daily. After putting in the drops, I would place a cotton pledget just inside your ear to prevent leakage of the solution when your head is in an upright position. I am giving you this instruction sheet on using ear drops to give you some extra guidance. (See Fig. 27.1.) If your condition shows no improvement or gets worse, contact Ms. Thompson or Dr. Osgood. Keep the container tightly closed, in a cool dry place, and out of the reach of children. Discard any unused portion after 2 weeks. This prescription does not have any refills, so you will need to contact Dr. Osgood's office or me if you need a refill. If you are not relieved in 2 weeks, you should see Ms. Thompson or Dr. Osgood again anyway. Once this infection is cleared up, I would recommend that you prevent a recurrence by dropping two to three drops of rubbing alcohol into each ear after you come out of the water from swimming. Do you have any questions?

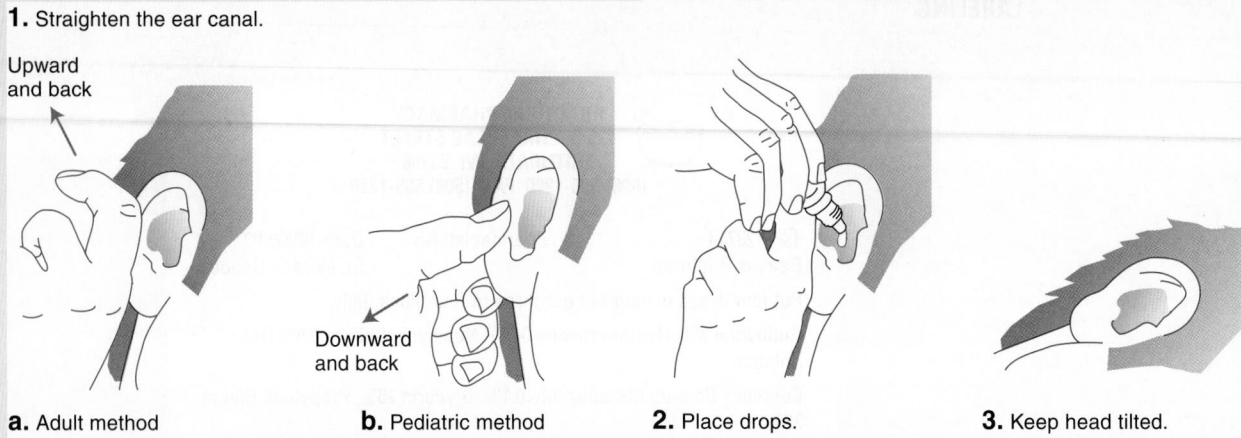

1. Straighten the ear canal.

Upward and back

a. Adult method

Downward and back

b. Pediatric method

2. Place drops.

3. Keep head tilted.

FIGURE 27.1 HOW TO USE EAR DROPS.
1. Wash your hands with soap and warm water.
2. Draw up a small amount of medication into the medicine dropper.
3. Lie on your side so that the affected ear points toward the ceiling.
4. Position the **tip** of the medicine dropper just inside the affected ear canal. Avoid touching the dropper against the ear or anything else. For adults, hold the earlobe up and back; for children, hold the earlobe down and back.
5. Squeeze the directed number of drops into your ear canal and allow the drops to run in.
6. Remain lying down for 3 to 5 minutes so that the medication has a chance to spread throughout the ear canal; you may gently massage the area around your ear to aid the spreading and distribution of the ear drops in the canal.
7. Place a clean cotton pledget just inside your ear to prevent leakage of the solution when your head is held in an upright position.
8. Replace the cap tightly on the bottle.

IMPORTANT
1. Never use ear drops if your eardrum has been damaged.
2. Avoid using very hot or very cold ear drops. The medication should be at room temperature or slightly warmer. If necessary, warm the drops by holding the bottle in your hand for a few minutes.

NOTE
It may be much easier to have someone else instill your ear drops.

(Image reprinted from Pray, SW. Nonprescription product therapeutics, 2nd ed. Baltimore, MD: Lippincott Williams & Wilkins, 2006.)

SAMPLE PRESCRIPTION 27.8

CASE: Jacob Stone is the 11-year-old male patient in Sample Prescription 25.4 who has undergone a multivisceral organ transplant. Originally, he was given his hydralazine in the form of powder packets, but now his mother has called Pharmacist Jennie Jackson and reported that Jacob does not like to take that powder in soft food. Mrs. Stone wants to know if there is a liquid product available. Jennie tells Mrs. Stone that there is no commercial product like this but that there is a compounded oral solution that she could make, and Jacob could try that. Jacob has a followup checkup this week, so Mrs. Stone brings in the prescription order shown here. Unfortunately, when Dr. Farrell wrote the prescription, he failed to specify a concentration, and he inadvertently wrote *mcg* when he meant *mg*. Dr. Jackson noticed this, called Dr. Farrell, and had the order clarified.

CONTEMPORARY PHYSICIANS GROUP PRACTICE
20 S. PARK STREET, TRITURATE, WI 53706
TEL: (608) 555-1333 FAX: (608) 555-1335

℞ # *123215*

NAME *Jacob Stone*   **DATE** *00/00/00*

ADDRESS *521 Lego Circle*

℞

Hydralazine HCl Oral Solution   *0.1% (5 mg/5 mL) J.J.*
Dispense   *60 mL*

Jennie Jackson 00/00/00

Change to 0.75 mg/kg/day
Sig: Give 0.75 mcg/kg/day po in four divided doses

Per phone consult with Dr. Farrell, dose was changed as indicated here. J.J.

REFILLS *2*   *R. Farrell*   **M.D.**

DEA NO. _____

MASTER COMPOUNDING FORMULATION RECORD

NAME, STRENGTH, AND DOSAGE FORM OF PREPARATION: Hydralazine HCl Oral Solution 0.1% (5 mg/5 mL)

QUANTITY: 60 mL

FORMULATION RECORD ID: SN008

THERAPEUTIC USE/CATEGORY: Antihypertensive

ROUTE OF ADMINISTRATION: Oral

INGREDIENTS:

Ingredient	Quantity Used	Physical Description	Solubility	Dose Comparison		Use in the Prescription
				Given	Usual	
Hydralazine HCl	60 mg	white powder	sol in water sl sol alcohol	0.75 mcg/kg/day changed to 0.75 mg/kg/day	0.75 mg/kg/day	antihypertensive
Sorbitol Solution 70%	18.7 mL	clear, colorless, viscous liquid	miscible with water or alcohol	40% w/v	—	sweetened vehicle
Propylene Glycol	5.8 mL	clear, colorless, viscous liquid	miscible with water or alcohol	10% w/v	varies	solvent, preservative
Methylparaben	39 mg	white powder	sl sol in water; fr sol in alcohol	0.065%	0.05%–0.25%	preservative
Propylparaben	21 mg	white powder	v sl sol in water; fr sol in alcohol	0.035%	0.02%–0.04%	preservative
Aspartame	30 mg	white powder	sp sol in water; sl sol in alcohol	0.05%	0.05%	sweetener
Purified Water	qs 60 mL	clear, colorless liquid	—	—	—	vehicle

COMPATIBILITY–STABILITY: This is an official *USP* formulation with known stability. This solution is made according to the compounding formula for Hydralazine Hydrochloride Oral Solution USP. The formula is given here. Hydralazine has compatibility and stability problems with some sugars and aldehydes, so it should not be made with sucrose-based syrups, and flavors should be avoided except at the time of administration (3). The formulation contains the paraben preservatives.

PACKAGING AND STORAGE: The *USP* monograph for this preparation recommends packaging in a light-resistant glass or plastic bottle with a child-resistant closure, and storage in the refrigerator.

BEYOND-USE DATE: The monograph recommends a beyond-use date of 30 days for this formulation (3).

CALCULATIONS

Dose/Concentration: Hydralazine HCl: The dose for this drug is 0.75 mg/kg/day in four divided doses rather than the 0.75 mcg/kg/day given in this prescription. Pharmacist Jackson called Dr. Farrell, who thanked Dr. Jackson for noticing the error and asked her to change the dose to the recommended amount.

$$\text{Weight of child in kg:} \frac{88 \text{ lb}}{2.2 \text{lb/kg}} = 40 \text{ kg}$$

$$\text{Dose in mg}: \left(\frac{0.75 \text{ mg}}{\text{kg/day}}\right)\left(\frac{40 \text{ kg}}{}\right)\left(\frac{\text{day}}{4 \text{ doses}}\right) = 7.5 \text{ mg/dose}$$

Ingredient Amounts

The *USP* formula for Hydralazine Hydrochloride Oral Solution is given here (3):

Hydralazine Hydrochloride		
for 0.1% Oral Solution	100 mg	
for 1.0% Oral Solution	1.0 g	
Sorbitol Solution (70%)		40 g
Methylparaben		65 mg
Propylparaben		35 mg
Propylene Glycol		10 g
Aspartame		50 mg
Purified Water, a sufficient quantity to make		100 mL

It is decided to make the 0.1% (1 mg/mL) solution because this would give a convenient 7.5-mL (1½-teaspoonful) dose. Reducing the preceding formula to make 60 mL of the 0.1% solution, we need the following:

Hydralazine HCl:	100 mg/100 mL × 60 mL = 60 mg
Sorbitol solution:	40 g/100 mL × 60 mL = 24 g
Methylparaben:	65 mg/100 mL × 60 mL = 39 mg
Propylparaben:	35 mg/100 mL × 60 mL = 21 mg
Aspartame:	50 mg/100 mL × 60 mL = 30 mg
Propylene glycol:	10 g/100 mL × 60 mL = 6 g

Sorbitol 70% solution has a specific gravity of 1.285. The volume of this solution equivalent to 24 g is calculated:

$$\left(\frac{\text{mL sorbitol solution}}{1.285 \text{ g sorbitol solution}}\right)\left(\frac{24 \text{ g sorbitol solution}}{}\right) = 18.7 \text{ mL sorbitol solution}$$

Propylene glycol has a specific gravity of 1.036. The volume of this solution equivalent to 6 g is calculated:

$$\left(\frac{\text{mL propylene glycol}}{1.036 \text{ g propylene glycol}}\right)\left(\frac{6 \text{ g propylene glycol}}{}\right) = 5.8 \text{ mL propylene glycol}$$

The *USP* monograph states that this preparation should be labeled by percent and, parenthetically, by milligrams per 5 mL, which, in this case, would be 0.1% (5 mg/5 mL).

MSDS AND SAFETY AND PERSONAL PROTECTIVE EQUIPMENT: Review MSDS for all components. Don a clean lab coat and disposable gloves.

SPECIALIZED EQUIPMENT: Electronic balance

COMPOUNDING PROCEDURE: Weigh 60 mg of hydralazine HCl, 39 mg methylparaben, 21 mg propylparaben, and 30 mg aspartame. Transfer the hydralazine and aspartame to a clean beaker. Add approximately 20 mL of Purified Water to the beaker and stir to completely dissolve the powder. Using a 20-mL syringe, measure 18.7 mL Sorbitol 70% Solution and add this to the beaker. Put the parabens in a separate small beaker. Using a 10-mL syringe, measure 5.8 mL propylene glycol and add this to the beaker containing the parabens; stir to dissolve. Transfer the paraben solution to the beaker containing the hydralazine solution. Use some Purified Water to completely rinse the propylene glycol–paraben stock solution into the beaker containing the hydralazine solution. Transfer the solution to a precalibrated 2-oz amber prescription bottle and add sufficient Purified Water to make the preparation measure 60 mL. Tightly cap the bottle and shake well to mix completely. Inspect the solution for clarity and test its pH with a portable pH meter. Label and dispense.

DESCRIPTION OF FINISHED PREPARATION: The preparation is a clear, colorless solution with apparent viscosity slightly greater than that of water.

QUALITY CONTROL: Check the pH of the preparation with a portable pH meter: pH = 4.5. (The *USP* monograph allows a pH range between 3.0 and 5.0.) The actual volume is checked and matches the theoretical volume of 60 mL.

MASTER FORMULA PREPARED BY: Jennie Jackson, PharmD

CHECKED BY: Mary Ann Kirkpatrick, RPh, PhD

COMPOUNDING RECORD

NAME, STRENGTH, AND DOSAGE FORM OF PREPARATION: Hydralazine HCl Oral Solution 0.1% (5 mg/5 mL)
QUANTITY: 60 mL   **DATE PREPARED:** mm/dd/yy   **BEYOND-USE DATE:** mm/dd/yy
CONTROL/RX NUMBER: 123215   **FORMULATION RECORD ID:** SN008

INGREDIENTS USED:

Ingredient	Quantity Used	Manufacturer Lot Number	Expiration Date	Weighed/ Measured by	Checked by
Hydralazine HCl	60 mg	JET Labs SN2611	mm/yy	bjf	jj
Sorbitol Solution 70%	18.7 mL	JET Labs SN2612	mm/yy	bjf	jj
Propylene Glycol	5.8 mL	JET Labs SN2613	mm/yy	bjf	jj
Methylparaben	39 mg	JET Labs SN2614	mm/yy	bjf	jj
Propylparaben	21 mg	JET Labs SN2615	mm/yy	bjf	jj
Aspartame	30 mg	JET Labs SN2616	mm/yy	bjf	jj
Purified Water	qs 60 mL	Sweet Springs AL0529	mm/yy	bjf	jj

QUALITY CONTROL DATA: The preparation is a clear, colorless solution with apparent viscosity slightly greater than that of water. The pH of the preparation was checked using a portable pH meter: pH = 4.5. The actual volume was checked and matches the theoretical volume of 60 mL.

LABELING

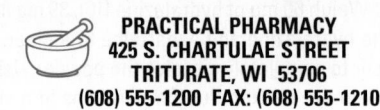

PRACTICAL PHARMACY
425 S. CHARTULAE STREET
TRITURATE, WI 53706
(608) 555-1200 FAX: (608) 555-1210

℞ 123215   Pharmacist: JJ   Date: 00/00/00
Jacob Stone   Dr. Farrell

Give 7.5 mL (one and one-half teaspoonfuls) by mouth four times daily. You may mix with juice or other beverage or soft food at the time of administration.

Hydralazine 0.1% Oral Solution (5 mg/5 mL)

Mfg: Compounded   Quantity: 60 mL

Refills: 2   Discard after: Give date

Auxiliary Label: Keep in the refrigerator. This medicine was compounded in our pharmacy for you at the direction of your prescriber.

PATIENT CONSULTATION: Good afternoon, Mrs. Stone. Good to see you again. Here is the new liquid hydralazine solution for Jacob. As you know, this medication is to help control his blood pressure. You are to give him 7.5 mL or one and one-half teaspoonfuls four times a day. Do you have an oral syringe to measure this amount? Do you feel comfortable with measuring this or would you like to go over that just to make sure? You may mix this with some fruit juice or other beverage or with soft food just prior to giving it to Jacob. If you forget to give a dose, give it as soon as you remember, but if it's close to the next dose, just skip it; do not double doses. Just as with the powder packets of this drug, this could make Jacob a little dizzy or give him a headache. If this becomes a problem, I suggest you call Dr. Farrell. I know that Jacob gets regular checkups to make sure everything is going well. Store this in the refrigerator and discard any unused contents after 1 month; I have put that date on this bottle. Keep this out of the reach of children. This may be refilled two times. Because this takes a little time to prepare, I suggest that you call ahead when you need a refill. Do you have any questions?

REFERENCES

1. The United States Pharmacopeial Convention, Inc. Chapter ⟨1151⟩. 2008 USP 31/NF 26. Rockville, MD: Author, 2007; 618–623.
2. CDER Data Standards Manual. Rockville, MD: Food and Drug Administration, 2006: Data Element Name: Dosage Form, http://www.fda.gov/cder/dsm/DRG/drg00201.htm.
3. The United States Pharmacopeial Convention, Inc. USP monographs. 2008 USP 31/NF 26. Rockville, MD: Author, 2007.
4. Marshall K, Foster TS, Carlin HS, Williams RL. Development of a compendial taxonomy and glossary for pharmaceutical dosage forms. Pharmacopeial forum. Rockville, MD: The United States Pharmacopeial Convention, Inc., 2003; 29(5).
5. The United States Pharmacopeial Convention, Inc. General notices. 2008 USP 31/NF 26. Rockville, MD: Author, 2007; 9–11.
6. The United States Pharmacopeial Convention, Inc. Chapter ⟨795⟩. 2008 USP 31/NF 26. Rockville, MD: Author, 2007; 316–317.
7. Kim MJ, Lim BS, Chang WG, et al. Phosphoric acid incorporated with acidulated phosphate fluoride gel etchant effects on bracket bonding. Angle Orthod 2005 Jul; 75(4): 678–684.
8. Connors KA, Amidon GL, Stella VJ. Chemical stability of pharmaceuticals, 2nd ed. New York: John Wiley & Sons, 1986; 264–273.
9. Trissel LA. Trissel's stability of compounded formulations, 3rd ed. Washington, DC: American Pharmacists Association, 2005; 108–111.
10. Trissel LA. Trissel's stability of compounded formulations, 3rd ed. Washington, DC: American Pharmacists Association, 2005; 35–36.
11. Trissel LA. Trissel's stability of compounded formulations, 3rd ed. Washington, DC: American Pharmacists Association, 2005; 307–309.
12. Connors KA, Amidon GL, Stella VJ. Chemical stability of pharmaceuticals, 2nd ed. New York: John Wiley & Sons, 1986; 483–490.

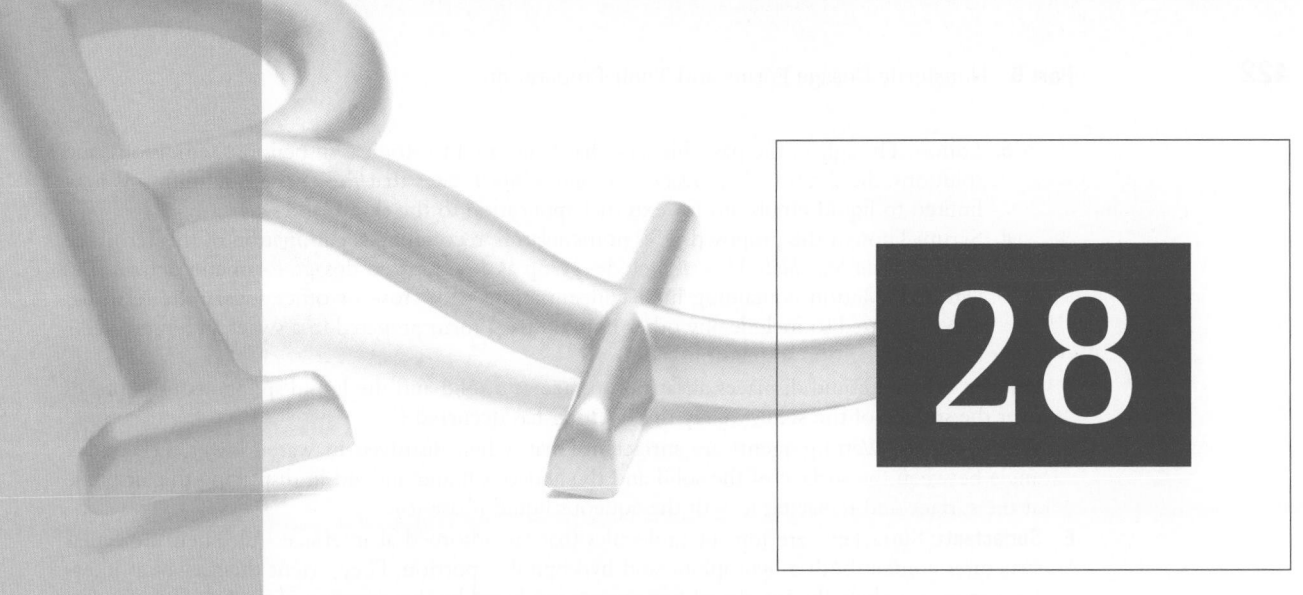

Suspensions

I. DEFINITIONS AND SUSPENSION NOMENCLATURE

A. **Suspensions:** "Suspensions are liquid preparations that consist of solid particles dispersed throughout a liquid phase in which the particles are not soluble" (1).

B. Other suspension nomenclature

1. Though the word *suspension* is now the *USP*-designated term for dosage forms that are solid-liquid dispersions, historically various other terms such as milk (e.g., milk of magnesia), magma (e.g., bentonite magma), lotion (e.g., hydrocortisone lotion), and syrup (e.g., doxycycline syrup) have been used as names for suspensions. Some terms, such as *milk* and *magma*, named specific types of suspensions, whereas some other terms were nonspecific as to physical system. For example, the term *lotion* has been used for solutions, suspensions, and liquid emulsions, and *syrup* could refer to either a solution or a suspension.

2. As was discussed at the beginning of Chapter 27, in 2002 the USP formed a group to work on simplifying and clarifying dosage form nomenclature. Under the system proposed by this group, dosage forms would be named by their route of administration (e.g., oral, topical) plus their physical system (e.g., tablet, solution, suspension) (2). For example, as of July 2007, the name White Lotion USP was changed to the more descriptive Zinc Sulfide Topical Suspension USP (3).

3. Because development and acceptance of and transition to a new nomenclature system will undoubtedly take many years, it is important for pharmacists and pharmacy technicians to understand new nomenclature but also recognize the various traditional terms used as names for dosage forms.

   a. Milk: A traditional term used for some oral aqueous suspensions (1). The name comes from the fact that the dispersed solid was usually a white-colored inorganic compound that made the suspension appear like milk.

   b. Magma: An older term used for suspensions of inorganic solids with a strong affinity for hydration, which resulted in a suspension with gel-like, thixotropic rheology (1). The solid could be a clay such as bentonite or kaolin or an inorganic/organic salt such as bismuth subsalicylate.

    c. Lotion: Though in the past this term has been used for topical suspensions, emulsions, and solutions, the 2006 *CDER Data Standards Manual* states that the current definition is now limited to liquid emulsions for external application to the skin (4).

    d. Syrup: Though the proposed *USP* nomenclature recommends elimination of this term, the *CDER Data Standards Manual* includes syrup as a designated dosage form and defines it as "an oral solution containing high concentrations of sucrose or other sugars; the term has also been used to include any other liquid dosage form prepared in a sweet and viscid vehicle, including oral suspensions" (2,4).

C. Wetting: When a liquid displaces air at the surface of a solid and the liquid spontaneously spreads over the surface of the solid, we say that wetting has occurred (5).

D. Wetting agents: Wetting agents are surfactants that, when dissolved in water, lower the contact angle between the surface of the solid and the aqueous liquid and aid in displacing the air phase at the surface and replacing it with the aqueous liquid phase (6).

E. Surfactants: Surfactants are ions or molecules that are adsorbed at interfaces (6). Their molecular structures contain both a hydrophilic and hydrophobic portion. They orient themselves at interfaces so as to reduce the interfacial free energy produced by the presence of the interface (7). For a detailed discussion of surfactants, see Chapter 20, Surfactants and Emulsifying Agents.

II. USES OF SUSPENSIONS

A. Oral suspensions

1. There is often a need to administer solid drugs orally in liquid form to patients who cannot swallow tablets or capsules. These patients include adults who cannot swallow solid dosage forms, infants or children who have not yet learned how to swallow whole tablets or capsules, nonambulatory patients with nasogastric tubes, and geriatric patients who no longer have the ability to swallow solid oral dosage units.

2. A manufactured liquid product should be used if available because the manufacturer has conducted stability and bioavailability testing on the product. Though pharmaceutical companies now manufacture a large number of oral liquid drug products, many therapeutic agents are still not available in liquid dosage forms. Furthermore, in recent years there have been significant problems with product shortages, including oral liquids. When a manufactured product is unavailable, pharmacists are often asked to compound oral liquid preparations for their patients who need them.

3. Liquid preparations can be made as solutions, suspensions, or emulsions, depending on the physical state and solubility properties of the active ingredients. For drugs that are soluble in water or a cosolvent system that is appropriate for oral use, oral solutions are made; oral and topical solutions are discussed in Chapter 27. If the active ingredient is an immiscible liquid, a liquid emulsion may be formulated; liquid emulsions are described in Chapter 29. When a liquid preparation is needed for a drug that is an insoluble solid, a suspension is formulated. In some cases, an insoluble form of a drug is made intentionally because the drug in soluble form has poor stability or a bad taste.

B. Suspensions for topical use and for administration to mucous membranes

1. As with oral suspensions, a manufactured product should be used if available.

2. Often, topical liquid preparations require compounding by the pharmacist because dermatologists find it desirable therapeutically to create formulas customized for a specific patient with a particular skin condition. Often these preparations are liquid-dispersed systems; numerous examples of dermatologic suspensions are given in this chapter, and two topical liquid emulsions are described in Chapter 29.

3. Suspensions are also administered to mucous membranes, including nasal, eye, ear, and rectal tissues. Though otic and rectal suspensions can be made with relative ease in the pharmacy, nasal and ophthalmic suspensions are not commonly compounded because these are required to be sterile, and this requires steam sterilization as bacterial filtration would remove the active suspended ingredients.

C. Injectable suspensions

1. As with ophthalmic and nasal products, injectable suspensions are required to be sterile, and most of these products are furnished by the manufacturer as sterile suspensions ready for administration.

2. In some cases, the manufacturer furnishes the active ingredient(s) and necessary excipients in a sterile, sealed vial, and the pharmacist, pharmacy technician, or nurse reconstitutes the suspension by adding sterile water or other sterile diluent to the vial at the time of dispensing or administration.

<table>
<tr><td>**III.**</td><td>**DESIRED PROPERTIES OF A SUSPENSION**</td></tr>
</table>

III. DESIRED PROPERTIES OF A SUSPENSION

A. Fine, uniform-sized particles

1. Very fine particles are desirable for both topical and oral suspensions. Particles in suspensions usually range from 0.5 to 3 microns (μm) in diameter.

   a. Uniform, finely divided particles give optimal dissolution and absorption. This is particularly important for suspensions that are intended for systemic use.

   b. A smooth, nongritty preparation is essential for patient acceptance. This is true for both topical and internal-use preparations.

   c. Small, uniform-sized particles are also needed to give suspensions with acceptable rates of settling.

2. Desired particle size is achieved through choice of drug form, selection of appropriate compounding equipment, and good compounding techniques.

   a. Choice of drug form

   (1) If a prescription or drug order specifies a certain form of a drug, that form must be used unless the prescriber is consulted. For example, if the prescription lists precipitated sulfur as an ingredient, that form should be used in the formulation.

   (2) In general, if a drug or chemical is available in more than one form and no form is specified in the drug order, choose the form that has the finest particle size (e.g., boric acid powder rather than boric acid crystals, colloidal sulfur rather than precipitated sulfur). Remember, however, that very fine particles have a high degree of surface-free energy, and very fine particles have an increased tendency to aggregate and eventually fuse together into a nondispersible cake (8). For a complete discussion of this subject and factors to consider and control, consult a book on physical pharmacy.

   (3) The form of drug or chemical used in compounding should be specified on the face of the prescription document or on the master formulation record and the record of compounding. This ensures product uniformity with each prescription refill.

   b. Compounding equipment and technique

   (1) Suspensions are usually made in the pharmacy using mortars and pestles. Choice of mortar type depends on both the characteristics of the ingredients and the volume of the preparation.

   (2) Proper technique for reducing particle size is discussed in section V. B. of Chapter 25, Powders.

   (3) Some pharmacists have found that they can ensure more uniform particles of the desired size for dispersions by passing the prepared powder through a sieve. A mesh size of the range 35 to 45 is considered adequate for suspensions. An example of this is in the *USP* compounding monograph for Ketoconazole Oral Suspension, which states, "If Tablets are used, finely powder the Tablets such that they pass through a 40-mesh or 45-mesh sieve" (3). Pharmaceutical sieves and mesh sizes are described and discussed in section IV. E. of Chapter 25. Small sieve nests with mesh sizes suitable for compounding can be ordered from some vendors of compounding supplies.

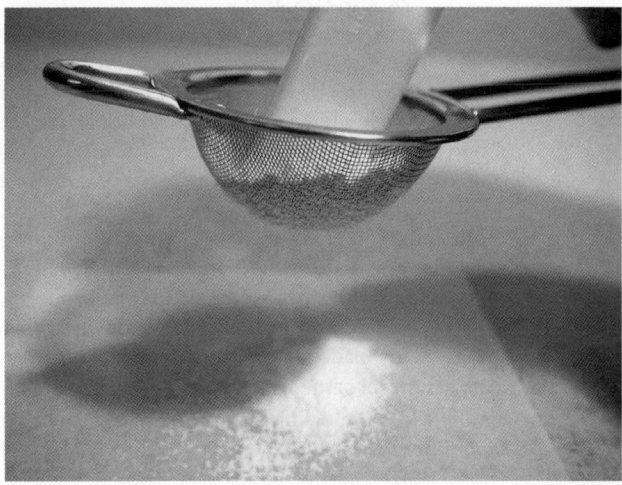

SIEVING A POWDER

B. Uniform dispersion of the particles in the liquid vehicle

Because, in a suspension, the solid does not dissolve, the solid should be evenly dispersed in the liquid vehicle. This ensures a uniform mixture and a uniform dose. To accomplish this, (i) the insoluble powder must be properly wet: that is, the air on the surface of the powder particles must be displaced by liquid, and (ii) any powder aggregates must be broken down to fine, primary particles and these coated with vehicle.

1. If the liquid vehicle is one with a low surface tension, the liquid will easily wet the solid.

2. In most situations, however, water constitutes all or part of the dispersing liquid; water has a high surface tension and does not easily wet many solids, especially hydrophobic drugs or chemicals. When water is a component of the liquid vehicle, special additives, techniques, or order of mixing may be needed to create a uniform suspension. The ingredients and procedure depend on the nature of the solid phase, the other ingredients in the formulation, and the intended route of administration.

    a. **Insoluble, hydrophilic powders:** These are easily wet by water and other water-miscible liquids used for pharmaceutical preparations. Though no special additives are necessary for wetting, the usual procedure is to initially mix the powders with a small amount of liquid vehicle to form a thick paste. In compounding, this is usually done by trituration using a mortar and pestle. This facilitates the desired efficient shearing of the solid particles, the breakup of powder aggregates, and the intimate mixing with the vehicle to give a smooth uniform suspension.

    (1) Two common examples of bulk powders in this class are zinc oxide and calamine. The procedure for suspending these powders is illustrated with Calamine Topical Suspension USP, which is described in Sample Prescription 28.1.

    (2) Most manufactured tablets, when used as ingredients for suspensions, are also easily wet by water. They have been formulated with tablet disintegrants, which absorb water to enhance the breakup of the tablet in the gastrointestinal tract. Tablet material is readily wet by a small amount of water or glycerin. After the tablets are allowed to soften, they are triturated to a smooth paste using a mortar and pestle. This is illustrated in Sample Prescription 28.5, which is described in this chapter and demonstrated on the CD that accompanies this book.

    b. **Insoluble, hydrophobic powders:** These powders are not easily wet by water. To wet such a solid, either a water-miscible liquid with a low surface tension may be used, or a wetting agent may be added to the water to reduce its surface tension. In both cases, remember to consider the route of administration when selecting an additive to improve wetting; additives to oral suspensions must be approved for internal use.

    (1) Use of water-miscible liquids with low surface tension for wetting solids: Because water has a surface tension of 72.8 dynes/cm (at 20°C) and glycerin has a surface tension of 63.4 dynes/cm, glycerin is a better wetting medium for hydrophobic drugs than is water. Examples of liquids used for wetting hydrophobic solids include glycerin, alcohol, propylene glycol, polyethylene glycol, any liquid surfactant, or an ingredient containing a surfactant. The use of liquids of this type for wetting a hydrophobic powder is illustrated on Color Plate 5 and with the compounding procedures for Sample Prescriptions 28.2 and 28.4.

    (2) Use of wetting agents: A wetting agent is a surfactant that, when added to water, improves its ability to wet hydrophobic powders. Examples include soaps such as sodium stearate, detergents such as sodium lauryl sulfate and dioctyl sodium sulfosuccinate (docusate sodium), and nonionic surfactants such as polysorbate 80 (Tween 80). These are described in Chapter 20, Surfactants and Emulsifying Agents.

    c. If possible, an ingredient that is already in the drug order should be used for wetting the insoluble solid. If there is no suitable liquid or surfactant in the formulation, use professional judgment to decide what, if anything, should be added. A small amount of glycerin, alcohol, or propylene glycol is often helpful. A convenient source of surfactant in a pharmacy is the stool softener docusate sodium. Docusate sodium is available formulated both in a liquid and in soft-gelatin capsules. To use a capsule, cut through the soft-gelatin with a razor blade and express the contents into a small amount of water.

C. Slow settling of particles (that is, slow sedimentation rate)

Though it is impossible to completely prevent settling of solid particles in a suspension, the rate of sedimentation can be controlled. Stokes' Law provides useful information in determining what

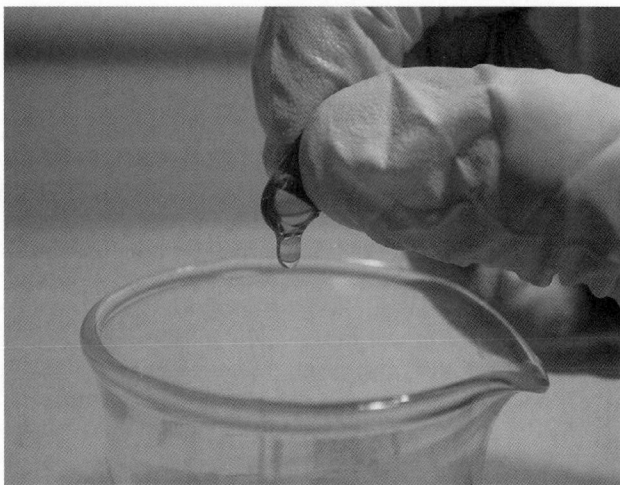

EXTRACTING SURFACTANT DOCUSATE NA FROM A SOFT-SHELL CAPSULE

parameters of a suspension may be controlled to retard the sedimentation rate of particles in a suspension.

$$v = \frac{2r^2(\rho_s - \rho_l)\, g}{9\eta}$$

where:

v = velocity of sedimentation
g = gravitational acceleration
ρ_s = density of the solid
ρ_l = density of the liquid
r = radius of the particles
η = viscosity of the liquid

Though gravitational acceleration (g) is a constant and the density of the solid (ρ_s) cannot be changed, the other factors in Stokes' Law can be manipulated to minimize sedimentation rate (v):

1. r: The particle size should be as small and uniform as possible. As discussed previously, this is controlled through choice of drug form and through proper use of compounding equipment and technique.
2. ρ_l: The density of the liquid may be increased. If the density of the liquid could be made equal to the density of the solid, the term ($\rho_s - \rho_l$) becomes zero, the sedimentation rate becomes zero, and the suspended particles do not settle. Though this is rarely achieved (e.g., zinc oxide has a density of 5.6 g/cm^3, whereas water has a density of 1.0 g/cm^3), the density of the medium can be manipulated to improve the sedimentation rate.
   a. For oral suspensions, the density of the liquid can be increased by adding sucrose, glycerin, sorbitol, or other soluble or miscible, orally acceptable additives. Glycerin has a density of 1.25 g/cm^3, Syrup NF has a density of 1.3 g/cm^3, and Sorbitol 70% has a density of 1.285 g/cm^3.
   b. For topical suspensions, any inactive, soluble, or miscible ingredient that is approved for topical use and that would increase density is acceptable.
3. η: The viscosity of the liquid medium may be increased by adding a viscosity-inducing agent, such as acacia, tragacanth, methylcellulose, sodium carboxymethylcellulose, carbomer, colloidal silicon dioxide, bentonite, or Veegum. Detailed information on viscosity-inducing agents and their use is given in Chapter 19, Viscosity-Inducing Agents.

D. **Ease of redispersion when the product is shaken**
   1. Solids should not form a hard "cake" on the bottom of the bottle when the preparation is allowed to stand.
      a. As was stated previously, very fine particles have an increased tendency to aggregate and eventually fuse together into a nondispersible cake because of the high surface-free energy

associated with very fine particles. This factor should be considered in selecting ingredients for suspensions.

    b. Because caking requires time to develop, a conservative beyond-use date should be considered for suspensions at risk for this problem.

2. The preparation should be sufficiently fluid so that redispersion of settled particles is easily accomplished with normal shaking of the container. The liquid should also pour freely from the container when a dose is to be administered or applied. Judicious use of viscosity-inducing ingredients when formulating suspensions is important in achieving this goal.

3. One special formulation technique, **flocculation,** is useful in producing suspensions that readily redisperse.

    a. Flocculation gives a controlled lacework-like structure of particles held together by weak bonds. These weak bonds hold the particles in the structure when the suspension is at rest but break apart easily when the suspension is shaken.

    b. This technique is often used in the pharmaceutical industry for manufactured suspension products. Some viscosity-inducing agents, such as bentonite and xanthan gum, form flocculated systems; these are available to the pharmacist and are useful as suspending agents in compounding.

    c. Various manufactured suspending vehicles, such as Ora-Plus and Suspendol-S, and the official NF suspending vehicles, Vehicle for Oral Suspension, Bentonite Magma, Suspension Structured Vehicle, and Sugar-Free Suspension Structured Vehicle, are examples of flocculated systems that are helpful in making suspensions that settle slowly but that are easily redispersed on shaking. A sample of manufactured suspension vehicles for compounding is illustrated in Color Plate 6.

IV. BASIC STEPS IN COMPOUNDING A SUSPENSION

A. Check all doses and concentrations for appropriateness.

B. Review Material Safety Data Sheets (MSDSs) for each bulk ingredient to determine safety procedures and recommended personal protective equipment to use when compounding the preparation.

C. Select the desired form for each solid ingredient. In some cases, this form depends on availability. For example, some drugs may be available only as manufactured tablets or capsules.

D. Calculate the amount of each ingredient required for the formulation. If tablets or capsules are used as a source for an active ingredient, the necessary calculations and procedure vary depending on the need for either a whole number or a fractional number of units.

1. If a **whole number** of tablets or capsules is needed, determine the correct number of dosage units to add. There is no need to first weigh the tablets or capsule contents. For an illustration of this procedure, see Sample Prescription 28.5, which is also demonstrated on the CD that accompanies this book.

2. If a **fractional number** of dosage units are needed, follow the steps given here. Remember that tablets and capsule powder contain added formulation ingredients, and this must be considered when determining the weight of tablet or capsule material to use in making the suspension. (See Sample Prescriptions 25.5 and 25.6 in Chapter 25 and Sample Prescription 28.6 in this chapter for examples of this procedure.)

    a. Determine the average weight of a tablet or the powder contents of a capsule. If only one unit is needed, weigh that unit or, for a capsule, the contents of that unit. Remember, for capsules you will not be adding the capsule shell to the suspension, so this should not be weighed.

    b. Use the equation given here to determine the amount of crushed tablet or capsule powder needed:

$$\frac{\text{Amt of drug per tablet or capsule}}{\text{wt. of one tablet or capsule contents}} = \frac{\text{Amt of drug needed}}{x \text{ wt. of tablet or capsule powder needed}}$$

$$x = \text{mg or g of tablet or capsule powder needed}$$

E. Weigh, measure, or count (for tablets or capsules) the calculated amount of each ingredient needed. If using a fractional number of tablets or capsules, crush or empty the appropriate number of units and weigh the amount calculated earlier.

F. Use the techniques for reducing particle size and mixing the powders as described in Chapter 25, Powders.

G. Wet the powders by adding a small amount of liquid vehicle to the powders in a mortar and triturating so that a thick, uniform paste is obtained. Steps **F** and **G** may be combined if appropriate.

H. Add additional liquid vehicle in portions with trituration until a smooth, uniform preparation is obtained.

I. Transfer the suspension to its dispensing container. To ensure complete transfer of the suspended solid active ingredients, use some of the remaining vehicle to rinse the material from the mortar into the dispensing container. A powder funnel with a large diameter stem may be used to facilitate the transfer.

J. Add sufficient vehicle to the dispensing container to make the preparation the desired volume.

K. Some pharmacists recommend that suspensions be homogenized for maximum uniformity and improved physical stability. This can be accomplished by passing the suspension through a hand homogenizer or by using a high-speed blender or homogenizer. If this is done, you will need to make extra suspension to allow for loss of preparation in the equipment.

V. STABILITY AND BEYOND-USE DATING

A. Physical stability of the system: Both maintenance of small particles and ease of redispersion are essential to the physical stability of the system. Because suspensions are physically unstable systems, beyond-use dates for these preparations should be conservative.

B. Chemical stability of the ingredients

1. For ingredient-specific information, check references such as those listed in Chapter 37. Examples are illustrated with the prescription ingredients in each of the sample prescriptions at the end of this chapter.

2. *USP* Chapter ⟨795⟩ recommends a **maximum 14-day beyond-use date** for water-containing liquid preparations made with ingredients in solid form when the stability of the ingredients in that specific formulation is not known (9). This assumes that the preparation will be stored at cold temperature (e.g., a refrigerator) (9); though this works well for oral suspensions, topical preparations are usually stored at room temperature, and the beyond-use date may need adjustment to compensate for this higher storage temperature. Concerns for chemical stability of labile drugs may necessitate greater limits on beyond-use dates.

3. *USP* Chapter ⟨1151⟩ states that suspensions should be stored and dispensed in tight containers (1).

4. Though technically it is very easy to make oral suspensions from crushed tablets and available suspending vehicles, care should always be used in checking and verifying the stability and the beyond-use date of the compounded preparation.

C. Microbiologic stability

1. *USP* Chapter ⟨1151⟩ states that suspensions should contain preservatives to protect against bacteria, yeasts, and molds (1). If antimicrobial ingredients are part of the prescribed formulation, extra preservatives are not needed.

2. Antimicrobial agents and their proper use are discussed in Chapter 16, and consideration of preservatives is presented in each of the following sample prescription formulations.

3. Though solubility of the preservative is a major concern when selecting a preservative for a solution, suspensions are disperse systems, so precipitation of a preservative in a suspension is acceptable; a saturated solution of the preservative will be maintained, and this should be sufficient for preservation.

VI. SPECIAL LABELING REQUIREMENTS FOR SUSPENSIONS

A. All suspensions are disperse systems and require a "**SHAKE WELL**" auxiliary label.

B. External use suspensions should be labeled "**FOR EXTERNAL USE ONLY**."

Sample Prescriptions

SAMPLE PRESCRIPTION 28.1

CASE: Professor George Helmholtz is a 160-lb, 5'11" tall, 68-year-old man who has recently retired from his university faculty position. He and his wife have purchased a lake cottage, and today, within a few hours of wading in the lake as he put in the pier for his boat, he found multiple small, defined red bites on his feet, ankles, and calves, and he reports that they itch "like crazy." He has gone to a local physician who has diagnosed "lake itch." This is caused by a fluke that is common to the lakes in the area. Though self-limiting, the bites are highly irritating, and the only therapy is symptomatic treatment of the itching with a soothing lotion that contains on effective local anesthetic.

CONTEMPORARY PHYSICIANS GROUP PRACTICE
20 S. PARK STREET, TRITURATE, WI 53706
TEL: (608) 555-1333 FAX: (608) 555-1335

℞ # *123655*

NAME *Prof. George Helmholtz*　　　　　**DATE** *00/00/00*

ADDRESS *2160 Electron Circle*

℞

　　　　　　Calamine Lotion with Lidocaine 2%

　　　　　　Dispense　　　　　　*180 mL*

　　　　　　　　　　　　　　　　　　　J. Joyous 0/00/00

　　　Sig: Apply to "lake itch" bites q 4 hr prn

REFILLS *3*　　　　　　*Marcy Dacy*　　　　　**M.D.**

　　　　　　　　DEA NO. _____

MASTER COMPOUNDING FORMULATION RECORD

NAME, STRENGTH, AND DOSAGE FORM OF PREPARATION: Calamine Topical Suspension with Lidocaine 2%

QUANTITY: 180 mL

FORMULATION RECORD ID: SS001

THERAPEUTIC USE/CATEGORY: Antiseptic/local anesthetic

ROUTE OF ADMINISTRATION: Topical

INGREDIENTS:

Ingredient	Quantity Used	Physical Description	Solubility	Dose Comparison		Use in the Prescription
				Given	Usual	
Lidocaine as lidocaine HCl monohydrate	4.439 g equivalent to 3.6 g lidocaine	white needles	insol in water, sol in alcohol	2%	1%–5%	local anesthetic
Calamine	14.4 g	pink powder	insol in water and alcohol	8%	5–20%	astringent, antiseptic; protective
Zinc Oxide	14.4 g	white powder	insol in water and alcohol	8%	5–20%	astringent, antiseptic; protective
Glycerin	3.6 mL	clear, viscous liquid	misc w/ water and alcohol	2%	—	humectant, wetting, levigating agent
Bentonite Magma	45 mL	grayish suspension	bentonite is insol in water and alcohol	—	—	suspending medium
Calcium Hydroxide Solution	qs 180 mL	cloudy solution	—	—	—	astringent, vehicle

COMPATIBILITY–STABILITY: The Calamine Lotion (now officially Calamine Topical Suspension) is an official *USP* formulation (3) that is known to be very stable. Lidocaine is available as the free base (MW = 234.3) and the hydrochloride salt-monohydrate (MW = 288.8). The base form is insoluble in water, and the hydrochloride monohydrate is soluble in water. Its pK_a = 7.86 (10). Lidocaine is an amide that is subject to hydrolysis. At neutral pH it is reported to be quite stable in aqueous solution (10), but the current preparation has a high pH = 12. At this pH, the drug is entirely in the insoluble base form, which would increase its stability; however, amides are less stable to hydrolysis at high pH. Therefore, care should be exercised in establishing a beyond-use date. In this formulation, the 2% refers to the quantity of base; if the base is unavailable and the hydrochloride monohydrate is used, an equivalent amount can be calculated by multiplying the base quantity by the ratio of their molecular weights, 288.9/234.3. Irrespective of the form used, the powder should be treated as an insoluble drug and combined with the other insoluble powders (calamine and zinc oxide) because the soluble hydrochloride salt will immediately precipitate if added to calcium hydroxide solution, and some drug could be inadvertently lost owing to sedimentation in the bottom of the solution vessel. No added preservative is needed for this preparation because the formula contains the antiseptics calamine and zinc oxide, and the preparation has a high pH that is unfavorable to microbial growth.

PACKAGING AND STORAGE: The *USP* monographs for both Calamine Topical Suspension and lidocaine solutions recommend storage in tight containers (3). As this is a topical preparation, storage should be at controlled room temperature.

BEYOND-USE DATE: Use the recommended maximum 14-day beyond-use date for compounded water-containing liquid formulations prepared from ingredients in solid form when there is no stability information for the formulation (9).

CALCULATIONS

Dose/Concentration: All concentrations okay

Ingredient Amounts

Lidocaine (in g): $\qquad$ $2\% \times 180\ \text{mL} = 0.02 \times 180\ \text{mL} = 3.6\ \text{g}$

The form available to this pharmacy is lidocaine HCl monohydrate. The quantity of this ingredient that is equivalent to 3.6 g of lidocaine is calculated:

$$\frac{234.3\ \text{g lidocaine}}{288.9\ \text{g lidocaine HCl}\cdot\text{H}_2\text{O}} = \frac{3.6\ \text{g lidocaine}}{x\ \text{g lidocaine HCl}\cdot\text{H}_2\text{O}};\ x = 4.439\ \text{g}$$

The formula for Calamine Topical Suspension USP is (3):

Calamine	80 g
Zinc Oxide	80 g
Glycerin	20 mL
Bentonite Magma	250 mL
Calcium Hydroxide Topical Solution a sufficient quantity to make	1,000 mL

Reducing this formula to make 180 mL:

Calamine and zinc oxide: $\qquad \dfrac{80\ \text{g}}{1{,}000\ \text{mL}} = \dfrac{x\ \text{g}}{180\ \text{mL}};\ x = 14.4\ \text{g}$

Glycerin: $\qquad \dfrac{20\ \text{mL glycerin}}{1{,}000\ \text{mL lotion}} = \dfrac{x\ \text{mL glycerin}}{180\ \text{mL lotion}};\ x = 3.6\ \text{mL glycerin}$

Bentonite Magma USP: $\dfrac{250\ \text{mL Bentonite Magma}}{1{,}000\ \text{mL lotiom}} = \dfrac{x\ \text{mL Bentonite Magma}}{180\ \text{mL lotion}};\ x = 45\ \text{mL Bentonite Magma}$

Calcium Hydroxide Topical Solution USP: This saturated solution, also known as *lime water*, is usually made in the pharmacy using calcium hydroxide powder and Purified Water. The clear supernatant solution is decanted at the time of use. The formula is in the *USP* but is also given in Chapter 29 of this book under the topic of Nascent Soap Emulsions. For this prescription, the Calcium Hydroxide Topical Solution is available in the pharmacy.

MSDS AND SAFETY AND PERSONAL PROTECTIVE EQUIPMENT: Review MSDS for all components. Don a clean lab coat, disposable gloves, and safety glasses. Avoid inhaling powders.

SPECIALIZED EQUIPMENT: Wedgwood mortar; all weighing is done on a class III torsion balance.

COMPOUNDING PROCEDURE: Measure 45 mL of Bentonite Magma and dilute with an equal volume of Calcium Hydroxide Topical Solution. Weigh 4.439 g of lidocaine HCl monohydrate and 14.4 g each of calamine and zinc oxide. Place the lidocaine in a Wedgwood mortar and add the calamine and zinc oxide using geometric dilution and triturate well in the mortar. Add 3.6 mL of glycerin and about 18 mL of diluted Bentonite Magma to the powders in the mortar; triturate until a smooth paste is formed. Gradually add the remainder of the diluted Bentonite Magma with trituration. Add 20 to 30 mL of Calcium Hydroxide Topical Solution to the mortar to dilute to a pourable suspension. Pour into a precalibrated 6-oz prescription bottle and use sufficient Calcium Hydroxide Topical Solution to rinse the mortar and qs to 180 mL mark. Tightly cap the bottle and shake well; label and dispense.

Note: An easy alternative for making this preparation would be to use commercially available Calamine Lotion. In this case, weigh the designated quantity of lidocaine and place it in the mortar. Add a small quantity of Calamine Lotion and triturate this to a smooth paste. Gradually add additional Calamine Lotion in portions with trituration to obtain a uniform, pourable suspension. Pour into a precalibrated 6-oz prescription bottle and use sufficient Calamine Lotion to rinse the mortar and qs to 180 mL mark.

DESCRIPTION OF FINISHED PREPARATION: The preparation is a pink suspension with a viscosity that is similar to thick syrup. The dispersed particles settle minimally on standing, and the preparation is easily redispersed with shaking.

QUALITY CONTROL: Volume = 180 mL; check pH with range 1 to 14 pH paper: pH = 12

MASTER FORMULA PREPARED BY: Jerilyn Joyous, PharmD   **CHECKED BY:** Pat Schoenfeld, RPh

COMPOUNDING RECORD

NAME, STRENGTH, AND DOSAGE FORM OF PREPARATION: Calamine Topical Suspension with Lidocaine 2%
QUANTITY: 180 mL   **DATE PREPARED:** mm/dd/yy   **BEYOND-USE DATE:** mm/dd/yy
FORMULATION RECORD ID: SS001   **CONTROL/RX NUMBER:** 123655

INGREDIENTS USED:

Ingredient	Quantity	Manufacturer Lot Number	Expiration Date	Weighed/ Measured by	Checked by
Lidocaine HCl monohydrate	4.439 g (contains 3.6 g lidocaine)	JET Labs SS2815	mm/yy	bjf	jj
Calamine14.4 g	JET Labs SS2811	mm/yy	bjf	jj	
Zinc Oxide	14.4 g SS2812	JET Labs	mm/yy	bjf	jj
Glycerin3.6 mL	JET Labs SS2813	mm/yy	bjf	jj	
Bentonite Magma	45 mL SS2814	JET Labs	mm/yy	bjf	jj
Calcium Hydroxide Solution	qs 180 mL JT1143	Prac. Pharm.	mm/yy	bjf	jj

QUALITY CONTROL DATA: The preparation is a pink suspension. It has a medium viscosity with minimal settling in 2 hours. The preparation is easily redispersed with shaking and pours easily. The pH of the preparation is checked with pH paper, range 1 to 14; pH = 12. Volume = 180 mL.

LABELING

PRACTICAL PHARMACY
425 S. CHARTULAE STREET
TRITURATE, WI 53706
(608) 555-1200 FAX: (608) 555-1210

℞   123655   Pharmacist: JJ   Date: 00/00/00
Prof. George Helmholtz   Dr. Marcy Dacy
Apply to "lake itch" bites every four hours as needed.
Calamine Topical Suspension with Lidocaine 2%
Mfg: Compounded   Quantity: 180 mL
Refills: 3   Discard after: Give date

Auxiliary Labels: <u>Shake well</u>. <u>For external use only</u>. This medicine was compounded in our pharmacy for you at the direction of your prescriber.

PATIENT CONSULTATION: Hello, Prof. Helmholtz, I'm Jerilyn Joyous, your pharmacist. Do you have any drug allergies? Are you currently taking or using any other medications? I see that you have been initiated as a full member of this lake community with a case of "Lake Itch." This prescription contains the local anesthetic lidocaine in a soothing calamine lotion; it should help with the itching and irritation. Apply it to the bites every 4 hours as needed. Try not to scratch the bites; the itching usually subsides rather soon, but if you break the skin, you may introduce an infection which will take a lot longer to resolve. If the bites seem to be getting worse or if this is irritating to your skin, discontinue use and contact Dr. Dacy. Shake the bottle well before using. You may want to pour some lotion on a cotton ball and use that to dab the lotion on the affected areas, but be careful not to get this in your eyes or mouth. Wash your hands thoroughly before and after application. Store this at room temperature out of the reach of children, and keep this container tightly closed. Discard any unused contents after 2 weeks (give date). This may be refilled three times. I know you want to avoid this in the future. I have been swimming in these lakes for many years, and my advice to you is towel off briskly after leaving the water; this physically removes the flukes before they get a chance to burrow into your skin. If you are swimming for a long time, you might want to come out of the water periodically and towel off. Also, when you are working along the shoreline, I would wear a pair of waders, if you have them. Do you have any questions?

SAMPLE PRESCRIPTION 28.2

CASE: Laura Lovely is a 145-lb, 5′3″-tall, 42-year-old woman who has seen Dr. Felz for contact dermatitis that he has diagnosed as poison ivy. Laura has just returned from a camping trip with her family and reports that she went for several hikes in a wooded area. She thinks that is where she came in contact with the poison ivy. Laura has had type 1 diabetes for 15 years, and it is well controlled using an insulin pump. She is also taking nabumetone for an arthritic condition in her lower spine. Laura's poison ivy is characterized by patches of red rash on her hands, arms, and calves, and she complains of intense itching of these areas. Currently, the rash is dry with no weeping. Dr. Felz has instructed Laura to immediately shower and shampoo her hair and carefully clean under her fingernails to make sure there is no residual toxin that could be spread to other areas of her body. She should also wash the clothing she has been wearing.

CONTEMPORARY PHYSICIANS GROUP PRACTICE
20 S. PARK STREET, TRITURATE, WI 53706
TEL: (608) 555-1333 FAX: (608) 555-1335

℞ #   *123687*

NAME *Laura Lovely*   DATE *00/00/00*

ADDRESS *9 Woodmont Circle*

℞

Hydrocortisone		*1%*
Menthol		*1/8%*
Calamine		*3 g*
Isopropyl Alcohol		*10%*
Cetaphil		*40 mL*
Purified Water	*q s ad*	*60 mL*

J. Junco 00/00/00

Sig: Apply to affected areas q 4 to 6 hr prn itching

REFILLS *1*   *Kenneth Felz*   M.D.

DEA NO. _____

MASTER COMPOUNDING FORMULATION RECORD

NAME, STRENGTH, AND DOSAGE FORM OF PREPARATION: Hydrocortisone 1%, Menthol 0.125%, Calamine 5%, Isopropyl alcohol 10%, Cetaphil 67% Topical Suspension

QUANTITY: 60 mL

FORMULATION RECORD ID: SS002

THERAPEUTIC USE/CATEGORY: Corticosteroid/Antipruritic

ROUTE OF ADMINISTRATION: Topical

INGREDIENTS:

Ingredient	Quantity Used	Physical Description	Solubility	Dose Comparison		Use in the Prescription
				Given	Usual	
Hydrocortisone	0.6 g	white powder	v sl sol water 1 g/40 mL alcohol	1%	0.5–2.5%	anti inflammatory
Menthol	150 mg weighed- 75 mg used	fine crystals with menthol odor	sl sol water v sol alcohol	0.125%	1–3%	antipruritic local analgesic
Calamine	3 g	pink powder	Insol in water and alcohol	5%	1–20%	protective
IPA 70%	8.6 mL	clear liquid w/ odor of alcohol	misc with water	10%	varies	disinfectant, solvent drying agent
Cetaphil	40 mL	liquid emulsion	misc w/water, alcohol	67%	—	emollient vehicle
Purified Water	qs 60 mL	clear liquid	—	—	—	vehicle

COMPATIBILITY-STABILITY: Topical shake lotions of this type that contain Hydrocortisone have been evaluated and reported in the literature. A good review of this subject can be found in the hydrocortisone monograph in *Trissel's Stability of Compounded Formulations* (11). Hydrocortisone suspensions that contain zinc oxide–type ingredients (calamine is essentially zinc oxide with 0.5% to 1% ferric oxide to impart the pink color) have limited stability. One study showed a 7% loss of hydrocortisone in 1 week and a 10% loss in 2 weeks (12). The other ingredients in this preparation are quite stable in a liquid suspension formulation. No additional preservative is needed for this preparation because the formula contains 10% isopropyl alcohol (IPA); also, Cetaphil contains paraben preservatives.

PACKAGING AND STORAGE: *USP* Chapter ⟨1151⟩ recommends that suspensions be packaged in tight containers (1). Because this is a topical preparation, store at controlled room temperature.

BEYOND-USE DATE: Using the literature cited earlier as a guide, use a 14-day beyond-use date for this preparation.

CALCULATIONS

Dose/Concentration

Calamine concentration (in w/v %):

$$\frac{3 \text{ g calamine}}{60 \text{ mL suspension}} = \frac{x \text{ g calamine}}{100 \text{ mL suspension}}; x = 5\text{g}/100 \text{ mL} = 5\%$$

Cetaphil concentration (in v/v %):

$$\frac{40 \text{ mL Cetaphil}}{60 \text{ mL suspension}} = \frac{x \text{ mL Cetaphil}}{100 \text{ mL suspension}}; x = 66.7 \text{ mL}/100 \text{ mL} = 67\%$$

All concentrations okay

Ingredient Amounts

Hydrocortisone (in g): $\qquad$ 1% × 60 mL = 0.6 g

Menthol (in g and mg): $\qquad$ 1/8% × 60 mL = 0.125% × 60 mL = 0.075 g = 75 mg

The amount of menthod is below the MWQ for a class III torsion balance. As menthol is soluble in one of the prescription ingredients, isopropyl alcohol (IPA), a solid-liquid aliquot using IPA would be most convenient. The quantities for one possible aliquot can be determined using the dilution factor method as described in Chapter 10. In this case, a dilution factor of 2 would be convenient: Weigh two times the amount of menthol needed, 75 mg × 2 = 150 mg; dissolve this in a portion of the required 70% IPA volume (4 mL would be a good amount), and measure the reciprocal of the dilution factor: ½ × 4 mL = 2 mL.

IPA (in mL): $\qquad$ 10% × 60 mL = 6 mL

IPA is available in the pharmacy as a 70% v/v solution. Following are the calculations for obtaining 6 mL of IPA from the 70% solution:

$$\frac{70 \text{ mL IPA}}{100 \text{ mL 70\% IPA}} = \frac{6 \text{ mL IPA}}{x \text{ mL 70\% IPA}}; x = 8.6 \text{ mL of 70\% IPA}$$

MSDS AND SAFETY AND PERSONAL PROTECTIVE EQUIPMENT: Review MSDS for all components. Don a clean lab coat, disposable gloves, and safety glasses. Avoid inhaling powders.

SPECIALIZED EQUIPMENT: Wedgwood mortar; all weighing is done on a class III torsion balance.

COMPOUNDING PROCEDURE: Weigh 150 mg of menthol, 600 mg of hydrocortisone, and 3 g of calamine. Dissolve the menthol in 4 mL of IPA 70% measured in a 10-mL graduated cylinder. Place the hydrocortisone in a mortar and add the calamine geometrically. Measure 2 mL of the menthol-IPA solution and an additional 6.6 mL of IPA 70% (for a total of 8.6 mL) and gradually add this to the powders in the mortar with trituration to wet the powders and form a smooth, uniform paste. Gradually, with trituration, add about 10 mL of Purified Water to the paste. This is to dilute the IPA content in the mortar before adding the Cetaphil because Cetaphil has components that are soluble in IPA; too high an IPA concentration will break down the emulsion structure of Cetaphil. Gradually add 40 mL of Cetaphil (measured in a 50-mL graduated cylinder) in small portions with trituration. Do not over-triturate the preparation because the Cetaphil contains surfactants that facilitate the introduction of air bubbles ("suds") into the preparation. Use additional small portions of Purified Water to rinse the graduated cylinder used to measure the Cetaphil and add the rinsings to the mortar; add a sufficient amount to dilute the preparation to give a pourable suspension. Transfer the suspension to a precalibrated 2-oz prescription bottle. Use additional Purified Water to rinse the mortar and to facilitate transfer to the prescription bottle; then qs with Purified Water to the 60-mL mark. Tightly cap the bottle and shake well; label and dispense.

DESCRIPTION OF FINISHED PREPARATION: The preparation is a pink, viscous suspension. The dispersed particles settle minimally on standing, and the preparation is easily redispersed with shaking.

QUALITY CONTROL: Volume = 60 mL; check pH with range 2 to 9 test strips: pH = 7

MASTER FORMULA PREPARED BY: Juliette Junco, PharmD $\qquad$ **CHECKED BY:** Pat Schoenfeld, RPh

COMPOUNDING RECORD

NAME, STRENGTH, AND DOSAGE FORM OF PREPARATION: Hydrocortisone 1%, Menthol 0.125%, Calamine 5%, Isopropyl alcohol 10%, Cetaphil 67% Topical Suspension

QUANTITY: 60 mL **DATE PREPARED:** mm/dd/yy **BEYOND-USE DATE:** mm/dd/yy

FORMULATION RECORD ID: SS002 **CONTROL/RX NUMBER:** 123687

INGREDIENTS USED:

Ingredient	Quantity Used	Manufacturer Lot Number	Expiration Date	Weighed/ Measured by	Checked by
Hydrocortisone	0.6 g	JET Labs SS2821	mm/yy	bjf	jj
Menthol	150 mg weighed – 75 mg used	JET Labs SS2822	mm/yy	bjf	jj
Calamine	3 g	JET Labs SS2823	mm/yy	bjf	jj
IPA 70%	8.6 mL	JET Labs SS2824	mm/yy	bjf	jj
Cetaphil	40 mL	Galderma JN9636	mm/yy	bjf	jj
Purified Water	qs 60 mL	Sweet Springs AL0529	mm/yy	bjf	jj

QUALITY CONTROL DATA: The preparation is a pink suspension with medium viscosity. There was minimal settling in 2 hours. The preparation is easily redispersed with shaking and pours easily. The pH of the preparation was checked with range 2 to 9 test strips: pH = 7. Volume = 60 mL.

LABELING

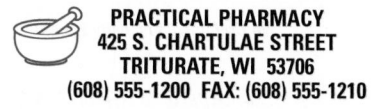

PRACTICAL PHARMACY
425 S. CHARTULAE STREET
TRITURATE, WI 53706
(608) 555-1200 FAX: (608) 555-1210

℞ 123687 Pharmacist: JJ Date: 00/00/00
Laura Lovely Dr. Kenneth Felz

Apply to affected areas every four to six hours as needed for itching.

Hydrocortisone 1%, Menthol 0.125%, Calamine 5% Topical Suspension

Contains Isopropyl Alcohol 10%, Cetaphil 67%

Mfg: Compounded Quantity: 60 mL

Refills: 1 Discard after: Give date

Auxiliary Labels: Shake well. For external use only. This medicine was compounded in our pharmacy for you at the direction of your prescriber.

PATIENT CONSULTATION: Hello, Ms. Lovely, I'm your pharmacist Juliette Junco. Do you have any drug allergies? Did Dr. Felz explain the purpose of this lotion and how to use it? This is a specially formulated lotion for your poison ivy; it contains hydrocortisone and several other ingredients that will help stop inflammation and itching, act as an antiseptic, and protect, cleanse, and lubricate the skin. Shake the bottle well before using, then apply the lotion to the affected areas every 4 to 6 hours as needed for itching. Be careful not to get this in your eyes or mouth. If your condition gets worse or you experience additional irritation, contact Dr. Felz. This is in a childproof container, but it should be kept out of the reach of children. Store it at room temperature and keep the bottle tightly closed. Discard any unused portion after 2 weeks (give date). This may be refilled once. I understand from Dr. Felz that he explained to you how you should shower and wash your clothes and any items that may still have residues of the poison ivy toxin. Do you know how to identify poison ivy for the future? As they say, "Leaflets three, let it be." You might want to get pictures of poison ivy at the library or the county extension office, or on the Internet. Do you have any questions?

SAMPLE PRESCRIPTION 28.3

CASE: Deborah Summit is a 140-lb, 5′6″ tall, 16-year-old female patient who has seen Dr. Pasmak for treatment of her acne. She has tried the usual over-the-counter products with limited success. She has inflamed papules on her face, lower neck, and upper back. Dr. Pasmak wants to try this compounded suspension of finely divided sulfur and phenol before employing antibiotics. Deborah's medication profile shows that she is currently taking fluoxetine 20 mg daily for depression. She reports that she also takes over-the-counter ibuprofen for headaches and menstrual pain.

CONTEMPORARY PHYSICIANS GROUP PRACTICE
20 S. PARK STREET, TRITURATE, WI 53706
TEL: (608) 555-1333 FAX: (608) 555-1335

℞ #   *123633*

NAME *Deborah Summit*   DATE *00/00/00*

ADDRESS *857 Triangle Parkway*

℞

Phenol	*1%*
White Lotion	
~~Methylcellulose 1500 cps 2%~~	*aa qs ad 60 mL*

Na CMC med. viscosity 2% gel

J. Junco 00/00/00

Sig: Apply to affected areas q am and hs

Called Dr. Pasmak to change Methylcellulose to Na CMC due to compatibility concerns. JJ

REFILLS *3*   *R. Pasmak*   M.D.

DEA NO. _____

MASTER COMPOUNDING FORMULATION RECORD

NAME, STRENGTH, AND DOSAGE FORM OF PREPARATION: Phenol 1% in Modified Zinc Sulfide Topical Suspension

QUANTITY: 60 mL

THERAPEUTIC USE/CATEGORY: Acne Antibacterial

FORMULATION RECORD ID: SS003

ROUTE OF ADMINISTRATION: Topical

INGREDIENTS:

Ingredient	Quantity Used	Physical Description	Solubility	Dose Comparison		Use in the Prescription
				Given	Usual	
Phenol	0.6 g	clear, light beige crystals w/ phenol odor	1 g/15 mL water; v. sol in alcohol	1%	0.5–2%	antiseptic; local anesthetic;
Na CMC med visc. 2% soln	30 mL	clear, viscous liquid	misc w/water and alcohol	—	—	viscosity inducer, vehicle
ZnSO₄ (to make 30 mL White Lotion)	1.2 g	white powder	sol in water	—	—	To make 30 mL White Lotion
Sulfurated Potash (to make 30 mL White Lotion)	1.2 g	yellowish brown large chunks	sol in water	—	—	To make 30 mL White Lotion
White Lotion (now Zinc Sulfide Topical Suspension)	30 mL	white suspension	forms insol ZnS & S plus sol K_2SO_4	half-strength	full strength	antibacterial, antifungal, keratolytic
Purified Water	qs	clear liquid	—	—	—	solvent, vehicle

COMPATIBILITY–STABILITY: White Lotion is an official *USP* formulation, which is now called Zinc Sulfide Topical Suspension. It is fairly stable, though the monograph states that it should be freshly made (3). Phenol is also fairly stable, but it is subject to oxidation. It is necessary to change the methylcellulose 1,500 cps to medium-viscosity sodium carboxymethylcellulose (Na CMC) because methylcellulose is reported to be incompatible with phenol (13). Both phenol and Zinc Sulfide Topical Suspension USP have antimicrobial properties, so no additional preservative is needed.

PACKAGING AND STORAGE: The *USP* monograph for Zinc Sulfide Topical Suspension recommends that it be dispensed in tight containers (3). Because this is a topical product, it should be stored at controlled room temperature.

BEYOND-USE DATE: Use the *USP* recommended maximum 14-day beyond-use date for a compounded water-containing liquid formulation prepared from ingredients in solid form when there is no stability information for the formulation (9).

CALCULATIONS

Dose/Concentration: All concentrations okay

Ingredient Amounts

Phenol (in g):   1% × 60 mL = 0.01 × 60 mL = 0.6 g

Na CMC medium viscosity (in g):   2% × 30 mL = 0.02 × 30 mL = 0.6 g

White Lotion (Zinc Sulfide Topical Suspension) USP:

The formula for 1,000 mL of Zinc Sulfide Topical Suspension, as given in the *USP*, states that 40 g each of sulfurated potash and zinc sulfate ($ZnSO_4$) are needed. Reducing this formula to make 30 mL:

$$\frac{40\ g}{1{,}000\ mL\ suspension} = \frac{x\ g}{30\ mL\ suspension};\ x = 1.2\ g\ of\ each$$

MSDS AND SAFETY AND PERSONAL PROTECTIVE EQUIPMENT: Review MSDS for all components. Don a clean lab coat, disposable gloves, and safety glasses. Use extreme caution when handling phenol because contact with skin may cause serious burns.

SPECIALIZED EQUIPMENT: Wedgwood mortar; funnel and filter paper; all weighing is done on a class III torsion balance.

COMPOUNDING PROCEDURE: Weigh 0.6 g each of phenol and Na CMC med viscosity. Place 30 mL of Purified Water (any temperature) in a small beaker and sprinkle the Na CMC on the surface. Stir with a glass stirring rod, then allow the liquid to stand until it clears (approximately 2 hours). Next make 30 mL of Zinc Sulfide Topical Suspension. Weigh 1.2 g each of $ZnSO_4$ and sulfurated potash, and dissolve each in 13.5 mL of water in separate beakers. Separately filter each of these two solutions; then add the sulfurated potash solution to the $ZnSO_4$ solution (the "stink" to the "zinc") slowly with constant stirring. Pour this suspension into a 2-oz prescription bottle that been precalibrated at 30 mL and 60 mL. Use extra Purified Water to completely rinse the suspension into the bottle and qs to the 30-mL mark. Transfer the phenol to this prescription bottle; tightly cap the bottle and shake well to dissolve the phenol. Add the Na CMC solution, and use additional Purified Water to completely rinse the Na CMC solution into the prescription bottle and qs to the 60-mL mark. Tightly cap the bottle and shake well. Label and dispense.

DESCRIPTION OF FINISHED PREPARATION: The preparation is a milky white suspension with very fine white particles. The suspension particles start to settle into a flocculated system in 20 to 30 minutes; at 2 hours, the bottom two-thirds of the product shows a flocculated powder structure. The preparation is easily redispersed with shaking.

QUALITY CONTROL: Volume = 60 mL; check pH with range 2 to 9 test strips: pH = 7.5

MASTER FORMULA PREPARED BY: Justiens Junco, RPh   **CHECKED BY:** Pat Schoenfeld, RPh

COMPOUNDING RECORD

NAME, STRENGTH, AND DOSAGE FORM OF PREPARATION: Phenol 1% in Modified Zinc Sulfide Topical Suspension
QUANTITY: 60 mL   **DATE PREPARED:** mm/dd/yy   **BEYOND-USE DATE:** mm/dd/yy
FORMULATION RECORD ID: SS003   **CONTROL/RX NUMBER:** 123633

INGREDIENTS USED:

Ingredient	Quantity Used	Manufacturer Lot Number	Expiration Date	Weighed/ Measured by	Checked by
Phenol	0.6 g	JET Labs SS2831	mm/yy	bjf	jj
Na CMC med visc. 2% soln	30 mL	Prac. Pharmacy XX2832	mm/yy	bjf	jj
ZnSO$_4$ (to make 30 mL White Lotion)	1.2 g	JET Labs SS2833	mm/yy	bjf	jj
Sulfurated Potash (to make 30 mL White Lotion)	1.2 g	JET Labs SS2834	mm/yy	bjf	jj
White Lotion (Zinc Sulfide Topical Suspension)	30 mL	—	—	bjf	jj
Purified Water	qs	Sweet Springs AL0529	—	bjf	jj

QUALITY CONTROL DATA: The preparation is a white suspension with fine, white particles. The suspension particles started to settle into a flocculated system at 25 minutes; at 2 hours, the bottom two-thirds of the product showed a flocculated structure with a cloudy zone at the top. The preparation was easily redispersed with shaking. The pH of the preparation was checked with range 2 to 9 pH test strips: pH = 7.5. Volume = 60 mL.

LABELING

PRACTICAL PHARMACY
425 S. CHARTULAE STREET
TRITURATE, WI 53706
(608) 555-1200 FAX: (608) 555-1210

℞ 123633   Pharmacist: JJ   Date: 00/00/00
Deborah Summit   Dr. R. Pasmak
Apply to affected areas every morning and every evening at bedtime.
Phenol 1% in Zinc Sulfide Topical Suspension 50%
Mfg: Compounded   Quantity: 60 mL
Refills: 3   Discard after: Give date

Auxiliary Labels: Shake well. For external use only. This medicine was compounded in our pharmacy for you at the direction of your prescriber.

PATIENT CONSULTATION: Hello, Miss Summit, I'm your pharmacist, Justiens Junco. Do you have any drug allergies? Are you currently using any prescription or over-the-counter medication? What did your physician tell you about this prescription? This lotion contains several ingredients, including phenol and sulfur, that are used to treat acne. Shake this well before using it, and apply it to the affected areas each morning and at bedtime daily. Be careful not to get this in your mouth or eyes. You may want to use a cotton ball to apply it. Be sure to wash the affected areas well before application, and wash your hands after applying the lotion. If your condition gets worse or you experience additional irritation, discontinue use and contact Dr. Pasmak. This is in a childproof container, but it is still best to keep it out of the reach of children. It should be stored at room temperature. Discard any unused portion after 2 weeks (give date). This may be refilled three times. Do you have any questions?

SAMPLE PRESCRIPTION 28.4

CASE: Dr. Kenneth Arrhenius is a 170-lb, 5′10″ tall, 32-year-old man. He recently took a position as assistant professor at State University. Since his teenage years, Dr. Arrhenius has a history of sporadic seborrheic dermatitis, occurring especially during time of stress. The recent flare-up of the condition has coincided with starting his new job, setting up his lab, and his first semester of teaching. At this time, his disorder presents as red, flaking, greasy areas on his scalp and several patches on his face. Dr. Gayle has had good success in treating this condition with the custom compounded suspension (given here) applied at bedtime, followed in the morning with 2.5% selenium sulfide shampoo and Cetaphil cleanser and application of 1% Hydrocortisone Lotion. Dr. Arrhenius' medication profile record shows that he is also taking omeprazole 20 mg at bedtime for gastroesophageal reflux disease. He also reports that he takes Tums as needed for chronic gastritis.

CONTEMPORARY PHYSICIANS GROUP PRACTICE
20 S. PARK STREET, TRITURATE, WI 53706
TEL: (608) 555-1333 FAX: (608) 555-1335

℞ #　*123632*

NAME *Dr. Kenneth Arrhenius*　　　　**DATE** *00/00/00*

ADDRESS *258 Kinetic Hill*

℞

Sulfur		9 g
Resorcinol monoacetate		3 mL
LCD		9 mL
Dermabase		qs
Purified Water	qs ad	90 mL

Sig: Apply to affected areas at bedtime

B. Beastly 00/00/00

REFILLS *1*　　　　　　　　*R. F. Gayle*　　　　　　**M.D.**

DEA NO. _____

MASTER COMPOUNDING FORMULATION RECORD

NAME, STRENGTH, AND DOSAGE FORM OF PREPARATION: Sulfur 10%, LCD 10%, Resorcinol monoacetate 3.3%, Dermabase 11%Topical Suspension

QUANTITY: 90 mL

THERAPEUTIC USE/CATEGORY: Antibacterial/antiseborrheic

FORMULATION RECORD ID: SS004

ROUTE OF ADMINISTRATION: Topical

INGREDIENTS:

Ingredient	Quantity Used	Physical Description	Solubility	Dose Comparison		Use in the Prescription
				Given	Usual	
Sulfur Colloidal	9 g	pale yellow, very fine powder	prac. insol. in water; v. sl. sol in alcohol	10% (w/v)	10% (w/v)	antibacterial; antifungal; keratolytic
Resorcinol Monoacetate	3 mL	viscous, pale amber liquid	spar. sol. in water; sol. in alcohol	3.3% (v/v)	1.5–3% (v/v)	antibacterial; antifungal
Coal Tar Topical Solution (LCD)	9 mL	dark brown mobile liquid	misc w/ water and alcohol	10% (v/v)	varies	antiseborrheic; antipsoriatic
Dermabase	10 g	white cream	insol in water and alcohol	11% (w/v)	varies	viscosity induction; emollient
Purified Water	qs ad 90 mL	clear liquid	—	—	—	vehicle

COMPATIBILITY–STABILITY: The sulfur and the tar ingredient (Coal Tar Topical Solution, also known as *LCD* or *liquor carbonis detergens*) in this preparation are compatible and very stable when in a suspension. The resorcinol monoacetate is somewhat more difficult to assess. It is an ester that undergoes hydrolysis, but the result is the active principle resorcinol. A lotion containing sulfur and resorcinol monoacetate is described in the resorcinol monoacetate monograph in the sixteenth edition of *Remington's Pharmaceutical Sciences*, but no stability data are given. No extra preservative is needed because both sulfur and resorcinol monoacetate have antimicrobial activity. In addition, the alcohol content is 8.4%.

PACKAGING AND STORAGE: The *USP* monographs for Coal Tar Topical Solution and for Resorcinol and Sulfur Topical Suspension recommend storage in tight containers; the *USP* monograph Resorcinol Monoacetate recommends storage in tight, light-resistant containers (3). Because this is a topical preparation, controlled room temperature will be the recommended storage conditions.

BEYOND-USE DATE: Use the recommended maximum 14-day beyond-use date for compounded water-containing liquid formulations prepared from ingredients in solid form when there is no stability information for the formulation (9).

CALCULATIONS

Dose/Concentration:

Sulfur (in w/v %):

$$\frac{9 \text{ g sulfur}}{90 \text{ mL lotion}} = \frac{x \text{ g sulfur}}{100 \text{ mL lotion}}; x = 10\text{g}/100 \text{ mL} = 10\%$$

Resorcinol monoacetate (RM) (in v/v %):

$$\frac{3 \text{ mL RM}}{90 \text{ mL lotion}} = \frac{x \text{ mL RM}}{100 \text{ mL lotion}}; x = 3.3 \text{ mL}/100 \text{ mL} = 3.3\%$$

Coal Tar Topical Solution USP (LCD) (in v/v %):

$$\frac{9 \text{ mL LCD}}{90 \text{ mL lotion}} = \frac{x \text{ mL LCD}}{100 \text{ mL lotion}}; x = 10 \text{ mL}/100 \text{ mL} = 10\%$$

Alcohol Content:

We are adding 9 mL of LCD, which contains 84% alcohol. The content of C_2H_5OH in mL is:

$$84\% \times 9 \text{ mL} = 7.56 \text{ mL}$$

The v/v % concentration of C_2H_5OH in the final preparation is calculated to be:

$$\frac{7.56 \text{ mL } C_2H_5OH}{90 \text{ mL lotion}} = \frac{x \text{ mL } C_2H_5OH}{100 \text{ mL lotion}}; x = 8.4 \text{ mL}/100 \text{ mL} = 8.4\%$$

All concentrations are okay for the intended use.

Ingredient Amounts

All ingredient amounts are given in the prescription order except for the Dermabase. Dermabase is a manufactured, nonmedicated o/w semisolid cream. It is sometimes added as an ingredient to topical suspensions to serve as a suspending and viscosity-inducing agent and to provide a smooth lotion with some emollient properties. The amount of Dermabase per volume of suspension is somewhat arbitrary and varies with the amount and type of solid ingredients and the desired preparation viscosity. For this preparation, 15 g of Dermabase was tried, and the result was a soft, semisolid cream-type preparation that did not pour easily from a standard liquid prescription bottle. Use of 10 g of Dermabase (11% w/v) gave a pourable liquid with good suspending qualities.

MSDS AND SAFETY AND PERSONAL PROTECTIVE EQUIPMENT: Review MSDS for all components. Don a clean lab coat, disposable gloves, and safety glasses. Avoid inhaling the sulfur powder.

SPECIALIZED EQUIPMENT: Wedgwood mortar; all weighing is done on an electronic balance.

COMPOUNDING PROCEDURE: Weigh 9 g of colloidal sulfur and transfer to a glass mortar. Using a 3-mL syringe, measure 3 mL of resorcinol monoacetate. Add the resorcinol monoacetate to the sulfur and triturate well to give a dry paste. Weigh 10 g of Dermabase and add with trituration to the sulfur paste. Measure 20 mL of Purified Water in a 25-mL graduated cylinder and **very** gradually add to the sulfur mixture with careful trituration. Measure 9 mL of LCD in a 10-mL graduated cylinder and gradually add it in portions with trituration to sulfur mixture. Add 15 mL of Purified Water with trituration and then additional water until the preparation thins to a pourable suspension. Transfer to a precalibrated 3-oz prescription bottle. Using successive water, rinse out the mortar and qs to the 90-mL mark on the bottle. Tightly cap the bottle and shake well. Label and dispense.

Note: Any change in the order of mixing affects the viscosity and appearance (sometimes significantly) of the finished preparation.

DESCRIPTION OF FINISHED PREPARATION: The suspension is a beige, creamy liquid. It is fairly thick but pours adequately after shaking. There is no significantly settling of solid particles on standing, and the preparation is easily redispersed with shaking.

QUALITY CONTROL: Volume = 90 mL; check pH with range 1 to 12 pH paper: pH = 5.

MASTER FORMULA PREPARED BY: Bing Beastley, PharmD   **CHECKED BY:** Pat Schoenfeld, RPh

COMPOUNDING RECORD

NAME, STRENGTH, AND DOSAGE FORM OF PREPARATION: Sulfur 10%, LCD 10%, Resorcinol monoacetate 3.3%, Dermabase 11% Topical Suspension

QUANTITY: 90 mL   **DATE PREPARED:** mm/dd/yy   **BEYOND-USE DATE:** mm/dd/yy

FORMULATION RECORD ID: SS004   **CONTROL/RX NUMBER:** 123632

INGREDIENTS USED:

Ingredient	Used	Quantity Lot Number	Manufacturer Date	Expiration Measured by	Weighed/ Checked by
Sulfur Colloidal	9 g	JET Labs SS2841	mm/yy	bjf	bb
Resorcinol Monoacetate	3 mL	JET Labs SS2842	mm/yy	bjf	bb
Coal Tar Topical Solution (LCD)	9 mL	JET Labs SS2843	mm/yy	bjf	bb
Dermabase	10 g	Paddock Labs UV5692	mm/yy	bjf	bb
Purified Water	qs ad 90 mL	Sweet Springs AL0529	mm/yy	bjf	bb

QUALITY CONTROL DATA: This is a beige, creamy-looking suspension. It is moderately thick but pours adequately after shaking. There is no visible settling of solid particles in 2 hours.

The pH of the preparation was checked with range 1 to 12 pH paper: pH = 5. Volume = 90 mL.

LABELING

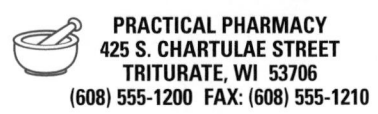

PRACTICAL PHARMACY
425 S. CHARTULAE STREET
TRITURATE, WI 53706
(608) 555-1200 FAX: (608) 555-1210

R̥ 123632   Pharmacist: BB   Date: 00/00/00
Dr. Kenneth Arrhenius   Dr. R. F. Gayle

Apply to affected areas at bedtime.

Sulfur 10%, Resorcinol Monoacetate 3.3% LCD 10%, Dermabase 11%
Topical Suspension

Alcohol content: 8.4%

Mfg: Compounded   Quantity: 90 mL

Refills: 1   Discard after: Give date

Auxiliary Labels: Shake well. For external use only. This medicine was compounded in our pharmacy for you at the direction of your prescriber.

PATIENT CONSULTATION: Hello, Dr. Arrhenius. I'm your pharmacist, Bing Beastly. Do you have any known drug allergies? Are you using any other medications, either nonprescription or prescription? Do you know the purpose of this medicine and how to use it? This is a specially formulated suspension to treat your seborrhea. It contains sulfur, resorcinol, and coal tar solution in a pleasant lotion. You are to apply this to the affected areas at bedtime. Be sure the cap is tightly on the bottle, then shake well before applying. You may want to use a cotton ball to apply it, being careful not to get any in your eyes or mouth. Be sure to wash the areas well before application, and wash your hands after applying it. Dr. Gayle has told me that you will also be using Selsun shampoo in the morning, but he said that you have a bottle of this on hand from a previous flare-up of this condition. If you run out of that, call us, and we will fill a prescription that Dr. Gayle has called in. Also you are to purchase some nonprescription Cetaphil for cleansing the area and hydrocortisone 1% lotion to apply in the morning after your shower. I can help you with that if you like. If this regimen does not seem to be helping, if the condition gets worse, or if the area becomes irritated or inflamed, call Dr. Gayle, and we can try something else. Be careful not to spill this or get any of the lotion on your clothes because this suspension contains a tar-type ingredient that will stain. This is in a childproof bottle, but it's still a good idea to keep it out of reach of children. This may be stored at room temperature, and any unused portion should be discarded after 2 weeks (give date). Dr. Gayle has authorized one refill if you need it. Do you have any questions?

SAMPLE PRESCRIPTION 28.5

CASE: Joseph Wilding is a 175-lb, 6′-tall, 75-year-old man. He was recently diagnosed with a brain tumor; it was successfully removed surgically, but Mr. Wilding suffered a stroke during the surgery. He has undergone rehabilitation therapy at a local center and is now at home recuperating. A visiting nurse and a physical therapist come to his home several times a week, and a nurse's aid provides daily assistance with care. Mr. Wilding has a 5-year history of hypertension, which has been well-controlled up to this time with enalapril 10 mg daily. His blood pressure has recently been elevated to 140/90, and he has some edema in his ankles. Dr. Wurtz wants to try adding hydrochlorothiazide 25 mg once a day to his regimen. Since his stroke, Mr. Wilding has had difficulty with swallowing tablets and capsules, so Dr. Wurtz has asked pharmacist Judy Thompson to make a hydrochlorothiazide oral suspension.

CONTEMPORARY PHYSICIANS GROUP PRACTICE
20 S. PARK STREET, TRITURATE, WI 53706
TEL: (608) 555-1333 FAX: (608) 555-1335

℞ # *123667*

NAME *Joseph Wilding*   **DATE** *00/00/00*

ADDRESS *568 Mockingbird Lane*

℞

Hydrochlorothiazide	*25 mg/5 mL*	
M & Ft Suspension	*60 mL*	

JET 00/00/00

Sig: one tsp (5 mL) by mouth q am

REFILLS *11 X*   *Ozzie Wurtz*   **M.D.**

DEA NO. _____

MASTER COMPOUNDING FORMULATION RECORD

NAME, STRENGTH, AND DOSAGE FORM OF PREPARATION: Hydrochlorothiazide Oral Suspension 25 mg/5 mL

QUANTITY: 60 mL

THERAPEUTIC USE/CATEGORY: Antihypertensive

FORMULATION RECORD ID: SS005

ROUTE OF ADMINISTRATION: Oral

INGREDIENTS USED:

Ingredient	Quantity Used	Physical Description	Solubility	Dose Comparison		Use in the Prescription
				Given	Usual	
Hydrochloro-thiazide as 50 mg tablets	300 mg (6 × 50 mg tabs)	peach-colored tablets	sl sol in water, sol in alcohol	25 mg daily	25–200 mg/day	Antihyper-tensive; diuretic
Citrucel	2 g	orange powder	MC sol in water, insol in alcohol	3.33%	variable	suspending agent
Sodium Benzoate	120 mg	white powder	1 g/1.8 mL water, 75 mL alcohol	0.2%	0.1–0.3%	preservative
Purified Water	qs 60 mL	clear liquid	—	—	—	vehicle

COMPATIBILITY–STABILITY: The stability of hydrochlorothiazide is described in *The Chemical Stability of Pharmaceuticals*. The drug is most stable at pH 4, with a half-life of 720 days at 25°C (14). Citrucel powder has been selected as the suspending agent for crushed hydrochlorothiazide tablets. Citrucel is an orange-flavored methylcellulose product marketed as an OTC bulk laxative. It is available sweetened with sucrose or as a sugar-free product sweetened with Aspartame. It makes a convenient suspending medium for extemporaneous suspensions. It does not contain a preservative, so a preservative should be added to provide protection from growth of bacteria, yeasts, and molds. Either Potassium Sorbate or Sodium Benzoate would be effective because suspensions made with Citrucel have a pH of approximately 4. This formulation uses sodium benzoate 0.2%.

PACKAGING AND STORAGE: Dispense in a tight container. Because this is an oral preparation, it should be stored in the refrigerator. This will enhance its stability, both chemical and microbiological, and also its taste.

BEYOND-USE DATE: Because this is a formulation with some known stability information, there is some flexibility in assigning a beyond-use date. Though the formulation is most likely stable for at least 6 months, the amount dispensed is only a 12-day supply, so use a conservative 30-day beyond-use date.

CALCULATIONS

Dose/Concentration: Dose of 25 mg hydrochlorothiazide (HCTZ) daily is okay for an elderly patient.

Ingredient Amounts

HCTZ (in mg): $\qquad$ 25 mg/5 mL × 60 mL = 300 mg

HCTZ is available as 50-mg tablets. Exactly six tablets are needed for 300 mg.

Citrucel: Recommended amount is 2 g for 60 mL of suspension.

Preservative: Sodium benzoate is selected. The amount (in mg) is calculated to be:

$$0.2\% \times 60 \text{ mL} = 0.002 \times 60 \text{ mL} = 0.12 \text{ g} = 120 \text{ mg}$$

MSDS AND SAFETY AND PERSONAL PROTECTIVE EQUIPMENT: Don a clean lab coat and disposable gloves.

SPECIALIZED EQUIPMENT: Glass mortar; all weighing is done on an electronic balance.

COMPOUNDING PROCEDURE: Place six 50-mg HCTZ tablets in a glass mortar and moisten the tablets with a small amount of Purified Water to facilitate crushing. On an electronic balance, weigh 120 mg of sodium benzoate and 2 g of Citrucel powder. Transfer the Citrucel and sodium benzoate to the mortar with the crushed HCTZ tablets and gradually add about 40 mL of Purified Water in portions with trituration. Transfer to a 60-mL precalibrated prescription bottle. Using more Purified Water, rinse out the mortar and transfer the rinsings to the prescription bottle. Add Purified Water to the calibration mark on the bottle. Cap the bottle tightly and shake well; label and dispense.

DESCRIPTION OF FINISHED PREPARATION: The preparation is an orange suspension; it is fairly viscous, and there is minimal settling on standing. The preparation pours adequately after shaking.

QUALITY CONTROL: Volume = 60 mL; check the pH of the preparation with range 1 to 12 pH paper: pH = 4

MASTER FORMULA PREPARED BY: Judith Thompson, RPh   **CHECKED BY:** Pat Schoenfeld, RPh

COMPOUNDING RECORD

NAME, STRENGTH, AND DOSAGE FORM OF PREPARATION: Hydrochlorothiazide Oral Suspension 25 mg/5 mL
QUANTITY: 60 mL   **DATE PREPARED:** mm/dd/yy   **BEYOND-USE DATE:** mm/dd/yy
FORMULATION RECORD ID: SS005   **CONTROL/RX NUMBER:** 123667

INGREDIENTS USED:

Ingredient	Quantity	Manufacturer Lot Number	Expiration Date	Weighed/ Measured by	Checked by
Hydrochlorothiazide as 50 mg tablets	300 mg (6 × 50 mg tabs)	BJF Generics XY5739	mm/yy	bjf	jet
Citrucel	2 g	SK-Beecham XX2852	mm/yy	bjf	jet
Sodium Benzoate	120 mg	JET Labs SS2851	mm/yy	bjf	jet
Purified Water	qs 60 mL	Sweet Springs AL0529	mm/yy	bjf	jet

QUALITY CONTROL DATA: The preparation is an orange suspension It is moderately viscous, and there is no visible settling on standing. The suspension becomes sufficiently fluid with shaking. The pH of the preparation was checked with range 1 to 12 pH paper: pH = 4. Volume = 60 mL.

LABELING

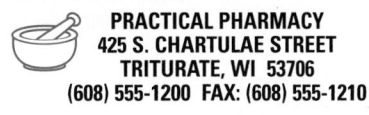

PRACTICAL PHARMACY
425 S. CHARTULAE STREET
TRITURATE, WI 53706
(608) 555-1200 FAX: (608) 555-1210

R̸ 123667   Pharmacist: JET   Date: 00/00/00
Joseph Wilding   Dr. Ozzie Wurtz

Take one teaspoonful (5 mL) by mouth every morning.

Hydrochlorothiazide 25 mg/5 mL Oral Suspension

Mfg: Compounded   Quantity: 60 mL

Refills: 11X   Discard after: Give date

Auxiliary Labels: Shake well. Keep in the refrigerator. This medicine was compounded in our pharmacy for you at the direction of your prescriber.

PATIENT CONSULTATION: Hello, Mrs. Wilding, I'm your pharmacist, Judy Thompson. Here is the prescription for Mr. Wilding. How are things going at home with his care? What did Dr. Wurtz tell you about this drug? It is called hydrochlorothiazide, and it should lower Mr. Wilding's blood pressure and reduce the swelling in his ankles. He is to take this in addition to the blood pressure drug enalapril that he has been taking for a number of years. He should take one teaspoonful or 5 mL of this liquid every morning. If you forget to give a dose, give it as soon as you remember, but if you miss his dose one day, do not double the dose the next day, just skip it. Mr. Wilding's potassium will need to be checked on a regular basis because this medicine can cause loss of potassium. This medication should increase his urine output, especially now when he is starting therapy; that is why he should take it in the morning, so he (and you) are not up frequently during the night with him going to the bathroom. Though uncommon, side effects from this medication may include upset stomach, dizziness, lightheadedness, and loose stools. If side effects occur and become bothersome, contact Dr. Wurtz. I remember that I gave you an oral syringe for his enalapril suspension; do you need another one, or is a measuring teaspoon more convenient for you to use? Store this in the refrigerator for best stability and taste. Shake the bottle well before measuring the dose. Discard any unused contents after a month. Keep out of reach of children. This may be refilled 11 times. Do you have any questions?

SAMPLE PRESCRIPTION 28.6

CASE: Peter Childs is a 68-lb (fiftieth percentile), 54″-tall (fortieth percentile), 10-year old white boy with type 1 diabetes diagnosed at age 5. He is currently using the following insulin regimen: NPH 4 units in the AM and 2 units at bedtime with lispro on a sliding scale (0.5 to 1.5 units) at breakfast and dinner. In addition to closely monitoring Peter's blood glucose, his parents keep tabs on his renal function by periodically collecting a 24-hour urine sample and measuring the volume to evaluate urinary output. The last sample was 950 mL and within the normal range of 1 to 2 mL/kg/hr. At a recent checkup, Peter's blood pressure was found to be 121/81 (elevated over the ninety-fifth percentile for a boy of his age and height). On his return checkup today, it was again elevated at 120/82, so Dr. Wurtz has decided to start him on an initial dose of captopril, 300 mcg/kg three times a day. Peter's parents will keep a close check on his renal function and will monitor his blood pressure. He is not on any other medications except for the occasional antibiotic for an infection and acetaminophen for fever.

CONTEMPORARY PHYSICIANS GROUP PRACTICE
20 S. PARK STREET, TRITURATE, WI 53706
TEL: (608) 555-1333 FAX: (608) 555-1335

℞ #   *123625*

NAME *Peter Childs*   **DATE** *00/00/00*

ADDRESS *2530 Souffle Circle*

℞

      Captopril   *300 mcg/kg/dose*
      Flavored Sugar-free Syrup   *qs*
          Give enough for 10 days

JRA 00/00/00

      Sig: Give one dose tid, one hr ac

REFILLS *1*   *Ozzie Wurtz*   **M.D.**

DEA NO. _____

MASTER COMPOUNDING FORMULATION RECORD

NAME, STRENGTH, AND DOSAGE FORM OF PREPARATION: Captopril Oral Suspension 9 mg/5 mL
QUANTITY: 150 mL   **FORMULATION RECORD ID:** SS006
THERAPEUTIC USE/CATEGORY: antihypertensive   **ROUTE OF ADMINISTRATION:** Oral

INGREDIENTS USED:

Ingredient	Quantity Used	Physical Description	Solubility	Dose Comparison		Use in the Prescription
				Given	Usua	
Captopril as 50 mg tablets	270 mg drug from 1,156 mg crushed tablet powder	white tablets	1 g/6 mL water; fr sol in alcohol	300 mcg/kg t.i.d. or 9 mg t.i.d.	300 mcg/kg t.i.d. or 9 mg t.i.d.	antihypertensive
Ora-Sweet SF	75 mL	colorless, clear, viscous liquid	mis w/water and alcohol	—	—	sweet, viscous vehicle
Ora-Plus	75 mL	colorless, cloudy, viscous liquid	mis w/water and alcohol	—	—	suspending vehicle

COMPATIBILITY–STABILITY: Captopril has limited stability in aqueous solution. It degrades by oxidation and is quite sensitive to conditions, including pH, temperature, and the presence of metal ions (15). Research published in *AJHP* found that a suspension made with crushed tablets in a 50:50 mixture of Ora-Sweet SF and Ora-Plus had a remaining content of 93% when stored for 10 days at 5°C (16). Both Ora-Sweet SF and Ora-Plus are preserved so an additional preservative is not needed.

PACKAGING AND STORAGE: This preparation should be dispensed in a tight, light-resistant container and stored in the refrigerator. The research article cited earlier found that in the chosen vehicle, the captopril content was diminished to 86% in 10 days when stored at 25°C, so proper storage temperature is essential. Refrigeration will also enhance the taste of the preparation.

BEYOND-USE DATE: Because this is a formulation with some known stability information, there can be some confidence when assigning a beyond-use date of 10 days. As noted, appropriate storage temperature is important; however, even when refrigerated, the study showed that the content of the suspension had dropped to 90% by 14 days.

CALCULATIONS

Dose/Concentration: Captopril: 300 mcg/kg t.i.d is an appropriate dose

Dose (in mg):

$$\text{Weight of child in kg: } \frac{68 \text{ lb}}{2.2 \text{ lb/kg}} = 31 \text{ kg}$$

$$300 \text{ mcg/kg} \times 31 \text{ kg} = 9,300 \text{ mcg} = 9.3 \text{ mg} \approx 9 \text{ mg/dose}$$

Ingredient Amounts

Captopril:

Amount of drug for 10 days: 9 mg/dose $\times$ 3 doses/day $\times$ 10 days = 270 mg

Captopril is available as 50-mg tablets. The number of tablets needed is calculated as:

$$\frac{270 \text{ mg catopril needed}}{50 \text{ mg catopril/tablet}} = 5.4 \text{ or 6 tablets}$$

Six 50-mg captopril tablets (300 mg of captopril) are found to weigh 1,284 mg. The quantity of crushed tablet powder that will contain 270 mg of Captopril is calculated as:

$$\frac{300 \text{ mg catopril}}{1,284 \text{ mg tablet powder}} = \frac{270 \text{ mg catopril}}{x \text{ mg tablet powder}}; x = 1,156 \text{ mg crushed tablet powder}$$

Volume of Suspension for 10 days using 5 mL/dose:

$$5 \text{ mL/dose} \times 3 \text{ doses/day} \times 10 \text{ days} = 150 \text{ mL}$$

MSDS AND SAFETY AND PERSONAL PROTECTIVE EQUIPMENT: Don a clean lab coat and disposable gloves.

SPECIALIZED EQUIPMENT: Glass mortar; all weighing is done on an electronic balance.

COMPOUNDING PROCEDURE: Weigh six tablets of Captopril 50 mg (total weight 1,284 mg or 214 mg per tablet). Crush the six tablets in a glass mortar and weigh 1,156 mg of this crushed tablet powder. Place the weighed tablet powder in a clean mortar. In a graduated cylinder, measure 75 mL each of Ora-Sweet SF and Ora-Plus, combine the two, and stir to mix well. Gradually with trituration add approximately 20 to 40 mL of the mixed vehicle to the mortar. Transfer the suspension to a 6-oz prescription bottle precalibrated at 150 mL. Using additional vehicle, rinse out the mortar and transfer the rinsings to the prescription bottle to qs to the 150-mL calibration mark on the bottle. Tightly cap the bottle and shake well; label and dispense.

DESCRIPTION OF FINISHED PREPARATION: The preparation is a cloudy, colorless suspension. The suspension has a medium viscosity, and there is minimal settling on standing. The preparation is easily redispersed with shaking.

QUALITY CONTROL: Volume = 150 mL; check the pH of the preparation using range 4.0 to 7.0 pH test strips: pH = 4.2.

MASTER FORMULA PREPARED BY: John Albers, PharmD   **CHECKED BY:** Pat Schoenfeld, RPh

COMPOUNDING RECORD

NAME, STRENGTH, AND DOSAGE FORM OF PREPARATION: Captopril Oral Suspension 9 mg/5 mL

QUANTITY: 150 mL   **DATE PREPARED:** mm/dd/yy   **BEYOND-USE DATE:** mm/dd/yy

FORMULATION RECORD ID: SS006   **CONTROL/RX NUMBER:** 123625

INGREDIENTS USED:

Ingredient	Quantity	Manufacturer Lot Number	Expiration Date	Weighed/ Measured by	Checked by
Captopril as 50 mg tablets	270 mg drug from 1,156 mg crushed tablet powder	BJF Generics XY3692	mm/yy	bjf	jra
Ora-Sweet SF	75 mL	Paddock Labs SS2862	mm/yy	bjf	jra
Ora-Plus	75 mL	Paddock Labs SS2863	mm/yy	bjf	jra

QUALITY CONTROL DATA: The preparation is a cloudy, colorless suspension. It has a medium viscosity with minimal, if any, settling in 2 hours. The preparation is easily redispersed with shaking and pours easily. The pH of the preparation was checked using range 4.0 to 7.0 pH test strips pH = 4.2. Volume = 150 mL.

LABELING

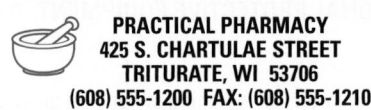

PRACTICAL PHARMACY
425 S. CHARTULAE STREET
TRITURATE, WI 53706
(608) 555-1200 FAX: (608) 555-1210

℞ 123625   Pharmacist: JRA   Date: 00/00/00
Peter Childs   Dr. Ozzie Wurtz

Take one teaspoonful (5 mL) of syrup three times daily, one hour before each meal.

Captopril 9 mg/5 mL Oral Suspension

Mfg: Compounded   Quantity: 150 mL

Refills: 1   Discard after: Give date

Auxiliary Labels: Shake well. Keep in the refrigerator. This medicine was compounded in our pharmacy for you at the direction of your prescriber.

PATIENT CONSULTATION: Hello, Mrs. Childs, I'm your pharmacist, John Albers. Here is the prescription for Peter. Is he allergic to any medications that you know of? I know that he uses insulin, but is he currently taking any other medications? What did Dr. Wurtz tell you about this drug and how to use it? This drug is known as *captopril*, and it should lower his blood pressure. It is important to give him one teaspoonful or 5 mL three times a day, approximately 1 hour before each meal. If you forget to give a dose, give it as soon as you remember, but if it is close to the next dose, skip it. Though uncommon, this medication may cause dizziness or lightheadedness, cough, and some skin reactions such as rash or itching. If these or any other adverse effects occur and become bothersome, contact Dr. Wurtz. The most common side effect is a cough; so if Peter develops a persistent cough, talk to Dr. Wurtz. Do notify Dr. Wurtz immediately if Peter experiences swelling of the face, lips, or tongue and difficulty breathing, as this could indicate a rare but serious reaction to this drug. I know that you monitor Peter's blood glucose. Will you also be checking his blood pressure? If you need assistance with that, let me know, as I would be happy to help you. Do you have something to accurately measure the dose of this liquid medicine? This is one drug for which storage of the suspension in the refrigerator is essential for stability. Shake the bottle well before measuring the dose. Discard any unused contents after 10 days. Even though there is a safety cap on the bottle, keep this out of reach of children. This may be refilled one time. Do you have any questions?

REFERENCES

1. The United States Pharmacopeial Convention, Inc. Chapter ⟨1151⟩ 2008 USP 31/NF 26. Rockville, MD: Author, 2007; 623.
2. Marshall K, Foster TS, Carlin HS, Williams RL. Development of a compendial taxonomy and glossary for pharmaceutical dosage forms. Pharmacopeial Forum. Rockville, MD: The United States Pharmacopeial Convention, Inc., 2003; 29(5).
3. The United States Pharmacopeial Convention, Inc. 2008 USP 31/NF 26. USP Monographs. Rockville, MD: Author, 2007.
4. Food and Drug Administration. CDER Data Standards Manual. Rockville, MD: 2006. Data Element Name: Dosage Form, http://www.fda.gov/cder/dsm/DRG/drg00201.htm.
5. Bummer PM. Interfacial phenomena. In: University of the Sciences in Philadelphia, ed. Remington: The science and practice of pharmacy, 21st ed. Philadelphia: Lippincott Williams & Wilkins, 2006; 283.
6. Sinko PJ. Martin's physical pharmacy and pharmaceutical sciences, 5th ed. Philadelphia: Lippincott Williams & Wilkins, 2006; 447–461.
7. Zografi G. Interfacial phenomena. In: Gennaro AR, ed. Remington: The science and practice of pharmacy, 19th ed. Easton, PA: Mack Publishing Co., 1995; 247.
8. Sinko PJ. Martin's physical pharmacy and pharmaceutical sciences, 5th ed. Philadelphia: Lippincott Williams & Wilkins, 2006; 499–500.
9. The United States Pharmacopeial Convention, Inc. Chapter ⟨795⟩ 2008 USP 31/NF 26. Rockville, MD: Author, 2007; 316–317.
10. Trissel LA. Trissel's stability of compounded formulations, 3rd ed. Washington, DC: American Pharmacists Association, 2005; 253–255.
11. Trissel LA. Trissel's stability of compounded formulations, 3rd ed. Washington, DC: American Pharmacists Association, 2005; 212–215.
12. Timmons P, Gray EA. Degradation of hydrocortisone in a zinc oxide lotion. J Clin Hosp Pharm 1983; 8:79–85.
13. Reilly WJ Jr. Pharmaceutical necessities. In: University of the Sciences in Philadelphia, ed. Remington: The science and practice of pharmacy, 21st ed. Philadelphia: Lippincott Williams & Wilkins, 2006; 1074.
14. Connors KA, Amidon GL, Stella VJ. Chemical stability of pharmaceuticals, 2nd ed. New York: John Wiley and Sons, 1986; 478–482.
15. Connors KA, Amidon GL, Stella VJ. Chemical stability of pharmaceuticals, 2nd ed. New York: John Wiley and Sons, 1986; 284–289.
16. Allen LV Jr, Erickson MA III. Stability of baclofen, captopril, diltiazem hydrochloride, Dipyridamole, and flecainide acetate in extemporaneously compounded oral liquids. Am J Health-Syst Pharm 1996; 53: 2179–2184.

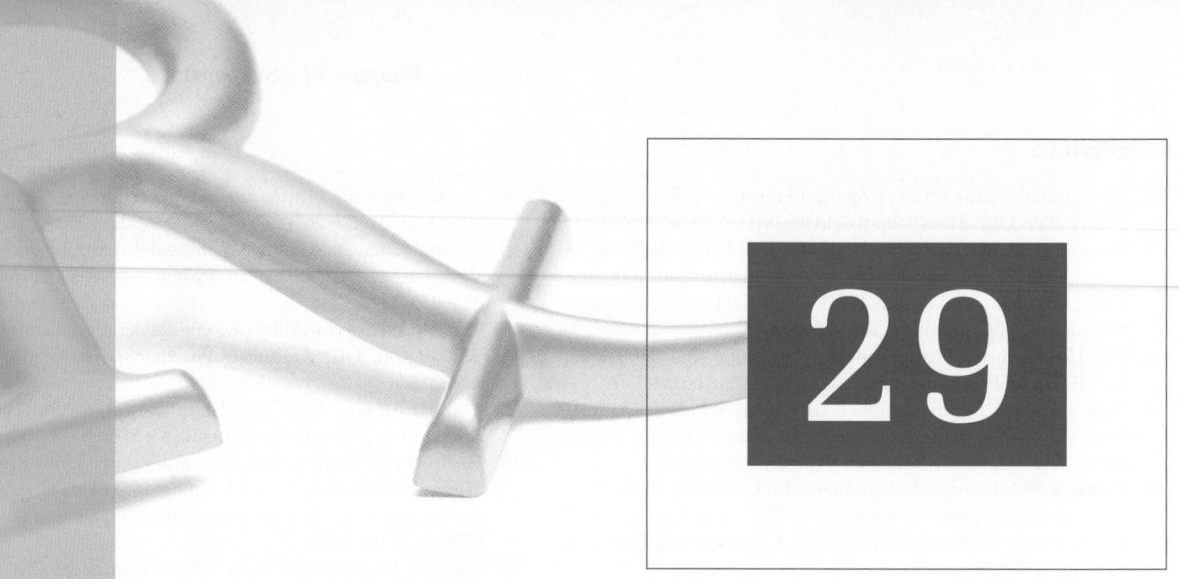

Liquid Emulsions

I. DEFINITIONS

A. **Emulsions:** "Emulsions are two-phase systems in which one liquid is dispersed throughout another liquid in the form of small droplets" (1).

1. All emulsions for oral administration are liquids, but emulsions for topical administration may be either liquid or semisolid. This chapter covers liquid emulsions; semisolid emulsions are discussed in Chapter 30, Semisolids: Ointments, Creams, Gels, Pastes, and Collodions.

2. It should be noted that general terms, such as *lotion*, *liniment*, and *liquid*, have been used to name topical liquids, which could be solutions, suspensions, or emulsions. As was discussed in Chapter 27, in 2002, USP formed a group to clarify pharmaceutical dosage form nomenclature. In 2006, FDA revised its dosage form terminology to help users of drug products in differentiating between topical dosage forms such as lotions, creams, ointments, and pastes (2). According to the 2006 FDA *CDER Data Standards Manual*, the following definitions apply:

   a. **Lotion:** "An emulsion, liquid dosage form. This dosage form is generally for external application to the skin" (2). A footnote states that this term will be restricted to emulsions and will no longer be used for solutions or suspensions (2).

   b. **Liniment:** "A solution or mixture of various substances in oil, alcoholic solutions or soap, or emulsions intended for external application" (2).

B. **Miscible/immiscible:** When two liquids are completely soluble (that is, molecularly dispersed) in each other in all proportions, they are said to be miscible; examples include water and alcohol, and olive oil and cottonseed oil. Some liquid pairs, such as castor oil and alcohol, are partially miscible, which means that they are soluble in each other in definite proportions. Immiscible liquid pairs are imperceptibly soluble in each other in any proportion; examples include water and mineral oil, and alcohol and mineral oil. Specific miscibility information for common pharmaceutical solvents is given in Chapter 15, Pharmaceutical Solvents and Solubilizing Agents; for a general discussion of miscibility, see section IV. C. 2. in Chapter 27, Solutions.

C. **Emulsification:** Emulsification is the process of creating an emulsion from two immiscible liquid phases. It can be accomplished when energy is applied to the system (e.g., trituration or homogenization) to create small droplets and cause a physical and/or electrostatic barrier to form around the droplets to prevent them from coalescing. This is accomplished by the use of emulsifying agents. The dispersed droplets are collectively termed the *internal phase*, and the continuous liquid is called the *external phase*.

D. **Emulsifying agents:** Emulsifying agents are surfactants that concentrate at the interface of the two immiscible phases, reduce the interfacial tension between the immiscible phases, provide a barrier around the droplets as they form, and prevent coalescence of the droplets. Some emulsifying agents also increase the viscosity of the system, slowing aggregation of the droplets and decreasing the rate of creaming. Surfactants and emulsifying agents commonly used for compounding purposes are described and discussed in Chapter 20, Surfactants and Emulsifying Agents.

E. **Creaming:** Creaming is the migration of the droplets of the internal phase to the top or bottom of the emulsion. The migration is caused by the difference in density between the two phases, and the direction of the movement depends on whether the internal phase is more or less dense than the continuous or external phase.

F. **Coalescence:** Coalescence is the merging of small droplets into larger droplets with eventual complete separation of phases so that the droplets cannot be re-emulsified by simple shaking of the preparation. With coalescence, the barrier formed by the emulsifying agent(s) is broken or destroyed. This irreversible coalescence of the droplets is also called *cracking*.

II. USES OF LIQUID EMULSIONS

A. **Oral emulsions:** As discussed in the chapters on solutions and suspensions, there are times when oral liquid preparations are needed. Generally, oral liquid emulsions are less acceptable to patients than are solutions or suspensions because of the objectionable oily feel of emulsions in the mouth. Therefore, an oral emulsion is formulated only when it is necessary to make a liquid preparation of an oil or when the solubility or bioavailability characteristics of a drug make this dosage form clearly superior.

B. **Topical emulsions:** Topical emulsions are more common. Emollient (soothing of the skin) or protective properties are often desired of topical preparations, and oils can serve these functions. When the oils are emulsified, they feel less greasy and are more aesthetically appealing to patients.

III. EMULSION TYPE

A. **Oil-in-water** (o/w): In this type, the oil is dispersed as droplets in an aqueous solution. This is the most common emulsion type. It is always preferred for oral preparations where an oily feel in the mouth is objectionable. It is also used for external preparations when ease of removal and/or a non-greasy-feeling preparation is desired.

B. **Water-in-oil** (w/o): In this type, the water is dispersed as droplets in an oil or oleaginous material. This type is used for external preparations when emollient, lubricating, or protective properties are desired.

C. **Factors that determine emulsion type**
1. Emulsifier
   As described in Chapter 20, some emulsifiers will form either w/o or o/w emulsions; others form only one type.
2. Phase ratio (that is, relative amounts of oil and water)
   All other things being equal, the phase that is present in the greater concentration tends to be the external phase, but an emulsifying agent that strongly favors a particular emulsion type and that forms a good barrier at the interface can overcome an unfavorable phase ratio.
3. Order of mixing
   Because the phase that is present in the greater concentration tends to be the external phase, the phase that is being added, usually by portions, tends to be the internal phase. The bulk external phase will continue to accommodate added internal phase as small droplets until either the bulk phase becomes completely packed or there is no longer sufficient emulsifying agent to serve as a barrier to coalescence. Then, if more internal phase is added, either it will fail to be emulsified and will remain as separate droplets or the emulsion will coalesce; or, if the emulsifier will allow it, phase inversion will occur. The external phase, which was the continuous phase, now becomes the dispersed droplets, the internal phase.

IV. DESIRED PROPERTIES OF A LIQUID EMULSION

A. Fine droplets

Emulsions with fine droplet size are desired. Many factors can contribute to small droplets.

1. One factor is the mechanical method used for mixing and shearing the two immiscible liquids. The pharmaceutical industry has specialized equipment for this task. For extemporaneous compounding, a rough-sided Wedgwood mortar is usually used for the emulsification process. Simple, relatively inexpensive hand-homogenizers and high-speed blenders are available, which may give finer and more uniform droplets.
2. Certain techniques, such as phase inversion, can be used to give fine, uniform-sized droplets.
3. Finally, some emulsifying agents give finer emulsions. For example, amino-soaps are better-balanced emulsifiers than are the alkali soaps and give more stable emulsions of finer droplet size (3).

B. Slow aggregation of the droplets and creaming of the preparation

1. Though almost all emulsions eventually cream, the rate of creaming should be slow enough to ensure accurate measurement of a dose or application of a uniform preparation.
2. Aggregation and creaming can be slowed through proper emulsification and through the use of various additives, such as viscosity-increasing agents. To control the rate of creaming, you can adjust some of the parameters found in Stokes' Law. Though this equation was developed for particles settling in a suspension, many of the same factors affect the rate of creaming for droplets in an emulsion. These include droplet size, viscosity of the continuous phase, and relative density difference of the droplets and the continuous phase. For a more complete discussion of Stokes' Law, see section III. C. in Chapter 28, Suspensions.

C. Ease of redispersion when shaken

Though aggregation and creaming are usually unavoidable, the preparation should be formulated so that the internal phase readily redisperses to give a uniform emulsion when the preparation is shaken. Furthermore, coalescence should not occur.

V. COMPOUNDING BASIC EMULSION TYPES

A. Acacia emulsions:
Acacia is unique among the polymer emulsifiers in its ability to form emulsions using only a Wedgwood mortar and pestle. It is therefore a useful ingredient for extemporaneous compounding of emulsions and is usually the first emulsifying agent considered when a compounded emulsion is needed.

1. The emulsification process for acacia emulsions requires the formation of a primary emulsion. The term *primary emulsion* is used to describe the initial emulsion formed with a prescribed ratio of ingredients. This prescribed set of ingredients gives a system of optimal viscosity and consistency so that the shearing force exerted in the mortar is maximized to allow the formation of an emulsion.
2. Ingredient ratio for primary acacia emulsions
   a. For fixed oils, such as vegetable oils, and for mineral oil, the oil-to-water-to-acacia ratio (o:w:a) is 4:2:1. In general, fixed oils (e.g., vegetable oils) form acacia emulsions more readily than does mineral oil, so if there is a choice of oils, select one of the fixed oils.
   b. The ratio for volatile and essential oils is 3:2:1 or 2:2:1.
   c. The absolute ingredient amounts calculated from the appropriate ratio are predicated on the total amount of oil in the formulation. Because acacia forms o/w emulsions, the oil is the internal phase. Therefore, all of the oil in the formulation must be emulsified when making the primary emulsion. After the primary emulsion is formed, the emulsion may be diluted with any extra water or water-miscible phase, as required.
3. Methods of forming the primary emulsion
   a. **Dry gum method.** The dry gum method usually is the preferred method. Its steps are given next and are illustrated with a set of four photographs in Color Plate 7.
      (1) The calculated amount of acacia and all the oil contained in the formulation are put in a Wedgwood mortar and triturated until a smooth slurry results and all the acacia is properly wet by the oil.
      (2) The amount of the aqueous phase, which is calculated from the ratio given earlier, is measured in a **clean, dry** graduated cylinder and is added, all at once, with **hard and fast** trituration.

(3) Trituration is continued until the primary emulsion is formed. You know this has occurred when the system changes from a translucent, oily-appearing liquid into a thick, white liquid. The sound of trituration also changes to give a crackling sound.

(4) Once the primary emulsion is formed, other ingredients may be added.

b. Wet gum method. With the wet gum method, the order of mixing is as follows:

(1) The appropriate amount of acacia is put in a Wedgwood mortar, and a small amount of water-miscible wetting agent, such as glycerin, is added to wet the acacia. This is necessary because powdered acacia gets lumpy when water is added directly to it.

(2) The calculated amount of water is then gradually added in portions with trituration.

(3) The oil is then gradually added with trituration until all the oil has been added and the primary is formed.

(4) As with the dry gum method, once the primary emulsion is formed, water or other ingredients may be added.

4. Order of mixing for acacia emulsions

a. Make the primary emulsion first using all the oil(s), the acacia, and Purified Water, in the appropriate ratio.

b. Additional water, water-miscible liquids, including flavored syrups, and water-soluble drugs or chemicals may then be added directly to the primary emulsion. Soluble ingredients that are in solid form may be dissolved first in water or another appropriate solvent before being added to the emulsion.

c. Insoluble ingredients, such as zinc oxide and calamine, should be put in a separate mortar, and the primary emulsion should be added to the powders in portions with trituration. This is done to wet the powders and reduce their particle size so that a smooth preparation results. This process is illustrated in Sample Prescription 29.1.

d. In some cases, oil-soluble ingredients may be dissolved in the oil phase before the formation of the primary emulsion. This is illustrated with the active ingredients avobenzone and oxybenzone in Sample Prescription 29.1. If the primary emulsion fails to form with the extra ingredient or ingredients in the oil phase, the ingredients should be handled as described in c. preceding.

5. Preservation and storage

a. *USP* Chapter ⟨1151⟩ states that preservatives are required for all emulsions (1). This is especially important with acacia emulsions because they are very susceptible to microbial (especially mold) growth.

b. Acacia emulsions have a pH in the range of 4.5 to 5.0, unless the formulation contains an ingredient that alters the pH. Therefore, preservatives that require a slightly acid pH, such as benzoic acid or sorbic acid, are effective preservatives for acacia emulsions. For the official acacia emulsion, Mineral Oil Emulsion USP, the use of either benzoic acid 0.2% or alcohol 4% to 6% is recommended. The benzoic acid may be added as its sodium salt. Methylparaben 0.2% with propylparaben 0.02% is also an acceptable preservative system. The quaternary ammonium preservatives, such as benzalkonium chloride, benzethonium chloride, and cetylpyridinium chloride, are not recommended because they are inactivated through binding with acacia.

c. For reasons of improved stability and taste, internal preparations should be stored in a refrigerator. External preparations are generally stored at controlled room temperature.

6. A complete description of acacia, including its incompatibilities and limitations, is given in Chapter 19, Viscosity-Inducing Agents.

B. Nascent soap emulsions: The term *nascent* means beginning to exist or to develop. As the name implies, the emulsifier is formed as these emulsions are made. These emulsifiers are the hard and soft soaps, which are discussed in Chapter 20, Surfactants and Emulsifying Agents. The current section concentrates on a prototype of this emulsion type, so-called lime water emulsions, in which the emulsifier, calcium oleate, is formed when saturated solution of calcium hydroxide (lime water) is added to a vegetable oil containing oleic acid.

1. Oil phase

a. Olive oil was the original oil used in these emulsions because, of all the vegetable oils, it has the largest amount of free fatty acid necessary for forming the soap-emulsifying agent.

b. Olive oil may be replaced by other vegetable oils; however, in this case, extra free fatty acid in the form of oleic acid must be added.

c. Depending on its source, olive oil may also need fortification with extra oleic acid. It may be advisable to add 3 to 5 drops of oleic acid per 30 mL of olive oil or 1 to 1.5 mL oleic acid per 30 mL of any other vegetable oil before the emulsification process is begun. Extra oleic acid may be added drop-wise during emulsification if necessary. This is illustrated in Sample Prescription 29.2.

2. Lime water should be freshly prepared. The formula can be found in the *USP* under Calcium Hydroxide Topical Solution. It is reproduced here (4):

    | Calcium hydroxide | 3 g |
    | Purified Water | 1,000 mL |

    Add the calcium hydroxide to 1,000 mL of cool Purified Water, and agitate the mixture vigorously and repeatedly during 1 hour. Allow the excess calcium hydroxide to settle. Dispense only the clear, supernatant.

3. Methods of preparation

    a. Bottle method: With this method, equal amounts of oil (containing adequate oleic acid) and lime water are placed in a bottle. The bottle is shaken vigorously to form the emulsion. The emulsion can then be used as a wetting agent for any solid insoluble ingredients. This method is illustrated on Color Plate 8, and the procedure is demonstrated on the CD that accompanies this book.

    b. Mortar method: The mortar method is often preferred when the formulation contains solid insoluble ingredients, such as zinc oxide or calamine. These solids concentrate at the oil–water interface as the emulsion is being formed and enhance the interfacial barrier, which improves the stability of the system. With this method, the solids are placed in a mortar. The oil (containing oleic acid) is added in portions with trituration until all the oil has been added and a smooth slurry of oil-powders is obtained. The lime water is then added in portions with trituration to form the emulsion.

4. Order of mixing: This depends somewhat on the method of emulsification as described earlier.

    a. With either method, water-miscible liquids and water-soluble drugs or chemicals should be added to the lime water before it is added to the bottle or mortar for emulsification. This is because water is the internal phase.

    b. Because oil is the external phase, oil-soluble and oil-miscible ingredients can be added to the oil before emulsification or to the emulsion after the water phase is emulsified.

    c. Any insoluble ingredients should be placed in a mortar. If the bottle method is used, the formed emulsion can serve as a wetting agent in triturating and incorporating these solids. Insoluble solids should never be merely added to the bottle with shaking. As described previously, when the mortar method is used, insoluble ingredients may be placed in the mortar at the beginning of the compounding process. In all cases, the wetting liquid should be added in portions with trituration to ensure the formation of a smooth preparation.

5. Handling incompatibilities: As indicated in section III. C. on soaps in Chapter 20, adding acidic ingredients to emulsions using soap emulsifiers shifts the equilibrium from the salt form of the soap, which is the surface active form, toward the undissociated acid form, which is oil-soluble. This destroys the barrier necessary for maintaining the emulsion.

    a. Examples of acidic ingredients commonly used in topical preparations that may be prescribed in nascent soap emulsions include phenol, resorcinol, menthol, salicylic acid, lactic acid, acetic acid, aluminum acetate solution (Burow's solution), and aluminum subacetate solution.

    b. The soap emulsifier may be protected from these pH-lowering ingredients by incorporating the offending ingredient or ingredients in 2 to 4 grams of an absorption base (e.g., lanolin, Hydrophilic Petrolatum USP, Aquabase, Aquaphor) per 30 mL of oil phase before the ingredients are incorporated in the formulation. This procedure is illustrated in Sample Prescription 29.2.

6. Preservation and storage

    a. Preservatives are not usually required for lime water emulsions because the calcium hydroxide generates a high pH that is not favorable for microbial or mold growth. Furthermore, these are external-use emulsions that often contain antiseptic or antimicrobial active ingredients.

    b. If a preservative is needed, alcohol or the parabens are suitable agents. Benzoic acid/sodium benzoate and sorbic acid/potassium sorbate are not effective because of the alkaline pH of these emulsions.

    c. As external use preparations, nascent soap emulsions are stored at controlled room temperature.

C. **Nonionic surfactant emulsions:** The most common nonionic emulsifying agents for liquid emulsions are combinations of polysorbates with sorbitan esters, the so-called Span-Tween surfactants.

1. Total amount of emulsifier needed
   a. A 2% to 5% w/v emulsifier combination has been recommended for liquid emulsions. Some sources report that using an amount in the upper range gives more stable preparations. This means that for 100 mL of a preparation, 5 g total of a polysorbate-sorbitan ester combination would be used.
   b. Other references recommend that the amount of emulsifier used should depend on the amount of internal phase to be emulsified. In this case, 10% to 20% w/v of the internal phase is a suggested guideline.
2. Relative amounts of emulsifier combinations
   a. A system was needed to aid formulators in making systematic decisions for amounts and types of surfactants to use in giving emulsions of maximum stability. Griffin addressed this problem by developing the hydrophile-lipophile balance (HLB) system (5). It is based on the fact that all surfactant molecules have both hydrophilic (water-loving) and lipophilic (oil-loving) portions. The balance between these two parts varies with the surfactant. Numbers from 1 to 20 were assigned to surfactants based on this balance, with the lower numbers given to lipophilic compounds and the higher numbers assigned to hydrophilic compounds. The former Atlas Powder Company, the firm that originally developed and marketed a number of nonionic surfactants, including Span, Tween, Arlacel, Brij, and Myrj, further developed and advocated this system.
   b. Span and Arlacel surfactants are considered lipophilic, with HLB numbers in the range of 1.8 to 8.6. They tend to form w/o emulsions. Tween emulsifiers have HLB numbers in the range of 9.6 to 16.7; they are more hydrophilic and favor o/w emulsions. Table 29.1 gives HLB values for some common nonionic surfactants used in compounding.
   c. Experimental work was also done to determine "required HLB" values for various types of formulations and ingredients. Table 29.2 gives some of these "required" values for both o/w and w/o emulsions with common pharmaceutical ingredients. Some sample calculations using HLB values are given later, and Sample Prescription 29.3, which is also demonstrated on the CD that accompanies this book, gives an additional illustration.
   d. When a formulation contains a blend of oil/wax ingredients, the final "required HLB" is calculated by summing the HLB contributions of all the oil/wax ingredients. The HLB contribution for an individual ingredient is determined by multiplying its required HLB times its weight fraction of all oil-type ingredients.
   e. Some formulators maintain that using a 50:50 blend of Span and Tween gives emulsions that are as satisfactory as those made using Span-Tween blends calculated from the HLB system.

Table 29.1	**HLB VALUES OF SOME SURFACTANTS**

SURFACTANT	HLB
Sorbitan trioleate (Span 85)*	1.8
Sorbitan tristearate (Span 65)*	2.1
Sorbitan sesquioleate (Arlacel 83)*	3.7
Glyceryl monostearate, N.F.	3.8
Sorbitan monooleate, N.F. (Span 80)*	4.3
Sorbitan monostearate, N.F. (Span 60)*	4.7
Sorbitan monopalmitate, N.F. (Span 40)*	6.7
Sorbitan monolaurate, N.F. (Span 20)*	8.6
Polyoxyethylene sorbitan tristearate (Tween 65)*	10.5
Polyoxyethylene sorbitan trioleate (Tween 85)*	11.0
Polyethylene glycol 400 monostearate	11.6
Polysorbate 60, N.F. (Tween 60)*	14.9
Polyoxyethylene monostearate (Myrj 49)*	15.0
Polysorbate 80, N.F. (Tween 80)*	15.0
Polysorbate 40, N.F. (Tween 40)*	15.6
Polysorbate 20, N.F. (Tween 20)*	16.7

*ICI Americas, Inc., Wilmington, Delaware.

Table 29.2	"REQUIRED HLB" VALUES OF SOME INGREDIENTS	

	EMULSION	
INGREDIENT	w/o	o/w
Acid, Lauric	—	15–16
Acid, Oleic	—	17
Acid, Stearic	6	15
Alcohol, Cetyl	—	15
Alcohol, Lauryl	—	14
Alcohol, Stearyl	—	14
Lanolin, Anhydrous	8	10
Oil, Castor	6	14
Oil, Cottonseed	5	10
Oil, Mineral	5	12
Oil, Olive	6	14
Petrolatum	5	12
Wax, Beeswax	4	12
Wax, Paraffin	4	11

Though this is often true for o/w systems, it may fail for w/o emulsions. The reason for this is readily apparent if the HLB values of common Spans and Tweens are observed. A 50:50 blend of many polysorbate-sorbitan ester combinations gives a final HLB of 10 or greater; this is a desirable HLB for most o/w emulsions. Such a resultant HLB is, however, often too high for stable w/o systems.

  f. Phase ratio also plays an important role in the type of emulsion formed using these emulsifiers.

3. Measurement of polysorbate-sorbitan ester emulsifiers: All are customarily measured by weight, not by volume. This is because, at room temperature, some of these emulsifiers are solids, and others are thick liquids.

4. Order of mixing

  a. Though some sources recommend dissolving the oil-soluble sorbitan ester portions (e.g., the Spans) in the oil and the water-soluble polysorbate part (e.g., the Tweens) in the water, many compounders find it much easier to dissolve or disperse both emulsifiers in the oil phase. Though the polysorbate compound eventually dissolves in water, it tends to "lump up" initially, making it difficult to work with.

  b. If no solid ingredients are present in the formulation, the emulsion can easily be made directly in the dispensing bottle. Put all ingredients in the bottle and shake well. A more uniform preparation, with finer emulsion droplets, may be achieved by passing the emulsion through a hand homogenizer or by processing the emulsion in a blender.

  c. If solids are to be added, this must be done in a mortar. Either use the bottle method to first make the emulsion and then add the emulsion, in portions with trituration, to the solids in the mortar, or put the solids in a Wedgwood mortar, add the oil-emulsifier with trituration, and then **gradually** add the water phase in portions with trituration.

5. Unlike gums, nonionic surfactants are not viscosity-inducing agents. When using these emulsifiers, it may be necessary to add a viscosity-inducing agent or a viscous vehicle to retard the rate of creaming. This, of course, depends on the consistency of the preparation, which is a function of both the phase ratio of the ingredients and the physical state (liquid, semisolid, solid) of the oil phase. For example, an emulsion with a high concentration of internal phase will be more viscous than a preparation with a small amount of dispersed phase. Likewise, emulsions that contain waxes for all or part of the oil phase will be more viscous than an emulsion made solely with a liquid oil. For an o/w oral preparation, flavored syrup, such as orange or cherry syrup, may be substituted for all or part of the water because it will serve the dual functions of flavoring and increasing the viscosity and density of the external phase.

Example 29.1	**6.** Sample calculations

℞

Mineral oil	50 mL
Span 60	qs
Tween 40	qs
Cherry syrup	40 mL
Purified Water	qs ad 120 mL

Total amount of emulsifier needed: 5% $\times$ 120 mL = 0.05 $\times$ 120 mL = 6 g

This is a preparation for internal use, so an o/w emulsion is preferred. Mineral oil has a "required" HLB of 12 (some sources give 10) for an o/w emulsion.

HLB of Span 60: 4.7 HLB of Tween 40: 15.6

If a 50:50 mixture is used, weigh 3 g each of Span 60 and Tween 40.

This combination has an HLB of:

$$
\begin{array}{ll}
50\% \times 4.7 &= 2.35 \\
50\% \times 15.6 &= \underline{7.8} \\
\text{Total HLB} &= 10.15
\end{array}
$$

This value is between the recommended HLBs of 10 and 12 and would give a perfectly satisfactory emulsion.

The amount of Span 60 and Tween 40 based on "required" HLB can be calculated using either alligation or algebra.

■ By algebra:

$$\mathrm{HLB} = f_T(\mathrm{HLB_T}) + f_S(\mathrm{HLB_S})$$

where:

$$
\begin{array}{l}
\mathrm{HLB} = \text{Total desired HLB} \\
\mathrm{HLB_T} = \text{HLB of the Tween} \\
\mathrm{HLB_S} = \text{HLB of the Span} \\
f_T \ \& \ f_S = \text{weight-fractions of Tween and Span respectively}
\end{array}
$$

because $f_T + f_S = 1$, then $f_T = 1 - f_S$

$$
\begin{array}{l}
\therefore\ 12 = (1 - f_S)(15.6) + f_S(4.7) \\
\quad\ 12 = 15.6 - (f_S)(15.6) + f_S(4.7) \\
\quad\ 10.9 f_S = 3.6 \\
\quad\ f_S = 0.33 \text{ This is the weight-fraction of Span.}
\end{array}
$$

The weight-fraction of Tween is:

$$f_T = 1 - f_S = 1 - 0.33 = 0.67$$

The weight in grams of Span 60 for 6 g of total emulsifier is:

$$0.33 \times 6\ g = 1.98\ g$$

The weight in grams of Tween 40 for 6 g of total emulsifier is:

$$0.67 \times 6\ g = 4.02\ g$$

■ By alligation:

15.6	7.3 parts of Tween 40
12	
4.7	3.6 parts of Span 60
	10.9 parts total

$$\frac{7.3 \text{ g Tween } 40}{10.9 \text{ g total emulsifier}} = \frac{x \text{ g Tween } 40}{6 \text{ g total emulsifier}} \; ; \; x = 4.02 \text{ g Tween } 40$$

$$\frac{3.6 \text{ g Span } 60}{10.9 \text{ g total emulsifier}} = \frac{x \text{ g Span } 60}{6 \text{ g total emulsifier}} \; ; \; x = 1.98 \text{ g Span } 60$$

VI. COMPATIBILITY, STABILITY, AND BEYOND-USE DATING

A. **Physical stability of the system:** Maintenance of small droplets and ease of redispersion are both essential to the physical stability of emulsion systems. Because emulsions are by nature physically unstable systems, beyond-use dates for these preparations should be conservative even with ingredients that are chemically stable.

B. **Chemical compatibility and stability of the ingredients**
1. Compatibility issues with the various emulsifying agents have been discussed previously in this chapter and in Chapters 19 and 20.
2. Because the preparation beyond-use date depends on the stability of each of the formulation ingredients, check ingredient stability using suitable references, such as those listed in Chapter 37. Examples are illustrated with the Sample Prescriptions that follow.
3. The *USP* chapter on pharmacy compounding, Chapter ⟨795⟩, recommends a maximum 14-day dating for all water-containing liquid preparations, such as emulsions, made with ingredients in solid form when the stability of the ingredients in the formulation is unknown (6). When ingredients of questionable stability are present, more conservative dating should be considered. Many external-use preparations are formulated from ingredients, such as zinc oxide and calamine, that are known to be very stable; for these preparations, a 1-month beyond-use date would be satisfactory.

C. **Microbiologic stability:** *USP* Chapter ⟨1151⟩ states that all emulsions should contain an antimicrobial agent because the aqueous phase is vulnerable to the growth of microorganisms (1). This is especially true of o/w emulsions and emulsions made with natural gums. Growth of fungi (molds) and yeasts is especially problematic, so the preservative chosen should have fungistatic as well as bacteriostatic properties. Bacteria have been shown to degrade glycerin, non-ionic and anionic surfactants, and especially natural gums such as acacia and tragacanth (1). When using a lipophilic preservative, an extra amount may be needed to allow for partitioning from the water phase (the component most vulnerable to microbiologic growth) into the oil phase. If antimicrobial ingredients are present in the formulation, extra preservatives may not be needed. For acceptable preservatives, see the previous discussion of individual emulsions types and Chapter 16, Antimicrobial Preservatives.

VII. SPECIAL LABELING REQUIREMENTS FOR EMULSIONS

A. All emulsions are disperse systems and need a "**SHAKE WELL**" auxiliary label.
B. External-use emulsions should be labeled "**FOR EXTERNAL USE ONLY.**"

Sample Prescriptions

SAMPLE PRESCRIPTION 29.1

CASE: Laurie Mower is a 26-year-old woman who is planning a climbing trip on Mt. Shasta in California. The last time she was there, she suffered rather severe sunburn, which was intensified by sun reflection off the snow at the high altitude. The area underneath her chin and the bottom inside of her nose was actually blistered. She wants to avoid a recurrence of this, so she has requested sunscreen and skin protection advice from her pharmacist, Ted Fence. Dr. Fence asks Laurie whether she has any allergies, and Laurie replies that she is allergic to aspirin, Pepto-Bismol, and other salicylates. Dr. Fence advises Laurie to use zinc oxide paste as a thick, opaque protective for the especially vulnerable areas that blistered on her previous experience. Then, he offers to work with her physician to formulate a special sunscreen that would protect the rest of her face and other exposed areas of her hands, arms, and the like. Dr. Fence wants ingredients that are not salicylates but that cover both the UVA and UVB spectra. He finds that oxybenzone (also known as *benzophenone-3*) absorbs light throughout the UVB range and also some UVA and UVC light, whereas avobenzone absorbs primarily in the UVA range. By using these two agents, Laurie would be protected from both sunburn (primarily resulting from UVB) and photosensitivity and deeper skin damage from the more deeply penetrating UVA wavelengths. Calamine and Zinc Oxide will provide some physical protection.

CONTEMPORARY PHYSICIANS GROUP PRACTICE
20 S. PARK STREET, TRITURATE, WI 53706
TEL: (608) 555-1333 FAX: (608) 555-1335

R # *123466*

NAME *Laurie Mower*   **DATE** *00/00/00*

ADDRESS *905 Chickadee Lane*

R

Calamine	5%	
Zinc Oxide	5%	
Avobenzone	3%	
Oxybenzone	3%	
Almond Oil	45 mL	
Acacia	qs	
Rose Water	qs ad	90 mL

Ted Fence 00/00/00

Sig: Apply to exposed areas of skin 30 min prior to sun exposure, then q 4 hr during the outing.

REFILLS *5*   *Jackson Parker*   **M.D.**

DEA NO. _____

MASTER COMPOUNDING FORMULATION RECORD

NAME, STRENGTH, AND DOSAGE FORM OF PREPARATION: Zinc Oxide 5%, Calamine 5%, Avobenzone 3%, Oxybenzone 3% Topical Sunscreen Emulsion

QUANTITY: 90 mL

THERAPEUTIC USE/CATEGORY: Sunscreen

FORMULATION RECORD ID: EM001

ROUTE OF ADMINISTRATION: Topical

INGREDIENTS USED:

Ingredient	Quantity Used	Physical Description	Solubility	Dose Comparison		Use in the Prescription
				Given	Usual	
Almond Oil	45 mL	clear, pale yellow oil	immisc w/ water, alcohol	—	—	oil phase of emulsion
Zinc Oxide	4.5 g	white powder	insol. in water and alcohol	4.4%	5–20%	protective, antiseptic
Calamine	4.5 g	pink powder	insol. in water and alcohol	4.4%	5–20%	protective, antiseptic
Avobenzone	2.7 g	yellow powder	pr. insol in water; sl. sol in alcohol	3%	3%	sunscreen
Oxybenzone	2.7 g	pale yellow powder	pr. insol in water; sol. in alcohol	3%	3%	sunscreen
Acacia	11.25 g	beige-colored powder	1 g/2 mL water; insol. in alcohol	—	—	emulsifying agent
Rose Water	qs ad 90 mL	clear, colorless liquid with rose scent	—	—	—	water phase of emulsion
Alcohol USP	5.7 mL	clear, colorless mobile liquid	miscible w/ water	6%	6%	preservative

COMPATIBILITY-STABILITY: The calamine and zinc oxide in this preparation are compatible and very stable in an acacia emulsion. The stabilities of the oxybenzone and the avobenzone are more difficult to assess. There are manufactured sunscreen products that contain these two ingredients, but the prescribed preparation contains extra ingredients that could affect the stability of these compounds. With respect to a preservative for this emulsion, though the zinc oxide and calamine have antimicrobial properties, an extra preservative will be added because of the susceptibility to microbial growth of acacia emulsions. One traditional preservative for acacia emulsions is benzoic acid, which works well in the usual pH of 4.5 to 5 for these emulsions; however, the pH of the final preparation was checked because the zinc oxide is a basic compound that might impart a higher pH to the emulsion. The pH was found to be 7, too high for using benzoic acid. Therefore, alcohol 6% is selected as the preservative.

PACKAGING AND STORAGE: The *USP* monographs for oxybenzone and avobenzone recommend storage in tight, light-resistant containers (4). Because this is a topical preparation, controlled room temperature will be the recommended storage conditions.

BEYOND-USE DATE: Use the *USP* recommended maximum 14-day beyond-use date for compounded water-containing liquid formulations prepared from ingredients in solid form when there is no stability information for the formulation (6).

CALCULATIONS

Dose/Concentration: All concentrations okay

Ingredient Amounts

Zinc oxide and calamine (in g): $5\% \times 90\ \text{mL} = 0.05 \times 90\ \text{mL} = 4.5\ \text{g}$

Avobenzone and oxybenzone (in g): $3\% \times 90\ \text{mL} = 0.03 \times 90\ \text{mL} = 2.7\ \text{g}$

Calculation of oil:water:acacia content for primary emulsion:

$$\text{oil:water:acacia} = 4{:}2{:}1 = 45\ \text{mL}{:}22.5\ \text{mL}{:}11.25\ \text{g}$$

Preservative: alcohol 6% is used. The volume of pure ethanol (C_2H_5OH) is calculated here.

$$6\% \times 90\ \text{mL} = 0.06 \times 90\ \text{mL} = 5.4\ \text{mL ethanol}$$

Ethanol is available as Alcohol USP, which is 95% ethanol. The volume of Alcohol USP that contains 5.4 mL of ethanol is calculated to be:

$$\frac{95\ \text{mL ethanol}}{100\ \text{mL Alcohol USP}} = \frac{5.4\ \text{mL ethanol}}{x\ \text{mL Alcohol USP}}\ ;\ x = 5.7\ \text{mL Alcohol USP}$$

MSDS AND SAFETY AND PERSONAL PROTECTIVE EQUIPMENT: Review MSDS for all components. Don a clean lab coat, disposable gloves, and safety glasses. Avoid inhaling powders.

SPECIALIZED EQUIPMENT: Wedgwood mortar; all weighing is done on a class III torsion balance.

COMPOUNDING PROCEDURE: Weigh 11.25 g of acacia and put it in a dry Wedgwood mortar. Gradually add 45 mL of almond oil and triturate well. Weigh 2.7 g each of avobenzone and oxybenzone and add these to the almond oil–acacia mixture and triturate to disperse and dissolve the drugs. In a clean 25-mL graduated cylinder, measure 22.5 mL of rose water. Add this all at once to the oil-drug-acacia mixture in the mortar and triturate rapidly to form the primary emulsion. Add some extra rose water to reduce the viscosity of the emulsion. Weigh 4.5 g each of zinc oxide and calamine and place in a mortar. Wet the powders by adding the previously formed emulsion to them with trituration. If the emulsion gets too thick, small amounts of additional rose water may be added. Using a 10-mL graduated cylinder, measure 5.7 mL of Alcohol USP and add it to the emulsion. Pour the emulsion into a precalibrated 3-oz prescription bottle with a child-resistant closure. For complete transfer of the emulsion to the bottle, use successive rinses of the mortar with rose water and use this to qs to the 90-mL mark. Cap tightly. Shake the bottle well; label and dispense.

DESCRIPTION OF FINISHED PREPARATION: A pink, viscous, o/w emulsion with a slight rose scent

QUALITY CONTROL: Volume = 90 mL. Check pH with range 2 to 9 test strips: pH = 7.

MASTER FORMULA PREPARED BY: Ted Fence, PharmD   **CHECKED BY:** Robert Fifrick, RPh

COMPOUNDING RECORD

NAME, STRENGTH, AND DOSAGE FORM OF PREPARATION: Zinc Oxide 5%, Calamine 5%, Avobenzone 3%, Oxybenzone 3% Topical Sunscreen Emulsion

QUANTITY: 90 mL

DATE PREPARED: mm/dd/yy

BEYOND-USE DATE: mm/dd/yy

FORMULATION RECORD ID: EM001

CONTROL/RX NUMBER: 123466

INGREDIENTS USED:

Ingredient	Quantity	Manufacturer Lot Number	Expiration Date	Weighed/ Measured by	Checked by
Almond Oil	45 mL	JET Labs EM2911	mm/yy	bjf	trf
Zinc Oxide	4.5 g	JET Labs XY1153	mm/yy	bjf	trf
Calamine	4.5 g	JET Labs SS2811	mm/yy	bjf	trf
Avobenzone	2.7 g	JET Labs EM2912	mm/yy	bjf	trf
Oxybenzone	2.7 g	JET Labs EM2913	mm/yy	bjf	trf
Acacia	11.25 g	JET Labs EM2914	mm/yy	bjf	trf
Rose Water	qs ad 90 mL	JET Labs EM2915	mm/yy	bjf	trf
Alcohol USP	5.7 mL	JET Labs EM2916	mm/yy	bjf	trf

QUALITY CONTROL DATA: The preparation is a pink o/w emulsion. It is fairly viscous, and no creaming or settling occurs in 2 hours. The preparation pours easily after shaking. The pH of the preparation was checked with pH range 2 to 9 test strips; pH = 7. Volume = 90 mL.

LABELING

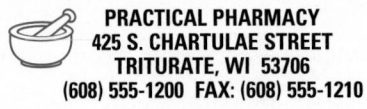

PRACTICAL PHARMACY
425 S. CHARTULAE STREET
TRITURATE, WI 53706
(608) 555-1200 FAX: (608) 555-1210

℞ 123466   Pharmacist: TRF   Date: 00/00/00
Laurie Mower   Dr. Jackson Parker

Apply to exposed areas of skin 30 minutes prior to sun exposure, then every four hours during outing.

Calamine 5%, Zinc Oxide 5%, Avobenzone 3%, Oxybenzone 3% Topical Emulsion

Contains Alcohol 6%

Mfg: Compounded   Quantity: 90 mL

Refills: 5   Discard after: Give date

Auxiliary Labels: Shake well. For external use only. This medicine was compounded in our pharmacy for you at the direction of your prescriber.

PATIENT CONSULTATION: Hi, Ms. Mower, I have your sunscreen lotion ready for you. As you know, Dr. Parker and I formulated this special sunscreen for you to use in your upcoming trip, though you can use it anytime you need a good sunscreen. Approximately 30 minutes prior to sun exposure, apply this lotion to areas of your skin that are not covered with clothing and that therefore will be exposed to the sun's rays; then reapply every 4 hours during your outing. As I mentioned to you before, I would use a complete blocking product such as zinc oxide paste for areas that you found were particularly vulnerable to the sun reflection off the snow on the mountain. This lotion will also lubricate and protect your skin. If you experience any type of skin reaction or allergy, discontinue use and contact Dr. Parker. I would try this out sometime before you leave for Mt. Shasta, so if you should have an adverse skin reaction, we can make a change in the formula; obviously you don't want to have problems on the mountain. Be sure to shake the bottle well before applying. This is for external use only. Store this out of the reach of children and when possible at moderate temperature, 65°F to 75°F. Discard any unused portion after 2 weeks (give date). This may be refilled five times.

SAMPLE PRESCRIPTION 29.2

CASE: Fr. Paul Saint is a 55-year-old male patient who lives at a local rural monastery. He recently was clearing brush from a nearby wooded area and was exposed to poison ivy. As a result, he has developed contact dermatitis that is red and itching. As yet there are no watery blisters. Dr. Largay has decided to use a w/o emulsion formulation because he believes that this system will act as a reservoir and hold the active ingredients in contact with Fr. Saint's skin for a longer time than would a suspension dosage form. Dr. Largay wants Fr. Saint to have ingredients that will act to both soothe and relieve the itching and prevent any secondary infection.

CONTEMPORARY PHYSICIANS GROUP PRACTICE
20 S. PARK STREET, TRITURATE, WI 53706
TEL: (608) 555-1333 FAX: (608) 555-1335

Rx # *123462*

NAME *Fr. Paul Saint*   **DATE** *00/00/00*

ADDRESS *926 Holy Lane*

Rx

Phenol		1.2 g
Menthol		0.3 g
Zinc Oxide		8 g
Lime water		60 mL
Cottonseed Oil	qs ad	120 mL

B. Bellfree 00/00/00

Sig: Apply to affected areas prn ut dict

REFILLS *1*   *J. T. Largay*   **M.D.**

DEA NO. _____

MASTER COMPOUNDING FORMULATION RECORD

NAME, STRENGTH, AND DOSAGE FORM OF PREPARATION: Phenol 1%, Menthol 0.25%, Zinc Oxide 6.7% Topical Emulsion

QUANTITY: 120 mL

THERAPEUTIC USE/CATEGORY: Antipruritic/Antiseptic

FORMULATION RECORD ID: EM002

ROUTE OF ADMINISTRATION: Topical

INGREDIENTS USED:

Ingredient	Quantity Used	Physical Description	Solubility	Dose Comparison		Use in the Prescription
				Given	Usual	
Menthol	300 mg	fine, colorless needle-like crystals w/ a mint-like scent	sl. sol. water; v. sol. alcohol	0.25%	1–3%	antipruritic, counterirritant
Phenol	1.2 g	colorless to light pink crystals w/ phenol odor	1 g/15 mL water; v. sol. alcohol	1.0%	0.5–2.0%	antipruritic, antiseptic, topical anesthetic
Zinc Oxide	8 g	white powder	insol in water and alcohol	6.7%	5–20%	astringent, protective, antiseptic
Calcium Hydroxide Solution	60 mL	colorless, cloudy liquid	misc w/water and alcohol	—	—	aqueous phase/ part of emulsifier
Cottonseed Oil	qs ad 120 mL	pale yellow oil	immisc w/water and alcohol	—	—	emollient, oil phase of emulsion
Oleic Acid	1.8 mL	pale yellow oily liquid	Prac insol in water; misc w/ alcohol & oils	—	—	part of emulsifier
Aquabase	4 g	semisolid ointment	insol in water and alcohol	—	—	auxiliary emulsifier

COMPATIBILITY–STABILITY: Menthol and phenol will potentially form a liquid eutectic mixture when triturated together in a mortar; however, this is an advantage with this formulation because it aids in breaking down the hard crystalline structure of the phenol prior to incorporation in the liquid and gives a smooth liquid preparation. Menthol and phenol are somewhat subject to oxidation, but they are sufficiently stable in this emulsion, which is similar in content to the *USP* preparation Phenolated Calamine Topical Suspension (4). There is one compatibility problem that must be addressed: The calcium oleate soap emulsifier, which is formed by the reaction of calcium hydroxide and oleic acid, will be destroyed by the addition of ingredients such as phenol and menthol (see the discussion of this incompatibility in the sections on nascent soap emulsions in this chapter and in Chapter 19). The calcium oleate can be protected from these ingredients by first incorporating the phenol and menthol in an adsorption base. Therefore, add 4 g of Aquabase. Though preservatives are required in all emulsions, no added preservative is needed in this formulation because phenol is an excellent antimicrobial agent, and menthol and zinc oxide also act as antiseptics.

PACKAGING AND STORAGE: Following the example of Phenolated Calamine Topical Suspension, this preparation should be packaged in a tight container (4). Because this is a topical preparation, storage should be in controlled room temperature.

BEYOND-USE DATE: Though this is probably a fairly stable preparation, use the *USP* recommended maximum 14-day beyond-use date for compounded water-containing liquid formulations prepared from ingredients in solid form when there is no stability information for the formulation (6).

CALCULATIONS

Dose/Concentration

Phenol (in w/v%):

$$\frac{1.2 \text{ g phenol}}{120 \text{ mL emulsion}} = \frac{x \text{ g phenol}}{100 \text{ mL emulsion}}; x = 1 \text{ g phenol/100 mL} = 1\%$$

Menthol (in w/v%):

$$\frac{0.3 \text{ g menthol}}{120 \text{ mL emulsion}} = \frac{x \text{ g menthol}}{100 \text{ mL emulsion}}; x = 0.25 \text{ g menthol/100 mL} = 0.25\%$$

Zinc Oxide (in w/v%):

$$\frac{8 \text{ g zinc oxide}}{120 \text{ mL emulsion}} = \frac{x \text{ g zinc oxide}}{100 \text{ mL emulsion}}; x = 6.7 \text{ g zinc oxide/100 mL} = 6.7\%$$

All concentrations are okay for the intended use.

Ingredient Amounts

For this sample prescription, it is assumed that the pharmacy has fresh Calcium Hydroxide Topical Solution (lime water) in stock. If this solution has to be made, the following calculations and procedure illustrate how to make l50 mL of lime water, which would provide enough to make the prescribed preparation twice.

$$\frac{3 \text{ g calcium hydroxide}}{1{,}000 \text{ mL water}} = \frac{x \text{ g calcium hydroxide}}{150 \text{ mL water}}; x = 0.45 \text{ g calcium hydroxide}$$

Weigh 450 mg of calcium hydroxide, transfer it to a graduated cylinder, and qs to 150 mL with Purified Water; stir occasionally over 1 hour, and then allow any solid to settle. Use the clear supernatant.

MSDS AND SAFETY AND PERSONAL PROTECTIVE EQUIPMENT: Review MSDS for all components. Don a clean lab coat, disposable gloves, and safety glasses. Avoid inhaling zinc oxide powder. Use extreme caution with phenol, as contact with skin may cause serious burns.

SPECIALIZED EQUIPMENT: Wedgwood mortar; all weighing is done on a class III torsion balance.

COMPOUNDING PROCEDURE: Weigh 300 mg of menthol, 1.2 g of phenol, and 8 g of zinc oxide. Place menthol and phenol in a Wedgwood mortar and triturate to force liquefaction of the eutectic mixture. Weigh 4 g of Aquabase and transfer to the mortar; incorporate the eutectic mixture in the Aquabase with trituration. Measure 45 to 50 mL of cottonseed oil in a graduated cylinder and draw 3 mL of oleic acid into a syringe. Add 1.5 mL of the oleic acid to the cottonseed oil. Add alternating portions of the zinc oxide and cottonseed oil to the eutectic/base mixture with trituration. Continue adding these alternately to maintain a proper consistency for making a smooth preparation until all the zinc oxide and cottonseed oil are added. Decant 60 mL of lime water from its container and add it in portions with trituration to the Wedgwood mortar. If the emulsion appears to be coalescing, add several more drops of oleic acid, keeping track of the total amount of oleic acid added (0.3 mL extra was added). Transfer the preparation to a precalibrated 4-oz prescription bottle with child-resistant closure. Use some cottonseed oil to rinse the mortar and to qs to the 120-mL mark on the prescription bottle. Cap tightly and shake well. Label and dispense.

DESCRIPTION OF FINISHED PREPARATION: A white, viscous, w/o emulsion with a scent of phenol and menthol

QUALITY CONTROL: Volume = 120 mL. Check pH with range 1 to 14 pH paper: pH = 12.

MASTER FORMULA PREPARED BY: Batziner Bellfree, PharmD   **CHECKED BY:** Robert Fifrick, RPh

COMPOUNDING RECORD

NAME, STRENGTH, AND DOSAGE FORM OF PREPARATION: Phenol 1%, Menthol 0.25%, Zinc Oxide 6.7% Topical Emulsion

QUANTITY: 120 mL   **DATE PREPARED:** mm/dd/yy   **BEYOND-USE DATE:** mm/dd/yy

FORMULATION RECORD ID: EM002   **CONTROL/RX NUMBER:** 123462

INGREDIENTS USED:

Ingredient	Quantity	Manufacturer Lot Number	Expiration Date	Weighed/ Measured by	Checked by
Menthol	300 mg	JET Labs SS2822	mm/yy	bjf	bb
Phenol	1.2 g	JET Labs SS2831	mm/yy	bjf	bb
Zinc Oxide	8 g	JET Labs SS2812	mm/yy	bjf	bb
Calcium Hydroxide Topical Solution	60 mL	Prac. Pharmacy JT1143	mm/yy	bjf	bb
Cottonseed Oil	qs ad 120 mL	JET Labs EM2911	mm/yy	bjf	bb
Oleic Acid	1.8 mL	JET Labs XY2918	mm/yy	bjf	bb
Aquabase	4 g	Paddock Labs RA012	mm/yy	bjf	bb

QUALITY CONTROL DATA: This preparation is a white w/o emulsion. It is fairly viscous, and there is no apparent creaming or settling in 2 hours. Though viscous, the preparation pours smoothly after shaking. The pH of the preparation was checked with pH paper, range 1 to14, and recorded; pH = 12. Volume = 120 mL.

LABELING

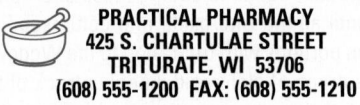

PRACTICAL PHARMACY
425 S. CHARTULAE STREET
TRITURATE, WI 53706
(608) 555-1200 FAX: (608) 555-1210

℞ 123462   Pharmacist: BB   Date: 00/00/00
Fr. Paul Saint   Dr. J. T. Largay

Apply to affected areas as needed as directed.

Phenol 1%, Menthol 0.25%, Zinc Oxide 6.7% Topical Emulsion

Mfg: Compounded   Quantity: 120 mL

Refills: 1   Discard after: Give date

Auxiliary Labels: Shake well. For external use only. This medicine was compounded in our pharmacy for you at the direction of your prescriber.

PATIENT CONSULTATION: Hello, Fr. Saint, I'm your pharmacist, Batziner Bellfree. Do you have any drug allergies? What did Dr. Largay tell you about this lotion? This is to treat the poison ivy that Dr. Largay diagnosed. The directions say to apply the lotion to affected areas as needed as directed. You will probably find that using it every 4 to 6 hours gives adequate relief, but you may use it more frequently if that helps. It will help with the itching and should prevent any infection. If the condition doesn't improve, or if it gets worse, contact Dr. Largay, because there are other things we can try. It is important not to scratch the affected area because that can damage the skin and could possibly allow introduction of an infection. To use the preparation, first shake the bottle well before using, then apply a thin layer over the area that is red and itching. Be sure to wash your hands before and after applying the lotion, and be careful not to get any in your eyes. This should be stored at room temperature away from heat and light. Discard any unused portion after 2 weeks (give date). You may have one refill. One last thing: You may now be more sensitive to plants such as poison ivy, so really try to avoid contact with those plants. You may want to get in touch with the county extension agent to find out how to rid the monastery property of the poison ivy without exposure to yourself or the other brothers or custodial staff. Do you have any questions?

SAMPLE PRESCRIPTION 29.3

CASE: Mildred Stauffacher is a 60-year-old woman who is scheduled for a colonoscopy. She has these tests every 3 years because she has some risk factors for colon cancer. In the past, she has used the purgative GoLYTELY, but she has told her doctor that she wants to try something different because the GoLYTELY makes her rectal area very raw and painful. They agree to try a castor oil laxative and want to use an emulsion to make it more palatable. Ms. Stauffacher says that she doesn't really like the flavor of mint or lemon of the commercial products, so Dr. Quacky says that he knows a pharmacist who can make one with cherry syrup that she might find more acceptable.

CONTEMPORARY PHYSICIANS GROUP PRACTICE
20 S. PARK STREET, TRITURATE, WI 53706
TEL: (608) 555-1333 FAX: (608) 555-1335

℞ #   *123465*

NAME *Mildred Stauffacher*   DATE *00/00/00*

ADDRESS *88 1/3 Third Avenue*

℞

Castor Oil		*45 mL*
Tween 80		*qs*
Span 20		*qs*
Cherry Syrup	*qs ad*	*90 mL*

J. Jupiter 00/00/00

Sig: Take entire contents of bottle at 4 PM on afternoon before procedure. Follow in 4 hours with X-Prep

REFILLS *0*   *Olive Quacky*   M.D.

DEA NO. _____

MASTER COMPOUNDING FORMULATION RECORD

NAME, STRENGTH, AND DOSAGE FORM OF PREPARATION: Castor Oil Oral Emulsion 2.5 mL/5 mL

QUANTITY: 90 mL

THERAPEUTIC USE/CATEGORY: Laxative

FORMULATION RECORD ID: EM003

ROUTE OF ADMINISTRATION: Oral

INGREDIENTS USED:

Ingredient	Quantity Used	Physical Description	Solubility	Dose Comparison		Use in the Prescription
				Given	Usual	
Castor Oil	45 mL	pale yellowish, transparent, viscid liquid	immis with water; misc with alcohol	45 mL	15–60 mL	laxative
Tween 80	3.8 g	light gold viscous liquid	misc with water, alcohol, oils	—	—	emulsifying agent
Span 20	0.7 g	amber-colored viscous liquid	insol in water, misc w/ oils	—	—	emulsifying agent
Cherry Syrup	qs ad 90 mL	red syrupy liquid	miscible with water	—	—	flavored vehicle

COMPATIBILITY-STABILITY: This is a very simple preparation containing just castor oil in an emulsion, and it should be very stable. There is an official *USP* Castor Oil Emulsion, but no formulation information is given (4). No extra preservative is needed because the commercially available cherry syrup comes preserved with sodium benzoate, and the pH of the emulsion is found to be 3.

PACKAGING AND STORAGE: The *USP* monograph for Castor Oil Emulsion recommends storage in tight containers (4). Because it is an oral emulsion, it should be stored in the refrigerator; this will enhance the taste and improve microbiologic stability.

BEYOND-USE DATE: Though there are manufactured versions of this formulation with expiration dates of several years, use a more conservative 1-month beyond-use date for this compounded preparation.

CALCULATIONS

Dose/Concentration: Dose of Castor Oil is appropriate for this use.

Ingredient Amounts

Total emulsifier concentration is 5%. This amount (in g) is:

$$5\% \times 90 \text{ mL} = 4.5 \text{ g}$$

Span 20 and Tween 80 are the emulsifiers. The amount of each in grams is calculated using the HLB system and alligation as shown here. (See the chapter text for an example using algebra.)

Because this is an oral emulsion, an o/w system is desired. The "required HLB" for a castor oil o/w emulsion is 14.

Using Span 20 and Tween 80 for emulsifiers, calculate the number of grams of each necessary to compound this prescription. Span 20 has an HLB of 8.6, and Tween 80 has an HLB of 15.

15.0		5.4	parts of Tween 80

| | 14 | | |

8.6		1.0	parts of Span 20
		6.4	parts total

Tween 80 (in g): 　　　　　　　$\dfrac{5.4}{6.4} \times 4.5\,g = 3.8\,g$ Tween 80

Span 20 (in g): 　　　　　　　$\dfrac{1.0}{6.4} \times 4.5\,g = 0.7\,g$ Span 20

MSDS AND SAFETY AND PERSONAL PROTECTIVE EQUIPMENT: Review MSDS for all components. Don a clean lab coat and disposable gloves.

SPECIALIZED EQUIPMENT: Wedgwood mortar; all weighing is done on an electronic balance.

COMPOUNDING PROCEDURE: Using the electronic balance, tare out the weight of a 5-mL syringe, then draw Tween 80 into the syringe to a weight of 3.8 g. Repeat using a 3-mL syringe and weigh 0.7 g of Span 20. Using a 3-oz prescription bottle that has been precalibrated at 45 mL and at 90 mL, pour castor oil into the bottle to the 45-mL mark. Squirt the Tween and the Span into the bottle and agitate to mix. Add cherry syrup to the 90-mL mark. Cap the bottle tightly, and shake well to form the emulsion. Label and dispense.

DESCRIPTION OF FINISHED PREPARATION: This preparation is a reddish pink o/w emulsion. It has moderate viscosity; there is slight creaming after standing undisturbed for 2 hours.

QUALITY CONTROL: Volume = 90 mL. Check pH with range 1 to 12 pH paper: pH = 3.

MASTER FORMULA PREPARED BY: Jor-el Jupiter, RPh 　　　　　**CHECKED BY:** Robert Fifrick, RPh

COMPOUNDING RECORD

NAME, STRENGTH, AND DOSAGE FORM OF PREPARATION: Castor Oil Oral Emulsion 2.5 mL/5 mL
QUANTITY: 90 mL 　　　　　**DATE PREPARED:** mm/dd/yy 　　　　　**BEYOND-USE DATE:** mm/dd/yy
FORMULATION RECORD ID: EM003 　　　　　**CONTROL/RX NUMBER:** 123465

INGREDIENTS USED:

Ingredient	Quantity	Manufacturer Lot Number	Expiration Date	Weighed/ Measured by	Checked by
Castor Oil	45 mL	JET Labs EM2919	mm/yy	bjf	jj
Tween 80	3.8 g	JET Labs EM2920	mm/yy	bjf	jj
Span 20	0.7 g	JET Labs EM2921	mm/yy	bjf	jj
Cherry Syrup	qs ad 90 mL	Fantasia CP2229	mm/yy	bjf	jj

QUALITY CONTROL DATA: This preparation is a red-pink o/w emulsion. It has moderate viscosity; after 2 hours, there appears a slightly transparent zone of cherry syrup at the bottom of the bottle, indicating some creaming. The preparation is very easily redispersed with shaking. The pH of the preparation was checked with pH paper, range 1 to 12, and recorded; pH = 3. Volume = 90 mL

LABELING

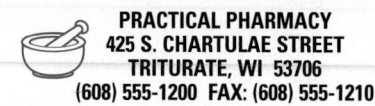

PRACTICAL PHARMACY
425 S. CHARTULAE STREET
TRITURATE, WI 53706
(608) 555-1200 FAX: (608) 555-1210

℞ 123465   Pharmacist: JJ   Date: 00/00/00
Mildred Stauffacher   Dr. Olive Quacky

Take the entire contents of this bottle at 4 PM on the afternoon
before the procedure. Follow in four hours with X-Prep.

Castor Oil 45 mL/90 mL Oral Emulsion

Mfg: Compounded   Quantity: 90 mL

Refills: 0   Discard after: Give date

Auxiliary Labels: Shake well. Keep in the refrigerator. This medicine was
compounded in our pharmacy for you at the direction of your prescriber.

PATIENT CONSULTATION: Hello, Ms. Stauffacher, I'm your pharmacist, Jor-el Jupiter. Do you have any drug allergies? Are you currently using any other prescription or over-the-counter drug products? What has your physician told you about using the medication? This is a laxative/purgative to prepare your gastrointestinal tract for your scheduled examination. Dr. Quacky told me that you did not like the GoLYTELY laxative that you used the last time you had a colonoscopy, so we will try this new method of preparation for this exam. Have you ever used castor oil before? This is rather fast-acting and may cause stomach cramps and diarrhea. I recommend that you don't wander too far from a bathroom after you have taken this medication. You should take the entire contents of this bottle at 4 PM on the afternoon before your test; then 4 hours after taking this, take a full dose of X-Prep liquid. If needed, they will give you an enema at the hospital before your procedure. Shake this bottle well before taking the contents. Keep it in the refrigerator until the day you have to take it—it will taste somewhat better if it is cold. You might want to have a little something like 7-Up or Sprite to rinse your mouth and wash this down. This is good for 1 month (give date), but if your appointment gets changed to a date beyond the expiration date of this preparation, contact Dr. Quacky for a new prescription order. Do you have any questions?

REFERENCES

1. The United States Pharmacopeial Convention, Inc. 2008 USP 31/NF 26. Rockville, MD: Author, 2007; 618.
2. Food and Drug Administration. CDER Data Standards Manual. Rockville, MD: Author, 2006: Data Element Name: Dosage Form, http://www.fda.gov/cder/dsm/DRG/drg00201.htm.
3. Spalton LM. Pharmaceutical emulsions and emulsifying agents. Brooklyn, NY: Chemical Publishing, Inc., 1950; 10.
4. The United States Pharmacopeial Convention, Inc. 2008 USP 31/NF 26. USP Monographs. Rockville, MD: Author, 2007.
5. Swarbrick J. Coarse Dispersions. In: Hoover JE, et. Remington's Pharmaceutical Sciences, 14th ed. Easton, PA: Mack. Publishing Co., 1970; 344.
6. The United States Pharmacopeial Convention, Inc. Chapter ⟨795⟩ 2008 USP 31/NF 26. Rockville, MD: Author, 2007; 316–317.

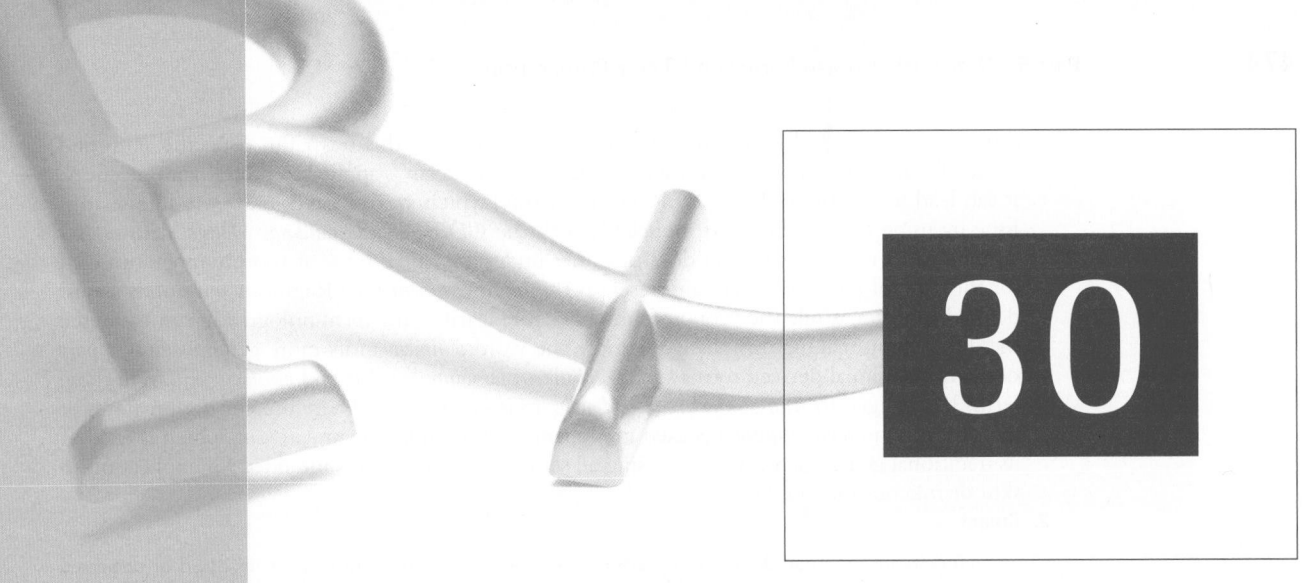

30

Semisolids: Ointments, Creams, Gels, Pastes, and Collodions

I. DEFINITIONS AND NOMENCLATURE FOR SEMISOLIDS

A. As was described in the beginning section of Chapter 27, the nomenclature for pharmaceutical dosage forms is in transition between use of traditional terms and definitions and a more systematic approach that has been proposed to more accurately and consistently describe drug products and preparations. During the period when traditional terms are still used but new terms and definitions are being suggested, it is important that pharmacists and pharmacy technicians understand proposed dosage form taxonomy and nomenclature but also recognize the various traditional terms used to describe dosage forms. The definitions and descriptions in this section should help in this regard. The quoted definitions below that are printed in regular font are the traditional ones from *USP 31/NF 26* Chapter ⟨1151⟩ Pharmaceutical Dosage Forms (1); the definitions in italic type are taken from the FDA *CDER Data Standards Manual* (2).

B. Definitions

   1. Ointment

   Ointments are semisolid preparations intended for external application to the skin or mucous membranes (1).

   A semisolid dosage form, usually containing <20% water and volatiles and >50% hydrocarbons, waxes, or polyols as the vehicle. This dosage form is generally for external application to the skin or mucous membranes (2).

   The problem with the first definition is that, although the word *ointment* has this general meaning, which applies to any semisolid dosage form for external application (e.g., oleaginous ointments, creams, gels), pharmaceutical manufacturers use this term for a specific semisolid dosage form type, oleaginous ointments. When the same term is applied to more than one entity, it can lead to confusion. The CDER nomenclature, which was adopted in 2006, addresses this issue by using the general term *semisolid* [which the *CDER Data Standards Manual* defines as a system that is not pourable and does not flow under low shear stress at room temperature (2)] for the type of physical system and reserves the term *ointment* for oleaginous semisolids as just defined in italics. While the proposed nomenclature clarifies the terminology, you can easily see the difficulty in making this change because the word *ointment* in its more general sense is part of many traditional derived terms such as *ointment jar*, *ointment slab*, and *ointment mill*. Will these terms be changed to *semisolid jar*, *semisolid slab*, *semisolid mill*, etc.? Therefore, for the purposes of this chapter, the term *semisolid* is used interchangeably with the term *ointment*, which is used in its traditional general sense, encompassing all semisolid dosage forms intended for application to skin or mucous membranes.

2. Cream

Creams are semisolid dosage forms containing one or more drug substances dissolved or dispersed in a suitable base. The term has traditionally been applied to semisolids that possess a relatively fluid consistency formulated as either water-in-oil (e.g., Cold Cream) or oil-in-water (e.g., Fluocinolone Acetonide Cream) emulsions. However, more recently the term has been restricted to products consisting of oil-in-water emulsions or aqueous microcrystalline dispersions of long-chain fatty acids or alcohols that are water-washable and more cosmetically and aesthetically acceptable (1).

An emulsion, semisolid dosage form, usually containing >20% water and volatiles and/or <50% hydrocarbons, waxes, or polyols as the vehicle. This dosage form is generally for external application to the skin or mucous membranes (2).

Notice the new CDER definition applies to any semisolid emulsion, not just water-washable (o/w) types.

3. Gel

Gels (sometimes called Jellies) are semisolid systems consisting of either suspensions made up of small inorganic particles or large organic molecules interpenetrated by a liquid (1).

A semisolid dosage form that contains a gelling agent to provide stiffness to a solution or a colloidal dispersion. A gel may contain suspended particles (2).

4. Paste

Pastes are semisolid dosage forms that contain one or more drug substances intended for topical application. One class is made from a single-phase aqueous gel (e.g., Carboxymethylcellulose Sodium Paste). The other class, the fatty pastes (e.g., Zinc Oxide Paste), consists of thick, stiff ointments that do not ordinarily flow at body temperature, and therefore serve as protective coatings over the areas to which they are applied (1).

A semisolid dosage form, containing a large proportion (20–50%) of solids finely dispersed in a fatty vehicle. This dosage form is generally for external application to the skin or mucous membranes (2).

5. Collodion

Although there are collodion dosage forms in the *USP*, this term is not defined in Chapter ⟨1151⟩, and it is not in the *CDER Data Standards Manual*. Traditionally, collodions have been considered solutions but, because they are very viscous systems applied to the skin, in the proposed *USP* taxonomy (described in Chapter 27), collodions are under the topical semisolid classification. Basically, a collodion is a thick solution composed of pyroxylin (a breakdown product of cellulose) that is dissolved in a solvent mixture of alcohol and ether. An example is given in Sample Prescription 30.8.

C. In *USP 31*, four general classes of ointment (semisolid) bases are defined and briefly described: hydrocarbon, absorption, water-removable, and water-soluble. These base types, their composition, and their characteristics are discussed in Chapter 23, Ointment Bases.

II.   USES OF SEMISOLID DOSAGE FORMS

A. To protect skin or mucous membrane from chemical or physical irritants in the environment and to permit rejuvenation of the tissue

B. To provide hydration of the skin or an emollient effect

C. To provide a vehicle for applying a medication either for local or systemic effect (e.g., local—a topical antibiotic; systemic—a nitroglycerin ointment for treating angina)

III. CHOICE OF A BASE

A. The choice of a base depends on the following factors:
  1. The action or effect desired (see preceding section, II)
  2. The nature of the incorporated medication
     a. Bioavailability
     b. Stability
     c. Compatibility
  3. The area of application
B. If a prescription order specifies a particular semisolid base and a change of base is necessary for compatibility or stability reasons, the prescriber should be consulted.

IV. PRINCIPLES OF COMPOUNDING OINTMENTS

A. **Compounding equipment**
  1. **Ointment slabs or pads**
     a. In the United States, ointments are commonly made using a spatula and an ointment slab or pad. In some other countries, mortars and pestles are the preferred compounding equipment.
     b. Although ointment pads offer the advantage of easy cleanup, they do have some limitations. Ointment slabs are preferred when a liquid ingredient must be incorporated into the ointment, especially if the liquid is an aqueous solution. Liquids soak into the parchment paper of ointment pads, and excess weight can be lost. Very sticky or thick ointments are often more easily made on a slab. Loss is usually less when an ointment is compounded on an ointment slab rather than on a pad. Ointment slabs and pads are pictured and are described in greater detail in the compounding equipment section of Chapter 13.
  2. **Spatulas**
     a. Generally, the large metal spatulas are used for levigation, spatulation, and incorporation of solid and liquid ingredients. Smaller metal spatulas are useful for removing a preparation from the large spatula and for transferring a preparation from the ointment slab or pad to the ointment jar.
     b. Black rubber or plastic spatulas are special-purpose spatulas that are used when an ingredient (e.g., iodine) reacts with a metal spatula. They are not for general use in compounding ointments because they do not have the proper combination of flexibility and strength to give efficient shear and mixing.
     c. Various types of spatulas are pictured and are described in greater detail in the compounding equipment section of Chapter 13.
  3. For pharmacies that compound a significant number of customized semisolid preparations, small-scale ointment mills and specialized electric ointment mixers are available. This sort of equipment can produce smooth, elegant preparations with minimal effort and have the added advantage of minimizing exposure of compounding personnel to the drugs and other components of preparations being compounded.

B. **Amount of excess preparation to make to compensate for loss during compounding**
  1. The amount of excess preparation needed depends on factors such as compounding technique, number and type of ingredients, and difficulty of the compounding process. When using traditional equipment, such as an ointment slab and spatula, between 2 and 4 g of an ointment may be lost in the compounding process when preparing a moderate amount of ointment (e.g., 15 to 120 g).
  2. Either a percentage of excess (e.g., **10%**) or a given amount of excess preparation (e.g., **3 g**) is usually made to compensate for this loss. The amount of excess made is based on the compounder's own experience and professional judgment.

C. **Incorporation of solid drugs and chemicals**
  1. **General principles**
     a. Because a smooth, nongritty preparation is desired, any solids incorporated into an ointment base should be either solubilized or in the finest state of subdivision possible.
     b. Auxiliary agents, such as levigating agents and solvents, are sometimes added during the formulation of an ointment to facilitate making a smooth, elegant preparation. Auxiliary agents that make a substantive change in the preparation's properties should be avoided. For example, if a stiff, paste-like ointment is desired, avoid adding an auxiliary agent that would significantly decrease the viscosity of the formulation.
  2. **Choice of drug form**
     a. If possible, pick a form of the drug that is a fine powder (e.g., boric acid powder rather than boric acid crystals, or colloidal sulfur rather than precipitated sulfur).

b. If the prescription order specifies a certain form, that form should be used unless the prescriber is consulted.

c. If a drug or chemical is available in more than one form, the selected form should be specified on the face of the prescription document or in the compounding record.

3. **Levigation**

   a. As described in Chapter 25, Powders, levigation is the process of reducing particle size of a solid by triturating it in a mortar or spatulating it on an ointment slab or pad with a small amount of a liquid or melted base in which the solid is not soluble. This process is illustrated on Color Plate 9 and is demonstrated on the CD that accompanies this book.

   b. Optimally, the liquid, called a **levigating agent,** is somewhat viscous and has a low surface tension to improve ease of wetting the solid. When solids are added directly to a semisolid base, a certain amount of energy is required just to overcome the high resistance to flow of the semisolid. This resistance to flow makes it difficult to provide adequate shear to reduce the particle size of a solid when the manual techniques used in compounding are employed. Levigating agents act as lubricating agents. They make incorporating solids easier, and they usually give smoother preparations.

   c. Often, the ointment formulation contains an ingredient that can be used as a levigating agent. This is the preferred situation. If the prescribed formula does not contain an ingredient that may be used for this purpose, it is generally acceptable to add an auxiliary agent, provided it is bland and nontoxic and does not make a substantive change in the preparation's physical or therapeutic properties.

   d. It is important to remember that auxiliary levigating agents are added to facilitate making a smooth, elegant preparation. A levigating agent is generally not added when

   (1) The solid being incorporated has very fine particles.

   (2) The quantity of solid to incorporate is small.

   (3) The ointment base is soft.

   (4) The final preparation is intended to be a stiff paste.

   e. Types of levigating agents

   (1) Commonly used levigating agents are listed in Table 30.1; their specific gravities, miscibilities, and general uses are given. More complete descriptions of the oils and solvents can be found in Chapter 15, Pharmaceutical Solvents and Solubilizing Agents, and the surfactant polysorbate 80 is described in Chapter 20, Surfactants and Emulsifying Agents.

   (2) Melted ointment base may also be used.

   (3) Special levigating agents are sometimes required for compatibility or stability reasons.

   f. Choosing a levigating agent

   (1) If the formulation already contains an ingredient that can function as a levigating agent, that liquid should be used.

   (2) When adding a levigating agent, check for compatibility with the other formulation ingredients and with the ointment base. Fortunately, most levigating agents are fairly nonreactive and cause few compatibility problems.

   (3) **General Rule:** Assuming that there are no compatibility problems with other ingredients in the formulation, levigating agents are usually chosen to be chemically similar to the ointment base. For example, mineral oil is the levigating agent of choice for oleaginous bases, such as hydrocarbon, absorption, and water-in-oil emulsion bases (see Sample Prescription 30.1). Glycerin, which is miscible with water, is usually used for water-removable and water-soluble bases.

   (4) Some active ingredients require special levigating agents. Several of these are listed here.

      (a) Polysorbate 80 (Tween 80) is used as the levigating agent for coal tar. Coal Tar Ointment USP contains an amount of polysorbate 80 equal to half the weight of coal tar (see Sample Prescription 30.3). Coal tar can be directly incorporated into some semisolid bases, but polysorbate 80's surfactant properties provide the advantage of facilitating removal of the preparation when this is desired. Coal tar will not mix with mineral oil or glycerin.

      (b) Castor oil has been recommended for levigating Peruvian balsam. This stems from the fact that the resinous part of Peruvian balsam separates from semisolid preparations that also contain sulfur unless an equal quantity of castor oil is used as the levigating agent for the Peruvian balsam (3).

      (c) Although ichthammol is a black, tarry substance, it is water-washable. Because it mixes with glycerin and fixed oils, these are suitable levigating agents. Some compounders think they get a better preparation by levigating ichthammol with an absorption base

Table 30.1	LEVIGATING AGENTS		

LEVIGATING AGENTS	SPECIFIC GRAVITY	MISCIBILITY	USES
Mineral Oil (also known as Heavy Mineral Oil)	0.88	Miscible with fixed oils* except castor oil	– Oleaginous bases – Absorption bases
	Light: 0.85	Immiscible with water, alcohol, glycerin, propylene glycol, PEG 400, and castor oil	– Water-in-oil emulsion bases
Glycerin	1.26	Miscible with water, alcohol, propylene glycol, and PEG 400	– Oil-in-water emulsion bases – Water-soluble bases – Ichthammol
		Immiscible with mineral oil and fixed oils*	
Propylene Glycol	1.04	Miscible with water, alcohol, glycerin, and PEG 400	– Oil-in-water emulsion bases – Water-soluble bases
		Immiscible with mineral oil and fixed oils*	
PEG 400	1.13	Miscible with water, alcohol, glycerin, and propylene glycol	– Oil-in-water emulsion bases – Water-soluble bases
		Immiscible with mineral oil and fixed oils*	
Cottonseed Oil	0.92	Miscible with mineral oil and other fixed oils,* including castor oil	– Cottonseed or any other vegetable oil can be used as a substitute for mineral oil when a vegetable oil is preferred or when the solid to be incorporated is more soluble or mixes more smoothly with a vegetable oil than with mineral oil
		Immiscible with water, alcohol, glycerin, propylene glycol, and PEG 400	
Castor Oil	0.96	Miscible with alcohol and other fixed oils*	– Ichthammol or Balsam of Peru – Same uses as described previously with cottonseed oil
		Immiscible with water, glycerin, propylene glycol, PEG 400, and mineral oil	
Polysorbate 80 (Tween 80)	1.06–1.09 (usually weighed)	Miscible with water, alcohol, glycerin, propylene glycol, PEG 400, mineral oil, and fixed oils*	– Coal tar – Other instances when a surfactant is desired – May be incompatible with some water-in oil emulsion bases

* Fixed oils consist of glyceryl esters of fatty acids that are liquids at room temperature and nonvolatile under ordinary conditions. Examples of fixed oils are cottonseed oil, castor oil, olive oil, sesame oil, and corn oil.

such as Hydrophilic Petrolatum USP, Aquabase, or Aquaphor. In this case, the amount of absorption base used is equal to the amount of ichthammol in the prescription order.

(5) Some levigating agents have compatibility problems with certain semisolid bases or additives. Some examples are listed here.

  (a) Some nonionic surfactants are incompatible with certain emulsion bases if the surfactant favors the opposite emulsion type. For example, polysorbate 80, which forms o/w emulsions, can cause a phase inversion and breakdown when mixed with some w/o emulsion bases.

(b) Depending on the relative amounts, castor oil may be incompatible with a semisolid base or formulation that contains a significant amount of mineral oil. This is because castor oil is immiscible with mineral oil.

(6) Levigating agents should be nonsensitizing and nonallergenic. The prescriber and patient should be consulted before lanolin-type compounds are added to a compounded preparation, because some patients are allergic to these compounds (whereas a much smaller percentage are allergic to purified derivatives such as wool-wax alcohol present in Aquaphor and Aquabase).

g. Amount of levigating agent to use

(1) Factors that determine the amount of levigating agent needed include

(a) The quantity and properties of the solids to be incorporated.

(b) The levigating agent selected.

(c) The properties of the ointment base.

(d) The desired spreading consistency of the ointment.

(2) Amounts of levigating agents used in official preparations can serve as a guide, but these vary considerably. Several examples illustrate this point.

(a) Zinc Oxide Ointment USP calls for 15% mineral oil to be used for 20% zinc oxide in White Ointment USP. (White Ointment contains the stiffening agent white wax 5% in white petrolatum.)

(b) Zinc Oxide Paste USP uses no levigating agent for 50% solids (25% zinc oxide and 25% starch) in white petrolatum.

(c) Sulfur Ointment USP uses 10% mineral oil for 10% sulfur in white petrolatum.

(3) **General rule:** Unless a prescription order specifically calls for a given amount of levigating agent, the **minimum amount** of levigating agent necessary to lubricate the powders is generally recommended.

(a) To give you some idea of how much this is, 3 g of zinc oxide (10% zinc oxide for a 30-g semisolid preparation) requires approximately 1.5 to 2 mL of mineral oil or 1 to 1.25 mL of glycerin to get adequate lubrication of the powder for levigation.

(b) In both of these cases, the percent w/w concentration of levigating agent for a 30-g ointment is 4% to 6%, which is an average amount to use. You can easily see, however, that the amount really depends on the amount of powder to be levigated.

(4) If an auxiliary levigating agent is used, the weight must be determined, and there should be a corresponding decrease in the weight of the ointment base to bring the preparation to the desired final weight. When added by volume, the amount of levigating agent used should be measured in a syringe or graduate. The weight of the levigating agent that is used should then be calculated using the agent's specific gravity and the volume incorporated. Specific gravities of various levigating agents are given in Table 30.1.

h. Documentation: The name of the levigating agent and the quantity used should be noted on the face of the prescription order or the compounding record.

4. Dissolution

a. Under certain circumstances, dissolving a solid ingredient in a solvent or oil and subsequent incorporation of the solution into the ointment base is the preferred treatment. Certain crystalline ingredients such as urea and camphor are difficult or impossible to levigate to a fine powder and should be dissolved in a suitable solvent before incorporation in the ointment base. Testosterone is an example of a compound that gives gritty ointments unless it is first dissolved in an appropriate vegetable oil. It is not soluble in mineral oil.

b. Types of solvents

(1) Water-miscible solvents include water, alcohol, isopropyl alcohol, glycerin, propylene glycol, and polyethylene glycol 400. Descriptions of these solvents appear in Chapter 15, Pharmaceutical Solvents and Solubilizing Agents.

(2) Lipophilic solvents include mineral oil and the various fixed oils, including castor oil, cottonseed oil, olive oil, and corn oil. Descriptions of these oils can also be found in Chapter 15.

c. Choosing a solvent

(1) Check a reference such as *Remington: The Science and Practice of Pharmacy, The Merck Index,* or *Martindale—The Complete Drug Reference* for solubility information on the ingredient(s) to be dissolved.

(2) If the formulation already contains an ingredient that would be a suitable solvent, that liquid should be used to dissolve the solid.

(3) Check for compatibility of the potential solvent with the semisolid base and the other formulation ingredients.

d. Capacity of various ointment bases to absorb solvents

Based on their makeup, ointment bases have varying capacities to absorb liquids.

(1) **Hydrocarbon bases** absorb no water and only very limited amounts of alcoholic solutions. Most oils mix easily with hydrocarbon bases, but they reduce the viscosity of the preparation.

(2) **Anhydrous absorption bases** can absorb large quantities of aqueous solutions and lesser amounts of alcoholic solutions.

(a) Hydrophilic Petrolatum USP and its branded commercial counterparts such as Aquabase and Aquaphor absorb an equal weight of water with relative ease and up to several times their weight of water with adequate spatulation and patience.

(b) These bases absorb less alcohol and isopropyl alcohol, possibly up to an equal weight, because these alcohols eventually dissolve the emulsifiers in these absorption bases and destroy their ability to emulsify extra hydroalcoholic liquid.

(c) As with hydrocarbon bases, absorption bases easily incorporate most oils, with a corresponding decrease in the viscosity of the system.

(3) **Water-in-oil emulsion bases** accept varied amounts of water and alcoholic solutions.

(a) Cold Cream and Rose Water Ointment USP are w/o emulsion bases that can absorb very little water.

(b) Two commercially available w/o emulsion bases, Hydrocream and Eucerin, absorb much more water than these but much less than their counterpart anhydrous absorption bases, Aquabase and Aquaphor.

(c) Although w/o emulsions bases easily accept most oils, as with hydrocarbon and absorption bases, their consistency may be decreased, depending on the amount of oil added.

(4) **Water-removable oil-in-water emulsion bases** accept water or water-miscible liquids in their external phase but eventually thin to a liquid emulsion with the addition of significant amounts of these liquids.

(a) The o/w emulsion base Hydrophilic Ointment USP and its commercial counterparts such as Dermabase and Aquaphilic Ointment take up about 30% of their weight of water without thinning. They will accept a somewhat lesser amount of alcohol and will eventually break down if too much alcohol is added.

(b) These ointment bases emulsify some amount of added oil because there is usually some excess emulsifying agent in the formulation. Larger quantities of oil may require the addition of a small amount of an o/w emulsifier, such as polysorbate 80 (Tween 80).

(5) As their name indicates, **water-soluble bases** are soluble in water. They are also soluble in alcohol.

(a) They accept a very limited amount of water or alcohol without loss of viscosity.

(b) Addition of an oil may require prior levigation with a liquid of intermediate chemical properties, such as glycerin or propylene glycol.

e. Strategies for adding solvents to nonabsorbing bases

If an aqueous or alcoholic solution must be added to a base that will not absorb it, the compounder may use one of the following strategies.

(1) Change the ointment base, in part or whole, to an absorption base or other base that will take up the liquid. If it is possible, stay within the same base class. For example, change from Cold Cream to Hydrocream, both w/o emulsion bases, rather than to Aquabase, an anhydrous absorption base. The prescriber should be consulted about base changes. This is illustrated with Sample Prescription 30.4.

(2) Add a nonionic auxiliary emulsifier or emulsifier combination.

(a) Fatty alcohols such as cetyl or stearyl alcohol can be added to hydrocarbon bases for this purpose. For example, when 5% cetyl alcohol is added to white petrolatum, the combination will absorb 40% to 50% of its weight in water (4). Because these fatty alcohols are waxy substances, the combination must be melted and then allowed to congeal so that a smooth base results.

(b) Stearyl or cetyl alcohol can also be added to water-soluble polyethylene glycol bases to improve their water or alcohol absorption properties. The Polyethylene Glycol Ointment monograph in the *National Formulary* notes that if 5% of the PEG 3350 is replaced with an equal quantity of stearyl alcohol, 6% to 25% of an aqueous solution can be incorporated in Polyethylene Glycol Ointment (5).

(c) Span nonionic surfactants are very useful for this purpose. For example, 2% to 5% Span 80, when directly incorporated into a hydrocarbon base, will enable the base to take up a significant amount of aqueous solution. This is illustrated with Sample Prescription 30.5.

    (3) Spatulate the solution and ointment base until a sufficient amount of the solvent evaporates.

  f. Be cautious when adding water to formulations containing drugs that are subject to hydrolysis. It may affect the stability of the preparation. Also, water-containing preparations must contain an antimicrobial ingredient or a preservative.

  g. Amount of solvent to add

    (1) General rule: Unless a prescription order specifically calls for a given amount of the solvent, use the **minimum amount** necessary to dissolve the solid ingredients.

    (2) If a solvent is added to the formulation, the weight must be determined, and there should be a corresponding decrease in the weight of the ointment base to bring the preparation to the desired final weight. The volume of solvent used should be measured in a syringe or graduate; the weight of this volume can then be calculated using the solvent's specific gravity and the volume incorporated. This is illustrated with Sample Prescriptions 30.4 and 30.5. Specific gravities of pharmaceutical solvents are given in the solvent descriptions in Chapter 15, and specific gravities for solvents and some liquids that are commonly added to compounded semisolids are given in Table 30.2.

  h. Documentation: The name of the solvent and the quantity used should be noted on the face of the prescription order or in the compounding record.

D. Incorporation of liquids

  1. Formulations that include liquids require semisolid bases that will absorb the liquid. If a liquid must be added to a base that will not absorb it, one of the strategies given earlier (in section C. 4.e.) for incorporating solutions may be used.

  2. When adding a nonviscous liquid such as an aqueous or hydroalcoholic solution, good technique and care must be used during incorporation. Because we are working with semisolids, even those bases that can take up a significant amount of liquid do not just absorb the liquid; the liquid must be carefully spatulated or triturated into the base.

Table 30.2	DENSITIES OF SELECTED LIQUIDS
LIQUID	**DENSITY**
Acetic Acid, Glacial	1.05
Acetone	0.79
Alcohol	0.82
Benzoin Tincture	0.85
Castor Oil	0.96
Chloroform	1.48
Coal Tar Solution (LCD)	0.87
Compound Benzoin Tincture	0.91
Cottonseed Oil	0.92
Glycerin	1.26
Hydrochloric Acid	1.18
Isopropyl Alcohol	0.78
Lactic Acid	1.20
Liquefied Phenol	1.06
Methyl Salicylate (Oil of Wintergreen)	1.18
Mineral Oil, Heavy	0.88
Mineral Oil, Light	0.85
Peppermint Oil	0.91
Phosphoric Acid	1.71
Polyethylene Glycol 400	1.13
Propylene Glycol	1.04
Resorcinol Monoacetate	1.20
Soluble Rose	1.16
Witch Hazel	0.98

    a. One method is to place the semisolid base on an ointment slab and create a depression in the base mass; then carefully pour the liquid that is to be incorporated into that depression to keep the liquid contained during the process. The liquid is then carefully spatulated in small portions into the base. This is illustrated in Color Plate 10.

    b. A second method is to put the semisolid base in a mortar and gradually add the liquid in portions with trituration until all has been added.

3. Certain thick liquids are measured by weight rather than by volume. Examples include coal tar, Peru balsam, ichthammol, and the polysorbate-sorbitan type emulsifiers. For thick and sticky liquids, it works well to wipe the weighing paper first with the chosen levigating agent before taring out the weight of the paper and adding the sticky liquid. The thick liquid is then easier to transfer completely from the weighing paper onto the ointment slab because the thick liquid slides more readily off the slippery surface created by the levigating agent on the weighing paper.

4. Some liquids require special levigating agents. Several of these are listed previously in the section on levigating agents (see IV.C.3).

5. Some liquids, especially aqueous and alcoholic solutions, soak into the paper of ointment pads. Ointment slabs are the preferred equipment for these preparations.

V. COMPATIBILITY AND STABILITY

A. Physical stability

1. Ointments are semisolid dosage forms and are therefore naturally more physically stable than are liquid preparations such as solutions, suspensions, or emulsions; sedimentation, caking, creaming, and precipitation of solids are not problems we encounter with ointments. This allows more flexibility with assigning beyond-use dates.

2. The strategies for achieving uniform, smooth, nongritty ointments and for incorporating liquid ingredients in ointment bases have been discussed previously in this chapter.

3. "Bleeding" of liquid ingredients and phase separation can occur. Special levigating agents, as outlined previously, may be helpful.

4. Glycerin or propylene glycol may be added as humectants to ointment bases containing water, to retard evaporation of the water and prevent drying out of the ointment base.

B. Chemical stability

1. Ingredients

    a. Check suitable references for information on chemical stability of the active ingredients and other formulation components. Issues of chemical stability are discussed in Chapter 37, and specific illustrations are given with sample prescriptions in this chapter and in the other dosage form chapters. The general topic of beyond-use dating is discussed in Chapter 4.

    b. Professional judgment is needed in applying *USP* Chapter ⟨795⟩ beyond-use dating (BUD) recommendations to semisolids because they are not specifically mentioned. Obviously, when stability information is known for a specific formulation and storage conditions, that information can be applied in setting the BUD for the preparation. In the absence of such information, the following information from *USP* Chapter ⟨795⟩ can act as a guideline (6).

        (1) If there is no water in the formulation, the standard for nonaqueous liquids and solid formulations could be applied to semisolids. This allows a 6-month BUD if the active ingredient(s) is a *USP* or *NF* substance, or 25% of the time remaining on the expiration date of a manufactured product used as an ingredient, whichever is less.

        (2) If a formulation contains water, the standard for water-containing liquid preparations would be prudent in many circumstances. This allows a maximum BUD of 14 days when the preparation is stored in the refrigerator. Since most topical preparations are stored at room temperature, this variable should be considered in setting a BUD for the preparation.

        (3) The third possibility in *USP* Chapter ⟨795⟩ uses the classification "all other formulations." This limits the BUD to the length of time for the intended therapy or 30 days, whichever is earlier.

        (4) Finally, when there are concerns for chemical stability of known labile active ingredient(s), this must be considered and may further limit the BUD.

2. Emulsifiers: For general compatibility information on emulsifiers, see Chapter 20, Surfactants and Emulsifying Agents. Soap-type emulsifiers cause most of the compatibility problems. Some specific ointment base examples include the following:

    a. Oil-in-water emulsions: Traditional vanishing creams used stearate soap-type emulsifiers, which are sensitive to pH and multivalent ions. Some manufacturers have reformulated vanishing creams to use nonionic surfactants. The formula of a cream should be checked if compatibility problems are suspected. Some oil-in-water emulsions, such as Hydrophilic

Ointment USP, do not have these compatibility problems because the emulsifying agent is the detergent sodium lauryl sulfate plus nonionic emulsifiers stearyl and cetyl alcohol.

b. Water-in-oil emulsions: Again, emulsion ointments that have soap-type emulsifiers may have problems. Two examples are Cold Cream and Rose Water Ointment. Both have emulsifiers formed by the reaction of sodium borate with the fatty acids in cetyl esters wax. This emulsion is sensitive to acid ingredients such as salicylic acid or phenolic compounds. Eucerin and Hydrocream are water-in-oil emulsion bases that contain nonionic emulsifiers. These bases are stable to acid ingredients.

C. Microbiologic stability

1. Ointments that contain water are subject to microbial growth. *USP* Chapter ⟨1151⟩ specifically states that **all emulsions** require an antimicrobial agent because the aqueous phase is favorable to the growth of microorganisms (1). This is especially true of ointments in which water is the external phase. For information on acceptable preservatives, see Chapter 16, Antimicrobial Preservatives.

2. If antimicrobial ingredients are present in the formulation, either for therapeutic purposes or as part of the preservative system of an ingredient, extra preservatives may not be needed. For example, Hydrophilic Ointment USP and manufactured emulsion ointment bases such as Dermabase, Acid Mantle Cream, Aquaphilic Ointment, Velvachol, and Dermovan contain preservatives.

3. It is important to remember that some preservatives, such as parabens and benzoic acid, are highly lipophilic; a significant portion of these may partition into the oil phase of the ointment and leave the water phase with an insufficient preservative concentration. Extra preservative may be needed.

Sample Prescriptions

The first two prescription orders given below are for *USP* formulations and are available as manufactured products from various sources. They would, therefore, not normally be compounded in the pharmacy. They are given here in an abbreviated format as examples of basic ointment preparations, one using a levigating agent for incorporation of insoluble powder and one using direct incorporation of a large quantity of powder to give a paste. The procedure for Sample Prescription 30.1 is also demonstrated on the CD that accompanies this book. Neither of these *USP* formulations have stability or compatibility issues. The manufactured products would have expiration dates of at least 2 years as assigned by the manufacturer following stability testing of the product. If such a preparation were compounded, a beyond-use date of 6 months for a nonaqueous preparation made with USP ingredients would be acceptable. Sample Prescription 30.3 is also for a *USP* preparation, but it is currently not available commercially and requires compounding. The other sample prescriptions in this section are custom formulations.

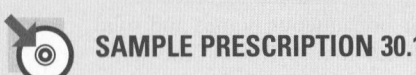

SAMPLE PRESCRIPTION 30.1

CONTEMPORARY PHYSICIANS GROUP PRACTICE
20 S. PARK STREET, TRITURATE, WI 53706
TEL: (608) 555-1333 FAX: (608) 555-1335

℞ #   *123310*

NAME *Basil Hoepe*   **DATE** *00/00/00*

ADDRESS *612 Companion Lane*

℞

Zinc Oxide Ointment USP
Disp 30 g

J. Jensen 00/00/00

Sig: Apply to affected areas qid ut dict

REFILLS *1*   *Linus Ashman*   **M.D.**

DEA NO. _____

INGREDIENTS USED:

Ingredient	Quantity Used	Physical Description	Solubility	Dose Comparison		Use in the Prescription
				Given	Usual	
Zinc Oxide	6.6 g	white powder	insol in water and alcohol	20%	varies from 1–25%	astringent, protective, antiseptic
Mineral Oil	5.6 mL	viscous, clear, oily liquid	immisc w/ water and alcohol	—	—	levigating agent
White Ointment USP	21.45 g	white semisolid	immisc with water & alcohol	—	—	base

CALCULATIONS

Dose/Concentration: Zinc Oxide is often used as a protectant, which is defined as a substance that protects injured or exposed skin surfaces from harmful or annoying stimuli. The concentration range specified by the FDA for zinc oxide as a protectant is 1% to 25%. Using the *USP* formula given below, the concentration of zinc oxide in this preparation can be calculated as:

$$\frac{200 \text{ g ZnO}}{1,000 \text{ g ointment}} = \frac{x \text{ g ZnO}}{100 \text{ g ointment}} \; ; x = 20 \text{ g}/100 \text{ g} = 20\,\%$$

Ingredient Amounts

Zinc Oxide Ointment USP has the following formula (7):

Zinc oxide	200 g
Mineral oil	150 g
White Ointment	650 g
To make	1,000 g

Amounts of each ingredient (in g) to make 33 g of ointment (3 g excess):

Zinc oxide:
$$\left(\frac{200 \text{ g zinc oxide}}{1,000 \text{ g ointment}}\right)\left(\frac{33 \text{ g ointment}}{}\right) = 6.6 \text{ g zinc oxide}$$

Mineral oil:
$$\left(\frac{150 \text{ g mineral oil}}{1,000 \text{ g ointment}}\right)\left(\frac{33 \text{ g ointment}}{}\right) = 4.95 \text{ g mineral oil}$$

White Ointment:
$$\left(\frac{650 \text{ g White Oint.}}{1,000 \text{ g oint.}}\right)\left(\frac{33 \text{ g oint.}}{}\right) = 21.45 \text{ g White Ointment}$$

The quantity of mineral oil is given in grams but, in small-scale compounding, it is usually measured volumetrically. Using the specific gravity (s.g.) of mineral oil, the number of milliliters needed for this prescription is calculated:

s.g.: between 0.860 and 0.905   avg. s.g. = 0.88

$$\left(\frac{\text{mL mineral oil}}{0.88 \text{ g mineral oil}}\right)\left(\frac{4.95 \text{ g mineral oil}}{}\right) = 5.6 \text{ mL}$$

White Ointment is an official *USP* preparation. Its formula and method of preparation is given in Table 23.2 in Chapter 23, Ointment Bases, and is demonstrated with this sample prescription on the CD that accompanies this book.

COMPOUNDING PROCEDURE: On a class III torsion or electronic balance, weigh 6.6 g of zinc oxide. With a 10-mL syringe or graduated cylinder, measure 5.6 mL of mineral oil. Place the zinc oxide on an ointment pad or slab. Add the mineral oil stepwise in small portions with levigation to the zinc oxide to form a smooth paste.

Weigh 21.45 g of White Ointment, and incorporate the zinc oxide–mineral oil paste into the White Ointment. Do this by adding the White Ointment stepwise in portions with spatulation to the paste. Spatulate the ointment well to achieve a smooth, uniform preparation.

DESCRIPTION OF FINISHED PREPARATION: The preparation should be a smooth, white opaque ointment of moderate consistency and with a slight sheen. The actual weight should be within the range of 30 g ± 10%.

LABELING

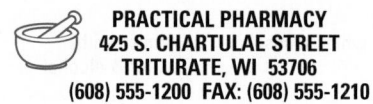

PRACTICAL PHARMACY
425 S. CHARTULAE STREET
TRITURATE, WI 53706
(608) 555-1200 FAX: (608) 555-1210

℞ 123310   Pharmacist: JJ   Date: 00/00/00
Basil Hoepe   Dr. Linus Ashman

Apply to affected areas four times a day as directed.

Zinc Oxide Ointment USP

Mfg: Compounded   Quantity: 30 g

Refills: 1   Discard after: Give date

Auxiliary Labels: For External Use Only. This medicine was compounded in our pharmacy for you at the direction of your prescriber.

SAMPLE PRESCRIPTION 30.2

CONTEMPORARY PHYSICIANS GROUP PRACTICE
20 S. PARK STREET, TRITURATE, WI 53706
TEL: (608) 555-1333 FAX: (608) 555-1335

℞ # *123311*

NAME *Justiens Case*   **DATE** *00/00/00*

ADDRESS *532 Lazy Acres Road*

℞

    Zinc Oxide
    Starch   aa   *15 g*
    White Petrolatum   qs ad *60 g*

G. Giles 00/00/00

Sig: Apply after each diaper change prn

REFILLS *prn*   *Ozzie Wurtz*   **M.D.**

          DEA NO. _____

INGREDIENTS USED: (For 10% excess, 66 g)

Ingredient	Quantity Used	Physical Description	Solubility	Dose Comparison		Use in the Prescription
				Given	Usual	
Zinc Oxide	16.5 g	white powder	insol in water and alcohol	25%	1–25%	protective astringent antiseptic
Starch	16.5 g	white powder	insol cold water and alcohol	25%	varies	absorbent protective demulcent
White Petrolatum	33 g	white, translucent semisolid	immisc with water and alcohol	—	—	base

CALCULATIONS

Dose/Concentration

This formulation is actually Zinc Oxide Paste USP. All concentrations are okay for the intended use.

Percent concentrations of zinc oxide and starch:

$$\frac{15\text{ g zinc oxide/starch}}{60\text{ g ointment}} = \frac{x\text{ g zinc oxide/starch}}{100\text{ g}}; x = 25\text{ g/100 g} = 25\,\%$$

Ingredient Amounts

Because this preparation is for treatment of diaper rash, a very thick, stiff formulation (such as a paste) is desired. For this reason, no levigating agent is added. The weights (in g) of all ingredients except the ointment base are given in the prescription order. The amount of white petrolatum is calculated by subtracting the weights of all the other ingredients from the total weight desired.

Weight of zinc oxide:	15 g
Weight of starch:	15 g
Total weight of powder ingredients:	30 g
Weight of white petrolatum:	60 g − 30 g = 30 g

To make excess ointment to compensate for loss during compounding, a 10% excess of each ingredient can be calculated and used:

Zinc oxide and starch: 15 g × 110% = 15 g × 1.1 = 16.5 g

White petrolatum: 30 g × 110% = 30 g × 1.1 = 33 g

COMPOUNDING PROCEDURE: On a class 3 torsion or electronic balance, weigh 16.5 g each of zinc oxide and starch and 33 g of white petrolatum. Transfer the powders to an ointment slab and spatulate them together until the combined powders are thoroughly mixed. Incorporate the powders directly into the white petrolatum in small portions with careful spatulation until a smooth paste is produced. Making such a preparation with a smooth, nongritty texture requires extra time and skill. It is best done by incorporating a small amount of powder at a time in a small amount of base until all the powder has been added and a smooth paste is obtained. Transfer to a 2-oz ointment jar, label, and dispense.

DESCRIPTION OF FINISHED PREPARATION: The preparation should be a smooth, white, opaque semisolid of very stiff consistency and with a "dry" matte appearance. The actual weight should be 60 g ±10%.

LABELING

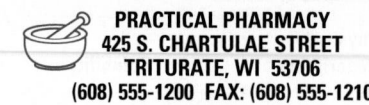

PRACTICAL PHARMACY
425 S. CHARTULAE STREET
TRITURATE, WI 53706
(608) 555-1200 FAX: (608) 555-1210

℞ 123311   Pharmacist: GG   Date: 00/00/00
Justiens Case   Dr. Ozzie Wurtz

Apply after each diaper change as needed.

Zinc Oxide 25% and Starch 25% Topical Paste (or may be labeled
Zinc Oxide Paste USP)

Mfg: Compounded   Quantity: 60 g

Refills: 1 year   Discard after: Give date

Auxiliary Label: External Use Only. This medicine was compounded in our
pharmacy for you at the direction of your prescriber.

SAMPLE PRESCRIPTION 30.3

CASE: P. Sandra Smith is a 130-lb, 5′1″-tall, 24-year-old patient with moderate psoriasis. Dr. Pixce has treated Ms. Smith's condition with several therapies, including topical corticosteroids and commercially available coal tar products. In each case, the results were not satisfactory or were unsustained. Before trying the Goeckerman regimen, which uses a combination of crude coal tar (CCT) and ultraviolet light therapy, Pharmacist Jolson suggests they try a traditional coal tar preparation, because reportedly these give better results than some of the newer refined coal tar products (8). The Goeckerman regimen is quite effective and gives sustained relief, but it is usually administered through treatment centers and requires daily ultraviolet light therapy followed by application of CCT for 8 hours (9); it is therefore messy, time consuming, and expensive. The following prescription order is for a *USP* formulation, but it is not currently available commercially, so Dr. Jolson will compound it in her pharmacy.

CONTEMPORARY PHYSICIANS GROUP PRACTICE
20 S. PARK STREET, TRITURATE, WI 53706
TEL: (608) 555-1333 FAX: (608) 555-1335

℞ # *123312*

NAME *P. Sandra Smith*   DATE *00/00/00*

ADDRESS *2530 Hosta Haven*

℞   *Coal Tar Ointment USP*

Dispense 1 oz

*Sig: Apply to affected areas after dinner and leave on for 4 hours,
then remove before bedtime for psoriasis*

J. Jolson 00/00/00

REFILLS *3*   *Penelope Pixce*   M.D.

DEA NO. _____

MASTER COMPOUNDING FORMULATION RECORD

NAME, STRENGTH, AND DOSAGE FORM OF PREPARATION: Coal Tar Ointment USP

QUANTITY: 30 g (plus 3 g excess)

THERAPEUTIC USE/CATEGORY: Psoriasis

FORMULATION RECORD ID: OT001

ROUTE OF ADMINISTRATION: Topical

INGREDIENTS USED:

Ingredient	Quantity Used	Physical Description	Solubility	Dose Comparison		Use in the Prescription
				Given	Usual	
Coal Tar	330 mg	black, tarry, thick liquid	sl sol in water; part sol in alcohol	1%	varies	antipruritic antieczema keratoplastic
Polysorbate 80	165 mg	yellow, oily, viscous liquid	misc with water, oils	0.5%	$^1/_2$–1 times the amount of coal tar	dispersing, emulsifying agent
Zinc Oxide Paste	32.505 g	white, semisolid paste	immisc with water	full strength	full strength	protective, vehicle

COMPATIBILITY–STABILITY: This is an official USP formulation that is known to be very stable. No preservative is needed because the zinc oxide in the Zinc Oxide Paste is an antiseptic and there is no water present in this formula.

PACKAGING AND STORAGE: The *USP* monograph for this preparation recommends storage in tight containers (7). Use a 1-oz ointment tube.

BEYOND-USE DATE: Although manufactured versions of this formulation are given expiration dates of several years, use a more conservative 6-month beyond-use date for this nonaqueous compounded preparation made with *USP* ingredients (6).

CALCULATIONS

Dose/Concentration: This is a USP formulation; all concentrations are appropriate.

Ingredient Amounts

Coal Tar Ointment USP has the following formula (7):

Coal Tar	10 g
Polysorbate 80	5 g
Zinc Oxide Paste	985 g
To make	1,000 g

Amounts of each ingredient (in g) to make 33 g of ointment (3 g excess to compensate for loss during compounding):

Coal Tar:
$$\left(\frac{10 \text{ g coal tar}}{1,000 \text{ g}} \right) \left(\frac{33 \text{ g}}{} \right) = 0.33 \text{ g coal tar}$$

Polysorbate 800:
$$\left(\frac{5 \text{ g polysorbate 80}}{1,000 \text{ g}} \right) \left(\frac{33 \text{ g}}{} \right) = 0.165 \text{ g polysorbate 80}$$

Zinc Oxide Paste: Use commercially available Zinc Oxide Paste USP

$$\left(\frac{985 \text{ g Zinc Oxide Paste}}{1,000 \text{ g}} \right) \left(\frac{33 \text{ g}}{} \right) = 32.505 \text{ g Zinc Oxide Paste}$$

MSDS AND SAFETY AND PERSONAL PROTECTIVE EQUIPMENT: Review MSDS for all components. Don a clean lab coat and disposable gloves. Handle coal tar with care because it stains.

SPECIALIZED EQUIPMENT: Ointment slab. All weighing is done on an electronic balance.

COMPOUNDING PROCEDURE: Weigh 330 mg of coal tar, 165 mg of polysorbate 80, and 32.505 g of Zinc Oxide Paste. Because the coal tar is thick and sticky, it works well to wipe the weighing paper first with polysorbate 80 before taring out the weight of the paper and adding the coal tar. This makes the paper slippery, so the coal tar is then more easily transferred completely onto the ointment slab with a metal spatula. Levigate the polysorbate 80 and coal tar together on an ointment slab and then incorporate this mixture into the Zinc Oxide Paste by spatulation using geometric dilution. Tare a 1-oz ointment tube, then transfer the ointment to the tube and note and record the weight of the preparation. Label and dispense.

DESCRIPTION OF FINISHED PREPARATION: The preparation is a smooth, grayish black opaque ointment with a moderately stiff consistency and with a slight sheen. There should be no apparent white particles in the ointment. It has the characteristic odor of coal tar.

QUALITY CONTROL: Check the actual weight; it should be within the range of ±10% of the prescribed weight of 30 g, and the loss from the theoretical weight of 33 g should be reasonable.

MASTER FORMULA PREPARED BY: Jennifer Jolson, PharmD   **CHECKED BY:** John Dopp, PharmD

COMPOUNDING RECORD

NAME, STRENGTH, AND DOSAGE FORM OF PREPARATION: Coal Tar Ointment USP
QUANTITY: 30 g (plus 3 g excess)   **DATE PREPARED:** mm/dd/yy   **BEYOND-USE DATE:** mm/dd/yy
FORMULATION RECORD ID: OT001   **CONTROL/RX NUMBER:** 123312

INGREDIENTS USED:

Ingredient	Quantity Used	Manufacture Lot Number	Expiration Date	Weighed/ Measured by	Checked by
Coal Tar	330 mg	JET Labs ON3031	mm/yy	bjf	jj
Polysorbate 80	165 mg	JET Labs ON3032	mm/yy	bjf	jj
Zinc Oxide Paste USP	32.505 g	Quality Generics XN8975	mm/yy	bjf	jj

QUALITY CONTROL DATA: The preparation is a smooth, grayish black opaque ointment with a moderately stiff consistency and with a slight sheen. When spread in a thin layer, there are no apparent white particles in the ointment. It has the odor of coal tar. The actual weight is checked and is 31.1 g, which is within the range of ±10% of the prescribed weight of 30 g and normal limits for expected loss from the theoretical weight of 33 g.

LABELING

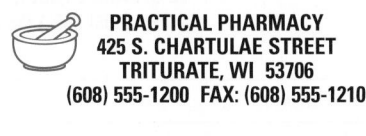

PRACTICAL PHARMACY
425 S. CHARTULAE STREET
TRITURATE, WI 53706
(608) 555-1200 FAX: (608) 555-1210

℞ 123312   Pharmacist: JJ   Date: 00/00/00
P. Sandra Smith   Dr. Penelope Pixce

Apply to affected areas after dinner and leave on for 4 hours, then
remove at bedtime for treatment of psoriasis.

Coal Tar Ointment USP

Mfg: Compounded   Quantity: 30 g

Refills: 3   Discard after: Give date

Auxiliary Label: For External Use Only. Photosensitivity Warning. This
medicine was compounded in our pharmacy for you at the direction of your
prescriber.

PATIENT CONSULTATION: Hello, Ms. Smith. I'm your pharmacist, Jennifer Jolson. Are you allergic to any drugs? Are you currently using (orally or topically) any other medications? What did Dr. Pixce tell you about this medication? This Coal Tar Ointment is to treat your psoriasis. Apply it to the affected areas each night right after dinner and leave it on for 4 hours, then remove it just before you go to bed. The goal is to have this ointment on the affected areas for 4 hours each day; Dr. Pixce thought that this schedule would provide 4 hours of treatment with the least interruption of your work and life activities. She and I discussed the fact that this schedule may not always be the best, so if this same goal can be accomplished with a different schedule, that is fine. It is recommended that you apply the ointment parallel with the growth of your hair shafts; for example, downward strokes on your arm. This is done to minimize irritation of the places where you hair shafts exit from your skin. Cover the areas of application with some clean, disposable material, such as plastic food wrap, because this ointment definitely does stain fabric: I remember one of my pharmacy professors telling our class that the only way to remove coal tar from fabric is with a scissors! I think the easiest way to remove this ointment from your skin at the end of the 4-hour application period is to moisten a tissue with some mineral oil and use that to gently remove the ointment; then gently wash the area with mild soap and warm water. Dispose of the tissue in a plastic sandwich bag and discard it in your garbage. This preparation might make the affected areas more sensitive to sunlight, causing redness of the skin. Do not use this in the anogenital areas and don't get this in or near your eyes. If your condition seems to be getting worse, or if other types of irritation occur, contact Dr. Pixce. This medication should be kept at room temperature, out of the reach of children. Discard any unused contents after 6 months. Dr. Pixce has authorized three refills. Do you have any questions?

SAMPLE PRESCRIPTION 30.4

CASE: Rudiger Simpson is a 165-lb, 5'10"-tall, 22-year-old male patient with a diagnosis of allergic dermatitis. Six months ago he earned his degree as a physician's assistant and started work as a surgical assistant to an orthopedic surgeon. He recently developed red, dry, very irritated skin on his wrists and the upper parts of his hands at the place where the elastic cuffs of his surgical gown contact his skin. He thinks that he is allergic to the elastic in those cuffs and has ordered a different type of surgical gown, but he has asked Dr. Stark for some sort of ointment to treat his skin condition. Dr. Stark wants to use a hydrocortisone–urea ointment with an oleaginous base because this will give superior protection and emollient therapy, but the commercial products all have water-washable cream bases. As a result, Dr. Stark prescribed the custom ointment described here. Pharmacist B. Bunny called Dr. Stark to request a change of ointment base to an absorption base (Aquabase brand of anhydrous hydrophilic petrolatum) so he can achieve a smooth, nongritty preparation by incorporating the urea as a solution. Dr. Stark has agreed as long as the ointment provides a good protective emollient base.

CONTEMPORARY PHYSICIANS GROUP PRACTICE
20 S. PARK STREET, TRITURATE, WI 53706
TEL: (608) 555-1333 FAX: (608) 555-1335

℞ #   *123365*

NAME *Rudiger B. Simpson*   DATE *00/00/00*

ADDRESS *951 Lisa Lane*

℞

Hydrocortisone	*0.6 g*
Urea	*6 g*
~~*White Petrolatum*~~ *qs ad*	*60 g*

Per telephone consult with Dr. Stark, changed White

Petrolatum to Aquabase   *B. Bunny 00/00/00*

Sig: Apply to affected area up to qid

REFILLS *4*   *Art Stark*   M.D.

DEA NO. _____

MASTER COMPOUNDING FORMULATION RECORD

NAME, STRENGTH, AND DOSAGE FORM OF PREPARATION: Hydrocortisone 1% and Urea 10% Topical Ointment
QUANTITY: 60 g (plus 6 g excess)   **FORMULATION RECORD ID:** OT002
THERAPEUTIC USE/CATEGORY: Anti-inflammatory/emollient   **ROUTE OF ADMINISTRATION:** Topical

INGREDIENTS USED:

Ingredient	Quantity Used	Physical Description	Solubility	Dose Comparison		Use in the Prescription
				Given	Usual	
Hydrocortisone	0.66 g	white powder	v sl sol in water; 1 g/40 mL alcohol	1.0%	0.25–2.5%	anti-inflammatory antipruritic
Paraben–Propylene Glycol Stock	1.32 mL (1.368 g)	clear, colorless liquid	misc w/ water, alcohol	0.18% MP 0.02% PP 2% PG	0.18% MP 0.02% PP 2% PG	Preservative
Urea	6.6 g	white crystalline powder	1 g/1.5 mL water; 10 mL alcohol	10%	5–30%	mild keratolytic; hydrates skin; removes scales
Purified Water	10 mL	clear, colorless liquid	—	—	—	solvent
Aquabase	47.372 g	white, translucent semisolid	insol in water and alcohol	—	—	vehicle; emollient

MP = methylparaben; PP = propylparaben; PG = propylene glycol

COMPATIBILITY–STABILITY: No stability data for this specific formulation is available and, because of the multiple ingredients in this formulation, its stability is somewhat difficult to evaluate. Because urea is a hard crystalline substance that is difficult to levigate to a fine powder, it is usually first dissolved in water before incorporation into the ointment base. Therefore, the stability of urea in aqueous solution is important. Compounded urea preparations have been evaluated and reported in the literature, but with mixed results. A good review of the subject can be found in *Chemical Stability of Pharmaceuticals*, which reports the calculated half-life of urea solution at 25°C and pH 7 to be 29 years (10). Because white petrolatum will not absorb the water needed to dissolve the urea, the white petrolatum should be replaced in whole or part with an absorption base such as Hydrophilic Petrolatum USP or a similar branded absorption base. (Another alternative would be to add 2% to 5% of Span 80 to emulsify the urea solution.) For the purpose of this formulation, the base was changed to Aquabase, a brand of Hydrophilic Petrolatum. The stability of hydrocortisone in this preparation is also difficult to assess. In aqueous solution, hydrocortisone undergoes oxidation and other complex degradation reactions. It is most stable at pH 3.5 to 4.5, and its stability is quite dependent on pH, with steep slopes for its pH-rate profile in both the acidic and basic regions (11). Although the hydrocortisone is not in solution, it may have contact with the water droplets of the urea aqueous solution, and *The Merck Index* reports that 10% solutions of urea in water have a pH of 7.2, a condition not favorable to the stability of hydrocortisone. Finally, because of the addition of water, a preservative must be added, and the combination 0.18% methylparaben and 0.02% propylparaben in propylene glycol has been selected.

PACKAGING AND STORAGE: Packaging should be in a tight, light-resistant ointment jar with recommended storage at controlled room temperature.

BEYOND-USE DATE: Use the *USP*-recommended maximum 14-day beyond-use date for compounded water-containing formulations prepared from ingredients in solid form when there is no stability information for the formulation (6).

CALCULATIONS

Dose/Concentration

Concentration (in %) for each active ingredient is calculated here.

Hydrocortisone:
$$\frac{0.6 \text{ g HC}}{60 \text{ g oint.}} = \frac{x \text{ g HC}}{100 \text{ g oint.}}; \; x = 1 \text{ g}/100 \text{ g} = 1\%$$

Urea:
$$\frac{6 \text{ g urea}}{60 \text{ g oint.}} = \frac{x \text{ g urea}}{100 \text{ g oint.}}; \; x = 10 \text{ g}/100 \text{ g} = 10\%$$

Both concentrations are appropriate for the condition.

Ingredient Amounts

The hydrocortisone and the urea are solids, and the prescription order gives the amounts of each in grams. To make excess ointment to compensate for loss during compounding, a 10% excess of each ingredient can be calculated and used:

Hydrocortisone: $\qquad\qquad 0.6 \text{ g} \times 110\% = 0.6 \text{ g} \times 1.1 = 0.66 \text{ g}$

Urea: $\qquad\qquad\qquad\quad 6 \text{ g} \times 110\% = 6 \text{ g} \times 1.1 = 6.6 \text{ g}$

As discussed earlier, urea has a hard crystalline structure that requires dissolution in water for a smooth ointment preparation. The solubility of urea in water is 1 g/1.5 mL. The amount of water required to dissolve the urea can be calculated:

$$\left(\frac{1.5 \text{ mL water}}{1 \text{ g urea}} \right)\left(\frac{6.6 \text{ g urea}}{} \right) = 9.9 \approx 10 \text{ mL water}$$

This addition of water means that a preservative should be added. Practical Pharmacy uses the stock solution (described in Chapter 16, Antimicrobial Preservatives) containing methylparaben and propylparaben in propylene glycol:

Methylparaben (MP)		9 g
Propylparaben (PP)		1 g
Propylene Glycol (PG)	qs ad	100 mL

A volume of 2 mL of this solution per 100 g of preparation provides the recommended 0.18% MP and 0.02% PP with approximately 2% PG. For our 66 g ointment, the volume needed is calculated to be:

$$\frac{2 \text{ mL stock soln}}{100 \text{ g ointment}} = \frac{x \text{ mL stock soln}}{66 \text{ g ointment}}; x = 1.32 \text{ mL stock solution}$$

That this volume gives the correct percent concentration of preservative is verified by calculation. For example, for MP:

$$\left(\frac{9 \text{ g MP}}{100 \text{ mL stock}}\right)\left(\frac{1.32 \text{ mL stock}}{}\right) = 0.119 \text{ g MP}$$

$$\frac{0.119 \text{ g MP}}{66 \text{ g ointment}} = \frac{x \text{ g MP}}{100 \text{ g ointment}}; x = 0.18 \text{ g MP}/100 \text{ g} = 0.18\%$$

The weight of this stock solution must be calculated to determine the weight of Aquaphor to give 66 g of ointment. PG has a specific gravity of 1.036. Because the small powder volume of the parabens is insignificant, you may use this as the specific gravity of the stock solution. Calculate the weight of 1.32 mL of the stock solution:

$$\left(\frac{1.036 \text{ g stock soln}}{\text{mL stock soln}}\right)\left(\frac{1.32 \text{ mL stock soln}}{}\right) = 1.368 \text{ g stock soln}$$

As discussed previously, the ointment base was changed from white petrolatum to an anhydrous absorption base, Aquabase. The amount of base is calculated by subtracting the weights of all the other ingredients from the total weight desired. The first step is to determine the actual weights of all the ingredients. The weights (in g) for hydrocortisone, urea, and the paraben–PG stock solution have been calculated previously. The weight of 10 mL of Purified Water used for dissolving the urea is 10 g (which assumes the density of water is 1 g/mL).

Weight of all ingredients:

Weight of hydrocortisone:	0.66 g
Weight of paraben-PG	1.368 g
Weight of urea:	6.6 g
Weight of water:	10. g
Total weight of ingredients:	18.628 g

Weight of Aquabase: 66 g − 18.628 g = 47.372 g

MSDS AND SAFETY AND PERSONAL PROTECTIVE EQUIPMENT: Review MSDS for all components. Don a clean lab coat and disposable gloves.

SPECIALIZED EQUIPMENT: Ointment slab. All weighing is done on an electronic balance.

COMPOUNDING PROCEDURE: Weigh 6.6 g of urea and measure 10 mL of Purified Water in a 10-mL graduated cylinder. Transfer both to a small beaker and stir to dissolve the urea in the water. With a 3-mL syringe, measure 1.32 mL of paraben–PG stock solution and add it to the urea solution. Weigh 47.372 g of Aquabase and 0.66 g of hydrocortisone powder. Place the hydrocortisone powder on an ointment slab and levigate this with a small amount of the Aquabase; then geometrically incorporate the rest of the Aquabase. Form a small "well" in the hydrocortisone-Aquabase and pour a small amount of the urea-paraben solution into the well. Using a spatula, carefully incorporate the urea solution into the ointment, being careful not to lose any of the solution. Continue this process in a stepwise manner until all the urea solution is added and spatulate to obtain a uniform ointment. Tare out the weight of a 2-oz ointment jar and transfer the finished ointment to this container. Note and record the weight of the ointment. Label and dispense.

DESCRIPTION OF FINISHED PREPARATION: The preparation should be a smooth, white, slightly translucent ointment of moderate consistency havng a slight sheen.

QUALITY CONTROL: Check the actual weight of the ointment; it should be within 60 g ± 10% and should be consistent with the theoretical weight of 66 g and the anticipated loss during compounding.

MASTER FORMULA PREPARED BY: B. Bunny, PharmD   **CHECKED BY:** John Dopp, PharmD

COMPOUNDING RECORD

NAME, STRENGTH, AND DOSAGE FORM OF PREPARATION: Hydrocortisone 1% and Urea 10% Topical Ointment
QUANTITY: 60 g (plus 6 g excess)   **DATE PREPARED:** mm/dd/yy   **BEYOND-USE DATE:** mm/dd/yy
FORMULATION RECORD ID: OT002   **CONTROL/RX NUMBER:** 123365

INGREDIENTS USED:

Ingredient	Quantity Used	Manufacturer Lot Number	Expiration Date	Weighed/ Measured by	Checked by
Hydrocortisone	0.66 g	JET Labs SS2821	mm/yy	bjf	bb
Paraben– Propylene Glycol Stock	1.32 mL (1.368 g)	Prac. Pharm. JT4872	mm/yy	bjf	bb
Urea	6.6 g	JET Labs ON3041	mm/yy	bjf	bb
Purified Water	10 mL	Sweet Springs AL0529	mm/yy	bjf	bb
Aquabase	47.372 g	Paddock Labs ON3042	mm/yy	bjf	bb

QUALITY CONTROL DATA: Preparation is a smooth, white, slightly translucent ointment of moderate consistency having a slight sheen. The actual weight was checked and is 62.9 g, which is within the range of ±10% of the prescribed weight of 60 g and consistent with the theoretical weight of 66 g.

LABELING

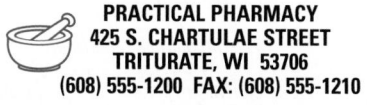

PRACTICAL PHARMACY
425 S. CHARTULAE STREET
TRITURATE, WI 53706
(608) 555-1200 FAX: (608) 555-1210

℞ 123365   Pharmacist: BB   Date: 00/00/00
Rudiger Simpson   Dr. Art Stark
Apply to affected area up to four times a day.
Hydrocortisone 1% and Urea 10% Topical Ointment
Mfg: Compounded   Quantity: 60 g
Refills: 4   Discard after: Give date

Auxiliary Labels: For External Use Only. This medicine was compounded in our pharmacy for you at the direction of your prescriber.

PATIENT CONSULTATION: Hello, Mr. Simpson. I'm your pharmacist, Dr. Bunny. Are you allergic to any drugs? Are you currently using or taking any other medications? What has Dr. Stark told you, or what do you know about, this ointment? This ointment contains the anti-inflammatory drug hydrocortisone plus the softening agent urea in a special ointment base that should reduce the dryness of your skin. Apply this to affected areas four times a day and rub it in well. If the condition doesn't seem to respond to the treatment or if the condition gets worse, contact Dr. Stark or me and we can try another treatment. I understand that you speculate that your surgical gown has caused this dermatitis and that you have already taken steps to get a different brand of garment. I hope that helps. As you know, this ointment is for external use only. It should be stored at room temperature, away from light and heat, and out of the reach of children. Discard any unused portion after 2 weeks (give date). This may be refilled four times. Do you have any questions?

SAMPLE PRESCRIPTION 30.5

CASE: Millie Butler is a 165-lb, 5′8″-tall 45-year-old patient with a 15-year history of plaque psoriasis. In the past, she has had exacerbations treated with a variety of topical emollients, keratolytic agents, and corticosteroids. She currently has some thick, scaly plaques on her hands, arms, and especially her elbows. She has recently earned her realtor's license and has started a new job, and she thinks that the stress of this has been a contributing factor to her current exacerbation. Because she deals daily with customers and thinks the psoriasis is "unslightly," she is especially concerned right now with getting a rapid remission. Dr. Sprague has prescribed the custom formula shown later. The lactic acid and urea are intended to reduce the scaling, particularly the thick lesions on her elbows. He wants to use the moderately potent corticosteroid triamcinolone in an oleaginous ointment base, because this is reported to be more effective in cases of this type (8,9). Pharmacist Wayne Thompson has informed Dr. Sprague that making a smooth ointment with urea requires the addition of a small amount of water, which will give the formulation a slightly creamlike consistency. Dr. Sprague agrees that this is acceptable, and he prefers this to the triamcinolone cream.

CONTEMPORARY PHYSICIANS GROUP PRACTICE
20 S. PARK STREET, TRITURATE, WI 53706
TEL: (608) 555-1333 FAX: (608) 555-1335

℞ # *123321*

NAME *Millie Butler*   **DATE** *00/00/00*

ADDRESS *624 Cottage Grove Rd.*

℞

Urea		*10%*
Lactic Acid		*5%*
Triamcinolone Acetonide		
Ointment 0.1%	*qs ad*	*15 g*

Sig: Apply sparingly to affected area bid for 2 weeks.

W. Thompson 00/00/00

REFILLS *1*   *Conway Sprague*   **M.D.**

DEA NO. _____

MASTER COMPOUNDING FORMULATION RECORD

NAME, STRENGTH, AND DOSAGE FORM OF PREPARATION: Urea 10%, Lactic Acid 5% and Triamcinolone 0.065% Topical Ointment

QUANTITY: 15 g (plus 1.5 g excess)

THERAPEUTIC USE/CATEGORY: Psoriasis

FORMULATION RECORD ID: OT003

ROUTE OF ADMINISTRATION: Topical

INGREDIENTS USED:

Ingredient	Quantity Used	Physical Description	Solubility	Dose Comparison		Use in the Prescription
				Given	Usual	
Urea	1.65 g	white crystalline powder	1 g/1.5 mL water, 10 mL alcohol	10%	5–30%	keratolytic; softens skin
Lactic Acid USP	0.76 mL (0.912 g)	clear, viscous liquid	misc w/ water, alcohol	5%	1–10%	increases hydration of skin
Purified Water	2.5 mL	clear liquid	—	—	—	solvent
Paraben– Propylene Glycol Stock	0.33 mL (0.342 g)	clear liquid	miscible w/ water and alcohol	0.18% MP 0.02% PP 2% PG	0.18% MP 0.02% PP 2% PG	Preservative
Sorbitan Monooleate (Span 80)	330 mg	viscous, amber-colored oily liquid	insol in/water and PG, miscible w/oil	2%	—	emulsifying agent
TCNL oint 0.1%	10.766 g	white, translucent semisolid	immisc w/ water, alcohol	0.065%	0.025–0.5%	topical corticosteroid

COMPATIBILITY–STABILITY: No stability data for this specific preparation is available. Because of the multiple ingredients, evaluation of this formulation is somewhat complex. From the viewpoint of physical compatibility, making a smooth ointment with urea requires the addition of water, but the prescribed oleaginous ointment base does not absorb water. Because the base ointment contains the active ingredient triamcinolone acetonide, a simple base change cannot be made. (Sample Prescription 30.4 is similar, but the base ointment in that preparation did not contain an active ingredient, so the hydrocarbon base could be changed to an absorption base.) Therefore, an emulsifying system must be added to the formulation so the aqueous solution can be incorporated into the triamcinolone acetonide ointment. Span 80 in a concentration of 2% w/w works well for this. In terms of chemical stability, compounded urea topical preparations have been evaluated and reported in the literature but with mixed results. A good review of the subject can be found in *Chemical Stability of Pharmaceuticals* (10). *The Merck Index* reports that 10% solutions of urea in water have a pH of 7.2. The addition of lactic acid to the urea solution will lower the pH, and this is reported to have a pH-stabilizing effect on urea (12). The lactic acid itself is a stable chemical in solution. The stability of the triamcinolone acetonide in this complex preparation is difficult to assess. According to the review of triamcinolone in *Analytical Profiles of Drug Substances*, this drug is very stable as a solid but, in aqueous or alcoholic solutions, it is similar to hydrocortisone and other corticosteroids in that it undergoes complex oxidative rearrangements with decomposition at alkaline pH (13). Although in this preparation the triamcinolone acetonide is not in a water or alcohol environment, it will be in contact with the emulsified droplets of the urea–lactic acid solution. This should have a limited effect, because the pH of the droplets are in a favorable acidic/neutral range and contact will be minimal, so the triamcinolone should be relatively stable in this preparation. Because of the addition of water to this ointment, a preservative must be added; the combination 0.18% methylparaben and 0.02% propylparaben in propylene glycol will be used.

PACKAGING AND STORAGE: Packaging should be in a tight, light-resistant, 1/2-oz ointment jar with recommended storage at controlled room temperature.

BEYOND-USE DATE: Use the *USP*-recommended maximum 14-day beyond-use date for compounded water-containing formulations prepared from ingredients in solid form when there is no stability information for the formulation (6). (Since this is a semisolid, it would also be permissible to use a 30-day beyond-use date recommended in *USP* Chapter ⟨795⟩ for "other formulations," but the expiration date on the triamcinolone acetonide ointment should be checked and the beyond-use date of the compounded preparation may not exceed 25% of the time remaining on the expiration date.)

CALCULATIONS

Dose/Concentration: All concentrations are appropriate for expected use.

Ingredient Amounts

Because this is a rather complex ointment, there is a good chance of material loss in the compounding process. Furthermore, the amount prescribed is relatively small so that even a small loss would mean a significant percent decrease in the amount dispensed. Therefore, prepare 10% excess. The following calculations for 16.5 g of ointment reflect this excess.

Urea (in g): $10\% \times 16.5 \text{ g} = 0.1 \times 16.5 \text{ g} = 1.65 \text{ g}$

Lactic Acid (in g): $5\% \times 16.5 \text{ g} = 0.05 \times 16.5 \text{ g} = 0.825 \text{ g}$

This amount of Lactic Acid is subject to interpretation. Lactic Acid is available as the USP liquid, which is 90% w/w with respect to the chemical lactic acid, and it has a density of 1.20 g/mL. The 0.825 g in this prescription could be interpreted as 0.825 g Lactic Acid USP (the liquid), or 0.825 g of lactic acid as the pure chemical. In either case, it would usually be measured volumetrically, so the 0.825 g should be converted to a volume.

For example:

1. For the 0.825 g of Lactic Acid USP interpretation, calculate the volume to measure as follows:

$$\left(\frac{\text{mL L.A. USP}}{1.20 \text{ g L.A. USP}} \right) \left(\frac{0.825 \text{ g L.A. USP}}{} \right) = 0.69 \text{ mL Lactic Acid USP}$$

2. For the 0.825 g of the pure chemical interpretation, calculate the volume to measure as follows:

$$\left(\frac{\text{mL L.A. USP}}{1.20 \text{ g L.A. USP}} \right) \left(\frac{100 \text{ g L.A. USP}}{90 \text{ g lactic acid}} \right) \left(\frac{0.825 \text{ g lactic acid}}{} \right) = 0.76 \text{ mL Lactic Acid USP}$$

Note: Another interpretation is also possible. Since Lactic Acid USP is a liquid, the original calculation could also be: $5\% \times 16.5 \text{ g} = 0.825 \text{ mL}$, in which case 0.825 mL of Lactic Acid USP would be measured.

Fortunately for this situation, the amounts are all close, and this is not a potent drug that requires a precise quantity. Dr. Sprague was consulted, and it was decided that interpretation 2, 0.825 g of the pure lactic acid chemical, would be used, with a volume of 0.76 mL of Lactic Acid USP. This volume can be measured in a 1-mL syringe. The weight of this volume of Lactic Acid USP is as follows:

$$1.20 \text{ g/mL} \times 0.76 \text{ mL} = 0.912 \text{ g}$$

As stated in Sample Prescription 30.4, because urea is difficult to pulverize, it is usually dissolved first in water and the solution is incorporated. The solubility of urea is 1 g/1.5 mL. The amount of water required to dissolve the urea can be calculated:

$$\left(\frac{1.5 \text{ mL water}}{1 \text{ g urea}} \right) \left(\frac{1.65 \text{ g urea}}{} \right) = 2.5 \text{ mL water}$$

This addition of water means that a preservative should be added. As shown in Sample Prescription 30.4, Practical Pharmacy uses the stock solution (described in Chapter 16, Antimicrobial Preservatives) containing methylparaben and propylparaben in propylene glycol:

Methylparaben (MP)		9 g
Propylparaben (PP)		1 g
Propylene Glycol (PG)	qs ad	100 mL

A volume of 2 mL of this solution per 100 g of preparation provides the recommended 0.18% MP and 0.02% PP with approximately 2% PG. For our 16.5 g of ointment, the volume needed is calculated as follows:

$$\frac{2 \text{ mL stock soln}}{100 \text{ g ointment}} = \frac{x \text{ mL stock soln}}{16.5 \text{ g ointment}} \; ; x = 0.33 \text{ mL stock solution}$$

That this volume gives the correct percent concentration of preservative is verified by calculation. For example, for MP:

$$\left(\frac{9 \text{ g MP}}{100 \text{ mL stock}} \right) \left(\frac{0.33 \text{ mL stock}}{} \right) = 0.030 \text{ g MP}$$

$$\frac{0.030 \text{ g MP}}{16.5 \text{ g ointment}} = \frac{x \text{ g MP}}{100 \text{ g ointment}} \; ; x = 0.18 \text{ g MP}/100 \text{ g} = 0.18\%$$

The weight of this stock solution must be calculated to determine the weight of triamcinolone acetonide ointment needed to qs ad 16.5 g of ointment. Propylene glycol has a specific gravity of 1.036. Because the small powder volume of the parabens is insignificant, you may use this as the specific gravity of the stock solution. Calculate the weight of 0.33 mL of the stock solution:

$$\left(\frac{1.036 \text{ g stock soln}}{\text{mL stock soln}} \right) \left(\frac{0.33 \text{ mL stock soln}}{} \right) = 0.342 \text{ g stock soln}$$

As discussed earlier, an emulsifying system must be added to enable the aqueous solutions to be incorporated into the triamcinolone acetonide ointment. Span 80 in a concentration of 2% w/w will be used. The weight (in g) of Span 80 needed is calculated:

$$2\% \times 16.5 \text{ g} = 0.02 \times 16.5 = 0.33 \text{ g}$$

To determine the amount of triamcinolone acetonide ointment needed, add the weights of all ingredients (including the water and emulsifying agent) and subtract this from the final desired ointment weight.

Urea	1.65 g
Water to dissolve the urea	2.5 g
Lactic Acid USP	0.912 g
PG–paraben solution	0.342 g
Span 80	0.33 g
Total ingredient weight:	5.734 g

Weight of triamcinolone acetonide 0.1% Ointment: 16.5 g − 5.734 g = 10.766 g

Weight (in g) of triamcinolone acetonide (T.A.) in final ointment:

$$0.1\% \text{ T.A.} \times 10.766 \text{ g} = 0.001 \text{ T.A.} \times 10.766 \text{ g} = 0.0108 \text{ g T.A.}$$

Final % w/w of triamcinolone acetonide in the final preparation:

$$\frac{0.0108 \text{ g T. A.}}{16.5 \text{ g oint.}} = \frac{x \text{ g T. A.}}{100 \text{ g oint.}} \; ; x = 0.065 \text{ g}/100 \text{ g} = 0.065\%$$

MSDS AND SAFETY AND PERSONAL PROTECTIVE EQUIPMENT: Review MSDS for all components. Don a clean lab coat and disposable gloves.

SPECIALIZED EQUIPMENT: All weighing is done on an electronic balance.

COMPOUNDING PROCEDURE: Weigh 1.65 g of urea and dissolve it in 2.5 mL of Purified Water in a beaker. Using 1-mL syringes, measure 0.76 mL of Lactic Acid USP and 0.33 mL of the propylene glycol–paraben stock solution. Add these to the urea solution. Weigh 330 mg of Span 80 and 10.766 g of triamcinolone 0.1% ointment. On an ointment slab, first incorporate the Span into the triamcinolone ointment, then incorporate the urea–lactic acid–paraben solution, levigating well with each addition to ensure uniform mixing and absorption of the solution by the base. Tare a ½-oz ointment jar and transfer the ointment to this container; note and record the weight of the ointment. Label and dispense.

DESCRIPTION OF FINISHED PREPARATION: Preparation is a smooth, whitish, slightly translucent ointment having a soft consistency and moderate sheen.

QUALITY CONTROL: Check the actual weight. It should be within the range of ±10% of the prescribed weight of 15 g, and the loss of material from the theoretical weight of 16.5 g should be reasonable.

MASTER FORMULA PREPARED BY: Wayne Thompson, PharmD   **CHECKED BY:** John Dopp, PharmD

COMPOUNDING RECORD

NAME, STRENGTH, AND DOSAGE FORM OF PREPARATION: Urea 10%, Lactic Acid 5%, and Triamcinolone Acetonide 0.065% Topical Ointment

QUANTITY: 15 g (plus 1.5 g excess)   **DATE PREPARED:** mm/dd/yy   **BEYOND-USE DATE:** mm/dd/yy

FORMULATION RECORD ID: OT003   **CONTROL/RX NUMBER:** 123321

INGREDIENTS USED:

Ingredient	Quantity Used	Manufacturer Lot Number	Expiration Date	Weighed/ Measured by	Checked by
Urea	1.65 g	JET Labs ON3041	mm/yy	bjf	wt
Lactic Acid USP	0.76 mL (0.912 g)	JET Labs SN2672	mm/yy	bjf	wt
Purified Water	2.5 mL	Sweet Springs AL0529	mm/yy	bjf	wt
Paraben– Propylene Glycol Stock	0.33 mL (0.342 g)	Prac. Pharm. JT4872	mm/yy	bjf`	wt
Sorbitan Monooleate (Span 80)	330 mg	JET Labs ON3042	mm/yy	bjf	wt
TCNL oint 0.1%	10.766 g	BJF Generics JF4985	mm/yy	bjf	wt

QUALITY CONTROL DATA: Preparation is a smooth, whitish, slightly translucent ointment having a soft consistency and moderate sheen. The actual weight is checked and is 14.9 g, which is an expected loss of material from the theoretical weight of 16.5 g. It is within the range of ±10% of the prescribed weight of 15 g.

LABELING

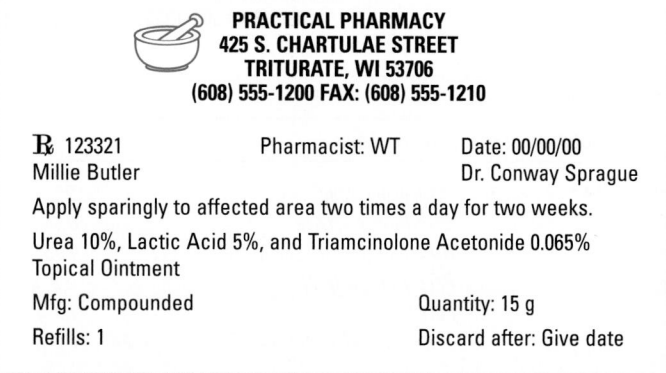

PRACTICAL PHARMACY
425 S. CHARTULAE STREET
TRITURATE, WI 53706
(608) 555-1200 FAX: (608) 555-1210

℞ 123321   Pharmacist: WT   Date: 00/00/00
Millie Butler   Dr. Conway Sprague

Apply sparingly to affected area two times a day for two weeks.

Urea 10%, Lactic Acid 5%, and Triamcinolone Acetonide 0.065%
Topical Ointment

Mfg: Compounded   Quantity: 15 g

Refills: 1   Discard after: Give date

Auxiliary Labels: For External Use Only. This medicine was compounded in
our pharmacy for you at the direction of your prescriber.

PATIENT CONSULTATION: Hello Ms. Butler. I'm Wayne Thompson, your pharmacist. Do you have any drug allergies? Are you taking or using any nonprescription or prescription medications? What has Dr. Sprague told you about this prescription? I know that you have previously used some similar medications for your psoriasis. This ointment contains triamcinolone, a more potent steroid ingredient than you have used before, and that is why the directions say to apply this sparingly. This is a custom formula that was made in our pharmacy, and it also contains lactic acid and urea, agents to help remove the scale and plaque, and it should soften and moisturize your skin. You are to apply this in a thin layer to the affected area two times a day for 2 weeks. At that time, Dr. Sprague wants to see you and re-evaluate your condition. If the condition gets worse, or if you don't seem to be getting any relief, contact Dr. Sprague. You should store this at room temperature, out of the reach of children. This may be refilled one time. Discard any unused portion after 2 weeks (give date). Do you have any questions?

SAMPLE PRESCRIPTION 30.6

CASE: Jeff Diaz is a 145-lb, 5'11″-tall 21-year-old college student with red, flaking, greasy areas on his face and scalp and with some pruritus. He is very self-conscious about this condition, feels it is affecting his self-confidence and social life, and just wants it to go away. He is hoping that Dr. Dacy can treat this with some kind of medication that will be inconspicuous on his face and hair. Dr. Dacy has diagnosed seborrheic dermatitis (SD) and has prescribed selenium sulfide 2.5% shampoo to be used daily until the SD on Jeff's scalp is under control, followed by regular use of the shampoo several times a week to maintain remission of symptoms. Dr. Dacy asked Pharmacist Juan Valdez to formulate a hydrocortisone 2% gel that will be unnoticeable when applied to the lesions on Mr. Diaz's face and scalp. Dr. Valdez has suggested the formulation on the prescription order shown. It should clear the lesions in 1 to 2 weeks. If the condition is not in remission by that time, Dr. Dacy wants to see Mr. Diaz for follow-up and possible treatment with topical tacrolimus.

CONTEMPORARY PHYSICIANS GROUP PRACTICE
20 S. PARK STREET, TRITURATE, WI 53706
TEL: (608) 555-1333 FAX: (608) 555-1335

R # *123712*

NAME *Jeff Diaz*   DATE *00/00/00*

ADDRESS *2396 Rosario Lane*

R

Hydrocortisone	2%
Disodium edetate	0.1%
Hydroxypropyl Cellulose	1.05 g
Propylene Glycol	2.5 g
Polysorbate 80	1.3 g
Isopropyl Alcohol 70% qs ad	60 g

Juan Valdez 00/00/00

Sig: Apply to affected areas on face and scalp 2 times daily ut dict

REFILLS *1*   *Marcy Dacy*   M.D.

DEA NO. _____

MASTER COMPOUNDING FORMULATION RECORD

NAME, STRENGTH, AND DOSAGE FORM OF PREPARATION: Hydrocortisone 2% Topical Gel
QUANTITY: 60 g   **FORMULATION RECORD ID:** OT004
THERAPEUTIC USE/CATEGORY: Anti-inflammatory   **ROUTE OF ADMINISTRATION:** Topical

INGREDIENTS USED:

Ingredient	Quantity Used	Physical Description	Solubility	Dose Comparison		Use in the Prescription
				Given	Usual	
Hydrocortisone	1.2 g	white powder	v sl sol in water; 1 g/40 mL alcohol	2%	0.5–2.5%	anti-inflammatory, antipruritic
Hydroxypropyl Cellulose	1.05 g	white granular powder	sol in water and alcohol	—	—	suspending agent
Propylene Glycol	2.5 g (2.4 mL)	clear, colorless liquid	misc with water and alcohol	—	—	solvent, preservative, humectant
Polysorbate 80	1.3 g	light yellow, viscous, oily liquid	v sol in water and alcohol	—	—	wetting and dispersing agent
Disodium Edetate (as dihydrate)	60 mg (66 mg)	white crystalline powder	sol in water; sl sol in alcohol	0.1% w/w	0.1% w/w/	chelating agent
Isopropyl Alcohol (IPA) 70%	61.2 mL	clear, colorless mobile liquid	miscible with water	56% w/w IPA	—	antiseptic and vehicle

COMPATIBILITY–STABILITY: No stability data for this specific formulation is available. The formulation was patterned after a Piroxicam gel formulation in the *International Journal of Pharmaceutical Compounding* (14). The stability of hydrocortisone in preparations such as these is not easy to predict. Hydrocortisone undergoes oxidation and other complex degradation reactions in aqueous solutions. It is most stable at pH 3.5 to 4.5, and its stability is quite dependent on pH, with steep slopes for its pH profile in both the acidic and basic regions (11). Aqueous solutions of hydroxypropyl cellulose are neutral, with a pH in the range of 5 to 8.5. Trace metals are reported to catalyze degradation reactions for hydrocortisone, and chelating agents such as disodium edetate offer some protection (11); therefore, 0.1% disodium edetate is added to this formulation. No additional preservative is needed because of the high content of isopropyl alcohol in the formula.

PACKAGING AND STORAGE: Packaging should be in a tight, light-resistant container, with recommended storage at controlled room temperature.

BEYOND-USE DATE: Use the *USP*-recommended maximum 14-day beyond-use date for compounded water-containing liquid formulations prepared from ingredients in solid form when there is no stability information for the formulation (6).

CALCULATIONS

Dose/Concentration

Hydrocortisone: The 2% concentration is appropriate for the use.

Isopropyl alcohol: Any preparation containing either ethyl or isopropyl alcohol should have the final percent concentration of the alcohol specified on the prescription label. Although this would seem to be simple enough, when a semisolid dosage form is involved, we are dealing with conflicting formats for expressing concentration. The prototype for expressing alcohol concentration in liquid preparations is given for ethanol in the General Notices of the *USP*. This is discussed with numerous examples in section V of Chapter 8. Basically, the standard for alcohol in liquid preparations is a v/v% of the pure alcohol in the preparation. Juxtaposed with this standard are the General Notices standards for expressing percent concentrations, which give w/w% for mixtures of solids and semisolids, w/v% for solids in liquids, and v/v% for liquids in liquids. Unfortunately, we have no direction for percent concentration of liquids in semisolids. Obviously we would want to select a format that is most meaningful.

According to the *USP* monographs, pure IPA has a s.g. of 0.78; 70% IPA is a 70% v/v solution of IPA in water with a s.g. of 0.88. As can be seen from the calculations in the ingredient amounts section (see later), the 60-g preparation contains 53.88 g or 61.2 mL of 70% IPA. Using these numbers, we can calculate a final percent concentration in one of the following ways:

1. w/w% of the 70% IPA solution in the preparation:

$$\frac{53.9\text{ g }70\%\text{ IPA}}{60\text{ g ointment}} = \frac{x\text{ g }70\%\text{ IPA}}{100\text{ g}}; \ x = 89.8\% \approx 90\%$$

2. v/w% of the 70% IPA solution in the preparation:

$$\frac{61.2\text{ mL }70\%\text{ IPA}}{60\text{ g ointment}} = \frac{x\text{ mL }70\%\text{ IPA}}{100\text{ g}}; \ x = 102\%$$

Note that a percent greater than 100% is an anomaly that results from using a v/w% and the fact that 70% IPA has a density less than 1.0.

3. w/w% of pure IPA in the preparation:

$$\left(\frac{70\text{ mL IPA}}{100\text{ mL }70\%\text{ IPA}}\right)\left(\frac{61.2\text{ mL }70\%\text{ IPA}}{}\right) = 42.8\text{ mL pure IPA}$$

$$\left(\frac{0.78\text{ g IPA}}{\text{mL IPA}}\right)\left(\frac{42.8\text{ mL IPA}}{}\right) = 33.4\text{ g IPA}$$

$$\frac{33.4\text{ g IPA}}{60\text{ g ointment}} = \frac{x\text{ g IPA}}{100\text{ g}}; \ x = 55.7\%$$

4. v/w% of pure IPA in the preparation:

$$\left(\frac{70 \text{ mL IPA}}{100 \text{ mL 70\% IPA}}\right)\left(\frac{61.2 \text{ mL 70\% IPA}}{}\right) = 42.8 \text{ mL pure IPA}$$

$$\frac{42.8 \text{ mL IPA}}{60 \text{ g ointment}} = \frac{x \text{ mL IPA}}{100 \text{ g}}; \ x = 71.3\%$$

It is apparent that the numbers vary considerably from approximately 56% to 102%. Methods 1 and 4 (although, by definition, there is no such thing as a v/w%) are probably most commonly used by pharmacists. For a semisolid preparation, method 3 may be the most correct method, but it is also the most laborious to calculate.

Ingredient Amounts

No excess was calculated for this preparation, but excess could be made if desired.

Hydrocortisone (in g):	$2\% \times 60 \text{ g} = 0.02 \times 60 \text{ g} = 1.2 \text{ g}$
Disodium edetate (in g):	$0.1\% \times 60 \text{ g} = 0.001 \times 60 \text{ g} = 0.06 \text{ g}$

Disodium edetate is available as the dihydrate. The equivalent quantity can be calculated using the molecular weights of the base compound (336.2) and the dihydrate (372.24):

$$\frac{60 \text{ mg Na}_2\text{edetate}}{336.2 \text{ mg Na}_2\text{edetate}} = \frac{x \text{ mg Na}_2\text{edetate dihydrate}}{372.24 \text{ mg Na}_2\text{edetate dihydrate}}; \ x = 66 \text{ mg Na}_2\text{edetate dihydrate}$$

Propylene glycol (PG): The amount given in the prescription order is in grams, but this is usually measured in volume. The volume can be calculated using the specific gravity of the PG. s.g. = 1.036.

$$\left(\frac{\text{mL PG}}{1.036 \text{ g PG}}\right)\left(\frac{2.5 \text{ g PG}}{}\right) = 2.4 \text{ mL propylene glycol}$$

The hydroxypropyl cellulose and the polysorbate 80 are given in grams and are weighed.

To determine the amount of 70% IPA needed, add the weights of all ingredients and subtract this from the final desired gel weight:

Hydrocortisone	1.2 g
Na$_2$ edetate dihydrate	0.066 g
Propylene Glycol	2.5 g
Hydroxypropyl Cellulose	1.05 g
Polysorbate 80 (Tween 80)	<u>1.3 g</u>
Total ingredient weight:	6.116 g

Weight of 70% IPA: 60 g − 6.116 g = 53.88 g

Isopropyl alcohol 70% has a specific gravity = 0.88. The volume of 70% IPA to measure can be calculated:

$$\left(\frac{\text{mL 70\% IPA}}{0.88 \text{ g 70\% IPA}}\right)\left(\frac{53.88 \text{ g 70\% IPA}}{}\right) = 61.2 \text{ mL 70\% IPA}$$

MSDS AND SAFETY AND PERSONAL PROTECTIVE EQUIPMENT: Review MSDS for all components. Don a clean lab coat and disposable gloves. Avoid inhaling powders.

SPECIALIZED EQUIPMENT: Glass mortar. All weighing is done on an electronic balance.

COMPOUNDING PROCEDURE: Weigh 1.05 g of hydroxypropyl cellulose and sprinkle in portions over 61.2 mL of 70% IPA, allowing each portion to become thoroughly wetted without stirring. Once the powder is wetted, stir gently. Allow this to sit overnight (at least 8 to 10 hours), stirring occasionally. Weigh 1.2 g of hydrocortisone and place in a glass mortar. Measure 2.4 mL of PG and weigh 1.3 g of polysorbate 80 and 66 mg of disodium edetate dihydrate. Add these with trituration to the hydrocortisone. Slowly, with trituration, add the hydroxypropyl cellulose gel to the mortar. Triturate well to a uniform consistency. Tare the weight of a 2-oz ointment jar and transfer the gel to this container. Note and record the weight of the preparation. Label and dispense.

DESCRIPTION OF FINISHED PREPARATION: Preparation is a colorless to slightly whitish transparent gel with a soft consistency.

QUALITY CONTROL: Check the actual weight of the preparation; it should be within the range of ±10% of the prescribed weight of 60 g, which in this case is also the theoretical weight.

MASTER FORMULA PREPARED BY: Juan Valdez, PharmD   **CHECKED BY:** Anna Legreid Dopp, Pharm D

COMPOUNDING RECORD

NAME, STRENGTH, AND DOSAGE FORM OF PREPARATION: Hydrocortisone 2% Topical Gel
QUANTITY: 60 g   Date Prepared: mm/dd/yy   **BEYOND-USE DATE:** mm/dd/yy
FORMULATION RECORD ID: OT004   **CONTROL/RX NUMBER:** 123712

INGREDIENTS USED:

Ingredient	Quantity Used	Manufacturer Lot Number	Expiration Date	Measured/ Weighed by	Checked by
Hydrocortisone	1.2 g	JET Labs SS2821	mm/yy	bjf	jv
Hydroxypropyl -cellulose	1.05 g	JET Labs ON3071	mm/yy	bjf	jv
Propylene Glycol	2.5 g (2.4 mL)	JET Labs SN2662	mm/yy	bjf	jv
Polysorbate 80	1.3 g	JET Labs ON3032	mm/yy	bjf	jvs
Disodium Edetate (as dihydrate)	60 mg (66 mg)	JET Labs ON6874	mm/yy	bjf	jv
Isopropyl Alcohol 70%	61.3 mL	JET Labs SS2824	mm/yy	bjf	jv

QUALITY CONTROL DATA: Preparation is a colorless to slightly whitish transparent gel with a soft consistency. The actual weight is checked and is 59.1 g, which is an expected loss of material from the theoretical weight of 60 g and is within ±10% of the prescribed weight of 60 g.

LABELING

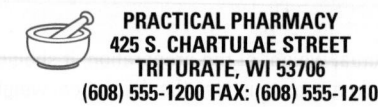

PRACTICAL PHARMACY
425 S. CHARTULAE STREET
TRITURATE, WI 53706
(608) 555-1200 FAX: (608) 555-1210

℞ 123712   Pharmacist: JV   Date: 00/00/00
Jeff Diaz   Dr. Marcy Dacy

Apply to affected areas on face and scalp two times a day as directed.

Hydrocortisone 2% Topical Gel; Contains Isopropyl Alcohol 56% w/w

Mfg: Compounded   Quantity: 60 g

Refills: 1   Discard after: Give date

Auxiliary Labels: Caution. Flammable. For External Use Only. Keep out of the reach of children. This medicine was compounded in our pharmacy for you at the direction of your prescriber.

PATIENT CONSULTATION: Hello, Mr. Diaz. I'm your pharmacist, Juan Valdez. Are you currently using any other medications? Are you allergic to any drugs? What has Dr. Dacy told you about this medication? This is a hydrocortisone gel that has been custom made for you to treat the seborrheic dermatitis on your face and scalp. Apply it to the affected areas two times daily as directed by Dr. Dacy. It is a clear gel and is not greasy so you should be able to use it during the day without it being noticeable. Because it contains isopropyl alcohol, it may sting. If your condition seems to be showing no improvement or seems to be getting worse, contact Dr. Dacy. Keep the container tightly closed, in a cool dry place. This is in a nonsafety container so be sure to keep it out of the reach of children. Because of the high alcohol content, it is flammable, so do not use it around any flame or lighted smoking material. Discard any unused portion after 2 weeks. This prescription has one refill, but Dr. Dacy indicated that she would like to see you in 2 weeks if the condition has not cleared. She has also prescribed a shampoo for you, and I have that ready also. Do you have any questions?

SAMPLE PRESCRIPTION 30.7

CASE: Lacey Bindl is a 115-lb, 5′4″-tall, 18-year-old high school senior. She is seeing Dr. Tacky for sunburn that she sustained using a local tanning salon. She has been anticipating her senior trip to Cancun, Mexico, and wanted to get a base tan before leaving on the trip. She is blond with fair skin and reports that she has had problems in the past with sunburn. Unfortunately, Lacey overused the tanning booth. She has erythema but no blistering. She reports that the burning is especially painful on her face, her neck and upper chest area, and the anterior surfaces of her arms. She would like something to relieve the burning and assist the sunburn in healing as rapidly as possible, but she doesn't want anything that will look "greasy" when she is at school. Dr. Tacky has prescribed a combination local anesthetic–antihistamine gel for the pain and inflammation. She is to use this three times a day as needed during the school day. At night and as often as possible during the day, Dr. Tacky has advised her to apply A&D ointment; although it may look greasy on her skin, it will help to rehydrate and heal the damaged skin. Dr. Tacky has told her to apply the prescribed gel sparingly because there have been some serious and even fatal accidents when patients have overused products like this. She should stay away from the tanning salon and use a good sunscreen, at least SPF 30, when she goes to Cancun. Dr. Tacky says that the pharmacist at Practical Pharmacy can advise her on a sunscreen product that will be effective.

CONTEMPORARY PHYSICIANS GROUP PRACTICE
20 S. PARK STREET, TRITURATE, WI 53706
TEL: (608) 555-1333 FAX: (608) 555-1335

℞ #   *123383*

NAME   *Lacey Bindl*   DATE   *00/00/00*

ADDRESS   *256 River Valley Lane*

℞   *Lidocaine HCl*   *600 mg*

         Diphenhydramine HCl   *300 mg*

         Poloxamer Lecithin Organogel   *q s ad*   *30 g*

                                                    C. Kraemer 00/00/00

                    Sig: Apply to affected areas tid prn sunburn

REFILLS   *4*

                                        Louise Tacky   M.D.

                        DEA NO.   _____

MASTER COMPOUNDING FORMULATION RECORD

NAME, STRENGTH, AND DOSAGE FORM OF PREPARATION: Lidocaine HCl 2% and Diphenhydramine HCl 1% Topical Gel
QUANTITY: 30 g (plus 3 g excess)   **FORMULATION RECORD ID:** OT005
THERAPEUTIC USE/CATEGORY: Anesthetic/Antihistamine   **ROUTE OF ADMINISTRATION:** Topical

INGREDIENTS USED:

Ingredient	Quantity Used	Physical Description	Solubility	Dose Comparison		Use in the Prescription
				Given	Usual	
Lidocaine HCl	660 mg	white powder	v sol in water and alcohol	2%	1–5%	local anesthetic
Diphenhydramine HCL	330 mg	white crystalline powder	1g/mL water or 2 mL alcohol	1%	1–2%	antihistamine
Lecithin/ Isopropyl palmitate	6.4 g	thick yellow liquid	dispersible in water	—	—	penetration enhancer, emollient, emulsifier
Poloxamer Gel 20%	25.6 g	clear liquid at cold temp; viscous gel at RT	misc with water and alcohol	—	—	vehicle

COMPATIBILITY–STABILITY: No stability data for this specific preparation are available. This formulation was patterned after a similar gel formulation in the *International Journal of Pharmaceutical Compounding* (15) but, while both formulations contain lidocaine, the prescribed preparation contains diphenhydramine HCl, and it does not include ketoprofen and cyclobenzaprine. Furthermore, that article states that no stability studies have been performed. Both diphenhydramine HCl and lidocaine HCl are available in manufactured aqueous and alcoholic solutions and are reported to be quite stable (16,17). No additional preservative is needed because this formulation uses commercial brands of lecithin–isopropyl palmitate solution (LIPS) and poloxamer 20% gel; both are preserved with sorbic acid and parabens. (See section IV. C in Chapter 19, Viscosity-Inducing Agents, for a more complete description.)

PACKAGING AND STORAGE: Packaging should be in a tight, light-resistant container, with recommended storage at controlled room temperature.

BEYOND-USE DATE: Use the *USP*-recommended maximum 14-day beyond-use date for compounded water-containing formulations prepared from ingredients in solid form when there is no stability information for the formulation (6).

CALCULATIONS

Dose/Concentration

Lidocaine HCl: w/w% is calculated as follows:

$$\frac{0.6 \text{ g lidocaine HCl}}{30 \text{ g gel}} = \frac{x \text{ g lidocaine HCl}}{100 \text{ g gel}}; \ x = 2 \text{ g}/100 \text{ g} = 2\%$$

Diphenhydramine HCl (DPH): w/w% is calculated as follows:

$$\frac{0.3 \text{ g DPH}}{30 \text{ g gel}} = \frac{x \text{ g DPH}}{100 \text{ g gel}}; \ x = 1 \text{ g}/100 \text{ g} = 1\%$$

These concentrations are appropriate for the intended use.

Ingredient Amounts

Prepare 3 g excess to compensate for loss on compounding.

Lidocaine HCl (in g) for 33 g of gel is calculated to be:

$$\frac{0.6 \text{ g lidocaine}}{30 \text{ g gel}} = \frac{x \text{ g lidocaine}}{33 \text{ g gel}}; \ x = 0.66 \text{ g lidocaine}$$

Diphenhydramine HCl (in g) for 33 g of gel is calculated to be:

$$\frac{0.3 \text{ g DPH}}{30 \text{ g gel}} = \frac{x \text{ g DPH}}{33 \text{ g gel}}; \ x = 0.33 \text{ g DPH}$$

Poloxamer lecithin organogel (PLO) can be made from the individual ingredients, or the 20% poloxamer gel and the combined lecithin–isopropyl palmitate solution may be purchased. These two liquids are then mixed together in a ratio of four parts of the poloxamer gel with one part of the LIPS. For this formulation, the purchased prepared gel and LIPS are used.

First, the weight (in g) of the PLO is calculated by subtracting the weight of all the other ingredients from the total preparation weight of 33 g:

$$33 \text{ g} - (0.33 \text{ g DPH} + 0.66 \text{ g lidocaine HCl}) = 33 \text{ g} - 0.99 \text{ g} = 32.01 \text{ g} = 32 \text{ g}$$

Second, using the ratio of four parts to one part for a total of five parts, calculate the weight (in g) of poloxamer gel 20% and of LIPS:

$$\frac{1 \text{ part LIPS}}{5 \text{ parts organogel}} = \frac{x \text{ g LIPS}}{32 \text{ g organogel}}; \ x = 6.4 \text{ g LIPS}$$

$$\frac{4 \text{ parts polox. 20\% gel}}{5 \text{ parts organogel}} = \frac{x \text{ g polox. 20\% gel}}{32 \text{ g organogel}}; \ x = 25.6 \text{ g poloxamer 20\% gel}$$

[If made from the individual ingredients, the 20% w/v poloxamer gel is made from poloxamer 407 (Pluronic F 127) as described in Chapter 19. This requires overnight storage in a refrigerator for the clear gel to form. The LIPS is made by adding 10 g of soya lecithin to 10 g of isopropyl palmitate and allowing the mixture to set overnight. Neither preparation is difficult to make, but both have to be made ahead of time because they require setting overnight. Furthermore, the manufactured solutions come already buffered and preserved but, if the solutions are made in the pharmacy, a preservative system and possibly a buffer must be added.]

MSDS AND SAFETY AND PERSONAL PROTECTIVE EQUIPMENT: Review MSDS for all components. Don a clean lab coat and disposable gloves. Avoid inhaling powders.

SPECIALIZED EQUIPMENT: Glass mortar. All weighing is done on an electronic balance.

COMPOUNDING PROCEDURE: Weigh 660 mg of lidocaine HCl and 330 mg of diphenhydramine HCl and place in a glass mortar. Triturate the powders to mix. Tare a small beaker and weigh 6.4 g of the LIPS and, in another tared beaker, weigh 25.6 g of poloxamer gel 20%. Add the LIPS to the poloxamer gel and stir to mix until a uniform gel is obtained. Slowly add a small portion of this to the powders in the mortar to make a smooth paste. Using trituration, continue to slowly add the PLO mixture until it is all blended together and you have obtained a uniform gel. Tare a 1-oz ointment jar and transfer the gel to this container; note and record the weight of the gel. Label and dispense.

DESCRIPTION OF FINISHED PREPARATION: Preparation is a cream-colored translucent gel. It is a viscous liquid when refrigerated but is more gel-like in consistency when at room temperature.

QUALITY CONTROL: Check the actual weight; it should be within the range of $\pm 10\%$ of the prescribed weight of 30 g, with a reasonable expected loss of material from the theoretical weight of 33 g.

MASTER FORMULA PREPARED BY: Chelsea Kraemer, RPh   **CHECKED BY:** Anna Legreid Dopp, PharmD

COMPOUNDING RECORD

NAME, STRENGTH, AND DOSAGE FORM OF PREPARATION: Lidocaine HCl 2% and Diphenhydramine HCl 1% Topical Gel
QUANTITY: 30 g (plus 3 g excess)   **DATE PREPARED:** mm/dd/yy   **BEYOND-USE DATE:** mm/dd/yy
FORMULATION RECORD ID: OT005   **CONTROL/RX NUMBER:** 123383

INGREDIENTS USED:

Ingredient	Quantity Used	Manufacturer Lot Number	Expiration Date	Weighed/ Measured by	Checked by
Lidocaine HCl	660 mg	JET Labs ON3081	mm/yy	bjf	ck
Diphenhydramine HCL	330 mg	JET Labs ON3082	mm/yy	bjf	ck
Lecithin/Isopropyl palmitate	6.4 g	JET Labs ON3083	mm/yy	bjf	ck
Poloxamer Gel 20%	25.6 g	JET Labs ON3084	mm/yy	bjf	ck

QUALITY CONTROL DATA: Preparation is a cream-colored translucent gel. It is a viscous liquid when refrigerated but is more gel-like in consistency when at room temperature. The actual weight is checked and is 30.9 g, which is an expected loss of material from the theoretical weight of 33 g, and is within the range of $\pm 10\%$ of the prescribed weight of 30 g.

LABELING

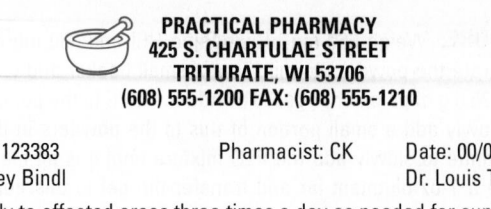

PRACTICAL PHARMACY
425 S. CHARTULAE STREET
TRITURATE, WI 53706
(608) 555-1200 FAX: (608) 555-1210

℞ 123383   Pharmacist: CK   Date: 00/00/00
Lacey Bindl   Dr. Louis Tacky

Apply to affected areas three times a day as needed for sunburn.

Lidocaine HCl 2% and Diphenhydramine HCl 1% Topical Gel

Mfg: Compounded   Quantity: 30 g

Refills: 4   Discard after: Give date

Auxiliary Label: For External Use Only. This medicine was compounded in our pharmacy for you at the direction of your prescriber.

PATIENT CONSULTATION: Hello, Lacey. I'm Chelsey Kraemer, your pharmacist. Do you have any drug allergies? Are you using any OTC or prescription medications? What has Dr. Tacky told you about the use of this gel? This is a custom formula containing the local anesthetic lidocaine and antihistamine diphenhydramine that should give you both relief of the burning and healing of your sunburn. You are to apply the gel sparingly three times daily as needed to the affected areas. If you don't seem to be getting any relief, contact Dr. Tacky. This is for external use only. You may store this at room temperature, but it is thinner and may apply better if it has been refrigerated. This gel has the unique property of being a liquid when at cool temperature, but it firms up when it is applied to a warm skin surface. This means that it stays in place on the applied skin area. Keep this out of the reach of children. This may be refilled four times. You should discard any unused portion after 2 weeks. Dr. Tacky also indicated that you should use A&D ointment at night and other times when convenient to help in the healing process and to moisturize your skin. I can help you with that if you like. Also, if you need some suggestions for a sunscreen product before leaving for Cancun, let me know and I can help you pick something out. You will want something that gives good protection from both UVA and UVB light and an SPF of at least 30. Do you have any questions?

SAMPLE PRESCRIPTION 30.8

CASE: Bobby Armstrong is a 98-lb, 5'-tall, 13-year-old middle schooler. He recently has noticed some warts on his right hand, and he is of that age when he is quite self-conscious about such things. However, he is afraid to have them removed with cryotherapy. Dr. Nock has told Bobby that he has a special wart remover liquid that is pain-free and that works really well. Dr. Nock has prescribed the formulation shown and has told Bobby that he should see improvement in a week or two, but it could take up to several months for complete removal so Bobby may need a little patience. Dr. Nock did warn Bobby that warts are contagious and can be spread to other areas of his own body or to others, so Bobby should avoid touching the warts unnecessarily and should wash his hands if he does touch them. He should also use single-use towels or a hand dryer at school and a separate towel just for drying those areas at home.

CONTEMPORARY PHYSICIANS GROUP PRACTICE
20 S. PARK STREET, TRITURATE, WI 53706
EL: (608) 555-1333 FAX: (608) 555-1335

R # 123745

NAME *Bobby Armstrong*   DATE *00/00/00*

ADDRESS *689 Spartan Circle*

R

Acetic Acid		*5%*
Lactic Acid		
Salicylic Acid	*aa*	*10%*
Flexible Collodion qs ad		*30 mL*

Hank Hound 00/00/00

Sig: *Apply to warts on your right hand daily at bedtime until resolved*

REFILLS *1*   *Ralph Nock*   M.D.

DEA NO. _____

MASTER COMPOUNDING FORMULATION RECORD

NAME, STRENGTH, AND DOSAGE FORM OF PREPARATION: Acetic Acid 5%, Lactic Acid 10%, and Salicylic Acid 10% Topical Collodion

QUANTITY: 30 mL

THERAPEUTIC USE/CATEGORY: Wart remover

FORMULATION RECORD ID: OT006

ROUTE OF ADMINISTRATION: Topical

INGREDIENTS USED:

Ingredient	Quantity Used	Physcial Description	Solubility	Dose Comparison		Use in the Prescription
				Given	Usual	
Acetic Acid (as Glacial Acetic Acid)	1.5 g (1.4 mL)	viscous, clear, colorless liquid	miscible with water and alcohol	5% (w/v)	2–100%	caustic, keratolytic
Lactic (as Lactic Acid USP)	3 g (2.8 mL)	viscous, clear, colorless liquid	miscible with water and alcohol	10% (w/v)	5–20%	caustic, keratolytic
Salicylic Acid	3 g	white crystalline powder	1 g/460 mL water or 2 mL alcohol	10% (w/v)	5–20%	caustic, keratolytic
Flexible Collodion	q.s. 30 mL	viscous, clear, colorless liquid	misc with alcohol immis with water	—	—	vehicle, protectant

COMPATIBILITY–STABILITY: This preparation is similar to Salicylic Acid Collodion USP (7), and the following procedure is patterned after that monograph. The salicylic acid and other organic acid ingredients in this preparation are quite stable in this nonaqueous solvent formulation. It is important to note that the acetic acid prescribed here means the chemical entity acetic acid, which is available in pure form as Glacial Acetic Acid USP. The NF article Acetic Acid contains 64% water and would be incompatible with Flexible Collodion. Collodion preparations should not be made in open containers because the flexible collodion contains very volatile solvents such as ether, acetone, and alcohol. Furthermore, flexible collodion is very incompatible with water so it is best to make these preparations directly in the dispensing container. Flexible collodion should not be put in graduated cylinders, beakers, mortars, or sinks! No added preservative is needed for this preparation, because the formulation ingredients are sufficiently hostile to microorganisms.

PACKAGING AND STORAGE: The *USP* monograph for Salicylic Acid Collodion recommends storage in tight containers, at controlled room temperature, and away from fire (7). These conditions would be recommended for this preparation.

BEYOND-USE DATE: Because this formulation contains no water and is made from USP ingredients, a 6-month beyond-use date would be acceptable. However, because of the volatile solvents in Flexible Collodion, a more conservative 1-month date will be used.

CALCULATIONS

Dose/Concentration: All are appropriate for the intended use.

Ingredient Amounts

Note: The percent concentration of the acetic acid and lactic acid can be interpreted in several ways. [This is discussed in the Concentrated Acid section (section VI) of Chapter 8.] If a v/v% interpretation is used, the gram amounts given here would be in milliliters; that is, 1.5 mL acetic acid and 3 mL lactic acid. The alternate interpretation of w/v% of pure chemical in solution is shown here and is used in this prescription order. For these ingredients, the difference in amounts is negligible, but that is not always the case; it depends on the w/w% of the concentrated acid and its density.

Acetic acid (in g): $5\% \times 30\ \text{mL} = 0.05 \times 30\ \text{mL} = 1.5\ \text{g}$ acetic acid

Salicylic acid and lactic acid (in g): $10\% \times 30\ \text{mL} = 0.1 \times 30\ \text{mL} = 3\ \text{g}$ of each

Volume of Glacial Acetic Acid:

Glacial Acetic Acid USP is 100% w/w acetic acid with a density of 1.05 g/mL.

$$\left(\frac{1\ \text{mL Gl. AA}}{1.05\ \text{g Gl. AA}} \right) \left(\frac{100\ \text{g Gl. AA}}{100\ \text{g AA}} \right) \left(\frac{1.5\ \text{g AA}}{} \right) = 1.4\ \text{mL Glacial Acetic Acid}$$

Volume of Lactic Acid:

Lactic Acid USP is 90% w/w lactic acid with a density of 1.20 g/mL.

$$\left(\frac{1\ \text{mL L.A. USP}}{1.20\ \text{g L.A. USP}} \right) \left(\frac{100\ \text{g L.A. USP}}{90\ \text{g L.A.}} \right) \left(\frac{3\ \text{g L.A.}}{} \right) = 2.8\ \text{mL Lactic Acid USP}$$

MSDS AND SAFETY AND PERSONAL PROTECTIVE EQUIPMENT: Review MSDS for all components. Don a clean lab coat, disposable gloves, and safety glasses. Avoid breathing the fumes; work in a well-ventilated area or, preferably, a fume or containment hood if available.

SPECIALIZED EQUIPMENT: All weighing is done on a class III torsion balance.

COMPOUNDING PROCEDURE: Calibrate a 1-oz applicator bottle at 30 mL using Alcohol. Weigh 3 g of salicylic acid. Using a 3-mL syringe, measure 1.4 mL of Glacial Acetic Acid. Using a separate 3-mL syringe, measure 2.8 mL of Lactic Acid. Place all of these ingredients in the applicator bottle and add approximately three-fourths of the needed volume of Flexible Collodion and swirl to mix and dissolve the Salicylic Acid. Add the remainder of the Flexible Collodion to qs to the calibration mark on the applicator bottle. Replace the applicator cap and carefully tighten; then agitate to thoroughly mix the solution. Label and dispense.

DESCRIPTION OF FINISHED PREPARATION: The preparation is a clear, colorless or slightly yellow, viscous solution with the odor of ether.

QUALITY CONTROL: The actual volume of the preparation is checked and matches the theoretical volume of 30 mL. (**Note:** Because this is not an aqueous solution, pH has no meaning and is not measured.)

MASTER FORMULA PREPARED BY: Hank Hound, PharmD   **CHECKED BY:** Anna Legreid Dopp, PharmD

COMPOUNDING RECORD

NAME, STRENGTH, AND DOSAGE FORM OF PREPARATION: Acetic Acid 5%, Lactic Acid 10%, and Salicylic Acid 10% Topical Collodion

QUANTITY: 30 mL   **DATE PREPARED:** mm/dd/yy   **BEYOND-USE DATE:** mm/dd/yy

FORMULATION RECORD ID: OT006   **CONTROL/RX NUMBER:** 123745

INGREDIENTS USED:

Ingredient	Quantity Used	Manufacturer Lot Number	Expiration Date	Weighed/ Measured by	Checked by
Acetic Acid (as Glacial Acetic Acid)	1.5 g (1.4 mL)	JET Labs SN2671	mm/yy	bjf	bb
Lactic Acid (as Lactic Acid USP)	3 g (2.8 mL)	JET Labs SV2672	mm/yy	bjf	bb
Salicylic Acid	3 g	JET Labs SN2641	mm/yy	bjf	bb
Flexible Collodion	q.s. 30 mL	JET Labs SN2673	mm/yy	bjf	bb

QUALITY CONTROL DATA: The preparation is a clear, colorless or slightly yellow, viscous solution with the odor of ether. The actual volume of the preparation was checked and matches the theoretical volume of 30 mL.

LABELING

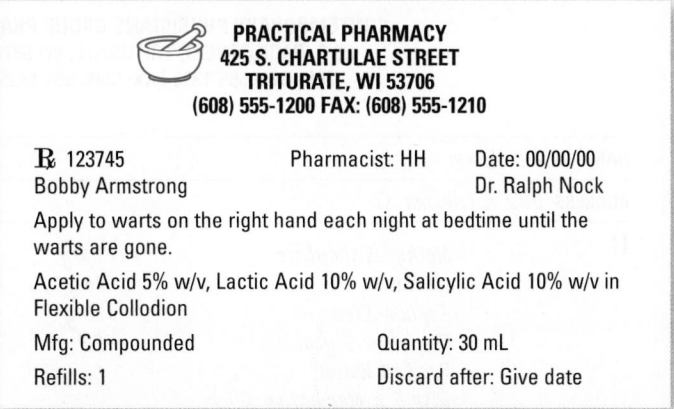

PRACTICAL PHARMACY
425 S. CHARTULAE STREET
TRITURATE, WI 53706
(608) 555-1200 FAX: (608) 555-1210

℞ 123745   Pharmacist: HH   Date: 00/00/00
Bobby Armstrong   Dr. Ralph Nock

Apply to warts on the right hand each night at bedtime until the warts are gone.

Acetic Acid 5% w/v, Lactic Acid 10% w/v, Salicylic Acid 10% w/v in Flexible Collodion

Mfg: Compounded   Quantity: 30 mL

Refills: 1   Discard after: Give date

Auxiliary Labels: Caution. Flammable. For External Use Only.
Keep out of the reach of children. This medicine was compounded in our pharmacy for you at the direction of your prescriber.

PATIENT CONSULTATION: Hello, Bobby. I'm your pharmacist, Hank Hound. Do you have any drug allergies? Are you using any other medications? What did Dr. Nock tell you about this medication? This liquid is a specially formulated liquid that is used to remove warts. It contains some acid ingredients that can be corrosive and irritating to normal skin, so you need to be very careful with it. In fact, before applying this liquid, you may want to put something like Vaseline around the warts to protect the surrounding skin. Use the applicator tip that is in the bottle to dab this liquid on the warts on your right hand each night at bedtime. Dr. Nock says to use this until they are removed.

It usually takes just a week or so, but it could take longer. To increase its effectiveness, you might want to soak your hand in warm water for about 5 minutes before application and put a covering, such as an adhesive bandage, over the area during the night. Wash the medication off in the morning. Be very careful not to get this near your eyes or other sensitive areas on your face or genital areas. Wash your hands immediately after applying this solution and be sure to immediately replace the container cap tightly. Use this in a well-ventilated area and be careful not to inhale the fumes. Also, keep it away from flames or lighted smoking materials, because this is a very flammable mixture. I'm sure that Dr. Nock warned you that warts are contagious, so try not to touch them and, if you do, wash your hands, then dab the warts dry with a towel that you keep only for that purpose. This preparation is obviously for external use only. It should be stored at room temperature and out of the reach of children. You may get one refill. Discard any unused contents after 1 month by placing the tightly capped bottle in a zip-lock plastic bag and disposing of it in the trash. Definitely do not pour the liquid in the sink or toilet as it will clog the drain. Do you have any questions?

SAMPLE PRESCRIPTION 30.9

CASE: Abbie Hamm is a 145-lb, 5′5″-tall, 63-year-old retired professor. She is in the process of revising her textbook for a new edition and is spending many hours each day at the computer. Over the last several weeks, she has been noticing increasing pain in her right elbow and radiating down her arm, and the symptoms persist (and even seem most bothersome) when she is trying to sleep at night. She thinks this is the result of using her computer mouse, which she has always found difficult. She has already taken some steps to alleviate the problem by reconfiguring her computer setup and putting her mouse on the left side. Dr. Clyde has diagnosed a repetitive strain injury and has referred her to a physical therapist for treatment. In the meantime, Professor Hamm would like some relief for the pain, but she is unable to take nonsteroidal anti-inflammatory drugs because of a long-standing problem with gastrointestinal reflux disorder and chronic gastritis. Dr. Clyde has recommended that she take acetaminophen, 500 mg every 6 hours, when needed for the pain and has prescribed a topical counterirritant medication stick for her to apply locally to her elbow in the area that seems to be the source of her pain. Pharmacist Jillian Woodruff at Practical Pharmacy provided Dr. Clyde with the medication stick formula given here.

CONTEMPORARY PHYSICIANS GROUP PRACTICE
20 S. PARK STREET, TRITURATE, WI 53706
TEL: (608) 555-1333 FAX: (608) 555-1335

℞ # *123950*

NAME *Abbie Hamm*　　　　　　　　　　　　　　**DATE** *00/00/00*

ADDRESS *202 E. Lansing St.*

℞

Methyl Salicylate	3.5 g
Menthol	1.5 g
Sodium Stearate	1.3 g
Propylene Glycol	2.5 g
Purified Water	1.2 g
Disp 5 g Medication Stick	

J. Woodruff 00/00/00

Sig: Apply to painful areas of right elbow and arm tid prn pain

REFILLS *prn*　　　　　　　　　　　　　*Emil Clyde*　　　　　　　**M.D.**

DEA NO.

MASTER COMPOUNDING FORMULATION RECORD

NAME, STRENGTH, AND DOSAGE FORM OF PREPARATION: Methyl Salicylate 35% and Menthol 15% Topical Medication Stick

QUANTITY: 5 g (plus 5 g excess)

THERAPEUTIC USE/CATEGORY: Counterirritant

FORMULATION RECORD ID: OT007

ROUTE OF ADMINISTRATION: Topical

INGREDIENTS USED:

Ingredient	Quantity Used	Physical Description	Solubility	Dose Comparison		Use in the Prescription
				Given	Usual	
Methyl Salicylate	3.5 g (3 mL)	light yellow, oily liquid; odor of wintergreen	1 g/1,500 mL water, misc w/ alcohol	35%	10–60%	counterirritant, local analgesic
Propylene Glycol	2.5 g (2.4 mL)	clear, colorless liquid	misc w/ water, alcohol	—	—	solvent, preservative, humectant
Menthol	1.5 g	colorless needlelike crystals; odor of menthol	sl sol water, v sol alcohol	15%	1.25–16%	counterirritant, local analgesic
Purified Water	1.2 g (1.2 mL)	clear, colorless liquid	misc w/ alcohol	—	—	solvent
Sodium Stearate	1.3 g	white powder	readily sol in hot water and alchool	—	—	emulsifier, stiffening agent

COMPATIBILITY–STABILITY: No stability data for this specific formulation is available, but the methyl salicylate and menthol should be quite stable in this formulation. There are numerous commercial nonprescription products with similar formulations. This formulation was patterned after a similar medication stick formulation given on the Internet site for Paddock Labs under Professional Publications, Secundum Artem, vol. 5, no. 3, Compounding Medication Sticks (18). No additional preservative is needed because of the presence of propylene glycol (25%), menthol, and methyl salicylate, all of which have preservative and antiseptic properties.

PACKAGING AND STORAGE: Packaging will be in a special medication stick tube container. Storage should be at controlled room temperature.

BEYOND-USE DATE: Use the *USP*-recommended maximum 30-day beyond-use date for compounded other formulations prepared from ingredients in solid form when there is no stability information for the formulation (6).

CALCULATIONS

Dose/Concentration

The active ingredients in this formulation are methyl salicylate and menthol. For this topical preparation, a w/w% concentration is calculated for these ingredients.

Methyl salicylate: w/w% is calculated as follows:

$$\frac{3.5 \text{ g methyl sal.}}{10 \text{ g preparation}} = \frac{x \text{ g methyl sal.}}{100 \text{ g preparation}}; \ x = 35 \text{ g}/100 \text{ g} = 35\%$$

Menthol: w/w% is calculated as follows:

$$\frac{1.5 \text{ g menthol}}{10 \text{ g preparation}} = \frac{x \text{ g menthol}}{100 \text{ g preparation}}; \ x = 15 \text{ g}/100 \text{ g} = 15\%$$

These concentrations are with normal ranges for this use: When used in nonprescription counterirritant external analgesics, FDA dosage range guidelines are 10% to 60% for methyl salicylate and 1.25% to 16% for menthol (19).

Ingredient Amounts

The medication stick applicator tubes have a volume capacity of 4.5 mL and hold approximately 5 g of materials such as methyl salicylate that have densities greater than 1.0. The formula on the prescription order is for 10 g, which gives 5 g excess to compensate for loss on compounding. The weights of all the ingredients are given for the 10-g formula. The water, methyl salicylate, and propylene glycol are liquids and would more conveniently be measured by volume. The volumes can be calculated using the specific gravities of each of these ingredients. Because water has a density of 1.0, 1.2 g of water has a volume of 1.2 mL and need not be calculated.

Methyl salicylate has a s.g. of 1.18; the volume of 3.5 g is calculated to be:

$$\left(\frac{\text{mL methyl sal.}}{1.18 \text{ g methyl sal.}}\right)\left(\frac{3.5 \text{ g methyl sal.}}{}\right) = 3.0 \text{ mL methyl salicylate}$$

Propylene Glycol has a s.g. of 1.036; the volume of 2.5 g is calculated to be:

$$\left(\frac{\text{mL PG}}{1.036 \text{ g PG}}\right)\left(\frac{2.5 \text{ g PG}}{}\right) = 2.4 \text{ mL propylene glycol}$$

MSDS AND SAFETY AND PERSONAL PROTECTIVE EQUIPMENT: Review MSDS for all components. Don a clean lab coat and disposable gloves.

SPECIALIZED EQUIPMENT: All weighing is done on an electronic balance.

COMPOUNDING PROCEDURE: Weigh 1.5 g of menthol and 1.3 g of sodium stearate. Place the sodium stearate in a small beaker. Measure 1.2 mL of Purified Water and 2.4 mL propylene glycol using 3-mL syringes and add to the beaker containing the sodium stearate. Heat this mixture in a microwave oven for about 10 seconds. Place the menthol in another small beaker. Measure 3 mL of methyl salicylate in a 3-mL syringe and add it to the beaker containing the menthol; stir to mix until the menthol is completely dissolved. Add this to the melted base in the other beaker and stir thoroughly. Allow this to cool slightly until it begins to become more viscous. Tare the weight of the medication tube, then pour the molten medication into the tube and note and record the weight of the medication. Allow it to solidify, then label and dispense.

DESCRIPTION OF FINISHED PREPARATION: Preparation is a colorless to slightly whitish, transparent, soft solid stick.

QUALITY CONTROL: Check the actual weight of the medication stick by weighing the medication stick tube before and after the preparation is added to the tube; the weight of the preparation should be within the range of ±10% of the prescribed weight of 5 g. The amount of preparation in the tube plus the loss observed in the beaker should be reasonable for the theoretical weight of 10 g.

MASTER FORMULA PREPARED BY: Jillian Woodruff, PharmD

CHECKED BY: Anna Legreid Dopp, PharmD

COMPOUNDING RECORD

NAME, STRENGTH, AND DOSAGE FORM OF PREPARATION: Methyl Salicylate 35% and Menthol 15% Topical Medication Stick

QUANTITY: 5 g (plus 5 g excess) **DATE PREPARED:** mm/dd/yy **BEYOND-USE DATE:** mm/dd/yy

FORMULATION RECORD ID: OT007 **CONTROL/RX NUMBER:** 123950

INGREDIENTS USED:

Ingredient	Quantity Used	Manufacturer Lot Number	Expiration Date	Weighed/ Measured by	Checked by
Methyl Salicylate	3.5 g (3 mL)	JET Labs ON3091	mm/yy	bjf	jw
Propylene Glycol	2.5 g (2.4 mL)	JET Labs SN2662	mm/yy	bjf	jw
Menthol	1.5 g	JET Labs ON3092	mm/yy	bjf	jw
Purified Water	1.2 g (1.2 mL)	Sweet Springs AL0529	mm	bif	jw
Sodium Stearate	1.3 g	JET Labs ON3093	mm/yy	bjf	jw

QUALITY CONTROL DATA: Preparation is a colorless to slightly whitish, transparent, soft solid stick. The actual weight of the stick was checked: the weight of the preparation is 5.4 g, which is an expected weight for the 4.5-mL tube and is within the range of ±10% of the prescribed weight of 5 g. The observed excess material in the beaker is reasonable for the theoretical weight of 10 g.

LABELING

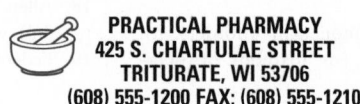

PRACTICAL PHARMACY
425 S. CHARTULAE STREET
TRITURATE, WI 53706
(608) 555-1200 FAX: (608) 555-1210

℞ 123950 Pharmacist: JW Date: 00/00/00
Abbie Hamm Dr. Emil Clyde

Apply to painful areas of right elbow and arm three times a day as needed for pain.

Methyl Salicylate 35% and Menthol 15% Topical Medication Stick

Mfg: Compounded Quantity: 5 g

Refills: As needed for 1 year Discard after: Give date

Auxiliary Labels: For External Use Only. Keep out of reach of children. This medicine was compounded in our pharmacy for you at the direction of your prescriber.

PATIENT CONSULTATION: Hi, Prof. Hamm. I'm your pharmacist, Jillian Woodruff. Do you have any drug allergies? Are you using any prescription or nonprescription medications? What has Dr. Clyde told you about the use of this medication stick? This is a custom-formulated preparation containing methyl salicylate and menthol and should give you some relief for the tendon and muscle pain in your arm. You are to apply this three times daily as needed to the painful areas of your right elbow and arm. To use this, remove the cap and turn the bottom of the tube counter-clockwise and then rub the medication stick over the area. You will probably have a sensation of either warmth or cooling, and this is normal. Two important precautions with this medication: (1) Do not use a heating pad or similar device on the area after you have applied the medication, and (2) do not wrap the area tightly with an elastic bandage or wrap or any type of occlusive dressing. If you develop a rash or hives after you start using this medication, or if the pains does not improve or gets worse, contact Dr. Clyde. This is for external use only. You should store this in a cool, dry place. It is especially important to keep this out of the reach of children; it contains methyl salicylate, which smells like wintergreen, and some children may mistake it for candy. This may be refilled as needed for a year, but I would suggest that you call ahead when you need a new tube since this is a custom-made preparation and it takes a little while to make it. You should discard any unused portion after a month. Do you have any questions?

REFERENCES

1. The United States Pharmacopeial Convention, Inc. Chapter ⟨1151⟩. 2008 USP 31/NF 26. Rockville, MD: Author, 2007; 617–621.
2. CDER Data Standards Manual. Rockville, MD: Food and Drug Administration, 2006: Data Element Name: Dosage Form, http://www.fda.gov/cder/dsm/DRG/drg00201.htm.
3. Gelone S, Gennaro AR. Topical drugs. In: University of the Sciences in Philadelphia, ed. Remington: the science and practice of pharmacy, 21st ed. Baltimore, MD: Lippincott Williams & Wilkins, 2006; 1285–1286.
4. Unvala HM. Cetyl alcohol. In: Kibbe AH, ed. Handbook of pharmaceutical excipients, 3rd ed. Washington, DC: American Pharmaceutical Association, 2000; 117.
5. The United States Pharmacopeial Convention, Inc. Official NF monographs. 2008 USP 31/NF 26. Rockville, MD: Author, 2007.
6. The United States Pharmacopeial Convention, Inc. Chapter ⟨795⟩. 2008 USP 31/NF 26. Rockville, MD: Author, 2007; 316–317.
7. The United States Pharmacopeial Convention, Inc. Official USP monographs. 2008 USP 31/NF 26. Rockuille, MD: Auther, 2007.
8. Ellsworth A. Psoriasis. In: Koda-Kimble MA, Young LY, eds. Applied therapeutics, 7th ed. Baltimore, MD: Lippincott Williams & Wilkins, 2001; 38.2–38.3.
9. Boettger RF, Fukushima LH. Common skin disorders. In: Helms RA, Quan DJ, Herfindal DR, eds. Textbook of therapeutics, 8th ed. Philadelphia: Lippincott Williams & Wilkins, 2006; 237–241.
10. Connors KA, Amidon GL, Stella VJ. Chemical stability of pharmaceuticals, 2nd ed. New York: John Wiley & Sons, 1986; 780–786.
11. Connors KA, Amidon GL, Stella VJ. Chemical stability of pharmaceuticals, 2nd ed. New York: John Wiley & Sons, 1986; 483–490.
12. Jejurkar P, Nash RA. The pH value of urea solutions in purified water. IJPC 1998; 2: 76.
13. Florey K, ed. Analytical profiles of drug substances, vol. 1. New York: Academic Press, 1972; 383.
14. Allen LV, Jr., ed. Piroxicam 0.5% in an alcoholic gel. IJPC 1997; 1: 181.
15. Allen LV, Jr., ed. Ketoprofen 10%, cyclobenzaprine 1% and lidocaine 5% in poloxamer lecithin organogel. IJPC 1998; 2: 154.
16. Trissel LA. Trissel's stability of compounded formulations, 3rd ed. Washington, DC: American Pharmacists Association, 2005; 148–149.
17. Trissel LA. Trissel's stability of compounded formulations, 3rd ed. Washington, DC: American Pharmacists Association, 2005; 253–255.
18. Allen LV, Jr. Compounding medication sticks. Secundum Artem 5(3), www.paddcocklabs.com. Accessed December 2007.
19. Federal Register. 1979; 44: 69874.

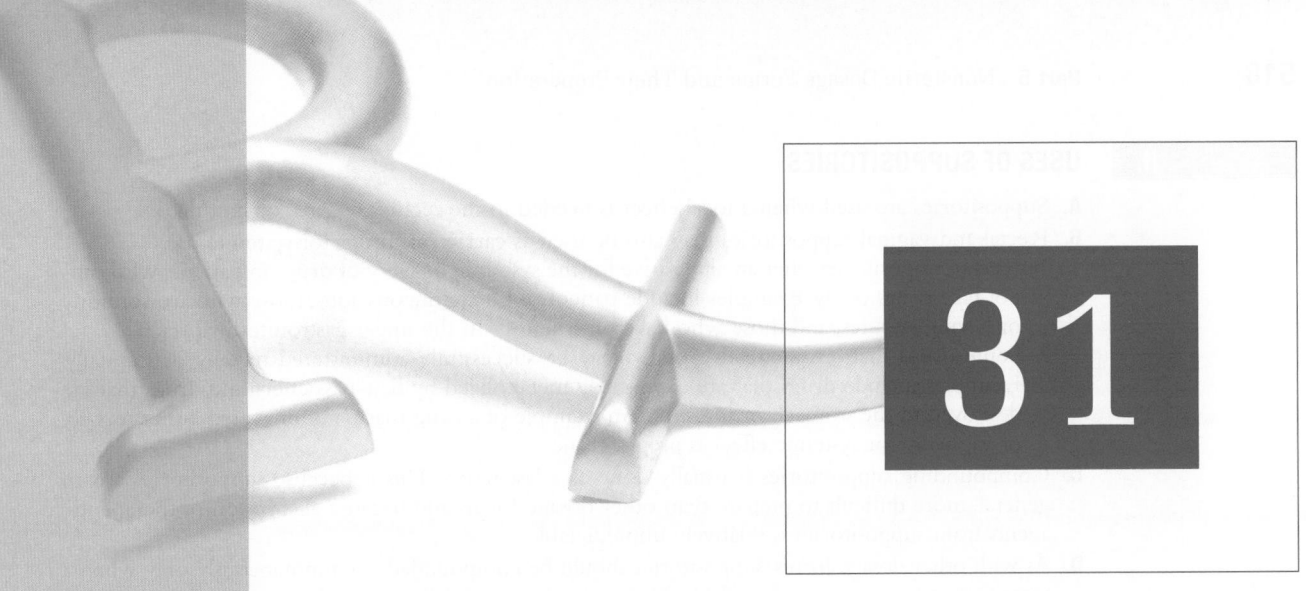

31

Suppositories

I. DEFINITIONS AND SUPPOSITORY NOMENCLATURE

A. **Suppositories:** "Suppositories are solid bodies of various weights and shapes, adapted for introduction into the rectal, vaginal, or urethral orifice of the human body. They usually melt, soften, or dissolve at body temperature. A suppository may act as a protectant or palliative to the local tissues at the point of introduction or as a carrier of therapeutic agents for systemic or local action" (1).

B. Other suppository nomenclature
1. As was discussed at the beginning of Chapter 27, in 2002 the USP formed a group to work on simplifying and clarifying dosage form nomenclature. Under the proposed system, the term *suppository* is used only for rectal administration, and similar dosage forms for administration vaginally or urethrally are termed *inserts* (2). The definitions in FDA's 2006 *CDER Data Standards Manual* have this same distinction and are similar to the proposed *USP* definitions given here:
   a. **Suppository:** "A solid dosage form in which one or more actives is dispersed in a suitable base and molded or otherwise formed into a suitable shape for insertion into the rectal area to provide local or systemic effect" (2).
   b. **Insert:** "A solid dosage form which is inserted into a body cavity, such as the urethra or vagina. See also SUPPOSITORY, a term used to describe inserts into the rectal region" (2).
2. The proposed nomenclature scheme uses the following format to name preparations: [drug substance] [route of administration] [physical state] [release pattern], so that, for example, the suppositories for Sample Prescription 31.1 would be named: Indomethacin 25 mg Rectal Suppositories. An immediate-release pattern is understood unless otherwise stated.

C. For this chapter, the term *suppository* will be used in the traditional sense and will include rectal suppositories and vaginal and urethral inserts.

II. USES OF SUPPOSITORIES

A. Suppositories are used when a local effect is needed in the rectum, vagina, or urethra.

B. Rectal and vaginal suppositories may also be used as carriers of drugs for systemic use.

    1. Rectal suppositories offer an alternative for the systemic delivery of drugs in patients who cannot take drugs orally. Examples include patients who are unconscious, those who are vomiting or having seizures, and those who have obstructions in the upper gastrointestinal tract.

    2. Some drugs that are ineffective orally may be successfully administered rectally or vaginally. Examples include drugs that are extensively metabolized by first-pass effect and drugs that are destroyed in the stomach or intestine. An example of a drug that is administered either rectally or vaginally for systemic effect is progesterone.

C. Compounding suppositories is usually done as a last resort. This is because suppositories are, in general, more difficult to prepare than other dosage forms and because absorption of therapeutic agents from suppositories is relatively unpredictable.

D. As with other dosage forms, suppositories should be compounded extemporaneously only when a manufactured product is not available. This principle is especially true with suppositories containing drugs needed for a systemic effect, because of the unpredictable absorption from suppositories.

III. SELECTING THE SUPPOSITORY BASE MATERIAL

A. To release drug for systemic action or to make drug available for local effect, the suppository base must melt, soften, or dissolve in the body orifice. Of the two most common suppository base materials, polyethylene glycol (PEG) dissolves, while fatty bases, such as cocoa butter and its synthetic substitutes, melt at body temperature. A detailed description of suppository bases and their properties is given in Chapter 24, Suppository Bases. Consult this chapter when selecting a suppository base for a compounded drug preparation.

B. The selection of suppository base material depends both on the intended use (systemic versus local effect) and the route of administration (rectal, vaginal, or urethral). Other factors to consider include patient comfort, and compatibility and stability of components in the base.

    1. Patient comfort

        a. In general, fatty-type bases are more comfortable for patients than are PEG bases.

        b. Fatty bases are bland and nonirritating to the sensitive tissues of the rectum, vagina, and urethra, whereas PEG bases can give a stinging or burning sensation. PEG bases also can cause a defecating reflex when used rectally. These effects can be minimized by adding 10% water to the PEG base and by moistening the suppository with water before insertion (3).

    2. Compatibility and stability

        a. In most cases, fatty bases are less reactive than PEG bases, so they have fewer compatibility and stability problems with incorporated therapeutic agents.

        b. One compatibility problem of fatty bases is the lowering of their melting point with the addition of drugs or other components that form eutectic mixtures with lower melting points. Chloral hydrate in cocoa butter is the classic example of this effect. A small amount of white wax or of cetyl esters wax can be added to overcome this problem; however, adding too much wax may produce a suppository that does not melt at body temperature.

        c. Because PEG bases are designed to dissolve rather than melt at the site of action, they can be formulated so that they will not melt on storage, even at fairly warm temperatures. In contrast, fatty bases are formulated to melt at body temperature and are therefore much more sensitive to warm temperatures; they must be stored at controlled room temperature or in the refrigerator.

    3. Route of administration

        a. Fatty bases are preferred for rectal suppositories because rectal tissues are especially sensitive to the irritating effects of PEG bases. As stated previously, PEG suppositories may also cause a defecating reflex.

        b. PEG bases are often preferred over fatty bases for vaginal and urethral suppositories; the vagina and urethra do not have sphincter muscles to prevent leakage from these body orifices, and the oily material of fatty bases is less desirable in this regard.

        c. Soft, rubbery suppository bases, such as glycerinated gelatin, are suitable for vaginal administration but are generally not firm enough for rectal or urethral use.

    4. Systemic effects

        a. In general, systemic absorption of drugs from suppositories is unpredictable. This is due both to the poor environment for absorption in the rectum and vagina (urethral inserts are used solely for local effect) and to the physical-chemical nature of the suppository base material coupled with the properties of the active ingredient(s).

(1) The amount of aqueous fluid in the rectum and vagina is variable but small. This affects the release of drug from the base. Although this influences both local action and systemic absorption, its major impact is on systemic absorption.

　　(a) Because PEG bases require dissolution for release of the drug from the dosage form, systemic effect depends on the amount of dissolving fluid present in the rectum or vagina. This is part of the rationale for recommending that patients moisten PEG suppositories before insertion; this puts a layer of water in contact with the suppository to help hasten dissolution upon insertion. Even in excess water, PEG bases dissolve slowly, taking up to 1 hour (2).

　　(b) Although fatty bases melt rather than dissolve, the incorporated drug must partition out of the base into the aqueous medium at the site of action before absorption can occur. This, too, requires a sufficient amount of aqueous media at the administration site.

(2) As was discussed in Chapter 24, fatty bases generally give poor release of hydrophobic drugs. Because many organic drug molecules are water-insoluble and hydrophobic except when present in their ionized salt or water-soluble complex form, this must be considered when choosing both the drug form and the suppository base.

　　(a) The release of a drug from a fatty, lipophilic suppository base to the aqueous medium in the rectum or vagina depends on the water/base partition coefficient of the drug.

　　(b) For this reason, from a bioavailability point of view, water-soluble ionized (salt) forms of drugs (which have high water/base partition coefficients) should be used when possible with fatty bases. For example, codeine phosphate is preferred over codeine base for systemic absorption when a fatty suppository base is being used. Some drugs such as acetaminophen and diazepam do not have water-soluble forms and give slow and unpredictable release from most fatty bases.

　　(c) Some commercially available fatty-acid suppository bases, such as Fattibase, contain surfactants and emulsifying agents that overcome, at least partially, the problem of poor bioavailability of hydrophobic drugs. The free acid indomethacin, which is illustrated in Sample Prescription 31.1, was studied in various suppository bases, and it showed poor release from fatty-acid bases unless surfactants were added to the base material (4).

(3) When formulated with an appropriate blend of polymers, PEG suppositories dissolve in body cavity fluids and release the active ingredient(s), both hydrophilic and hydrophobic drugs. Provided there are sufficient aqueous secretions in the body cavity, PEG suppositories provide more reliable release of hydrophobic drugs from the dosage form than do fatty bases.

b. Suppositories made with bases that contain a dispersing agent, such as silicon dioxide, silica gel, or bentonite, and/or a surfactant or emulsifying agent may break apart more easily and spread more effectively over the target tissue or absorbing surfaces.

c. Because of the unpredictability of release of drug from suppository bases, it is important to monitor the effectiveness of the drug delivery system by frequent monitoring of therapeutic results. Drugs with narrow therapeutic windows should be administered in compounded suppositories only with the greatest of caution.

5. Local action

a. Choice of a base is not as critical when local action is desired, because nearly any base holds the active ingredient in contact with the affected tissue.

b. Suppositories made with bases that contain a dispersing agent and/or a surfactant may break apart more easily, and the active ingredients may be spread more effectively on the target tissue.

c. When an emollient local effect is desired, a fatty base is preferred.

IV. SELECTING A COMPOUNDING METHOD

A. Suppositories are now almost always made by fusion. The method of hand-rolling suppositories, while seldom used, is discussed and illustrated in this chapter because it offers a truly extemporaneous method that can be used in any pharmacy when a customized suppository is needed and the molds and equipment for the fusion method are not immediately available. At one time, suppositories were also made by compression, but this method is no longer used in extemporaneous compounding.

B. Depending on the compounding method selected, special calculations, compounding techniques, and equipment may be required to give accurate doses of suppositories.

C. Hand-rolling suppositories

  1. Advantages

    a. Hand-rolled suppositories do not require special calculations.

    b. Special equipment is not required for this method. A pill roller is useful, but a broad-bladed spatula or any stiff, flat piece of nonreactive material can be used for this purpose.

    c. Cocoa butter is the base used for hand-rolled suppositories. It is readily available in bars or push-up tubes from any drug wholesaler. It is also available in grated form from suppliers of compounding ingredients and equipment.

  2. Disadvantages

    a. Preparing and forming hand-rolled suppositories requires experience and good technique.

    b. Even when well made, hand-rolled suppositories do not have the elegant appearance of suppositories made by fusion.

D. Fusion

  1. Advantages

    a. The fusion method does not require well-developed manual compounding technique.

    b. Suppositories made by fusion have an elegant, professional appearance.

  2. Disadvantages

    a. Special suppository molds are required to make suppositories by fusion.

    b. Caution must be used when incorporating drugs sensitive to heat.

    c. Because the components are dosed and measured by weight but compounded by volume, density calculations, mold calibrations, or double-casting procedures are required to give accurate doses.

      (1) Because suppositories are semisolid at room temperature, most of the base components and active ingredients are solids and are measured by weight.

      (2) The components are then combined, melted, and poured into suppository mold cavities. This means that the dosage unit is measured by volume—the volume of the mold cavity. The final amount of drug in a dosage unit therefore depends on two factors: the w/w concentration of active ingredient in the base material and the weight of the mixture contained in each mold cavity. The weight of mixture in the mold cavity depends on the volume of the cavity and the density of the molten mixture.

      (3) Consider the following example: The usual volume of a suppository mold cavity is 2 mL. Depending on the density of the melted mixture of ingredients, the weight of a 2-mL suppository can vary considerably. To calculate the weight per suppository, multiply the density (d) or specific gravity (s. g.) of the mixture times the volume of the mold cavity.

        For example:

$$\text{Water, } d = 1 \text{ g/mL}: 1 \text{ g/mL} \times 2 \text{ mL} = 2 \text{ g}$$

$$\text{Cocoa butter, } d = 0.86 \text{ g/mL}: 0.86 \text{ g/mL} \times 2 \text{ mL} = 1.72 \text{ g}$$

$$\text{PEG 400, } d = 1.125 \text{ g/mL}: 1.125 \text{ g/mL} \times 2 \text{ mL} = 2.25 \text{ g}$$

      (4) Obviously, the density of the material has a significant effect on the final weight of the dosage unit. To determine the quantity of base and active ingredients(s) to weigh when compounding suppositories by fusion, it is necessary to either calibrate the mold cavities for the desired base or use a double-casting procedure. There are other factors to consider as well. Examples (31.1 through 31.4) are given and discussed in section V. B of this chapter on fusion compounding methods.

V.   **CALCULATIONS AND PROCEDURES FOR COMPOUNDING SUPPOSITORIES**

A. Hand-rolling of suppositories

This method is limited to suppositories made using cocoa butter as the base material, because cocoa butter is the only suppository base that can be molded without the use of heat. The procedure for hand-rolling suppositories is described here and is illustrated with Sample Prescription 31.2.

  1. Check the doses of the active ingredients.

  2. Check the compatibility and stability of the active ingredients and the formulation.

3. Decide on the desired finished weight per suppository. The usual weight per unit for various suppository types are as follows:
   a. Adult rectal: 2 g
   b. Vaginal: 2 to 5 g
   c. Pediatric rectal: 1 g
   d. Male urethral: 4 g
   e. Female urethral: 2 g
4. Calculate the quantity of each ingredient needed for compounding the preparation. Make enough material for two extra suppositories to compensate for loss of material during the compounding process.
   a. Multiply the dose per unit times the number of units to determine the amount of each active ingredient.
   b. Multiply the finished weight per unit times the number of units.
   c. Subtract the total weight of active ingredients from the total weight of the suppositories to determine the amount of base (cocoa butter) needed.
5. If the cocoa butter is in a bar or in large pieces, grate or reduce the cocoa butter to very small pieces.
6. Weigh the calculated amount of active ingredient(s) and cocoa butter.
7. Place the active ingredients(s) in a **glass** mortar and triturate to a fine powder.
8. Add a small amount of cocoa butter and triturate, using pressure to soften and/or liquefy the cocoa butter so that it acts as a levigating agent for the active ingredient(s).
9. Add the rest of the cocoa butter by geometric dilution, triturating and scraping down the sides of the mortar regularly.
10. Using a metal spatula, remove the mass from the mortar and place the material in a clean piece of white filter paper. Put on a pair of clean plastic disposable gloves. Knead the mass in the filter paper until it is pliable but not soft and sticky.
11. While it is still in the filter paper, start to shape the mass into a cylindric pipe by rolling it in the filter paper between your hands (in the same manner as you made "snakes" out of modeling clay when you were in preschool).
12. Put the cylindric mass on an ointment slab and, using a **clean** pill roller or a broad-bladed spatula, roll the mass into a smooth cylindric pipe. Use the gauge on the ointment slab or a ruler for determining the proper length of the pipe so that equal pieces of appropriate length can be cut. The approximate dimensions per suppository are as follows:
    a. 1 to $1\frac{1}{2}$ inches long with a diameter of approximately 3/8 inch for adult rectal and vaginal suppositories
    b. Proportionate but smaller for pediatric rectal suppositories
    c. 4 inches long by 3/16 inch in diameter for male urethral inserts
    d. 2 to 3 inches long by 3/16 inches in diameter for female urethral inserts
13. As you roll the mass, use the pill roller or spatula to keep the ends of the pipe as blunt and square as possible; you may wish to roll the pipe slightly longer than necessary and cut off the irregular ends of the pipe before cutting it into equal pieces. (Remember that you made enough material for two extra suppositories to compensate for loss such as this during compounding.)
14. Using a razor blade, cut the pipe into equal-length pieces. After you cut the first piece, check its weight to be sure that you are in the approximate desired weight range per suppository.
15. Form a point on one end of each suppository. Suppositories should be bullet-shaped for ease of insertion.
16. Weigh each suppository; if necessary, adjust each to the proper weight by slicing thin pieces from the blunt end. The suppositories should each be the target weight (e.g., 2 g ±10%).
17. Wrap each suppository in foil or seal in individual plastic bags.

B. **Fusion**
1. Suppository molds
   a. A wide assortment of suppository molds is available from vendors of compounding supplies. Depending on the company, aluminum molds for rectal and vaginal suppositories are available with either 1- or 2-mL capacity cavities and with 10 to 1,000 cavities per mold. Urethral molds, both male and female, are also available. A wide variety of disposable molds can also be purchased.
   b. Although preference for disposable versus aluminum molds depends on the individual using them, the type of suppository base being used, and the intended use of the

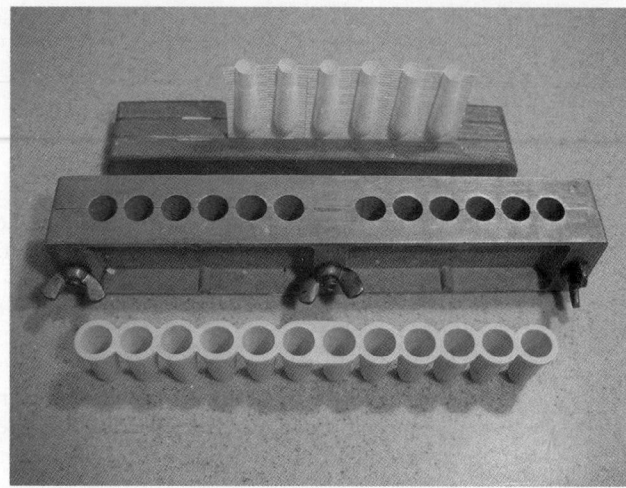

ALUMINUM AND DISPOSABLE SUPPOSITORY MOLDS

suppository, in general, aluminum molds give more uniform, accurate dosage units than do plastic disposable molds.

  c. Mold lubrication

    (1) Disposable molds have the advantage of not requiring any prior lubrication because the suppositories are just popped out or the plastic material peeled off at the time of use.

    (2) Although aluminum molds usually require lubrication before use, this is relatively easy with the use of spray vegetable oils. Just a light coating is needed; any excess should be wiped off with a tissue.

  d. Suppository wrappers

    (1) Disposable molds also have the advantage of providing the wrapping material for the suppositories; the suppositories are dispensed in the plastic shell that is used as the mold.

    (2) Suppositories that have been made in a nondisposable mold should have a protective covering applied before being placed in the dispensing container. They should either be wrapped individually in aluminum foil or sealed in small polyethylene plastic bags. The foil can be purchased precut in small squares (and it even comes in colors), or the 3" × 3" squares can be cut from a sheet of aluminum foil. Alternatively, small polyethylene bags, zipper-lock or plain, can be purchased for a nominal price.

  e. Although aluminum molds have a greater initial investment cost, in the long term they may be less expensive to use than disposable molds.

2. Suppository base materials for the fusion method

  a. All four suppository base types that are recognized in the *USP* (1) may be used with the fusion method. These bases and their properties are discussed in Chapter 24.

  b. Melting fatty bases

    (1) Microwave ovens are not recommended for melting fatty bases because these devices do not provide the carefully controlled temperature required. Similarly, although these bases could be carefully melted by direct heat on a hot plate, the more controlled temperature provided by a warm-water bath is preferred. This is especially true when melting cocoa butter.

    (2) If the base is in a bar or in large solid blocks, grate or shred the base into very small pieces. This increases the efficiency of the melting process. Furthermore, overheating the melt is less likely when there are no large chunks that require melting.

    (3) Place the base in a beaker or crucible and carefully heat this on a warm-water bath until the base has just turned to a fluid. If available, use a warm-water bath with a thermostat (such as the one pictured in Chapter 13), because this makes the process of controlled heating much easier.

    (4) If the base is cocoa butter, have the water bath temperature at approximately 55°C and melt the base carefully. Melted cocoa butter should maintain an opalescent, creamy appearance with a temperature of approximately 34°C. You can tell visually if the critical temperature has been exceeded for cocoa butter because the fluid changes to a clear, golden color. One recommendation to avoid overheating cocoa butter is to add it in portions to the heating vessel. Then, if the critical temperature is exceeded and the fluid becomes clear, the vessel can be removed from the heat source and extra grated cocoa butter can be added to reduce the temperature of the melt and provide new β-crystals for the desired polymorph.

(5) If a cocoa butter substitute base such as Fattibase is used, follow the manufacturer's instructions for the heating temperature. For example, the recommended melting temperature for Fattibase is approximately 50°C, and this base should not be heated above 60°C.

c. Preparing and melting PEG and glycerinated gelatin bases

(1) Both PEG and glycerinated gelatin bases can be made using either a microwave oven or a hot plate. In either case, care must be exercised so that the material is not overheated.

(2) Preformulated blends of PEG, such as Polybase, and typical solid PEG base components melt at between 37° and 63°C, but they may be heated up to 100°C without danger of decomposition. The melting points of commonly used PEGs are given in Table 24.1 of Chapter 24.

(3) The formula and method of preparation for glycerinated gelatin suppository base is the same as the pediatric chewable gummy gel base given in Table 26.3 of Chapter 26.

3. Compounding procedures

Four examples are given here to show the necessary calculations and compounding procedures for making suppositories by fusion. These principles are used in Sample Prescriptions 31.1 and 31.3 at the end of this chapter.

Example 31.1

Fusion Method When Precalibrating the Suppository Mold:

$\textbf{R}$ Aspirin   100 mg

   Suppository base   qs

   Dispense 6 suppositories

Procedure:

1. Select the base material for this preparation. In this case, cocoa butter is selected because this is a comfortable base for rectal administration. A synthetic fatty-acid base such as Fattibase would also be acceptable, but a PEG base should not be used because aspirin is reported to be unstable in this type of base (5).

2. Select a suitable suppository mold. If an aluminum mold is used, permanently inscribe an identifying mark on the mold and record this with the calibration information for the base selected. If a disposable mold is used, record the manufacturer and the lot number of the mold with the calibration information.

3. Calibrate the suppository mold for the base being used—cocoa butter, in this example. This is done by carefully melting the grated cocoa butter, pouring it into five suppository mold cavities, trimming and removing each suppository from its mold cavity, and weighing each suppository. Using this weight data, calculate the mean suppository calibration weight for cocoa butter in this mold. Because the density of a base may vary depending on temperature of the melt, note and record the temperature of the melt so that this fusion temperature is used each time this calibration weight is used with this mold and base. In this example, the temperature of the melt is 34°C (the target temperature for melted cocoa butter), and the average weight per suppository is 1.72 g. If another base is used, follow the manufacturer's instructions for heating temperature.

4. Calculate the amount of active ingredient(s) for the prescription order plus two extras to compensate for loss of material during the compounding process.

$$8 \times 100 \text{ mg} = 800 \text{ mg aspirin}$$

5. Using the suppository calibration weight and the desired number of suppositories, calculate the final weight for all suppositories:

$$8 \times 1.72 \text{ g} = 13.76 \text{ g total weight for 8 suppositories}$$

6. Calculate the quantity of cocoa butter needed by subtracting the weight of the active ingredient(s) from the total weight of the eight suppositories.

$$\text{Quantity of cocoa butter} = 13.76 \text{ g} - 0.8 \text{ g} = 12.96 \text{ g cocoa butter}$$

7. Prepare the powdered active ingredient(s). If the powder is very finely divided (e.g., micronized), weigh it directly. Otherwise, weigh a small excess of the quantity of the active ingredient needed, reduce this to a fine powder by trituration in a mortar, and then weigh the calculated quantity of powder. In this example, weigh approximately 825 mg of aspirin, triturate it to a fine powder in a mortar, and weigh 800 mg of this powder.

8. Prepare the suppository base material—cocoa butter, in this case. If it is in a bar or in large pieces, grate or reduce it to small pieces. Weigh the calculated amount of suppository base—in this case, 12.96 g of cocoa butter.

9. Before melting the base and combining the ingredients, prepare the suppository mold. Be certain it is clean. Apply a lubricant to the mold if needed.

10. Put a small portion of the base in a beaker or crucible and carefully heat this on a warm-water bath until the base has just turned to a fluid. If the base is cocoa butter, melt it very carefully on a warm-water (approximately 55°C) bath. The cocoa butter should be heated to approximately 34°C, as that is the temperature used when calibrating the mold.

11. Add the powdered drug to the melted base and stir well to mix.

12. Add the remainder of the grated base in portions with stirring, being careful not to overheat. Stir to ensure a uniform mixture. The temperature of the melt should be the same as the temperature for the base when the calibration was done (e.g., 34°C in this example).

13. Pour the molten mixture into six or seven suppository mold cavities. Overfill the cavities slightly because the base will contract somewhat as it cools.

14. Allow the suppositories to solidify at room temperature, then place the mold in the refrigerator for about 30 minutes to allow the suppositories to harden. Do not put the mold in the refrigerator until the suppositories have congealed, or the base will contract too rapidly and a thin cavity will form down the center of each suppository.

15. Trim any excess material from the top of the mold using a warm spatula or a razor blade.

16. Perform a quality control check on the suppositories by weighing the finished suppositories. If a large batch of suppositories is molded at one time, a random sample of suppositories can be weighed. Reject any suppositories that are out of the allowed tolerance of target weight ±10%.

17. If you are using a disposable mold as the dispensing wrapper, place the suppositories in a dispensing container. If a reusable mold is used, carefully remove the suppositories from the mold cavities. Wrap each suppository in foil or put in individual small plastic bags and place the suppositories in a dispensing container.

Example 31.2

Procedure when using a density displacement factor:

The preceding procedure assumes that 800 mg of aspirin occupies the same volume as 800 mg of cocoa butter. This is not exactly accurate. In Table 31.1, check the density displacement factor for aspirin with cocoa butter. Notice that aspirin has a density factor (DF) of 1.1 (or 1.3, depending on the reference) with cocoa butter; that is, 1.1 or 1.3 g of aspirin will displace 1 g of cocoa butter. This should be taken into account in calculating the amount of cocoa butter needed for these suppositories.

Procedure:

1. Using the DF for the drug, calculate the amount of base (e.g., cocoa butter) that is displaced by the amount of drug used (e.g., 800 mg aspirin). In this example, because there are two density displacement factors given for aspirin in Table 31.1, an average DF of 1.2 is used.

$$\frac{1.2 \text{ g aspirin}}{1 \text{ g cocoa butter}} = \frac{0.8 \text{ g aspirin}}{x \text{ g cocoa butter}}; x = 0.667 \text{ g cocoa butter displaced by 0.8 g aspirin}$$

2. Based on this amount, calculate the weight of cocoa butter needed for the prescription order:

$$13.76 \text{ g} - 0.667 \text{ g} = 13.093 \text{ g cocoa butter}$$

Therefore, the amount of cocoa butter to weigh in the procedure just given is 13.093 g rather than 12.96 g.

Table 31.1	DENSITY FACTORS FOR COCOA BUTTER SUPPOSITORIES

MEDICATION	FACTOR
Aloin[a]	1.3
Alum	1.7
Aminophylline	1.1
Aminopyrine	1.3
Aspirin[a]	1.3
Aspirin	1.1
Barbital	1.2
Belladonna extract	1.3
Benzoic acid	1.5
Bismuth carbonate	4.5
Bismuth salicylate	4.5
Bismuth subgallate	2.7
Bismuth subnitrate	6.0
Boric acid	1.5
Castor oil	1.0
Chloral hydrate	1.3
Cocaine hydrochloride	1.3
Codeine phosphate[a]	1.1
Digitalis leaf	1.6
Dimenhydrinate[a]	1.3
Diphenhydramine hydrochloride[a]	1.3
Gallic acid	2.0
Glycerin	1.6
Ichthammol	1.1
Iodoform	4.0
Menthol	0.7
Morphine hydrochloride	1.6
Opium	1.4
Paraffin	1.0
Pentobarbital[a]	1.2
Peruvian Balsam[b]	1.1
Phenobarbital	1.2
Phenol[b]	0.9
Potassium bromide	2.2
Potassium iodide	4.5
Procaine	1.2
Quinine hydrochloride	1.2
Resorcinol	1.4
Salicylic acid	1.3
Secobarbital sodium[a]	1.2
Sodium bromide	2.3
Spermaceti	1.0
Sulfathiazole	1.6
Tannic acid	1.6
White wax	1.0
Witch hazel fluid extract	1.1
Zinc oxide	4.0
Zinc sulfate	2.8

[a]From King RE. Dispensing of medication, 9th ed. Easton, PA: Mack Publishing Co., 1984; 96.

[b]Density adjusted taking into account white wax in mass.
Sources: Davis H. Bentley's textbook of pharmaceutics, 5th ed. Baltimore, MD: Williams & Wilkins, 1949; Büchi J, Pharm Acta Helv 1940; 20: 403.

When should you be concerned with compensating for differences in volume displacement? Density factors are important when the following conditions are met:

a. The drug has a quantity dose and is being used for systemic effect. If the drug is being used topically, we just want a certain concentration in contact with the tissue in the body cavity; in this case, very precise quantities per dosage unit are usually not clinically significant.

b. The quantity of drug is a relatively significant portion of the dosage form. For example, if the quantity of drug is 500 mg in a 2-g (2,000-mg) dosage unit, a difference in displacement volume could affect the potency of the finished preparation, but a 5-mg quantity is so small that displacement differences are not significant.

c. A density difference exists between the base and the drug. If the DF for a drug in a base is 1.0, a density displacement calculation is not needed because there is equal displacement of drug for base.

Because we often do not have a DF for the drug and base in question (most of the published factors were determined experimentally long ago and were primarily for cocoa butter and older drugs), it is helpful to analyze the possibilities mathematically so that we can make informed judgments about when to compensate for displacement differences. For example, take the case of cocoa butter and look at the DFs for various drugs with cocoa butter in Table 31.1.

a. Notice that for inorganic substances such as zinc oxide and salts such as sodium bromide, the DFs are all at least 2.0 and many are 4.0 or more. For such a drug as this, unless it is being used topically (as, for example, zinc oxide), the displacement factor should be considered.

b. Now notice organic drugs such as diphenhydramine HCl and codeine phosphate; the DFs for these drugs are lower, in the range of 0.7 to 2.0, with a mean value of 1.3, much closer to the neutral value of 1.0.

c. Now pick a dosage amount per suppository and a reasonable DF and calculate the difference in amount of cocoa butter base per suppository.

Drug amount/suppository = 100 mg   DF = 1.3

Calibration weight of base/suppository = 2.000 g

Calculate the weight of cocoa butter displaced by 100 mg of drug if the DF of the drug with cocoa butter is 1.3:

$$\frac{1.3 \text{ g drug}}{1 \text{ g cocoa butter}} = \frac{0.1 \text{ g drug}}{x \text{ g cocoa butter}}; x = 0.077 \text{ g cocoa butter displaced by 0.1 g drug}$$

Calculate the weight of cocoa butter per suppository if not compensating for DF:

2.000 g weight of suppository

−0.100 g drug

1.900 g cocoa butter needed per suppository

Calculate the weight of cocoa butter per suppository when considering DF:

2.000 g weight of suppository

−0.077 g drug displacement

1.923 g cocoa butter needed/suppository

The difference in weight of cocoa butter per suppository is 23 mg. To put this in perspective, the standard deviation (SD) for suppositories made in aluminum molds was determined by a group of laboratory students to be ±17 mg for cocoa butter and ±22 mg for a PEG base. Weight differences of this magnitude represent a small percent difference, 1% for a 20-mg difference with a 2-g suppository (e.g., 1% × 2,000 mg = 20 mg). Suppositories, because of their method of preparation, do not have exceedingly precise final weights per unit, and small differences in the amount of base material are expected. Fortunately, because their gross weight per unit is relatively large, these small differences are acceptable. In contrast, a 20-mg difference for a 200-mg capsule would represent a 10% difference and would be on the borderline for acceptability.

This exercise can be repeated for various weights of active ingredients and different DFs: For example, when repeated for a DF of 2.0, the base weight difference is approximately double or 50 mg. These values should give you some idea of the point at which it becomes important to consider density displacement. The question then becomes, what can be done when you have a drug for systemic use that has a dose of 100 mg or greater and you have no estimate for its DF? The double-casting method, which is shown next, can be used in this circumstance.

| **Example 31.3** | **Fusion method using a double-casting procedure:** |

The following is an example of a suppository prescription in which the drug makes up a considerable amount of the dosage unit, but the pharmacist does not have a DF for the drug in this base. In such cases as this, a double-casting procedure should be used.

℞	Progesterone	200 mg
	Suppository base	qs
	Dispense 6 vaginal suppositories	

Procedure:

1. Select the base material for this preparation. PEG bases are recommended for vaginal suppositories. Base 5 in Table 24.2 of Chapter 24 has been reported to give good results, and manufactured preformulated PEG suppository bases such as Polybase are acceptable and readily available. The one chosen for this example is PEG base 4 in Table 24.2; this base is 40% PEG 8,000 and 60% PEG 400.

2. Calculate the amount of PEG 8,000 and PEG 400 needed. Because of the loss that will occur in the compounding procedure, an excess amount of base material must be made. In this case, for PEG base with an approximate density of 1.125 g/mL, the minimum needed for eight suppositories (two extras) would be:

$$2 \text{ mL/mold cavity} \times 1.125 \text{ g/mL} \times 8 \text{ suppositories} = 18 \text{ g}$$

Make 30 g of base using the amounts determined below.

PEG 8,000: 40% × 30 g = 12 g PEG 8,000

PEG 8,000 is a solid and can be weighed.

PEG 400: 60% × 30 g = 18 g PEG 400

PEG 400 is a liquid and is usually measured volumetrically. s.g. = 1.125 g/mL.

$$\frac{1.125 \text{ g PEG 400}}{1 \text{ mL PEG 400}} = \frac{18 \text{ g PEG 400}}{x \text{ mL PEG 400}}; x = 16 \text{ mL PEG 400}$$

3. Calculate the amount of active ingredient(s) and excipients needed for the prescription order. Remember to calculate for two extras.

$$8 \times 200 \text{ mg} = 1,600 \text{ mg progesterone}$$

4. If particle size reduction is needed, weigh an excess amount of drug, triturate, and weigh the amount just calculated.

5. Before melting the base and combining the ingredients, prepare the suppository mold. Be certain it is clean. Apply a lubricant to the mold if needed.

6. Put the measured PEGs in a beaker and melt for approximately 1 minute in the microwave oven, or use a warm–water bath and heat to approximately 60°C.

7. Put the weighed drug (1,600 mg progesterone) in a small beaker and add approximately **one-third** of the melted PEG base. The progesterone may melt or dissolve, giving a clear liquid. For drugs that do not melt or dissolve, disperse and suspend the drug throughout the melted base.

8. Pour the drug-base liquid in the **bottoms** of eight or fewer mold cavities. Be sure to get complete transfer of all this material to the mold cavities, because this contains the active ingredient.

9. Qs all eight cavities with extra melted PEG base. Overfill the cavities slightly, because the base will contract somewhat as it cools.

10. Allow the suppositories to solidify at room temperature for about 15 to 20 minutes and then in the refrigerator.

11. Carefully trim and discard excess material from the top of the mold with a razor blade; this trimmed material is extra melted base used to completely fill the cavities and does not contain any drug.

12. Remove the suppositories from the mold cavities. We now have eight suppositories that in total contain 1,600 mg of drug and enough base material for the eight suppositories, but the drug is not uniformly distributed: there may be 150 mg in one suppository and 10 mg or even no drug in another suppository.

13. Put the eight suppositories in a clean beaker and remelt the material. Stir to obtain a homogeneous mixture.

14. Now repour the homogeneous mixture. If there were no loss of material in the beaker, you would get exactly eight suppositories. This is never possible and, furthermore, you need to overfill the cavities to compensate for contraction on cooling. Therefore, pour six or seven nicely filled suppository cavities and repeat the congealing and trimming procedure.

15. If using a disposable mold as a dispensing wrapper, place six suppositories in a dispensing container. If a reusable mold is used, remove the suppositories from the mold cavities, select the six best suppositories, and wrap each suppository in foil or put in individual, small plastic bags and place the suppositories in a dispensing container.

| **Example 31.4** | **Using the double-casting method to determine density displacement factors:** |

In the aforementioned example, if the suppository mold is calibrated with pure PEG base to obtain a mean weight of PEG base per cavity, and the completed suppositories (containing drug) are now weighed to get a mean weight with drug, a density factor for the drug in this PEG base can be calculated. This is useful information because it means that future suppositories of this type can be made with a single casting.

Procedure:

1. Calibrate the mold for the base by pouring five suppositories with pure base, trimming and removing each suppository from its mold cavity, and weighing each. As with example 31.1, note and record the temperature of the melt so that this fusion temperature is used each time suppositories are made with this base and mold and with this calibration weight. In this example, the temperature of the melt is the same as in example 31.3, 60°C, and the average weight per suppository with just PEG base is found to be 2.371 g.

2. Weigh the six progesterone suppositories and calculate a mean weight per suppository. For this example, the mean weight is 2.341 g. Of this 2.341 g, 0.2 g is progesterone and the rest, 2.141 g, is PEG base:

$$2.341 \text{ g progesterone/PEG} - 0.2 \text{ g progesterone} = 2.141 \text{ g PEG}$$

Note: If progesterone had a 1.0 DF, 0.2 g of progesterone would have displaced 0.2 g of PEG and the weight of the progesterone suppositories would have been the same as that of the suppositories made with just PEG base, 2.371 g.

3. Calculate the number of grams of PEG base that was displaced by 0.2 g of progesterone. This is the amount of PEG base in the pure base suppositories minus the amount of PEG base in the progesterone suppositories:

$$2.371 \text{ g} - 2.141 \text{ g} = 0.23 \text{ g of PEG base displaced by 0.2 g progesterone}$$

4. Calculate the DF for progesterone in PEG base. This is the number of grams of drug that will displace 1 g of base.

$$\frac{0.2 \text{ g progesterone}}{0.23 \text{ g PEG base}} = \frac{x \text{ g progesterone}}{1 \text{ g PEG base}}; x = 0.87 \text{ g progesterone displaces 1 g PEG base}$$

Note: The preceding example uses fictitious numbers to illustrate a process for calculating a DF. The actual experimental DFs for progesterone are 1.0 with PEG base and 1.25 in cocoa butter. These known DFs for progesterone in two different bases together with published DFs for drugs in cocoa butter (such as those listed in Table 31.1) have been used to estimate DFs for these other drugs in PEG base. For example, the DF listed for boric acid in cocoa butter is 1.5. The DF of boric acid in PEG base is estimated as follows:

$$\frac{1.0 \text{ DF progesterone in PEG base}}{1.25 \text{ DF progesterone in cocoa butter}} = \frac{x \text{ DF boric acid in PEG base}}{1.5 \text{ DF boric acid in cocoa butter}};$$

$$x = 1.2 \text{ DF for boric acid in PEG base}$$

This value matches closely the DF for boric acid that was experimentally determined to be 1.22. These estimated values should always be verified experimentally.

VI. COMPATIBILITY, STABILITY, AND BEYOND-USE DATING

A. Physical stability: Because suppositories are solid mixtures, this dosage form is quite stable physically. There are few potential problems.

1. The most notable physical stability problem for suppositories involves cocoa butter. It exists in several polymorphic forms that have melting points at or below room temperature. One of these low-melting-point polymorphs can result when cocoa butter is overheated even slightly during the fusion process. Cocoa butter also can have its normal melting point lowered by the addition of some drugs. For more information on cocoa butter incompatibilities, see Chapter 24, Suppository Bases.

2. For all suppositories, but especially those made using bases with low melting points (such as cocoa butter or synthetic fatty-acid bases), a potential physical problem is melting during storage. Proper labeling and patient instructions for storage conditions can address this problem.

B. Chemical stability

1. For suppositories made by fusion, degradation of active ingredients can occur during the heating process. If an active ingredient is labile to this type of instability, consider using a suppository base such as cocoa butter that melts at low temperature or use the hand-rolling method of compounding.

2. PEG bases are incompatible with a large number of drugs, especially those prone to oxidation. PEG also interacts with some plastics such as polystyrene, which is used in some prescription vials, so suppositories dispensed in this type of plastic should first be wrapped in foil or placed in polyethylene plastic bags. Additional information on PEG incompatibilities can be found in the descriptions of PEG in Chapters 23 and 24.

3. Each sample prescription at the end of this chapter considers the chemical stability of each ingredient in the given dosage form and uses this information in assigning a beyond-use date to the preparation. Examples are given that illustrate the use of various reference resources to determine stability and assign beyond-use dates. The topic of chemical stability of drugs and chemicals is addressed in Chapter 37.

C. Beyond-use dating

1. A general discussion on assigning beyond-use dates for solid dosage forms can be found in Chapter 4.

2. For *USP* compounded formulations, a beyond-use date is given in the formulation monograph. Examples include Progesterone Vaginal Suppositories and Morphine Sulfate Suppositories (6).

3. *USP* Chapter ⟨795⟩ has the following general guidelines for compounded solid dosage forms.

> In the absence of stability information that is applicable to a specific drug and preparation, the following maximum beyond-use dates are recommended for nonsterile compounded drug preparations that are packaged in tight, light-resistant containers and stored at controlled room temperature unless otherwise indicated.
>
> **For Nonaqueous Liquids and Solid Formulations—**
> *Where the Manufactured Drug Product is the Source of Active Ingredient*—The beyond-use date is not later than 25% of the time remaining until the product's expiration date or 6 months, whichever is earlier.
> *Where a USP or NF Substance is the Source of Active Ingredient*—The beyond-use date is not later than 6 months. (7)

VII. PATIENT CONSULTATION

A. With suppositories, it is especially important to give the patient or caregiver good instructions on the use and storage of this dosage form. When suppositories are dispensed in foil or plastic wrapping, instruct the patient to remove the wrapping before inserting the suppository. Though this may seem intuitive, there are now special drug delivery devices, such a transdermal systems, that are applied with foil or plastic membranes in place, so explicit instructions are needed.

B. A patient instruction sheet on the proper administration techniques for rectal suppositories is given in Fig. 31.1.

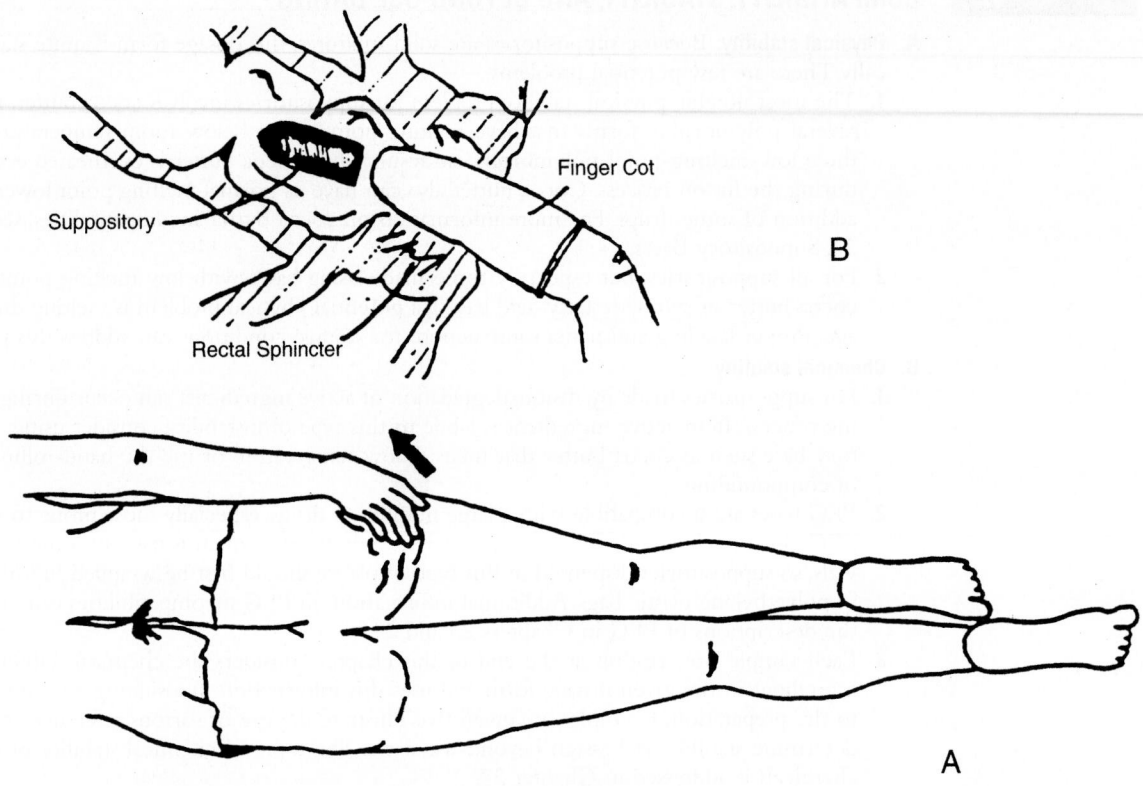

FIGURE 31.1 HOW TO INSERT A RECTAL SUPPOSITORY
1. Wash your hands carefully with soap and warm water.
2. Remove all foil or other wrappings from the suppository to be inserted.
3. Lubricate the tapered (pointed) end of the suppository with a small amount of K-Y Jelly or other type of lubricating gel but *not* petroleum jelly (e.g., Vaseline). If such a lubricant is not available, moisten suppository with a small amount of water.
4. Lie on your side with your lower leg straightened out and upper leg bent forward, toward the stomach. (See drawing A.)
5. Lift upper buttocks to expose rectal area.
6. Gently insert the suppository into your rectum until it passes the sphincter. (About 1/2 to 1 inch in infants and 1 inch in adults.) (See drawing B.)
7. Gentle, persistent pressure allows the suppository to remain in place without discomfort.
8. Hold buttocks together for a few seconds and remain lying down for about 15 minutes.
9. Avoid excessive movement or exercise for approximately 1 hour.
10. Wash your hands after inserting the suppository.
NOTE
Suppositories should be kept in a tightly closed container and stored in a cool place. See package for any further storage instructions.

(Adapted from the Michigan Pharmacists Association's Patient Education Program.)

Sample Prescriptions

SAMPLE PRESCRIPTION 31.1

CASE: Bonnie Toehouse is a 115-lb, 5′1″-tall, 55-year-old patient with a diagnosis of rheumatoid arthritis. An initial trial with ibuprofen was not sufficiently effective, so indomethacin was prescribed. Ms. Toehouse is currently taking indomethacin 25-mg capsules tid, with breakfast, lunch, and dinner, and indomethacin 50-mg suppositories, one-half suppository inserted at bedtime. Her symptoms are currently satisfactorily controlled with this regimen, and she is tolerating the drug well. She has expressed some dissatisfaction with the suppositories: It is difficult and inconvenient to split them in half and she complains of some rectal irritation. On consulting with Pharmacist Billy Butterfield, Dr. Ozzie Wurtz has learned that manufactured indomethacin suppositories are available only in the 50-mg strength, and these suppositories are formulated in a polyethylene glycol base that is irritating to the rectal tissues of some patients. Dr. Butterfield tells Dr. Wurtz that he could make 25-mg suppositories in a blander synthetic cocoa butter base for Ms. Toehouse; however, because indomethacin is generally not as well released from the bland base, they will need to monitor Ms. Toehouse's response. If need be, the dose can be increased and/or the formulation can be modified. Dr. Wurtz feels that it is well worth doing a trial with the compounded suppositories.

CONTEMPORARY PHYSICIANS GROUP PRACTICE
20 S. PARK STREET, TRITURATE, WI 53706
TEL: (608) 555-1333 FAX: (608) 555-1335

R # *123903*

NAME *Bonnie Toehouse*   **DATE** *00/00/00*

ADDRESS *2530 Talbott Trail*   **AGE**   **WT/HT**

R

Indomethacin	*25 mg*	
Fattibase	*qs*	

Dispense 6 suppositories

Sig: Insert 1 supp pr at bedtime for arthritis

B. Butterfield 00/00/00

REFILLS *3*   *Ozzie Wurtz*   **M.D.**

DEA NO. _____

MASTER COMPOUNDING FORMULATION RECORD

NAME, STRENGTH, AND DOSAGE FORM OF PREPARATION: Indomethacin 25 mg Rectal Suppositories

QUANTITY: 6 (plus 2 extra for loss on compounding)　　　**FORMULATION RECORD ID:** SP001

THERAPEUTIC USE/CATEGORY: Nonsteroidal antiinflammatory drug　　**ROUTE OF ADMINISTRATION:** Rectal

INGREDIENTS USED:

Ingredient	Quantity Used	Physical Description	Solubility	Dose Comparison		Use in the Prescription
				Given	Usual	
Indomethacin 25-mg Capsules	8 × 25 mg capsules	white powder	Pract insol in water; 1 g/ 50 mL alcohol	25 mg qid (including oral dose)	25–50 mg 2–3 times daily	arthritis
Fattibase	qs	waxy, white solid	immisc w/water and alcohol	—	—	base

COMPATIBILITY–STABILITY: Indomethacin Suppositories are official in the *USP*, but no suppository base material is specified (6). Indomethacin has been well studied. It undergoes hydrolysis in aqueous solution, and the drug in both solid form and in solution is sensitive to light. Its photodegradation is decreased by storage in light-resistant containers and the use of antioxidants (8). The manufactured suppositories, which use a PEG base, contain the antioxidants butylated hydroxyanisole, butylated hydroxytoluene, and the chelating agent edetic acid (9). The bioavailability of indomethacin in various suppository bases has been studied in rabbits; the fatty-acid base that showed satisfactory release of the drug contained the surfactants sorbitan fatty-acid esters and polyoxyl 40 stearate (4). The commercial fatty-acid base Fattibase contains similar emulsifying and suspending agents, glyceryl monostearate and polyoxyl stearate (10). This suppository preparation is made with just Fattibase, but a sorbitan ester such as Span 80 (sorbitan monooleate) can be added in the future if needed to improve performance of the dosage form. The prescribed suppositories contain no water, so a preservative is not needed.

PACKAGING AND STORAGE: Because indomethacin is photosensitive, these suppositories should be stored in tight, light-resistant containers. Fattibase has a melting point of 96° to 99°F, and the manufacturer of Fattibase recommends storage in the refrigerator.

BEYOND-USE DATE: These suppositories are a solid formulation made with a manufactured dosage form, so use the beyond-use date recommended in *USP* Chapter ⟨795⟩ for such compounded preparations: 6 months or 25% of the time remaining until the product's expiration date, whichever is earlier (7).

CALCULATIONS

Dose/Concentration: The daily dose of three 25-mg capsules and one 25-mg suppository is at target levels and is below the recommended maximum daily dose of 200 mg.

Ingredient Amounts

The procedure for this preparation uses the double-casting method. Although the quantity of drug per suppository is only 25 mg, this prescription uses the material in indomethacin capsules, which contains excipients in addition to the drug, and the powder per unit weighs more than 100 mg. Because the double-casting method is used, no precalibration of the mold cavities for the base is needed unless Pharmacist Butterfield wants to calculate a DF for indomethacin capsule powder with Fattibase. Because this preparation is for an initial trial, a DF will not be calculated at this time.

Because a whole number of capsules is needed (25 mg of indomethacin per dose and indomethacin available as 25-mg capsules), there are no necessary calculations for amount of active ingredients: Use the contents of eight indomethacin 25-mg capsules for eight suppositories.

An estimation of total weight of Fattibase is needed so that a sufficient amount of Fattibase can be melted. In this case, because material for eight suppositories is being made and a standard mold for rectal suppositories with 2 mL per mold cavity is used, an amount in excess of 14.24 g of Fattibase should be melted:

Fattibase has a s.g. of 0.89 at 37°C (10).

$$8 \text{ supp} \times 2 \text{ mL/supp} \times 0.89 \text{ g/mL} = 14.24 \text{ g Fattibase at minimum needed}$$

In the procedure that follows, 20 g of Fattibase is melted.

MSDS AND SAFETY AND PERSONAL PROTECTIVE EQUIPMENT: Don a clean lab coat and disposable gloves.

SPECIALIZED EQUIPMENT: Aluminum suppository mold; all weighing is done on a class III torsion balance.

COMPOUNDING PROCEDURE: Open a rectal suppository mold and spray the interior very lightly with vegetable oil spray. Reassemble the mold. Empty the contents of eight indomethacin 25-mg capsules and place the powder in a small beaker. Weigh approximately 20 g of Fattibase, put it in a clean beaker or crucible, and melt the Fattibase on a hot-water bath to 50° to 53°C. Add about one-third of the melted Fattibase to the indomethacin powder in the beaker and stir to mix. It may be necessary to stir until the mixture is near its congealing point so that the indomethacin capsule powder remains suspended and maintains a uniform, homogeneous mixture. Note and record the temperature on the melt, 48°C. Pour the mixture into the bottom of eight or fewer mold cavities. If necessary, reheat the mixture and add some extra Fattibase so that all of the mixture with indomethacin can be poured into mold cavities. Fill the eight cavities with extra Fattibase that is at the same temperature as is recorded for the indomethacin–Fattibase mixture. Let the suppositories solidify and then finish hardening them in the refrigerator. Remove and trim excess Fattibase material from the top of the mold with a razor blade. Remove the eight suppositories from the mold and remelt. Stir the mixture to obtain a homogeneous mix. When the melt is at the recorded temperature of 48°C, repour it into six or seven cavities. As before, let the suppositories solidify and then put them in a refrigerator for 15 to 20 minutes to harden. Trim the excess material from the top of the mold with a razor blade and remove the suppositories. Select the six best suppositories; weigh each and record the weight. Wrap each suppository in foil and dispense in a tight, light-resistant container.

DESCRIPTION OF FINISHED PREPARATION: The suppositories are opaque white with a smooth surface.

QUALITY CONTROL: Weigh and record the weight of each suppository; the mean weight should be close to the estimated weight of 1.78 g for 2-mL suppositories made with base material having a specific gravity of 0.89. The temperature of the melt at pouring is recorded as 48°C.

MASTER FORMULA PREPARED BY: Billy Butterfield, PharmD   **CHECKED BY:** Robert Schwartz, RPh

COMPOUNDING RECORD

NAME, STRENGTH, AND DOSAGE FORM OF PREPARATION: Indomethacin 25 mg Rectal Suppositories
QUANTITY: 6 (plus 2 extras)   **DATE PREPARED:** mm/dd/yy   **BEYOND-USE DATE:** mm/dd/yy
FORMULATION RECORD ID: SP001   **CONTROL/RX NUMBER:** 123903

INGREDIENTS USED:

Ingredient	Quantity Used	Manufacturer Lot Number	Expiration Date	Weighed/ Measured by	Checked by
Indomethacin 25-mg Capsules	8 × 25 mg capsules	BJF Generics SP3111	mm/yy	bjf	bb
Fattibase	qs	Paddock Labs SP3112	mm/yy	bjf	bb

QUALITY CONTROL: The suppositories are opaque white with a smooth surface. Each suppository was weighed and the weight was recorded as shown in the chart that follows.

1.786 g	1.779 g	1.792 g	1.796 g	1.764 g	1.777 g	$\bar{X}$ = 1.782 g

The mean weight was 1.782 g, which is very close to the estimated weight of 1.78 g for 2-mL suppositories made with base material having a specific gravity of 0.89. The temperature of the melt at pouring was recorded at 48°C.

LABELING

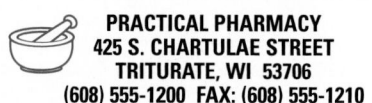

PRACTICAL PHARMACY
425 S. CHARTULAE STREET
TRITURATE, WI 53706
(608) 555-1200 FAX: (608) 555-1210

℞ 123903   Pharmacist: BB   Date: 00/00/00
Bonnie Toehouse   Dr. Ozzie Wurtz
Insert one suppository rectally at bedtime for arthritis.
Indomethacin 25 mg Rectal Suppositories
Mfg: Compounded   Quantity: 6 suppositories
Refills: 3   Discard after: Give date

Auxiliary Labels: For rectal use. Keep in the refrigerator. May cause drowsiness, dizziness. Keep out of the reach of children. This medicine was compounded in our pharmacy for you at the direction of your prescriber.

PATIENT CONSULTATION: Hello, Ms. Toehouse. I'm your pharmacist, Billy Butterfield. Do you have any drug allergies? Are you taking any other medications? What did Dr. Wurtz tell you about these suppositories? These are indomethacin suppositories for your arthritis. They have been specially formulated for you with a nonirritating suppository base ingredient that hopefully will be more comfortable for you. They are also exactly the correct strength so that you will not have to cut these in half. You are to unwrap and insert one suppository rectally at bedtime. I know that you have been using suppositories. Do you have any questions about how to use these? As I mentioned, these are custom-made suppositories, and we can make changes to the formula if you think that they are not adequately controlling your arthritis: Please call Dr. Wurtz or me if you have any concerns. As you know, for arthritis you should be sure to use these and your indomethacin capsules on a regularly scheduled basis to reduce the pain and inflammation in your joints. Have you experienced any side effects with indomethacin, such as drowsiness, dizziness, or stomach or intestinal upset? If you get hives, shortness of breath, tightness in your chest, or any unusual reaction including headaches and skin rash, call Dr. Wurtz immediately, as this could indicate a rare but more serious side effect. Keep these in the refrigerator and out of the reach of children. Discard any unused suppositories after 6 months (or 25% rule). You may have this prescription refilled three times. Because these have to be specially made in our pharmacy, it would be helpful if you would call in advance of when you need them so we can have them ready when you need them. Do you have any questions?

SAMPLE PRESCRIPTION 31.2

CASE: Joseph Draheim is a 37-lb, 40″-tall, 3-year-old with a diagnosis of viral laryngotracheobronchitis (viral croup). He has a fever, stridor, and the cough typical of this disease. Although viral croup is self-limiting and usually resolves in several days without treatment, the cough and stridor are difficult for the child and the parents; it is frightening and no one gets much rest while the symptoms persist. Supportive treatment is appropriate, and systemic corticosteroids can be used to alleviate the inflammatory edema and the resulting airway narrowing that causes the stridor and hoarse cough. The usual treatment is dexamethasone, 0.6 mg/kg in a single dose (11). Dr. Hokey has asked Pharmacist Bobby Schwartz to compound the dexamethasone in suppository form because the standard manufactured elixir is 0.5 mg/5 mL, which gives a volume too large (100 mL) for Joseph to comfortably consume and, while the concentrated oral solution (0.5 mg/0.5 mL) gives a more reasonable volume (10 mL), the alcohol content is too high (30%) for this child.* An IM injection would be another alternative, but Dr. Hokey and Joseph's mother want to avoid giving Joe "a shot." Making a powder packet (chartulae) by crushing an appropriate amount of dexamethasone tablets and giving this powder with soft food offers one reasonable alternative to the suppository.

---

*The American Academy of Pediatrics Committee on Drugs has recommended that the quantity of ethanol contained in a single dose of a drug product or preparation should not be able to cause a blood concentration greater than 25 mg/100 mL. Their published article, "Ethanol in Liquid Preparations Intended for Children" gives equations and tables of values that allow prescribers and pharmacists to calculate the volumes and concentrations of preparations containing alcohol that will result in safe blood concentrations in children. The equation used is:

$$\text{Dose } (D) = \text{Plasma concentration } (Cp) \times \text{Volume of distribution } (Vd)$$

where D is quantity of alcohol in mg, Cp is blood ethanol concentration of 250 mg/L, and Vd is 0.6 L/kg $\times$ patient body weight (in kg) (12).

For our patient, D is calculated to be:

$$\left(\frac{250 \text{ mg}}{L}\right)\left(\frac{0.6 \text{ L}}{\text{kg}}\right)\left(\frac{\text{kg}}{2.2 \text{ lb}}\right)\left(\frac{37 \text{ lb}}{1}\right) = 2{,}523 \text{ mg ethanol}$$

Using the $d_4^{20} = 0.789$ g/mL value for absolute ethanol, this equates to 3.2 mL of ethanol. The dose of dexamethasone concentrate for our patient is 10 mL and, with an ethanol concentration of 30%, this gives 3 mL of absolute ethanol, much too close to the maximum allowed volume of 3.2 mL.

CONTEMPORARY PHYSICIANS GROUP PRACTICE
20 S. PARK STREET, TRITURATE, WI 53706
TEL: (608) 555-1333 FAX: (608) 555-1335

℞ #   *123906*

NAME *Joseph Draheim*   **DATE** *00/00/00*

ADDRESS *623 San Francisco Circle*

℞
Dexamethasone   10 mg
Cocoa Butter   qs

Disp. 1 Supp.

Sig: Insert 1 supp pr for symptoms of croup

B. Schwartz 00/00/00

REFILLS *NR*   *Hokey*   **M.D.**

DEA NO.

MASTER COMPOUNDING FORMULATION RECORD

NAME, STRENGTH, AND DOSAGE FORM OF PREPARATION: Dexamethasone 10 mg Rectal Suppositories (as Dexamethasone Sodium Phosphate)

QUANTITY: 6 (plus 2 extra for loss on compounding)   **FORMULATION RECORD ID:** SP002

THERAPEUTIC USE/CATEGORY: Corticosteroid   **ROUTE OF ADMINISTRATION:** Rectal

INGREDIENTS USED:

Ingredient	Quantity Used	Physical Description	Solubility	Dose Comparison		Use in the Prescription
				Given	Usual	
Dexamethasone as Dexamethasone Sodium Phosphate	80 mg dexamethasone as 104 mg dex Na phos	white crystalline powder	0.5 g/mL in water; sl sol in alcohol	0.6 mg/kg 1×	0.6 mg/kg 1×	antiinflammatory agent
Cocoa Butter	7.896 g	light yellow, waxy solid	insol. in water; sl sol in alcohol	—	—	base, vehicle

COMPATIBILITY–STABILITY: Dexamethasone and its salts are sensitive to heat (13), so hand-rolled suppositories will be compounded. The parent drug dexamethasone is hydrophobic and practically insoluble in water, but the sodium phosphate salt is freely soluble in water (13). As a result, free dexamethasone would be predicted to have poor and variable release and absorption from the lipophilic cocoa butter, while release of the soluble salt from this suppository base should be more satisfactory, and so this will be the form used. Because the dose is based on the quantity of the free dexamethasone, a calculation must be made to determine the equivalent quantity of the salt form. This is a nonaqueous formulation, so a preservative is not needed.

PACKAGING AND STORAGE: Packaging for dexamethasone in tight, light-resistant containers is recommended (13). Cocoa butter suppositories should be stored at controlled room temperature or in a cold place. Package the suppository in a tight, amber vial and label that the package be stored in the refrigerator.

BEYOND-USE DATE: These suppositories are a solid formulation made with a *USP* active ingredient, so use the beyond-use date recommended in *USP* Chapter ⟨795⟩ for such compounded preparations: 6 months (7).

CALCULATIONS

Dose/Concentration: The pediatric dose of dexamethasone for croup is 0.6 mg/kg given in one dose.

This patient has a body weight of 37 lb; his weight (in kg) is:

$$\text{Body weight (in kg):} \frac{37 \text{ lb}}{2.2 \text{ lb/kg}} = 16.8 \text{ kg}$$

Dose of dexamethasone (in mg): 0.6 mg/kg $\times$ 16.8 kg = 10 mg

The active ingredient to be used is dexamethasone sodium phosphate (MW = 516). The quantity of this salt that is equivalent to 10 mg dexamethasone (MW = 392) is calculated to be:

$$\frac{392 \text{ mg dexameth}}{516 \text{ mg dexameth} - \text{Na PO}_4} = \frac{10 \text{ mg dexameth}}{x \text{ mg dexameth} - \text{Na PO}_4}; x = 13 \text{ mg dexameth} - \text{Na PO}_4$$

Ingredient Amounts

Although only one suppository is needed for this prescription, a small batch will be made and kept in the pharmacy for other anticipated prescription orders. A 6-month beyond-use date will be given to this stock supply.

These suppositories are being made by the hand-rolling method. They are made to be 1 g each because they are for a 3-year-old child.

Total weight for eight suppositories:

$$1 \text{ g/supp} \times 8 \text{ suppositories} = 8 \text{ g total}$$

Weight (in mg) of dexamethasone sodium phosphate for eight suppositories:

$$13 \text{ mg/supp} \times 8 \text{ suppositories} = 104 \text{ mg dexamethasone sodium phosphate}$$

The dexamethasone sodium phosphate is available as the pure powder.

Weight (in g) of cocoa butter base for eight suppositories:

$$8 \text{ g} - 0.104 \text{ g dexamethasone sodium phosphate} = 7.896 \text{ g cocoa butter}$$

MSDS AND SAFETY AND PERSONAL PROTECTIVE EQUIPMENT: Review MSDS for all components. Don a clean lab coat and disposable gloves. Avoid inhaling dexamethasone sodium phosphate powder.

SPECIALIZED EQUIPMENT: All weighing is done on an electronic balance.

COMPOUNDING PROCEDURE: Weigh 104 mg of dexamethasone sodium phosphate powder and transfer to a glass mortar. Weigh 7.896 g of cocoa butter. Add a small amount of finely shaved cocoa butter to the dexamethasone powder and triturate well. Add the rest of the finely shaved cocoa butter by geometric dilution and triturate well to form a plastic mass. Remove the mass from the mortar and place it in a piece of clean white filter paper. Knead the material to form a plastic mass. Transfer the mass to an ointment slab and, using a clean pill roller, roll the mass into a cylindric pipe that is slightly longer than 6 inches. Using a clean razor blade, cut off the irregular ends of the pipe and then cut the pipe into six equal pieces. Shape with one pointed end and weigh each piece (each should weigh 1 g ±10%). Cut off any excess with a razor blade. Put each suppository in a zipper-closure bag. Dispense one unit in an amber vial with a tight, child-resistant closure. Put the other suppositories in a similar container that is labeled appropriately (drug name and quantity, date compounded, and control number), and store in the refrigerator.

DESCRIPTION OF FINISHED PREPARATION: The suppositories are light yellow cylinders with a tapered point on one end.

QUALITY CONTROL: Weigh and record the weight of each suppository. Each should weigh 1 g ±10%.

MASTER FORMULA PREPARED BY: Bobby J. Schwartz, PharmD

CHECKED BY: Robert W. Schwartz, RPh

COMPOUNDING RECORD

NAME, STRENGTH, AND DOSAGE FORM OF PREPARATION: Dexamethasone 10 mg Rectal Suppositories (as Dexamethasone Sodium Phosphate)

QUANTITY: 6 (plus 2 extra for loss)   **DATE PREPARED:** mm/dd/yy   **BEYOND-USE DATE:** mm/dd/yy

FORMULATION RECORD ID: SP002   **CONTROL/RX NUMBER:** 123906

INGREDIENTS USED:

Ingredient	Quantity Used	Manufacturer Lot Number	Expiration Date	Weighed/ Measured by	Checked by
Dexamethasone as Dexamethasone Sodium Phosphate	80 mg examethasone as 104 mg dex Na phos	JET Labs SP3121	mm/yy	bjf	bs
Cocoa Butter	7.896 g	JET Labs SP3122	mm/yy	bjf	bs

QUALITY CONTROL: The suppositories are light yellow cylinders with a tapered point on one end. Each suppository is approximately 1″ long, and the weight of each was recorded in the chart given here. All were within tolerance of 1 g ±10%

1.086 g	1.058 g	0.972 g	0.996 g	1.064 g	1.077 g	$\bar{X}$ = 1.042 g

LABELING

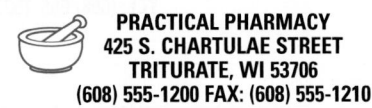

PRACTICAL PHARMACY
425 S. CHARTULAE STREET
TRITURATE, WI 53706
(608) 555-1200 FAX: (608) 555-1210

℞ 123906   Pharmacist: BS   Date: 00/00/00
Joseph Draheim   Dr. Hokey

Insert one suppository rectally for croup.

Dexamethasone 10 mg Rectal Suppositories (as Dexamethasone
Sodium Phosphate)

Mfg: Compounded   Quantity: 1 suppository

Refills: None   Discard after: Give date

Auxiliary Labels: For rectal use. Keep in the refrigerator.
This medicine was compounded in our pharmacy for you
at the direction of your prescriber.

PATIENT CONSULTATION: Hello, Mrs. Draheim, I'm Bobby Schwartz, the pharmacist who prepared Joseph's prescription. Does Joseph have any drug allergies? Is he taking any other medications? What did Dr. Hokey tell you about this medicine and how to use it? This is a dexamethasone suppository to treat the inflammation and swelling in Joe's throat that is causing his cough and wheezing. To use this, unwrap the suppository and insert it rectally. Hold it in place for a few moments to allow it to melt. Have you used suppositories before? I will give you an instruction sheet that will give you some helpful hints on administration techniques (see Fig. 31.1). Joe should need only one dose, and he should be feeling better in 1 to 3 days. If he does not seem to be experiencing relief, or if his condition does not improve in a few days, contact Dr. Hokey. These suppositories are sensitive to heat and will melt above about 85°F, so if you do not give this immediately, store it in a cool place or the refrigerator and out of reach of children. There are no refills but, as I say, you should not need any additional medication for this. Joe should be better soon. Do you have any questions?

SAMPLE PRESCRIPTION 31.3

CASE: Rod Robinson is a 170-lb, 5′10″-tall 72-year-old man with a diagnosis of metastatic prostate cancer. Until now, his pain has been controlled by a combination of medications including oral oxycodone 5 mg with acetaminophen 325 mg, fentanyl patches and, more recently, with oral hydromorphone 4 to 6 mg q3h. Now Mr. Robinson is no longer able to swallow his medications. Dr. Paque wants more control than is possible with fentanyl patches, and he wants to avoid using parenteral (IM or IV) therapy as long as possible. Dr. Paque would like to switch Mr. Robinson's hydromorphone to rectal suppositories 6 mg q3h prn for pain. Because this drug is available commercially only as 3-mg suppositories, Pharmacist Jean Jones has agreed to compound the 6-mg hydromorphone suppositories for Mr. Robinson.

CONTEMPORARY PHYSICIANS GROUP PRACTICE
20 S. PARK STREET, TRITURATE, WI 53706
TEL: (608) 555-1333 FAX: (608) 555-1335

℞ # *123932*

NAME *Rod Robinson*   DATE *00/00/00*

ADDRESS *312 Campfire Trail*

℞
                          Hydromorphone HCl   6 mg
                          Fattibase   qs

                          #6 Suppositories

                                                        Jean Jones 00/00/00

                    Sig: Insert 1 supp pr q 3 hr prn pain

REFILLS *NR*   *Henry Paque*   M.D.

                              DEA NO.   *AP3296577*

MASTER COMPOUNDING FORMULATION RECORD

NAME, STRENGTH, AND DOSAGE FORM OF PREPARATION: Hydromorphone HCl 6 mg Rectal Suppositories
QUANTITY: 6 (plus 2 extra for loss on compounding)   **FORMULATION RECORD ID:** SP003
THERAPEUTIC USE/CATEGORY: Narcotic analgesic   **ROUTE OF ADMINISTRATION:** Rectal

INGREDIENTS USED:

Ingredient	Quantity Used	Physical Description	Solubility	Dose Comparison		Use in the Prescription
				Given	Usual	
Hydromor-phone HCl	120 mg weighed, 48 mg used	white powder	1 g/3 mL water	6 mg rectally q3h	3–6 mg rectally q3h	narcotic analgesic
Silica Gel	240 mg weighed, 96 mg used	fine, white granular powder	insol in water and alcohol	—	—	diluent, suspending agent, disintegrant
Fattibase	15.2 g	white waxy solid	immis w/ water and alcohol	—	—	base, vehicle

COMPATIBILITY–STABILITY: Although not an official *USP* product, manufactured Hydromorphone HCl suppositories are available; these suppositories are in a cocoa butter base with silicon dioxide (14). The chemical structure of hydromorphone (with a phenolic group) would indicate that it may be subject to oxidation, and the manufactured aqueous solutions of the drug contain antioxidants and chelating agents. The drug appears to be quite stable, as it is available commercially in aqueous solution. In this formulation, the hydromorphone HCl is in a nonaqueous, inert type of suppository base, Fattibase, and should be compatible and stable. This is a nonaqueous formulation, so a preservative is not needed.

PACKAGING AND STORAGE: The *USP* monograph for Hydromorphone HCl Tablets recommends storage in tight, light-resistant containers (6), so dispense these suppositories in a suitable tight, amber vial. Fattibase has a melting point of 96° to 99°F, and the manufacturer of Fattibase recommends storage in the refrigerator (9).

BEYOND-USE DATE: These suppositories are a nonaqueous solid dosage form made with a *USP* ingredient, so use the *USP* Chapter ⟨795⟩ recommended beyond-use date of 6 months (7).

CALCULATIONS

Dose/Concentration: Dose okay for the intended purpose.

Ingredient Amounts: Amounts are for eight suppositories, including two extra. This method uses fusion with a calibrated mold.

Determine the mean weight of Fattibase per mold cavity:

On a warm-water bath, slowly heat the Fattibase to approximately 50° to 53°C to completely melt the base. Remove the container from the warm-water bath and allow the base to cool to 48°C; record this temperature. Pour the pure Fattibase into five mold cavities. Allow this to solidify and then trim and remove the suppositories. Weigh each suppository on digital balance (see weights recorded here). Calculate the mean weight of Fattibase per cavity.

Suppository 1	1.911 g
Suppository 2	1.918 g
Suppository 3	1.923 g
Suppository 4	1.903 g
Suppository 5	<u>1.934 g</u>
	9.589 g

Mean weight per suppository:

$$9.589 \text{ g Fattibase/5 suppositories} = 1.918 \text{ g Fattibase/suppository}$$

Weight of hydromorphone HCl (in mg): 6 mg/suppository $\times$ 8 suppositories = 48 mg

This amount is below the MWQ for a class III torsion balance, so a dilution and aliquot must be made. Hydromorphone HCl is a controlled substance, so a minimum amount should be weighed, 120 mg. Silica gel may be used as the diluent so that it can also serve as a suspending and dispersing agent. A convenient amount of silica gel to use would be 240 mg.

Total amount of dilution:

$$120 \text{ mg hydromorphone} + 240 \text{ mg silica gel} = 360 \text{ mg dilution}$$

Amount of dilution that will contain 48 mg of hydromorphone HCl:

$$\frac{120 \text{ mg hydromorphone}}{360 \text{ mg dilution}} = \frac{48 \text{ mg hydromorphone}}{x \text{ mg dilution}}; x = 144 \text{ mg dilution}$$

Weight of Fattibase for eight suppositories:

Note: Because the amount of hydromorphone HCl–silica gel dilution is small in comparison to the weight of the base (18 mg in 2 g), any difference in displacement on a gram-for-gram basis is negligible. Therefore, neither a DF nor the double-casting method is needed.

Multiply the mean weight per cavity by the number of suppositories desired and subtract the weight of the hydromorphone HCl aliquot. This is the amount of Fattibase needed for the preparation.

Total weight for eight suppositories:

$$8 \text{ suppositories} \times 1.918 \text{ g/suppository} = 15.344 \text{ g for 8 suppositories}$$

Weight of Fattibase for eight suppositories:

$$15.344 \text{ g} - 0.144 \text{ g hydromorphone aliquot} = 15.2 \text{ g Fattibase needed}$$

Because hydromorphone HCl is a controlled substance in C-II, it is required to have an accurate accounting of the drug weighed, dispensed, and discarded in making excess material to compensate for loss during compounding:

Amount weighed: 120 mg

Amount dispensed: 36 mg

Amount discarded: 84 mg

MSDS AND SAFETY AND PERSONAL PROTECTIVE EQUIPMENT: Review MSDS for all components. Don a clean lab coat and disposable gloves.

SPECIALIZED EQUIPMENT: Aluminum suppository mold; all weighing is done on a class III torsion balance.

COMPOUNDING PROCEDURE: Open a rectal suppository mold and spray the interior very lightly with vegetable oil spray. Reassemble the mold. Weigh 120 mg of hydromorphone HCl and 240 mg of silica gel. Put the hydromorphone in a mortar and add the silica gel using geometric dilution. Weigh 144 mg of this mixture and place it in a beaker. Weigh 15.2 g of grated Fattibase. Place the beaker containing the hydromorphone aliquot on a warm-water bath and add the grated Fattibase to the beaker in portions, melting the Fattibase with each addition. When all the Fattibase has been added, stir to mix and continue stirring until the mixture is 50°C and the mixture is uniform. Remove the container of melt from the warm-water bath and stir the mixture while allowing the melt to reach 48°C. Pour the melt into seven mold cavities, overfilling slightly. Let the mixture solidify at room temperature, then place in the refrigerator to harden. When hardened, trim excess material from the top of the mold with a razor blade. Remove the suppositories from the mold cavities. Select the six best suppositories and weigh and record the weight of each as a quality control measure. Seal each suppository individually in a zipper-closure polyethylene bag. Dispense in an amber prescription vial with a tight, child-resistant closure.

DESCRIPTION OF FINISHED PREPARATION: The suppositories are opaque, white with a smooth surface.

QUALITY CONTROL: Weigh and record the weight of each suppository; the weight of each suppository should be close to the calibrated weight of 1.918 g. Record the temperature of the melt at pouring (should be approximately 48°C).

MASTER FORMULA PREPARED BY: Jean Jones, PharmD   **CHECKED BY:** Robert Schwartz, RPh

COMPOUNDING RECORD

NAME, STRENGTH, AND DOSAGE FORM OF PREPARATION: Hydromorphone HCl 6 mg Rectal Suppositories

QUANTITY: 6 (plus 2 extras) **DATE PREPARED:** mm/dd/yy **BEYOND-USE DATE:** mm/dd/yy

FORMULATION RECORD ID: SP003 **CONTROL/RX NUMBER:** 123932

INGREDIENTS USED:

Ingredient	Quantity Used	Manufacturer Lot Number	Expiration Date	Weighed/ Measured by	Checked by
Hydromorph-one HCl	120 mg weighed, 48 mg used	JET Labs SP3131	mm/yy	bjf	jj
Silica Gel	240 mg weighed, 96 mg used	JET Labs SP3132	mm/yy	bjf	jj
Fattibase	15.2 g	Paddock Labs SP3112	mm/yy	bjf	jj

QUALITY CONTROL: The suppositories are opaque, white with a smooth surface. Each suppository was weighed and the weight was recorded in the chart that follows.

1.956 g	1.979 g	1.892 g	1.896 g	1.884 g	1.877 g	$\bar{X}$ = 1.914 g

All units are within the allowed tolerance of 1.918 g $\pm$10% (1.726 to 2.11 g). The temperature of the melt at pouring was recorded at 48°C.

LABELING

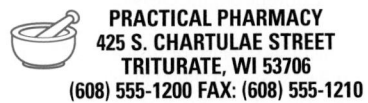

PRACTICAL PHARMACY
425 S. CHARTULAE STREET
TRITURATE, WI 53706
(608) 555-1200 FAX: (608) 555-1210

Rx 123932 Pharmacist: JJ Date: 00/00/00
Rod Robinson Dr. Henry Paque

Insert one suppository rectally every three hours as needed for pain.

Hydromorphone HCl 6 mg Rectal Suppositories

Mfg: Compounded Quantity: 6 suppositories

Refills: None Discard after: Give date

Auxiliary Labels: For rectal use. Keep in the refrigerator May cause drowsiness, dizziness. Federal do not transfer label. This medicine was compounded in our pharmacy for you at the direction of your prescriber.

PATIENT CONSULTATION: Hello, Mrs. Robinson. I'm your pharmacist, Jean Jones. Does Mr. Robinson have any drug allergies? I know that Mr. Robinson has been taking several other medications. Can you please tell me what he currently is using; I want to make sure these new suppositories do not interact or interfere with any of his other medications. What did Dr. Paque tell you about this medication? These are hydromorphone suppositories, and they will act similarly to the oral tablets Mr. Robinson has been taking recently. These should give him good relief from his pain. As with his other pain medications, this drug usually causes drowsiness, so don't be alarmed if he feels this effect. On the positive side, these will help him to sleep; however, we want him to feel comfortable and sufficiently alert when he wants to be awake. Other medications, either prescription or nonprescription, that cause drowsiness will intensify this effect, so be sure to consult Dr. Paque or me before using something like that. For example, if you have any hydromorphone tablets or fentanyl patches left, you would not want to use them with these suppositories unless you first check with Dr. Paque. Medications such as this one sometimes cause stomach upset, even if taken rectally. If this should happen, call Dr. Paque. To administer a dose, unwrap and insert one suppository rectally. This may be repeated every 3 hours if needed for pain. Have you ever given suppositories before? Here is a sheet of helpful instructions (see Fig. 31.1). Do not exceed the prescribed dose; if these are not controlling Mr. Robinson's pain for 3 hours, call Dr. Paque. Store these in a refrigerator and out of the reach of children. Discard unused medication after 6 months (give date), but be sure to remove the identifying label from the container first. While there are no refills indicated on the label, Dr. Paque wants to be sure that Mr. Robinson's pain is controlled, so when you need more please contact Dr. Paque or me. Because these are specially made in our pharmacy for Mr. Robinson, it would be best to call ahead when you are close to running out. Do you have any questions?

REFERENCES

1. The United States Pharmacopeial Convention, Inc. Chapter ⟨1151⟩. 2008 USP 31/NF 26. Rockville, MD: Author, 2007; 622–623.
2. Marshall K, Foster TS, Carlin HS, Williams RL. Development of a compendial taxonomy and glossary for pharmaceutical dosage forms. Pharmacopeial forum. Rockville, MD: The United States Pharmacopeial Convention, Inc., 2003; 29(5).
3. Plaxco Jr JM. Suppositories. In: King RE, ed. Dispensing of medications, 9th ed. Easton, PA: Mack Publishing Co., 1984; 93.
4. Yamazaki M, Soichi I, Sasaki N, et al. Comparison of three test methods for suppositories. Pharmacopeial forum. Rockville, MD: The United States Pharmacopeial Convention, Inc., 1991; Sept–Oct; 2427–2437.
5. Connors KA, Amidon GL, Stella VJ. Chemical stability of pharmaceuticals, 2nd ed. New York: John Wiley & Sons, 1986; 229.
6. The United States Pharmacopeial Convention, Inc. USP monographs. 2008 USP 31/NF 26. Rockville, MD: Author, 2007.
7. The United States Pharmacopeial Convention, Inc. Chapter ⟨795⟩. 2008 USP 31/NF 26. Rockville, MD: Author, 2007; 316–317.
8. Connors KA, Amidon GL, Stella VJ. Chemical Stability of Pharmaceuticals, 2nd ed. New York: John Wiley & Sons, 1986; 509–516.
9. Physicians' Desk Reference, 58th ed. Montvale, NJ: Thomson PDR, 2004; 2000.
10. Fattibase™ Product Data Sheet. Paddock Laboratories, Minneapolis, MN.
11. Blanchard N. Pediatric infectious diseases. In: Koda-Kimble MA, Young LY, eds. Applied therapeutics, 7th ed. Baltimore, MD: Lippincott Williams & Wilkins, 2001; 94.18.
12. American Academy of Pediatrics Committee on Drugs. Ethanol in liquid preparations intended for children. Pediatrics 1984; 73: 405–407.
13. Trissel LA. Trissel's stability of compounded formulations, 3rd ed. Washington, DC: American Pharmacists Association, 2005; 135–138.
14. Physicians' Desk Reference, 58th ed. Montvale, NJ: Thomson PDR, 2004; 446–450.

Part 6

*Sterile Dosage Forms
and Their Preparation*

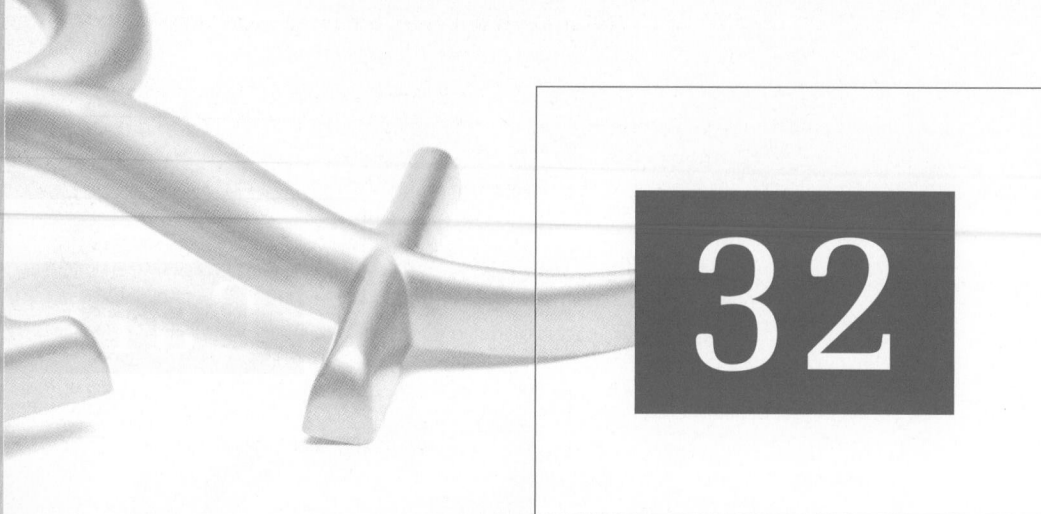

32

General Principles of Sterile Dosage Form Preparation

Gordon S. Sacks, PharmD, BCNSP

I. INTRODUCTION

A primary responsibility of the pharmacist is to ensure safe sterile dosage form preparation. Compounding an accurate formulation free of microbial and particulate matter is an essential component of this process. A number of procedures have been developed by such organizations as the USP and the American Society of Health-System Pharmacists (ASHP) to assist pharmacists in complying with sterile preparation admixture guidelines. As was described in Chapter 12 of this book, the USP is a private, nonprofit organization recognized by the federal government as the official group responsible for setting national standards for drug purity and safety. Most recently, the USP has become involved with issuing standards on the pharmaceutical compounding of sterile preparations. On January 1, 2004, the USP formally adopted Chapter ⟨797⟩, the first official chapter enforceable by regulatory agencies concerning the procedures and requirements for compounded sterile preparations (CSPs). Much of the same information was previously published as recommendations in nonenforceable materials including *USP* Chapter ⟨1206⟩, which focused on dispensing for home care, and *ASHP Guidelines on Quality Assurance for Pharmacy-Prepared Sterile Products*, which gave standards and procedures for sterile dosage form preparation in hospitals and institutional settings. Since 2005, Chapter ⟨797⟩ has undergone major revision and, in December 2007, a new and expanded document was posted on the USP's Internet Web site. These revised standards take effect on June 1, 2008; they were published in the *2008 USP Pharmacists' Pharmacopeia* and are scheduled for publication in the *2009 USP 32/NF 27*.

The following is a summary of guidelines necessary for accurate and safe preparation of CSPs. For a more complete discussion of this topic, refer to *USP* Chapter ⟨797⟩, which is now considered to be the standard of practice for this area of pharmaceutical compounding (1).

II.   DEFINITIONS

A. **Ante-area:** an area adjacent to the clean room, which, although of high quality, may have a lesser air cleanliness classification than does the clean room. The ante-area should be maintained as an International Organization for Standardization (ISO) Class 8 or higher (see Table 32.1 for ISO classifications). Activities in the ante-area include such things as hand washing and gowning and unpacking of clean-room supply packages. Cardboard boxes and other packaging materials are not brought into clean rooms, because opening and handling them introduces particulates into the environment.

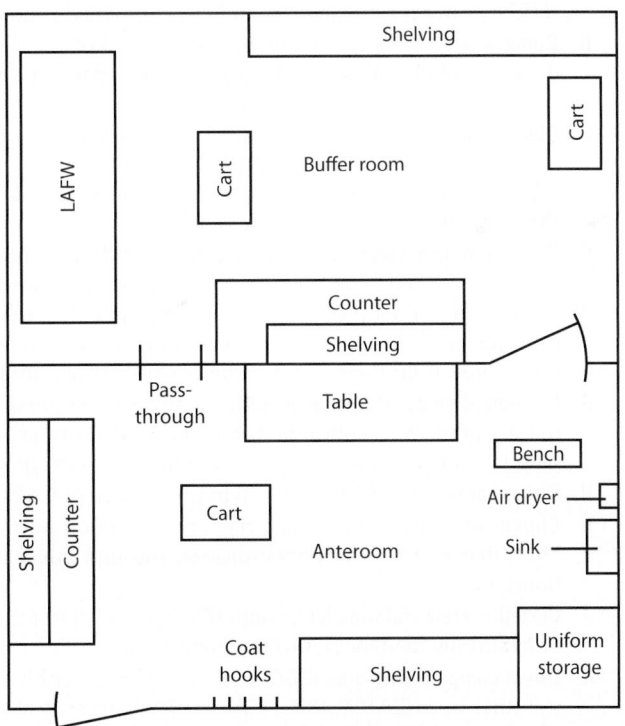

SAMPLE FLOOR PLAN FOR A CLEAN ROOM AND ANTE-AREA

B. **Beyond-use date (BUD):** the time and date after which a CSP should not be stored or transported. It is determined from the time and date the CSP is compounded. The BUD definition in *USP* Chapter ⟨797⟩ also references *USP* General Notices and Chapter ⟨795⟩ Pharmaceutical Compounding—Nonsterile Preparations. The General Notices defines BUD as, "the date after which a compounded preparation may not be used" (2) (See Chapter 4, Expiration and Beyond-Use Dating, of this book for additional information on this topic.)

Table 32.1	ISO CLASSIFICATION OF PARTICULATE MATTER IN ROOM AIR[a]		
CLASS NAME		**PARTICLE COUNT**	
ISO CLASS	U.S. FS 209E	ISO (m³)	FS 209E (ft³)
3	Class 1	35.2	1
4	Class 10	352	10
5	Class 100	3,520	100
6	Class 1,000	35,200	1,000
7	Class 10,000	352,000	10,000
8	Class 100,000	3,520,000	100,000

Reprinted with permission from Chapter ⟨797⟩ 2009 USP 32/NF 27. Rockville, MD. The United States Pharmacopeial Convention, Inc., 2008: http://www.usp.org/USPNF/pf/generalChapter797.html, Accessed February 2008; adapted from former Standard No. 209E, General Services Administration, Washington, DC, 20407 (September 11, 1992) and ISO 14644-1:1999, Cleanrooms and associated controlled environments—Part I: Classification of air cleanliness. For E

C. **Biological safety cabinet (BSC):** a cabinet that provides an environment for aseptic preparation of CSPs. It has an open front with inward vertical airflow to protect the worker from contamination by hazardous drugs and a downward airflow blown through a high-efficiency particulate air (HEPA) filter for preparation and environmental protection.

D. **Buffer area:** ISO Class 7 environment that houses devices used in aseptic compounding. Such devices include, but are not limited to, laminar airflow workbenches (LAFWs), BSCs, or compounding aseptic isolators (CAIs).

E. **Clean room:** a room that is designed and maintained to meet a specified airborne particulate cleanliness class, such as Class 1,000 (ISO Class 6) or Class 10,000 (ISO Class 7). Clean rooms contain LAFWs in order to prevent particulate and microbiologic contamination of drug preparations as they are being prepared or processed.

F. **Compounding aseptic containment isolator (CACI):** a compounding aseptic isolator (CAI) designed to protect the worker from cytotoxic or hazardous airborne drug particles during the compounding or material transfer process. Air should first pass through a microbially retentive HEPA filter before exchange with the surrounding environment. The air exhaust from the isolator should be properly vented from the building when volatile drugs are processed within the isolator.

G. **Compounding aseptic isolator (CAI):** an isolator designed for the aseptic compounding and material transfer of pharmaceutical preparations. A HEPA filter should be used with a CAI for air exchange with the surrounding environment. These devices are sometimes referred to as *barrier isolators*.

H. **Critical area:** an ISO Class 5 environment where CSPs, containers, and closures are processed.

I. **Critical site:** any surface (e.g., vial septa, injection port) or opening (e.g., opened ampules, needle hubs) that is at risk for contamination through direct contact with air, moisture (e.g., oral secretions), or touch.

J. **Closed-system vial transfer devices (CSTDs):** vial transfer systems that allow no venting or exposure of hazardous substances into the environment.

K. **Direct compounding area (DCA):** the critical area within an ISO Class 5 primary engineering control (that is, an LAFW, BSC, CAI, etc.) where critical sites are exposed to unidirectional HEPA-filtered air, also know as *first air*.

L. **Disinfectant:** a chemical or physical agent used to eliminate harmful pathogens. These agents may not necessarily kill microorganisms or fungal spores.

M. **Endotoxin:** a pyrogenic product present in bacterial cell walls. These substances are lipopolysaccharides that can be found anywhere live or dead bacteria have been present. As large molecules, they are not destroyed by steam sterilization or bacterial filtration. They can be destroyed on glassware using dry heat sterilization. The most common source of endotoxin material is water that has contained bacterial contamination; the endotoxin can remain after any bacteria are removed or killed. When a solution containing the endotoxin in injected into a patient, it can cause fever and even death.

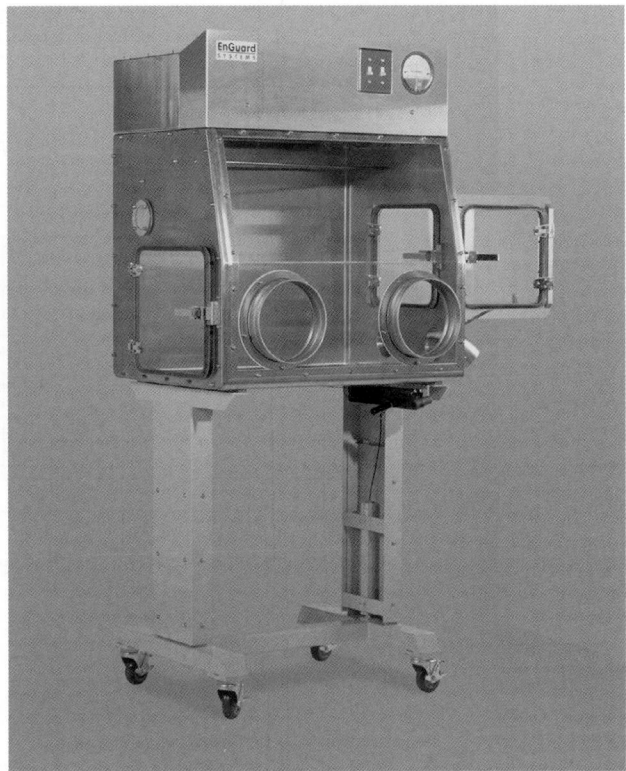

COMPOUNDING ASEPTIC ISOLATOR
(Photo Courtesy of Containment Technologies Group, Inc.)

N. **First air:** refers to the air that has passed through a unidirectional HEPA filter that is free of contaminants.

O. **HEPA filter:** a filter that provides a HEPA (or high-efficiency particulate air) environment, which is an essential component of both horizontal and vertical laminar airflow workbenches and other aseptic processing areas. For these purposes, the HEPA filters are certified to provide air that is filtered with a minimum 0.3-μm particle retaining efficiency of 99.97%.

P. **Laminar airflow workbench (LAFW):** also known as *laminar flow hoods,* workbenches that provide an environment of specially filtered air that sweeps the work area and provides an aseptic work area. Regular room air is drawn through a gross filter into an intake opening in the hood; the air then goes through a plenum where the airflow is equalized and is then passed in a unidirectional parallel flow pattern (laminar flow) through a HEPA filter. The air is forced through the HEPA filter and over the work area at a velocity of 90 ft/min, which is sufficient to sweep particulate matter away from the work area.

    With **horizontal** flow hoods, the HEPA filter takes up the back, vertical surface of the hood space, and the laminar air blows from the HEPA filter horizontally across the work area and directly at the worker who is standing at the front edge of the hood and working on the workbench surface.

    With **vertical** flow hoods, the HEPA filter takes up the top, horizontal surface of the hood space, and the laminar air blows from the HEPA filter downward through the hood space and into intake grills located along the front and back edges of the workbench surface. Vertical flow hoods, also called **biological safety cabinets (BSCs)**, can be used for any aseptic processing, but they are required for working with cytotoxic or other hazardous drugs. They have a clear glass or plastic shield that comes partway down the front of the hood space; the clear front shield and the vertical flow pattern with air contained within the hood protect the worker from contamination by drugs being processed within the hood.

Q. **Media fill:** a procedure in which personnel who do aseptic processing of CSPs prepare a simulated preparation using microbiologic growth medium, such as Soybean-Casein Digest Medium. The simulated preparation is then incubated to determine whether the preparation was contaminated during the procedure. The media-fill procedure attempts to simulate as closely as possible the exact environmental and process-related conditions and intensity level (e.g., time during the work shift

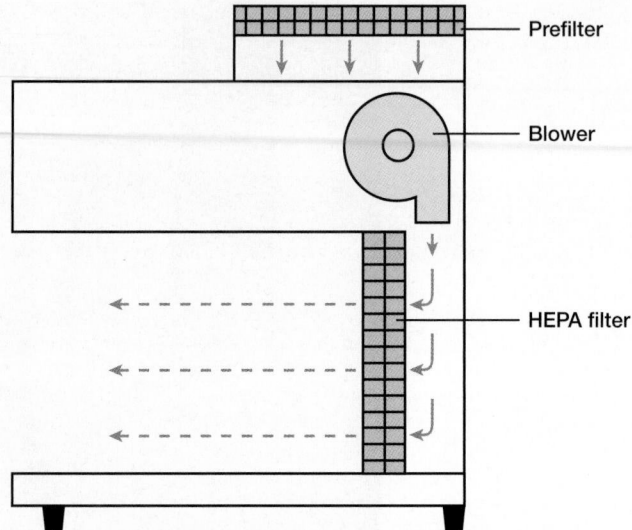

HORIZONTAL LAMINAR AIRFLOW WORKBENCH (LAFW)

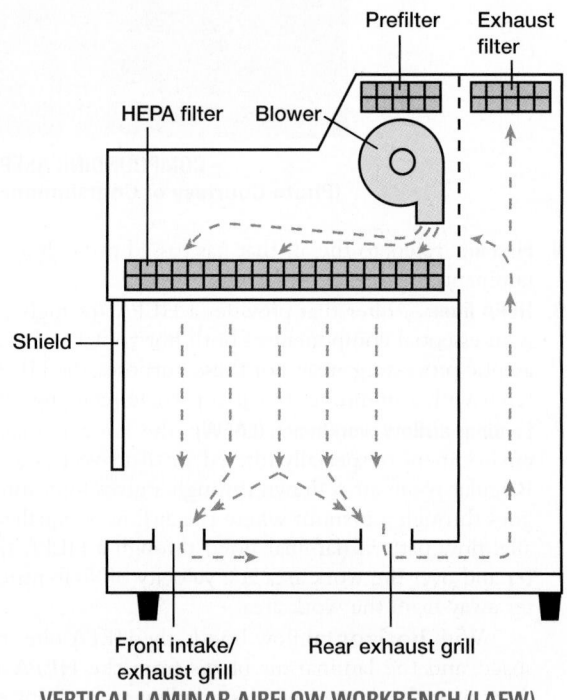

VERTICAL LAMINAR AIRFLOW WORKBENCH (LAFW)

and number of transfers or manipulations required to create a preparation) of actual practice; the verification procedure should be representative of the greatest risk that might be experienced in an actual practice situation.

R. Multiple-dose container: a container with antimicrobial preservatives consisting of several doses of a preparation that is intended to be used multiple times. A beyond-use date (BUD) of 28 days (based on the day the container is first opened or entered) is given for multiple-dose containers with antimicrobial preservatives unless a shorter date is specified by the manufacturer.

S. Negative-pressure room: a room that is at a lower pressure than the adjacent spaces so that the net flow of air is *into* the room (3).

T. Pharmacy bulk package: a container that holds many single doses of a sterile preparation intended for parenteral administration or the compounding of parenteral admixtures only. The closure of the pharmacy bulk package should be penetrated only once for transfer and should be manipulated only in a clean room. Pharmacy bulk packages must be labeled as "Pharmacy Bulk Package—Not for Direct Infusion," contain information referring to the safe use of the preparation, and list detailed information about the time period in which the preparation may be used once it has been entered, given that it has been stored in accordance with the labeled conditions.

U. **Primary engineering control (PEC):** an ISO Class 5 device or room that provides the proper environment for preparation of CSPs. Such devices include, but are not limited to, LAFWs, BSCs, CAIs, and CACIs.

V. **Preparation:** a sterile or nonsterile pharmaceutical dosage form or nutrient that is compounded in a licensed pharmacy or healthcare-related facility in accordance with an order from a licensed prescriber.

W. **Product:** a drug, pharmaceutical dosage form, or nutrient that is commercially manufactured in an FDA-approved facility. Such a product has been evaluated by the FDA for safety and efficacy, and FDA-approved labeling and product information accompanies the product.

X. **Positive-pressure room:** a room that is at a higher pressure than adjacent spaces so that the net airflow *is out* of the room (3).

Y. **Pyrogen:** a substance that induces a fever in a patient.

Z. **Single-dose container:** a container holding a preparation intended for a single use and for parenteral administration only. One such example is a prefilled syringe.

AA. **Segregated compounding area:** a separate designation area (but not an ISO Class 7 environment) containing an ISO Class 5 PEC used for the preparation of low-risk level CSPs with a BUD of 12 hours or less.

BB. **Sterility:** the absence of viable microorganisms. Because sterility cannot usually be confirmed with absolute certainty, statistical probability is used to describe it.

CC. **Sterilizing-grade membranes:** filter membranes that "retain 100% of a culture of 10^7 microorganisms of a strain of *Brevundimonas (Pseudomonas) diminuta* per square centimeter of membrane surface under a pressure of not less than 30 psi (2.0 bar). Such filter membranes are nominally at 0.22-μm or 0.2- μm porosity" (1).

DD. **Terminal sterilization:** a lethal procedure that is carried out at the end of processing, when a product or preparation is in its final sealed container, with the purpose of achieving a sterility assurance level of less than 10^{-6} (that is, the probability of a nonsterile unit is greater than one in a million) (4).

EE. **Unidirectional flow:** air flowing in a single and uniform manner that sweeps the work area and provides an aseptic processing area.

III.   TRAINING, EVALUATION, AND RESPONSIBILITY OF COMPOUNDING PERSONNEL IN ASEPTIC MANIPULATION SKILLS

A. "Compounding personnel are responsible for ensuring that CSPs are accurately identified, measured, diluted, and mixed and are correctly purified, sterilized, packaged, sealed, labeled, stored, dispensed, and distributed"(1).

B. Health care professionals who supervise compounding personnel shall ensure the following:
   1. Personnel are adequately trained and educated.
   2. Ingredients are correctly identified, in terms of quality and purity.
   3. Open or partially used containers are properly stored.
   4. Proper sterilization techniques are used for CSPs.
   5. Compounding equipment and devices are kept clean and maintained as accurate.
   6. CSPs are evaluated for potential harm from added substances prior to dispensing and administration.
   7. Appropriate packaging for CSPs is used to maintain sterility and stability.
   8. Compounding environments maintain purity or sterility of CSPs.
   9. CSP labels are accurate and complete.
   10. BUDs are valid based on scientific criteria or direct testing.
   11. Compounding procedures are in accordance with established criteria.
   12. Compounding deficiencies can be identified rapidly and corrected.
   13. Compounding procedures are separate from quality review.

C. Personnel involved in the preparation of CSPs must be trained through didactic instruction in the theory of sterile compounding and by practical skills to perform aseptic manipulations.

D. Compounding personnel must pass written and media-fill testing initially and at least annually for low- and medium-risk level conditions and semiannually for high-risk level conditions.

E. Should compounding personnel fail written tests or produce gross microbial colonization within media-fill test vials, expert compounding personnel will immediately retrain and reevaluate these personnel to correct all deficiencies in aseptic practices.

F. **Cleaning and disinfection of sterile compounding areas**
   1. Food, drinks, and other similar products must never be brought into areas where components and ingredients used for the preparation of CSPs are present. This includes ante-areas, buffer areas, and segregated compounding areas.
   2. Surfaces of LAFWs, BSCs, CAIs, and CACIs must be cleaned and disinfected at the beginning of each work shift, prior to each batch preparation, every 30 minutes during prolonged periods of CSP preparation, and during heavy surface contamination such as a spill.
   3. When no compounding of CSPs is occurring, floors of all ISO Class 7 and 8 areas, buffer areas, and ante-areas must be cleaned and disinfected by mopping.
   4. Cleaning materials used in the compounding areas, such as wipers and sponges, must be non-shedding and remain in these areas until disposal.
   5. If it is deemed acceptable to reuse specific cleaning materials (e.g., mops) based on manufacturer recommendations, procedures must be developed to ensure the efficacy of these materials while preventing contamination of the area on repeated use.
   6. A suitable disinfecting agent [e.g., sterile isopropyl alcohol (IPA)] must be used to wipe clean compounding supplies and equipment when removed from shipping boxes.
   7. Sterile IPA should remain on compounding surfaces at least 30 seconds to allow complete disinfection prior to initiating CSP preparation.

G. **Personnel cleansing and garbing**
   1. Personnel must be properly trained about the use of protective equipment (i.e., gloves, gowns, head covers, facemasks) to ensure aseptic preparation of CSPs.
   2. Personnel experiencing health problems that may increase the burden of airborne particulates must not be allowed to participate in aseptic compounding procedures. Examples of such health conditions include rashes, weeping sores, and active respiratory infections.
   3. All personal outer garments (e.g., hats, sweaters), cosmetics, jewelry, body piercings, and artificial nails must be removed prior to entering the buffer or compounding areas as these materials can increase particulates into the air or interfere with the effectiveness of protective equipment.
   4. Personnel garbing and cleansing must be performed in an order considered to progress from the dirtiest to the cleanest activity, such as placement of (i) shoe covers, (ii) hair covers and face-masks, (iii) eye shields, (iv) fingernail cleaning, (v) hand and forearm washing, (vi) nonshedding gown, and (vii) sterile gloves.
   5. Prior to donning sterile gloves, personnel must clean their hands with an alcohol-based surgical scrub possessing persistent activity and wait until their hands are completely dry.
   6. Gloves must be routinely disinfected with sterile 70% IPA during the compounding process and must be inspected for holes or punctures.
   7. On exiting the compounding area, a person's gown may be retained for reuse if not visibly soiled, but shoe covers, hair covers, facemasks, and gloves must be replaced with new ones prior to reentry.
   8. The preceding activities are not required for preparation of immediate-use CSPs when using a CAI if written manufacturer documentation is available to show that such personnel procedures are not required to ensure an aseptic environment.

H. **Competency evaluation of garbing and aseptic work practices**
   1. Glove fingertip sampling must be used as a tool to evaluate personnel involved in compounding of all CSP risk levels, because touch contamination is the most common breach in aseptic technique.
   2. All personnel must be visually observed to confirm competency in hand hygiene, garbing procedures, and routine disinfection of gloved hands.
   3. All personnel must pass three gloved fingertip-sampling procedures, with no growth on sterile contact agar plates, prior to being allowed to compound CSPs.
   4. After completing the hand hygiene, gowning, and gloving procedures, a gloved fingertip and thumb sample from each hand of the compounder must be collected by having him/her lightly press into the appropriate agar plates.
   5. Gloves should not be disinfected with sterile 70% IPA just prior to sampling.
   6. Media-fill tests must be used to evaluate aseptic technique of all compounding personnel involved in the preparation of CSPs.
   7. Commercially available sterile fluid culture media (i.e., Soybean-Casein Digest Medium) may be used and incubated at 30° to 35°C for 14 days to detect microbial contamination.

Table 32.2	USP CHAPTER <797>, RISK LEVEL ASSESSMENT				

CLASSIFICATION OF RISK LEVEL	REQUIREMENTS	EXAMPLES	STORAGE DATING RECOMMENDATIONS BASED ON TEMPERATURE		
			ROOM (20–25°C)	REFRIGERATION (2–8°C)	FREEZER (≤ –10°C)
Low risk	Simple admixtures using closed-system transfer methods; CSPs prepared in ISO Class 5 air quality	Vancomycin reconstitution, insulin drip, fluorouracil syringe, potassium chloride dialysate	≤48 hr	≤14 days	≤45 days
Medium risk	Admixtures using multiple additives, small volumes, or batch preparations; process involves long duration; CSPs prepared in ISO Class 5 air quality	Parenteral nutrition (PN), batch preparations	≤30 hr	≤7 days	≤45 days
High risk	Admixtures using nonsterile ingredients or open-system transfers; CSPs prepared in ISO Class 5 air quality	Phenol in glycerin, L-glutamine	≤24 hr	≤3 days	45 days

CSP, compounded sterile preparation; ISO, International Organization for Standardization.
Source: The United States Pharmacopeial Convention, Inc. Chapter ⟨797⟩. 2009 USP 32/NF 27. Rockville, MD: Author, 2008: http://www.usp.org/USPNF/pf/generalChapter797.html (accessed February 2008).

I. **Surface cleaning and disinfection sampling and assessment**
   1. Sampling of work surfaces for microbial contamination must be performed in all ISO classified areas on a periodic basis.
   2. Evaluation of work surfaces may be in the form of contact plates or swabs following specific compounding activities.
      a. Plates are generally used for sampling flat surfaces.
      b. Swabs are used for sampling irregular surfaces and equipment.
   3. The amount of microbial contamination is reported as colony-forming units (cfu), and corrective actions should be taken when the number of cfu exceed the guidelines outlined in Table 32.2.

IV. **CSP MICROBIAL CONTAMINATION RISK LEVELS**

A. **Risk levels** refer to the potential risk to patients caused by the introduction of microbial contamination into a finished sterile preparation and subsequent opportunity for growth of inadvertently added contaminants.

B. The USP designates three risk level conditions—low, medium, or high—during the compounding of CSPs.
   1. In assigning risk levels, source and quality of ingredients and environmental and processing factors are considered.
   2. The source of CSP contamination may be in the form of microbial (i.e., microorganisms, spores, endotoxins) or physical or chemical substances (i.e., foreign chemicals, physical matter).
   3. The determination of compounding risk levels applies to CSPs immediately after the final aseptic mixing or sterilization procedure.
   4. The ultimate responsibility of assigning the appropriate risk level lies with the licensed health care professional supervising the compounding of the CSP.

Table 32.3	RECOMMENDED ACTION LEVELS FOR MICROBIAL CONTAMINATION

ISO CLASSIFICATION	AIR SAMPLE (cfu per cubic meter of air per plate)
5	>1
7	>10
≥8	>100

Reprinted with permission from Chapter ⟨797⟩ 2009 USP 32/NF 27. Rockville, MD. The United States Pharmacopeial Convention, Inc., 2008: http://www.usp.org/USPNF/pf/generalChapter797.html, Accessed February 2008; source: Guidance for Industry—Sterile Drug Products Produced by Aseptic Processing—Current Good Manufacturing Practice—US HHS, FDA September 2004.

C. The characteristics of the various risks levels are described as follows:
1. **Low-risk** level conditions
   a. Compounding occurs within an ISO Class 5 PEC that is within an appropriate environment such as an ISO Class 7 buffer area.
   b. Compounding activities involve only simple transfers or mixing with three or fewer sterile commercially available products and no more than two entries into any one sterile container.
   c. See Table 32.2 for further examples of low-risk level assessment and storage period information.
   d. When the PEC cannot be located in an ISO Class 7 buffer area (or other specified placement for CAIs or CACIs), the maximum BUD is 12 hours or less and they must comply with the following four criteria:
      (1) All PECs are ISO Class 5 located in a segregated compounding area.
      (2) The segregated compounding area must be in an area that will minimize the risk of contamination: sealed windows that do not connect to outdoors and low-traffic areas.
      (3) Sinks must be separated from the ISO Class 5 PEC device.
      (4) All aseptic work practices and cleaning and disinfection procedures are strictly followed.
   e. Quality assurance practices are performed, including, but not limited to
      (1) Maintenance of ISO Class 5 air quality.
      (2) Visual confirmation of compounding personnel wearing appropriate protective garb.
      (3) Review of ingredients to ensure correct identity and amounts compounded.
      (4) Visual inspection to ensure particulate-free preparations and accurate labeling.
   f. Media-fill testing is performed at least annually by compounding personnel.
2. **Medium-risk** level conditions
   a. Compounding occurs within an ISO Class 5 environment.
   b. Compounding activities include multiple complex manipulations or activities of prolonged duration with more than three sterile products and entries into any one container.
   c. Compounding process involves pooling ingredients from multiple sterile products for administration to multiple patients or one patient on multiple occasions.
   d. All quality assurance procedures specified for low-risk level conditions are followed.
   e. Media-fill testing is performed at least annually by compounding personnel.
   f. See Table 32.2 for further examples of medium-risk level assessment and storage period information.
3. **High-risk** level conditions
   a. Nonsterile ingredients or products not intended for administration by sterile routes or use of nonsterile devices prior to terminal sterilization is involved.
   b. Sterile ingredients, devices, and containers are exposed for more than 1 hour to air quality worse than an ISO Class 5 environment.
   c. Improper compounding garb and glove procedures are followed.
   d. Nonsterile water-containing ingredients or preparations are stored for more than 6 hours prior to terminal sterilization.
   e. Ingredient strength and purity do not meet their original specifications.
   f. All high-risk level CSP preparations must undergo sterilization by filtration with a filter having a nominal pore size not larger than 0.2 μm within an air quality environment of ISO Class 5 or better.

g. A media-fill test should be performed at least semiannually by compounding personnel.

h. See Table 32.2 for further examples of high-risk level assessment and storage period information.

V. CONSIDERATIONS FOR CSP

A. Immediate-use CSPs

1. Immediate-use CSPs are intended only for emergency situations, such as cardiopulmonary resuscitation.

2. In order to be considered an immediate-use CSP, all of the following six criteria must be met:

a. The compounding process involves simple transfer manipulations.

b. Duration of the compounding procedure is less than 1 hour.

c. The preparation is compounded in accordance with aseptic techniques.

d. The CSP is administered not later than 1 hour after initiation of the compounding process.

e. The CSP shall be discarded if administration does not begin within 1 hour after initiation of the compounding process.

f. The CSP shall be properly labeled, identifying names and amounts of all ingredients, initials of compounding personnel, and patient identification information.

B. Single-dose and multiple-dose containers

1. Single-dose containers (i.e., bags, bottles, syringes) opened or exposed to air quality worse than ISO Class 5 should be used within 1 hour.

2. Single-dose containers opened or exposed to ISO Class 5 air quality or cleaner air may be used up to 6 hours after initial opening or entry.

3. Single-dose containers (e.g., ampuls) may not be stored after entry or opening.

4. Multiple-dose containers must be used within 28 days after initial opening or entry.

C. Hazardous drugs

1. Health care workers must prepare hazardous drugs only under conditions that minimize their risk of exposure and adverse events.

2. Hazardous drugs must be stored separately from other inventory to reduce the risk of contamination and exposure.

3. The storage area for hazardous drugs should have sufficient general exhaust ventilation [i.e., at least 12 air changes per hour (ACPH)] in non–clean rooms in which CACIs are located.

4. Appropriate personnel protective equipment (PPE) must be worn when hazardous drugs are prepared in a BSC or CACI, including the following:

a. Gowns.

b. Facemasks.

c. Hair covers.

d. Chemo-type gloves.

e. Shoe covers or dedicated shoes.

f. Eye protection.

5. Appropriate PPE must also be used at all times when hazardous drugs are handled during receiving, distributing, stocking, inventory, preparing for administration, and disposal.

6. All hazardous drugs must be prepared in an ISO Class 5 environment, maintaining a negative pressure of 0.01-inch water column and a minimum of 12 ACPH.

7. CSTDs must be used within the ISO Class 5 environment of a BSC or CACI.

8. Access must be limited to areas where hazardous drugs are prepared.

9. Personnel compounding hazardous drugs must be fully trained with annual verification in techniques, including:

a. Safe aseptic manipulation practices.

b. Negative-pressure techniques when using a BSC or CACI.

c. Correct use of CSTDs.

d. Containment, cleanup, and disposal procedures in case of spills or breakages.

e. Treatment of personnel on physical contact or inhalation exposure of hazardous substances.

10. Compounding personnel of reproductive capability must acknowledge in writing an understanding of the risks associated with handling hazardous drugs.

11. All applicable federal and state regulations must be adhered to for disposal of hazardous drug wastes.

D. Radiopharmaceuticals

1. Appropriate PECs, radioactivity containment, and shielding procedures must be used for compounding of all radiopharmaceutical CSPs.

2. Radiopharmaceuticals compounded with volumes of less than 100 mL from a sterile single-dose injection (or less than 30 mL from a multiple-dose container) are considered low-risk CSPs.

3. Appropriately shielded vials and syringes must be used for compounding in an ISO Class 5 environment PEC located in an ISO Class 8 environment or cleaner air quality.

4. Multiuse radiopharmaceutical vials punctured by needles with no direct contact contamination, compounded with technetium-99m, and exposed to an ISO Class 5 environment may be used up until the time indicated by manufacturers' recommendations.

5. Technetium-99m/molybdenum-99 generator systems must be eluted in an ISO Class 8 environment or cleaner air.

6. Low-risk radiopharmaceutical CSPs with a 12-hour or briefer BUD must be prepared in a separate compounding area with a demarcated line defining this specific area.

7. Handling of shielded radiopharmaceutical CSP vials may take place in a limited-access ambient environment with no specific ISO class designation.

E. Allergen extracts

Allergen extracts are not subject to personnel, environmental, and storage requirements for all CSP microbial contamination risk levels when all of the following criteria are met:

1. The compounding process involves a simple transfer.

2. The preparation contains preservatives to prevent microbial growth.

3. Proper hand-cleansing procedure is followed by personnel prior to the compounding activity.

4. Proper PPE are used (i.e., hair covers, facial hair covers, gowns).

5. Antiseptic hand-cleansing procedures (i.e., alcohol-based hand scrub) are performed throughout the compounding activity.

6. Proper powder-free sterile gloves are used during the activity.

7. Sterile 70% IPA is used to disinfect gloves during allergen extract CSP preparation.

8. Proper aseptic technique is used with ampul necks and vial stoppers.

9. Direct contact contamination of critical sites (i.e., needles, opened ampuls) is minimized.

10. Each multiple-dose vial of allergen extract prepared is properly labeled with patient name, BUD, and storage temperature range.

11. No single-dose allergen extract CSP is stored for future use.

VI. VERIFICATION OF COMPOUNDING ACCURACY AND STERILITY

A. To ensure patient safety and efficacy of a CSP, the quality of the compounding procedure must be verified in terms of accuracy and sterility.

B. A verification process includes preplanned testing, monitoring and, above all, documentation, to show compliance with environmental guidelines, personnel procedures, and policies ensuring the accuracy and purity of CSPs.

C. After CSPs are compounded, the finished labeled preparations must be visually evaluated for the accuracy of ingredient purity, amounts, and concentrations.

D. The compounding processes must be reviewed to ensure that appropriate standardized devices were used and calibrated, with the correct measurements being properly recorded.

E. When ingredients or compounding processes cannot be verified (i.e., unlabeled syringes, incomplete labeling, uncalibrated devices), the CSP must be discarded and cannot be administered to any patient.

F. A quantitative chemical assay of the finished CSP is recommended, although not required, to verify the correct identity and strength of ingredients.

G. Sterilization methods for high-risk level CSPs

1. Filtration

   a. Pharmaceutical fluids that require sterilization for human use can be sterilized through use of commercially available sterile filters that are approved for human use.

   b. CSPs must be chemically and physically compatible with the sterile membrane filter that is used.

   c. Filters with a nominal pore size of 0.2 or 0.22 μm that are pyrogen-free must be used for purposes of sterilization.

   d. Filtration must allow the sterilization process to occur rapidly without requiring the filter to be replaced during the process.

   e. Filters must undergo the manufacturer's recommended integrity test (e.g., bubble point test) after filtering CSPs.

2. Steam
   a. The preferred method for sterilizing aqueous preparations is saturated steam under pressure, otherwise know as *autoclaving*.
   b. To ensure sterility, all ingredients and surfaces must be exposed to steam at 121°C for between 20 and 60 minutes.
   c. Prior to sterilization, solutions are passed through a 1.2-μm or smaller filter to remove particulate matter.
3. Dry heat
   a. When moisture will damage the material or the material is impermeable to steam, a dry-heat sterilization process must be employed.
   b. Higher temperatures and prolonged exposure times are used with dry heat vs. steam sterilization.
   c. During the dry-heat sterilization process, an even distribution of dry air throughout the chamber is accomplished with the assistance of a blower device.
   d. Effectiveness of the dry-heat process must be verified with appropriate biologic indicators, such as temperature-sensing devices.
4. Depyrogenation
   a. Glassware or vials must be sterilized with dry-heat depyrogenation.
   b. To ensure sterility, all containers are exposed to dry heat at 250°C for 30 minutes. Glass and metal devices are typically covered with aluminum foil during exposure to dry heat.
   c. Effectiveness of the depyrogenation process must be verified using endotoxin challenge vials.
   d. At least a 3 log reduction in endotoxin indicates that the dry heat depyrogenation process is successful in rendering containers free of pyrogens and viable microbes.

VII.   ENVIRONMENTAL QUALITY AND CONTROL

A. **Exposure of critical sites**
   1. The risk of contamination increases with exposure to air quality worse than ISO Class 5.
   2. The surface of a critical site may increase the risk of contamination; for example, rough, permeable surfaces retain microorganisms more readily than do smooth glass surfaces.
   3. During the preparation of CSPs, the highest priority of the compounding personnel must be given to the avoidance of physical contact and airborne contamination with critical sites.
B. **ISO Class 5 air sources, buffer areas, and ante-areas**
   1. Buffer areas must provide air quality of at least ISO Class 7.
   2. Devices or objects that are not essential to CSP compounding (i.e., computers, carts, cabinets) may be placed in buffer areas, but the environment must be monitored for effects on air quality.
   3. Every compounding facility is expected to verify that all PECs are properly located, maintained, and monitored.
C. **Facility design and environmental controls**
   1. Compounding facilities are environmentally controlled (e.g., temperature of 20°C) to provide comfortable conditions for compounding personnel while wearing the required compounding garb.
   2. Compounding facilities include PECs that are designed to minimize exposure of critical sites to airborne contamination.
   3. PECs may include LAFWs, BSCs, CAIs, and CACIs, all of which maintain ISO Class 5 air quality for 0.5-μm particles during the preparation of CSPs.
   4. Buffer areas, which typically act as the core location of the PEC, are designed to provide at least ISO Class 7 air quality for 0.5-μm and larger particles.
   5. PECs control airborne contamination through the use of HEPA-filtered unidirectional airflow in the work environment.
   6. Appropriate policies and procedures must be developed and adhered to in order to ensure the desired environmental conditions.
   7. The work environment for compounding CSPs is designed to provide the cleanest critical sites (i.e., ISO Class 5).
   8. For buffer areas with a physical separation (e.g., walls, doors) from ante-areas, a minimum difference of 0.02- to 0.05-inch water column of positive pressure is mandatory.
   9. Displacement airflow or an air velocity of 40 ft/min across a line of demarcation may be used for buffer areas not physically separated from ante-areas.

10. PECs should be located out of areas with high traffic flow in order to avoid conditions that could disrupt airflow.
11. Appropriate airflow for the various air quality classifications are determined through the number of ACPH.
    a. ACPH of 30 or more is required for ISO Class 7 buffer areas and ante-areas with HEPA-filtered airflow.
    b. ACPH of 15 or more is required for ISO Class 5 areas with a recirculating device for HEPA-filtered air.
12. Factors that influence air exchange requirements include the following:
    a. Total number of compounding personnel working in the room.
    b. Specific compounding procedures that produce particulates.
    c. Temperature in the room.
13. A HEPA-filtered air supply for buffer areas should be introduced at the ceiling, with return vents low on the walls.
14. The efficiency of all HEPA filters should be verified via particle size testing after installation.
15. Only those activities and tasks essential to the preparation and staging of components for compounding of CSPs are to be performed in the buffer area.
16. Only furniture, supplies, and equipment essential for compounding activities can be placed in the buffer area.
17. To minimize microorganism colonization, the surfaces of ceilings, wall, floors, and so on within the buffer area must be smooth, free from cracks, nonporous, cleanable, and impermeable to disinfectants.
18. Junctures of ceilings to walls must be repaired to prevent accumulation of dirt.
19. Ceiling tiles must be sealed to the support frame to prevent dislodgment, which could serve as a port of entry for contaminants.
20. The exterior lens surface of ceiling lighting fixtures should be sealed, smooth, and cleanable with disinfectants.
21. No sources of water (e.g., sinks or drains) can be located within the buffer area.
22. All work surfaces must be designed to be smooth and composed of materials that promote effective cleaning and disinfection.

D. Placement of PECs

1. All PECs for preparation of CSPs must be located within an ISO Class 7 buffer area unless both of the following conditions apply:
   a. The CAIs maintain ISO Class 5 air quality during compounding operations when particle counts are sampled 6 to 12 inches upstream of the critical site exposure.
   b. No more than 3520 particles are counted during material transfer.
2. Compounding procedures for high-risk level CSPs, such as weighing and mixing, must be performed in environments where background particle counts do not exceed ISO Class 8.
3. The recovery time to achieve ISO Class 5 air quality during preparation of CSPs in isolators must be clearly documented.

E. Viable and nonviable environmental air sampling testing

1. At a minimum, environmental sampling must occur at the following times:
   a. During commissioning and certification of new facilities and equipment.
   b. After any facility or equipment is serviced.
   c. During recertification of facilities or equipment.
   d. When problems with compounding techniques or end-preparation integrity have been identified.
   e. When CSPs are suspected as a source of infection in patients.
2. Sampling programs differ for nonviable and viable airborne particles: The intention for nonviable particles is to directly verify the performance of engineering controls used for measuring different levels of air cleanliness.
3. PECs (LAFWs, BSCs, CAIs, and CACIs) must be certified by qualified individuals at least every 6 months and whenever the device or room is serviced, relocated, or altered in any way.
4. Secondary engineering controls (buffer and ante-areas) must also undergo certification at least every 6 months under conditions similar to those outlined for PECs.
5. Qualified individuals performing the certification testing should follow procedures as outlined in the CETA Certification Guide for Sterile Compounding Facilities (*CAG-003-2006*).
6. Pressure differential or airflow between buffer and ante-areas as well as the ante-area and general environment must be monitored by a pressure gauge.

7. Pressure differential monitoring results must be documented and posted on a log with a minimum daily frequency (preferably every work shift).

8. A pressure differential not less than 5 Pa must exist between the ISO Class 7 and general pharmacy areas.

9. For preparation of low- and medium-risk level CSPs, the differential airflow between the buffer area and ante-area must have a minimum velocity of 40 ft/min (0.2 m/s).

10. An appropriate environmental sampling plan for viable airborne particles must be predicated on the risk associated with the compounding activities performed.

    a. Sampling sites must include locations within each ISO Class 5, 7, and 8 area, as well as areas with the greatest potential for breaches in sterility (e.g., counters near doors, pass-through boxes).

    b. Sample location, collection method, sampling frequency, air volume sampled, and time of sampling must be documented as part of the sampling plan.

11. Use of growth medium, such as Soybean-Casein Digest Medium (also known as *trypticase soy broth* or *agar*), is required for testing of airborne particles.

    a. In high-risk level compounding, sample testing for fungi must be performed, and malt extract agar should be used.

    b. When testing for surface contamination, media must be supplemented with additives (i.e., trypticase soy agar with lecithin and polysorbate 80) to prevent disinfectants from interfering with the results.

    c. Media plate covers must be secured, placed in an inverted position, and incubated at an appropriate temperature for a time period that will promote adequate replication of microorganisms.

       (1) Trypticase soy agar is recommended to incubate at 30° to 35°C for 48 to 72 hours

       (2) Malt extract agar is recommended to incubate at 26° to 30°C for 5 to 7 days

    d. If excessive levels of microbial growth are detected, an investigation of compounding processes is performed. This may include personnel compliance with hygiene and garbing, cleaning procedures, standard operating procedures, and quality of environmental controls.

    e. The amount of microbial contamination is reported as colony-forming units (cfu), and corrective actions should be taken when the number of cfu exceeds the guidelines outlined in Table 32.3.

12. Viable air sampling

    a. Volumetric collection methods are required for determining the contamination of controlled air environments with viable microorganisms.

    b. Impaction, a type of volumetric air sampling, is the preferred method used for air sampling, because it is the most accurate.

    c. Other methods, such as settling plates, are more likely to be affected by particle size and airflow and may not necessarily reflect the concentration of viable particles in the environment.

    d. Air sampling must be performed in zones that are prone to contamination at all risk levels (i.e., low, medium, high) during the entire compounding process, such as gowning, staging, labeling, and cleanup.

    e. Air sampling must be performed inside the ISO Class 5 environment for low-risk level CSPs with a 12-hour or briefer BUD during the certification of the PEC.

13. Air-sampling devices

    a. To obtain the most accurate results, 400 to 1,000 liters of air must be collected by air-sampling devices at each location.

    b. *USP* Chapter ⟨1116⟩, Microbiological Evaluation of Clean Rooms and Other Controlled Environments, is recommended for compounding personnel to obtain further in-depth information on the use of volumetric air-sampling devices.

    c. During the recertification process for compounding facilities and equipment (i.e., every 6 months), air sampling must also be performed.

    d. If any equipment is serviced or any location within the compounding facility undergoes construction, air sampling should be repeated.

VIII. SUGGESTED STANDARD OPERATING PROCEDURES

All facilities involved in the preparation of CSP must have written standard operating procedures (SOPs) to ensure quality control of the compounding environment. For a more complete discussion of this topic, refer to *USP* Chapter ⟨797⟩, which is now considered to be the standard of practice for this area of pharmaceutical compounding (1). The SOPs may address some of the following issues.

   A. Personnel access to the buffer area

   B. Decontamination of compounding supplies

   C. Minimization of traffic flow in and out of the buffer area

   D. Personnel cleansing and garbing

   E. Cleaning procedures for critical sites in the DCA

IX. VERIFICATION OF AUTOMATED COMPOUNDING DEVICES FOR PARENTERAL NUTRITION COMPOUNDING

   A. Automated compounding devices (ACDs) were developed to assist with the accuracy and precision of preparation of parenteral nutrition (PN) formulations, which may contain 20 or more individual additives.

   B. A pharmacist other than the compounding personnel is preferred for confirming that the measured volumes in syringes correspond with the PN order.

   C. The two major methods used for verifying the accuracy of the compounding process by ACDs are volumetric and gravimetric analysis.

   D. Each ACD has its own set of internal surveillance checks that have the capability to measure each nutrient volume added to the final PN container.

   E. If the weight of the final PN container is different from the theoretical weight calculated by the automated system (sum of the volume for each ingredient multiplied by its specific gravity), then the pharmacist is alerted to a possible error in the admixture process.

   F. Gravimetric analysis may also be used to assess the precision of the final PN admixture.

      1. An analytical balance is used to determine the weight of individual additive containers that have a narrow margin of safety.

      2. For example, if overfill for a final PN formulation was supplied solely from a potassium chloride container, the consequences of this error could be fatal.

   G. Refractometry also is used to determine whether PN formulations have been compounded properly.

      1. The refractive index of dextrose and amino acids can be measured with a refractometer and compared to values established for known concentrations of dextrose and amino acids in PN base formulations.

      2. If the measured refractive indices differ substantially from predicted values, then the base formulation may have been improperly admixed. Refractometers cannot be used with IV fat emulsion, so alternative methods must be used to assess the integrity of total nutrition admixture (TNA) systems, which contain this component.

      3. Research has shown that factors other than incorrect preparation can result in refractive indices deviating from predicted values.

      4. In contrast to indirectly measuring final dextrose concentrations with refractometric analysis, certain instruments use chemical analysis to directly measure final dextrose concentrations. Although dextrose concentrations of PN formulations administered in clinical practice may exceed the range of detection, samples can be diluted and compared against control solutions to determine whether the formulation is within an acceptable margin of error.

X. FINISHED PREPARATION RELEASE CHECKS AND TESTS

   A. Physical inspection

      1. All CSPs must be visually inspected for particulates on conclusion of the compounding procedure and prior to dispensing of the preparation.

      2. A lighted white or black background should be used for the detection of particulates, and closure of package containers and seals should be checked.

   B. Compounding accuracy checks

      1. Written procedures must be developed to verify accuracy of ingredient identities, amounts, sterility, stability, packaging, and labeling.

      2. Sterility testing must be performed on all high-risk level CSPs prepared in batches of more than 25 identical containers, exposed longer than 12 hours to temperatures between 2° and 8°C or for greater than 6 hours at a temperature of 8°C or higher.

      3. Procedures must be developed requiring the ongoing monitoring of high-risk level CSPs for evidence of microbial growth if these preparations are dispensed prior to receiving the results of sterility tests.

      4. If sterility tests are positive for microbial contamination, policies must be in place for immediate recall of the dispensed CSP and notification of the patient and physician.

5. Bacterial endotoxin testing must be performed on all high-risk level CSPs, excluding inhalation and ophthalmic preparations, prepared in batches of more than 25 identical containers, exposed longer than 12 hours to temperatures between 2° and 8°C or for greater than 6 hours at a temperature of 8°C or higher.
6. Written procedures must be developed to verify the following information:
    a. CSP labels identify correct amounts of ingredients.
    b. CSP labels match with original written order for ingredient identities, purities, and amounts.
    c. Fill volumes or quantities in CSPs are correct.

XI. STORAGE AND BEYOND-USE DATING

A. **BUDs versus expiration dates**
1. The BUD refers to the date and time after which a CSP must not be stored or transported.
2. BUDs for CSPs are based on the potential for microbial growth and pyrogen formation with regard to risk level and duration of storage (see Table 32.2).
3. Expiration dates are determined from rigorous analytical assays and testing for the chemical and physical stability of manufactured sterile products.
4. Information that should be considered during the assignment of BUDs for CSPs include the following:
    a. Stability of ingredients.
    b. Compatibility of ingredients.
    c. Degradation mechanism of ingredients.
    d. Container type and material.
    e. Fill volume.
5. CSPs exposed to temperatures of at least 40°C for longer than 4 hours should be discarded.
6. The only valid methods for establishing BUDs for CSPs are semiquantitative procedures such as thin-layer chromatography and quantitative stability-indicating assays such as high-performance liquid chromatography.
7. The BUD for multiple-dose containers used in the preparation of CSPs after they are initially entered or opened is 28 days.

B. **Monitoring of controlled storage areas**
1. Compounding personnel are responsible for monitoring the drug storage areas within the facility.
2. Categories of controlled temperature areas
    a. Room temperature: 20° to 25°C
    b. Cold temperature: 2° to 8°C
    c. Freezing temperature: −10° to −25°C
3. Controlled temperature areas should be monitored at least once daily.

XII. MAINTAINING STERILITY, PURITY, AND STABILITY OF DISPENSED AND DISTRIBUTED CSP

A. **Packaging, handling, and transport**
1. Compounding personnel are responsible for ensuring the quality and integrity of CSPs during transit after release from the preparation area.
2. Methods must be developed to avoid alteration in the positioning of syringe plungers or tips.
3. Foam padding should be used when CSPs are transported via pneumatic tube systems.
4. Alternative transport methods should be considered for CSPs with unique stability requirements (e.g., instability due to shaking or on exposure to extremes in temperature or light).
5. Special transportation methods must be developed for hazardous CSPs in order to protect the personnel and environment that come into contact with these agents.
6. When shipping CSPs to recipients outside the compounding facility, labels must clearly identify BUDs as well as instructions for storage and disposal after expiration.
7. Compounding facilities may need to provide a functioning refrigerator or freezer to the recipient if required for CSP storage.

B. **Use and storage**
1. Proper storage directions and BUD information must be displayed on CSP labeling to ensure the quality and integrity of the dispensed CSP.
2. Expired and partially used CSPs must be returned to the compounding facility for discarding.
3. CSP storage in patient-care areas must be designed in such a way as to prevent access by unauthorized personnel.

C. Readying for administration
1. Procedures must be developed to ensure sterility during CSP administration to patients.
2. Techniques may include proper hand hygiene, replacement of administration sets, in-line filtration sets, and operation of infusion control devices.
3. CSP stability and sterility must be confirmed if the CSP has been exposed to temperatures of 30°C or more for longer than 1 hour.

D. Redispensed CSPs
1. CSPs returned to the compounding facility may be redispensed only when integrity of the final preparation can be verified in terms of purity, stability, and sterility.
2. Confirmation of the following conditions may assist compounding personnel in determining the integrity of returned CSPs:
   a. Storage in an environment of controlled cold temperature (i.e., refrigeration).
   b. Protection from exposure to light (if applicable).
   c. No evidence of package or container tampering.
3. CSPs must not be redispensed if the original BUD has been exceeded.

XIII.   PATIENT OR CAREGIVER TRAINING

A. The compounding facility must develop a formal training program to ensure that the patient or caregiver is knowledgeable and trained in the handling and use of the CSP.

B. The training program is expected to include such information about CSPs so that the patient or caregiver understands the following:
1. Intended use, therapeutic goals, and duration of therapy.
2. Methods for determining CSP integrity on receipt (e.g., visual inspection for container leakage, particulates, or discoloration).
3. Proper techniques for CSP administration, handling, and storage.
4. Process for verification of labels to ensure accurate identity, dose, and administration of the CSP.
5. Proper techniques for aseptic preparation of the CSP.
6. Proper methods for catheter and dressing care.
7. Signs and symptoms that may indicate complications from CSP administration.
8. Mechanism for responding to equipment malfunctions (e.g., catheter breakage).
9. Mechanism for obtaining emergency services.
10. Procedures for disposal of biohazardous waste materials (e.g., syringes or needles).

XIV.   PATIENT MONITORING AND ADVERSE EVENTS REPORTING

A. Compounding facilities must develop programs to monitor a patient's response to CSPs.

B. Programs for documenting adverse events of patients in response to CSP administration must include a feedback mechanism by which patients and caregivers can report concerns.

C. Supervisors of compounding facilities must review CSP adverse event reports in order to implement corrective actions and avoid future events.

XV.   QUALITY ASSURANCE PROGRAM

A. Compounding facilities must develop a formal quality assurance (QA) program to monitor compliance with policies, processes, and procedures used in the preparation of CSPs.

B. Elements that should be considered when developing a QA program include the following:
1. Formal written policies.
2. All phases of CSP preparation, such as maintenance of the compounding environment.
3. Specific details for conducting monitoring and evaluation programs.
4. Descriptions for reporting the results of monitoring and evaluation programs.
5. Development of plans to ensure follow-up on recommended action levels.
6. Identification of personnel accountable for various aspects of the QA program.

REFERENCES

1. The United States Pharmacopeial Convention, Inc. Chapter ⟨797⟩. 2009 USP 32/NF 27. Rockville, MD: Author, 2008: http://www.usp.org/USPNF/pf/generalChapter797.html. Accessed February 2008.
2. The United States Pharmacopeial Convention, Inc. General notices. 2008 USP 31/NF 26. Rockville, MD: Author, 2007; 12.
3. American Society of Heating, Refrigerating and Air-Conditioning Engineers, Inc. (ASHRAE), Laboratory Design Guide.
4. Center for Drug Evaluation and Research. Sterile Drug Products Produced by Aseptic Processing. Rockville, MD: Food and Drug Administration, September 2004: http://www.fda.gov/cder/guidance/5882fnl.htm. Accessed February 2008.

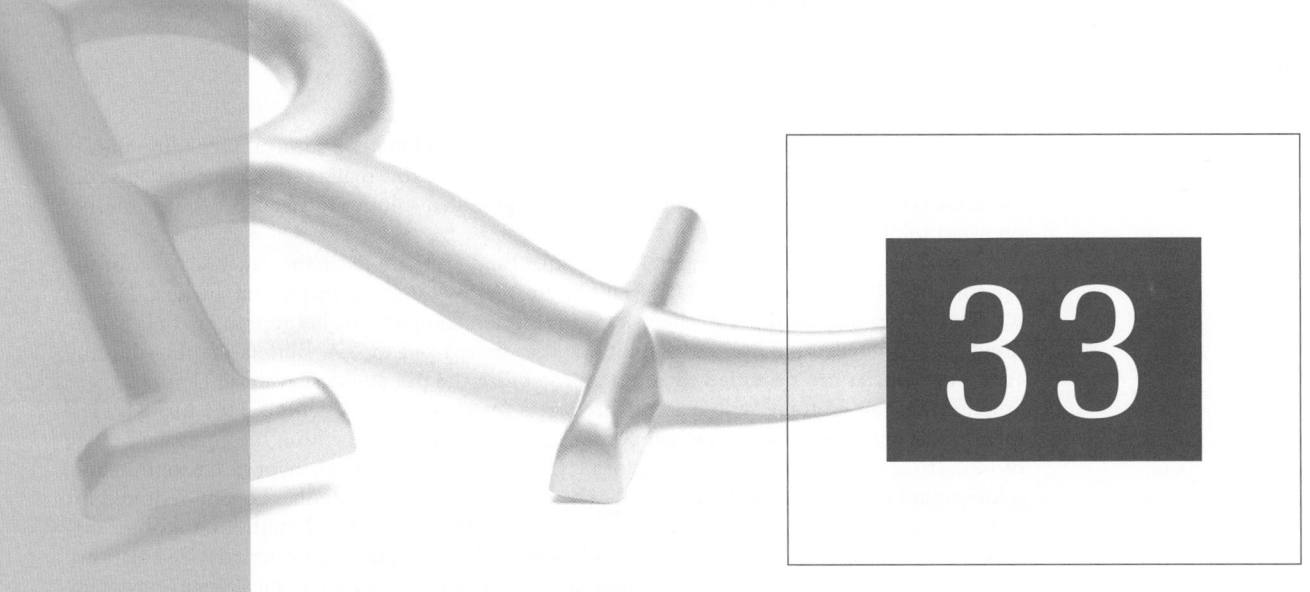

Ophthalmic, Nasal, Inhalation, and Irrigation Solutions

I. OPHTHALMIC SOLUTIONS

A. **Definition:** "Ophthalmic solutions are sterile solutions, essentially free from foreign particles, suitably compounded and packaged for instillation into the eye" (1).

B. **Special cautions** As stated in the definition, ophthalmic solutions must be sterile and free from particulates. Because of the inherent danger of causing serious eye infection and even loss of eyesight through the use of contaminated ophthalmic preparations, the greatest care must be used in preparing these solutions. Unfortunately, there have been a number of accidents in recent years in which preparations that were intended to be sterile were compounded in pharmacies and were not processed properly and so were not sterile. In one case, the preparations were ophthalmic solutions, and several patients were injured and two patients lost eyes (2). Ophthalmic solutions should be compounded extemporaneously only if the following conditions apply:

1. There are no available commercial product alternatives.
2. The compounder possesses the appropriate knowledge and technique.
3. The necessary equipment and supplies are available to make sterile solutions.

C. **Desired properties**

1. Sterility and clarity are not just desired properties; they are absolute requirements for ophthalmic solutions.
2. When the solution is dispensed in a multidose container that is to be used over a period of time longer than 24 hours, a preservative must be added to ensure microbiologic safety over

563

the period of use. If the solution is to be used during or following a surgical procedure on the eye, the solution should not contain a preservative because this may be irritating or damaging to exposed ocular tissues (1). In this case, if a compounded solution is needed, a sterile, freshly prepared solution should be used.

3. Although solutions with the same pH as lacrimal fluid (7.4) are ideal, the outer surfaces of the eye tolerate a larger range, 3.5 to 8.5 (1). The normal useful range to prevent corneal damage is 6.5 to 8.5 (3). The final pH of the solution is often a compromise, because many ophthalmic drugs have limited solubility and stability at the desired pH of 7.4. Buffers or pH-adjusting agents or vehicles can be added to adjust and stabilize the pH at a desired level (1).

4. Solutions that are isotonic with tears are preferred. An amount equivalent to 0.9% NaCl is ideal for comfort and should be used when possible. The eye can tolerate within the equivalent range of 0.6% to 2% NaCl without discomfort (1). There are times when hypertonic ophthalmic solutions are necessary therapeutically or when the addition of an auxiliary agent, required for reasons of stability, supersedes the need for isotonicity. There are several methods useful for calculating isotonicity. These are described and illustrated in Chapter 11, Isotonicity Calculations.

5. As with all pharmaceutical solutions, ophthalmic solutions must be chemically and physically stable. This subject is discussed in Chapter 27, Solutions, and in Chapter 37, Compatibility and Stability of Drug Products and Preparations.

6. The active ingredient(s) should be present in the most therapeutically effective form. This goal must often be compromised for reasons of solubility or stability of the active ingredient or comfort for the patient. For example, though most drugs are most active in their undissociated form, they are least soluble in this form. They may also be less stable at pH values that favor the undissociated form (1).

7. Ophthalmic solutions should be free of chemicals or agents that cause allergy or toxicity to the sensitive membranes and tissues of the eye. Auxiliary agents, such as preservatives and antioxidants, should be added with care, because many patients are sensitive to these substances. Before adding an auxiliary agent, check with the patient about allergies and sensitivities.

D. Active ingredients and components

1. The easiest way to compound an ophthalmic solution is to use sterile water or sterile isotonic saline solution to dissolve or dilute a manufactured sterile, solid drug or concentrated, aqueous solution of the drug. If the active ingredient is not available in a sterile form, a nonsterile but high-quality pure powder may be used. Use of each type of ingredient is illustrated in the sample prescriptions at the end of this chapter.

2. In deciding whether other components are needed, the compounder must use knowledge of chemistry, pharmaceutics, microbiology, and therapeutics. Possible auxiliary agents include buffers, tonicity adjustors, preservatives, antioxidants, and viscosity-inducing agents.

3. Buffers

   a. Formulas for a variety of ophthalmic buffering vehicles are given in Chapter 18, Buffers and pH Adjusting Agents. The most widely used ophthalmic buffer solutions are Boric Acid Vehicle and Sorensen's Modified Phosphate Buffer.

   b. Boric Acid Vehicle

      (1) Boric Acid Vehicle is a 1.9% aqueous solution of boric acid. This concentration is approximately isotonic with tears, but it is not iso-osmotic with red blood cells. This is because the membrane on red blood cells is permeable to boric acid. Therefore, although boric acid is a common ingredient in ophthalmic preparations, it may not be used parenterally.

      (2) Boric Acid Vehicle has a pH of approximately 5. Though this vehicle does not possess large buffer capacity, it will stabilize the pH of a drug solution close to pH 5. This, of course, depends on the pH generated by the drug itself and on the buffer capacity of the drug.

      (3) Because Boric Acid Vehicle does not have strong buffering capacity, it is useful when extemporaneously compounding ophthalmic solutions of drugs that are most stable at acid pH. Boric Acid Vehicle will stabilize the pH of the solution at approximately 5 for the short expiratory periods used for compounded solutions. At the same time, its weak buffer capacity is easily overcome by the natural buffers in lacrimal fluid, so its acidic solutions are not uncomfortable when instilled in the eye.

      (4) Boric acid is available as crystals and powder. The crystals are preferred for making Boric Acid Vehicle, because they give more crystal-clear solutions than does the powder.

      (5) According to the *USP XXI*, Boric Acid Vehicle is useful for making ophthalmic solutions of the salts of the following drugs: benoxinate, cocaine, dibucaine, phenylephrine,

piperocaine, procaine, proparacaine, tetracaine, and zinc (4). King's *Dispensing of Medication* adds ethylmorphine, neostigmine, ethyl hydrocupreine, and phenacaine to the list (5).

(6) A modified Boric Acid Vehicle can be made for drugs that are especially sensitive to oxidation. The antioxidants sodium bisulfite and sodium metabisulfite in a concentration of 0.1%, or the chelating agent disodium edetate in a concentration of 0.1%, may be added to retard oxidation. This modified vehicle is useful for drugs prone to oxidation. Examples include physostigmine and epinephrine (5).

c. Sorensen's Modified Phosphate Buffer

(1) Sorensen's Phosphate Buffer is made using two stock solutions: one acidic, containing NaH_2PO_4, and one basic, containing Na_2HPO_4. The formulas for the stock solutions are given in Table 18.3 of Chapter 18, Buffers and pH Adjusting Agents. Each solution is 1/15 or 0.067 M. The stock solutions are mixed in an appropriate ratio to give a desired pH. Table 18.3 also shows the volume ratios to mix to give a desired pH.

(2) When mixed as directed, these buffer solutions are not isotonic. If an isotonic buffer is desired, a solute must be added for tonicity adjustment. Examples of possible solutes include sodium chloride, sodium nitrate, and dextrose. The choice of a tonicity adjusting solute depends on the compatibility of the solute with the other ingredients in the formulation. Table 18.3 shows the weight in grams of sodium chloride that must be added to 100 mL of buffer solution to give an isotonic buffer. If a different solute is desired, the amount of this solute can be calculated using its sodium chloride equivalent (see section III of Chapter 11 for sample calculations).

(3) Sorensen's Modified Phosphate Buffer has a significant buffer capacity and should not be used outside the pH range of 6.5 to 8.0.

(4) According to the *USP XXI,* Sorensen's Modified Phosphate Buffer is useful for making ophthalmic solutions of the salts of the following drugs: pilocarpine, eucatropine, scopolamine, and homatropine (4). King's *Dispensing of Medication* adds atropine, ephedrine, and penicillin to this list (5).

d. An alternative way of adding a buffering vehicle is to use a manufactured artificial tears product that contains an appropriate buffer. Caution must be exercised in using these products, because they may also contain other ingredients, such as viscosity-inducing agents and preservatives that could cause compatibility problems. *Drug Facts and Comparisons*, the *PDR for Ophthalmology*, and the product prescribing information (product package insert) list the ingredients of artificial tears products.

e. Amount of buffer solution to use

(1) The buffer solution is often used as the tonicity adjustor for the ophthalmic solution. Under these circumstances, isotonicity calculations determine the amount of buffer solution to use.

(2) A minimum amount of buffer is needed to provide a buffering effect. One general rule states that the concentration of the buffer should be ten times that of the drug, the concentrations of both expressed in molar quantities (6). Another recommendation states that a concentration of 0.05 to 0.5 M of buffer gives sufficient buffering capacity (7). Both of these general rules are somewhat arbitrary; they are based on buffer solutions that are made from conjugate pairs with a pK_a within one unit of the desired pH. Although Boric Acid Vehicle has a higher molar concentration (approximately 0.3 M) than has Sorenson's Modified Phosphate Buffer (0.067 M), Sorensen's buffer has significantly greater buffering capacity because it consists of a conjugate pair, whereas Boric Acid Vehicle is merely a solution of a mild acid.

(3) Because the aforementioned general rules require a bit of calculation, a more simplified recommendation, which gives a "ballpark" figure, is for the volume of the buffer solution to be one-third of the volume of the finished product. If isotonicity calculations show that less than one-third of the final volume should be buffer solution, a compromise between isotonicity and buffering is needed. The one-third of the volume is an oversimplified but convenient figure (6).

4. Tonicity adjustor

a. As indicated earlier, the buffer solution is convenient to use as the tonicity adjustor.

b. In circumstances when a buffer is not needed, any compatible salt or nonelectrolyte that is approved for ophthalmic preparations may be used. Sodium chloride, sodium nitrate, sodium sulfate, and dextrose are common neutral tonicity adjustors.

5. Antimicrobial preservatives

a. *USP* Chapter ⟨1151⟩ states the following concerning the use of preservatives in ophthalmic solutions:

> Each solution must contain a suitable substance or mixture of substances to prevent the growth of, or to destroy, microorganisms accidentally introduced when the container is opened during use. Where intended for use in surgical procedures, ophthalmic solutions, although they must be sterile, should not contain antibacterial agents, since they may be irritating to the ocular tissues (1).

b. The authors of *Extemporaneous Ophthalmic Preparations* give the following advice on the use of antimicrobial preservatives in ophthalmic solutions (8):

(1) Because of preservative toxicity, especially following ocular surgery, avoid preservatives, if possible, and use either unpreserved Sterile Water for Injection or Sodium Chloride Injection 0.9% as vehicles for ophthalmic drugs. This means that the solution should be discarded after 24 hours because of the danger of contamination by microorganisms. This practice is practical only in a hospital or institutional setting where fresh solution can be furnished every day, so it is useful primarily for inpatients.

(2) For ambulatory patients and when hospitalized patients are discharged, it can be assumed that the eye has sufficiently healed so that it is less vulnerable to irritation and toxicity due to preservatives. At this time, the solution vehicle can be changed to Bacteriostatic Water for Injection or Bacteriostatic Sodium Chloride Injection. The beyond-use date is then based on the chemical stability of the active ingredient(s). (**Note:** A recent revision to *USP* Chapter ⟨797⟩ puts additional time limits on the beyond-use dates of these compounded sterile preparations; see the section later in this chapter on beyond-use dates.)

(3) Manufactured multidose artificial tears products contain one or more preservatives; they provide another alternative ophthalmic vehicle for ambulatory patients. When using these products for vehicles, consideration must be given to the volume of any added solution so that the preservative in the product is not diluted beyond its effective concentration.

c. Agents: Although more than a dozen preservatives are approved for ophthalmic solutions (see Table 16.2 in Chapter 16, Antimicrobial Preservatives), there is no ideal ophthalmic preservative.

(1) Benzalkonium chloride (BAC), phenylmercuric acetate (PMA) or phenylmercuric nitrate (PMN), thimerosal, and chlorobutanol are the most commonly used ophthalmic preservatives. Information on each of these agents, including official articles, solubilities, effective concentrations, and information on incompatibilities, can be found in Chapter 16.

(2) Benzyl alcohol and the parabens are not often used in manufactured ophthalmic products, but they are approved for ophthalmic use (9). They are the preservatives most commonly found in Bacteriostatic Water for Injection and Bacteriostatic Sodium Chloride Injection.

d. Before adding a preservative, always check on patient sensitivity, on compatibility of the preservative with all other ingredients in the formulation, and on recommended preservative concentration. *Martindale: The Complete Drug Reference* and *Handbook of Pharmaceutical Excipients* are two excellent resources for compatibility information.

e. Table 33.1 gives the maximum concentrations of some common preservatives approved for use in nonprescription ophthalmic products (10).

Table 33.1	MAXIMUM CONCENTRATIONS OF PRESERVATIVES APPROVED FOR USE IN OPHTHALMIC PRODUCTS[a]	
AGENT	**MAXIMUM LEVEL (%)**	
Benzalkonium chloride	0.013	
Benzethonium chloride	0.01	
Chlorobutanol	0.5	
Phenylmercuric acetate	0.004	
Phenylmercuric nitrate	0.004	
Thimerosal	0.01	

[a]Maximum levels are for direct contact with eye tissues and not for ocular devices such as contact lens products.
Source: FDA Advisory Review Panel on OTC Ophthalmic Drug Products. Final report, December 1979.

Table 33.2	MAXIMUM CONCENTRATIONS OF OPHTHALMIC ADDITIVES FOR USE IN OPHTHALMIC PRODUCTS[a]

AGENT	MAXIMUM LEVEL (%)
ANTIOXIDANTS	
Sodium bisulfite	0.1
Sodium metabisulfite	0.1
Thiourea	0.1
Ethylenediaminetetraacetic acid	0.1
WETTING/CLARIFYING AGENTS	
Polysorbate 80	1.0
Polysorbate 20	1.0
VISCOSITY AGENTS	
Polyvinyl alcohol	1.4
Polyvinylpyrrolidone	1.7
Methylcellulose	2.0
Hydroxypropyl methylcellulose	1.0
Hydroxyethylcellulose	0.8

[a]Maximum levels are for direct contact with eye tissues and not for ocular devices such as contact lens products.
Source: FDA Advisory Review Panel on OTC Ophthalmic Drug Products. Final report, December 1979.

6. Antioxidants
    a. Check references and use your general knowledge of chemistry to decide whether the active ingredient or ingredients are subject to oxidation. If oxidation is a problem, an antioxidant may be necessary or recommended. If an antioxidant is recommended, check references for compatibility information. Maximum concentrations of antioxidants approved for use in nonprescription ophthalmic products are given in Table 33.2 (10).
    b. Agents: Although several antioxidants are approved for ophthalmic solutions, as with preservatives, they all have some disadvantages. Sodium bisulfite, sodium metabisulfite, and disodium edetate are commonly used antioxidants for ophthalmic products. Information on each of these agents, including descriptions of official articles, solubilities, and effective concentrations, can be found in Chapter 17, Antioxidants.
        (1) As reported in Chapter 17, sulfites must be used with caution because of reported incidents of allergic reactions to these compounds. Even though they have been used as antioxidants in solutions of epinephrine, they are reported to inactivate this compound. The reaction is pH dependent, and boric acid has a stabilizing effect (11).
        (2) As discussed in Chapter 17, disodium edetate is technically not an antioxidant but a chelator of heavy metal ions. It serves as an antioxidant for drugs that have their oxidation catalyzed by heavy metals. Edetate is reported to have a synergistic effect on the preservative effectiveness of BAC (12); this may be a reason for its presence in many commercial ophthalmic products preserved with BAC. Although edetic acid is also an effective antioxidant, it is not often used in compounding ophthalmic solutions because of its poor water solubility; disodium edetate is the preferred form because it is water-soluble.
7. Other agents: When needed, wetting, clarifying, and viscosity-inducing agents may be added to ophthalmic solutions. Maximum concentrations of these components approved for use in nonprescription ophthalmic products are given in Table 33.2.

II.   NASAL SOLUTIONS

A. **Definition:** These solutions are sprayed or instilled into the nasal cavity. Although they are not specifically mentioned as a class in *USP* Chapter ⟨1151⟩, there are official USP nasal solutions, such as Naphazoline Hydrochloride Nasal Solution. Nasal solutions are most often used for local action, but they may also be used for systemic effect.

B. Special cautions

1. While not quite as critical as for ophthalmic solutions, nasal solutions should be sterile, and compounders should make this dosage form only when they have the knowledge and necessary equipment and when there is no alternative commercial product.

2. At one time, nasal solutions were used almost exclusively for local action but, in recent years, this route of administration has also been used for systemic effects. Compounding and dispensing nasal solutions for systemic administration should be done with the greatest caution. Although procedures have been described in the literature for calibration of droppers and nasal sprays, results in practice have not been encouraging. In one study of nasal droppers, ten physicians acted as the test subjects; all ten overused the drug by a range of 41% to 338% (13). Similar results were found during an informal study conducted by pharmacy students using a procedure recommended for calibration of nasal spray bottles in which nasal solution was sprayed into a tared plastic bag and the bag then reweighed to determine quantity per spray. For systemic nasal drug administration, metered-dose drug delivery systems are recommended, especially when potent drugs are involved. Nasal actuators that deliver 0.1 mL per pump are available from some vendors of compounding supplies.

C. Desired properties and components

1. The FDA Center for Drug Evaluation and Research (CDER) has issued *Guidance for Industry: Nasal Spray and Inhalation Solution, Suspension, and Spray Drug Products—Chemistry, Manufacturing, and Controls Documentation* (available on the FDA Internet site at http://www.fda.gov/cder/guidance/4234fnl.htm, accessed February 2008) (14). This guidance was written for the pharmaceutical industry, and while the information and recommendations do not impose mandatory requirements either on the industry or on pharmacies that compound these preparations, the information provided is very useful.

2. Nasal solutions should be sterile when dispensed. The section on nasal solutions in the FDA *Guidance for Industry* states that microbial quality should be controlled by tests and criteria as given in *USP* Chapter ⟨61⟩, Microbial Limit Tests (14). Though there is no absolute requirement for sterility of nasal solutions in the *USP* (15) or the FDA *Guidance for Industry* (14), sterility is considered to be an important safety issue, so it is recommended that pharmacists who compound nasal solutions render them sterile at the time of dispensing (16).

3. Multidose containers of nasal solutions should contain an antimicrobial preservative or other agent(s) that will prevent the growth of microorganisms, which may be introduced in the preparation during use.

4. Normal nasal secretions have a pH in the range of 5.5 to 6.5. Because nasal secretions lack significant natural buffer capacity, highly buffered solutions, especially outside the normal pH range, should be avoided (17).

5. The cilia in nasal passages are sensitive to osmotic pressure, so nasal solutions should be as close to isotonic as is possible. Nasal solutions with osmolarity comparable to aqueous 0.5% to 2% sodium chloride solutions are relatively comfortable and should not harm nasal cilia.

D. Active ingredients and components

1. As with ophthalmic solutions, active ingredients for nasal solutions may be bulk powders or liquids or sterile manufactured products.

2. The vehicle for nasal solutions is usually water, but it may be a cosolvent system, provided the other solvent or solvents are approved for internal use.

3. Buffers

   a. If a buffer is desired with a pH in the neutral range, a dilute phosphate buffer at pH 6.5 is recommended (16). The isotonic Sorenson's Modified Phosphate Buffer Solution at pH 6.5, as given in Table 18.3 in Chapter 18, would be a good choice.

   b. If a buffer is needed for purposes of drug stability or solubility with a pH that is outside the normal range, a buffer or pH-adjusting agent that has low buffer capacity should be selected. See Chapter 18 for more information on this subject.

4. Antimicrobial preservatives

   a. Antimicrobial preservatives that are approved for internal use would be suitable for preserving nasal solutions. These are listed and described in Chapter 16.

   b. When selecting a preservative, check for compatibility with active ingredients and other necessary added excipients. Also check to be sure that the preservative is active at the pH of the finished nasal solution.

5. Tonicity adjustors: Sodium chloride and dextrose are recommended tonicity adjustors for nasal solutions (17).
6. Other components
   a. In addition to preservatives, buffers, and tonicity adjusting agents, nasal solutions may also contain antioxidants, surfactants, and viscosity-inducing agents.
   b. The effect of tonicity and the specific effects of various drugs, salts, surfactants, cosolvents, oils, and preservatives was investigated in the late 1940s and early 1950s by Proetz (18). Sample Prescription 33.5 uses a formula developed by Proetz for a nasal preparation. A summary of this work can be found in the seventh edition of *Dispensing of Medication*, pages 913–915. Some findings helpful in formulating compounded nasal solutions are given here (19).
      (1) Although nasal passages can tolerate a relatively wide range of tonicity without pain, isotonicity is important. Highly hypertonic solutions (4% to 4.5% sodium chloride solutions) and hypotonic solutions (0.3% or less sodium chloride solutions) were found to cause damage to nasal cilia.
      (2) Alcohol in concentrations up to 10%, when in an isotonic solution, caused no problems.
      (3) BAC in concentrations up to 0.1%, if incorporated into an isotonic saline solution, showed no damage to cilia.
      (4) Anionic surfactants such as sodium lauryl sulfate and docusate sodium could be used in concentrations of 0.01% without pain or a burning sensation, but concentrations of 0.05% caused some discomfort. Nonionic surfactants were acceptable at much higher concentrations.

III. INHALATION SOLUTIONS (1,20)

A. **Definition:** Inhalations are dosage forms "designed to be dispersed in a current of air and drawn into the airways when the patient breathes in" (20). They are administered either by the nasal or oral route, with the respiratory tract as the intended site for local effect or for systemic absorption of an active ingredient. They may be drugs, solutions, or suspensions (1).

B. **Cautions:** As with ophthalmic and nasal dosage forms, inhalations should be compounded with great care and only when there is no alternative commercial product available.

C. **Desired properties and components**
   1. Inhalation solutions are required to be sterile: Section III.F.2.f of the FDA *Guidance for Industry* states, "All aqueous-based oral inhalation solutions, suspensions, and spray drug products must be sterile" (14). Although this guidance was written for the pharmaceutical industry, compounded inhalation solutions must also be sterile.
   2. The usual vehicles for inhalation solutions are Sterile Water for Inhalation and Sodium Chloride Inhalation Solution 0.9%. Both meet the sterility standards in *USP* Chapter ⟨71⟩, Sterility Tests. Neither contains an antimicrobial preservative, so if either of these is used as the vehicle for a compounded inhalation solution, it must be packaged and labeled for single use (15), or a preservative must be added. Sodium Chloride Injection 0.9% and Sterile Water for Injection are also acceptable vehicles. Small quantities of cosolvents such as alcohol or glycerin may be added when needed (20).
   3. As with ophthalmic and nasal solutions, inhalation solutions should be as close to isotonic as is possible. Sodium chloride is the most common tonicity–adjusting agent.
   4. An antimicrobial preservative is required for any inhalation solution dispensed in a multidose container (21). Preservatives that are approved for internal use would be suitable for preserving inhalation solutions; these are listed and described in Chapter 16. When selecting a preservative, check for compatibility with active ingredients and other necessary added excipients. Also check to be sure that the preservative is active at the pH of the finished inhalation solution.
   5. Inhalation solutions may contain additives similar to those used in nasal solutions, but agents such as preservatives, antioxidants, buffers, and surfactants should be used only as necessary, and the concentration of these additives should be as low as possible. These solutions are delivered to very sensitive tissues in the lungs, and this should always be considered in formulating a solution for inhalation.

6. For proper delivery of solution to the respiratory tract, inhalation solutions must first be nebulized to form very small, uniform droplets that will pass through the mouth or nose, throat, and bronchial tree to the bronchioles and alveoli of the lungs. Hand-held nebulizers and intermittent positive-pressure breathing (IPPB) machines are available for this purpose (1).

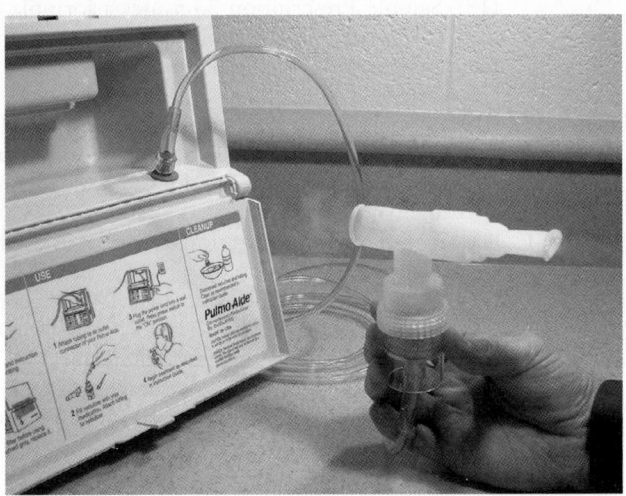

NEBULIZER

IV.   IRRIGATION SOLUTIONS

A. **Definition:** These are sterile solutions used to soak, flush, or irrigate wounds or body cavities, such as the bladder (1,20).
B. **Cautions:** As with the other sterile solutions discussed in this chapter, irrigation solutions should be compounded with great care and only when there is no alternative commercial product available. In 1990, the FDA issued an "alert letter" to pharmacists after the death of two hospital patients; the incident involved incorrectly prepared irrigation solutions for surgical procedures (2). Such solutions are administered to vulnerable body tissues and must be sterile; they should be handled in the same fashion as parenteral products.
C. **Desired properties and components**
   1. Irrigation solutions must be sterile.
   2. They are not for parenteral use and should be labeled "not for injection" and "for irrigation only."
   3. The usual vehicle for irrigating solutions is water.
   4. Because irrigating solutions come in contact with open wounds and delicate body tissues and membranes, special consideration must be given to isotonicity and pH of the solution. Additives may be necessary to achieve these objectives, but they must be chosen with great care.

V.   COMPOUNDING PROCEDURES

A. Follow the usual compounding procedures with respect to checking doses and concentrations, general stability and compatibility of the formulation ingredients, selection of ingredients and equipment, and so on as outlined in Chapter 12, General Guidelines for Preparing Compounded Drug Preparations, and as illustrated in the sample prescriptions that follow. For ophthalmic solutions, the *ASHP* Technical Assistance Bulletin on Pharmacy-Prepared Ophthalmic Products gives good general instructions on preparing these solutions (22). (Available on the American Society of Health-System Pharmacists' Internet site at http://www.ashp.org/, Accessed December 2007).
B. Because these are sterile dosage forms, their preparation and packaging should be done in a sterile environment such as a laminar airflow workbench or a barrier isolator. A sterile, particle-free solution can be achieved by one of the following methods.
   1. Using sterile parenteral drug products as the solution ingredients, prepare the solution as you would a parenteral preparation, using aseptic technique and packaging the solution in a clean, particle-free, sterile container. See Chapter 32, General Principles of Sterile Dosage Form

Preparation, and Chapter 34, Parenteral Preparations, for a discussion of the principles and sample prescriptions using techniques for this type of aseptic processing. Sample Prescriptions 33.3 and 33.4 in this chapter illustrate the use of sterile manufactured products for making compounded ophthalmic solutions.

2. Prepare the solution using nonsterile but high-quality ingredients, and filter the solution using a 0.2- or 0.22-μm bacterial filter into a dispensing container that is clean, particle-free, and sterile. For solutions sterilized by bacterial filtration, a small excess is often prepared to allow for loss during the filtration process. Compatibility and stability of the preparation ingredients should be considered, because some bacterial filters adsorb certain types of drug molecules; large molecules such as peptides or proteins are particularly vulnerable. Sample Prescriptions 33.1, 33.2, and 33.5 illustrate the use of a bacterial membrane filter unit.

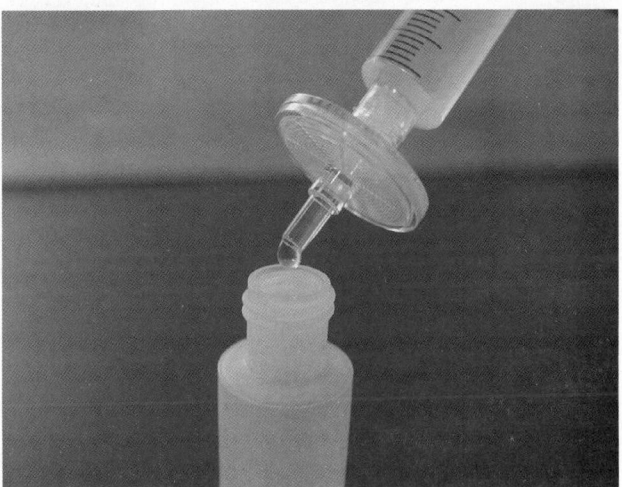

STERILIZATION OF A COMPOUNDED SOLUTION USING A BACTERIAL MEMBRANE FILTER

3. If an autoclave is available, terminal steam sterilization can be used. In this case, the solution may be prepared using nonsterile but high-quality ingredients and packaged in an appropriate clean, particle-free container that is stable to the elevated temperature and pressure needed for steam sterilization. The preparation is then autoclaved in the dispensing container.

   a. Usual quality control procedures for steam sterilization must be used. Monitoring devices that track and record time, temperature, and pressure are used, as is verification of the autoclave cycle through use of biologic and other indicators. For pharmacies that have access to autoclaves in institutional settings such as hospitals, the methods are well controlled and

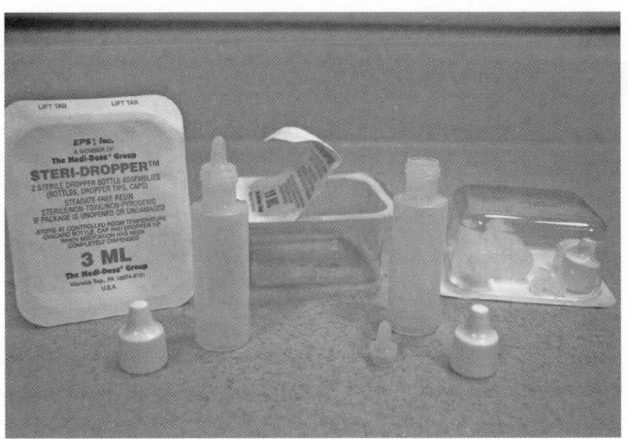

STERILE DROPPER BOTTLES

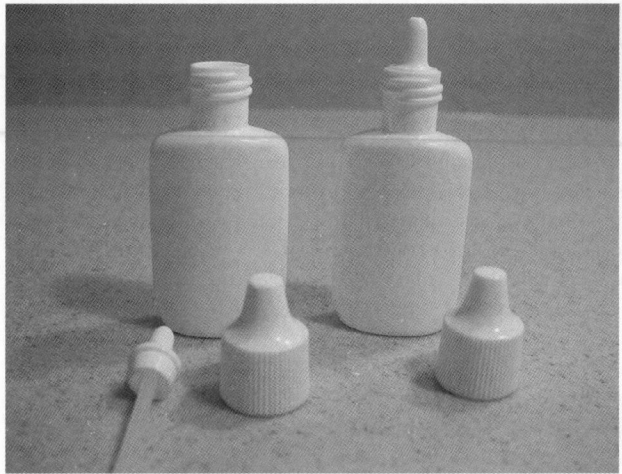

NASAL SPRAY BOTTLES

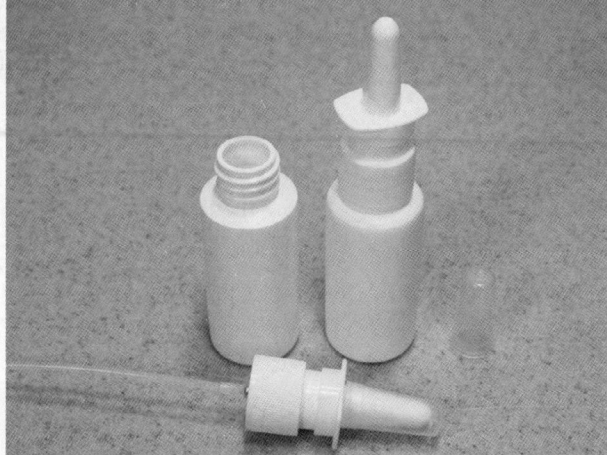

NASAL ACTUATOR

documented as required by accreditation standards. Pharmacists using their own equipment should employ standard operating procedures that assure that the equipment and methods give preparations that are sterile. The accidents with nonsterile ophthalmic solutions, which were discussed at the beginning of this chapter, involved steam sterilization procedures that were inadequate (2).

    b. Because steam sterilization uses elevated temperature and pressure, consider drug and container stability under these conditions before using this method.

4. Packaging must be in a sterile container.

    a. For small volumes of solution, presterilized dropper containers, in sizes 3 mL, 7 mL, and l5 mL, are available for purchase from vendors of compounding supplies.

    b. An alternative for an ophthalmic or nasal preparation is to empty the contents from the container of a manufactured sterile product (such as artificial tears for an ophthalmic solution or sterile saline nasal mist for a nasal solution), rinse the sterile container with sterile water, and use this container for the compounded preparation.

    c. Dropper bottles, nasal spray bottles, and nasal actuators (with controlled volume per spray) are available from compounding suppliers. If these are not sterile as purchased, they should be sterilized before use.

    d. Most often, sterile irrigation solutions are prepared by adding ingredients to a bottle of Sterile Water for Irrigation or Sodium Chloride Irrigation. This then also provides the sterile container.

    e. Nonsterile containers can be sterilized using either an autoclave or an ethylene oxide sterilizer. Before using one of these methods, check to be sure that the container and closure materials will withstand the required sterilization conditions.

VI.   **BEYOND-USE DATING**

A. Manufactured products

    1. Even for multidose manufactured products that contain antimicrobial preservatives, shorter beyond-use dates (BUDs) are recommended for these products than for nonsterile dosage forms because of the danger of contamination during use and the serious consequences of using a nonsterile product. Research has been done and papers have been published on loss of sterility of ophthalmic solutions under conditions of use (23). As a result, some hospitals and nursing homes use a policy of discarding ophthalmic products 30 days after unsealing. The nurse or caregiver dates the sealed ophthalmic container when the seal is broken and the bottle is entered for the first time, and any unused portion is discarded after 30 days. For sterile multidose products, *USP* Chapter ⟨797⟩ recommends a 28-day BUD after first entry; this recommendation is for sterile, manufactured, preserved solutions handled by health care professionals (24). The pharmacist should consider the expected storage and handling conditions for dispensed sterile products when assigning a BUD.

2. For unpreserved sterile manufactured products that are available in single-dose or single-use quantities, manufacturers recommend immediate use on unsealing the container and discarding any unused solution. *USP* Chapter ⟨797⟩ recommends a 1-hour limit if the container is opened outside a controlled ISO Class 5 environment and a 6-hour limit if the container is opened and maintained within a Class 5 or cleaner air space (24). (See Chapter 32 for a discussion of ISO classes.)

B. Compounded solutions

Compounded sterile solutions are discussed in both *USP* Chapter ⟨795⟩ and *USP* Chapter ⟨797⟩; using these two chapters as guides, the most conservative recommended BUD should be used.

1. *USP* Chapter ⟨795⟩
Chapter ⟨795⟩ on pharmacy compounding of nonsterile preparations recommends a maximum 14-day dating for all water-containing liquid preparations made with ingredients in solid form when the stability of the ingredients in the formulations is not known (25). Obviously, for drugs that are labile to chemical degradation, a shorter dating must be used.

2. *USP* Chapter ⟨797⟩
Standards for BUDs specific to compounded sterile preparations are given in Chapter ⟨797⟩. In this case, the BUD is dependent both on the chemical stability of the preparation components and on sterility issues that are addressed by risk levels in Chapter ⟨797⟩. (See Chapter 32 of this book for details of Chapter ⟨797⟩.)

Assuming adherence to all personnel and environmental controls described in Chapter ⟨797⟩ (e.g., compounding done in an ISO Class 5 hood that is located in an ISO Class 7 buffer area), the maximum storage periods by risk level are as follows:

a. Low-risk level: 48 hours at controlled room temperature; 14 days at cold temperature (e.g., refrigerator); and 45 days in frozen state (e.g., freezer between −25° and −10°C).

b. Medium-risk level: 30 hours at controlled room temperature; 7 days at cold temperature (e.g., refrigerator); and 45 days in frozen state (e.g., freezer between −25° and −10°C).

c. High-risk level: 24 hours at controlled room temperature; 3 days at cold temperature (e.g., refrigerator); and 45 days in frozen state (e.g., freezer between −25° and −10°C) (24).

VII. PATIENT CONSULTATION

A. For outpatient use, be sure to give the patient or caregiver good instructions on how to administer these solutions, including techniques to avoid contamination of the solution and the administration device such as the dropper or nasal actuator.

B. Guides for instructing a patient on the proper administration and use of ophthalmic solutions and ointments are given in Figures 33.1 and 33.2.

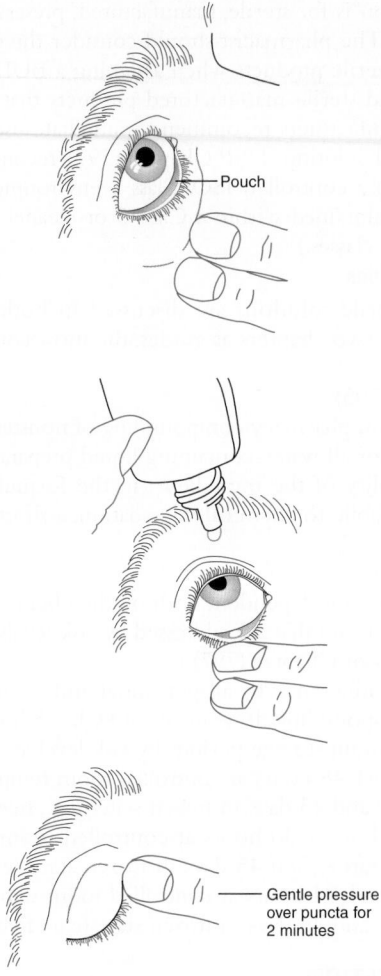

FIGURE 33.1. HOW TO USE EYE DROPS.
1. Wash your hands carefully with soap and warm water.
2. If the product container is transparent, check the solution before use. If it is discolored or has changed in any way since it was purchased (e.g., particles in the solution, color change), do not use the solution. Return it to the pharmacy.
3. If the product container has a depressible rubber bulb, draw up a small amount of medication into the eye dropper by first squeezing and then relieving pressure on the bulb.
4. Place the head back with chin tilted up and look toward the ceiling.
5. With both eyes open, gently draw down the lower lid of the affected eye with your index finger (see top illustration).
6. In the "gutter" formed, drop the directed number of drops (see middle illustration).
   IMPORTANT: The dropper or administration tip should be held as near as possible to the lid without actually touching the eye. DO NOT allow the dropper or administration tip to touch any surface.
7. If possible, hold the eyelid open and do not blink for 30 seconds.
8. You may want to press your finger against the inner corner of your eye for one minute. This will keep the medication in your eye (see bottom illustration).
9. Tightly cap the bottle.

REMEMBER
- This is a **sterile** solution. Contamination of the dropper or eye solution can lead to a serious eye infection. If you accidentally touch the dropper to any surface, wipe the dropper with a clean tissue. If you think you have contaminated the dropper or solution, consult your physician or pharmacist for instructions.
- If irritation persists or increases, discontinue use and consult your physician immediately.
- Generally, eye makeup should be avoided while using eye solutions. If you have questions about this, consult your pharmacist or physician.
- You may want to use a mirror when applying the drops, or it may be much easier to have someone help you instill your eye drops.

(Image reprinted with permission from Pray, SW. Nonprescription Product Therapeutics, Second Edition. Baltimore, Maryland: Lippincott Williams & Wilkins, 2006.)

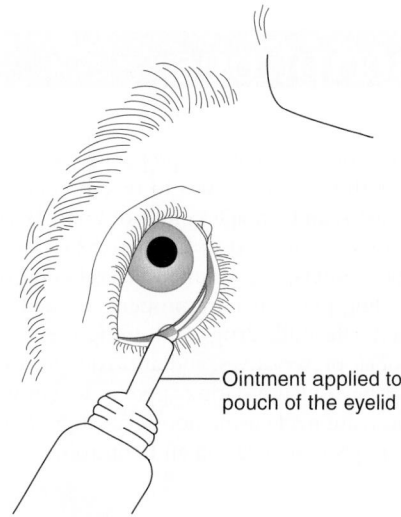

Ointment applied to
pouch of the eyelid

FIGURE 33.2. HOW TO USE EYE OINTMENT.
1. Wash your hands carefully with soap and warm water.
2. You may want to hold the ointment tube in your hand for a few minutes to warm and
   soften the ointment.
3. Gently cleanse the affected eyelid with warm water and a soft cloth before applying the
   ointment.
4. This procedure should be done in front of a mirror.
5. With the affected eye looking upward, gently pull the lower eyelid downward with your
   index finger to form a pouch.
6. Squeeze a thin line (approximately ¼–½ inch) of ointment from the tube along the pouch.
   IMPORTANT: Be very careful when applying this ointment. DO NOT allow the tip of the
   ointment tube to touch the eyelid, the eyeball, your finger, or any surface.
7. Close the eye gently and rotate the eyeball to distribute the ointment. You may blink
   several times to evenly spread the ointment.
8. Replace the cap on the ointment tube.
9. After you apply the ointment, your vision may be blurred temporarily. Do not be alarmed.
   This will clear up in a short while, but do not drive a car or operate machinery until your
   vision has cleared.

REMEMBER:
- This is a **sterile** ointment. Contamination of the tip or the cap of the tube can lead to a serious eye infection. If you accidentally touch the tip to any surface, wipe it with a clean
  tissue. If you think you have contaminated the tip or the ointment, consult your physician
  or pharmacist for instructions.
- If irritation persists or increases, discontinue use and consult your physician immediately.
- Generally, eye makeup should be avoided while using eye ointments. If you have
  questions about this, consult your pharmacist or physician.
- It may be much easier to have someone help you apply your eye ointment.

(Image reprinted with permission from Pray, SW. Nonprescription Product Therapeutics,
Second Edition. Baltimore, Maryland: Lippincott Williams & Wilkins, 2006.)

Sample Prescriptions

As indicated previously, sterile preparations should be made only when necessary and with the utmost care and with strict adherence to recommended environmental conditions, personnel training, aseptic procedures, and storage conditions and BUDs for finished preparations. As indicated previously, these topics are discussed in Chapter 32 of this book and in *USP* Chapter ⟨797⟩. For the following prescription orders, it is assumed that all conditions described in Chapter ⟨797⟩ are in place and that compounding personnel are properly trained. The first two samples prescriptions, which are made with nonsterile bulk drugs and components, are included to illustrate the use of added buffers, antimicrobial preservatives, and antioxidants; methods for tonicity adjustment; and necessary procedures and beyond-use dating specific to compounding with nonsterile ingredients. Because these preparations are made using nonsterile ingredients, they are in the *USP* Chapter ⟨797⟩ high-risk level, which requires extra caution and controls.

SAMPLE PRESCRIPTION 33.1

CASE: Chelsea Von Katrinca is a 146-lb, 5′5″-tall, 63-year-old female patient who was diagnosed 3 weeks ago with glaucoma. Ms. Von Katrinca has a long medical history of moderate persistent asthma for which she uses a betamethasone inhaler 2 puffs bid, theophylline SR 300 mg q12h, and albuterol MDI prn. She has experienced bronchospasm in response to OTC ibuprofen and sulfites in wine. Because of her history with asthma and bronchospasm, Dr. Paque does not want to risk using a β-blocker ophthalmic solution, which is considered first-line therapy for glaucoma. He initially started Ms. Von Katrinca on a topical carbonic anhydrase inhibitor, brinzolamide 1% bid. Now she has returned to the eye clinic for a follow-up check, and her intraocular pressure is still elevated. Dr. Paque wants to add epinephrine eye drops to her regimen and has prescribed epinephrine HCl 1% ophthalmic solution. Pharmacist Jorge calls Dr. Paque because Ms. Von Katrinca's medication profile indicates that she is allergic to sulfites, and Dr. Jorge informs Dr. Paque that all the available commercial epinephrine products contain sodium metabisulfite as an antioxidant. Dr. Paque and Pharmacist Jorge agree that a compounded sulfite-free epinephrine solution should be made for this patient.

CONTEMPORARY PHYSICIANS GROUP PRACTICE
20 S. PARK STREET, TRITURATE, WI 53706
TEL: (608) 555-1333 FAX: (608) 555-1335

℞ #   *123237*

NAME *Chelsea Von Katrinca*   DATE *00/00/00*

ADDRESS *512 Poodle Lane*

℞

Epinephrine HCl   *1%*

Buffer, preserve, and make isotonic, but make sulfite-free
Dispense 15 mL **Use 5 × 3-mL bottles JJ**

J. Jorge 00/00/00

Sig: 1 drop in each eye bid

REFILLS *5*   *Paque*   **M.D.**

DEA NO. _____

MASTER COMPOUNDING FORMULATION RECORD

NAME, STRENGTH, AND DOSAGE FORM OF PREPARATION: Epinephrine HCl 1% Ophthalmic Solution
QUANTITY: 20 mL (5 mL excess)
THERAPEUTIC USE/CATEGORY: Antiglaucoma

FORMULATION RECORD ID: OP001
ROUTE OF ADMINISTRATION: Ophthalmic

INGREDIENTS:

Ingredient	Quantity Used	Physical Description	Solubility	Dose Comparison		Use in the Prescription
				Given	Usual	
Epinephrine HCl	200 mg	white powder	readily sol in water	1%	0.25–2%	lower intraocular pressure
Benzalkonium Chloride (BAC) 17% w/v Solution	1 mL (170 mg) measured; 0.012 mL (2 mg) used	clear, colorless liquid	v sol in water and alcohol	0.01%	0.01%	antimicrobial preservative
Disodium Edetate Injection 150 mg/mL	0.13 mL for 20 mg	clear, colorless liquid	soluble in water	0.1%	0.1%	chelating agent
Boric Acid (crystals)	224 mg	clear, colorless crystals	soluble in water and alcohol	1.2%	—	buffer and tonicity adjuster
Sterile Water for Injection	qs ad 20 mL	clear, colorless liquid	—	—	—	vehicle- solvent

COMPATIBILITY-STABILITY: Epinephrine is an old, established ophthalmic drug that has been well studied (11,26). When in aqueous solution, the drug is subject to oxidation, racemization, and reactions with bisulfite, an antioxidant that is often added to epinephrine solutions to retard oxidation of the drug. Epinephrine is most stable at a pH of 3 to 4. It should be protected from light and, as much as is possible, from oxygen. Boric acid has a protective effect against oxidation and bisulfite reactions. When these conditions are met, the drug is quite stable in solution (11). The pHs of aqueous solutions of epinephrine HCl are in the range 2.2 to 5.0 (26). For this prescription preparation, boric acid is recommended as a buffer and tonicity-adjusting agent (5), and BAC 0.01% is a useful preservative for hydrochloride salts. Because this solution is to be made sulfite-free, disodium edetate is added as a chelating agent to protect against oxidation and to enhance the preservative effectiveness of BAC (12).

PACKAGING AND STORAGE: The *USP* monograph for Epinephrine Ophthalmic Solution recommends storage in tight, light-resistant containers (15). The monograph also states that manufactured Epinephrine Ophthalmic Solutions should be labeled to indicate that the solution should not be used if it is pinkish or darker than slightly yellow or if it contains a precipitate. As discussed previously in this chapter, *USP* Chapter ⟨797⟩ guidelines for sterile preparations have BUDs linked to risk level and storage conditions (24). This preparation is in the high risk level because it is made with nonsterile ingredients. This means the maximum BUD is 3 days in the refrigerator and 45 days in frozen state. Using these guidelines, the 15 mL of solution will be packaged in five separate 3-mL sterile ophthalmic dropper bottles with instructions to the patient to store the bottle in current use in the refrigerator and discard after 3 days. The other bottles should be stored in the freezer and removed one by one every 3 days for current use and storage in the refrigerator.

BEYOND-USE DATE: Although properly prepared epinephrine solutions are quite stable, *USP* Chapter ⟨797⟩ guidelines for sterile preparations made with nonsterile ingredients dictate a maximum of 3 days when stored in the refrigerator and 45 days when stored in the freezer (24). Use a conservative 30-day BUD with storage in the freezer and 3-day BUD with storage in the refrigerator.

CALCULATIONS

Dose/Concentration: Concentration is appropriate for intended use.

Ingredient Amounts

Amounts are for 20 mL of solution to allow for loss in the filtering process.

Active ingredient: Epinephrine HCl (EPI): 1% $\times$ 20 mL = 0.01 $\times$ 20 mL = 0.2 g

Preservative: BAC 0.01% is used to preserve this solution. The amount needed to preserve the solution: 0.01% $\times$ 20 mL = 0.0001 $\times$ 20 mL = 0.002 g = 2 mg

Practical Pharmacy has BAC as the 17% w/v concentrate. Expressed in more convenient units, this is 17 g/100 mL = 17,000 mg/100 mL = 170 mg/mL. This solution is too concentrated to allow the needed amount, 2 mg, to be measured directly. A liquid-liquid aliquot is most practical. One possible aliquot would be as follows: With a 1-mL syringe, withdraw 1 mL (170 mg) of the 17% BAC concentration. Transfer to a 20-mL syringe or a 25-mL graduated cylinder and qs to 17 mL with sterile water. This gives a solution with a convenient concentration of 170 mg/17 mL or 10 mg/mL. You can see by inspection that 0.2 mL is needed for 2 mg. This should be verified by calculation:

$$\left(\frac{10 \text{ mg}}{\text{mL}}\right)\left(\frac{0.2 \text{ mL}}{}\right) = 2 \text{ mg}$$

Antioxidant: As stated previously, an antioxidant is usually added to epinephrine solutions because the drug is labile to oxidation. Sodium metabisulfite is the usual antioxidant used but, in this case, the patient is allergic to that compound. Pharmacist Jorge has decided to use the chelating agent disodium edetate (EDTA) in a concentration of 0.1% to enhance the stability of the epinephrine. The calculations for obtaining the required amount of this chelating agent are as follows:

$$0.1\% \times 20 \text{ mL} = 0.001 \times 20 \text{ mL} = 0.02 \text{ g} = 20 \text{ mg}$$

The pharmacy has disodium edetate as the sterile injection 150 mg/mL. The volume needed is as follows:

$$\frac{150 \text{ mg}}{\text{mL}} = \frac{20 \text{ mg}}{x \text{ mL}}; x = 0.13 \text{ mL}$$

Isotonicity Calculation

Note: For this example, the Sodium Chloride Equivalent method is used to determine the amount of tonicity adjustor needed. Boric acid crystals are used as both the tonicity adjustor and the buffering agent. (The Sodium Chloride Equivalent values for epinephrine HCl (EPI) and boric acid (BA) can be found in Appendix D, and this method is described and illustrated in Chapter 11, Isotonicity Calculations.) Because of their small concentrations in this preparation, the contributions to isotonicity of the BAC and EDTA are disregarded.

The Sodium Chloride Equivalent for EPI = 0.29 (i.e., 0.29 g NaCl/g EPI).

The quantity (in g) of NaCl equivalent to 0.2 g EPI:

$$\frac{0.29 \text{ g NaCl}}{1 \text{ g EPI}} = \frac{x \text{ g NaCl}}{0.2 \text{ g EPI}}; x = 0.058 \text{ g NaCl}$$

Because 0.9% NaCl in water is isotonic, the quantity of NaCl needed to make 20 mL of water isotonic is as follows:

$$0.9\% \times 20 \text{ mL} = 0.009 \times 20 \text{ mL} = 0.18 \text{ g}$$

The quantity of NaCl needed to make 1% EPI solution isotonic is:

$$0.18 \text{ g} - 0.058 \text{ g} = 0.122 \text{ g NaCl}$$

The Sodium Chloride Equivalent of BA = 0.5.

The quantity of BA osmotically equivalent to 0.122 g NaCl is:

$$\frac{0.5 \text{ g NaCl}}{1 \text{ g BA}} = \frac{0.122 \text{ g NaCl}}{x \text{ g BA}}; x = 0.224 \text{ g BA}$$

This is the quantity of BA that needs to be added to the 0.2 g of EPI to make 20 mL of solution isotonic. This should be sufficient for buffering. BA has a MW of 62, so that a solution that is 0.224 g/20 mL is approximately 0.2 M.

MSDS AND SAFETY AND PERSONAL PROTECTIVE EQUIPMENT: Review MSDS for all components. Use aseptic technique for preparing this sterile preparation. Remove jewelry and wash hands and forearms with germicidal soap. Don foot covers, hair covers, a face mask, and a clean, low-shedding gown. Apply an alcohol-based hand cleaner, allow to dry, and put on sterile, powder-free protective gloves.

SPECIALIZED EQUIPMENT: Electronic balance; laminar airflow workbench (LAFW). Wipe the surfaces of the LAFW with sterile 70% isopropyl alcohol using a lint-free cloth.

COMPOUNDING PROCEDURE: Weigh 200 mg of EPI and 224 mg of BA crystals. Place the following items in the LAFW: EPI; BA; Sterile Water for Injection vials; BAC concentrated solution; EDTA vial; clean, 50-mL beaker (that has been rinsed with sterile water for injection and air-dried); 1-mL, 3-mL, and 20-mL syringes; filter needle; regular needles; bacterial membrane filter; and five 3-mL sterile dropper bottles. Using a 20-mL syringe, withdraw 20 mL of Sterile Water for Injection from its vial and use to calibrate the 50-mL beaker at 20 mL. Empty the beaker and place the weighed EPI and BA in the beaker. Using a 1-mL syringe, withdraw 0.13 mL from the EDTA vial and transfer this to the beaker containing the EPI and BA. Using a 3-mL syringe, measure 1 mL of BAC 17% and inject this through the syringe tip of a 20-mL syringe. Put a needle on the 20-mL syringe and draw sterile water into the syringe to the 17-mL mark. Agitate to mix. Using a fresh 1-mL syringe, withdraw through the syringe tip 0.2 mL of this dilution and transfer to the beaker containing the EPI, BA, and EDTA. Using a 20-mL syringe, withdraw sterile water from its vial and use to qs to the 20-mL mark on the beaker; swirl to mix and completely dissolve the EPI and BA. Attach a 5 μm filter needle to a 20-mL syringe and use to draw up approximately 20 mL of solution. Remove the filter needle and apply a 0.22 μm bacterial filter to the syringe tip. With the syringe in an upright position (syringe tip up), express any air from the syringe and filter unit and then wet and fill the filter unit until a bead of solution is visible at the end of the unit. Now position the syringe with tip down and express a drop onto a pH test strip; then expel solution in excess of 20 mL onto sterile gauze or into the beaker. Finally, push out the desired five 3-mL portions of solution into five 3-mL sterile dropper bottles. Carefully apply the ophthalmic bottle tips and caps to the bottles and tighten the bottle caps to ensure that the dropper tips are snapped securely in place. Remove the preparations from the LAFW; label and dispense.

DESCRIPTION OF FINISHED PREPARATION: The preparation is a clear, colorless solution with an apparent viscosity of water.

QUALITY CONTROL: The pH of the preparation is checked with range 0 to 6 pH test strips: pH = 4.5. The final actual volumes are checked and match the theoretical volumes of 5×3 mL plus approximately 4 mL of excess waste solution.

MASTER FORMULA PREPARED BY: Jennie Jorge, PharmD   **CHECKED BY:** Larry Davidow, PhD, RPh

COMPOUNDING RECORD

NAME, STRENGTH, AND DOSAGE FORM OF PREPARATION: Epinephrine HCl 1% Ophthalmic Solution
QUANTITY: 20 mL (5 mL excess)   **DATE PREPARED:** mm/dd/yy   **BEYOND-USE DATE:** mm/dd/yy
FORMULATION RECORD ID: OP001   **CONTROL/RX NUMBER:** 123237

INGREDIENTS USED:

Ingredient	Quantity Used	Manufacturer Lot Number	Expiration Date	Weighed/ Measured by	Checked by
Epinephrine HCl	200 mg	JET Labs OS2711	mm/yy	bjf	jj
Benzalkonium Chloride (BAC) 17% w/v Solution	1 mL (170 mg) measured; 0.012 mL (2 mg) used	JET Labs OS2712	mm/yy	bjf	jj
Disodium Edetate Injection 150 mg/mL	0.13 mL for 20 mg	Sterile Labs PP2713	mm/yy	bjf	jj
Boric Acid (crystals)	224 mg	JET Labs OS2714	mm/yy	bjf	jj
Sterile Water for Injection	qs ad 20 mL	Sterile Labs PP2715	mm/yy	bjf	jj

QUALITY CONTROL DATA: The preparation is a clear, colorless solution with an apparent viscosity of water. The pH of the preparation is checked with range 0 to 6 pH test strips: pH = 4.5. The final actual volumes were checked and match the theoretical volumes of 5 × 3 mL plus approximately 4 mL of excess waste solution.

LABELING

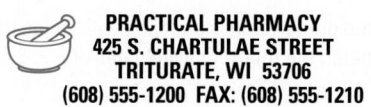

PRACTICAL PHARMACY
425 S. CHARTULAE STREET
TRITURATE, WI 53706
(608) 555-1200 FAX: (608) 555-1210

℞ 123237   Pharmacist: JJ   Date: 00/00/00
Chelsea Von Katrinca   Dr. Paque

Put one drop in each eye two times daily.

Epinephrine HCl 1%; Inactive Ingredients: Benzalkonium Cl 0.01% and Disodium edetate 0.1% as preservatives

Discard or return bottle to pharmacy if solution changes in color or clarity or if any particles are in the solution.

Mfg: Compounded   Quantity: 5 × 3 mL
Refills: 5   Discard after: Give date

Auxiliary Labels: For the eye. This medicine was compounded in our pharmacy for you at the direction of your prescriber. Store bottle being used in the refrigerator and discard after 3 days; store extra bottles in the freezer until the time of use.

PATIENT CONSULTATION: Hello, Ms. Von Katrinca. I think you know me; I'm your pharmacist Jennie Jorge. I have just specially formulated and compounded this solution for you. I know that you have had adverse reactions to sulfites, and drops of this sort that are manufactured usually contain sulfites, so Dr. Paque and I consulted on making these to be sulfite-free. Your medication profile says that you have also had an adverse reaction to ibuprofen; do you have any other drug allergies? I know that you are using several drugs for asthma. How is that therapy going? Have you been pretty free of asthma attacks? I also have on your medical record that you were recently diagnosed with glaucoma and started using brinzolamide or Azopt drops. Dr. Paque said that those drops have not quite controlled your glaucoma, so we are adding these drops, called epinephrine, to your regimen. What did Dr. Paque tell you about this medicine? You are to place one drop in each eye two times a day. You should space putting in these drops about 10 minutes after your other drops. This is to allow your eyes some time to stop any tearing so these drops do not just get washed out. I think that we talked when you got your Azopt drops about the correct technique for using eye drops in glaucoma. It involves applying slight pressure to the inner corner of your eye after putting in your drops to keep them in place so they can have the desired effect. How is that going? Would you like me to go over it with you again? I don't think you should have any problems with these drops, but call Dr. Paque if you develop any eye irritation that doesn't go away. I have packaged these drops in five separate 3-mL sterile ophthalmic dropper bottles. You should store the bottle in current use in the refrigerator and discard it after 3 days. Store the other bottles in the freezer and remove them one by one every 3 days for current use and storage in the refrigerator. These drops should be kept out of the reach of children. If you notice any change in color or clarity or any particles in the solution, do not use that solution and return it to me at the pharmacy. Discard any unused bottles after 1 month (give date). This prescription may be refilled five times, but I think that Dr. Paque wants to see you in 2 weeks to evaluate your condition and how the drops are working. Do you have any questions?

SAMPLE PRESCRIPTION 33.2

CASE: The prescription given here for Shelby Richards is for pilocarpine nitrate 2% ophthalmic solution. As with the epinephrine solution just discussed, this is used as second-line therapy in the treatment of glaucoma. It is generally available as a manufactured product so, unless it is temporarily not supplied or is discontinued, it would not normally be compounded in the pharmacy. A pilocarpine ophthalmic solution that occasionally must be compounded is for a concentration, usually a more dilute concentration, that is not commercially available. In that case, a manufactured pilocarpine (either the hydrochloride or nitrate) ophthalmic solution may be diluted with an appropriate commercial artificial tears solution. In selecting an artificial tears product, choose one that uses the same preservative system as the product containing the pilocarpine. This will avoid the problem of diluting the antimicrobial preservative beyond its effective concentration. Also check any other components in both products to be sure there are no incompatibility problems. This sample prescription is given here to illustrate the use of other auxiliary ingredients and an alternative method for determining isotonicity.

CONTEMPORARY PHYSICIANS GROUP PRACTICE
20 S. PARK STREET, TRITURATE, WI 53706
TEL: (608) 555-1333 FAX: (608) 555-1335

℞ #   *123248*

NAME *Shelby Richards*   DATE *00/00/00*

ADDRESS *982 Schweppe Road*

℞

Pilocarpine Nitrate   2%

Buffer, preserve, and make isotonic

Dispense 15 mL

Bernie Brewer 00/00/00

Use 5 × 3-mL bottles BB

Sig: One drop in each eye qid

REFILLS *2*   *P. V. Heider*   M.D.

DEA NO. _____

MASTER COMPOUNDING FORMULATION RECORD

NAME, STRENGTH, AND DOSAGE FORM OF PREPARATION: Pilocarpine NO_3 2% Ophthalmic Solution
QUANTITY: 20 mL (5 mL excess)   **FORMULATION RECORD ID:** OP002
THERAPEUTIC USE/CATEGORY: Antiglaucoma   **ROUTE OF ADMINISTRATION:** Ophthalmic

INGREDIENTS:

Ingredient	Quantity Used	Physical Description	Solubility	Dose Comparison		Use in the Prescription
				Given	Usual	
Pilocarpine Nitrate	0.4 g	white powder	1 g/4 mL water	2%	0.5–6%	glaucoma
Phenylmercuric Nitrate 1:10,000 solution	8 mL	clear, colorless liquid	v sl sol in water	0.004%	0.002–0.004%	preservative
Sorensen's acid stock solution	14 mL measured; 6.8 mL used	clear, colorless liquid	miscible with water	—	—	buffering agent, vehicle
Sorensen's base stock solution	6 mL measured; 2.9 mL used	clear, colorless liquid	miscible with water	—	—	buffering agent, vehicle
Sodium Nitrate	147 mg weighed; 71 mg used	white powder	1 g/1.1 mL water	—	—	isotonicity adjustor
Sterile water	2.3 mL	clear, colorless liquid	—	—	—	vehicle

COMPATIBILITY–STABILITY: Pilocarpine is an old, established ophthalmic drug that has been well studied (27,28). It is most stable at about pH 5. Pilocarpine is quite stable, even when autoclaved. Protection from light is recommended. Phenylmercuric Nitrate (PMN) 0.004% is chosen as the preservative because pilocarpine nitrate is incompatible with BAC. *USP XXI* recommends the use of Sorenson's phosphate buffer at pH 6.5 for pilocarpine ophthalmic solutions (4), but boric acid would also be satisfactory.

PACKAGING AND STORAGE: The *USP* monograph for Pilocarpine Nitrate Ophthalmic Solution recommends storage in tight, light-resistant containers (15). As discussed previously in this chapter, *USP* Chapter ⟨797⟩ guidelines for sterile preparations have BUDs linked to risk level and storage conditions (24). This preparation is in the high risk level because it is made with nonsterile ingredients. Using these guidelines, the 15 mL of solution will be packaged in five separate 3-mL sterile ophthalmic dropper bottles with instructions to the patient to store the bottle in current use in the refrigerator and discard after 3 days. The other bottles should be stored in the freezer and removed one by one every 3 days for current use and storage in the refrigerator.

BEYOND-USE DATE: Although this preparation is known to be quite stable, *USP* Chapter ⟨797⟩ guidelines for sterile preparations made with nonsterile ingredients dictate a maximum of 3 days when stored in the refrigerator and 45 days when stored in the freezer (24). Use a conservative 30-day BUD with storage in the freezer and 3-day BUD with storage in the refrigerator.

CALCULATIONS

Dose/Concentration: Concentration appropriate for the intended use.

Ingredient Amounts

Note: Calculate for 5 mL excess: 15 mL + 5 mL = 20 mL

Active Ingredient: Pilocarpine NO_3: 2% × 20 mL = 0.4 g

Preservative: PMN 0.004% is chosen as the preservative (as BAC is incompatible with pilocarpine nitrate). The amount needed to preserve the solution is calculated: 0.004% × 20 mL = 0.00004 × 20 mL = 0.0008 g.

The pharmacy has a 1:10,000 stock solution of PMN. The amount of this solution needed is calculated as follows:

$$\frac{1 \text{ g PMN}}{10{,}000 \text{ mL solution}} = \frac{0.0008 \text{ g PMN}}{x \text{ mL solution}} ; \ x = 8 \text{ mL solution}$$

Buffer: Sorensen's Modified Phosphate Buffer at pH 6.5 is chosen as the buffer. The pharmacy has the acid and basic stock solutions. Pharmacist Brewer has decided to make 20 mL of the buffer and will make it isotonic with sodium nitrate, because sodium chloride is incompatible with PMN. On consulting with Table 18.3 in Chapter 18 for the formula of Sorensen's Modified Phosphate Buffer, the pharmacist has determined that to obtain a pH of 6.5, the acid and basic stock solutions should be mixed in a ratio of 7:3.

Acid solution (Monobasic Sodium Phosphate solution):   20 mL × 0.7 = 14 mL

Basic solution (Dibasic Sodium Phosphate solution):   20 mL × 0.3 = 6 mL

From Table 18.3, the amount of NaCl needed to make 100 mL of this buffer solution isotonic is 0.5 g. For 20 mL, the amount is:

$$\frac{0.5 \text{ g NaCl}}{100 \text{ mL solution}} = \frac{x \text{ g NaCl}}{20 \text{ mL solution}} ; \ x = 0.1 \text{ g NaCl}$$

Sodium nitrate has a Sodium Chloride Equivalent of 0.68. The amount of sodium nitrate equivalent to 0.1 g of NaCl is as follows:

$$\frac{0.68 \text{ g NaCl}}{1 \text{ g NaNO}_3} = \frac{0.1 \text{ g NaCl}}{x \text{ g NaNO}_3} ; \ x = 0.147 \text{ g NaNO}_3$$

Isotonicity Calculation

With a mixed buffer system such as Sorenson's Modified Phosphate Buffer, the easiest method for isotonicity calculations is the USP (also called the Sprowls or White–Vincent) Method (which is discussed in Chapter 11, Isotonicity Calculations). Using values in Appendix D, the volume of water to make 1 g of pilocarpine NO_3 isotonic is 25.7 mL. The volume of water to make 0.4 g of pilocarpine NO_3 isotonic is as follows:

$$\frac{1 \text{ g Pilocarpine NO}_3}{25.7 \text{ mL water}} = \frac{0.4 \text{ g Pilocarpine NO}_3}{x \text{ mL water}} ; \ x = 10.3 \text{ mL water}$$

The approximate volume of isotonic Sorenson's Modified Phosphate Buffer needed is as follows:

$$20 \text{ mL} - 10.3 \text{ mL} = 9.7 \text{ mL}$$

Remember: From an isotonicity point of view, the PMN aliquot solution is like water because the PMN content is so small, so 8 mL of the 10.3 mL of water to make the 0.4 g of pilocarpine NO_3 isotonic comes from the PMN aliquot solution.

The following calculations are not needed for this preparation. They are shown here to illustrate the freezing point depression method for isotonicity calculations and the use of boric acid (BA) as the tonicity adjustor-buffer. (Isotonicity values are given in Appendix D, and this method is discussed in Chapter 11.)

Freezing point depression of a 1% solution of pilocarpine nitrate = 0.14°C.

Freezing point depression of a 2% solution of pilocarpine nitrate is calculated to be:

$$\frac{1\% \text{ pilocarpine NO}_3}{0.14°C} = \frac{2\% \text{ pilocarpine NO}_3}{x°C} ; \ x = 0.28°C$$

Amount of additional freezing point depression needed for isotonicity:

$$0.52°C - 0.28°C = 0.24°C$$

BA 1.9% solution is isotonic and has a freezing point depression of 0.52°C. The percent BA needed to give a freezing point depression of 0.24°C is calculated as follows:

$$\frac{1.9\% \text{ BA}}{0.52°C} = \frac{x \% \text{ BA}}{0.24°C} ; \ x = 0.88\% \text{ BA}$$

The number of grams of BA needed at this concentration for 20 mL of solution is calculated to be:

$$\frac{0.88 \text{ g BA}}{100 \text{ mL solution}} = \frac{x \text{ g BA}}{20 \text{ mL}}; x = 0.176 \text{ g BA}$$

MSDS AND SAFETY AND PERSONAL PROTECTIVE EQUIPMENT: Review MSDS for all components. Use aseptic technique for preparing this sterile preparation. Remove jewelry and wash hands and forearms with germicidal soap. Don foot covers, hair covers, a face mask, and a clean, low-shedding gown. Apply an alcohol-based hand cleaner, allow to dry, and put on sterile powder-free protective gloves.

SPECIALIZED EQUIPMENT: Electronic balance; laminar airflow workbench (LAFW). Wipe the surfaces of the LAFW with sterile 70% isopropyl alcohol using a lint-free cloth.

COMPOUNDING PROCEDURE: Prepare the isotonic buffer solution as follows: Weigh 0.147 g sodium nitrate and place in a clean beaker. Measure 14 mL Sorensen's acid stock solution and 6 mL Sorensen's base solution and add both to the sodium nitrate. Swirl to dissolve. Weigh 0.4 g pilocarpine nitrate. Place the following items in the LAFW: pilocarpine; isotonic buffer solution; PMN 1:10,000 solution; Sterile Water for Injection vials; clean, 50-mL beaker (that has been rinsed with Sterile Water for Injection and air-dried); 3-mL, 10-mL, and 20-mL syringes; filter needle; regular needles; bacterial membrane filter; pH test strip, and five 3-mL sterile dropper bottles. Using a 20-mL syringe, withdraw 20 mL of Sterile Water for Injection from its vial and use to calibrate the 50-mL beaker at 20 mL. Empty the beaker and place the weighed pilocarpine in the beaker. Using a 10-mL syringe, withdraw 8 mL of PMN 1:10,000 solution and add this to the pilocarpine in the beaker. Swirl to mix. Using a 3-mL syringe, withdraw 2.3 mL of sterile water from its vial and add this to the pilocarpine nitrate solution. Swirl to mix. Use the previously prepared buffer solution to qs the pilocarpine nitrate solution to 20 mL. Swirl to mix the solution well. Inspect for precipitation and place a drop of the solution on a pH test strip and record the pH. Attach a 5-μm filter needle to a 20-mL syringe and draw the 20 mL of drug solution into the syringe. Remove the filter needle and apply a 0.22-μm bacterial filter to the syringe tip. With the syringe in an upright position (syringe tip up), express any air from the syringe and filter unit, and wet and fill the filter unit until a bead of solution is visible at the tip of the filter unit. Now position the syringe with tip down and expel solution in excess of 15 mL onto sterile gauze or into the beaker. Finally, push out the desired 15 mL of solution into the five 3-mL sterile dropper bottles. Carefully apply the ophthalmic bottle tips and cap to the bottles and tighten the bottle cap to ensure that the dropper tip is snapped securely in place. Remove the preparation from the LAFW; label and dispense.

DESCRIPTION OF FINISHED PREPARATION: The preparation is a clear, colorless solution with an apparent viscosity of water.

QUALITY CONTROL: The pH of the preparation is checked using range 2 to 9 pH test strips: pH = 6.5. The final actual volumes are checked and match the theoretical volumes of 5 × 3 mL plus the approximately 4 mL of residual excess waste solution.

MASTER FORMULA PREPARED BY: Bernie Brewer, PharmD   **CHECKED BY:** Larry Davidow, PhD, RPh

COMPOUNDING RECORD

NAME, STRENGTH, AND DOSAGE FORM OF PREPARATION: Pilocarpine NO_3 2% Ophthalmic Solution
QUANTITY: 20 mL (5 mL excess)   **DATE PREPARED:** mm/dd/yy   **BEYOND-USE DATE:** mm/dd/yy
FORMULATION RECORD ID: OP002   **CONTROL/RX NUMBER:** 123248

INGREDIENTS USED:

Ingredient	Quantity Used	Manufacturer Lot Number	Expiration Date	Weighed/ Measured by	Checked by
Pilocarpine Nitrate	0.4 g	JET Labs OS2721	mm/yy	bjf	bb
Phenylmercuric Nitrate 1:10,000 Solution	8 mL	Prac. Pharmacy JD8422	mm/yy	bjf	bb
Sorensen's acid stock soln	14 mL measured; 6.8 mL used	Prac. Pharmacy JD8423	mm/yy	bjf	bb
Sorensen's base stock soln	6 mL measured; 2.9 mL used	Prac. Pharmacy JD8424	mm/yy	bjf	bb
Sodium Nitrate	147 mg weighed; 71 mg used	JET Labs OS2725	mm/yy	bjf	bb
Sterile water	2.3 mL	Sterile Labs PP2715	mm/yy	bjf	bb

QUALITY CONTROL DATA: The preparation is a clear, colorless solution with an apparent viscosity of water. The pH of the preparation was checked using range 2 to 9 pH test strips: pH = 6.5. The final actual volumes were checked and match the theoretical volume of 5 × 3 mL plus the approximately 4 mL of residual excess waste solution.

LABELING

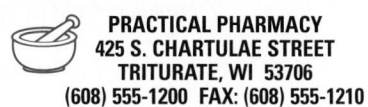

PRACTICAL PHARMACY
425 S. CHARTULAE STREET
TRITURATE, WI 53706
(608) 555-1200 FAX: (608) 555-1210

R̥ 123248   Pharmacist: BB   Date: 00/00/00
Shelby Richards   Dr. Patsy Heider

Place one drop in each eye four times daily.

Pilocarpine Nitrate 2%; Contains Phenylmercuric Nitrate 0.004% as a preservative

Mfg: Compounded   Quantity: 5 × 3 mL

Refills: 2   Discard after: Give date

Auxiliary Label: For the eye. This medicine was compounded in our pharmacy for you at the direction of your prescriber. Store bottle being used in the refrigerator and discard after 3 days; store extra bottles in the freezer until the time of use.

PATIENT CONSULTATION: Hello, Ms. Richards. I'm your pharmacist, Bernie Brewer. Do you have any drug allergies? (If so, what reaction did you have to the medication?) What do you know about this medication? Are you taking or using any other medications? Are you using any other eye drops? Do you wear contact lenses? This medication is pilocarpine nitrate eye drops, and it is used for glaucoma. Place one drop in each eye four times daily. I will give you an instruction sheet that will help you use these drops, and I will be happy to go over the procedure with you. Use this medication until your physician tells you to stop or for the length of time that he has told you. These drops may sting briefly. If they become too irritating or cause severe redness or swelling in your eyes, contact your doctor. Because these drops will contract your pupils, you may notice reduced vision at night or in other low-light conditions. These drops will cause blurred vision. I have packaged these drops in five separate 3-mL sterile ophthalmic dropper bottles. You should store the bottle in current use in the refrigerator and discard it after 3 days. Stored the other bottles in the freezer and remove them one by one every 3 days for current use and storage in the refrigerator. Keep out of reach of children. Each time you use the solution, check it to be sure it is still clear and contains no particles. If you notice anything, do not use it but return it to the pharmacy. Discard any unused bottles after 1 month (give date). This may be refilled two times. Do you have any questions?

SAMPLE PRESCRIPTION 33.3

CASE: Melvin Dean is a 170-lb, 5′10″-tall, 67 year-old man in whom a bacterial corneal ulcer of the right eye has been diagnosed. Dr. Smitby has found that the concentration of commercially available tobramycin is too low to effectively treat this condition and has consulted with pharmacist Patsy Wineswig about using a fortified ophthalmic solution. Dr. Wineswig has suggested a 1% tobramycin ophthalmic solution, which is in the middle of the range of 0.91% to 1.36% w/v that has been reported to be effective for this condition (29–31). Mr. Dean is currently taking pravastatin 20 mg daily for high cholesterol, and lisinopril 10 mg and hydrochlorothiazide 25 mg daily for hypertension.

CONTEMPORARY PHYSICIANS GROUP PRACTICE
20 S. PARK STREET, TRITURATE, WI 53706
TEL: (608) 555-1333 FAX: (608) 555-1335

℞ #   *123255*

NAME *Melvin Dean*   DATE *00/00/00*

ADDRESS *777 Highland Avenue*

℞   *Tobramycin Fortified Ophthalmic Solution 1%*

Dispense 5 mL

Sig: Put 1 drop in right eye every hour today, then q 4 hr × 7 days

P. Wineswig 00/00/00

REFILLS *0*   *Lance Smitby*   M.D.

DEA NO. _____

MASTER COMPOUNDING FORMULATION RECORD

NAME, STRENGTH, AND DOSAGE FORM OF PREPARATION: Tobramycin 1% Ophthalmic Solution

QUANTITY: 5 mL

THERAPEUTIC USE/CATEGORY: Antibiotic

FORMULATION RECORD ID: OP003

ROUTE OF ADMINISTRATION: Ophthalmic

INGREDIENTS: (for 5 mL, no excess made)

Ingredient	Quantity Used	Physical Description	Solubility	Dose Comparison		Use in the Prescription
				Given	Usual	
Tobramycin Ophthalmic Solution 0.3%	4 mL	clear, colorless liquid	misc with water	1% (Tobramycin)	0.3–1.4% (Tobramycin)	antibiotic
Tobramycin Injection 40 mg/mL	1 mL	clear, colorless liquid	misc with water	1% (Tobramycin)	0.3–1.4% (Tobramycin)	antibiotic

COMPATIBILITY–STABILITY: Fortified tobramycin ophthalmic solutions are usually made with commercial Tobramycin Ophthalmic Solution and Tobramycin Injection. In a concentration range of 9.1 to 13.6 mg/mL (0.91% to 1.36% w/v), these have been reported in the literature to be stable for at least 91 days when stored at 8°C (29,30). Tobramycin Ophthalmic Solution is available from various manufacturers; all are preserved with 0.01% BAC and contain boric acid. The injection products contain phenol, sodium bisulfite, and EDTA.

PACKAGING AND STORAGE: The *USP* monograph for Tobramycin Ophthalmic Solution recommends storage in tight containers and avoiding exposure to excessive heat (15). Storage in the refrigerator is recommended.

BEYOND-USE DATE: Although this preparation has been tested to be chemically stable for 91 days when stored at 8°C, the number and type of ingredients and manipulations places it in the *USP* Chapter ⟨797⟩ low-risk level, which allows a maximum BUD of 14 days. This BUD assumes that the preparation was made using recommended environmental controls and that the finished solution is stored in the refrigerator. Because this solution will be used in a home environment and will be frequently removed from the refrigerator when administering doses, a more conservative 10-day BUD will be used. This should be adequate because the duration of therapy is just 8 days.

CALCULATIONS

Dose/Concentration: Although the concentration of the commercial ophthalmic solution is 0.3%, there have been numerous reports of successful use of this antibiotic at 0.91% to 1.36% (29–31).

Ingredient Amounts

The available ingredients for this fortified solution are Tobramycin Ophthalmic Solution 0.3% and Tobramycin Injection 40 mg/mL. The volume of each is calculated using either algebra or alligation. Both methods are shown here. In either case, the concentrations of the solutions must be expressed in a single format, either as percent or as milligrams per milliliter. This conversion is shown first.

Tobramycin Ophthalmic Solution: 0.3% = 0.3 g/100 mL = 300 mg/100 mL = 3 mg/mL

Tobramycin Injection 40 mg/mL: 40 mg/mL = 0.04 g/mL = 4 g/100 mL = 4%

By algebra:

First, the volumes of the two solutions sum to the final preparation volume of 5 mL:

$$V_I + V_O = 5 \text{ mL or } \quad V_I = 5 \text{ mL} - V_O$$

where V_I = volume of the Injection (4% or 40 mg/mL)

V_O = volume of the 0.3% ophthalmic solution

Second, the sum of the percent of each solution times its volume is equal to the final percent desired times the final volume desired (this example using concentration in percent):

$$0.3\% \, (V_0) + 4\% \, (5 - V_0) = 1\%(5)$$

$$0.003 \, V_0 + 0.04(5 - V_0) = 0.01(5)$$

$$0.003 \, V_0 + 0.2 - 0.04 \, V_0 = 0.05$$

$$0.037 \, V_0 = 0.15$$

$$V_0 = 4.05 \approx 4 \text{ mL}$$

$$V_I = 5 \text{ mL} - 4 \text{ mL} = 1 \text{ mL}$$

By alligation:

4.0		0.7	parts 40 mg/mL injection (4%)
	1.0		
0.3		3.0	parts 0.3% ophthalmic solution
		3.7	parts total

The volume of the 0.3% Tobramycin Ophthalmic Solution is calculated to be:

$$\frac{3 \text{ parts } 0.3\% \text{ oph.}}{3.7 \text{ parts total}} = \frac{x \text{ mL } 0.3\% \text{ oph}}{5 \text{ mL total}}; x = 4.05 \text{ mL} \approx 4 \text{ mL } 0.3\% \text{ oph. solution}$$

The volume of the Tobramycin Injection 40 mg/mL (4%) is calculated to be:

$$\frac{0.7 \text{ parts injection}}{3.7 \text{ parts total}} = \frac{x \text{ mL injection}}{5 \text{ mL total}}; x = 0.95 \text{ mL} \approx 1 \text{ mL injection}$$

MSDS AND SAFETY AND PERSONAL PROTECTIVE EQUIPMENT: Review MSDS for all components. Use aseptic technique in all procedures for preparing this sterile preparation. Remove jewelry and wash hands and forearms with germicidal soap. Don foot covers, hair covers, a face mask, and a clean, low-shedding gown. Apply an alcohol-based hand cleaner, allow to dry, and put on sterile powder-free protective gloves.

SPECIALIZED EQUIPMENT: Laminar airflow workbench (LAFW); wipe the surfaces of the LAFW with sterile 70% isopropyl alcohol using a lint-free cloth.

COMPOUNDING PROCEDURE: Place the following items in the LAFW: the drug solutions, two 3-mL syringes, a filter needle, and regular needles. Remove the cap and dropper tip from the commercial bottle of Tobramycin 0.3% Ophthalmic Solution. The tip should be removed carefully to avoid contamination; this can be done by using the loosened bottle cap to bend the tip until it dislodges from the bottle. Let the dropper tip rest in the bottle cap in the LAFW so as to avoid contaminating any part of the tip. (**Note:** An alternative method is to use a fine-gauge needle to make the transfers through the dropper tip but, with this method, care must be used to avoid enlarging the dropper tip orifice.) Using a 3-mL syringe, withdraw 1 mL of the ophthalmic solution from its bottle and discard. Attach a 5-μm filter needle to a 3-mL syringe and withdraw a slight excess of 1 mL of drug solution from the Tobramycin 40 mg/mL Injection vial. Remove the filter needle and apply a regular needle. With the syringe positioned with the needle pointing upward, express any air bubbles and fill the new needle; then, with the needle pointing downward, express any excess drug solution onto sterile gauze or into a waste container so that the volume in the syringe is 1 mL. Transfer the 1 mL of injection to the ophthalmic bottle. Carefully, using the ophthalmic bottle cap, replace the ophthalmic bottle tip onto the bottle and snap the tip in place. Secure the bottle cap and agitate to completely mix the solution. Express a drop of solution onto the pH paper and record the pH of the solution. Remove the preparation from the LAFW; label and dispense.

DESCRIPTION OF FINISHED PREPARATION: The preparation should be a clear, colorless solution with an apparent viscosity of water.

QUALITY CONTROL: The pH of the preparation can be checked by expressing a drop of the finished solution from the dropper tip onto pH paper (range 4 to 9) while the finished container is still in the LAFW: pH = 7.5. The volume withdrawn from the injection vial into the syringe is verified at 1 mL, and the volume remaining in the 2-mL injection vial is observed to be approximately 1 mL. This matches the theoretical volume that should remain. The amount withdrawn from the ophthalmic solution bottle is verified at 1 mL, and the amount of final solution in the 5-mL ophthalmic bottle appears at the appropriate level.

MASTER FORMULA PREPARED BY: Patsy Wineswig, RPh   **CHECKED BY:** Larry Davidow, PhD, RPh

---

COMPOUNDING RECORD

NAME, STRENGTH, AND DOSAGE FORM OF PREPARATION: Tobramycin 1% Ophthalmic Solution
QUANTITY: 5 mL   **DATE PREPARED:** mm/dd/yy   **BEYOND-USE DATE:** mm/dd/yy
FORMULATION RECORD ID: OP003   **CONTROL/RX NUMBER:** 123255

INGREDIENTS USED:

Ingredient	Quantity Used	Manufacturer Lot Number	Expiration Date	Weighed/ Measured by	Checked by
Tobramycin Ophthalmic Solution 0.3%	4 mL	BJF Generics OB2726	mm/yy	bjf	pw
Tobramycin Injection 40 mg/mL	1 mL	Sterile Labs PP2715	mm/yy	bjf	pw

QUALITY CONTROL DATA: The preparation is a clear, colorless solution with an apparent viscosity of water. The pH of the preparation was checked by expressing a drop of the finished solution from the dropper tip onto range 4 to 9 pH paper: pH = 7.5. The volume from the injection vial in the syringe was verified at 1 mL, and the volume remaining in the 2-mL injection vial was approximately 1 mL, which matches the theoretical volume that should remain. The amount withdrawn from the ophthalmic solution bottle was verified at 1 mL, and the amount of final solution in the 5-mL ophthalmic bottle appears at the appropriate level.

LABELING

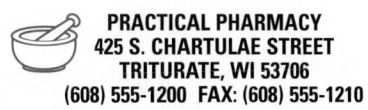

PRACTICAL PHARMACY
425 S. CHARTULAE STREET
TRITURATE, WI 53706
(608) 555-1200 FAX: (608) 555-1210

℞ 123255   Pharmacist: PW   Date: 00/00/00
Melvin Dean   Dr. Lance Smitby

Put one drop in the right eye every hour today and then every four hours for seven days.

Tobramycin Ophthalmic Solution 1%; Contains Benzalkonium Cl as a preservative.

Mfg: Compounded   Quantity: 5 mL
Refills: 0   Discard after: Give date

Auxiliary Label: For the eye. Keep in the refrigerator; do not freeze. This medicine was compounded in our pharmacy for you at the direction of your prescriber.

PATIENT CONSULTATION: Hello, Mr. Dean. I'm your pharmacist, Patsy Wineswig. Do you have any drug allergies? Your medication record says that you are taking pravastatin, lisinopril, and hydrochlorothiazide. Is this list current? Are you taking any other medications? Are you using any other eye drops? Do you wear contact lenses? What did Dr. Smitby tell you about this medication? This medication is tobramycin eye drops, which is being used to treat your eye infection. Place one drop in your right eye every hour today and then every 4 hours for 7 days. We would like to have you use these drops as much as possible around the clock without your waking especially to put drops in your eye, so put a drop in your eye as soon as you arise in the morning and space out the doses approximately every 4 hours so that you put a drop in your eye just before you go to bed at night. If you do get up in the night and it has been about 3 or 4 hours since your last dose, put a drop in at that time. Do you understand my meaning? I will give you an instruction sheet that will help you use these drops, and I will be happy to go over the procedure with you. Be very careful that you do not contaminate the dropper tip on the bottle by touching it to your eye or skin. If you have someone at home who can help you put the drops in your eye, this may work the best. Use this medication for the full 8 days of therapy. These drops may sting briefly. If they become too irritating or cause severe redness or swelling in your eye, contact Dr. Smitby immediately. Store these in the refrigerator, but protect from freezing. Take them out of the refrigerator a little while before you use them so they warm up a bit closer to room temperature. Keep them out of reach of children. Discard any unused portion as soon as your 8-day therapy is finished and certainly after 10 days (give date). You cannot save any leftover drops for future infections as they are not that stable and besides, you may unintentionally get some contamination in them, which would grow over time. There are no refills. When did Dr. Smitby want to see you for a recheck? Do you have any questions?

SAMPLE PRESCRIPTION 33.4

CASE: Dr. Jon Dropp is a 195-lb, 6′2″-tall, 32-year-old man who is being discharged from Medical Center Hospital following eye surgery. Dr. Barksen has been using nonpreserved cefazolin ophthalmic solution, which is compounded in the hospital pharmacy, since the surgery, and she wants to continue this therapy for several days to ensure that there is no infection at the surgical site during this critical time of her patient's recovery. Dr. Dropp is in good general health and is taking no other medications at this time.

CONTEMPORARY PHYSICIANS GROUP PRACTICE
20 S. PARK STREET, TRITURATE, WI 53706
TEL: (608) 555-1333 FAX: (608) 555-1335

℞ # *123229*

NAME *Dr. Jon Dropp*   DATE *00/00/00*

ADDRESS *7685 Turkish Lane*

℞

Cefazolin Ophthalmic Solution 0.33%

Make isotonic but preservative-free

Dispense 10 mL

Steve Hunter 00/00/00

Sig: 1 drop in left eye qid

REFILLS *2*   *R. Barksen*   M.D.

DEA NO. _____

MASTER COMPOUNDING FORMULATION RECORD

NAME, STRENGTH, AND DOSAGE FORM OF PREPARATION: Cefazolin 0.33% Ophthalmic Solution
QUANTITY: 10 mL   **FORMULATION RECORD ID:** OP004
THERAPEUTIC USE/CATEGORY: Antibiotic   **ROUTE OF ADMINISTRATION:** Ophthalmic

INGREDIENTS:

Ingredient	Quantity Used	Physical Description	Solubility	Dose Comparison		Use in the Prescription
				Given	Usual	
Cefazolin Sterile Powder for Injection 500-mg vial	33 mg as 0.26 mL of 125 mg/mL reconstituted injection	white powder	sol in water; v sl sol in alcohol	0.33% (Cefazolin)	0.3–1.3% (Cefazolin)	antibiotic
Sodium Chloride 0.9% Injection	3.8 mL for reconstitution; 9.74 to qs ad 10 mL	clear, colorless liquid	misc with water	—	—	sterile diluent

COMPATIBILITY–STABILITY: This sample prescription is typical of antibiotic ophthalmic solutions that are made using a manufactured sterile powder for injection. This preparation is prescribed to be made preservative-free, which would be recommended during and immediately after ocular surgery and at certain other times. A *USP* formulation, Cefazolin Ophthalmic Solution, is also 0.33% cefazolin, but it contains the preservative thimerosal. That preparation is stated to be stable for 5 days when stored in the refrigerator (15). Another similar ophthalmic preparation that is 0.5% cefazolin and is preservative-free is reported in *Extemporaneous Ophthalmic Preparations* to be stable for 10 days at 2° to 8°C (32). A preparation identical to this one (preservative-free, 0.33% cefazolin in Sodium Chloride Injection) is described in *Extemporaneous Ophthalmic Preparations*, and the recommended BUD is 24 hours because of use in an uncontrolled home environment (32). It is obvious from these various sources that cefazolin presents both issues of chemical stability and concerns about contamination of a nonpreserved ophthalmic solution. When the eye can tolerate a preservative, a preserved version of this solution can be made by using Bacteriostatic Sodium Chloride Injection. Alternatively, thimerosal 0.002% could be added as is indicated in the *USP* Cefazolin Ophthalmic Solution.

PACKAGING AND STORAGE: The *USP* monograph for Cefazolin Ophthalmic Solution requires packaging in a sterile ophthalmic container and storage in the refrigerator (15).

BEYOND-USE DATE: When prepared as described using sterile ingredients, this preparation is in Chapter ⟨797⟩ low-risk level, which allows a BUD of 48 hours at controlled room temperature or 14 days when stored in the refrigerator. However, this drug has limited chemical stability that allows a maximum 5-day BUD when the preparation is stored in the refrigerator (15). Furthermore, some pharmacists who practice in ophthalmology recommend a more conservative 24-hour BUD for nonpreserved compounded ophthalmic solutions; a fresh solution is made daily until the patient's eye can tolerate a preserved solution (8,32). For this preservative-free ophthalmic solution, a conservative 24-hour BUD will be used.

Note: Because studies have shown that reconstituted cefazolin, when frozen, is stable for 30 days to 12 weeks (depending on the concentration and diluent) (33), an alternative would be to make three 3-mL bottles of this solution and have the patient store the bottle in use in the refrigerator and the other bottles in the freezer; then each day the patient would discard the used bottle and remove another bottle from the freezer. This may be more convenient for the patient, as he would not have to get a fresh bottle from the pharmacy each day.

CALCULATIONS

Dose/Concentration: Concentrations of cefazolin in topical ophthalmic solutions in the range of 33 mg/mL (0.33%) to 133 mg/mL (1.33%) have been reported (32).

Ingredient Amounts

Cefazolin needed (in mg): $0.33\% \times 10 \text{ mL} = 0.0033 \times 10 \text{ mL} = 0.033 \text{ g} = 33 \text{ mg}$

Cefazolin is available as the sodium salt in vials containing the dry powder for reconstitution. Practical Pharmacy has available 500-mg vials that may be reconstituted with Sterile Water for Injection, Bacteriostatic Water for Injection, or Sodium Chloride Injection. The prescribing information that accompanies the vial states that when reconstituted with 3.8 mL of diluent, the result is 4 mL of solution with a concentration of 125 mg/mL. (Although the drug is present as the sodium salt, the milligram strength on the vial is in terms of the free acid form.)

Using the 500-mg vial and reconstituting it with 3.8 mL of diluent, the volume of the injection to contain the 33 mg of cefazolin is as follows:

$$\frac{125 \text{ mg cefazolin}}{1 \text{ mL solution}} = \frac{33 \text{ mg cefazolin}}{x \text{ mL solution}} \; ; x = 0.26 \text{ solution}$$

To obtain 10 mL of solution containing 33 mg of cefazolin (0.33%), the volume of additional diluent is calculated: 10 mL − 0.26 mL = 9.74 mL.

The choice between Sterile Water for Injection or Sodium Chloride Injection 0.9% as the diluent is made on the basis of obtaining a solution that is as close as possible to isotonic. Three methods for determining isotonicity values are shown here; any one of these methods may be used. The Sodium Chloride Equivalent, Freezing Point Depression, and USP Method numerical values can be found Appendix D. Note that the values in the table are for cefazolin **sodium**, which is the form of the drug we are using, and cefazolin sodium contains 2 mg of sodium per 33 mg of cefazolin. Therefore, for these calculations we will use the content of cefazolin sodium in our preparation, 35 mg rather than 33 mg, and a percent concentration of 0.35% rather than 0.33%.

USP Method

The easiest and most intuitive method to use in this case is the USP method. The V^{1g} value gives the volume of water that will make 1 g of the drug or chemical isotonic. The V^{1g} value for sodium cefazolin is 14.4 mL. The volume for 35 mg or 0.035 g is calculated as follows:

$$\frac{1 \text{ g Na cefazolin}}{14.4 \text{ mL water}} = \frac{0.035 \text{ g Na cefazolin}}{x \text{ mL water}} \; ; x = 0.5 \text{ mL water}$$

From an isotonicity point of view, 0.5 mL out of a 10-mL preparation is a negligible amount of water needed. We could use Sterile Water for Injection for the vial reconstitution and Sodium Chloride Injection 0.9% for the 9.74 mL of diluent, but it would also be acceptable to use all Sodium Chloride Injection 0.9%.

Sodium Chloride Equivalent Method

The Sodium Chloride Equivalent for sodium cefazolin = 0.13.

Amount of NaCl equivalent to 35 mg sodium cefazolin:

$$\frac{0.13 \text{ g NaCl}}{1 \text{ g Na cefazolin}} = \frac{x \text{ g NaCl}}{0.035 \text{ g Na cefazolin}} \; ; x = 0.0046 \text{ g NaCl}$$

The amount of NaCl needed to make 10 mL of sterile water isotonic:

$$0.9\% \times 10 \text{ mL} = 0.009 \times 10 \text{ mL} = 0.09 \text{ g NaCl}$$

Amount of NaCl needed to make 0.35% sodium cefazolin solution isotonic:

$$0.09 \text{ g} - 0.0046 \text{ g} = 0.0854 \text{ g NaCl}$$

As we can see, 0.0854 g is very close to 0.09 g. Since the contribution to isotonicity of the 35 mg of sodium cefazolin is so small, we could use Sterile Water for Injection for the vial reconstitution and Sodium Chloride Injection 0.9% for the 9.74 mL of diluent, but it would also be acceptable to use all Sodium Chloride Injection 0.9%.

Freezing Point Depression Method

Freezing point depression of a 1% solution of sodium cefazolin = 0.07°C.

Freezing point depression of a 0.35% solution of sodium cefazolin is calculated to be:

$$\frac{0.07°C}{1\% \text{ Na cefazolin}} = \frac{x°C}{0.35\% \text{ Na cefazolin}} \; ; x = 0.024°C$$

Amount of additional freezing point depression need for isotonicity:

$$0.52°C - 0.024°C = 0.496°C \approx 0.50°C$$

We can see that 0.50°C is very close to the isotonic freezing point depression of 0.52°C and that the contribution of the 35 mg of sodium cefazolin to isotonicity for our preparation is negligible. Once again, we come to the conclusion that we could use either Sterile Water for Injection for the vial reconstitution and Sodium Chloride Injection 0.9% for the 9.74 mL of diluent or use all Sodium Chloride Injection 0.9%.

MSDS AND SAFETY AND PERSONAL PROTECTIVE EQUIPMENT: Review MSDS for all components. Use aseptic technique in all procedures for preparing this sterile preparation. Remove jewelry and wash hands and forearms with germicidal soap. Don foot covers, hair covers, a face mask, and a clean, low-shedding gown. Apply an alcohol-based hand cleaner, allow to dry, and put on sterile, powder-free protective gloves.

SPECIALIZED EQUIPMENT: Laminar airflow workbench (LAFW); wipe the surfaces of the LAFW with sterile 70% isopropyl alcohol using a lint-free cloth.

COMPOUNDING PROCEDURE: Place in the LAFW the following items: the cefazolin drug vial, a Sodium Chloride Injection 0.9% vial, 5-mL and 10 mL syringes, a filter needle and regular needles, and a 15-mL sterile dropper bottle. Using a 5-mL syringe, withdraw 3.8 mL of Sodium Chloride Injection 0.9% from its vial and inject into the cefazolin sodium vial. Shake the vial to dissolve the drug and mix the solution. Attach a 5-μm filter needle to a 1-mL syringe and withdraw a slight excess of 0.26 mL of drug solution from the cefazolin sodium vial. Remove the filter needle and apply a regular needle. With the syringe positioned with the needle pointing upward, express any air bubbles and fill the new needle; then, with the needle pointing downward, express any excess drug solution onto sterile gauze or into a waste container so that the volume in the syringe is 0.26 mL. Transfer the 0.26 mL of injection to the sterile ophthalmic dropper bottle. Using a 10-mL syringe, transfer 9.74 mL of Sodium Chloride Injection 0.9% to the ophthalmic bottle. Carefully apply the ophthalmic bottle tip and cap to the bottle and tighten the bottle cap to ensure that the dropper tip is snapped securely in place. Agitate to completely mix the solution. Check the pH of the solution by expressing a drop of the finished solution from the dropper tip onto a range 2 to 9 pH test strip; then recap the bottle and remove the preparation from the LAFW. Label and dispense.

DESCRIPTION OF FINISHED PREPARATION: The preparation should be a clear, colorless solution with an apparent viscosity of water.

QUALITY CONTROL: While the finished container is still in the LAFW, the pH of the preparation should be checked by expressing a drop of the finished solution from the dropper tip onto a range 2 to 9 pH test strip: pH = 5. The volume from the injection vial that was drawn into the syringe is verified at 0.26 mL, and the volume remaining in the 4-mL injection vial should be approximately 3.74 mL, matching the theoretical volume that should remain in the vial. The amount of final solution in the ophthalmic bottle should be at the appropriate level for the bottle size.

MASTER FORMULA PREPARED BY: Steve Hunter, RPh   **CHECKED BY:** Larry Davidow, PhD, RPh

COMPOUNDING RECORD

NAME, STRENGTH, AND DOSAGE FORM OF PREPARATION: Cefazolin 0.33% Ophthalmic Solution
QUANTITY: 10 mL   **DATE PREPARED:** mm/dd/yy   **BEYOND-USE DATE:** mm/dd/yy
FORMULATION RECORD ID: OP004   **CONTROL/RX NUMBER:** 123229

INGREDIENTS USED:

Ingredient	Quantity Used	Manufacturer Lot Number	Expiration Date	Weighed/ Measured by	Checked by
Cefazolin Sterile Powder for Injection 500-mg vial	33 mg as 0.26 mL of 125 mg/mL reconstituted injection	Sterile Labs PP2728	mm/yy	bjf	sh
Sodium Chloride 0.9% Injection	3.8 mL for reconstitution; 9.74 to qs ad 10 mL	Sterile Labs PP2716	mm/yy	bjf	sh

QUALITY CONTROL DATA: The preparation is a clear, colorless solution with an apparent viscosity of water. The pH of the preparation was checked by expressing a drop of the finished solution from the dropper tip onto pH paper while the finished container was still in the LAFW: pH = 5. The volume from the injection vial that was drawn into the syringe was verified at 0.26 mL, and the volume remaining in the 4-mL injection vial was approximately 3.74 mL. The amount of final solution in the ophthalmic bottle appears at the appropriate level for the bottle size.

LABELING

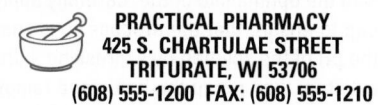

PRACTICAL PHARMACY
425 S. CHARTULAE STREET
TRITURATE, WI 53706
(608) 555-1200 FAX: (608) 555-1210

℞ 123229   Pharmacist: SH   Date: 00/00/00
Jon Dropp   Dr. Roberta Barksen
Place one drop in the left eye four times daily.
Cefazolin Ophthalmic Solution 0.33%, Preservative-free
Mfg: Compounded   Quantity 10 mL
Refills: 2   Discard after: Give date

Auxiliary Label: For the eye. Keep in the refrigerator; do not freeze. This medicine was compounded in our pharmacy for you at the direction of your prescriber.

PATIENT CONSULTATION: Hello, Dr. Dropp. I'm your pharmacist, Steve Hunter. Do you have any drug allergies? What did Dr. Barksen tell you about these eye drops? Do you wear contact lenses? Has your doctor discussed with you when you can start using them again? These are cefazolin eye drops, which are being used to prevent an eye infection following your eye surgery. Place one drop in your left eye four times a day. We would like to have you space out your doses as much as possible, so put a drop in your eye as soon as you arise in the morning and space out the doses so that you put a drop in your eye just before you go to bed at night. I will give you an instruction sheet that will help you use these drops, and I will be happy to go over the procedure with you. Be very careful that you do not contaminate the dropper tip on the bottle by touching it to your eye or skin. These drops should be comfortable to use, but if they become irritating or cause redness or swelling in your eyes, contact Dr. Barksen. Store these in the refrigerator, but take them out of the refrigerator a little while before you use them so they warm up a bit. Keep them out of reach of children. Because these drops do not contain a preservative, bacteria, viruses, or molds could grow in the solution if it should be contaminated during use. Because your eye is so sensitive to infection right now, we want to guard against this, so I will make a fresh solution for you every day. Discard any unused portion as soon as you pick up your new bottle. At the end of 3 days, Dr. Barksen has told me she wants to see you. We will then evaluate your situation. If she still thinks you need an antibiotic, we could compound the same type of drops with a preservative so you don't have to get a fresh solution every day. Right now, though, your eye is just too sensitive for ingredients such as preservatives. Do you have any questions?

SAMPLE PRESCRIPTION 33.5

CASE: Dr. Juliana Dias is a 105-lb, 5′-tall, 27-year-old woman who needs treatment for nasal dryness and irritation. She recently has moved from New York City to Santa Fe, New Mexico, where the air is very dry, and she is experiencing dry, inflamed nasal membranes with thick, crusty nasal secretions. Because of previous allergic reactions to preservatives in contact lens solutions, she knows she is allergic to several preservatives used in manufactured sterile saline nasal solutions. Dr. Quacky has had good success in treating similar situations with "tried and true" compounded Proetz Nasal Solution. Juliana's only other medical problem is allergies to various pollens and molds, which she usually self-treats with generic OTC loratadine 10-mg tablets, one daily. In the past, during seasons of high pollen count, she has used prescription fluticasone nasal spray, but she is hoping New Mexico will be a good climate for her allergies.

CONTEMPORARY PHYSICIANS GROUP PRACTICE
20 S. PARK STREET, TRITURATE, WI 53706
TEL: (608) 555-1333 FAX: (608) 555-1335

℞ # *123705*

NAME *Dr. Juliana Dias*   DATE *00/00/00*

ADDRESS *1593 Coyote Court*

℞

Proetz Nasal Solution:		
Glycerin		*20 mL*
Ethanol 70%		*40 mL*
Normal Saline Sol'n	*q s ad*	*500 mL*

Pat Butler 00/00/00

Dispense 60 mL
Sig: Spray in each nostril qid and prn for irritation
and dryness
Please label as Proetz Nasal Solution O.Q.

REFILLS *prn*   *Olive Quacky*   M.D.

DEA NO. _____

MASTER COMPOUNDING FORMULATION RECORD

NAME, STRENGTH, AND DOSAGE FORM OF PREPARATION: Proetz Nasal Solution (Glycerin 4%, Alcohol 5.6% in 0.9% Sodium Chloride Solution)

QUANTITY: 60 mL

THERAPEUTIC USE/CATEGORY: Nasal moisturizer

FORMULATION RECORD ID: NS001

ROUTE OF ADMINISTRATION: Nasal

INGREDIENTS:

Ingredient	Quantity Used	Physical Description	Solubility	Dose Comparison		Use in the Prescription
				Given	Usual	
Glycerin	2.4 mL	clear, colorless, viscous liquid	miscible with water and alcohol	4%	varies	humectant, vehicle, preservative
Alcohol USP 95% v/v	3.5 mL to make 4.8 mL 70% ethanol	clear, colorless, mobile liquid	miscible with water	5.6%	varies	vehicle, preservative, antiseptic
Sodium Chloride 0.9% Injection	qs 60 mL	clear, colorless iquid	miscible with alcohol and glycerin	—	—	vehicle

COMPATIBILITY–STABILITY: All ingredients in this preparation are compatible and very stable when in an aqueous solution. No extra preservative is needed because the alcohol (5.6%) acts as a preservative.

PACKAGING AND STORAGE: Dispense in a nasal spray bottle. Controlled room temperature is the recommended storage condition.

BEYOND-USE DATE: Because this is a nasal solution, it should be sterile as dispensed, but there are less stringent restrictions with regard to BUDs. Nasal solutions need not comply with Chapter ⟨797⟩. Because the ingredients in this preparation are known to be very stable, a longer BUD may be used than the 14-day dating recommended by *USP* Chapter ⟨795⟩ for compounded water-containing liquid formulations prepared from ingredients in solid form when there is no stability information for the formulation (25). However, because of the possibility of contamination during use of a nasal preparation, a moderate 30-day BUD will be used.

CALCULATIONS

Dose/Concentration

Glycerin (in v/v%):

$$\frac{20 \text{ mL Glycerin}}{500 \text{ mL solution}} = \frac{x \text{ mL Glycerin}}{100 \text{ mL solution}}; x = 4\% \text{ Concentration appropriate for use}$$

Alcohol (in v/v%): 70% × 40 mL = 28 mL

$$\frac{28 \text{ mL C}_2\text{H}_5\text{OH}}{500 \text{ mL solution}} = \frac{x \text{ mL C}_2\text{H}_5\text{OH}}{100 \text{ mL solution}}; x = 5.6\% \text{ Concentration appropriate for use}$$

Ingredient Amounts

Glycerin (in mL):

$$\frac{20 \text{ mL glycerin}}{500 \text{ mL solution}} = \frac{x \text{ mL glycerin}}{60 \text{ mL solution}}; x = 2.4 \text{ mL glycein}$$

The 70% ethanol must be made using Alcohol USP, which is 95% ethanol. The amount of Alcohol USP needed is calculated in the following steps.

70% ethanol (in mL) needed for 60 mL of preparation:

$$\frac{40 \text{ mL } 70\% \text{ ethanol}}{500 \text{ mL solution}} = \frac{x \text{ mL } 70\% \text{ ethanol}}{60 \text{ mL solution}} \text{ ; } x = 4.8 \text{ mL } 70\% \text{ ethanol}$$

Ethanol (C_2H_5OH) contained in this volume of 70% ethanol:

$$70\% \times 4.8 \text{ mL} = 3.36 \text{ mL}$$

Alcohol USP (in mL) that will contain this amount of ethanol:

$$\frac{95 \text{ mL } C_2H_5OH}{100 \text{ mL Alcohol USP}} = \frac{3.36 \text{ mL } C_2H_5OH}{x \text{ mL Alcohol USP}} \text{ ; } x = 3.5 \text{ mL Alcohol USP}$$

MSDS AND SAFETY AND PERSONAL PROTECTIVE EQUIPMENT: Review MSDS for all components. Use aseptic technique in all procedures for preparing this sterile preparation. Remove jewelry and wash hands and forearms with germicidal soap. Don foot covers, hair covers, a face mask, and a clean, low-shedding gown. Apply an alcohol-based hand cleaner, allow to dry, and put on sterile, powder-free protective gloves.

SPECIALIZED EQUIPMENT: Perform this compounding procedure in a laminar airflow workbench (LAFW); wipe the surfaces of the LAFW with sterile 70% isopropyl alcohol using a lint-free cloth.

COMPOUNDING PROCEDURE: Place the following in the LAFW: Alcohol USP; glycerin; Sterile Water for Injection vial; Sodium Chloride Injection vials; 3-mL, 5-mL, and 60-mL syringes; regular needles; 0.2-μm bacterial membrane filter unit, pH paper; and sterile nasal spray bottle. Using a 5-mL syringe, withdraw 3.5 mL of Alcohol USP; then withdraw into that syringe Sterile Water for Injection to the 4.8-mL mark. Pull back the plunger on a 60-mL syringe and transfer the alcohol solution to the syringe through the syringe tip. Measure 2.4 mL of glycerin with a 3-mL syringe and transfer this to the 60-mL syringe containing the alcohol solution. Agitate to mix. Put a fresh needle on the 60-mL syringe and, with the needle pointing upward, express all the air in the syringe and needle. Insert the needle into a vial of Sodium Chloride Injection 0.9% and withdraw this solution to the 60-mL mark on the syringe. Agitate to mix. Apply a 0.2-μm bacterial membrane filter unit to the 60-mL syringe tip. With the syringe in an upright position (filter unit tip up), wet and fill the filter unit. With the syringe tip pointing downward, expel one drip of solution onto a pH test strip and then transfer the completed solution to a 60-mL sterile nasal spray bottle. Label and dispense.

DESCRIPTION OF FINISHED PREPARATION: The preparation is a clear, colorless solution with apparent viscosity approximately that of water. It has a slight characteristic odor of alcohol.

QUALITY CONTROL: Volume = 60 mL. Check pH with pH range 2 to 9 test strips: pH = 5.

MASTER FORMULA PREPARED BY: Pat Butler, PharmD   **CHECKED BY:** Larry Davidow, PhD, RPh

COMPOUNDING RECORD

NAME, STRENGTH, AND DOSAGE FORM OF PREPARATION: Proetz Nasal Solution (Glycerin 4%, Alcohol 5.6% in 0.9% Sodium Chloride Solution)

QUANTITY: 60 mL   **DATE PREPARED:** mm/dd/yy   **BEYOND-USE DATE:** mm/dd/yy

FORMULATION RECORD ID: NS001   **CONTROL/RX NUMBER:** 123705

INGREDIENTS USED:

Ingredient	Quantity Used	Manufacturer Lot Number	Expiration Date	Weighed/ Measured by	Checked by
Glycerin	2.4 mL	JET Labs SS2813	mm/yy	bjf	Psb
Alcohol USP 95% v/v	3.5 mL to make 4.8 mL 70% ethanol	JET Labs SN2653	mm/yy	bjf	Psb
Sodium Chloride 0.9% Injection	qs 60 mL	Sterile Generics NS0529	mm/yy	bjf	Psb

QUALITY CONTROL DATA: The preparation is a clear, colorless solution with apparent viscosity approximately that of water. It has a slight odor of alcohol. The pH of the preparation was checked with pH range 2 to 9 test strips and recorded as pH = 5. The actual volume is checked and matches the theoretical volume of 60 mL.

LABELING

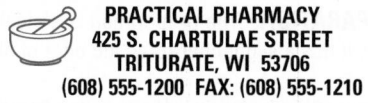

PRACTICAL PHARMACY
425 S. CHARTULAE STREET
TRITURATE, WI 53706
(608) 555-1200 FAX: (608) 555-1210

℞ 123705   Pharmacist: PSB   Date: 00/00/00
Dr. Juliana Dias   Dr. Olive Quacky

Spray into each nostril four times daily and as needed for irritation and dryness.

Proetz Nasal Solution Contains: Glycerin 4%; Alcohol 05.6% in 0.9% Sodium Chloride Solution

Mfg: Compounded   Quantity: 60 mL

Refills: until 00/00/01   Discard after: Give date

Auxiliary Label: For the Nose; This medicine was compounded in our pharmacy for you at the direction of your prescriber.

PATIENT CONSULTATION: Hello, Dr. Dias. I'm your pharmacist, Pat Butler. Welcome to Santa Fe. I hear that you are here on a postdoctoral fellowship at the Institute. We hope you like it here. Are you currently using any other medications? I know that you are allergic to some preservatives such as benzalkonium chloride and thimerosal, but are you allergic to any other drugs? What has Dr. Quacky told you about this medication? This is a nasal solution used for nasal stuffiness caused by low humidity. The directions are to spray into each nostril four times a day and as needed for irritation and dryness. Have you ever used a nasal spray before? Basically, you should keep your head straight or slightly tipped forward; then, with the tip of the nozzle just inside your nostril, squeeze the bottle firmly as you sniff gently. Remove the nozzle from your nostril before releasing the pressure on the bottle so that you do not aspirate material from your nostril into the spray bottle. After spraying, you should rinse the nozzle with water and wipe with a clean tissue before replacing the bottle cap. If your condition seems to show no improvement or seems to get worse, contact Dr. Quacky. Although this solution is very stable, you may eventually contaminate it because you are putting the spray nozzle into your nostrils, so discard any unused portion after 1 month. This prescription may be refilled any time for a year. Do you have any questions?

REFERENCES

1. The United States Pharmacopeial Convention, Inc. Chapter ⟨1151⟩. 2008 USP 31/NF 26. Rockville, MD: Author, 2007; 618–620.

2. Bloom MZ. Compounding in today's practice. Am Pharm 1991; 31: 31–37.

3. Gonnering R, et al. The pH tolerance of rabbit and human corneal endothelium. Invest Ophthalmol Vis Sci 1979; 18: 373–390.

4. The United States Pharmacopeial Convention, Inc. 1985 USP XXI/NFXVI. Rockville, MD: Author, 1985; 1338–1339.

5. Cadwallader DE. EENT preparations. In: King RE. Dispensing of medication, 9th ed. Easton, PA: Mack Publishing Co., 1984; 149–150.

6. Hanson AL. A practical guide to the compounding and dispensing of basic dosage forms. Madison, WI: University of Wisconsin, 1982; 97.

7. Martin A, Bustamante P. Physical pharmacy, 4th ed. Philadelphia: Lea & Febiger, 1993; 178.

8. Reynolds LA, Closson RG. Extemporaneous ophthalmic preparations. Vancouver, WA: Applied Therapeutics, Inc., 1993; 6–7.

9. Kibbe AH. Handbook of pharmaceutical excipients, 3rd ed. Washington DC: American Pharmaceutical Association and Pharmaceutical Press, 2000.

10. FDA Advisory Review Panel on OTC Ophthalmic Drug Products. Final report, December 1979.

11. Connors KA, Amidon GL, Stella VJ. Chemical stability of pharmaceuticals, 2nd ed. New York: John Wiley & Sons, 1986; 438–447.

12. Deardorff DL. Ophthalmic solutions. In: Hoover JE, ed. Remington's pharmaceutical sciences, 14th ed. Easton, PA: Mack Publishing Co., 1970; 1545–1577.

13. Gallagher G. Doctors and drops. Br Med J 1991; 303: 761.

14. FDA Center for Drug Evaluation and Research. Guidance for industry: nasal spray and inhalation solution, suspension, and spray drug products—chemistry, manufacturing, and controls documentation. http://www.fda.gov/cder/guidance/4234fnl.htm). Accessed February 2008.

15. The United States Pharmacopeial Convention, Inc. Official monographs. 2007 USP 30/NF 25. Rockville, MD: Author, 2006.

16. Allen Jr. LV. The art, science, and technology of pharmaceutical compounding, 3rd ed. Washington, DC: American Pharmacists Association, 2008; 296.

17. Cadwallader DE. EENT preparations. In: King RE, ed. Dispensing of medication, 9th ed. Easton, PA: Mack Publishing Co., 1984; 157–158.

18. Proetz AW. Essays on the applied physiology of the nose. St Louis: Annal Publishing Co., 1953.

19. Riegelman S, Sorby DL. EENT medications. In: Martin EW, ed. Dispensing of medication, 7th ed. Easton, PA: Mack Publishing Co., 1971; 913–915.

20. Marshall K, Foster TS, Carlin HS, Williams RL. Development of a compendial taxonomy and glossary for pharmaceutical dosage forms. Pharmacopeial forum. Rockville, MD: The United States Pharmacopeial Convention, Inc., 2003; 29(5).

21. Allen Jr. LV. The art, science, and technology of pharmaceutical compounding, 3rd ed. Washington, DC: American Pharmacists Association, 2008; 309.

22. American Society of Hospital Pharmacists. ASHP technical assistance bulletin on pharmacy-prepared ophthalmic products. Arn J Hosp Pharm 1993; 50:1462–1463.

23. Ford JL, Brown MW, Hunt PB. A note on the contamination of eye-drops following use by hospital out-patients. J Clin Hosp Pharm 1985; 10: 203–209.

24. The United States Pharmacopeial Convention, Inc. Chapter ⟨797⟩. 2009 USP 32/NF 27. Rockville, MD: Author, 2008. http://www.usp.org/USPNF/pf/generalChapter797.html. Accessed February 2008.

25. The United States Pharmacopeial Convention, Inc. Chapter ⟨795⟩. 2008 USP 31/NF 26. Rockville, MD: Author, 2007; 316–317.

26. Trissel LA. Trissel's stability of compounded formulations, 3rd ed. Washington, DC: American Pharmacists Association, 2005; 159–160.

27. Connors KA, Amidon GL, Stella VJ. Chemical stability of pharmaceuticals, 2nd ed. New York: John Wiley & Sons, 1986; 675–684.

28. Trissel LA. Trissel's stability of compounded formulations, 3rd ed. Washington, DC: American Pharmacists Association, 2005; 347–349.

29. Reynolds LA, Closson RG. Extemporaneous ophthalmic preparations. Vancouver, WA: Applied Therapeutics, Inc., 1993; 304–305.

30. McBride HA, et al. Stability of gentamicin sulfate and tobramycin sulfate in extemporaneously prepared ophthalmic solutions at 8°C. Am J Hosp Pharm 1991; 48: 507–509.

31. Abel SR, Sorensen SJ. Eye disorders. In: Koda-Kimble MA, Young LY, eds. Applied therapeutics, 7th ed. Baltimore, MD: Lippincott Williams & Wilkins, 2001; 49-18.

32. Reynolds LA, Closson RG. Extemporaneous ophthalmic preparations. Vancouver, WA: Applied Therapeutics, Inc., 1993; 81–84.

33. Trissel LA. Handbook of injectable drugs, 12th ed. Bethesda, MD: American Society of Health-System Pharmacists, 2003; 228–230.

34

Parenteral Preparations

Mary Swandby, RPh

I.   INTRODUCTION

Although most parenteral products are manufactured by the pharmaceutical industry, many pharmacists and pharmacy technicians—particularly those working in hospitals, clinics, or home health care practices or those servicing long-term care facilities—routinely handle and manipulate IV admixtures and injections. As was indicated previously, these pharmacy personnel require special knowledge and training. Most often, this begins in pharmacy school or technician training courses, but there is also on-the-job training plus elective courses, video and multimedia resources, special seminars, and much published literature on this subject. Such training is described in *USP* Chapter ⟨797⟩, Pharmaceutical Compounding—Sterile Preparations, as outlined in Chapter 32. Various professional organizations, such as the American Society of Health-System Pharmacists, National Home Infusion Association, and the National Association of Boards of Pharmacy, to name a few, have developed training materials and models for practice. A pharmacist practicing in this specialty area has a special responsibility for knowing and understanding the standards of practice for handling sterile drug products, as well as understanding the physiologic requirements of infusing medications safely. Sample medication orders are presented in this chapter under the presumption that the pharmacist or technician has the necessary training and experience to ensure that the principles of sterile technique presented in Chapter 32 are scrupulously followed.

II.   PREPARATION OF PARENTERAL DOSAGE FORMS

The procedures given here are very basic. Anyone compounding sterile preparations requires advanced instruction using the resources described previously.

A. Review the order for legibility and safety, including the following:
1. Clarification of unacceptable abbreviations.
2. Verification of completeness of information necessary to perform dose calculations.

B. Check the dose, including allowable
1. Route of administration.

   2. Volume of administration.

   3. Concentration of the solution.

   4. Rate of administration.

   A later section (V) on parenteral routes of administration gives guidance on some on these factors.

C. Check for stability and compatibility of the preparation. Verify the type of venous access (peripheral, central line, peripherally inserted central catheter, etc.) to ensure that the osmolality of the infusate is within acceptable ranges.

D. Perform any additional necessary calculations. Verify the correctness of all calculations performed by other health care professionals in supplying the order to the pharmacy.

E. Prepare the appropriate labels.

F. Remove any personal items known to increase particulate matter or to harbor microorganisms, such as jewelry, cosmetics, artificial nails, hats, and sweaters.

G. As previously described in Chapter 32, before entering the buffer area, perform body cleansing and don appropriate garb in order from dirtiest to cleanest areas as follows: (i) shoe covers, (ii) hair and beard covers, and (iii) eye shields.

H. Wash hands, fingernails, and forearms up to the elbows with an antimicrobial agent such as is described in the Center for Disease Control and Prevention *Guideline for Hand Hygiene in Healthcare Settings* (1).

I. Put on a nonshedding gown or chemoprotective gown as appropriate.

J. Enter the buffer zone. Disinfect hands with an alcohol-based surgical scrub demonstrating persistent activity. Allow hands to dry completely. Put on sterile gloves, being sure to cover the cuff of the gown so that no skin is exposed.

K. Disinfect the direct compounding area (DCA) using materials, techniques, and frequency as described in Chapter 32 and *USP* Chapter ⟨797⟩.

L. Assemble the supplies needed to make the preparation and disinfect any surfaces as directed in Chapter 32 and *USP* Chapter ⟨797⟩. This includes, but is not limited to, syringes, needles, drug products, IV solutions, and alcohol swabs.

M. Prepare the preparation, applying appropriate principles of sterile technique.

   1. If using a horizontal laminar airflow workbench (LAFW), be sure to work a minimum of 6" inside the front edge of the hood.

   2. If using a biological safety cabinet (BSC), work behind the front shield and above the area where the laminar airstream splits to enter the grills at the front and back edges of the work surface that allow the air to recirculate.

   3. If using a compounding aseptic isolator (CAI) or a compounding aseptic containment isolator (CACI), follow the manufacturer's guidelines for use and training materials.

   4. Be careful not to let anything come between a critical surface and the air coming from the high-efficiency particulate air (HEPA) filter. Be aware of placement of supplies and zones of turbulence created by articles in the laminar airflow stream.

   5. Be careful not to touch any critical surfaces such as the shaft or other parts of the needle except its cap, or the syringe tip or any part of the syringe plunger except the disk or lip that is used to move the plunger.

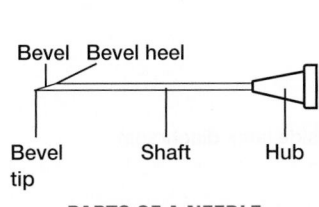

PARTS OF A NEEDLE

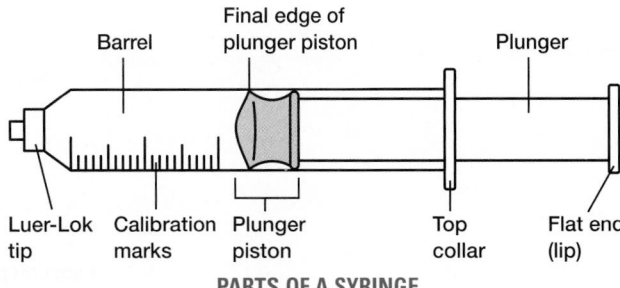

PARTS OF A SYRINGE

   6. Wipe all vials, ampuls, and injection ports with sterile alcohol wipes.

      a. Swab the diaphragms of vials from back to front before entering with a needle.

      b. Enter vial diaphragms with the needle bevel up and use slight lateral pressure so the needle tip and heel go in the same hole to prevent coring the diaphragm.

      c. Remember that vials are sealed systems, so it is important to maintain equalized pressure: volume of air or liquid in = volume of liquid or air withdrawn.

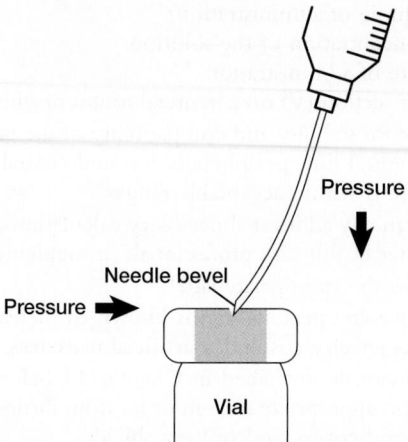

NEEDLE PENETRATION OF A VIAL TO PREVENT CORING

d. When using ampuls, eliminate any possible glass shards in the liquid withdrawn by using a filter needle.

e. When injecting drug solution through the injection port into a large-volume parenteral bag or a minibag, be sure that the needle penetrates both the exterior diaphragm and the inside diaphragm. Also use care to ensure that the needle does not puncture the IV bag.

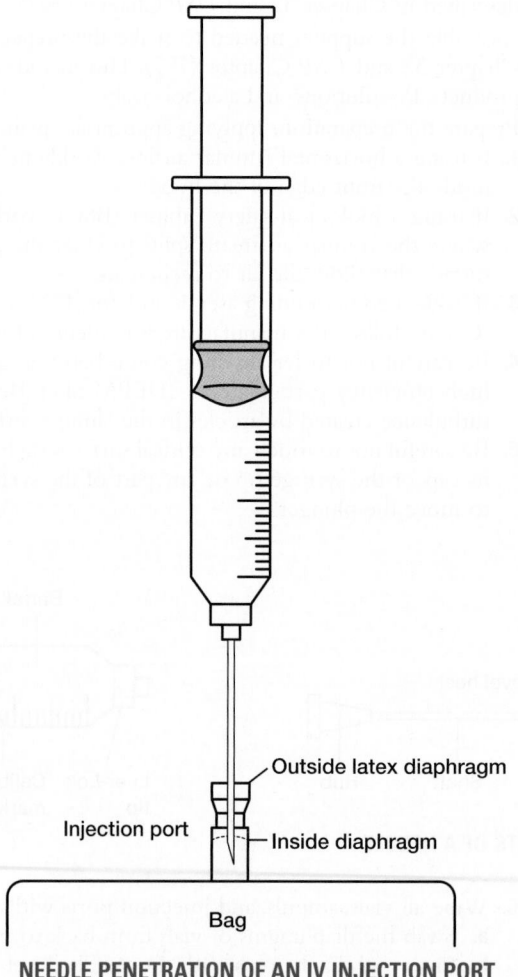

NEEDLE PENETRATION OF AN IV INJECTION PORT

N. Remove the product from the DCA and immediately apply the appropriate labels.

O. Properly dispose of sharps and other used supplies.

III.   USES OF PARENTERAL PRODUCTS

A. Parenteral administration offers one alternative when a patient is unable (e.g., unconscious, vomiting) to take medication by mouth.

B. Some drugs must be given parenterally because they are not therapeutically active when taken orally owing to inactivation in the gastrointestinal tract or first-pass metabolism by the liver.

C. The parenteral route may be necessary or preferred when drug action is required immediately.

D. In some cases, a drug must be injected because it requires direct delivery to an organ, a lesion, a muscle, or a nerve.

E. Fluids, electrolytes, and/or nutrients may be delivered parenterally for patients who cannot take these orally.

F. Depots of drugs in long-acting drug delivery systems injected into muscle masses may offer superior therapy or convenience.

G. Implantable pumps offer advantages in certain circumstances.

IV.   DISADVANTAGES OF PARENTERAL THERAPY

A. Manufactured parenteral products are more difficult and costly to produce than are nonsterile dosage forms. Because they must conform to strict requirements for microbiologic purity, particulate matter, and pyrogenicity, special equipment and facilities are needed.

B. In pharmacies and patient care, special equipment, devices, and techniques are also required for the safe preparation, handling, and administration of parenteral products. Specially trained personnel are needed.

C. Once administered, a parenteral product cannot be removed. Problems with drug, dose, or adverse effects may be difficult or impossible to reverse.

D. Any introduction of pathogens into the product during production, preparation, manipulation, or handling or during administration to the patient can have serious and even deadly consequences.

E. Because drug products are being injected directly into tissue, pain or tissue damage may be associated with the administration.

V.   PARENTERAL ROUTES OF ADMINISTRATION

Note: The size of a needle is designated using two numbers, the *length* in inches of the shaft and the *gauge*, which is the diameter of the needle bore.

A. Intradermal (ID)

1. Injection area: located just below the surface of the skin (at the interface between the epidermis and dermis). This route is most often used for skin tests in which systemic absorption is undesirable and could be dangerous (e.g., serious allergic reactions).

2. Volumes: limited to small quantities, usually 0.1 mL, but may be as small as 0.02 mL and as large as 0.5 mL.

3. Syringe size: 1-mL syringes, often labeled *tuberculin*, because these syringes were used to administer tuberculin skin tests. Unlike other syringes, these are available with and without needles attached. If a syringe is sent to a nursing unit with a needle attached, you **must** be certain the needle cover is snapped securely in place. If it is not sent with a needle, the syringe should be filled with 0.1 mL excess for priming the new needle. The syringe should then be labeled with a statement to this effect: "This syringe contains 0.1 mL excess for priming."

4. Needle sizes: 25 to 30 gauge, ⅜ to ⅝ inch long.

B. Subcutaneous (subcut or subcutaneous; see information on error-prone abbreviations in Table 1.1 of Chapter 1)

1. Injection area: subcutaneous fat tissue located beneath the skin between the dermis and muscle. When administering a drug subcutaneously, the skin may be pinched up to avoid giving the drug into the muscle. This route is used for insulin, injectable pain medication, and others where specified.

2. Volumes: limited to approximately 2.5 mL (these upper limits may be painful and the preparation must be injected over 1 to 5 minutes). For continuous subcutaneous infusions, the maximum volume per infusion site has been reported in various sources to be between 3 and 10 mL/hr depending on the therapy being delivered to the tissue. For example, in the text *Cancer Nursing: Principles and Practice*, infusion of opioid analgesics by subcutaneous infusion is recommended at rates not exceeding 5 to 10 mL/hr (2).

3. Syringes sizes: 1 or 3 mL.

4. Needle sizes: depends on use. Insulin syringes have ultrafine needles of 30 gauge (a 32-gauge needle is now available), ½ inch; "hypos" are often 25-gauge, ½ to ⅝ inch long. Insulin syringes come with the needle attached. It is left in place for administering the dose after withdrawing the drug from the product vial. For other drugs, the needle used for withdrawing the dose is usually removed, a Luer tip cap is applied, and the nurse or caregiver selects and attaches an appropriate needle at the time of injection. In this case, excess for priming the new needle should be included in the syringe and the syringe labeled to this effect. For continuous infusions, several catheters are available on the market to facilitate this method of drug delivery, from 25- to 27-gauge butterfly catheters to catheters using a Teflon infusion cannula inserted at right angles into the subcutaneous tissue.

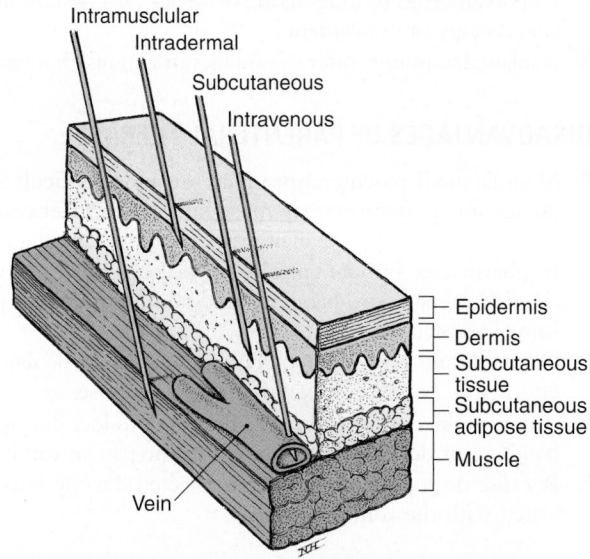

VARIOUS PARENTERAL ROUTES OF ADMINISTRATION.
(Reprinted from Stein SM. Drug administration. In: Boh LE, ed. Pharmacy practice manual: a guide to the clinical experience, 2nd edition. Philadelphia: Lippincott Williams & Wilkins, 2001.)

C. **Intramuscular (IM)**
  1. Injection area: muscle mass—deltoid (arm), gluteus maximus (buttocks), vastus lateralis (top of leg). Any nonirritating drug can be given by this route.
  2. Volumes: The volume administered is limited by the mass of the injected muscle. For adults, up to 2 mL may be given in the deltoid muscle of the upper arm, and up to 5 mL into the gluteal medial muscle of the buttock (these upper limits may be painful). For children, the volumes are more restricted. See Table 34.1 for guidelines. Notice that for small children, the vastus lateralis muscle is the recommended muscle because it is the largest muscle mass in children younger than 3 years, and it is free of major nerves and vessels. The gluteus maximus is not well developed until a child has walked for at least 1 year (3). It is also avoided because it has a major large nerve, the sciatic nerve, running through the middle. **Notice that for children up to 3 years, the maximum volume is 1 mL** (3). Be sure to keep this in mind when making IM injections for children.
  3. Syringes sizes: 1 to 5 mL.
  4. Needle sizes: 20 to 23 gauge, ½ to 1½ inches long.

D. **Intravenous (IV)**
  1. Injection areas: veins. This route is used for fluid, electrolyte, and nutrient replacement; for administration of any drug that needs to get into systemic circulation immediately; for irritating drugs; and for drugs that require carefully controlled blood levels.
  2. Volumes: Obviously, volume is less of a limitation with IV therapy. There are fluid restrictions—approximately 3 liters per day for adults and less for children. Certain disease states further restrict fluid load. The flow rate may also be restricted by the size of the vein chosen for administering the drug.
  3. Syringe sizes: 1 to 60 mL.

Table 34.1	GUIDELINES FOR MAXIMAL AMOUNTS OF SOLUTIONS TO BE INJECTED INTO MUSCLE TISSUES				
MUSCLE GROUP	BIRTH TO 1½ YR (cc)	1½ TO 3 YR (cc)	3 TO 6 YR (cc)	6 TO 15 YR (cc)	15 YR TO ADULTHOOD (cc)
Deltoid	Not recommended	Not recommended unless other sites are not available 0.5	0.5	0.5	1
Gluteus maximus	Not recommended	Not recommended unless other sites are not available 1	1.5	1.5–2	2–2.5
Ventrogluteal	Not recommended	Not recommended unless other sites are not available 1	1.5	1.5–2	2–2.5
Vastus lateralis	0.5–1	1	1.5	1.5–2	2–2.5

Reprinted with permission from Howry LB, Bindler RM, and Tso Y: *Pediatric Medications*. Philadelphia: Lippincott, 1981, p. 62.
Note: The accepted symbol for milliliter is now "mL" nor "cc."

4. Needle: 20 to 23 gauge, ½ to 1½ inches long.
5. Intravenous administration is further subdivided into continuous or constant infusion, intermittent infusion, and bolus or IV push. For calculations involving flow rate for continuous or intermittent infusions, see the next section (VI) on calculations.

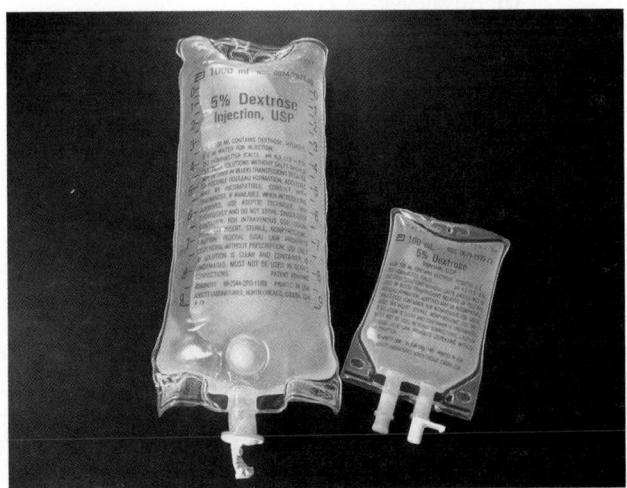

PICTURE OF LARGE-VOLUME PARENTERAL (LVP) AND SMALL-VOLUME PARENTERAL (MINIBAG)

a. **Continuous:** The drug is added to a large-volume parenteral (LVP) solution, and the solution is then slowly and continuously dripped into a vein.
   (1) Advantages
      (a) It allows fluid and drug therapy to be administered simultaneously.
      (b) It achieves continuous, constant blood levels for the drug.
      (c) It minimizes vein irritation and trauma because most drugs are less irritating when in dilute solutions.
      (d) Continuous infusion is usually a cost saver over intermittent or bolus administration, because fewer units are needed and less nursing and pharmacy staff time is involved in preparation, processing, and administration.

(2) Disadvantages
  (a) IV infusion requires greater monitoring because it runs continuously or requires a centrally inserted catheter or a peripherally inserted central catheter (PICC) to ensure infusion into the large vessels of the central vasculature (e.g., superior vena cava).
  (b) If the IV infiltrates and cannot be continued, part of the dose has not been administered.
  (c) It must be used with caution in fluid-restricted patients.
  (d) The extended run times cannot be used with certain unstable drugs.
  (e) In the event of an infusion device or tubing malfunction (free-flow), there is potential for a serious adverse event if the entire contents of the solution is infused over a short time period.

b. Intermittent: The drug is added to an intermediate volume (25 to 100 mL) and given in an intermediate period of time (15 to 60 minutes), at **spaced** intervals, such as every 6 hours.
  (1) Advantages
    (a) It requires less monitoring than does continuous infusion.
    (b) The complete dose is given in a moderate fluid volume and over a moderate period of time; therefore, there is less chance of toxicity than with bolus administration, without the disadvantages of continuous administration.
    (c) Many drugs are more stable at moderate concentrations than in the concentrated solutions required by bolus administration.
    (d) Some drugs are more effective when given by this method since they depend on high peak levels to achieve the desired outcome
  (2) Disadvantages:
    (a) Fluids and some electrolytes cannot be given this way.
    (b) Drug blood levels are less constant than with continuous administration, which may decrease the effectiveness of some medications.
    (c) The method cannot be used for direct administration to an organ or tissue.
    (d) It is sometimes impractical for immediate injection in emergency situations.

c. IV push or bolus: The drug solution is placed in a syringe and administered in a short period of time (minutes) directly into a vein or IV tubing that goes into a vein. This may be a one-time administration or it may be repeated at spaced intervals.
  (1) Advantages
    (a) IV push or bolus can be used for immediate injection in emergency situations.
    (b) It requires no ongoing monitoring of IV fluid administration.
    (c) It is less expensive than intermittent administration because there is no pump, controller, extra IV tubing, or bag.
  (2) Disadvantages
    (a) Many drugs are more irritating in the highly concentrated solutions used for IV push or bolus.
    (b) Some drugs are less stable in concentrated solutions.
    (c) Drug toxicity is a greater problem when a total dose is given in a bolus over a short period of time.
    (d) Drug blood levels fluctuate more than with either continuous or intermittent IV dosing.
    (e) When repeated doses are given, more staff time may be required, because at least 2 to 10 minutes may be needed at the bedside for each dose given.

VI.   CALCULATIONS FOR PARENTERAL PREPARATIONS AND ADMINISTRATION

A. For calculations of a general nature, see Chapters 7 through 11 on pharmaceutical calculations. Calculations specific to parenteral preparations and sample medication orders are given in the pages that follow.

B. Powder volume

Some parenteral products have limited stability when in solution and are furnished by the product manufacturer as dry powder for reconstitution. At the time the drug is to be administered, a sterile diluent, usually Sterile Water for Injection or Sodium Chloride for Injection, is added.

The volume that the powder occupies after it is dissolved in solution is called the *powder volume*. For some drug products, this volume is so small that it is considered negligible no matter what the dilution. For other products, it occupies an intermediate volume, in which case the powder volume must be considered when making calculations involving concentrated solutions but may be ignored with more dilute solutions. For other products, the powder volume is substantial and must always be taken into account.

Example 34.1

Although we usually think of powder volume in reference to parenteral products, all powders occupy a volume when dissolved. This is probably most obvious in the oral antibiotic powders for reconstitution. For example, a 100-mL bottle of amoxicillin for oral suspension requires the addition of 60 mL of Purified Water to give 100 mL of a suspension. In this case, the powder volume is 40 mL (100 mL − 60 mL = 40 mL). This information can be very useful. Suppose you wanted to give a dose of 165 mg for a product that has a concentration of 250 mg/5 mL when the product is reconstituted as directed on the bottle or package insert; the volume of the 165-mg dose would be:

$$\frac{250 \text{ mg}}{5 \text{ mL}} = \frac{165 \text{ mg}}{x \text{ mL}}; x = 3.3 \text{ mL}$$

If the pharmacist or prescriber thought that this volume would be difficult for the patient to measure and that a 1-teaspoonful (5-mL) volume would be more convenient, the product could be reconstituted to give 165 mg/5 mL. This could be done in the following manner:

1. Calculate the total number of milligrams of amoxicillin in the bottle:

$$\frac{250 \text{ mg}}{5 \text{ mL}} = \frac{x \text{ mg}}{100 \text{ mL}}; x = 5,000 \text{ mg/bottle}$$

2. Calculate the number of milliliters needed for this amount of drug to give a concentration of 165 mg/5 mL:

$$\frac{165 \text{ mg}}{5 \text{ mL}} = \frac{5,000 \text{ mg}}{x \text{ mL}}; x = 152 \text{ mL suspension}$$

3. Based on a powder volume of 40 mL, calculate the number of milliliters of Purified Water that must be added to the bottle to give a final volume of 152 mL:

$$152 \text{ mL} - 40 \text{ mL} = 112 \text{ mL}$$

4. It may be necessary to add the water in two steps, and the partially reconstituted product will probably have to be transferred to a larger bottle to accommodate the total volume of 152 mL.

These same principles may be applied to parenteral powders for reconstitution. The following example illustrates the use of powder volume in a therapeutic situation.

Example 34.2

Rocephin (ceftriaxone sodium) for Injection is available in 2-g vials for reconstitution. The product package insert states that when 7.2 mL of Sterile Water for Injection is added to this vial, the concentration of the resulting solution is 250 mg/mL. Your medical team wants to give this drug to a 10-month-old, 20-lb child. A drug information reference gives the following dosage information for infants and children: For serious infections (other than meningitis) in children 12 years of age or younger, the recommended dose is 50 to 75 mg/kg/day in divided doses every 12 hours.

1. The medical team is considering giving 75 mg/kg/day IM in two divided doses. The dose in milligrams of ceftriaxone is first calculated for this child.

$$\text{Weight of child (in kg): } \frac{20 \text{ lb}}{2.2 \text{ lb/kg}} = 9.09 \text{ kg}$$

Based on this weight, the dose for this child is calculated:

$$\text{Milligrams per day: } 9.09 \text{ kg} \times 75 \text{ mg/kg/day} = 682 \text{ mg/day}$$

$$\text{Milligrams per dose: } \frac{682 \text{ mg/day}}{2 \text{ doses/day}} = 341 \text{ mg/dose}$$

2. Next, the number of milliliters of Ceftriaxone for Injection reconstituted as recommended in the product package insert is calculated:

$$\frac{250 \text{ mg}}{\text{mL}} = \frac{341 \text{ mg}}{x}; x = 1.36 \text{ mL}$$

3. It is decided that this volume is too large to give IM to this child (see Table 34.1), and it is uncertain whether the powder for injection is sufficiently soluble to make a more concentrated IM

injection. An IV push administration is being considered. The physician asks if the drug can be made in a concentration of 100 mg/mL. You must now calculate the number of milliliters of Sterile Water for Injection to add to an unreconstituted 2-g vial to obtain this concentration.

a. First, calculate the powder volume of the drug in the 2-g vial.

The volume of injection when reconstituted as directed in the package insert:

$$\frac{250 \text{ mg}}{1 \text{ mL}} = \frac{2,000 \text{ mg}}{x \text{ mL}}; x = 8 \text{ mL}$$

Volume of diluent added when reconstituted as directed in the package insert: 7.2 mL

Powder volume: 8 mL − 7.2 mL = 0.8 mL

b. Now calculate the new volume of water to add for reconstitution to give a concentration of 100 mg/mL.

New volume of injection when reconstituted to give 100 mg/mL:

$$\frac{100 \text{ mg}}{\text{mL}} = \frac{2,000 \text{ mg}}{x \text{ mL}}; x = 20 \text{ mL}$$

Powder volume: 0.8 mL

New volume of diluent to give 100 mg/mL:

$$20 \text{ mL} − 0.8 \text{ mL} = 19.2 \text{ mL}$$

c. As with the previous example, it may be necessary to add the water in two portions, and the partially reconstituted product will probably have to be transferred to a larger sterile vial or 20-mL syringe to accommodate the total volume of 20 mL.

C. Calculation of IV flow rates

Intravenous administration, either continuous or intermittent, requires that the flow of the IV solution into the patient be regulated at a recommended rate or over a desired or recommended time interval.

1. One method for controlling rate of flow is to use an IV infusion set that has a drip chamber. (See the illustration of the IV infusion set with IV bag.)

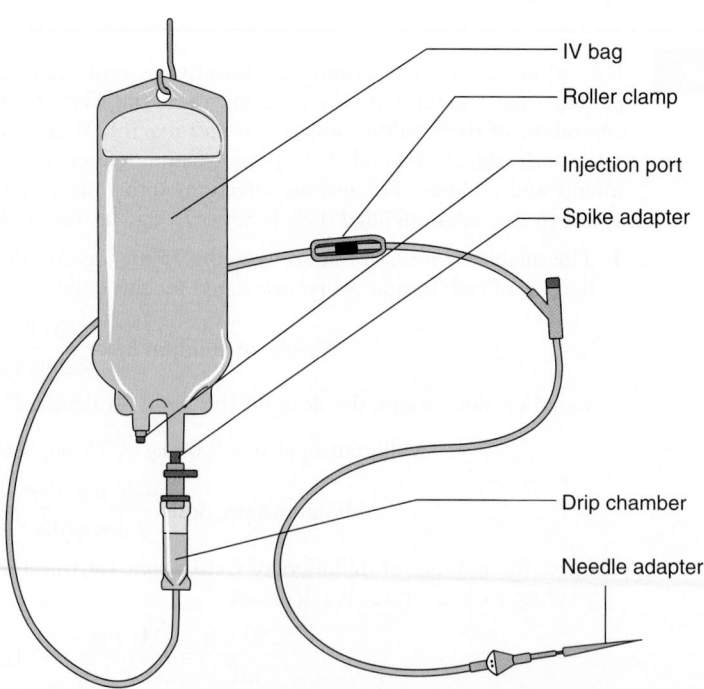

INTRAVENOUS INFUSION SET WITH IV BAG

a. An IV infusion set is plastic tubing that has a spike adapter on one end that is inserted into a port of the IV bag or bottle; the other end of the tubing has a needle or similar adapter that accesses the patient's vein. The IV set has a drip chamber of transparent plastic inserted in the tubing immediately below the spike adapter. The orifice from the bottom of the adapter into the drip chamber gives a controlled drop size (e.g., 0.05 mL/drop or 20 drops/mL).

b. The rate of flow is regulated using a roller clamp on the IV set that controls the number of drops per minute that flow into the drip chamber and through the rest of the tubing and into the patient.

c. There are several common IV sets: 10 drops/mL, 15 drops/mL, 20 drops/mL, and 60 drops/mL; the latter is sometimes called a micro-drip or a mini-drip set.

d. The nurse or caregiver counts the number of drops per minute entering the drip chamber and converts this to milliliters per minute using the drops-per-milliliter set size. If the rate of flow is either too fast or too slow, the rate is adjusted using the roller clamp. This process is illustrated with several examples given here and with several of the sample medication orders that follow.

2. In some circumstances, either precise administration rates or positive pressure are required; in these circumstances infusion devices such as controllers or IV pumps are needed. For infusion devices such as this, the desired rate in milliliters per hour or milliliters per minute is programmed into the device software.

Example 34.3

Given the following order:

KCl 20 mEq in 500 mL dextrose 5% in water (D5W). Infuse IV over 8 hours.

The administration set delivers 20 drops/mL.

1. What is the flow rate in milliliters per hour?

$$500 \text{ mL}/8 \text{ hr} = 62.5 \text{ mL/hr} = 63 \text{ mL/hr}$$

2. What is the flow rate in drops per minute?

By dimensional analysis:

$$\left(\frac{20 \text{ drops}}{\text{mL}}\right)\left(\frac{63 \text{ mL}}{\text{hr}}\right)\left(\frac{\text{hr}}{60 \text{ min}}\right) = 21 \text{ drops/min}$$

Example 34.4

Given the following order:

Ampicillin Na 175 mg in 100 mL 0.9 % NaCl Solution. Infuse IV piggyback over 15 minutes and repeat q6h.

The administration set delivers 15 drops/mL.

1. What is the flow rate in milliliters per **minute**?

$$100 \text{ mL}/15 \text{ minutes} = 6.7 \text{ mL/min}$$

2. What is the flow rate in drops per minute?

By dimensional analysis:

$$\left(\frac{15 \text{ drops}}{\text{mL}}\right)\left(\frac{6.7 \text{ mL}}{\text{min}}\right) = 101 \text{ drops/min}$$

By proportion:

$$\frac{15 \text{ drops}}{\text{mL}} = \frac{x \text{ drops}}{6.7 \text{ mL}}; x = 101 \text{ drops}$$

Notice in this last calculation that we calculate the number of drops per minute by calculating the number of drops in 6.7 mL. Because 6.7 mL is the volume given in each minute, the number of drops in 6.7 is the number of drops given in each minute (101 drops, in this case).

Example 34.5 Given the following order:

Nitroglycerin IV 50 mg in 250 mL Normal Saline Solution (NSS). Start at 5 mcg/min and titrate dose with respect to response.

The administration set delivers 60 drops/mL.

1. What is the flow rate of nitroglycerin (NTG) solution in milliliters per hour?

$$\left(\frac{250\ mL}{50\ mg\ NTG}\right)\left(\frac{mg}{1,000\ mcg}\right)\left(\frac{5\ mcg\ NTG}{min}\right)\left(\frac{60\ min}{hr}\right) = 1.5\ mL/hr$$

2. What is the flow rate in drops per minute?

$$\left(\frac{60\ drops}{mL}\right)\left(\frac{1.5\ mL}{hr}\right)\left(\frac{hr}{60\ min}\right) = 1.5\ drops/min$$

Note: When the administration set delivers 60 drops/mL, the milliliters per hour equal drops per minute.

D. **Mixing two or more drugs in one syringe**
1. Check the doses.
2. Check compatibility.
   a. Check the product package insert, the *Handbook on Injectable Drugs,* or the *King Guide to Parenteral Admixtures* for compatibility information.
   b. Consult prescriber concerning any substantive changes.
3. Special techniques for assuring proper dose volumes when one or more volumes are **small**
   a. Examples of common circumstances
      (1) Pediatric doses
      (2) Insulin
      (3) Biotech drugs
   b. Two issues that must be considered relative to the dose volumes under consideration
      (1) Amount of dead space in the syringe hub and needle lumen
      (2) Priming volume
   c. Dead space in syringe hub and needle lumen

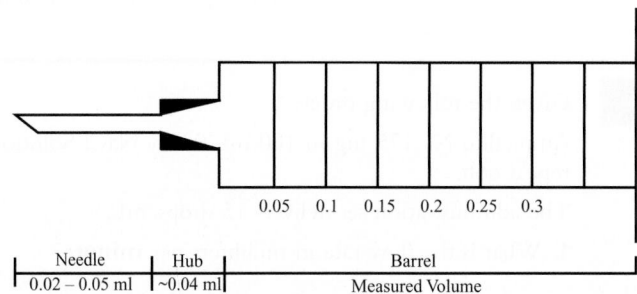

The volume in the syringe hub varies with the manufacturer and the syringe size. The volume in the needle lumen varies with the manufacturer and the needle gauge (ga) and length. Volumes were checked for various 1-mL syringes and several sizes of needles. The hub and lumen volumes for this sample are given here.

Volume in hub = 0.04 mL

Volume in the lumen of a 1-inch 22-ga needle = 0.03 mL

Volume in the lumen of a 1½-inch 19-ga filter needle = 0.05 mL

When you have a small volume for a dose and a serial multiple draw into the same syringe, you will get too much of the first drug (by the volume left in the hub and needle when the first drug is drawn) and not enough of the second drug (by that same volume). Potential errors are shown with the following examples.
(1) Filter needle used and not changed between draws: 0.09 mL

[0.04 mL (hub) + 0.05 mL (needle) = 0.09 mL]

(2) 22-ga 1-inch needle used and not changed between draws: 0.07 mL

[0.04 mL (hub) + 0.03 mL (needle) = 0.07 mL]

(3) Any needle used but changed between draws: 0.04 mL (just the volume in the syringe hub, as the needle was changed between the draws)

As you can see, for small dose volumes (less than 1.0 mL), dead space can make a significant difference. You can also see that even if you switch needles between draws, you may still get a substantial percent error (from the 0.04-mL dead space in the syringe hub) if one of the dose volumes is very small.

d. Methods of handling dead space with small dose volumes: There are two ways of handling this dead space, depending on the circumstances.

(1) If a precise dose is needed: If a particular dose of each drug is needed, the problem of dead space can be circumvented in the following way:

(a) Draw the proper dose of each drug into separate syringes.

(b) Remove the protective hub cap from the tip of a third syringe, draw back its plunger, and then, using aseptic technique, shoot each drug solution into that third syringe through the hub opening.

By drawing the proper dose volume of each drug into separate syringes and then injecting each into a third syringe, only the correct measured volume of each drug is in the third syringe. The extra dead-space volume remains in the original needles and syringes. This is illustrated with Sample Medication Order 34.4.

(2) For injections that are given routinely and adjusted based on monitoring parameters: There are some cases for which small volumes are drawn sequentially in the same syringe. A common example is the use of regular and long-acting insulins when given at the same time; administering both injections in one syringe allows the patient to take just one shot. In this case, the use of three syringes would be both complex and expensive for the patient. Because doses are given routinely and are adjusted based on blood glucose levels, as long as the same procedure and sequence of drawing is used, the concern about needle dead space is not germane. It is, however, very important always to use the same sequence and procedure, because the dead space still exists and affects the volumes drawn; in this case, this is compensated for by adjusting doses with monitoring outcomes. This method is illustrated with Sample Medication Order 34.5.

e. Priming volume: In the example given above in section d, where a precise dose is needed, extra volume of each drug solution obviously must be drawn to fill the hub of the third syringe and to prime the new needle that the nurse will apply when administering the drug solution to the patient. This is called *priming volume.*

(1) If the drug volumes are **equal**, the priming volume may be split equally, one-half for each drug. For example, if there are two drugs, and the desired priming volume is 0.1 mL, you would use 0.05 mL of each for the priming volume.

(2) If the drug volumes are **unequal**, the priming volume must have the same volume proportion of each drug solution as is in the dose volume. For example:

Drug A: 0.1-mL dose volume

Drug B: 0.2-mL dose volume

Total dose volume: 0.3 mL

If you desire a priming volume of 0.1 mL, one-third of this volume (0.1/0.3 = 1/3), or 0.033 mL, must be Drug A and two thirds of this volume (0.2/0.3 = 2/3), or 0.067 mL, must be Drug B.

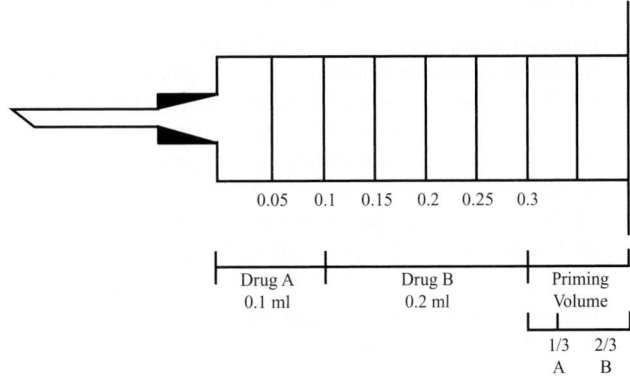

Therefore, to administer 0.1 mL of Drug A and 0.2 mL of Drug B in one syringe, draw 0.13 mL of Drug A in one syringe (0.1 mL for the dose and 0.03 mL for priming volume); draw 0.27 mL of Drug B in a second syringe (0.2 mL for the dose and 0.07 mL for priming volume); shoot these solutions into a third syringe and apply a Luer-tip cap. This syringe now contains 0.4 mL (0.13 mL of Drug A + 0.27 mL of Drug B = 0.4 mL). When the nurse gives the 0.3-mL dose, she will apply an appropriate needle to the syringe and will fill the syringe hub and the needle. She will then depress the syringe plunger to the 0.3-mL mark on the syringe before giving the dose. This is one reason that the volume to be administered should always be indicated on the syringe label.

Sample Medication Orders

Note: In the following sample medication orders, unless otherwise indicated, the product descriptions and stability information are taken from the product's package insert. Because this information varies with the manufacturer, always consult the product package insert or container label for the product you are using. Often this information changes over time even for the same product and manufacturer, so this information should be rechecked frequently.

SAMPLE MEDICATION ORDER 34.1

CASE: Darbie Potensky is a 5'11", 189-lb, 69-year-old man. He was working at his job as a chef when he began having chest pain and shortness of breath. After ambulance transport to Happy Valley Community Hospital, medical staff determined that he had a pulmonary embolus (PE). Darbie also is being treated for congestive heart failure, hypertension, and mild renal insufficiency. His physician, Dr. Prendergas, ordered a heparin drip. Hospital policy requires using manufactured bags in a standard concentration of heparin sodium 25,000 units in 250 mL D5W; however, the concentration usually purchased commercially is out of stock. The inpatient pharmacy prepares the same concentration so that when the shipment arrives, no changes in therapy need to be made.

HAPPY VALLEY COMMUNITY HOSPITAL
220 TANAGER WAY
BIRDVILLE, ILLINOIS 60644

PHYSICIAN ORDERS	**WEIGHT-BASED HEPARIN INFUSION PROTOCOL**
Patient Name: <u>Darbie Potensky</u>	Room # 315NW
Date & Time: 00/00/00 1830	Pt #: 5698765
Weigh patient on admission. <u>86 kg</u>	Diagnosis: <u>Pulmonary embolus</u>

HEPARIN

1) Heparin <u>lab</u> orders: PT/INR and hemogram on the first day, then hemogram every three days.
PTT 6 hours after starting heparin & every 6 hours for the first 24 hours, then daily.
After initial 24 hours, obtain PTT 6 hours after any adjustment in heparin rate.
If PTT is greater than 135 sec for two consecutive measurements, notify physician.

2) Heparin orders: cardiovascular treatment (e.g., DVT, PE):

Heparin loading dose = <u>70</u> units/kg IV push
Heparin maintenance infusion ≅ <u>15</u> units/kg/hr and monitor PTT in 6 hours
Use PTT to adjust heparin infusion rate using the following:
20–29 sec—increase heparin rate by 200 units/hr
30–49 sec—increase heparin rate by 100 units/hr
50–74 sec—no change in heparin rate
75–94 sec—decrease heparin rate by 100 units/hr
95–114 sec—decrease heparin rate by 200 units/hr
115 or greater—decrease heparin rate by 300 units/hr

Ordering Provider *I. Prendergas,* MD   Date: *00/00/00*
         Signature

ORDER REVIEW AND DOSING CALCULATIONS

Dose/Concentration

Heparin **bolus dose** in units:

$$\left(\frac{70 \text{ units}}{\text{kg}}\right)\left(\frac{86 \text{ kg}}{}\right) = 6{,}020 \text{ units} \approx 6{,}000 \text{ units}$$

Continuous infusion rate in units per hour:

$$\left(\frac{15 \text{ units}}{\text{kg/hr}}\right)\left(\frac{86 \text{ kg}}{}\right) = 1{,}290 \text{ units/hr} \approx 1{,}300 \text{ units/hr}$$

Concentration = total drug quantity/total volume

Concentration (in units/mL) = 25,000 units/250 mL = 100 units/mL

Dose Ordered

6,000 units [70 units/kg for this 189-lb (86-kg) man] IV push followed by continuous infusion at 1,300 units/hr and monitored using an activated partial thromboplastin time (aPTT) coagulation test.

$$\text{Continuous infusion dose per hour} = 1{,}300 \text{ units/hr}$$

Flow rate (in mL/hr) = dose per hour divided by concentration (in units/mL)

$$\text{Flow rate} = \frac{1{,}300 \text{ unit/hr}}{100 \text{ units/mL}} = 13 \text{ mL/hr}$$

Note: Incorrect dosing of Heparin has been implicated in numerous sentinel events. Many institutions have protocols for Heparin use, mandating standardized concentration of drug and consistent dosing protocols, to minimize errors. In addition, the abbreviation "u" should never be used. Always write all doses using the entire word "units."

IV Flow Rate Calculations

Milliliters per hour:

$$\left(\frac{250 \text{ mL}}{25{,}000 \text{ units}}\right)\left(\frac{1{,}300 \text{ units}}{\text{hr}}\right) = 13 \text{ mL/hr}$$

Drops per minute:

$$\left(\frac{60 \text{ drops}}{\text{mL}}\right)\left(\frac{13 \text{ mL}}{\text{hr}}\right)\left(\frac{\text{hr}}{60 \text{ min}}\right) = 13 \text{ drops/min}$$

Note: Although IV Heparin flow rates are often regulated using an infusion controller for which the rate is programmed in milliliters per hour, the preceding calculation is to give you additional practice in calculating IV flow rate using a drip chamber.

Length of time one bottle will last: $\dfrac{250 \text{ mL}}{13 \text{ mL/hr}} = 19.2 \text{ hr}$

Ingredient Amounts

Heparin Na injection concentration: 5,000 units/mL

Volume of heparin Na injection for IV infusion solution:

$$\frac{5{,}000 \text{ units}}{\text{mL}} = \frac{25{,}000 \text{ units}}{x \text{ mL}}; \ x = 5 \text{ mL}$$

COMPOUNDING RECORD

HAPPY VALLEY COMMUNITY HOSPITAL
220 TANAGER WAY
BIRDVILLE, IL 60644

Name: Darbie Potensky

Pt Number: 5698765

MD: Prendergas

Room: 315NW

Current weight: 86 kg

Rx: 101607-22

Ingredients	Amt	Mfg	Lot	Exp
Heparin Na vial 5,000 units/mL	25,000 units/5 mL	Hospira	2351356	mm/yy
In Dextrose 5% solution	250 mL	Baxter	BB25463	mm/yy

Compounding instructions: Use aseptic technique in all procedures for preparing this sterile preparation. Remove jewelry and wash hands and forearms with germicidal soap. Don foot covers, hair covers, a face mask, and a clean, low-shedding gown. Apply an alcohol-based hand cleaner, allow to dry, and put on sterile, powder-free protective gloves. Wipe the surfaces of the LAFW with sterile 70% isopropyl alcohol using a lint-free cloth. Assemble the materials needed, including needles and syringes needed. Using a sterile alcohol swab for each surface, disinfect all vial septa and injection port of D5W bag. Withdraw 5 mL of heparin sodium from vial and add to D5W 250-mL bag. Invert bag to mix thoroughly. Label appropriately.

Prepared at 1800 00/00/00

Do not hang after: 1800 00/02/00

Prepared by: MES, RPh

REFRIGERATE UNTIL USE

COMPATIBILITY-STABILITY/BEYOND-USE DATE

Stability-Compatibility: Heparin sodium is available as an injectable solution that is stable at room temperature. Although there are conflicting reports in the literature, heparin is considered to be physically compatible and stable in 5% Dextrose in Water Injection at the concentration of this constant infusion solution per the *Handbook of Injectable Drugs* (4) and the manufacturer's labeling for the premade infusion bags.

Packaging and Storage and Beyond-Use Date: The pharmacy will put a "Store in the refrigerator" label on this unpreserved LVP. The pharmacy will label the bag with its customary 48-hour beyond-use date, which is consistent with the policy of this hospital for IV solutions of this type when labeled for storage in the refrigerator.

FINAL PREPARATION CHECK: All volumes should be checked and confirmed. The solution should be inspected and found to be clear, colorless, and free of any particulates or turbidity.

LABELING

HAPPY VALLEY COMMUNITY HOSPITAL
220 TANAGER WAY
BIRDVILLE, IL 60644

Name: Darbie Potensky   Room: 315NW
Pt Number: 5698765   Current weight: 86 kg

MD: Prendergas   Rx: 101607-22

Heparin sodium   25,000 units

In Dextrose 5% solution   250 mL

Infuse initially at 15 units/kg/hr (1,300 units/hr) and adjust dose as
appropriate based on aPTT results.

Infusion rate: 13 mL/hr initially; adjust based on aPTT results.

Prepared at 1800 00/00/00   Prepared by: MES, RPh

Do not hang after: 1800 00/02/00

REFRIGERATE UNTIL USE

SAMPLE MEDICATION ORDER 34.2

CASE: Richard J. "RJ" Reynolds is a 5′5″, 44-year-old man weighing 133 lb with a 60-pack-per-year history of smoking. He was recently diagnosed with small-cell lung cancer and is receiving a cisplatin-based chemotherapy regimen. He presents to his primary care physician, Dr. Doctor, complaining of leg cramps. A complete metabolic panel reveals a serum potassium level of 2.6 and serum magnesium of 1.4 mg/dL. Dr. Doctor sends RJ to the clinic's infusion center for electrolyte replacement therapy.

BEST HEALTHCARE ONCOLOGY CLINIC
1100 EAST HEALTHCARE AVE., SUITE 200
POTOSI, WI 53820

Patient Name: Richard Reynolds   Patient Number: 1020162
Date of Birth: mm/dd/yyyy

Physician Orders:

Infuse Magnesium Sulfate 3 grams and Potassium Chloride 60 mEq intravenously over 6 hours per PICC line for electrolyte replacement. Flush line per clinic protocol after infusion.

Signature: *J. Doctor,* MD   Date: *00/00/0000*

ORDER REVIEW AND DOSING CALCULATIONS

The clinic pharmacy prepares all infusion center medications. According to references, the doses of both electrolytes are appropriate for this patient and his condition. The clinic protocols mandate that all potassium infusions must be given at a rate of 10 mEq/hr or slower. With an osmolality in the range of 4,000 mOsm/L, potassium chloride is extremely irritating to peripheral veins and must be diluted. While magnesium can be given as a direct IV injection in certain clinical situations such as eclampsia of pregnancy, it should be diluted for electrolyte replacement therapy. The pharmacy determines that the two electrolytes are compatible in 0.9% Sodium Chloride for Injection for 24 hours (4). Both electrolytes will be added to 1,000 mL of 0.9% Sodium Chloride for Injection and infused with an infusion pump to minimize the risk of free flow of potassium.

Dose/Concentration: Doses and concentrations appropriate and by protocol (see earlier)

Ingredient Amounts

Magnesium sulfate dose in grams = 3 grams

Magnesium sulfate injection concentration = 500 mg/mL or 0.5 g/mL

Volume of magnesium sulfate to add (in mL):

$$\frac{0.5\ g}{1\ mL} = \frac{3\ g}{x\ mL}; x = 6\ mL$$

Potassium chloride dose (in mEq) = 60 mEq

Potassium chloride injection concentration = 2 mEq/mL

Volume of potassium chloride to add (in mL):

$$\frac{2\ mEq}{1\ mL} = \frac{60\ mEq}{x\ mL}; x = 30\ mL$$

IV Flow Rate Calculations

Rate in milliliters per hour = total bag volume/total hours of infusion

Rate = 1,000 mL/6 hr, or 167 mL/hr

COMPOUNDING RECORD

BEST HEALTHCARE ONCOLOGY PHARMACY
1100 EAST HEALTHCARE AVE., SUITE 240
POTOSI, WI 53820

COMPOUNDING RECORD

Medications	Amt	Mfg	Lot #	Exp
Potassium Chloride inj 2 mEq/mL	30 mL	Hospira	12567841	mm/yy
Magnesium Sulfate inj 500 mg/mL	6 mL	Hospira	45512874	mm/yy
Sodium Chloride 0.9% bag	1,000 mL	Baxter	AB25415	mm/yy
Supplies	**# used**			
Syringe, 30 mL	1	BD	45212z5	mm/yy
Syringe, 10 mL	1	BD	58742a5	mm/yy
Needle 22-ga × 1"	2	BD	45552z4	mm/yy

Compounding instructions: Use aseptic technique in all procedures for preparing this sterile preparation. Remove jewelry and wash hands and forearms with germicidal soap. Don foot covers, hair covers, a face mask, and a clean, low-shedding gown. Apply an alcohol-based hand cleaner, allow to dry, and put on sterile, powder-free protective gloves. Wipe the surfaces of the LAFW with sterile 70% isopropyl alcohol using a lint-free cloth. Assemble the materials needed, including needles and syringes. Using a sterile alcohol swab for each surface, disinfect all vial septa and injection port of NSS bag. Withdraw potassium chloride 60 mEq/30 mL and add to NSS bag; invert bag to mix thoroughly. Withdraw magnesium sulfate 3 grams (24 mEq)/6 mL and add to bag. Invert bag and mix electrolytes thoroughly throughout solution. Label appropriately.

Patient Name: Reynolds, Richard
Prepared by: D. Gillis, CPT
Date: 00/00/00 1300

Ordering MD: Dr. J. Doctor
Checked by: M. Swandby, RPh
Beyond-use date: 1300 00/01/00

COMPATIBILITY-STABILITY/BEYOND-USE DATE

Stability-Compatibility: The pharmacy has both electrolytes available as solutions in multidose vials, and the primary IV solution, 0.9% Sodium Chloride Injection, in a polyvinyl chloride bag.

Potassium chloride injection has a neutral pH in the range of 4 to 8. The solution itself is chemically and physically very stable, and it is physically compatible in NSS with magnesium sulfate (4). The multidose vials used by this pharmacy contain methylparaben (0.05%) and propylparaben (0.005%) as a preservative system but, when diluted in the LVP solution, this would not provide sufficient preservative to protect the preparation from microbial growth. After adding potassium chloride injection to an IV solution, the bag should be inverted several times to ensure adequate mixing.

Magnesium sulfate is available as a 50% solution providing 500 mg/mL or 4.06 mEq/mL. The calculated osmolarity of the 50% solution is 4,060 mOsm/L, very similar to that of potassium chloride injection. The adjusted pH is in the 5 to 7 range (4).

Packaging and Storage and Beyond-Use Date: The pharmacy will label this unpreserved LVP "Store in the refrigerator; do not freeze." The pharmacy will label the bag with its customary 24-hour beyond-use date, which is consistent with the stability of the mixture as noted previously.

LABELING

BEST HEALTHCARE ONCOLOGY PHARMACY
1100 EAST HEALTHCARE AVE., SUITE 240
POTOSI, WI 53820

Name: Reynolds, RJ   Pt Number: 1020162
MD: Doctor, JM   Date: 00/00/00

Potassium Chloride   60 mEq
Magnesium Sulfate   3 grams (24 mEq)
In 0.9% Sodium Chloride Solution 1,000 mL

Infuse at 167 mL/hr over 6 hours.
Prepared at <u>1300 00/00/00</u>
Prepared by: D. Gillis, CPT   Checked by: <u>M. Swandby, RPh</u>
Do not hang after: <u>1300 00/01/00</u>

REFRIGERATE UNTIL USE. DO NOT FREEZE.

FINAL PREPARATION CHECK: All volumes should be checked and confirmed. The solution should be inspected and found to be clear, colorless, and free of any particulates or turbidity.

SAMPLE MEDICATION ORDER 34.3

CASE: Peter Leindurt is a 44-year-old patient with non-Hodgkin's lymphoma admitted to the hospital after spiking a temperature to 103° F. Blood cultures are drawn from his Groshong catheter and peripherally. Culture results show a *C. parapsilosis* systemic infection. The Groshong catheter is removed. In view of Peter's history of severe electrolyte imbalances and elevated serum blood urea nitrogen (BUN) and creatinine with a previous course of amphotericin B, Peter is started on Abelcet (amphotericin B lipid complex).

BEST HEALTHCARE HOSPITAL
1300 EAST HEALTHCARE AVENUE
POTOSI, WI 53820

PHYSICIAN ORDERS

Patient Name: <u>Leindurt, Peter</u>

Date & Time: 00/00/00 1100

Weigh patient on admission. <u>59.8 kg</u>

Room # 318NW

Patient number: 4586741

Diagnosis: <u>Fungal central line infection</u>

Amphotericin B lipid complex 300 mg in D5W intravenously over 2 hours once daily.
Flush IV line with Dextrose 5% before and after each infusion.

Ordering Provider: <u>D. Bugg</u>, MD
Signature

Date: <u>00/00/00 1100</u>

ORDER REVIEW AND DOSING CALCULATIONS

Amphotericin B lipid complex is a yellow opaque suspension available in a concentration of 5 mg/mL, 20-mL vials. According to the product labeling, it has a pH of 5 to 7 and is incompatible with saline-containing solutions. It is prepared to achieve a final concentration of 1 mg/mL. The drug will be added to a 250-mL D5W bag, and the pharmacy has determined that the 250-mL bags that they carry contain 25 mL of overfill. A 5-μm filter needle is supplied with the preparation.

Patient Dose Check

The usual dose as noted in the product package insert is 5 mg/kg.

Dose = patient weight (in kg) $\times$ dose (in mg/kg):

$$59.8 \text{ kg} \times 5 \text{ mg/kg} = 299 \text{ mg}$$

Therefore, a 300-mg dose is appropriate.

Ingredient Amounts

Volume of Amphotericin B lipid complex to add = dose/concentration of drug in vial:

$$\text{Volume to add} = \frac{300 \text{ mg}}{5 \text{ mg/mL}} = 60 \text{ mL}$$

The pharmacy has determined that the 250-mL D5W bags that they stock have 25 mL overfill. In order to achieve a final bag concentration of 1 mg/mL, the pharmacy must remove volume from the bag prior to adding the Amphotericin product to the bag.

Volume to remove = total bag volume + volume of drug being added − final desired bag volume

Volume to remove = 275 mL + 60 mL − 300 mL = 35 mL

COMPOUNDING RECORD

BEST HEALTHCARE HOSPITAL
1100 EAST HEALTHCARE AVENUE
POTOSI, WI 53820

COMPOUNDING RECORD

Medications	Amt	Mfg	Lot #	Exp
Amphotericin B lipid complex 20-mL vials, 5 mg/mL	60 mL	Hospira	12567841	mm/yy
Dextrose 5% in Water bag	250 mL	Hospira	45512874	mm/yy
Supplies	**# used**			
Syringe, 60 mL	2	BD	45212z5	mm/yy
Needle 18 ga × 1½″	2	BD	45552z4	mm/yy

Compounding instructions: Use aseptic technique in all procedures for preparing this sterile preparation. Remove jewelry and wash hands and forearms with germicidal soap. Don foot covers, hair covers, a face mask, and a clean, low-shedding gown. Apply an alcohol-based hand cleaner, allow to dry, and put on sterile, powder-free protective gloves. Wipe the surfaces of the LAFW with sterile 70% Isopropyl Alcohol using a lint-free cloth. Assemble the materials needed, including needles and syringes. Shake the three 20-mL vials of amphotericin B lipid complex gently to ensure complete suspension of drug. Using a sterile alcohol swab for each surface, disinfect all vial septa and injection port of D5W bag. Remove 35 mL D5W from bag and discard. Withdraw Amphotericin B lipid complex 300 mg/60 mL. Attach 5-μm filter needle to syringe and inject into D5W bag. Invert bag and rotate gently several times to disperse drug suspension.

Patient Name: Peter Leindurt
Prepared by: D. Gillis, CPT
Date: 00/00/00 1300

Ordering MD: Dr. D. Bugg
Checked by: M. Swandby, RPh
Beyond-use date: 1300 00/02/00

COMPATIBILITY-STABILITY/BEYOND-USE DATE

The product labeling indicates that amphotericin B lipid complex is stable for 48 hours refrigerated, with an additional 6 hours at room temperature. The pharmacy will label the preparation with a 48-hour beyond–use date and add appropriate auxiliary directions.

LABELING

BEST HEALTHCARE HOSPITAL
1300 EAST HEALTHCARE AVENUE
POTOSI, WI 53820

Name: Leindurt, Peter   Pt Number: 4586741
MD: D. Bugg   Date: 00/00/00

Amphotericin B Lipid Complex   300 mg
Dextrose 5% in Water   250 mL
Final concentration 1 mg/mL   Total volume: 300 mL

Infuse 300 mg intravenously over 2 hours. Pump rate 150 mL/hr.

Prepared at 1300 00/00/00   Do not use after: 1300 00/02/00
Prepared by: D. Gillis, CPT   Checked by: M. Swandby, RPh

Store in refrigerator. Do not freeze.
Shake bag gently to suspend drug prior to infusing.
Do not use in-line filter during infusion.
DO NOT MIX WITH SODIUM CHLORIDE-CONTAINING SOLUTIONS.

FINAL PREPARATION CHECK: All volumes should be checked and confirmed. The solution should be inspected and found to be a yellow suspension. Bag should be shaken gently to ensure that drug is free of large clumps and redistributes uniformly throughout the solution.

SAMPLE MEDICATION ORDER 34.4

CASE: Doremus Hogwart is a 34-year-old man who presents to his primary care physician with complaints of plantar foot pain due to a persistent plantar wart. Doremus has tried several over-the-counter remedies to remove the wart without success. His physician, Dr. Ellen McGonagall, decides to inject the wart with a combination of *Candida* skin test antigen and lidocaine 1%, in an effort to stimulate an immune response that will eradicate the wart. Dr. McGonagall calls in the order to the adjacent oncology clinic pharmacy.

BEST HEALTHCARE INTERNAL MEDICINE CLINIC
1100 EAST HEALTHCARE AVE., SUITE 260
POTOSI, WI 53820

Patient Name: <u>Doremus Hogwart</u>   Patient Number: <u>5645342</u>
Date of Birth: mm/dd/yyyy

Physician Orders:
Mix 0.1 mL of Candida Skin Test antigen with 0.9 mL lidocaine 1% injection in a syringe, for intralesional injection.

Signature: *E. McGonagall*, MD   Date: *00/00/0000*

ORDER REVIEW AND DOSING CALCULATIONS: A literature search reveals a review article in which this method was described (5). The pharmacist, Henrietta Fishwich, learns that the physician will take the prepared syringe and inject the area immediately under the plantar wart and then use the needle to stab the wart in several areas. Because an unspecified volume of the solution will be used, there is no need to overfill the syringe. The doses of each component are clearly spelled out in the order and correspond to the preparation described in the reference.

COMPOUNDING RECORD

BEST HEALTHCARE ONCOLOGY PHARMACY
1100 EAST HEALTHCARE AVE., SUITE 240
POTOSI, WI 53820

COMPOUNDING RECORD

Medications	Amt	Mfg	Lot #	Exp
Candida Skin Test Antigen	0.1 mL	Allermed	12567841	mm/yy
Lidocaine 10 mg/mL injection, 20-mL vial	0.9 mL	Hospira	45512874	mm/yy
Supplies	**# used**			
Syringe, 3 mL	2	BD	45212z5	mm/yy
Syringe, tuberculin 1 mL	1	BD	25521e3	mm/yy
Needle 23 ga × 5/8″	2	BD	45552z4	mm/yy

Compounding instructions: Use aseptic technique in all procedures for preparing this sterile preparation. Remove jewelry and wash hands and forearms with germicidal soap. Don foot covers, hair covers, a face mask, and a clean, low-shedding gown. Apply an alcohol-based hand cleaner, allow to dry, and put on sterile, powder-free protective gloves. Wipe the surfaces of the LAFW with sterile 70% Isopropyl Alcohol using a lint-free cloth. Assemble the materials needed, including needles and syringes. Using a sterile alcohol swab for each surface, disinfect all vial septa. Pull back plunger of a 3-mL syringe to 1 mL. Using the tuberculin syringe, withdraw 0.1 mL of *Candida* antigen and add to 3-mL syringe through the tip. Using the other 3-mL syringe, withdraw 0.9 mL of lidocaine 10 mg/mL and add through the syringe tip to the 3-mL syringe containing the *Candida* antigen. Cap syringe with a syringe tip cap, place in a zipper-lock bag, and label. After final check, transport immediately to Dr. McGonagall in the Internal Medicine Clinic.

Patient Name: Doremus Hogwart
Prepared by: D. Gillis, CPT
Date: 00/00/00 1000

Ordering MD: Dr. E. McGonagall
Checked by: H. Fishwich, RPh
Beyond-use date: 1100 00/00/00

COMPATIBILITY-STABILITY/BEYOND-USE DATE: *Candida* skin test antigen in Buffered Saline is a clear, colorless solution with a pH of 8.0 to 8.5. It is preserved with Phenol 0.4% . Pharmacist Fishwich can find no compatibility information about *Candida* antigen when mixed with lidocaine. The pharmacy stocks Lidocaine 1% for injection in a 20-mL multidose vial, preserved with methylparaben. Lidocaine has an adjusted pH of about 6.5. Lacking compatibility information, Pharmacist Fishwich decides to prepare the injection as ordered, observe for visible signs of incompatibility, and label the syringe with a "USE IMMEDIATELY" label and a 1-hour beyond-use date.

LABELING

BEST HEALTHCARE ONCOLOGY PHARMACY
1100 EAST HEALTHCARE AVE., SUITE 240
POTOSI, WI 53820

Name: Doremus Hogwart   Pt Number: 5645342
MD: E. McGonagall   Date: 00/00/00

Candida Skin Test Antigen   0.1 mL
Lidocaine 1% (10 mg/mL) Injection   0.9 mL
                                    Total volume: 1 mL

For use as intralesion injection.

Prepared at 1000 00/00/00   Do not use after: 1100 00/00/00
Prepared by: D. Gillis, CPT   Checked by: H. Fishwich, RPh

FOR IMMEDIATE USE; MUST BE DISCARDED AFTER 1100 00/00/00.
DELIVER IMMEDIATELY TO DR. MCGONAGALL IN INTERNAL
MEDICINE CLINIC.

FINAL PREPARATION CHECK: All volumes should be checked and confirmed. The solution should be inspected and found to be clear, colorless, and free of any particulates or turbidity.

PATIENT CONSULTATION: Hello, Mr. Hogwart. I understand that Dr. McGonagall sent you over to pick up this injection to treat your wart. Do you have any drug allergies? Has anyone ever told you that you are allergic to local anesthetics, or Novocain? No? That is good. This injection is a combination of a medication commonly used to test your immune system responses and a local anesthetic called *lidocaine*. If your immune system is working well, you will have an immune response in the area of the wart that is bothering you, and your own immune cells will attack the wart and take care of it. The medication can be used only immediately after it is prepared, so take it right back over to Dr. McGonagall. It may sting when injected, but that should last only a minute, until the anesthetic takes effect. The area may turn red and seem irritated. If that does not resolve after a few days, contact the doctor again. Good luck to you!

SAMPLE MEDICATION ORDER 34.5

CASE: Sugar McGee is a 54-year-old woman with type 2 diabetes who, immediately after meals, has been experiencing high blood glucose readings in the 300- to 350-mg/dL range, accompanied by blurred vision and frequent urination. Her endocrinologist, Dr. Honeydoo, prescribed a combination of a rapid-acting insulin analog added to her isophane insulin to provide better postprandial blood sugar control. Sugar presents the prescription to her pharmacist and requests help in drawing up the first dose, since she is on her way home to eat dinner shortly. Pharmacist Smith instructs Sugar in the order of mixing described here and prepares the first injection for Sugar to use immediately.

TIMBUKTU ENDOCRINOLOGY SPECIALISTS, SC
2999 WEST BELTLINE HWY.
TIMBUKTU, WI 53710
608-333-7171 FAX 608-333-7181

R # *6538*

NAME *Sugar McGee*   DATE *00/00/00*

ADDRESS *1325 Beyond the Bend Road Timbuktu, WI*

R

Insulin glulisine vial 100 units/mL   10 mL
Insulin isophane human vial 100 units/mL   10 mL

N. Smith 00/00/00

Sig: Inject 10 units of glulisine insulin and 55 units of isophane insulin 15 minutes before breakfast and 15 minutes before supper each day.

REFILLS *11*   *Ima D. Honeydoo, MD*

DEA

ORDER REVIEW AND DOSING CALCULATIONS

Stability-Compatibility: When vials of insulin are stored in the refrigerator but protected from freezing, the insulin is stable until the expiration date given on the bottle. Bottles of insulin stored at room temperature and protected from direct sunlight are stable for 28 days. These are multidose vials and contain a preservative.

Isophane (NPH) and Insulin glulisine must be given immediately after mixing. Although premixing results in some decrease in the maximum blood concentration (C_{max}) compared with separate simultaneous injections, the time to maximum concentration is not affected and bioavailability appears to be similar between separate injections and premixed injections. This applies to insulin lispro and insulin aspart, also rapid-acting insulins. All three can be mixed with NPH insulin but must be administered immediately and within 15 minutes before or immediately after a meal. Rapid-acting insulins cannot be mixed with any other long-acting insulin besides NPH.

When mixing insulin in a single syringe, the insulin glulisine (a clear solution) is drawn first and then the NPH (a cloudy solution). One way to remember the order of mixing is to think of a perfect summer day-clear to partly cloudy. Because air must be replaced in each vial equal to the volume removed, this means that mixing insulin in a single syringe requires a special sequence:

Example: Glulisine (or regular insulin) needed = x units
          NPH insulin needed = y units

Order of steps:

1. Swab NPH vial stopper with alcohol and allow to dry. Do not invert NPH vial. Using an insulin syringe, inject y units of air into NPH vial and take out needle without drawing any insulin into the syringe. Do not invert NPH vial prior to this step.
2. Swab insulin glulisine vial stopper with alcohol and allow to dry. Using the same syringe, inject x units of air into the glulisine insulin vial and withdraw x units of glulisine insulin.
3. Mix NPH by rolling vial gently in palms to disperse the particles; then swab vial stopper with alcohol and allow to dry. Insert the needle into the NPH vial, withdraw y units of NPH insulin (total units of insulin in the syringe is now $x + y$ units), and withdraw the needle.

Insulin is routinely drawn sequentially in the same syringe. Because of the small volumes involved and the dead space in the needle and hub of the syringe, it is important always to draw insulin in the same way and use the same brand of syringes. A different dose would also result if the two insulin types were drawn in separate syringes and either given separately or first pooled in a third syringe or vial.

CALCULATIONS

Dose/Concentration: Insulin dosage is dependent on the patient's blood glucose.

Ingredient Amounts: Insulin syringes are marked in units; draw 10 units of Insulin glulisine and 55 units of NPH Insulin for a total of 65 units.

COMPOUNDING RECORD

TIMBUKTU PHARMACY
428 LONELY ROAD
TIMBUKTU, WI 53710

COMPOUNDING RECORD

Medications	Amt	Mfg	Lot #	Exp
Insulin glulisine vial 100 units/mL	10 units (0.1 mL)	Sanofi-Aventis	12567841	mm/yy
Insulin Human isophane 100 units/mL	55 units (0.55 mL)	Lilly	45512874	mm/yy
Supplies	**# used**			
Syringe, U-100 Insulin	1	BD	45212z5	mm/yy

Compounding instructions: Use aseptic technique in all procedures for preparing this sterile preparation. Remove jewelry and wash hands and forearms with germicidal soap. Don foot covers, hair covers, a face mask, and a clean, low-shedding gown. Apply an alcohol-based hand cleaner, allow to dry, and put on sterile, powder-free protective gloves. Wipe the surfaces of the LAFW with sterile 70% Isopropyl Alcohol using a lint-free cloth. Assemble the materials needed, a U-100 insulin syringe, and one 10-mL bottle each of glulisine U-100 insulin and of human isophane U-100 insulin. Swab the insulin glulisine and isophane vial ports with an alcohol swab. Using the 1-mL insulin syringe with attached needle, pull the plunger back to 65 units (0.65 mL). Insert the needle into the isophane vial and push in 55 units (0.55 mL) of air so the plunger is now at the 10-unit mark. Withdraw the needle and insert it into the glulisine vial. Push the remaining volume of air into that vial and, with the vial inverted, draw back the syringe plunger to 10 units (0.1 mL) to withdraw that amount of insulin glulisine from the vial. Gently rotate the isophane vial to disperse the particles, and reswab the stopper with alcohol. Let dry. Next, using the same syringe and needle, reenter the isophane insulin vial and withdraw 55 units (0.55 mL) of insulin from the vial: The plunger should now be at the 65-units mark. Remove the needle from the vial and recap the needle. Draw back the plunger and rotate to mix. With the needle pointing upward, move the plunger back to the previous marking. Remove all materials from the hood and place a label on the syringe. Place the syringe in a labeled zipper-closure bag.

Patient Name: Sugar McGee
Prepared by: D. Gillis, CPT
Date: 00/00/00 1700

Ordering MD: I. Honeydoo, MD
Checked by: N. Smith, RPh
Beyond-use date: 1700 00/00/00

LABELING FOR SYRINGE

Sugar McGee   Log #101607-14
Insulin glulisine 10 units
Insulin Isophane human 55 units
Total dose 65 units
Rotate gently before injecting.
USE IMMEDIATELY.

QUALITY CONTROL: All volumes should be checked and confirmed. The suspension should appear cloudy but with no larger crystals or particulates. Inspect the Insulin glulisine vial to ensure that it is clear, without particles. Mark vial "FOR MIXTURES ONLY" and use this vial for mixed insulin doses to ensure that it is not used for doses intended for intravenous use, to avoid inadvertent injection of isophane particles.

PATIENT CONSULTATION: Good evening, Sugar. It is nice to see you again. Have you been having trouble with your blood sugars around mealtimes? You were using regular human insulin and NPH insulin before, correct? Are you still familiar with the signs of hypo- and hyperglycemia? Because this new synthetic insulin, insulin glulisine, is faster acting, let's review the signs of low blood sugar again. You may experience feelings of anxiousness, tremors, and shaking, as well as a racing heart and flushing or coldness. You may also have trouble thinking clearly, or experience changes in your vision or difficulty speaking. That all sounds familiar? That's good. I am going to give you these step-by-step instructions on how to draw up your insulin doses, but you still follow the same steps as you did with the regular human insulin/NPH combination. Yes, that's right; remember "Clear to partly cloudy." Don't forget to mark your glulisine vials as "for mixtures only," just like you did with the regular vials you used for mixtures before. Notice that the directions for use say to inject this insulin mixture 15 minutes before breakfast and 15 minutes before supper. It is important that you draw this mixture just before you inject it. Do you have any questions for me? As this is the first time you will be using this insulin, I am glad to see Mr. McGee is with you to drive home, just in case you should have any unexpected reaction on the way home. Okay, go ahead and give your dose now before dinner and remember to record your blood sugars in your planner so that you can report on the effectiveness of this combination to Dr. Honeydoo when you see him next week. Have a nice evening, Mrs. McGee.

SAMPLE MEDICATION ORDER 34.6

CASE: RJ Reynolds returns to the oncology clinic for his next cycle of chemotherapy. His current weight is 128 lb, and his laboratory parameters are stable, with a hemoglobin of 12.2 g/dL, white blood cell count of 6.8×10^9 per liter, and platelet count of 368×10^9 per liter. This is day 1 of his third course of cisplatin and etoposide, with orders written as follows:

BEST HEALTHCARE ONCOLOGY CLINIC
1100 EAST HEALTHCARE AVE., SUITE 200
POTOSI, WI 53820

Patient Name: Richard Reynolds   Patient Number: 1020162
Date of Birth: mm/dd/yyyy   Cycle 3   Day 1
Height in cm: 165.1 cm   Weight: 58.2 kg   BSA: 1.63 m²

Physician Orders:

Premedicate with ondansetron 10 mg and dexamethasone 10 mg given intravenously.
Hydration: 1,000 mL 0.9% Sodium Chloride with 20 mEq Potassium Chloride IV over 1 hour prior to initiating cisplatin.

122 mg/ BB

Cisplatin 75 mg/m² or ~~135~~ mg in 1,000 mL 0.9% Sodium Chloride with Mannitol 25 g IV over 2 hours.
Etoposide 100 mg/m² or 163 mg in 0.9% Sodium Chloride IV 500 mL IV over 2 hours.

Signature: *J. Doctor*, MD   Date: *00/00/0000*

ORDER REVIEW AND DOSING CALCULATIONS

Pharmacist Betty Bright reviews the orders for completeness and accuracy prior to initiating sterile compounding in the oncology pharmacy's negative-pressure chemotherapy preparation room containing the biological safety cabinet used for chemotherapy preparation. Betty notes that the body surface area (BSA) on the order is correct, using the Mosteller formula:

$$BSA\,(m^2) = \sqrt{\frac{Ht\,(cm)\ \times\ Wt\,(kg)}{3,600}}$$

$$BSA\,(m^2) = \sqrt{\frac{165.1\ \times\ 58.2}{3,600}} = 1.63\ m^2$$

However, the dose for the cisplatin that Betty is about to compound is 75 mg/m^2, which, for Mr. Reynolds, is

$$\left(\frac{75\ mg}{m^2}\right)\left(\frac{1.63\ m^2}{}\right) = 122\ mg,$$

not the 135 mg written on the order. Betty contacts Dr. Doctor, who agrees with the dose clarification as noted on the orders.

Ingredient Amounts

Volume of cisplatin injection: Product concentration is 1 mg/mL; for 122 mg, 122 mL are needed.

Volume of mannitol injection: Product is 25% w/v, 25 g/100 mL; for 25 g, 100 mL are needed.

The pharmacy has determined that the 1,000-mL NSS bags that they stock have 50 mL overfill. To achieve a final volume of 1,000 mL, the pharmacy must remove volume from the bag prior to adding the cisplatin and mannitol to the bag.

Volume to remove = total bag volume + volume of drugs being added − final desired bag volume

Volume to remove = 1,050 mL + 122 mL + 100 mL − 1,000 mL = 272 mL

BEST HEALTHCARE ONCOLOGY PHARMACY
1100 EAST HEALTHCARE AVE., SUITE 240
POTOSI, WI 53820

COMPOUNDING RECORD   102607-24

Medications	Amt	Mfg	Lot #	Exp
Cisplatin 1 mg/mL 100-mL vial	100 mL	BMS	12567841	mm/yy
Cisplatin 1 mg/mL 50-mL vial	22 mL	BMS	24551155	mm/yy
Mannitol 25% 50-mL vials	100 mL	Hospira	45512874	mm/yy
Sodium Chloride 0.9% bag	1,000 mL	Baxter	AB25415	mm/yy
Supplies				
Syringe, 60 mL	3	BD	45212z5	mm/yy
Needle 20-ga × 1″	3	BD	45552z4	mm/yy

Compounding instructions: Use aseptic technique in all procedures for preparing this sterile preparation. Remove jewelry and wash hands and forearms with germicidal soap. Don foot covers, hair covers, a face mask, and a clean, low-shedding chemoprotective gown. Apply an alcohol-based hand cleaner, allow to dry, and put on sterile chemotherapy gloves. Wipe the surfaces of the BSC with sterile 70% Isopropyl Alcohol using a lint-free cloth. Assemble the preparation materials needed. Using a separate sterile alcohol swab for each surface, disinfect all vial septa and injection port of NSS bag. Attach an injection port adapter to the injection port of the bag. Withdraw 272 mL from NSS bag and discard. Draw up a total of 122 mg/122 mL from cisplatin vials using a closed-system transfer device and add to bag. Draw up a total of 25 g/100 mL from mannitol vials and add to bag. Remove injection port adapter, invert bag, and mix medications thoroughly throughout solution. Dispose of all preparation materials in chemotherapy waste container.

Patient Name: Reynolds, Richard
Prepared by: D. Gillis, CPT
Date: 00/00/00 1300

Ordering MD: Dr. J. Doctor
Checked by: B. Bright, RPh
Beyond-use date: 1300 00/01/00

COMPATIBILITY-STABILITY/BEYOND-USE DATE: Cisplatin injection has a pH of 4.0, and mannitol injection 25% has a pH of 5.9, according to manufacturers' labeling. The combination of the two drugs in NSS is reported to be stable for 24 to 72 hours at various concentrations (4). The pharmacy will assign a beyond-use date of 24 hours at room temperature and apply appropriate chemotherapy disposal warning labels as well.

FINAL PREPARATION CHECK: The pharmacist checks to verify that the correct volumes of all medications are added to the bag and that the preparation is a clear, colorless solution free of any particulate matter.

LABELING

BEST HEALTHCARE ONCOLOGY PHARMACY
1100 EAST HEALTHCARE AVE., SUITE 240
POTOSI, WI 53820

Name: Reynolds, Richard J   Pt Number: 1020162
MD: Doctor, JM   Date: 00/00/00
Rx #: 10260724

Cisplatin   122 mg
Mannitol   25 g
In 0.9% Sodium Chloride Solution   1,000 mL total volume
Infuse at 500 mL/hr over 2 hours.
Prepared at <u>1300 00/00/00</u>
Prepared by: <u>D. Gillis, CPT</u>   Checked by: <u>B. Bright, RPh</u>
Do not hang after: <u>1300 00/01/00</u>

ANCILLARY LABELS: Store at room temperature. Chemotherapy—observe precautions for handling and disposal.

SAMPLE MEDICATION ORDER 34.7

CASE: Maura Hertz is a 58-year-old woman who is 5'4" tall and weighs 138 lb. She has psoriatic arthritis and presents at the Best Healthcare Rheumatology Clinic for an every 8-week infusion of infliximab. The orders are faxed to the oncology clinic pharmacy for preparation.

BEST HEALTHCARE RHEUMATOLOGY CLINIC
1100 EAST HEALTHCARE AVE., SUITE 246
POTOSI, WI 53820

Patient Name: <u>Maura Hertz</u>   Patient Number: <u>02041981</u>
Date of Birth: mm/dd/yyyy   Dose #7

Physician Orders:
Premedicate with diphenhydramine 50 mg PO and acetaminophen 650 mg PO 30 minutes prior to initiation of infusion.

Infuse 300 mg infliximab intravenously over 2 hours. Monitor temperature, blood pressure, respirations, and pulse prior to initiating infusion and every 30 minutes until 1 hour after infusion. Adjust rate as necessary to control symptoms. For severe infusion reactions, stop infusion and follow anaphylaxis protocol.

Signature: *M. Fezziwig,* MD   Date: *00/00/0000*

ORDER REVIEW AND DOSING CALCULATIONS

Pharmacist Betty Bright reviews the orders for completeness and accuracy prior to initiating sterile compounding in the oncology pharmacy's LAFW. Betty notes that the dose is correct at 5 mg/kg when rounded to the nearest 50 mg, the clinic's protocol.

Patient weight (in kg): $\dfrac{138 \text{ lb}}{2.2 \text{ lb/kg}} = 62.7 \text{ kg}$

Dose = 5 mg/kg × 62.7 kg = 313.6 mg, rounded to 300 mg per clinic protocol.

Ingredient Amounts

Infliximab is available as a 100-mg vial for reconstitution with 10 mL of Sterile Water for Injection to give a concentration of 10 mg/mL.

Volume of reconstituted infliximab 10 mg/mL needed:

$$\frac{10 \text{ mg}}{1 \text{ mL}} = \frac{300 \text{ mg}}{x \text{ mL}}; \, x = 30 \text{ mL}$$

Volume of IV solution: Withdraw 30 mL from NSS 250-mL bag to compensate for addition of 30 mL of reconstituted infliximab injection.

Concentration of infliximab in IV solution: 300 mg/250 mL = 1.2 mg/mL

BEST HEALTHCARE ONCOLOGY PHARMACY
1100 EAST HEALTHCARE AVE., SUITE 240
POTOSI, WI 53820

COMPOUNDING RECORD   102607-24

Medications	Amt	Mfg	Lot #	Exp
Infliximab 100-mg vials	300 mg	Centocor	215456	mm/yy
Sterile Water for Inj USP	30 mL	Hospira	24551335	mm/yy
Sodium Chloride 0.9% bag	250 mL	Baxter	AB25415	mm/yy
Supplies				
Syringe, 30 mL	2	BD	45212z5	mm/yy
Needle 22-ga × 1″	3	BD	45552z4	mm/yy

Compounding Instructions: Use aseptic technique in all procedures for preparing this sterile preparation. Remove jewelry and wash hands and forearms with germicidal soap. Don foot covers, hair covers, a face mask, and a clean, low-shedding gown. Apply an alcohol-based hand cleaner, allow to dry, and put on sterile gloves. Wipe the surfaces of the LAFW with sterile 70% Isopropyl Alcohol using a lint-free cloth. Assemble the preparation materials needed. Using a separate sterile alcohol swab for each surface, disinfect all vial septa and injection port of NSS bag. Withdraw 30 mL from NSS bag and discard. Add 10 mL sterile water for injection to each of three 100-mg infliximab vials, directing stream to glass wall of the vial. Do not use vial if vacuum is not present. Gently swirl solution by rotating the vial to dissolve the powder. DO NOT SHAKE. Allow solution to stand for 5 minutes. Solution is clear and yellow and may have translucent protein particles. Draw up a total of 300 mg/30 mL from three infliximab vials and add slowly to NSS bag. Gently mix medication throughout solution.

Patient Name: Hertz, Maura
Prepared by: D. Gillis, CPT
Date: 00/00/00 1000

Ordering MD: Dr. M. Fezziwig
Checked by: B. Bright, RPh
Beyond-use date: 1300 00/00/00

f. It should be used cautiously in patients with a history of hyperlipidemia.

g. It must be used cautiously in preterm infants, because they have immature hepatic function and therefore have poor clearance of lipid that can accumulate in the lungs. This may be fatal.

h. Questions exist regarding immunosuppressant activity of lipid emulsion when it is given by bolus infusion (i.e., over less than 6 hr). This does not seem to be a problem when IV lipid is given slowly by continuous IV infusion over a 12- to 24-hour period. On the other hand, when IV lipid emulsion is administered as a separate infusion in addition to dextrose and amino acids, it should be infused over no longer than 12 hours; this time limit is recommended to prevent the growth of microorganisms that can be inadvertently introduced into the manufacturer's original container during IV administration.

4. In 2004, the USP announced the development of Chapter ⟨729⟩, Globule Size Distribution in Lipid Injectable Emulsions, a proposal to define specific globule size limits in order to promote standardization in the quality of lipid emulsions produced by commercial manufacturers (2).

a. Two methods are identified for analyzing the size and dispersion of lipid globules, a critical factor determining the safety of lipid emulsions.

b. One method uses light-scattering techniques to determine the mean droplet size (MDS); this technique is viewed as a manufacturing parameter (3).

c. The upper limit for MDS is 500 nm or 0.5 μm.

d. The second method uses the light obscuration or light extinction method to identify the amount of fat globules in the large-diameter tail of globule populations for lipid injectable emulsions; this technique is viewed as a stability parameter (3).

e. The upper limit for this population of fat globules is a volume-weighted percent of fat >5 μm or expressed as $PFAT_5 < 0.05\%$.

f. The intent of the $PFAT_5$ limit is to identify coarse dispersions of lipid injectable emulsions that may alter lipid clearance from blood circulation as well as unstable lipid emulsions that may ultimately deposit in the lungs and cause respiratory failure.

g. From a clinical standpoint, studies of compounded TNAs have demonstrated obvious phase separation or "cracking" of formulations with $PFAT_5 > 0.4\%$ (i.e., approximately tenfold higher than the upper limit) (4).

h. In general, final concentrations of amino acids must exceed 4%, dextrose concentrations must be $>10\%$, and lipid emulsion concentrations must be $>2\%$ in order to maintain TNA stability (3).

F. Total kilocalories-per-day requirement

1. The general requirement for total kilocalories per day is 25 to 35 kcal/kg ABW.

2. As with the amino acid requirement, the amount of kilocalories per kilogram of ABW will depend on the patient's stress level, disease state, and level of body injury. This is based on the theory that in certain diseases states, more calories are expended.

3. There is some controversy about increasing the level of kilocalories per kilogram of ABW based on the level of stress—for example, 25 kcal/kg in mild stress, 30 kcal/kg with moderate stress, and 35 kcal/kg in severe stress. As dextrose is the major source of calories, you may ask, "Would there be any problem with giving too much dextrose?" Remember from biochemistry:

$$4\ C_6H_{12}O_6 \text{ (excess dextrose)} + O_2 \rightarrow C_{16}H_{32}O_2 \text{ (lipid)} + 8\ CO_2 + 8\ H_2O$$

Too much dextrose can result in the following:

a. Lipid deposited in the liver with the result of liver dysfunction.

b. Excess carbon dioxide production with the result of respiratory distress, especially a problem with patients on a ventilator or with chronic obstructive pulmonary disease (COPD). If extra calories are needed for a patient with respiratory problems, IV lipid should be given directly to avoid excess carbon dioxide production.

c. Generally, these problems develop when dextrose administration exceeds 7 mg/kg/min.

G. Electrolytes, vitamins, and trace elements

1. **Sodium:** The parenteral recommended daily intake (RDI) is determined by clinical need; the approximate usual range is 1 to 2 mEq/kg ABW.

a. **Sodium** is principally an extracellular cation with no established RDI. Its inclusion in the TPN is based upon clinical need.

b. For example, patients with end-stage liver disease or congestive heart failure or those with iatrogenic fluid overload may require severe sodium restriction.

c. Conversely, patients with large nasogastric fluid losses, high ileostomy or pancreatic fistula outputs, or significant small-bowel losses often require substantial quantities of sodium per day.

2. **Potassium:** The parenteral RDI is determined by clinical need; the approximate usual range is 1 to 2 mEq/kg ABW.

FDA SAFETY ALERT:

Hazards of Precipitation Associated with Parenteral Nutrition

April 18, 1994

To: Hospital Pharmacists
Hospital Risk Managers
Hospital Nutritional Support Teams
Home Health Care Nutrition Support Services
Hospital Directors of Nursing
Home Care Pharmacists
Home Care Nurses
Physicians

This is to alert you of a concern that precipitate formation in total parenteral nutrition (TPN) admixtures may present a life-threatening hazard to your patients.

The Food and Drug Administration has received a report from one institution of 2 deaths and at least 2 cases of respiratory distress, which developed during peripheral infusion of a three-in-one (amino acids, carbohydrate and lipids) TPN admixture. The admixture contained 10% FreAmine III, dextrose, calcium gluconate, potassium phosphate, other minerals, and a lipid emulsion all of which were combined using an automated compounder. The solution may have contained a precipitate of calcium phosphate. Autopsies revealed diffuse microvascular pulmonary emboli containing calcium phosphate. One literature report cites an adult case of subacute interstitial pneumonitis associated with calcium phosphate precipitates.

TPN solutions are made according to a variety of formulations and compounding protocols. Thus, there are possibilities of calcium phosphate precipitates and many other chemical incompatibilities. Precipitates could develop because of a number of factors such as: the concentration, pH, and phosphate content of the amino acid solutions; the calcium and phosphorous additives: the order of mixing; the mixing process: or the compounder. The presence of a lipid emulsion in the TPN admixture would obscure the presence of any precipitate.

Because of the potential for life threatening events, caution should be taken to ensure that precipitates have not formed in any parenteral nutrition admixtures.

There is a medical need for the use of parenteral nutrition in some patients. Until data can be developed and validated to support specific recommendations for TPN preparation, the FDA suggests the following steps to decrease the risk of additional injuries:

1. The amounts of phosphorous and of calcium added to the admixture are critical. The solubility of the added calcium should be calculated from the volume at <u>the time the calcium is added.</u> It should not be based upon the final volume.

    Some amino acid injections for TPN admixtures contain phosphate ions (as a phosphoric acid buffer). These phosphate ions and <u>the volume at the time the phosphate is added</u> should be considered when calculating the concentration of phosphate additives. Also, when adding calcium and phosphate to an admixture, the phosphate should be added first.

    The line should be flushed between the addition of any potentially incompatible components.

2. A lipid emulsion in a three-in-one admixture obscures the presence of a precipitate. Therefore, if a lipid emulsion is needed either. (1) use a two-in-one admixture with the lipid infused separately. or (2) if a three-in-one admixture is medically necessary, then add the calcium before the lipid emulsion and according to the recommendations in number 1 above.

    If the amount of calcium or phosphate which must be added is likely to cause a precipitate, some or all of the calcium should be administered separately. Such separate infusions must be properly diluted and slowly infuse to avoid serious adverse events related to the calcium.

FIGURE 35.1. FDA SAFETY ALERT FROM THE DEPARTMENT OF HEALTH AND HUMAN SERVICES.

3. When using an automated compounding device, the above steps should be considered when programming the device. In addition, automated compounders should be maintained and operated according to the manufacturer's recommendations. Any printout should be checked against the programmed admixture and weight of components.

4. During the mixing process, pharmacists who mix parenteral nutrition admixtures should periodically agitate the admixture and check for precipitates. Medical or home care personnel who start and monitor these infusions should carefully inspect for the presence of precipitates both before and during the infusion. Patients and caregivers should be trained to visually inspect for signs of precipitation. They also should be advised to stop the infusion and seek medical assistance if precipitates are noted.

5. A filter should be used when infusing either central or peripheral nutrition admixtures. At this time, data has not been submitted to document which size filter is most effective in trapping precipitates.

   Standards of practice vary, but the following is suggested: a 1.2 micron air eliminating filter for lipid containing admixtures and a 0.22 micron air eliminating filter for nonlipid containing admixtures.

6. Parenteral nutrition admixtures should be administered within the following time frames: if stored at room temperature, the infusion should be started within 24 hours after mixing: if stored at refrigerated temperatures, the infusion should be started within 24 hours of rewarming. Because warming parenteral nutrition admixtures may contribute to the formation of precipitates, once administration begins, care should be taken to avoid excessive warming of the admixture.

   Persons administering home care parenteral nutrition admixtures may need to deviate from these time frames. Pharmacists who initially prepare these admixtures should check a reserve sample for precipitates over the duration and under the conditions of storage.

7. If symptoms of acute respiratory distress, pulmonary embolus, or interstitial pneumonitis develop, the infusion should be stopped immediately and thoroughly checked for precipitates. Appropriate medical intervention should be instituted. Home care personnel and patients should immediately seek medical assistance.

   These recommendations represent the best advice that the FDA can provide at this time. The FDA recognizes there may be alternative safety measures which could be taken to prevent the infusion of precipitates in TPN admixtures. The FDA has requested that industry develop and submit data that will be used to revise relevant labeling (instructions for use) to clarify these issues.

   Practitioners who become aware of similar or other drug or device related deaths, serious illnesses and/or serious injuries are asked to notify the FDA. Please submit your reports to MedWatch, Medical Product Reporting Program, by phone at 1-800-FDA-1088 (also call for MedWatch information); by FAX at 1-800-FDA-0178; by modem at 1-800-FDA-7737; or by mail to MedWatch. HF-2. Food and Drug Administration, 5600 Fishers Lane, Rockvill, MD 20857.

   The Safe Medical Devices Act of 1990 (SMDA) requires hospitals and other facilities to report death, serious illness and injury associated with the use of medical devices. You should follow the procedures established by your facility for such mandatory reporting. Practitioners who become aware of any medical device related adverse event or product problem/malfunction should report to their Medical Device User Facility Reporting person. If it is not reportable under the SMDA. It may be reported directly to MedWatch.

FIGURE 35.1. FDA SAFETY ALERT FROM THE DEPARTMENT OF HEALTH AND HUMAN SERVICES. (*continued*)

a. Potassium is principally an intracellular cation with no established RDI; thus, its inclusion in the TPN is dictated by clinical need.

b. Potassium requirements can be greatly influenced by acid–base status.
   (1) During metabolic acidosis, an excess of hydrogen ions is present in the circulation, and potassium exchanges its intracellular position for hydrogen ions in an attempt to abate the acidemia, thus causing hyperkalemia.
   (2) Conversely, hypokalemia results during metabolic alkalosis.

3. **Calcium:** Parenteral RDI is approximately 10 mEq or 200 mg Ca ion per day.
   a. Up to 98% of total body calcium is in bone and can be readily mobilized in times of need under the influence of parathyroid hormone.
   b. Certain patients, such as those with severe short-bowel syndrome and those requiring massive blood transfusions, may require substantially greater quantities of calcium. Such increases given in the TPN admixture should be accomplished gradually.
   c. Dosage increases of 5 mEq/day up to a total maximum of 20 mEq/day for acute care are reasonable, and simultaneous monitoring of serum phosphorus is recommended during such times.
4. **Magnesium:** Parenteral RDI is approximately 10 mEq or 120 mg Mg ion per day.
   a. Magnesium plasma concentration affects parathyroid hormone secretion, so this ion is closely linked to calcium metabolism.
   b. Patients with short-bowel syndrome, alcoholics, and the like often require larger doses to achieve magnesium homeostasis. As with calcium, the increased dose can be advanced incrementally by 5 mEq/day up to a total maximum of 40 mEq/day.
5. **Phosphorus:** Parenteral RDI is approximately 30 mmol or 1,000 mg P per day.
   a. The role of phosphorus in physiologic processes is diverse; it influences respiration, myocardial function, and platelet and red and white blood cell functions.
   b. In the presence of normal renal function, if phosphate is omitted from TPN formulations, a potentially life-threatening hypophosphatemia can be induced within a week of initiating the TPN therapy.
6. **Trace elements**
   a. The normal daily requirements for trace elements are contained in each 3 mL of MTE-5, which provides 12 mcg of chromium, 1.2 mg of copper, 0.3 mg of manganese, 60 mcg of selenium, and 3 mg of zinc.
   b. In certain conditions, additional selenium (for long-term home TPN) and zinc (for patients with high ileostomy or diarrheal outputs) may be necessary.

IV.   SPECIAL TOPICS

A. Peripheral parenteral nutrition (PPN)

1. PPN is given through a peripheral vein, usually in the arm.
2. Because of the risk of phlebitis, these solutions should have an osmolarity approximately half that of central TPN solutions.
   Approximate osmolarities (in mOsmol/L):

Plasma	300
0.9% NaCl	300
D5W	250
D10W	500
IV lipid emulsion	300
TPN	1,800
PPN	900

3. In essence, the electrolyte and IV lipid emulsion contents of a PPN solution are similar to those for a central TPN, but the amino acid content is cut by approximately half, and the dextrose concentration is greatly reduced.
4. Uses of PPN
   a. PPN may be used to support patients who are able to ingest only a portion of their caloric and protein requirements orally or enterally and when central-vein TPN is not feasible.
   b. PPN is traditionally a short-term therapy (fewer than 10 days), because it does not provide total caloric and protein requirements, and these hypertonic solutions are not well tolerated by peripheral veins for extended periods.
   c. PPN is not recommended for patients with severe undernutrition, increased electrolyte needs (especially potassium), fluid restriction, or the need for prolonged IV nutrition support.

B. Special amino acid solutions

1. Formulas and descriptions of various specialty amino acid solutions can be found in *Drug Facts and Comparisons*. There are special formulations for patients under stress, those with hepatic failure, and those with renal disease.

2. The use of these specialty products is somewhat controversial. They are usually more expensive than standard formulas, and some practitioners think they offer little significant clinical advantage. Additional information on this subject can be found in the journal article, "Value of specialty intravenous amino acid solutions," in the March 15, 1996, issue of the *American Journal of Health-System Pharmacy*.

3. Amino acid solutions for patients with **hepatic failure**

   a. These amino acid solutions contain higher levels of branched-chain amino acids (BCAAs), such as isoleucine, leucine, and valine, and lower levels of aromatic amino acids (tryptophan, phenylalanine) and methionine. An example product is HepatAmine.

   b. This formula modification resulted from an analysis of the plasma content of patients with encephalopathy, a clinical complication found in patients with liver failure. It was noted that in the plasma of these patients, the ratio of aromatic amino acids to BCAAs is elevated. It was thought that the increased levels of aromatic amino acids may be contributing to the development of liver encephalopathy.

   c. Current recommendations support the use of BCAA formulations only in chronic encephalopathy unresponsive to standard amino acid products and pharmacotherapy.

C. **Factors affecting the precipitation of calcium phosphate in TPN solutions**

Calcium and phosphate, two nutritional requirements for TPN solutions, are conditionally compatible. Precipitation depends on numerous factors as described here (see also references 5–11). The chemical equation given here should aid in understanding these factors.

$$HPO_4^{-2} + Ca^{+2} \rightleftharpoons H_2PO_4^{-1} + Ca^{+2}$$
$$\downarrow \qquad\qquad\qquad \downarrow$$
$$CaHPO_4 \downarrow \qquad\qquad Ca(H_2PO_4)_2$$
$$\text{very insoluble} \qquad\qquad \text{relatively soluble}$$

1. **pH of the solution:** The pH dependence of the phosphate–calcium precipitation is illustrated in the preceding equation. Dibasic calcium phosphate ($CaHPO_4$) is very insoluble, whereas monobasic calcium phosphate ($Ca[H_2PO_4]_2$) is relatively soluble. At low pH, the soluble monobasic form ($H_2PO_4^{-1}$) predominates but, as the pH increases, more dibasic phosphate (HPO_4^{-2}) becomes available to bind with calcium and precipitate. Therefore, the lower the pH of the parenteral solution, the more calcium and phosphate that can be solubilized.

2. **Concentration of the calcium:** Because it is the free calcium that can form insoluble precipitates, enhanced precipitate formation is expected as the concentration of calcium is increased.

3. **Salt form of the calcium:** Although calcium gluconate is much more soluble than calcium chloride, calcium chloride has a much higher percent dissociation. The higher the dissociation, the more free calcium is available. The concentration of calcium available for precipitation when added as the gluconate salt is less than that available when an equimolar amount of calcium is added as the chloride salt. Calcium gluceptate has no real advantage over the gluconate salt form.

4. **Concentration of the phosphate:** As can be seen in the previous equations, it is the dibasic calcium phosphate salt that is insoluble. The concentration of dibasic phosphate in solution depends on both the total phosphate concentration and the pH of the solution. Potassium Phosphate Injection has a high pH (6.2 to 6.8) relative to that of dextrose or amino acid solutions. Addition of Potassium Phosphate Injection to a TPN solution not only increases the concentration of the phosphate but also may increase the pH of the solution and that favors precipitation.

5. **Concentration of amino acids:** Amino acids form soluble complexes with calcium and phosphate, reducing the amount of the free calcium and phosphate available for precipitation. Amino acids also appear to provide an intrinsic buffering system to a TPN solution. Amino acid formulations have pHs in the range of 4.5 to 6.5. Those containing higher concentrations of amino acids show less of an increase in pH when phosphate is added and, consequently, an increased tolerance for calcium addition.

6. **Composition of amino acid solutions:** Amino acid solutions formulated with electrolytes contain calcium and phosphate, and these must be considered in any projection of compatibility. Some amino acids contain cysteine hydrochloride, which may affect the solubility of calcium and phosphate. Cysteine hydrochloride lowers the pH of the solution, enabling the more soluble monobasic form of phosphate to exist. Therefore, adding cysteine hydrochloride can increase the solubility of calcium and phosphate in a TPN solution.

7. **Concentration of dextrose in the solution:** Dextrose also forms a soluble complex with calcium and phosphate. It can also act as a weak buffer. The pH of dextrose solutions is relatively low (4 to 5) owing to the presence of free sugar acids (e.g., gluconic acid) present and formed from the oxidation of the aldehyde moiety on dextrose during sterilization and storage of dextrose solutions. Studies have shown that higher concentrations of dextrose reduce the free calcium and phosphate that can form insoluble precipitates.

8. **Temperature of the solution:** Temperature of solution also plays a key role. As temperature is increased, the calcium salts (chloride or gluconate) are dissociated more completely and more calcium ions become available for precipitation. Therefore, an increase in temperature increases the amount or possibility of precipitation. Care must be exercised when transferring these solutions to warmer environments such as neonate nurseries and cribs.

9. **Presence of other additives:** The addition of other drugs to a TPN solution may alter the pH of the solution. Additives may also introduce the possibility of precipitation of other products or incompatibilities with other ions.

10. **Order of mixing:** The FDA recommends that phosphate should be the first electrolyte added to the TNA admixture and that calcium should be the last additive.

D. **Vitamins**

1. In April 2001, the FDA amended requirements for marketing of an "effective" adult parenteral multivitamin formulation and recommended changes to the 12-vitamin formulation that had been available for more than 20 years.

2. The new requirements for increased dosages of vitamins B_1, B_6, C, and folic acid as well as addition of vitamin K (creating a 13-vitamin formulation) are based on the recommendations from a 1985 workshop sponsored jointly by the American Medical Association's (AMA) Division of Personal and Public Health Policy and the FDA's Division of Metabolic and Endocrine Drug Products.

3. Specific modifications of the previous formulation include increasing the provision of ascorbic acid (vitamin C) from 100 mg/day to 200 mg/day, pyridoxine (vitamin B_6) from 4 mg/day to 6 mg/day, thiamine (vitamin B_1) from 3 mg/day to 6 mg/day, and folic acid from 400 mcg/day to 600 mcg/day, and adding phylloquinone (vitamin K) 150 mcg/day.

4. When using the 12-vitamin formulation, vitamin K can be given individually as a daily dose (0.5 to 1 mg/day) or a weekly dose (5 to 10 mg one time per week). Patients who are to receive warfarin for anticoagulation should be monitored more closely when receiving vitamin K to ensure the appropriate level of anticoagulation is maintained.

5. Multivitamins may come in several different forms. They may be packaged as a lyophilized powder intended for reconstitution and dilution in a TPN. They may also be manufactured in two separate vials or in special mix-o-vial units that have two chambers separated by a rubber stopper that can be pushed down when the solutions are to be mixed.

   a. These special formulations are necessary because of the limited compatibility and stability of several vitamins when combined.

   b. The multivitamin solutions are mixed together and added to the TPN just before use. Often if the TPN is made at a site that is remote from the care site (e.g., home health care, nursing home), the vitamin unit is sent with the TPN solution and is mixed and added just before the TPN solution is hung.

   c. The limited stability of the combined multivitamins should be considered in assigning a beyond-use date to a TPN solution that contains multivitamins.

E. **Trace elements**

1. Trace Elements are added to the TPN solution once each day. Trace elements are commercially available as single- or multiple-entity products and in both pediatric and adult formulations.

2. Standard trace element solutions contain Se, Cr, Cu, Mn, and Zn. There are various other trace element solutions that contain iodine or molybdenum, alone or in combination, added to the standard trace elements.

3. Patients who have sustained small-bowel or large-bowel fluid losses should receive supplemental zinc (5 to 10 mg/day) added separately in addition to the amount in the trace element cocktail (3 to 5 mg/day).

4. Patients who have hepatic cholestasis should have copper and manganese withheld from the TPN solution, because these trace elements are excreted in the bile. Neurologic damage from deposition of manganese in the basal ganglia has been reported in parenteral nutrition patients with chronic liver disease or cholestasis.

F. **Other additives:** Other components commonly added to TPN solutions include insulin, heparin, hydrocortisone, and histamine H_2-receptor antagonists.

G. **Aluminum contamination**

1. In 1990, the FDA published a proposal to regulate the aluminum content of parenteral solutions.

2. It was not until 10 years later that a final rule was published with a proposed effective date in 2001.

3. Due to manufacturer difficulties in achieving compliance with the regulation, the final effective date set for implementation was July 2004.

4. The FDA mandates that parenteral aluminum exposure be limited to less than 5 mcg/kg/day.

5. Large-volume parenteral solutions are required to contain less than 25 mcg/L aluminum.

6. Small-volume parenteral solutions are required to be labeled with the maximum aluminum content at expiration.

7. With regards to parenteral nutrition, products that are known to be lower in aluminum should be utilized, including substitution of sodium phosphate for potassium phosphate.

8. Patient safety should be the first and foremost concern when considering substitutions for products with higher aluminum concentration. Thus, owing to risk of precipitation between calcium and phosphorus, calcium gluconate should be used preferentially over calcium chloride, despite its higher aluminum content.

H. **Automated compounding devices**

1. Due to the complex nature of parenteral nutrition formulations, the majority of compounding pharmacies in the United States use automated compounding devices (ACD) for the parenteral nutrition preparation.

2. Each ACD has its own internal standards for ensuring the accuracy and precision of the compounding process.

3. Refer to section IX in Chapter 32 for a more in-depth discussion of the quality control methods used for ACDs.

I. **Monitoring**

1. For an excellent review article on parenteral nutrition monitoring, see "Parenteral nutrition monitoring in hospitalized patients" (12).

2. Monitoring parameters (See Table 35.1 for a sample TPN monitoring sheet.)

   a. **Temperature:** daily to detect infection or sepsis.

   b. **Weight:** daily to monitor fluid imbalance and maintenance and improvement of clinical condition. Generally, patients should gain only 1 to 2 lb per week. Larger weight gains are usually retained fluid or lipid from too many calories; a sudden weight gain usually reflects fluid retention.

   c. **Nitrogen balance (NB):** Nitrogen balance monitors nitrogen utilization to determine whether the patient's metabolic status is anabolic (buildup) or catabolic (breakdown). It is defined as the difference between the nitrogen intake and nitrogen excretion.

$$NB = NI - NO$$

NI is the nitrogen put into the body by TPN and other nutritional sources. NO is the nitrogen excreted by all routes. You may see two different, but equivalent, forms of this basic equation in the literature:

$$NB = NI_{(g/24\ hr)} - (UUN_{(g/24\ hr)} + 4\ g)$$

or

$$NB = Protein_{(g/24\ hr)}/6.25 - (UUN_{(g/24\ hr)} + 4\ g)$$

NI is obtained by calculating the number of grams of protein infused in the form of amino acids and multiplying that by 16% (the approximate amount of nitrogen in amino acids). Note that you get the same number by dividing the number of grams of protein or amino acids given by 6.25. The grams of nitrogen can also be determined from the specifications for the particular amino acid solutions being used. This information can be found in the product package insert or the product description in *Drug Facts and Comparisons.*

Urine urea nitrogen (UUN) is a standard lab test. Urea is the breakdown product of protein. Four grams of nitrogen is the estimated average loss by other routes, such as through the skin or in feces.

Table 35.1	TPN MONITORING SHEET

Patient Name: _____ Location: _____ Medical Records #: _____

ABW: _____ IBW: _____ Height: _____ Age: _____

Est. kcal Req./Day _____

Problems & Comments: _____

Freqency		Date	Date	Date	Date	Date	Date	Date	Date	Date
D	WEIGHT (KG)									
D	INPUT (ML/DAY)									
D	OUTPUT (ML/DAY)									
D	TPN INF (ML/DAY)									
D	LIPID INF (ML/DAY)									
D	KCAL (ENTERAL)									
D	TOTAL KCAL									
D	TOTAL PROTEIN (G)									
B	WBC (3.5–10.0)									
W	HCT (40–50)									
	% SEGS									
	% BANDS									
W	PLATELETS (140–380)									
B	PT/PTT (10–13/23–36)									
W	SODIUM (135–144)									
W	POTASSIUM (3.6–4.8)									
W	CHLORIDE (99–108)									
W	CO2 CONTENT (24–33)									
W	GLUCOSE (70–110)									
B	UREA NITROGEN (7–20)									
B	CREATININE (.6–1.3)									
B	CALCIUM (8.8–10.4)									
B	PHOSPHORUS (2.6–4.4)									
B	URIC ACID (4.0–8.0)									
W	CHOLESTEROL (160–310)									
W	TOTAL PROTEIN (6.3–8.0)									
W	ALBUMIN (3.9–5.1)									
W	TOTAL BILI (0–1.4)									
W	GG-TRANSPEP (0–65)									
W	ALKPHOS (35–130)									
W	GO-TRANSAM (0–50)									
W	LDH (90–200)									
W	TRIGLY (<200)									
B	MAGNESIUM (1.7–2.3)									
	Miscellaneous									

Frequency Key: W = weekly   φ No labs drawn   Parameters are the minimum required

D = daily   —Values (current rate) may be obtained more often

B = biweekly

| Example 35.1 | 1. | JS is a patient receiving a TPN solution that provides 102 g Protein per 24 hours. What is his $NI_{(g/24\ hr)}$? |

$$16\% \times 102 \text{ g Protein} = 16.3 \text{ g N}$$

or

$$102 \text{ g Protein}/6.25 = 16.3 \text{ g N}$$

2. The 24-hour UUN reported by the lab is 9.5 g/24 hr.
3. Calculate the NB for this patient:

$$NB = 16.3 - (9.5 + 4) = 2.8 \text{ g}$$

What is an acceptable value for NB? Although this depends on the clinical situation, a positive 4 to 6 g/day in unstressed patients is considered acceptable (13). If the NB is too low or is negative, the TPN formula can be changed to increase the amino acid content.

   d. **Plasma proteins:** Concentrations of serum plasma proteins can be used as a measure of nutritional status, because an increase in these reflects protein anabolism.

     (1) Serum albumin is the most commonly determined plasma protein, but its usefulness in monitoring nutritional status is limited because of its long half-life, because the body pool of albumin is large, and because its level in the serum is affected by so many other factors (12).

     (2) Two other plasma proteins, transferrin and prealbumin, have been found to be useful indicators (12).

   e. **Lab tests**

     (1) Table 35.1 shows a sample TPN monitoring sheet, including lab tests with a typical frequency of determination. The lab tests that are performed and their frequency and normal values vary with the hospital and the clinical condition of the patient. Notice that there are hematologic tests, electrolyte and glucose concentrations, lipid–cholesterol monitoring tests, and liver and renal function tests. For more detailed information on lab tests, see the article on monitoring TPN therapy (12).

     (2) It is important to realize that acceptable values for some lab tests may be different for patients on TPN than for normal healthy individuals. For example, acceptable blood glucose concentrations are much higher for patients receiving TPN.

     (3) Monitoring of lab values with adjustments of TPN formulas and therapy is becoming a focal point of pharmacist input and participation on the health care team.

   f. Clinical status: How is the patient doing? This is a very important monitoring parameter. A desired clinical outcome of therapy should be determined, and all efforts in TPN therapy should be geared toward this end.

Sample TPN Order

GD (Medical Record #200440, Room TLC-480) is a 52-year-old, 176-lb man who is 6′1″ tall. He is admitted to the trauma unit after an automobile accident. He is not expected to eat or take tube feedings for more than 7 days owing to multiple injuries to his small bowel. His physician, Dr. Solier, has written the following TPN order:

The prescribed 24-hour TPN is to contain:

Amino Acids	120 g
Dextrose	346 g
Lipid	55 g
Sodium Chloride	110 mEq

Potassium Acetate	80 mEq
Sodium Phosphate	30 mmol
Magnesium Sulfate	24 mEq
Calcium Gluconate	10 mEq
Ranitidine	150 mg
Multivitamins	10 mL
Multiple Trace Elements	3 mL

The flow rate for this TPN is 100 mL/hr.

1. Calculate GD's IBW and determine whether the TPN requirements should be based on GD's ABW or an adjusted body weight.
2. Determine whether all the nutrients, electrolytes, and fluid volume are within the normal range for GD. You may ignore the electrolyte contributions in the amino acid solution and in the IV lipid emulsion. See the text information in this chapter and Table 35.2, the TPN Requirement Worksheet, for the 24-hour requirements for electrolytes, trace elements, and vitamins. Sample calculations are given later, with the results in Table 35.2.
3. This pharmacy will dispense a 24-hour TPN in one IV bag. Calculate the volume in milliliters of each component for each 24-hour bag of this TPN solution. You have the following supplies:

   - Crystalline amino acid solution as Travasol 10%
   - Dextrose solution as Dextrose 70% in Water
   - IV Lipid as IV Lipid Emulsion 20%
   - Sterile Water for Injection
   - Various electrolytes and other additives, the concentrations of which are given in Figure 35.2, the Total Parental Nutrition Formula Record.

Sample calculations are given here, and the results are recorded in Table 35.2, the TPN Requirement worksheet.

Table 35.2	**TPN REQUIREMENT WORKSHEET**

Patient Name: GD   Age: 52

Height: 6'1"   Weight (ABW): 176 lb, 80 kg   IBW: 80 kg

AVERAGE 24-HOUR ADULT REQUIREMENTS FOR TPN COMPONENTS

COMPONENT	REQUIREMENT	AMOUNT ORDERED	EVALUATION
Fluid	30–35 mL/kg	30 mL/kg	OK
Protein (AA)	0.8–2.0 g AA/kg ABW	1.5 g AA/kg ABW	OK
Dextrose	3–5 mg/kg/min	3 mg/kg/min	OK
IV lipid	≤≤ 30% of total kcal	23%	OK
kcal/kg ABW	25–35 kcal/kg ABW	26.9 kcal/kg ABW	OK
Sodium	1–2 mEq/kg ABW	1.9 mEq/kg	OK
Potassium	1–2 mEq/kg ABW	1 mEq/kg	OK
Phosphate	20–40 mmol	30 mmol	OK
Magnesium	8–20 mEq	24 mEq	OK
Calcium	10–15 mEq	10 mEq	OK
Trace elements	3 mL	3 mL	OK
Vitamins	10 mL unit	10-mL unit	OK

AA, amino acids; ABW, actual body weight.

```
Patient Name: GD                          Location: TLC-480 Medical Record #200440
Dosing Weight: 80 kg                      Administration Date/Time: 00/01/00 @ 1,600
Expiration Date/Time: 00/02/00 @ 1,600    Bag ID #: 001
Infusion Volume Ordered: 2,400 mL         Infusion Rate: 100 mL/hr
```

Base Components	Concentration	Dose Ordered	Volume (mL)
Protein	Travasol 10%	120 g	1,200
Dextrose	D70W	346	494
Lipid Emulsion	20%	55	275

Additives	Concentration	Dose Ordered	Volume (mL)
Sodium Phosphate	3 mmol P/mL 4 mEq Na/mL	30 mEq	10
Sodium Chloride	4 mEq/mL	110 mEq	27.5
Potassium Acetate	2 mEq/mL	80 mEq	40
Magnesium Sulfate	4 mEq/mL	24 mEq	6
Calcium Gluconate	0.45 mEq/mL	10 mEq	22.2
Adult Multivitamins	—	10 mL	10
Trace Elements	—	3 mL	3
Ranitidine	25 mg/mL	150 mg	6

Additives per ion:

Na	150 mEq
K	80 mEq
Mg	24 mEq
Ca	10 mEq
Ac	80 mEq
Cl	110 mEq
P	30 mmol

FIGURE 35.2. TOTAL PARENTERAL NUTRITION FORMULA RECORD.

SAMPLE CALCULATIONS FOR 24-HOUR REQUIREMENTS FOR GD

1. **Body weight**
   a. Weight in pounds (given): 176 lb
   b. Actual weight in kilograms:

$$\frac{176\ lb}{2.2\ lb/kg} = 80\ kg$$

   c. IBW in kilograms: IBW = 50 kg + 2.3 (13″) = 79.9 kg
   GD's current ABW is appropriate for his height; no adjustment is needed.
2. **Fluid**
   a. Volume ordered per day:

$$100\ mL/hr \times 24\ hr/day = 2400\ mL$$

   b. Fluid requirements: 30 to 35 mL/kg/day

$$2,400\ mL/80\ kg = 30\ mL/kg—Okay$$

3. **Protein (amino acids)**
   a. Grams of protein ordered per day: 120 g amino acids (AA)
   b. Protein (AA) requirement: 0.8 to 2.0 g/kg ABW

$$120\ g\ AA/80\ kg\ ABW = 1.5\ g\ AA/kg\ ABW—Okay$$

   c. Kilocalories per day from ordered protein:

$$120 \text{ g AA/day} \times 4 \text{ kcal/g AA} = 480 \text{ kcal/day}$$

4. **Dextrose**
   a. Grams of dextrose ordered per day: 346 g
   b. General dextrose requirements: 3 to 5 mg/kg/min

$$\left(\frac{1,000 \text{ mg}}{\text{g}}\right)\left(\frac{346 \text{ g Dextrose}}{\text{day}}\right)\left(\frac{\text{day}}{1,440 \text{ min}}\right)\left(\frac{}{80 \text{ kg}}\right)$$

$$= 3 \text{ mg/kg/min} \text{ — Okay}$$

   c. Kilocalories per day from ordered dextrose:

$$346 \text{ g dextrose/day} \times 3.4 \text{ kcal/g dextrose} = 1,176 \text{ kcal/day}$$

5. **IV lipid emulsion**
   a. Grams of lipid ordered per day: 55 g
   b. General requirements for IV lipid: no greater than 30% of total kilocalories per day
   c. Kilocalories per day from ordered lipid:

$$55 \text{ g lipid/day} \times 9 \text{ kcal/g lipid} = 495 \text{ kcal/day}$$

   d. Total ordered kilocalories per day:

$$480 \text{ (AA)} + 1,176 \text{ (dextrose)} + 495 \text{ (lipid)} = 2,151 \text{ kcal/day}$$

   e. Percent of total kilocalories as IV lipid:

$$495 \text{ kcal}/2,151 \text{ kcal} = 23\% \text{ of total kcal as IV lipid—Okay}$$

6. Total kilocalories per kilogram ABW per day
   a. General requirements for total kilocalories per day: 25 to 35 kcal/kg ABW
   b. Total ordered kilocalories per kilogram ABW per day:

$$2,151 \text{ kcal}/ 80 \text{ kg ABW} = 26.9 \text{ kcal/kg/day—Okay}$$

7. **Electrolytes**
   a. Phosphorus: The parenteral RDI of ~30 mmol is sufficient for most TPN patients.

$$30 \text{ mmol is ordered—Okay}$$

   b. Sodium: Generally, most patients require 1 to 2 mEq/kg/day in the TPN.
The Sodium (Na) comes from two sources, the Sodium Chloride (110 mEq) and the Sodium Phosphate (NaP). The Na concentration of the NaP solution is 4 mEq/mL. The volume of NaP to be added to the TPN is based on the desired amount of phosphate, 30 mmol. The volume for this is 10 mL. Therefore the Na content from the NaP is calculated to be:

$$4 \text{ mEq/mL} \times 10 \text{ mL} = 40 \text{ mEq Na}$$

The total Na in the 24-hour TPN is calculated to be:

$$110 \text{ mEq (from the NaCl)} + 40 \text{ mEq (from the NaP)} = 150 \text{ mEq Na}$$

The amount of Na based on milliequivalents per kilogram per day is calculated to be:

$$150 \text{ mEq}/80 \text{ kg ABW} = 1.88 \text{ mEq/kg—Okay}$$

   c. Potassium: Generally most patients require 1 to 2 mEq/kg/day in the TPN.

$$80 \text{ mEq is ordered}$$
$$80 \text{ mEq}/80 \text{ kg ABW} = 1 \text{ mEq/kg—Okay}$$

   d. Calcium: The parenteral RDI of ~10 mEq/day is sufficient for most TPN patients. The range is 10 to 20 mEq/day.

$$10 \text{ mEq is ordered—Okay}$$

   e. Magnesium: The parenteral RDI of ~10 mEq/day is sufficient for most TPN patients. The range is 8 to 40 mEq/day.

$$24 \text{ mEq is ordered—This is within the acceptable range.}$$

SAMPLE CALCULATIONS FOR IV ADDITIVES FOR EACH 24-HOUR SUPPLY OF TPN

See Figure 35.2 for concentrations of ingredients.

1. **Amino acids**
   From Travasol 10%

$$\frac{10 \text{ g AA}}{100 \text{ mL Travasol}} = \frac{120 \text{ g AA}}{x \text{ mL Travasol}}; x = 1{,}200 \text{ mL Travasol}$$

2. **Dextrose**
   From Dextrose 70% (D70W):

$$\frac{70 \text{ g Dextrose}}{100 \text{ mL D70W}} = \frac{346 \text{ g Dextrose}}{x \text{ mL D70W}}; x = 494 \text{ mL D70W}$$

3. **IV lipid emulsion**
   From IV Lipid Emulsion 20%

$$\frac{20 \text{ g Fat}}{100 \text{ mL IV Fat Emulsion}} = \frac{55 \text{ g Fat}}{x \text{ mL IV Fat Emulsion}}; x$$
$$= 275 \text{ mL IV Fat Emulsion}$$

4. **Sodium phosphate**
   From Sodium Phosphate (NaP) 3 mmol P/mL:

$$\frac{3 \text{ mmol P}}{\text{mL NaP}} = \frac{30 \text{ mmol P}}{x \text{ mL NaP}}; x = 10 \text{ mL NaP}$$

5. **Potassium acetate**
   From Potassium Acetate (KAc) 2 mEq K/mL:

$$\frac{2 \text{ mEq K}^+}{\text{mL KAc}} = \frac{80 \text{ mEq K}^+}{x \text{ mL KAc}}; x = 40 \text{ mL KAc}$$

6. **Sodium chloride**
   From Sodium Chloride (NaCl) 4 mEq/mL:

$$\frac{4 \text{ mEq Na}^+}{\text{mL NaCl}} = \frac{110 \text{ mEq Na}^+}{\text{mL NaCl}}; x = 27.5 \text{ mL NaCl}$$

7. **Magnesium sulfate**
   From Magnesium Sulfate (MgSO$_4$) 4 mEq/mL:

$$\frac{4 \text{ mEq Mg}^{+2}}{\text{mL MgSO}_4} = \frac{24 \text{ mEq Mg}^{+2}}{x \text{ mL MgSO}_4}; x = 6 \text{ mL MgSO}_4$$

8. **Calcium gluconate**
   From Calcium Gluconate (CaGluc) 0.45 mEq/mL:

$$\frac{0.45 \text{ mEq Ca}^{+2}}{\text{mL CaGluc}} = \frac{10 \text{ mEq Ca}^{+2}}{x \text{ mL CaGluc}}; x = 22.2 \text{ mL CaGluc}$$

Note: See Figure 35.1 for safety alert.

9. **Trace elements**
   From MTE-5: 3 mL
10. **Multivitamins**
    From Infuvite: 10 mL
11. **Ranitidine**
    From Ranitidine Injection 25 mg/mL:

$$\frac{25 \text{ mg Ranitidine}}{\text{mL}} = \frac{150 \text{ mg Ranitidine}}{x \text{ mL}}; x = 6 \text{ mL}$$

12. Sterile Water for Injection

A total 24-hour fluid volume of 2,400 mL is needed to give the TPN at a rate of 100 mL/hr. Therefore, the volumes of all additives are added and the sum is subtracted from 2,400 mL to determine the amount of Sterile Water for Injection to add for the desired final volume of 2,400 mL.

The volumes of each additive were just calculated (see earlier) and are shown in the last column of Figure 35.2. The sum of these values is 2,093.7 mL ≈ 2,094 mL. Therefore, the volume of Sterile Water for Injection to add is 306 mL:

$$2,400 \text{ mL} - 2,094 \text{ mL} = 306 \text{ mL}$$

REFERENCES

1. McMahon MM, Farnell MB, Murray JM. Nutritional support of critically ill patients. Mayo Clin Proc 1993; 68: 911–920.
2. The United States Pharmacopeial Convention, Inc. Chapter ⟨729⟩. 2008 USP 31/NF 26. Rockville, MD: Author, 2007; 285–287.
3. Driscoll DF. Lipid injectable emulsions: 2006. Nutr Clin Pract 2006; 21: 381–386.
4. Driscoll DF, Bhargava HN, Zaim RH, et al. Physicochemical stability of total nutrient admixtures. Am J Health-Syst Pharm 1995; 52: 623–634.
5. Schuetz DH, King JC. Compatibility and stability of electrolytes, vitamins and antibiotics in combination with 8% amino acids solution. Am J Hosp Pharm 1978; 35: 33–44.
6. Henry RS, Jurgens RW, Sturgeon R, et al. Compatibility of calcium chloride and calcium gluconate with sodium phosphate in a mixed TPN solution. Am J Hosp Pharm 1980; 37: 673–674.
7. Eggert LD, Rusho WJ, MacKay MW, et al. Calcium and phosphorus compatibility in parenteral nutrition solutions for neonates. Am J Hosp Pharm 1982; 39: 49–53.
8. Fitzgerald KA, MacKay MW. Calcium and phosphate solubility in neonatal parenteral nutrition solutions containing Aminosyn PF. Am J Hosp Pharm 1987; 44: 1396–1400.
9. Mikrut BA. Calcium and phosphate solubility in neonatal parenteral nutrient solutions containing Aminosyn PF or Trophamine. Am J Hosp Pharm 1987; 44: 2702–2704.
10. Lenz GT, Mikrut BA. Calcium and phosphate solubility in neonatal parenteral nutrient solutions containing Aminosyn PF or Trophamine. Am J Hosp Pharm 1988; 45: 2367–2371.
11. Trissel LA, ed. Calcium and phosphate compatibility in parenteral nutrition. Houston: TriPharma Communications, 2001.
12. Manzo CB, Dickerson RN. Parenteral nutrition monitoring in hospitalized patients. Hosp Pharm 1993; 28: 561–568.
13. Dickerson RN. Using nitrogen balance in clinical practice. Hosp Pharm 2005; 40: 1081–1085.

Part 7

Veterinary Pharmacy

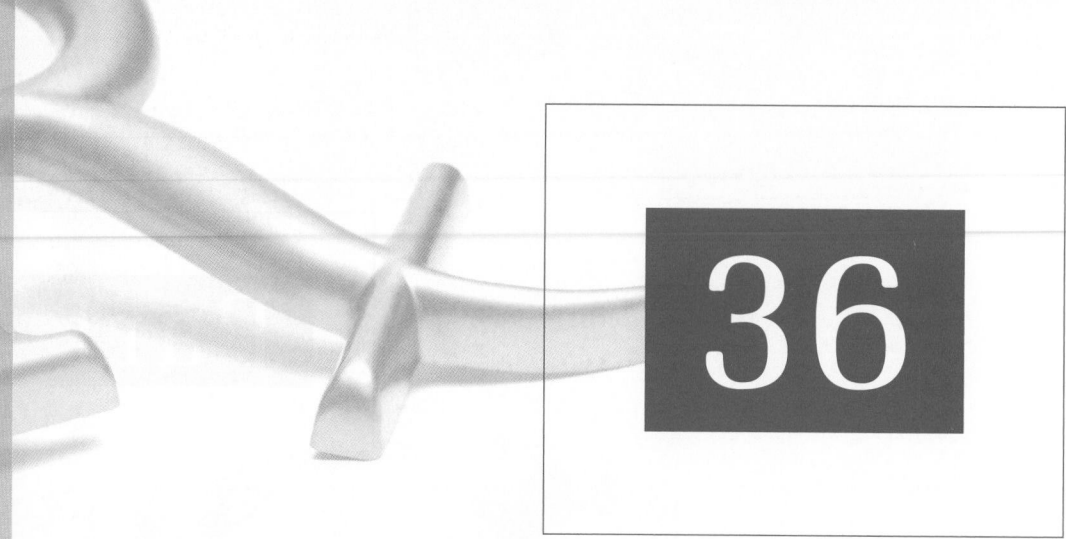

36

Veterinary Pharmacy Practice

Gigi Davidson, RPh, DICVP

I. INTRODUCTION

A pharmacist's responsibility for providing patients with high-quality pharmaceutical care extends beyond the human species. While colleges of pharmacy and licensing boards have focused almost exclusively on human pharmacotherapy, society expects an equally competent quality of pharmaceutical care and products to be provided for nonhuman family members. It behooves all pharmacists to be equipped with a working knowledge of veterinary pharmacotherapy and to develop a clinically and legally sound algorithm for processing veterinary prescriptions. True mastery of veterinary pharmacotherapy is a lifelong learning process, but all pharmacists can acquire a functional understanding of providing drugs and care for animal patients by considering the information outlined in this chapter.

II. INFORMATION RESOURCES

Many veterinary-specific information resources are not presented during undergraduate pharmacy education. Some of the most useful resources are listed here.

A. Texts
  1. **Veterinary Drug Information Monographs:** These monographs have been carefully prepared and approved by USP Committees of Experts for Veterinary Drugs, Veterinary Information and Pharmacy Compounding. All information presented is evidence-based and peer-reviewed.

    a. Information monographs: Similar to the former *USP-Dispensing Information* monographs for human patients, these monographs include useful information such as indications, extra-label use, species and dosage forms, dosing, label and extra-label withdrawal times, and relevant human data. Unfortunately, they are no longer included in printed copies of *USP/NF* but are available free of charge at the following URL: http://www.usp.org/audiences/veterinary/monographs/main.html.

    b. Substance monographs (e.g., Cisapride monohydrate)

    c. Compounding formulation monographs (e.g., Sodium Bromide Injection)

2. USP Pharmacists' Pharmacopoeia, beginning with 2nd edition, 2008 (1)

    a. Veterinary drug monographs (information, substance, formulation)

    b. Veterinary pharmacopeial stimuli articles

    c. Veterinary drug regulations

        (1) The Animal Medicinal Drug Use Clarification Act

        (2) Extra-label use of drugs in food-producing animals

    d. FDA Form 1932A for reporting adverse drug reactions, lack of efficacy or product defects, http://www.fda.gov/opacom/morechoices/fdaforms/FDA-1932a.pdf

    e. Important veterinary contacts

    f. List of potential food/drug/excipient toxins in animal species

3. Plumb's Veterinary Drug Handbook, by Donald Plumb (2): AHFS-style comprehensive, referenced drug monographs and important veterinary reference information, companion veterinary patient education information literature (*Veterinary Drug Handbook: Client Information Edition*)

4. Saunders Handbook of Veterinary Drugs, by Mark Papich (3): condensed drug monographs with phonetic guide and accompanying patient educational information

5. Veterinary Herbal Medicine, by Susan Wynn (4): comprehensive description of herbal and alternative medicines used in animal patients

6. Veterinary Pharmacology and Therapeutics, by Mark Papich and Jim Riviere (5): comprehensive veterinary pharmacology text for all species

7. Small Animal Clinical Pharmacology and Therapeutics, by Dawn Merton Boothe (6): comprehensive, illustrated veterinary pharmacology text for dogs and cats

B. Free-access Internet sites

1. Food and Drug Administration Center for Veterinary Medicine, www.fda.gov/cvm

    a. *FDA Veterinarian,* News and events in veterinary medicine: published bimonthly. Articles are free of copyright and may be reprinted. Editor Jon F. Scheid. Comments are invited: Phone 240-276-9110, fax 240-276-9115, or write to *FDA Veterinarian,* Center for Veterinary Medicine, Communications Staff (HFV-12), 7519 Standish Place, Rockville, MD 20855.

        (1) Scientific news

        (2) New drug approvals

        (3) Drug approval withdrawals

    b. *Compliance Policy Guides* (CPGs) for drug use in animals, http://www.fda.gov/ora/compliance_ref/cpg/cpgvet/default.htm: CPGs are printed guidance documents in an organized system for statements of FDA compliance policy, including those statements that contain regulatory action guidance information. These guides are internal guidance documents to assist FDA field inspectors during inspections. These CPGs do not create or confer any rights, privileges, or benefits on or for any private person but are intended for internal guidance.

    c. Adverse Drug Event Reporting for animals, http://www.fda.gov/cvm/adereporting.htm: Veterinarians and animal owners may report adverse experiences with animal drugs, feeds, and devices to the FDA by completing the information listed at the link provided (FDA Form 1932A).

    d. *Green Book* (FDA-approved veterinary drugs), http://www.fda.gov/cvm/Green_Book/elecgbook.html: The *Green Book* is a byproduct of The Generic Animal Drug and Patent Restoration Act (GADPTRA) enacted in 1988. The *Green Book* serves to fulfill the portion of the GADPTRA requiring that a list of all animal drug products approved for safety and effectiveness be made available to the public. The *Green Book* is updated in January of each calendar year. Pharmacists should consult the *Green Book* to determine approval status and availability of drug products used in animals.

    e. Freedom of Information Summaries (FOIS) for Veterinary Approved Drugs, http://www.fda.gov/cvm/FOI/foidocs.htm: A Freedom of Information (FOI) Summary summarizes the safety and effectiveness information submitted by the drug manufacturer to support the approval of a new animal drug. FOIS summarize the indications for use, dosage form, route of administration, and the recommended dosage. Pivotal and supplementary studies supporting safety and effectiveness of the drug in the target animal as well as human food safety are also presented in the FOIS.

f. Information for Consumers, http://www.fda.gov/cvm/consumer.html: These PDF brochures are intended to answer frequently asked questions regarding use of veterinary drugs, devices, and feeds. This page was used recently to answer questions from consumers who were concerned about melamine-contaminated batches of pet food.

g. Good Manufacturing Practices: This document contains a comprehensive description of federal requirements for manufacturers of drug products.

h. Regulatory activity regarding veterinary medicine, http://www.fda.gov/foi/warning.htm: Warning letters issued to firms pursuant to an FDA inspection are listed on this site and are searchable by company, subject, FDA office, date, and responses. Veterinarians search this site when choosing a compounding pharmacist with whom to work.

2. American Veterinary Medical Association, www.avma.org
   a. Guidance documents and position statements on veterinary issues
   b. Veterinary scientific news
   c. Peer-reviewed veterinary scientific articles
   d. Animal and human public health issues
3. Veterinary Support Personnel Network, www.vspn.org
   a. Veterinary continuing education
   b. Veterinary discussion forums and chat rooms
   c. Library holdings

C. Subscription services
   1. Journals
      a. The *Journal of the American Veterinary Medical Association (JAVMA)*, http://www.avma.org/journals/javma/javma_about.asp
         (1) Original peer-reviewed veterinary scientific research
         (2) Current veterinary news and events
         (3) Guidelines and position statements regarding animal health and welfare
            (a) AVMA Position Statement on Compounding For Animals
            (b) AVMA Guidelines on Euthanasia
            (c) Compendium of Animal Rabies Prevention and Control
      b. *The International Journal of Pharmaceutical Compounding (IJPC)*, http://www.ijpc.com/
         (1) Original research
         (2) Feature articles on veterinary medicine
         (3) Veterinary compounded preparation formulas
   2. Forums
      a. The Veterinary Information Network (VIN), www.vin.com
         (1) Message boards for veterinary practitioners moderated by expert veterinary consultants
         (2) Clinical rounds with continuing education credit
         (3) Library holdings
         (4) Scientific abstracts and manuscripts
         (5) Client educational materials
         (6) Scientific research forum proceedings
         (7) User-friendly search engine
      b. Veterinary Forum—Professional Compounding Centers of America
         (1) Moderated discussion of contemporary pharmacy issues
         (2) Focus on providing compounded preparations for animal patients
   3. Listservs
      a. American College of Veterinary Pharmacists, members@vetemeds.org
      b. Society of Veterinary Hospital Pharmacists, svhp_l@listserv.uga.edu
      c. *International Journal of Pharmaceutical Compounding*, NETWORK@LISTS.IJPC.COM

D. Veterinary colleges: directory of U.S. Colleges of Veterinary Medicine, academic pharmacists and pharmacologists for questions regarding veterinary pharmacotherapy, http://www.veterinaryschools.com/dvm-schools-colleges-programs.html

III.   PROFESSIONAL VETERINARY PHARMACY ORGANIZATIONS

A. International College of Veterinary Pharmacists (ICVP), www.svhp.org
   1. Board-certified veterinary academic teaching hospital pharmacists
   2. Certification via credentialing, continuing education, and examination

B. **American College of Veterinary Pharmacists** (ACVP), www.vetmeds.org

Monthly newsletters for practicing veterinarians, pharmacists, and pet owners

C. **Veterinary drug information hotline**

Board-certified veterinary pharmacy specialist consultants

D. **Veterinary Specialty Training programs to achieve certification**

80+-hours Accreditation Council for Pharmacy Education (ACPE) approved continuing education credits annually

1. Annual conference: ~12 hours ACPE credits
2. Mid-year conference: ~12 hours ACPE credits
3. 40-hour ACPE certificate program in advanced canine and feline pharmacotherapy
4. 20-hour ACPE certificate program in advanced exotic animal species pharmacotherapy
5. 20-hour ACPE certificate program in advanced equine pharmacotherapy
6. Diplomate in Veterinary Pharmacy specialty certification program

E. **Society of Veterinary Hospital Pharmacists (SVHP)**, www.svhp.org

1. Web site with current news, critical issues, and position statements
2. Newsletter: six issues annually
3. Annual conference: ~20 hours ACPE credits
4. Listserv

F. **Professional Compounding Centers of America** (PCCA), www.pccarx.com

1. ACPE-approved veterinary pharmacotherapy CE: ~40 hours
2. International Veterinary Symposium: ~20-hour ACPE credit
3. Online veterinary pharmacotherapy courses
   a. Introduction to Veterinary Pharmacotherapy: 20 hours ACPE or 2-hour college credit
   b. Advanced Veterinary Pharmacotherapy: 20 hours ACPE
4. Webinars
   a. Introduction to Veterinary Pharmacotherapy
   b. Veterinary Practice Builders: Small Animal Niches
   c. Veterinary Practice Builders: Equine Niches
   d. Providing Care and Compounds for Feline Patients
   e. Providing Care and Compounds for Canine Patients

IV. LEGAL CONSIDERATIONS

A. **Evolution of Animal Drug Law.** Humans consume some animal species as food. Because it is currently legal in the United States for a human to consume any species except another human, drug use laws for animal species evolved quite differently from laws for drug use in the human species. The following is a brief outline of legislation critical to the use of drugs in animal species.

1. **Food, Drug and Cosmetic Act, 1938**
   a. Mandated FDA approval for all drugs in the United States, except those qualifying for pharmacy practice exemption
   b. Did not address drug use in animal patients
   c. Did not create a veterinary practice exemption

2. **Animal Drug Amendment, 1968**
   a. From 1938 to 1968, there were increasing incidents of drugs accumulating in the human food chain through meat, milk, and eggs, causing human deaths and illnesses.
   b. Legal definition of a food animal species is problematic as animal use is determined by individual human preference. For example, rabbits may be kept as pets, performance animals (e.g., rabbit hopping, which is essentially stadium jumping for rabbits), pelt animals, meat animals, or laboratory animals or may be raised to serve as food for other nonhuman species (e.g., reptiles and raptors). Therefore, any nonhuman animal is potentially a food-producing animal in the United States.
   c. This Act codified restriction on drug use in nonhuman patients to only those products that were approved specifically for use in the target species. For example, amoxicillin labeled for humans could not be used in dogs, and antiinflammatory drugs labeled for dogs could not be used in cattle.
   d. An unintended consequence of this law was that use of human-labeled drugs and compounded preparations in animal patients became technically illegal.

3. **Animal Medicinal Drug Use Clarification Act, 1996** (AMDUCA), http://www.fda.gov/cvm/s340.htm
   a. This Act codified extra-label use of drugs by veterinarians within the context of a valid veterinarian–client–patient relationship (VCPR) while avoiding drug residues in the food chain.

    (1) VCPR is federally mandated and means as follows:

      (a) The veterinarian has assumed the responsibility for making clinical judgments regarding the health of the animal and the need for medical treatment, and the client has agreed to follow the veterinarian's instructions.

      (b) The veterinarian has sufficient knowledge of the animal to initiate at least a general or preliminary diagnosis of the medical condition of the animal. This means that the veterinarian has recently seen and is personally acquainted with the keeping and care of the animal either by virtue of an examination of the animal or by medically appropriate and timely visits to the premises where the animal is kept.

      (c) The veterinarian is readily available or has arranged for emergency coverage for follow-up evaluation in the event of adverse reactions or the failure of the treatment regimen.

    (2) A valid VCPR must be present before a veterinarian can prescribe any of the following:

      (a) Legend drugs

      (b) Off-label use of over-the-counter drugs

      (c) Compounded preparations

  b. AMDUCA prohibited extra-label drug use that would result in drug residues in the human food chain. AMDUCA banned use of the following drugs or chemicals in food-producing animals (http://www.fda.gov/cvm/Documents/530_41.pdf):

    (1) Chloramphenicol

    (2) Clenbuterol

    (3) Diethylstilbestrol (DES)

    (4) Dimetridazole

    (5) Furazolidone, nitrofurazone, other nitrofurans

    (6) Fluoroquinolones

    (7) Glycopeptide

    (8) Ipronidazole

    (9) Other nitroimidazoles

    (10) Phenylbutazone animal and human drugs in female dairy cattle 20 months of age or older

    (11) Sulfonamide drugs in lactating dairy cattle (except approved use of sulfadimethoxine, sulfabromomethazine, and sulfamethoxypyridazine)

  c. AMDUCA codifies compounding for animal patients as long as starting ingredients are FDA-approved drugs.

  d. *Compliance Policy Guides* are internal guidance documents for FDA inspectors that allow regulatory discretion in areas that are not provided for by law. Veterinary-related CPGs are continuously revised and posted at this link: http://www.fda.gov/ora/compliance_ref/cpg/cpgvet/default.htm.

B. Food animals: Defined as any animal patient, or a tissue or byproduct thereof, which can be consumed by humans.

  1. Any nonhuman species can be legally consumed by humans[1] in the United States.

  2. Some typical food animal species are as follows:

    a. Cattle

    b. Poultry

    c. Sheep

    d. Goats

    e. Pigs

    f. Fish

    g. Deer

  3. Species that may be consumed by humans include but are not limited to the following:

    a. Rabbits

    b. Buffalo

    c. Alligators

    d. Ostrich

    e. Rattlesnakes

C. Animal use: One other legal consideration of drug use in animal species involves the intended use of the animal.

  1. Companion: Drug use in pets is the least restrictive of the various uses.

  2. Performance: The animal has a "job" other than just being a pet.

---

[1]At the time of publication, a bill is being discussed in the U.S. Congress that would prohibit horses from being slaughtered or sold for the purpose of being used for food.

   a. Service animals
   Assistance animals for challenged humans (e.g., visually challenged, physically challenged, hearing-impaired, patients with epilepsy)
   b. Military and police animals
      (1) Mounted-police horses
      (2) Search-and-rescue dogs
      (3) Drug-detecting dogs
      (4) US Department of Agriculture customs dogs
      (5) Bomb-detection dogs
   c. Cart or plow horses
   d. Competitive sports
      (1) Equine sports (racing, showing, jumping, conformation, etc.)
         (a) Drug use is dictated by the rules of each discipline.
         (b) American Association of Racing Commissioners International (ARCI; www.arci.com) rules racing sports. Five classes of drug use in race horses are based on the following:
            (i) Eliminating unfair "doping" of horses.
            (ii) Ensuring safety for competing horses.
            (iii) Ensuring safety for competing riders.
      (2) Canine sports: Drug use is governed by the various canine sport disciplines (racing, showing, agility, etc.).
      (3) Rabbit sports (rabbit hopping): Drug use is governed by the discipline.
3. Food-producing: Drug use in food-producing animals is strictly regulated and carries serious penalties for violation drug residues.
   a. Labeled product withdrawal times (WDTs) for these products:
      (1) Meat
      (2) Milk
      (3) Eggs
   b. Calculating WDTs for extra-label drug use in food animals: Drugs may be administered to food producing animals only if a reasonable and accurate estimate can be made predicting the time when drug residues are below a legally acceptable limit in animal tissues consumed by humans. WDTs are included on the labels of drugs approved for use in food animal species, but if extra-label use occurs in a food-producing animal, the prescribing veterinarian must provide the WDT. For example, if a veterinarian chooses to use doxycycline in a dairy goat being treated for tick-borne disease, the veterinarian must provide an accurate time period during which the goat's owner must discard all milk produced by that goat to prevent doxycycline residues from entering the human food chain. Pharmacists may assist in determination of this WDT but should not provide it without consulting a veterinarian. For drugs for which the WDT cannot be accurately predicted, a minimum WDT of 180 days should be listed on the label of dispensed drugs.
      (1) Consider the United States' "tolerance" for drug residues.
         (a) Tolerances based on percent of drug remaining in tissues that has been determined to be safe for human consumption
            (i) 0.1% of dose remaining after 10 half-lives
            (ii) 0.01% of dose remaining after 13 half-lives
            (iii) 0% tolerance for drugs as banned in AMDUCA
         (b) Drug residue tolerances are usually stated in parts per million, which is equivalent to milligrams of drug per kilogram of tissue.
      (2) Food Animal Residue Avoidance Database (FARAD)
         (a) Available to veterinarians
         (b) Comprehensive database of WDTs for various drugs in various species
         (c) http://www.farad.org/
   c. Informed consent: Pharmacists and veterinarians who are uncertain of the ultimate disposition for food animal species treated with extra-label drugs should obtain written assurance from the animal's owner that treated animals shall never enter the food chain. For example, if a pet goat requires use of enrofloxacin to treat a urinary tract infection, the veterinarian should obtain, prior to prescribing the enrofloxacin, a written statement from the owner that the goat is a pet and none of its tissues will ever enter the human food chain. Pharmacists dispensing banned drugs should also obtain this informed consent as well as make notations on the label of the dispensed prescription that no tissues of the animal shall ever enter the human food chain.

V. IMPORTANT VETERINARY TERMINOLOGY

Veterinary prescription abbreviations and dosage forms evolved differently from those used for humans and can be quite confusing to pharmacists not familiar with veterinary abbreviations. Table 36.1 lists abbreviations and terminology important to practicing veterinary pharmacists. In addition to the terms listed in the table, the veterinary pharmacist should become familiar with anatomic terminology for the various veterinary species to completely understand drug administration instructions written by the veterinarian.

VI. DOSAGE FORMS USED IN ANIMAL PATIENTS

Large variations between the animal species' anatomy, physiology, and behavior necessitate the development of drug dosage forms for animals that are significantly different from those used in human patients. The veterinary pharmacist should be familiar with the various veterinary dosage forms and be prepared to assist veterinarians and pet owners in selecting the most appropriate dosage form when a compounded preparation is required for a given patient. Table 36.2 lists and briefly describes dosage forms used in animal patients.

Table 36.1	IMPORTANT ABBREVIATIONS USED IN VETERINARY MEDICINE

ABBREVIATION	MEANING
Avian	Bird species
BAR	Bright, alert, and responsive (used for monitoring patient status)
Bolus	A large, oral, solid dosage form (not parenteral)
Bovine	Cattle species
BSA	Body surface area
BW	Body weight (usually in kilograms but always confirm units)
Canine	Dog species
Caprine	Goat species
Drench	A volume of liquid medication administered orally to livestock
DLH	Domestic long hair, used to indicate long-haired cat breeds
DSH	Domestic short hair, used to indicate short-haired cat breeds
Fe—	Feline, (fe + a line) used to indicate that patient is a cat
Feline	Cat species
FeLV	Feline leukemia virus (usually followed by a + or − to indicate carrier status)
FHV	Feline herpesvirus
FIP	Feline infectious peritonitis
FIV	Feline immunodeficiency virus (usually followed by a + or − to indicate carrier status)
FLUTD	Feline lower urinary tract disease
FUS	Feline urologic syndrome (equivalent to FLUTD)
FS	Female, spayed
Intact	Used to indicate reproductive status of the animal, has not been neutered
KCS	Keratoconjunctivitis sicca (also known as *dry eye*)
K-9	Canine, shorthand to indicate that patient is a dog
KV	Killed virus vaccine
MLV	Modified live virus vaccine
MC	Male, castrated
Murine	Mouse species
Ovine	Sheep species
Paste	Viscous, oral dosage form usually delivered in dial-a-dose oral syringes or catheter-tip syringes (not topical)
PCV	Packed cell volume (similar to hematocrit)
Porcine	Pig species
Ruminant	Species possessing four-chambered stomachs containing a rumen
SID	Once daily
TPR	Temperature, pulse, and respiration (used for monitoring patient status)
WDT	Withdrawal time

Table 36.2	DOSAGE FORMS USED IN ANIMAL PATIENTS	

ROUTE OF ADMINISTRATION	DOSAGE FORM	COMMENTS
Oral	Tablet	Usually less than 1 inch in diameter and sized as appropriate for diameter of target species' esophagus
	Chewable treat	Flavored according to target species preference
	Capsule	Usually less than 0.75 inches and sized as appropriate for target species; dosage form most likely to adhere to esophageal mucosa if not followed with food or liquid
	Solution	Concentrations appropriate to deliver dose in a volume appropriate for target species
	Suspension	Concentrations appropriate to deliver dose in a volume appropriate for target species
	Drench	A concentrated oral liquid usually delivered to livestock
	Paste	A concentrated, viscous oral dosage form usually delivered by dial-a-dose syringes, not intended for topical application
	Bolus	Solid dosage form usually larger than 1 inch in diameter and intended for oral administration to large animals (e.g., horses, cattle, goats); not for parenteral administration
	Powder	Medication uniformly mixed in a suitably flavored powder trituration to allow for dosing into food via calibrated scoop or spoon
Buccal	Solution	pK$_a$ of drug must be compatible with pH of target species' saliva to facilitate transmucosal absorption
Parenteral	Sterile solution	Usually concentrated to allow for delivery of dose in volumes appropriate for route and species
	Sterile suspension	Usually concentrated to allow for delivery of dose in volumes appropriate for route and species; may provide for longer duration of drug activity
	Sterile implant	Solid dosage form or gel intended to provide a slow release of drug over a given time interval; usually in a biodegradable matrix or gel
Transdermal	Transdermal device	A patch or other matrix facilitating slow, constant release of drug across skin or other tissue
	Transdermal gel	Drug concentrated into small volumes that can be applied to vascular areas of skin for perfusion into systemic circulation
	Transdermal solution	Drug concentrated in vehicle that facilitates rapid percutaneous absorption into systemic circulation
Rectal	Suppository	Solid or semisolid dosage forms used in some exotic animal species; retention difficult to achieve in most species unless caregiver is willing to perform manual occlusion of the anus until dissolution or absorption is complete
	Enema	Solutions or suspensions usually intended to facilitate evacuation of rectal or colonic contents; not usually retained long enough to provide for absorption into systemic circulation
Topical	Dressing	Usually refers to topical medications applied to the feet of hoof stock, especially horses
	Poultice	Usually a soft, thick ointment or cream that is applied to a cloth and warmed for local application to the limbs of horses; may also be applied directly to the tissue under an occlusive wrap that is removed several hours later
	Sweat	Usually a solution or suspension of counterirritants and analgesics applied to limbs of horses to relieve edema

| VII. | SPECIES CONSIDERATIONS IN DRUG DELIVERY |

A. Anatomy

1. **Body size**
   a. Animal drug therapy is usually based on a milligram-per-kilogram dosage based on body weight.
   b. Very few empiric dosages exist for animal patients.
   c. Narrow therapeutic index drugs (e.g., cytotoxic agents) frequently are dosed on body surface area (BSA), which is calculated from body weight in kilograms based on unique formulas for each species. It is imperative to use the correct species' BSA chart when calculating dosages (see Table 36.3, Body Surface Area Values for Dogs and Cats).

2. **Horizontal orientation**
   a. An animal's horizontal orientation means it lacks the benefit of gravity to facilitate passage of solid dosage forms to its stomach.
   b. Animals do not swallow medications with a glass of liquid.

| Table 36.3 | BODY SURFACE AREA VALUES FOR DOGS AND CATS |

Dog Body Surface Area Conversion Chart Body Weight (kg) to Meters Squared (m²)

Calculated from the formula: $m^2 = \dfrac{10.1 \times \text{weight in grams}^{2/3}}{10{,}000}$

WEIGHT TO BODY SURFACE AREA CONVERSION CHART—DOGS

Kg	M²	Kg	M²	Kg	M²	Kg	M²	Kg	M²
0.5	0.064	10.0	0.469	20.0	0.744	30.0	0.975	40.0	1.181
1.0	0.101	11.0	0.500	21.0	0.759	31.0	0.997	41.0	1.201
2.0	0.160	12.0	0.529	22.0	0.785	32.0	1.018	42.0	1.220
3.0	0.210	13.0	0.553	23.0	0.817	33.0	1.029	43.0	1.240
4.0	0.255	14.0	0.581	24.0	0.840	34.0	1.060	44.0	1.259
5.0	0.295	15.0	0.608	25.0	0.864	35.0	1.081	45.0	1.278
6.0	0.333	16.0	0.641	26.0	0.886	36.0	1.101	46.0	1.297
7.0	0.370	17.0	0.668	27.0	0.909	37.0	1.121	47.0	1.302
8.0	0.404	18.0	0.694	28.0	0.931	38.0	1.142	48.0	1.334
9.0	0.437	19.0	0.719	29.0	0.953	39.0	1.162	49.0	1.352

Cat Body Surface Area Conversion Chart Body Weight (kg) to Meters Squared (m²)

Calculated from the formula: $m^2 = \dfrac{10.0 \times \text{weight in grams}^{2/3}}{10{,}000}$

WEIGHT TO BODY SURFACE AREA CONVERSION CHART—CATS

Kg	M²	Kg	M²	Kg	M²	Kg	M²	Kg	M²
0.1	0.022	1.4	0.125	3.6	0.235	5.8	0.323	8.0	0.400
0.2	0.034	1.6	0.137	3.8	0.244	6.0	0.330	8.2	0.407
0.3	0.045	1.8	0.148	4.0	0.252	6.2	0.337	8.4	0.413
0.4	0.054	2.0	0.159	4.2	0.260	6.4	0.345	8.6	0.420
0.5	0.063	2.2	0.169	4.4	0.269	6.6	0.352	8.8	0.426
0.6	0.071	2.4	0.179	4.6	0.277	6.8	0.360	9.0	0.433
0.7	0.079	2.6	0.189	4.8	0.285	7.0	0.366	9.2	0.439
0.8	0.086	2.8	0.199	5.0	0.292	7.2	0.373	9.4	0.445
0.9	0.093	3.0	0.208	5.2	0.300	7.4	0.380	9.6	0.452
1.0	0.100	3.2	0.217	5.4	0.307	7.6	0.387	9.8	0.458
1.2	0.113	3.4	0.226	5.6	0.315	7.8	0.393	10.0	0.464

    c. Irritating drugs lead to esophageal erosion and strictures. These drugs should be given with food or chased with at least 6 mL of a suitable liquid. Solid forms of doxycycline are well documented to cause esophagitis in cats.

3. Skin cover

    a. Fur

        (1) Drug absorption is proportional to the density of hair follicles on the animal's hair coat.

        (2) Hair follicle density varies according to species and anatomic region.

        (3) Shaving improves adhesion of drug delivery patches but also increases drug absorption owing to increased perfusion and disruption of hair follicles.

    b. Feathers

        (1) Feathers are required for thermoregulation in avian species; they act as insulation against heat and cold.

        (2) Disruption of feather integrity from topical drug administration can lead to the bird's inability to thermoregulate.

    c. Scales

        (1) Scales can be an obstacle to drug penetration (injection, topical).

        (2) They also can be an obstacle to restraint of the animal for drug administration (e.g., sharp spines or horns that can injure a caregiver).

4. Digestive organs

    a. Ruminant stomach (cattle, sheep, goats, deer)

        (1) Four chambers

            (a) Rumen

            (b) Omentum

            (c) Abomasum (true glandular stomach)

            (d) Reticulum

        (2) Heavily populated with microflora to facilitate cellulose digestion

            (a) Some drugs (e.g., trimethoprim, chloramphenicol) are degraded by rumen microflora and are inactive.

            (b) Some drugs (antibiotics) kill rumen microflora and cause enterotoxemia from gram-negative overgrowth.

    b. Cecum (horses, rabbits)

        (1) Heavily populated with microflora to facilitate digestion of food

        (2) Microflora break down undigested food passed from the stomach and small intestine into viable, usable nutrients.

        (3) Cecal microflora metabolize some drugs into toxins (e.g., ursodiol)

    c. Proventriculus or crop (birds)

        (1) This is a food storage organ.

        (2) It can stall drug dissolution and absorption.

        (3) Birds can regurgitate drugs from crop long after administration.

B. Physiology

    1. Dietary habit: impact on drug disposition as well as flavor preference

    a. Carnivores: Short, fast, gastrointestinal (GI) tract that causes sustained-release dosage forms designed for humans to pass to the large intestine and be eliminated before the drug is released.

    b. Herbivores

        (1) These species have a long, complex, relatively alkaline GI tract as compared to that of humans.

        (2) This GI tract is heavily populated with microflora, which can either destroy drugs or be destroyed by drugs.

        (3) Large volumes of fluid exert an effect on concentration gradients of drugs requiring passive diffusion.

        (4) Weak bases are relatively more bioavailable than weak acids, allowing for potentially lower doses relative to those for humans.

    2. Thermoregulatory capability

    (a) Homeothermic species: ability to raise body temperature

    (b) Poikilothermic species: inability to raise body temperature, so consider impact of topical drugs, vasodilators, vasoconstrictors, environment, etc.

    (c) Inability to sweat: reliance on panting/grooming to cool, so consider effect of respiratory depressants

3. **Ability to vomit:** impact on poison ingestion
   a. Vomiting species
      (1) Dogs
      (2) Cats
      (3) Ferrets
      (4) Pigs
   b. Nonvomiting species
      (1) Horses
      (2) Cattle
      (3) Rabbits
      (4) Goats
      (5) Sheep
4. **Glomerular filtration rate** (GFR): generally inversely proportional to body size; impact on renally eliminated drugs
   a. Dogs and cats: relatively higher GFR than humans
   b. Horses: relatively lower GFR than humans
5. **Hemoglobin structure**
   a. Most mammals: 4 sulfhydryl groups on hemoglobin molecules
   b. Cats: 8 to 20 sulfhydryl groups on hemoglobin molecules; very susceptible to oxidative injury and hypoxia

C. **Metabolic capacity:** Not all species are equivalent to humans in terms of biotransformation and drug elimination. Species-specific deficiencies are an essential part of the veterinary pharmacist's knowledge base.
   1. Glucuronide conjugation: limited in cats
   2. Acetylation: limited in dogs
   3. Sulfation: limited in pigs
   4. Ornithine conjugation: active in birds
   5. Variations in CYP 450 isoenzymes and drug metabolism from species to species, thus making drug interactions less predictable when compared to humans

D. **Behavior**
   1. Grooming effects on topical drug administration
      a. Topical drug therapy is equivalent to systemic drug therapy in cats.
      b. Cats may also groom topical medications off of other pets.
   2. Social hierarchy and dominance
      a. Alpha animals are difficult to medicate if they are dominant over the caregiver.
      b. Herd animals are extremely stressed by isolation from the herd for medical therapy.

E. **Habitat**
   1. **Controlled environment:** similar to human care situations
   2. **Outdoor habitat:** livestock, animals kept solely outside
      a. Effects of ultraviolet light
         (1) Topical drug degradation
         (2) Photosensitizing drugs
      b. Exposure to elements
         (1) Effect of rain on topically applied drugs
         (2) Effect of hot and cold temperatures
            (a) Faster drug elimination (e.g., aminoglycosides) in poikilothermic species at warmer temperatures
            (b) Respiratory and central nervous system depressants (e.g., opioids) interfere with panting and ability to cool.

F. **Species-specific toxins**
   Drug metabolism and disposition vary widely from species to species, and drug components and foods that are innocuous in humans may be toxic or fatal to nonhuman species. For this reason, pharmacists engaged in preparing medications for animal patients should be aware of species-specific drug and food toxicities. Certain toxic foods, drugs, and excipients should be avoided when preparing compounded therapies for animals. Not only should the actual agents be avoided, but also artificial versions of these toxins should never be used as they may cause an animal to develop an affinity for a toxic substance. For example, flavoring medications with artificial chocolate flavor does not pose a toxic threat to dogs but encourages those dogs to ingest real chocolate if given an opportunity. Pharmacists should routinely search the American Society for the Prevention of Cruelty to Animals

Table 36.4	DRUGS, EXCIPIENTS, AND FOODS WITH KNOWN TOXICITY IN ANIMAL SPECIES		
DRUG, EXCIPIENT, FOOD	**SPECIES AFFECTED**	**TOXICITY**	**REFERENCE**
Acetaminophen	Dogs, cats	Hepatotoxicity (dogs) and red blood cell oxidative injury (cats)	Campbell A, Chapman M. Handbook of poisoning in dogs and cats. Malden MA: Blackwell Science, 2000; 31, 205.
Alcohols	Dogs, cats, birds	Central nervous system toxicity	Osweiler G, Carson T, Buck W, Van Gelder G. Clinical and diagnostic veterinary toxicology, 3rd ed. Dubuque, IA: Kendall/Hunt, 1976; 388.
Avocado	Birds	Pulmonary congestion, nonsuppurative inflammation of the liver, kidney, pancreas, skin, and proventriculus	LaBonde J. Avian toxicology. In: Proceedings of the 2006 Association of Avian Veterinarians Meeting.
Benzocaine	Cats	Red blood cell oxidative injury, hemolytic anemia	Harvey J. Toxic hemolytic anemias. In: Proceedings of the American College of Internal Medicine Meeting 2006.
Chocolate	Dogs, birds	Cardiovascular and central nervous system stimulation	Campbell A, Chapman M. Handbook of poisoning in dogs and cats. Malden MA: Blackwell Science, 2000; 106.
Estrogen	Dogs	Bone marrow suppression	Campbell A, Chapman M. Handbook of poisoning in dogs and cats. Malden MA: Blackwell Science, 2000; 245.
Ethyl glycols (diethylene glycol, ethylene glycol)	Dogs, cats	Central nervous system toxicity, nephrotoxicity	Campbell A, Chapman M. Handbook of poisoning in dogs and cats. Malden MA: Blackwell Science, 2000; 22, 127.
Garlic/onions	Dogs, cats	Hemolytic anemia	Warman SM. Dietary intoxications. In: Proceedings of the British Small Animal Veterinary Congress, 2007.
Grapes/raisins	Dogs	Renal toxicity	Warman SM. Dietary intoxications. In: Proceedings of the British Small Animal Veterinary Congress, 2007.
Macadamia nuts	Dogs	Neurotoxicity	Warman SM. Dietary intoxications. In: Proceedings of the British Small Animal Veterinary Congress, 2007.
Macrolide antibiotics, oral route	Horses, rabbits	Diarrhea, enteritis, colic	Papich MG. Current considerations in antimicrobial therapy for horses. In: Proceedings of the American Academy of Equine Practitioners, vol 47, 2001.
Methylene blue	Cats	Red blood cell oxidative injury, hemolytic anemia	Harvey J. Toxic hemolytic anemias. In: Proceedings of the American College of Internal Medicine Meeting, 2006.
Nonsteroidal antiinflammatory agents for humans (naproxen, ibuprofen)	Dogs, cats	Gastrointestinal ulceration and perforation, nephrotoxicity	Campbell A, Chapman M. Handbook of poisoning in dogs and cats. Malden MA: Blackwell Science, 2000; 148, 192.
Pennyroyal	Cats	Hepatotoxicity	Wismer T. Toxicology of household products. In: Proceedings of the International Veterinary Emergency and Critical Care Symposium, 2007.

(continued)

Table 36.4	DRUGS, EXCIPIENTS, AND FOODS WITH KNOWN TOXICITY IN ANIMAL SPECIES (*continued*)

DRUG, EXCIPIENT, FOOD	SPECIES AFFECTED	TOXICITY	REFERENCE
Permethrin	Cats	Neuromuscular and central nervous system toxicity	Campbell A, Chapman M. Handbook of poisoning in dogs and cats. Malden MA: Blackwell Science, 2000; 238.
Phenazopyridine	Cats	Hepatotoxicity and red blood cell oxidative injury	Harvey J. Toxic hemolytic anemias. In: Proceedings of the American College of Internal Medicine Meeting, 2006.
	Dogs	Keratoconjunctivitis sicca	
Phosphate enemas	Cats	Profound hypocalcemia	Wismer T. ASPCA Poison Control Center.
Pseudoephedrine	Dogs, cats	Cardiovascular and central nervous system stimulation	Plumlee K. Poisons in the medicine cabinet. In: Proceedings of the Western Veterinary Conference, 2004.
Raw yeast dough	Dogs	Alcohol poisoning, gastrointestinal dilatation, and volvulus	Warman SM. Dietary intoxications. In: Proceedings of the British Small Animal Veterinary Congress, 2007.
Salt	Dogs, cats	hypernatremia, central nervous system toxicity	Campbell A, Chapman M. Handbook of poisoning in dogs and cats. Malden MA: Blackwell Science, 2000; 42.
Tobacco products	Dogs, cats	Muscle weakness, twitching, depression, tachycardia, shallow respiration, collapse, coma, and cardiac arrest	Plumlee K. Household poisons. In: Proceedings of the Western Veterinary Conference, 2004.
Xylitol	Dogs, birds	Profound hypoglycemia and hepatocellular necrosis	Wismer T. Hepatic toxins and the emergent patient. In: Proceedings of the International Veterinary Emergency and Critical Care Symposium, 2006.

(ASPCA) Poison Control Center Web page at http://www.aspca.org to maintain current knowledge of potential food and drug toxins in animals. Examples of drugs, excipients, and foods that are toxic to animal species can be found in Table 36.4.

VIII.   ALGORITHM FOR FILLING VETERINARY PRESCRIPTIONS

A. Check to see that all the components of the prescription are present:
  1. Printed or stamped name, address, and telephone number of the licensed practitioner
  2. Drug Enforcement Agency (DEA) registration number of the licensed practitioner, if a controlled substance
  3. Legal signature of the licensed practitioner
  4. Name and strength of drug
  5. Directions for use
  6. Full name and address of the client
  7. Animal identification (species and/or name)
  8. Cautionary statements including, if applicable, WDTs for food animals (meat, milk, eggs, honey)
  9. Number of refills, if any

B. Examine the species and breed of the animal. What is the animal's "job"?
  1. **Food animal**
    a. Is the drug banned?
    b. Is the drug approved for use in the target animal?
    c. If extra-label, is an accurate WDT listed on the prescription?
    d. If a food animal species but its job is as a pet, is informed consent in place to keep the animal out of the food chain?
  2. **Performance animal**
    a. Is the animal a service animal?
    b. Can the owner manage administration?

      c. Will the therapy impair the animal's ability to do its job?

      d. Are there drug prohibitions in the animal's discipline?

      e. Will the animal be tested for drugs?

      f. Will drugs mask the tests?

      g. Will drugs affect the animal's performance?

      h. Will drugs affect the safety of the animal? Of the handler/rider?

   3. Pet: Is this animal clearly a pet?

C. Examine the drug, dose, route, frequency, and duration of the drug therapy.

   1. Is the drug appropriate for use in this species? In this disease state?

   2. Are there any current medications or foods on the patient's profile that will interact with this drug or otherwise interfere with the administration of this drug?

   3. According to body weight, is the dose appropriate for this patient? Is dosing in milligrams per kilogram? Is dosing in milligrams per animal? Is weight provided?

   4. Has the drug been dosed on BSA? Consult a species-specific BSA chart to confirm accurate dosing.
Has the animal had this drug before? If so, what product and what dosage form? Will bioavailability be altered if a different dosage form is provided?

   5. Is the route appropriate for this patient? For this owner?

   6. Is the frequency appropriate?

   7. Is the duration appropriate?

   8. Is there evidence to support extra-label use in the target species?

   9. What is the drug's metabolic fate in this species? If not known, what is the metabolic fate in humans or known species?

   10. Is there an approved veterinary product for the target species?

   11. Is there an approved human product for the target species?

   12. Is there a likelihood of therapeutic failure from the commercially available product (e.g., poor bioavailability in target species)?

   13. What dosage forms are available as the commercially available product? Can the pet owner manipulate those dosage forms to accurately achieve the desired dose?

   14. Are there any inactive ingredients in the commercially available form that will be toxic or not tolerated by this species?

   15. Does the drug have to be compounded to achieve the desired dose?

   16. If a compounded preparation is indicated, do you have a reliable formula?

   17. What is the stability of the compounded preparation? Is the beyond-use date supported by evidence?

D. Examine the final product for proper labeling with instructions for administration, handling, and storage. Ensure that packaging is compatible with long-term stability of the drug.

E. Determine that the final product is properly packaged to prevent ingestion by children and other pets.

F. Determine appropriate counseling for the client.

   1. Ensure that he or she understands the following:

      a. Indications

      b. Instructions for use

      c. Storage and handling

      d. Caregiver protection

      e. Administration tips

   2. What are the adverse effects noted with the drug in the target species (to pet or owner or other pets)?

   3. For what signs will the owner monitor to detect possible toxicity?

   4. What should be done if a dose is missed?

   5. How is the owner monitoring the pet's response?

   6. How shall any unused drug be responsibly disposed of?

   7. Does the client have any questions?

   8. Does the client know how to reach you for more information?

Sample Prescriptions

SAMPLE PRESCRIPTION 36.1

CASE: "Lucy Caroline" is a 15-year-old spayed, domestic short-haired cat that weighs 4.3 kg. Lucy Caroline has been diagnosed with feline hypertension and requires amlodipine at an empiric dose of 0.625 mg orally once daily. Lucy Caroline's caregiver, Ruth Davis, presents with the prescription shown here. Lucy Caroline has had no other prescriptions filled at your pharmacy.

Contemporary Veterinarians Group Practice
20 S. Park Street, Triturate, WI 53706
Tel: (608) 555-1334 Fax: (608) 555-1336

℞ # *123047*

NAME *"Lucy Caroline" Davis 15 YO, DSH, FS 4.3kg BW*   **DATE** *00/00/00*

ADDRESS *713 Reed Street, Triturate, WI*

℞

Amlodipine 0.625 mg PO SID × 30 days

G. Jones 00/00/00

REFILLS *PRN*   *J. M. Herriot, DVM*

DEA NO. *AH1234567*

ALGORITHM

Lucy Caroline is not a food animal.

Lucy Caroline is not a performance animal.

All of the elements of the prescription are present for complete filling. (**Note:** although this is not the standard prescription writing format, it is the format largely used by veterinarians to allow the pharmacist and the pet owner to select the best dosage form for compliance.)

A veterinary drug reference is used to determine the appropriateness of the drug, dose, route, frequency, and duration of the therapy.

The pharmacist determines that FDA-approved, human-labeled amlodipine tablets (2.5 mg) are available to fill this prescription. The expiration date on the bottle of manufactured tablets is 18 months from the date dispensed, so a beyond-use date (BUD) of one year is appropriate for the prescription container label. (See section IV of Chapter 4, Expiration and Beyond-Use Dating.)

Ms. Davis is consulted to see if she is capable of quartering the commercially available amlodipine 2.5-mg tablets to achieve a 0.625-mg dose. She confirms that she is, and that Lucy readily accepts oral tablet medications.

After consultation, the pharmacist determines that this prescription can be filled with eight of the commercially available amlodipine 2.5-mg generic tablets.

The prescription is dispensed in a light-resistant, child-proof prescription vial.

On dispensing the medication, the pharmacist shows Ms. Davis how to quarter the tablets and instructs her to store the medication at controlled room temperature, to wash her hands after administration, and to watch Lucy for any signs of lethargy or fainting. The pharmacist tells

Ms. Davis that if she misses a dose, she should give it as soon as she remembers and then give the dose at the next scheduled administration time. Ms. Davis is then asked if she has any further questions and is directed to the phone number on the label of the dispensed prescription should she have questions at a later time.

LABELING

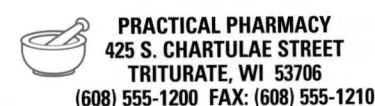

PRACTICAL PHARMACY
425 S. CHARTULAE STREET
TRITURATE, WI 53706
(608) 555-1200 FAX: (608) 555-1210

℞ 123047   Date: 00/00/00
Lucy Caroline Davis, cat   Dr. Herriot

Give one-fourth ($^1/_4$) tablet orally once daily for 30 days.

Amlodipine 2.5 mg tablets

Mfg: Eon   Quantity: 8 tablets

Refills: PRN   Discard after: 1 year

Dispensed by: G. Jones, RPh

SAMPLE PRESCRIPTION 36.2

CASE: Suppose Lucy Caroline's caregiver calls back 1 week later and states that she overestimated Lucy's willingness to take the tablets. She is wondering if amlodipine is available in a flavored liquid formulation. The pharmacist contacts Dr. Herriot and relays Ms. Davis's concerns. Dr. Herriot asks the pharmacist about possibilities. The pharmacist has located a referenced stability study for a 1-mg/mL amlodipine oral suspension used in human pediatric patients and feels it would be suitable for Lucy. Dr. Herriot faxes over to the pharmacy a new prescription for Lucy.

Contemporary Veterinarians Group Practice
20 S. Park Street, Triturate, WI 53706
Tel: (608) 555-1334 Fax: (608) 555-1336

℞ # *123048*

NAME *"Lucy Caroline" Davis 15 YO, DSH, FS 4.3kg BW*   **DATE** *00/00/00*

ADDRESS *713 Reed Street, Triturate, WI*

℞   *Amlodipine 1mg/ml oral suspension*

                0.625ml PO SID x 30 days

                                                G. Davidson 00/00/00

REFILLS *PRN*   *J. M. Herriot, DVM*

                        DEA NO.   *AH1234567*

MASTER COMPOUNDING FORMULATION RECORD

NAME, STRENGTH, AND DOSAGE FORM OF PREPARATION: Amlodipine 1mg/mL Oral Suspension

QUANTITY: 30 mL (extra for administration mishaps)

THERAPEUTIC USE/CATEGORY: Antihypertensive

FORMULATION RECORD ID: VT001

ROUTE OF ADMINISTRATION: Oral

INGREDIENTS:

Ingredient	Quantity Used	Physical Description	Solubility	Dose Comparison		Use in the Prescription
				Given	Usual	
Amlodipine 5-mg tablets	6	white tablets	sl sol in water; sp sol in alcohol	0.625 mg PO q24h	0.625 mg PO q24h	antihypertensive
Ora-Plus	15 mL	colorless, cloudy viscous liquid	misc w/water and alcohol	—	—	suspending agent
Ora-Sweet 30 mL	qs ad	colorless, clear viscous liquid	misc w/water and alcohol	—	—	flavoring agent

COMPATIBILITY–STABILITY: A stability study evaluating amlodipine 1 mg/mL oral suspension in Ora-Plus/Ora-Sweet (Nahata MC, et al. Stability of amlodipine besylate in two liquid dosage forms. J Am Pharm Assoc 1999 May–Jun; 39(3): 375–377) was located by the pharmacist (7). It stated that amlodipine 1 mg/mL oral suspension formulated in either methylcellulose/Syrup NF vehicle or Ora-Sweet/Ora-Plus vehicle is stable for 91 days when stored in the refrigerator.

PACKAGING AND STORAGE: To be dispensed in a plastic, brown prescription bottle and stored in the refrigerator. Shake well before use.

BEYOND-USE DATE: 90 days

CALCULATIONS

Dose/Concentration

Dose = 0.625 mg

Concentration = 1 mg/mL

Dose in mL: 0.625 mg $\times$ 1 mL/1 mg = 0.625 mL

Ingredient Amounts

Number of milliliters of suspension to prepare for 30 days:

$$0.625 \text{ mL} \times \text{once-daily dosing} \times 30 \text{ days} = 18.75 \text{ mL}$$

(The pharmacist will prepare 30 mL in anticipation that Lucy may resist taking the oral medication on some days.)

Number of amlodipine 5-mg tablets required to compound the prescription:

$$1 \text{ mg/mL} \times 30 \text{ mL suspension} = 30 \text{ mg required/5 mg per tablet} = 6 \text{ tablets}$$

MSDS AND SAFETY AND PERSONAL PROTECTIVE EQUIPMENT: Don a clean lab coat and disposable gloves.

SPECIALIZED EQUIPMENT: No special equipment is needed.

COMPOUNDING PROCEDURE: Count 6 × 5-mg amlodipine tablets into glass mortar. Triturate into fine powder with pestle. Serially add 15 mL Ora-Plus to the crushed amlodipine tablets and triturate until a uniform mixture is achieved. Add 10 mL Ora-Sweet to mortar and continue to triturate until a uniform suspension is achieved. Transfer all amlodipine suspension to a graduated container and add a quantity of Ora-Sweet sufficient to make a final total volume of 30 mL. Transfer resulting suspension into a 1-oz amber prescription bottle, label, and dispense. The prescription should be dispensed with a child-resistant cap, but accompanied by an oral syringe and appropriate dispensing cap (Adapta-Cap, BAXA Corporation) to facilitate removal of the suspension at the pet owner's home.

DESCRIPTION OF FINISHED PREPARATION: The preparation is a viscous, uniformly suspended, white liquid that is easily redispersed after shaking.

QUALITY CONTROL: The suspended particles start to settle into a flocculated system in 3 to 4 hours and are easily redispersed after shaking.

MASTER FORMULA PREPARED BY: Gigi Davidson, RPh   **CHECKED BY:** Laurel Kinosian, RPh

---

COMPOUNDING RECORD

NAME, STRENGTH, AND DOSAGE FORM OF PREPARATION: Amlodipine 1 mg/ml Oral Suspension
QUANTITY: 30 ml   **DATE PREPARED:** mm/dd/yy   **BEYOND-USE DATE:** 90 days refrigerated
FORMULATION RECORD ID: VT001   **CONTROL/RX NUMBER:** 123048

INGREDIENTS USED:

Ingredient	Quantity Used	Manufacturer Lot Number	Expiration Date	Weighed/ Measured by	Checked by
Amlodipine 5-mg tablets	6	Aeon 167893	mm/yy	bjf	gd
Ora-Plus	15 mL	Paddock 117988	mm/yy	bjf	gd
Ora-Sweet	qs ad 30 mL	Paddock 117007	mm/yy	bjf	gd

QUALITY CONTROL DATA: The preparation is a viscous, uniformly suspended, white liquid that is easily redispersed after shaking. The suspended particles started to settle into a flocculated system after 3 hours but were easily redispersed after shaking.

LABELING

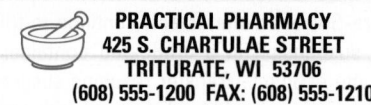

PRACTICAL PHARMACY
425 S. CHARTULAE STREET
TRITURATE, WI 53706
(608) 555-1200 FAX: (608) 555-1210

℞ 123048   Date: 00/00/00
Lucy Caroline Davis, cat   Dr. Herriot

Give 0.63 mL orally once daily for 30 days.

Amlodipine 1mg/mL Oral Suspension

Mfg: Compounded   Quantity: 30 mL

Refills: PRN   Discard after: 90 days

Store in refrigerator.

Shake well before using.

Dispensed by: G. Davidson, RPh

PATIENT CONSULTATION: Hello, Ms. Davis. I'm your pharmacist, Gigi Davidson. We have prepared a liquid form of amlodipine for Lucy Caroline. This medication is not commercially available as a liquid, but we have identified a recipe used in human children that will be appropriate for Lucy. The dose is the same as the oral tablets that you tried previously, 0.625 mg. When you get home, please remove the child-resistant cap and replace it with this blue dispensing cap. This will make it easier for you to remove doses using an oral dosing syringe. Shake the bottle well for a few seconds. Insert the syringe into the hole in the dispensing cap, turn the bottle upside down, and then withdraw 0.63 mL in the syringe. I have made a mark on the syringe with a marker to show you exactly where 0.63 mL is. Turn the bottle right-side up and remove the syringe. Insert the tip of the syringe into the side of Lucy's mouth and squirt it into her cheek pouch so that she cannot spit it back out. Give Lucy positive feedback—attention or perhaps a small treat—after you medicate her so that she will associate the medication with a pleasant experience. Replace the lid to the dispensing cap and then place the bottle back in the refrigerator out of the reach of children and other pets until the next use. There is more than 1 month's supply in this bottle, but I have dispensed a little extra in case Lucy spits out the medication. If you forget to give a dose, give it as soon as you remember it and then return to the regular dosing schedule the next day. Do not give two doses in less than 12 hours. This medication is refillable for the next year. Do you have any questions?

SAMPLE PRESCRIPTION 36.3

CASE: Letta Mae Draheim is a 4-year-old female, spayed Dachshund presenting to her veterinarian with lethargy and loss of appetite and history of exposure to ticks. Letta Mae has been diagnosed with canine ehrlichiosis, a tick-transmitted disease, which is successfully treated with doxycycline. Mr. Draheim initially had a prescription filled for doxycycline calcium 10 mg/mL oral suspension, but Letta Mae initially regurgitated on administration of the commercially available liquid and subsequently refused to accept it. Letta Mae's veterinarian, Dr. Calico Schmitt, has now prescribed a solid dosage form of doxycycline that will hopefully be more acceptable to Letta Mae.

Contemporary Veterinarians Group Practice
20 S. Park Street, Triturate, WI 53706
Tel: (608) 555-1334 Fax: (608) 555-1336

℞ #   *123890*

NAME *Letta Mae Draheim (dog) owner: G. W. Draheim*   **DATE** *00/00/00*

ADDRESS *15805 Mercury Drive*

℞

Doxycycline   5 mg/kg/dose
M & Ft Capsules for 21 days-Put in small capsules
Sig: Give one cap bid for 21 days

Note: Letta Mae weighs 15 lbs.

G. Davidson 00/00/00

REFILLS *0*   *Calico Schmitt*   **D.V.M.**

DEA NO. _____

MASTER COMPOUNDING FORMULATION RECORD

NAME, STRENGTH, AND DOSAGE FORM OF PREPARATION: Doxycycline 34 mg Oral Veterinary Capsules

QUANTITY: 42 (plus 2 extras for loss on compounding)   **FORMULATION RECORD ID:** VT002

THERAPEUTIC USE/CATEGORY: Antibiotic   **ROUTE OF ADMINISTRATION:** Oral

INGREDIENTS USED:

Ingredient	Quantity Used	Physical Description	Solubility	Dose Comparison		Use in the Prescription
				Given	Usual	
Doxycycline 50-mg Capsules (as hyclate)	30 × 50 mg	yellow/white powder	sol in water; sl sol in alcohol	5 mg/kg bid	Dogs: 5–10 mg/kg/day	broad-spectrum antibiotic
Lactose	623 mg	white powder	1 g/5 mL water; v sl sol in alcohol	—	—	diluent

COMPATIBILITY–STABILITY: Doxycycline in manufactured capsules is in the form of doxycycline hyclate, but the labeled amount and the dose is in terms of the parent drug. In a solid dosage form, doxycycline hyclate is quite stable. As we are adding only lactose, there should be no compatibility or stability concerns.

PACKAGING AND STORAGE: The *USP* monograph for Doxycycline Hyclate Capsules recommends storage in tight, light-resistant containers. Use a tight, amber prescription vial and store at controlled room temperature.

BEYOND-USE DATE: Because the source of the active ingredient is manufactured capsules, use the recommended beyond-use date as specified in *USP* Chapter ⟨795⟩ for solid formulations made with active ingredients from manufactured drug products: no later than 25% of the time remaining until the product's expiration date or 6 months, whichever is earlier.

CALCULATIONS

Dose/Concentration

The dose of doxycycline in dogs was confirmed in *Plumb's Veterinary Drug Handbook* (2)

$$\text{Weight (in kg) of dog: } \frac{15\text{ lb}}{2.2\text{ lb/kg}} = 6.8\text{ kg}$$

$$\text{Dose (in mg): } \left(\frac{5\text{ mg doxycycline}}{\text{kg/dose}}\right)\left(\frac{6.8\text{ kg}}{}\right) = 34\text{ mg doxycycline/dose}$$

Ingredient Amounts

Calculations are for two extra capsules.

Doxycycline: 34 mg/capsule $\times$ 44 capsules = 1,496 mg

Active ingredient available: Doxycycline Hyclate Capsules, USP 50 mg (BJF Generics; Lot Y067G; Exp mm/yy)

Number of 50-mg capsules needed:

$$\frac{50\text{ mg doxycycline}}{\text{cap}} = \frac{1,496\text{ mg doxycycline}}{x\text{ caps}}; x = 29.92 \text{ or } 30 \text{ capsules}$$

Average content weight for each 50-mg capsule is 288 mg. Weight of doxycycline capsule powder needed for 44 doses:

$$\frac{50\text{ mg doxycycline}}{288\text{ mg capsule powder}} = \frac{1,496\text{ mg doxycycline}}{x\text{ mg capsule powder}}; x = 8,617\text{ mg capsule powder}$$

Weight of doxycycline capsule powder needed for each capsule:

$$8,617\text{ mg/44 caps} = 196\text{ mg/cap}$$

After Table 26.1 was consulted, capsule shell sizes 5 and 4 were tried. Unfortunately, there is too much powder for size 5 capsules and too little for size 4 capsules. Therefore, add a small amount of lactose to give 210 mg per capsule; this is the weight in milligrams given in Table 26.1 for lactose and size 4 capsules. For 44 capsules, the amount of extra lactose to add is calculated:

$$210\text{ mg/capsule} \times 44\text{ capsules} = 9,240\text{ mg}$$

$$9,240\text{ mg powder} - 8,617\text{ mg powder from doxycycline caps} = 623\text{ mg lactose}$$

MSDS AND SAFETY AND PERSONAL PROTECTIVE EQUIPMENT: Don a clean lab coat and disposable gloves.

SPECIALIZED EQUIPMENT: All weighing is done on an electronic balance.

COMPOUNDING PROCEDURE: Weigh the capsule powder for doxycycline hyclate 50-mg capsules. Each 50-mg capsule contains 288 mg of doxycycline capsule powder. Weigh 623 mg of lactose and transfer it to a glass mortar. Empty 30 doxycycline capsules and add this powder to the lactose in stepwise fashion with trituration to obtain a uniform mixture. Transfer the powder mixture to an ointment pad and punch 42 capsules using size no. 4 clear, colorless capsule shells. Tare out the weight of a weighing paper and an empty size 4 capsule shell; then weigh each filled capsule so that the powder contents weigh 210 mg. Label and dispense the capsules in a capsule vial with a child-resistant closure.

DESCRIPTION OF FINISHED PREPARATION: The preparation is fine, white powder encapsulated in no. 4 clear, colorless capsules.

QUALITY CONTROL: Each capsule is weighed to contain 210 mg $\pm$10% of powder. Adjust the content of any capsule that is outside this tolerance.

MASTER FORMULA PREPARED BY: Gigi Davidson, RPh   **CHECKED BY:** Laurel Kinosian, RPh

COMPOUNDING RECORD

NAME, STRENGTH, AND DOSAGE FORM OF PREPARATION: Doxycycline 34 mg Oral Veterinary Capsules

QUANTITY: 42 (plus 2 extra)   **DATE PREPARED:** mm/dd/yy   **BEYOND-USE DATE:** mm/dd/yy

FORMULATION RECORD ID: VT002   **CONTROL/RX NUMBER:** 123890

INGREDIENTS USED:

Ingredient	Quantity Used	Manufacturer Lot Number	Expiration Date	Weighed/ Measured by	Checked by
Doxycycline 50-mg Capsules	30 × 50 mg	BJF Generics Y067G	mm/yy	bjf	gd
Lactose	623 mg	JET Labs XY1159	mm/yy	bjf	gd

QUALITY CONTROL DATA: The powder in the capsules appears as fine, white powder. The size no. 4 clear, colorless gelatin capsules are full, with no dead space. Each capsule has been individually weighed to contain exactly 210 mg of powder.

LABELING

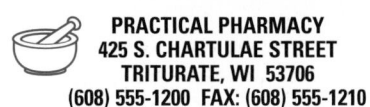

PRACTICAL PHARMACY
425 S. CHARTULAE STREET
TRITURATE, WI 53706
(608) 555-1200 FAX: (608) 555-1210

℞ 123890   Pharmacist: GD   Date: 00/00/00

Letta Mae Draheim (dog)   Dr. Calico Schmitt

owner: G. W. Draheim

Give one capsule by mouth two times daily for 21 days.

Doxycycline 34-mg Oral Veterinary Capsules

Mfg: Compounded   Quantity: 42

Refills: 0   Discard after: Give date

This medicine was compounded in our pharmacy for you at the direction of your prescriber.

PATIENT CONSULTATION: Hello, Mr. Draheim. I'm Gigi Davidson, your pharmacist. What did Dr. Schmitt tell you about this medication? This medication is the same antibiotic, doxycycline, that you tried previously in liquid form. It is used to treat infections, such as canine ehrlichiosis, that Letta Mae got from a tick. You should give Letta Mae one capsule two times a day for 21 days. You will need to open her mouth and put the capsule in the very back of her mouth at the top of her throat. Make sure she swallows the capsule and doesn't spit it out. It often helps to close her mouth and gently hold it shut while massaging her throat. Sometimes doxycycline capsules get stuck in the throat before they reach the stomach. This can cause severe burns of Letta Mae's throat, so please give her at least 6 mL—that is, a generous teaspoonful—of water to swallow or a small meatball of food to force the capsule to the stomach. You should also not let Letta Mae stay out in bright sunshine for long periods of time, because doxycycline may cause her to get sunburn on her ears and nose and any places where her fur may not completely cover her skin. It is important that you complete the full course of therapy. If her symptoms don't start to clear up within a few days, call Dr. Schmitt. Try not to miss any doses. If you should miss a dose, give it as soon as possible. However, if it is almost time for her next dose, skip the missed dose and go back to her regular dosing schedule. This medication should be stored in a cool, dry place away from children. Discard any unused portion after 6 months (or 25% of manufactured doxycycline capsule expiration date, whichever is less; give date), although you should not have any capsules left because you will be giving Letta Mae all of the capsules. There are no refills with this prescription. Do you have any questions or concerns?

REFERENCES

1. The United States Pharmacopeial Convention, Inc. USP pharmacists' pharmacopeia, 2nd ed. Rockville, MD: Author, 2008.
2. Plumb D. Plumb's veterinary drug handbook, 6th ed. Hoboken, NJ: Wiley-Blackwell, 2008.
3. Papich M. Saunders handbook of veterinary drugs, 2nd ed. Amsterdam, The Netherlands: Elsevier, 2006.
4. Wynn S. Veterinary herbal medicine. St. Louis, MO: Mosby Publishing, Inc., 2007.
5. Papich M, Riviere J, eds., Veterinary pharmacology and therapeutics, 9th ed. Hoboken, NJ: Wiley-Blackwell, 2009.
6. Boothe DM. Small animal clinical pharmacology and therapeutics. Amsterdam, The Netherlands: Elsevier, 2001.
7. Nahata MC, Morosco RS, Hipple TF. Stability of amlodipine besylate in two liquid dosage forms. J Am Pharm Assoc 1999; 39: 375–377.

Part 8

Compatibility and

Stability

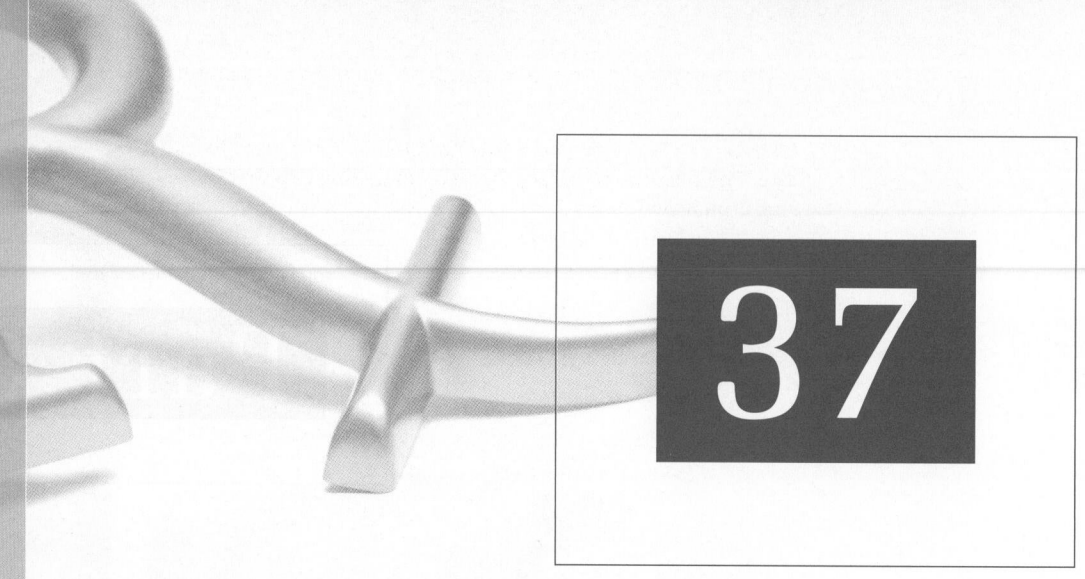

Compatibility and Stability of Drug Products and Preparations

Melgardt de Villiers, PhD

I. DEFINITIONS

A. Stability: In *USP* Chapter ⟨1191⟩ Stability Considerations in Dispensing Practice, stability is defined as "the extent to which a product retains, within specified limits, and throughout its period of storage and use (i.e., its shelf-life), the same properties and characteristics that it possessed at the time of its manufacture" (1). Chapter ⟨1191⟩ recognizes five types of stability: chemical, physical, microbiologic, therapeutic, and toxicologic (1).

Stability is determined by appropriate stability testing. The purpose of stability testing is to provide evidence on how the quality of a drug substance or drug product varies with time under the influence of a variety of environmental factors such as temperature, humidity, and light and to establish a shelf life for the drug product and recommended storage conditions.

B. Physical properties: These are the properties of drugs and dosage forms that we can see or test by physical means. Is the drug a solid, a liquid, or a gas? Is it dissolved, suspended, or emulsified, or is it adsorbed to the surface of a container? When a physical change occurs, the same drug or chemical is still present, but its physical state is altered. Pharmaceutical examples of physical changes include a drug precipitating out of solution; a drug adsorbing to the walls of a polyvinyl chloride (PVC) container; and two solid drugs forming a liquid eutectic mixture when triturated together in a mortar.

    1. From a pharmaceutical viewpoint, there are both desirable and undesirable physical changes. When we make a drug solution, we want the physical change of the solid drug dissolving in the chosen solvent. In contrast, when we have an intravenous drug solution, it is unacceptable, and perhaps lethal, for the drug to precipitate out of solution.

2. Chapter ⟨1191⟩ of the *USP* gives the following criteria for acceptable levels of physical stability: "The original physical properties, including appearance, palatability, uniformity, dissolution, and suspendability, are retained" (1).

C. **Chemical properties:** The chemical properties of drugs are those manifested by the drug's particular molecular structure. When a chemical change occurs, the original drug molecule is no longer present.

1. Recall from your study of general chemistry some of the types of reactions that occur with inorganic molecules. For example,

a. Acid-base neutralization reactions, such as:

$$NaOH + HCl \rightarrow Na^+ + Cl^- + H_2O$$

b. Oxidation-reduction reactions, such as:

$$4\,Fe + 3O_2 \rightarrow 2\,Fe_2O_3\ (rust)$$

c. Displacement reactions, such as:

$$NaCl + AgNO_3 \rightarrow Na^+ + NO_3^- + AgCl\downarrow$$

d. Release of gas, such as:

$$NaHCO_3 + HCl \rightarrow Na^+ + Cl^- + H_2O + CO_2$$

2. Most drugs are complex organic molecules, and chemical changes that occur with them are often more complicated than the simple types shown here; your study of organic and medicinal chemistry has provided you with the detailed knowledge you need to understand and to anticipate many of these changes.

3. Usually we buy drugs of a desired structure, and any change in that structure is undesirable. We then say that degradation or decomposition has occurred. Occasionally, however, we make use of a chemical change to prepare a desired drug preparation, as in making finely divided sulfur and potassium sulfide from solutions of zinc sulfate and sulfurated potash when compounding Zinc Sulfide Topical Suspension, also known as White Lotion:

$$K_2S_3 \cdot K_2S_2O_3 + ZnSO_4 \cdot 7H_2O \rightarrow ZnS + S_2 + K_2SO_4 + K_2S_2O_3 + 7H_2O$$

4. Chapter ⟨1191⟩ of the *USP* gives the following criteria for acceptable levels of chemical stability: "Each active ingredient retains its chemical integrity and labeled potency, within the specified limits" (1).

D. **Microbiologic properties:** Drug products should be free of microbiologic contamination and should resist any microbial growth.

1. Though certain products, such as parenterals and ophthalmics, are required to be sterile, all drug products should be free of microbiologic contamination.

2. For drug products that are labile to the growth of microorganisms introduced during use, preservatives should be added. Preservatives are discussed in Chapter 16, Antimicrobial Preservatives.

3. Chapter ⟨1191⟩ of the *USP* gives the following criteria for acceptable levels of microbiologic stability: "Sterility or resistance to microbial growth is retained according to the specified requirements. Antimicrobial agents that are present retain effectiveness within the specified limits" (1).

E. **References:** Table 37.1 gives a list of references that contain helpful information on compatibility and stability of drugs and drug products and preparations.

II. RESPONSIBILITY FOR PROVIDING QUALITY DRUG PRODUCTS

A. Providing the public with quality drug products is the joint responsibility of regulatory agencies such as the Food and Drug Administraiton (FDA), pharmaceutical manufacturers, and pharmacists.

B. Standards and guidelines for manufacturing, marketing, handling, and dispensing these products are set by the following:

1. Federal and state governments through agencies such as the FDA and state boards of pharmacy

2. Nonprofit groups and commissions, such as the United States Pharmacopeial Convention (USP), the National Association of Boards of Pharmacy, and the Joint Commission on Accreditation of Healthcare Organizations

Table 37.1	REFERENCES FOR COMPATIBILITY AND STABILITY INFORMATION

Books

Bing CM. *Extended Stability for Parenteral Drugs*
Connors KA, Amidon GL, Stella VJ. *Chemical Stability of Pharmaceuticals*, 2nd edition, 1986
Florey K. *Analytical Profiles of Drug Substances*
King JC. *King Guide to Parenteral Admixtures*
King RE. *Dispensing of Medication*, 1984
Nahata MC, Pai VB, Hipple TF. *Pediatric Drug Formulations*
Reynolds LA, Closson RD. *Extemporaneous Ophthalmic Preparations*
Trissel LA. *Handbook on Injectable Drugs*
Trissel LA. *Trissel's Stability of Compounded Formulations*
Trissel LA. *Trissel's Tables of Physical Compatibility*
AHFS Drug Information
ASHP Handbook on Extemporaneous Formulations, 1987 and 2003
Drug Facts and Comparisons
Drug Information Handbook
Handbook of Pharmaceutical Excipients
Martindale: The Complete Drug Reference (formerly The Extra Pharmacopoeia)
Mosby's Drug Consult
Physician Desk Reference
Remington: The Science and Practice of Pharmacy
Secundum Artem (Paddock Labs)
The Merck Index
United States Dispensatory (no longer in print)
United States Pharmacopeia/National Formulary
USP Dispensing Information (*USP/DI*), Volumes 1 and 3
USP Pharmacists' Pharmacopeia

Journals

*American Journal of Health-System Pharmacy**
Drug Development and Industrial Pharmacy
European Journal of Pharmaceutics
European Journal of Pharmaceutics and Biopharmaceutics
Hospital Formulary
Hospital Pharmacy (Lippincott Williams & Wilkins)
International Journal of Pharmaceutical Compounding
International Journal of Pharmaceutics
Journal of Pharmaceutical Sciences
Journal of Pharmacy Technology
Journal of Pharmacy and Pharmacology
*PDA Journal of Pharmaceutical Science and Technology***
Pharmaceutical Research
European Journal of Pharmaceutics
European Journal of Pharmaceutics and Biopharmaceutics

Notes: Many of these books are also available on CD-ROM or online.
Databases Searches: *International Pharmaceutical Abstracts; Medline; SciFinder Scholar from CAS Services, Micromedix.*
Information on compatibility and stability is also available from drug product manufacturers. The department to contact depends on the organization of the company: Listings of manufacturers with addresses and telephone numbers are given in the *PDR* and *Facts and Comparisons* and are also usually available on the Internet site for the company.
*Former titles include *American Journal of Hospital Pharmacy* and *Clinical Pharmacy*.
**Formerly *Journal of Parenteral Science and Technology*.

3. Professional associations, such as the American Pharmacists Association and the American Society of Health-System Pharmacists

C. Responsibility of the pharmacist

1. In its General Information Chapter ⟨1191⟩ Stability Considerations in Dispensing Practice, the *USP* clearly states that it is the pharmacist's responsibility to ensure that drug products provided to patients meet acceptable criteria of stability (1). Chapter ⟨1191⟩ is recommended reading for all pharmacy students, pharmacists, and pharmacy technicians.

   a. Chapter ⟨1191⟩ outlines those factors that affect product stability. The pharmacist should be conscious of these factors when handling and storing drug products (1).

   (1) Ingredients, whether therapeutically active or pharmaceutically necessary, can affect the stability of drug substances and dosage forms.

   (2) Environmental factors that can reduce stability include exposure to adverse temperatures, light, humidity, oxygen, and carbon dioxide.

   (3) Dosage form factors that influence drug stability include particle size (emulsions and suspensions), pH, solvent system composition (water and overall polarity), compatibility of anions and cations, solution ionic strength, primary container, chemical additives, and molecular binding between drugs and excipients.

   b. To help ensure that quality, stable pharmaceutical products are dispensed and used, the *USP* recommends that pharmacists do the following (1):

   (1) Watch for and comply with expiration dates, rotate stock, and use older products first.

   (2) Store drugs and drug products under recommended environmental conditions.

   (3) Observe products for evidence of instability.

   (4) Properly handle drugs and drug products that require extemporaneous manipulation.

   (5) Package products using recommended containers and closures.

   (6) Educate patients about the proper storage, use, and disposal of drug products and preparations.

2. The pharmacist shares a responsibility with pharmaceutical manufacturers for the stability of manufactured drug products, and pharmacists are encouraged to report to the manufacturer and to the FDA any problems with packaging, labeling, or evidence of instability in manufactured drug products. The report to the FDA can be done easily by going to its Web site at www.fda.gov. The home page has a selection for product problem reporting. A report may be submitted online or by telephone, or the paper report form can be downloaded and faxed to FDA or sent using a postage-paid addressed form. As of October 2008, the FDA program for reporting drug product problems is called *MedWatch,* but the agency changes or reorganizes its programs from time to time, so it is best to check their Web site for current information.

3. While the *USP* recognizes five types of stability, this chapter concentrates on chemical and physical stability because when these are maintained, the others follow. Microbiological stability has been discussed in previous chapters (see Chapter 17, Antimicrobial Preservations, and the Chapters in Part 6, Sterile Dosage Forms and their Preparation).

4. In the following discussion, the stability and compatibility of both manufactured products and extemporaneously compounded drug preparations are considered, but the major emphasis is on drug preparations made or manipulated by the pharmacist and pharmacy technician.

D. FDA regulation of product stability

1. The International Conference on Harmonization (ICH) of Technical Requirements for Registration of Pharmaceuticals for Human Use is a unique project that brings together the regulatory authorities of Europe, Japan, and the United States and experts from the pharmaceutical industry in the three regions to discuss scientific and technical aspects of product registration. The purpose is to make recommendations on ways to achieve greater harmonization in the interpretation and application of technical guidelines and requirements for product registration in order to reduce or obviate the need to duplicate the testing carried out during the research and development of new medicines. Within this context, ICH has developed a number of guidance documents for the stability testing of pharmaceutical products. The activities of the ICH are divided into four major topic categories, one being all the things related to chemical and pharmaceutical quality assurance of drug products. Within this category, ICH has published six guidance documents related to the stability of pharmaceutical products. These guidances include the following:

   a. Stability Testing of New Drug Substances and Products (2)

   b. Photostability Testing of New Drug Substances and Products (3)

   c. Stability Testing for New Dosage Forms (4)

2. The "Stability Testing for New Dosage Forms" is especially important for the pharmacist interested in stability testing (4). This guidance gives recommendations on what should be done

regarding stability testing of new dosage forms of known drugs that are already registered. A new dosage form is considered to be a drug product that is a different pharmaceutical product type that contains the same active substance as included in the existing approved drug product. These include products of different administration route (e.g., oral to rectal), new specific functionality/delivery systems (e.g., immediate release tablet to modified release tablet), and different dosage forms of the same administration route (e.g., capsule to tablet, solution to suspension).

III. PHYSICAL CHANGES

A. The *USP* (1) defines physical stability as the assurance that the product retains its original physical properties, including appearance, palatability, uniformity, dissolution, and suspendability, during its shelf-life.

B. Liquefaction of solid ingredients

1. Efflorescent powders: These powders contain water of hydration that may be released when the powders are triturated or when stored in an environment of low relative humidity. The water liberated when the drug or chemical is triturated may cause the powders to become damp or pasty. If water is released to the atmosphere because of low relative humidity, the drug loses its crystallinity and becomes powdery. Furthermore, if water of hydration is given off, a given weight of the resulting powder no longer contains the same amount of drug.

     a. For examples of efflorescent drugs, see Table 37.2.

     b. Strategies for handling these drugs include the following:

       (1) Store and dispense these powders in tight containers.

       (2) The anhydrous form of the drug may be substituted for the hydrate, but be sure to make appropriate dose corrections. For example, Sodium Sulfate USP is available as the decahydrate (Glauber's salt) with a molecular weight of 322. The laxative dose of Sodium Sulfate decahydrate is 15 g. If the anhydrous form is substituted (MW = 142), only 6.6 g should be used:

$$\frac{15 \text{ g Na}_2\text{SO}_4 \cdot 10 \text{ H}_2\text{O}}{322 \text{ g/mol}} = \frac{x \text{ g Na}_2\text{SO}_4 \text{ anhydrous}}{142 \text{ g/mol}} \; ; \; x = 6.6 \text{ g Na}_2\text{SO}_4 \text{ anhydrous}$$

2. Hygroscopic and deliquescent drugs: Hygroscopic drugs or chemicals are solids that absorb moisture from the air. The term deliquescent refers to hygroscopic powders that may absorb sufficient moisture to dissolve and form a solution.

     a. For examples of hygroscopic and deliquescent drugs, see Table 37.3.

     b. Strategies for handling these drugs include the following:

       (1) Store and dispense these drugs in tight containers. This means that powders dispensed as chartulae or divided powders should be sealed in plastic or foil and the packets put in tight containers. This is especially important in humid weather.

       (2) For solid compounded formulations, an inert, powdered ingredient that will preferentially absorb water may be added to the formulation. Often there are sufficient other suitable powders in the formulation to fulfill this function. If not, a suitable, inert, water-

Table 37.2	EFFLORESCENT POWDERS
Alums	Morphine acetate
Atropine sulfate	Quinine bisulfate
Caffeine	Quinine hydrobromide
Calcium lactate	Quinine hydrochloride
Citric acid	Scopolamine hydrobromide
Cocaine	Sodium acetate
Codeine	Sodium carbonate (decahydrate)
Codeine phosphate	Sodium phosphate
Codeine sulfate	Strychnine sulfate
Ferrous sulfate	Terpin hydrate

Reprinted from King RE, ed. Dispensing of medications, 9th ed. Easton, PA: Mack Publishing Co., 1984;40.

Table 37.3	**HYGROSCOPIC AND DELIQUESCENT POWDERS**
Ammonium bromide	Pepsin
Ammonium chloride	Phenobarbital sodium
Ammonium iodide	Physostigmine hydrobromide
Calcium bromide	Physostigmine hydrochloride
Calcium chloride	Physostigmine sulfate
Ephedrine sulfate	Pilocarpine alkaloid
Hydrastine hydrochloride	Potassium acetate
Hydrastine sulfate	Potassium citrate
Hyoscyamine hydrobromide	Sodium bromide
Hyoscyamine sulfate	Sodium iodide
Iron and ammonium citrate	Sodium nitrate
Lithium bromide	Zinc chloride

Reprinted from King RE, ed. Dispensing of medications, 9th ed. Easton, PA: Mack Publishing Co., 1984;40.

insoluble (e.g., not lactose) powder may be added. Light magnesium oxide is sometimes used for this purpose and is acceptable, provided the quantity needed is not sufficient to impart a therapeutic laxative effect. When you add extra ingredients, consult with the prescriber. If necessary, make adjustments to maintain the intended dose.

(3) Counsel the patient to store the product or preparation in its original tight container and in a low-humidity environment.

3. Pharmaceutical eutectic mixtures of drugs: A pharmaceutical eutectic mixture is defined as two or more substances that may liquefy when intimately mixed (as with trituration) at room temperature.

a. Under certain conditions, a "damp" powder, a pasty mass, or a liquid may result when two drugs or chemicals, which are solid at room temperature, are triturated together. This interesting phenomenon can easily be explained. It is well known that impurities present in chemicals impart melting points that are lower and less sharp than the melting point of the pure chemical. (Recall from organic chemistry lab that you checked for the purity of a compound by measuring its melting point; a clear, sharp melting point indicated pure compound.) If two or more drugs are triturated together, each may act as an impurity to the other and cause a mutual lowering of the original melting point of each individual compound. If the melting points of the pure compounds are low to begin with, the melting point of the mixture may be below room temperature, and a liquid or paste may result.

b. Whether liquefaction occurs or does not and the composition of the liquid or paste can both be analyzed using a phase diagram for the specific combination of compounds. For a more thorough discussion of this topic, consult a book of physical pharmacy (5,6). In general, liquefaction depends on the following:

(1) Ambient room temperature

(2) Original melting points of the substances

(3) Proportions in which the substances are mixed

(4) Extent and degree of pressure used in trituration

(5) Presence of other ingredients that may sorb any liquid formed

c. For examples of drugs that may form liquid eutectic mixtures, see Table 37.4.

d. There are some cases in which the formation of liquid eutectics is desirable.

(1) The local anesthetic EMLA Cream owes its success as a topical anesthetic, effective in preventing needle stick pain when drawing blood, to the high concentrations of lidocaine and prilocaine achieved by forming a liquid eutectic mixture of these two components.

(2) There are some solids that have hard crystalline structures that do not reduce to fine powder with direct trituration. An extra compounding step, known as *pulverization by intervention* (described in section V.B.2 of Chapter 25, Powders), is needed to make fine particles of this type of ingredient. However, if another ingredient in the formulation forms a liquid eutectic with this crystalline solid, the two can be triturated together, and the resulting liquid that is formed can either be adsorbed on an inert solid, as described later

Table 37.4	SUBSTANCES THAT LIQUEFY WHEN MIXED
Acetaminophen	Lidocaine
Acetanilid	Menthol
Aminopyrine	Phenacetin (Acetophenetidin)
Antipyrine	Phenol
Aspirin	Phenylsalicylate (Salol)
Benzocaine	Prilocaine
Betanaphthol	Resorcinol
Camphor	Salicylic Acid
Chloral hydrate	Thymol

or, if the formulation is a dispersed system or a semisolid, the liquid can be directly incorporated in the formulation. This circumvents the need for the pulverization by intervention step. This method is illustrated with Sample Prescription 25.2 and is demonstrated on the CD that accompanies this book.

  e. Strategies for handling drugs that form liquid eutectic mixtures include the following:

    (1) Force the liquid eutectic to form, then sorb the liquid onto an inert, high-melting, finely divided solid. This is done by triturating together the eutectic forming drugs to force the formation of the liquid; then an inert powder is added in portions with trituration to sorb the liquid. (As mentioned earlier, this method is illustrated with Sample Prescription 25.2.)

      (a) If possible, an ingredient already present in the formulation should be used to sorb the liquid.

      (b) If no suitable powder is in the formulation, an inert powder may be added. Magnesium carbonate is reported to be the agent of choice, but light or heavy magnesium oxide, calcium phosphate, starch, talc, and lactose may also be suitable (5,7).

    (2) An alternative method is to separately triturate each potential eutectic former with an inert powder, such as one of those given earlier; then the protected powders are mixed together by gentle spatulation.

    (3) When you add extra ingredients, consult with the prescriber. If necessary, make adjustments to maintain the intended dose.

C. Changes in crystal form

  1. Solid crystals are the most commonly encountered phase in pharmaceutical practice. Most pharmaceutical materials, either the active pharmaceutical ingredients or excipients, are in solid phase.

  2. The solid phase can be further classified into two major types of subphases based upon the order of molecular packing. Crystalline, in which the molecules aggregate together with both short-range and long-range orders, is probably the most well known. The amorphous form, or glass, conversely, only presents short-range order but no long-range order in the way of molecular packing.

  3. There are crystalline drugs that can exist in different crystalline structures in the solid state, although they are identical in the liquid or vapor state. Different polymorphic forms of the same substance will exhibit different physical properties, such as melting points and rates of dissolution.

    a. Examples include ampicillin, methylprednisolone, hydrocortisone, various sulfa drugs, and barbiturates.

    b. Because different polymorphs can give different dissolution rates, the use of different polymorphic forms in a solid dosage form can affect the drug's bioavailability. This is a problem that has long been recognized by the pharmaceutical industry and is one of the reasons behind bioequivalence testing to ensure equivalent therapeutic performance of solid dosage forms made by different manufacturers.

    c. The pharmacist should realize that metastable polymorphs are sometimes used in manufacturing solid dosage forms to give more rapid dissolution and improved bioavailability. Manipulation of these products in compounding may result in reversion to the more stable, less soluble, less available polymorph.

    d. One common pharmaceutical substance that is notorious because of the problems caused by its polymorphic reversions is cocoa butter. Cocoa butter has several polymorphic forms, with melting points of 18°, 24°, 28° to 31°, and 34°C. Cocoa butter is used as a base for making suppositories and must be melted when the suppositories are made by fusion. It can very easily be overheated, and when it is, it solidifies as one of the lower melting polymorphs, which may melt at room temperature, or the suppositories may liquefy when handled by the patient during insertion. To avoid this problem, cocoa butter must be melted slowly and carefully, with the temperature not exceeding 34°C. This is illustrated with Example 31.1 in Chapter 31, Suppositories.

4. Pseudopolymorphs, such as hydrates, solvates, and co-crystals, may also form when drug powder are exposed to water, solvent, or other excipients during processing. The situation with hydrates or solvates can be more complex. Compared to solvates and co-crystals, hydrates play a much more important role in drug development. A survey conducted in 1999 indicated that more than 90 hydrates were included in USP monographs (8). A similar survey done on compounds in the European Pharmacopoeia indicated that approximately 29% of 808 organic compounds can form hydrates (9).

5. The amorphous state, also called *glass,* has many important applications, and lots of intensive studies have been devoted to these solids. However, the structural elucidation of amorphous materials is still incomplete. Glasses are formed by temperature quenching, fast evaporation of solvents, lyophilization, vapor condensation, mechanical stress, and the like. Although these pathways are different, they all kinetically avoid crystallization (except for mechanical stress) and keep the molecules in the coordinations as they were in liquid state. Amorphous solids are thermodynamically less stable than are crystalline solids.

D. Precipitation from solution

  1. General principles

    a. As stated at the beginning of this chapter, unintended precipitation of an active ingredient or excipient from solution can be a major hazard with pharmaceutical solutions.

      (1) For oral or topical solutions, if an active ingredient precipitates, the particles will usually settle to the bottom of the container so that the initial doses poured from it will be subpotent and the later doses will be superpotent. This can result in either therapeutic failure or toxicity.

      (2) With intravenous solutions, the danger from precipitation can be even greater because insoluble particles can lodge in capillaries and block them, resulting in severe consequences and even death.

    b. Factors that can cause precipitation are discussed later, but it should be realized that pharmaceutical solutions are usually complex, and prediction of precipitation in them is never simple. Numerous reports in journal articles have pointed out that when reading and interpreting compatibility studies involving precipitation, all conditions of the study are relevant and may affect the outcome (10).

    c. When interpreting compatibility reports, it is important to note: (i) the manufacturers of the drugs, (ii) the drug concentrations, (iii) the base solution or diluents and their manufacturers, (iv) order of mixing, (v) time frames, (vi) temperature, and (vii) test methods. Changes in any of these factors can alter the results. Two examples:

      (1) The combination of injectable solutions of dopamine hydrochloride (12.8 mg/mL) and furosemide (5 mg/mL) had been reported to be compatible when mixed in usual IV solutions. It was later noticed that combining these same drugs in a Y-site administration gave a precipitate. It was subsequently learned that with this particular Y-site administration, one of the drug solutions was from a different manufacturer that used a different buffer, and a different pH resulted (10).

      (2) In a study testing the physical compatibility of a large number of pairs of drug solutions, it was found that while some combinations were always compatible and some combinations were always incompatible, there were some cases for which compatibility depended on the order of mixing the two drug solutions; for some, the length of time after mixing was a factor (initial, 1-hour, and 3-hour testing was done) (11).

  2. **Solvent effects:** When a drug is dissolved in a solvent and a second solvent, one in which the drug is poorly soluble, is added, the drug may precipitate.

    a. Typical examples of solvent effects:

    Topical: When water or an aqueous solution is added to an alcoholic solution of salicylic acid, precipitation may occur. (The solubility of salicylic acid is 1 g/2.7 mL of alcohol but only 1 g/460 mL water.)

Oral: When an aqueous solution or syrup is added to Phenobarbital Elixir, precipitation may occur. See Example 37.6 for information on the solubility of phenobarbital in various solvents. Injectables: Digoxin has a water solubility of 0.08 mg/mL. Digoxin Injection is available in a cosolvent system containing 40% propylene glycol and 10% alcohol. If it is diluted with an aqueous injectable solution, precipitation may occur.

Example 37.1

Another drug with similar problems is diazepam. Diazepam Injection has the following formula (12):

5 mg/mL Diazepam
40% Propylene Glycol
10% Ethanol
5% Benzoic acid/Na Benzoate
1.5% Benzyl Alcohol
qs Water pH = 6.4−6.9

Observe the data in Table 37.5 and note the following results if Diazepam Injection is diluted with an aqueous injection such as Dextrose 5% in Water (D5W). In each case, 1 mL of Diazepam Injection (that is, 5 mg of the drug) is used.

Dilute 50:50: 1 mL Diazepam Injection and 1 mL D5W (that is, 50% original), gives 5 mg/2 mL = 2.5 mg/mL, which is >0.41 mg/mL; result, precipitation.

Dilute 1:10: 1 mL Diazepam Injection and 9 mL D5W (that is, 10% original) gives 5 mg/10 mL = 0.5 mg/mL, which is >0.072 mg/mL; result, precipitation.

Dilute 1:100: 1 mL Diazepam Injection and 99 mL D5W: 5 mg/100 mL = 0.05 mg/mL, which is approximately equal to 0.056 mg/mL; result, just at the borderline.

---

b. Usually the problem occurs when water is added to an alcoholic solution of a drug that is poorly soluble in water. The reverse can also be true. For example, codeine phosphate is very soluble in water, but it is not very soluble in alcohol. If alcohol is added to an aqueous solution of codeine phosphate, the drug may precipitate. This is why cough syrups that contain a large percentage of alcohol to solubilize other water-insoluble ingredients contain codeine base rather than codeine phosphate.

c. Remember that the useful (though approximate) relationship between solubility and solvent volume-fraction is logarithmic, not linear:

$$log\ S_T = vf_{water} log\ S_{water} + vf_{sol} log\ S_{sol}$$

where:

S_T = total solubility of the drug or chemical
vf_{water} = volume fraction of water
S_{water} = solubility of the drug or chemical in water
vf_{sol} = volume fraction of the other cosolvent
S_{sol} = solubility of the drug or chemical in the cosolvent.

Table 37.5	SOLUBILITY OF DIAZEPAM IN VARYING DILUTIONS OF THE ORIGINAL FORMULATION SOLVENT AND IN WATER, D5W, AND NS
SOLVENT	**SOLUBILITY (MG/ML)**
100% original	5.2
80% original	1.6
50% original	0.41
20% original	0.11
10% original	0.072
Water	0.053
D5W	0.056
NS	0.045

Reprinted with permission from Stella VJ, Roberts RD. Unpublished results. In: Trissel LA, ed. Handbook of injectable drugs, 4th ed. Bethesda, MD: American Society of Hospital Pharmacists, 1986; XVII.

| **Example 37.2** | An acetaminophen solution is desired with a concentration of 325 mg/5 mL. The pharmacist finds the following solubility information for acetaminophen in *Remington: The Science and Practice of Pharmacy*: 1 g/70 mL water; 1 g/10 mL alcohol (13). |

1. Express the total desired solubility (S_T) and the solubility in water (S_{water}) and alcohol (S_{alc}) in common terms (e.g., mg/mL):

$$S_T = 325 \text{ mg}/5 \text{ mL} = 65 \text{ mg/mL}$$

$$S_{water} = 1 \text{ g}/70 \text{ mL} = 1,000 \text{ mg}/70 \text{ mL} = 14.3 \text{ mg/mL}$$

$$S_{alc} = 1 \text{ g}/10 \text{ mL} = 1,000 \text{ mg}/10 \text{ mL} = 100 \text{ mg/mL}$$

2. Recall that the sum of volume fractions = 1

   Therefore, $vf_{water} + vf_{alc} = 1$; and $vf_{alc} = 1 - vf_{water}$

3. Substituting in the log solubility equation just given and solving for vf_{water}:

$$\log 65 = (1 - vf_{water}) \log 100 + vf_{water} \log 14.3$$

$$1.813 = (1 - vf_{water}) (2) + vf_{water} (1.155)$$

$$1.813 = 2 - 2 \, vf_{water} + 1.155 \, vf_{water}$$

$$0.845 \, vf_{water} = 0.187$$

$$vf_{water} = 0.187/0.845 = 0.22, \text{ or } 22\% \text{ water and } 78\% \text{ alcohol}$$

Remember that this equation is for pure systems containing the drug and the cosolvent system and that the result is just a good estimate. In formulation situations, we usually have other ingredients present, such as sweeteners, flavors, and other active ingredients and excipients. These factors alter the conditions and the results. The use of this equation is illustrated in Sample Prescription 27.5 in Chapter 27, Solutions.

---

    d. Compounding strategies when adding additional solvents to a drug solution
        (1) To maintain a true solution, be sure you are using an appropriate solvent system.
            (a) For solubilities, consult appropriate references, such as *Remington: The Science and Practice of Pharmacy* or *The Merck Index*. If necessary, you may calculate approximate required solvent ratios using the log solubility equation given earlier.
            (b) If you need to make an aqueous dilution of an injectable drug solution that contains a drug in a cosolvent system, follow the manufacturer's instructions in the product package insert or recommendations in a reference, such as *Trissel's Handbook of Injectable Drugs*. For example, a manufacturer of Digoxin Injection recommends that it be diluted with at least a fourfold volume of Sterile Water for Injection or the equivalent.
            (c) If information is not available, make a reasonable dilution and observe the solution for a period of time, or dilute the product so that the final concentration of the drug is below its saturation concentration. In all cases, observe the solution and be sure to give sufficient time for redissolution if precipitation occurs.
            (d) Decrease the drug concentration so that the drug is soluble in the solvent system. For systemic medications, remember that if you change the concentration of the active ingredient(s) in the preparation, you must change the volume of the dose administered to give the same quantity of drug.
        (2) For oral or topical products, you may wish to make a suspension. A suspending agent may be required. Remember that a "Shake Well" label is required for dispersed systems.
        (3) If you make a substantive change, you should first consult the prescriber.
    3. **pH Effects:** Most drugs are weak electrolytes (weak acids or weak bases), and their degree of ionization (i.e., the relative concentration of drug in its salt [charged] form versus its neutral [uncharged] form) depends on the pH of the solution. When there is a large difference in the solubilities of the two forms, as is usually the case, a problem may occur when you alter the pH of the solution. This can happen when drug solutions with differing pH's are combined or when a drug that generates a different pH is added to the original drug solution.

| Example 37.3 | The two compounds shown here are examples of drugs that are weak electrolytes; chlorpromazine is a neutral weak base, and phenobarbital is a neutral weak acid. Solutions of these drugs and others like them are often given by injection where precipitation of the drug could be dangerous and even fatal. |

1. Chlorpromazine HCl (protonated salt form): solubility 1 g/2.5 mL water

   Chlorpromazine base (neutral uncharged form): insoluble in water

The foregoing chemical structure shows the neutral free base (water-insoluble) form of the drug; the hydrochloride salt form has a proton (H^+) on the amine nitrogen, giving a positively charged, water-soluble molecule. So here you have a drug with high water solubility in its salt form and low water solubility in its free base form. If you have an aqueous solution of Chlorpromazine HCl (e.g., Chlorpromazine HCl Injection, pH = 3 to 5) and you were to raise the pH of the solution, some of the salt form of the drug would be converted to the neutral free form. If the concentration of neutral form exceeds its water solubility, precipitation will occur.

2. Phenobarbital Na (salt form): 1 g/mL water

   Phenobarbital (neutral acid form): 1 g/1,000 mL water

This chemical structure shows the neutral free acid (water-insoluble) form of the drug; the sodium salt form is a water-soluble ionic compound with a Na^+ in place of one of the imide hydrogens. Again, you have a drug with high water solubility in its salt form and low water solubility in its neutral free form, but this time you have the opposite salt type—the salt of a weak acid rather than the salt of a weak base. In this case, if you have an aqueous solution of phenobarbital Na (e.g., Phenobarbital Na Injection, pH = 9.2 to 10.2) and were to lower the pH of the solution, some of the salt form of the drug would be converted to the neutral free acid form. If the concentration of phenobarbital acid exceeds its water solubility, precipitation will occur.

When working with drugs and drug products such as these, it is very important to determine the potential for problems if you need to combine, dilute, or manipulate these drugs. To make this determination, you need to look up information about the drug, use your knowledge of chemistry, and in some cases perform some calculations. Consider the following steps in this process.

    a. **Check the solubilities of all the drugs in the solvents involved** (that is, the solubilities of both the salt and free forms in the desired solvent or solvent system).

        (1) Even if you have a lot of experience with drugs and their solubilities, this information is not always intuitive; in fact, it can be rather surprising. For example, codeine and morphine have chemical structures that are quite similar, yet codeine base has a water solubility of 1 g/120 mL, whereas the water solubility of morphine base is 1 g/5,000 mL.

        (2) Sometimes both the salt and the free form are soluble in water and other pharmaceutical solvents, such as alcohol. If this is the case, precipitation will not be a problem with

a change in pH or solvent system. For example, both ephedrine base and ephedrine HCl are soluble in both water and alcohol.

(3) The solvent system involved is important. In the chlorpromazine and phenobarbital examples given earlier, there is a good possibility for precipitation if the pH is altered in an unfavorable direction. If, however, the solvent system contains sufficient alcohol, precipitation may not occur—even with a change in pH—if the neutral form is sufficiently soluble in the alcohol-water cosolvent system.

b. Determine the salt type of the drug: Is the drug in solution the salt of a neutral weak acid or a neutral weak base? In aqueous solutions, precipitation occurs when the salt form is converted to the neutral free form by a change in pH (that is, by raising the pH for the salts of weak bases and by lowering the pH for salts of weak acids). You need to know the salt type of your drug to know whether a pH change will be problematic. Because determination of salt type can be difficult, a brief discussion of this with some helpful hints is given in Figure 37.1. For a more thorough discussion of this topic, you may want to read the applicable section in the book *Thermodynamics of Pharmaceutical Systems: An Introduction for Students of Pharmacy* (14).

c. Estimate the resultant pH of the solution. This may be done by checking an appropriate reference or by actual measurement.

(1) If you are adding a pure chemical, check the monograph in *Remington: The Science and Practice of Pharmacy* or *The Merck Index* for the pH of an aqueous solution of that chemical.

(2) If you are adding a manufactured drug solution, the product package insert or a reference such as *Trissel's Handbook of Injectable Drugs* often gives helpful information. Drug products often are buffered for stability or solubility purposes, and the pH of their solutions is different than if just pure drug were present in solution.

(3) It is helpful to learn examples of widely used classes of drugs that have distinctly acid or basic pH's. This is especially true for pharmacists and pharmacy technicians who work with IV admixtures. The lists following give some examples of injectable drug solutions that have distinctly acidic or basic pH's:

Drug Solutions That Have Acid pH's

> Phenothiazines
> Tetracycline HCl
> Ascorbic Acid
> Glycopyrrolate
> Metaraminol Bitartrate
> Morphine Sulfate

Drug Solutions That Have Basic pH's

> Phenytoin Na
> Aminophylline
> Sodium Bicarbonate
> Sodium Barbiturates

(4) Though you should be careful when adding any vehicle or diluent that may affect the pH, be aware that buffer capacity is important. Most drugs and drug solutions have sufficient buffer capacity to overwhelm the pH effects of a neutral, unbuffered liquid vehicle or large-volume parenteral (LVP) solution. Relative amounts may be critical. Erythromycin lactobionate IV is a good example of a product in which solubility is very sensitive both to pH and to concentration when sterile diluent is added for reconstitution.

(5) The pH of the resultant solution under consideration can be checked using pH paper or strips or a pH meter.

d. Calculate the pH of precipitation. If it seems as if there may be a problem, you can calculate the pH of precipitation for the drug or drugs involved. First look up the pK_a(s) of the drug(s) under consideration. The Appendices section of the CD that accompanies this book has a long list of pK_a's for drugs and chemicals. Other useful references include books of medicinal chemistry, *Trissel's Stability of Compounded Formulations*, and *The Merck Index*. Then use this information to calculate the pH of precipitation using the appropriate equation given here. Compare this calculated limiting pH with the estimated pH in item **c.** heretofore.

First consider some common misconceptions about determining acid-base character of organic compounds.

Misconception #1:   If a drug solution has a pH below 7, the drug must be a neutral weak acid, and if the pH of the drug solution is above 7, the drug must be a neutral weak base.

Fact: You cannot tell whether the parent drug is a neutral weak acid or base from the pH of its solutions.

1. It is true that when a pure compound is dissolved in water, if it is a neutral weak acid, the solution will have a pH below 7, and a neutral weak base will give a pH above 7. However, often the neutral species has limited water solubility, so it is usually the salt form that is dissolved, and then the pH of a solution of the salt form varies with the compound.

Examples of some compounds and their salts with pH values of their solutions are given here. Note the variability.

   Benzoic Acid, a neutral weak acid, pH of 2.8.
   Salt form, Sodium Benzoate, pH of about 8.

   Salicylic Acid, a neutral weak acid, pH of 2.4.
   Salt form, Sodium Salicylate, pH of between 5–6.

   Phenol, a neutral weak acid, pH of approximately 6.

   Chlorpromazine, a neutral weak base with alkaline reaction.
   Salt form, Chlorpromazine HCl, pH of about 4.0–5.5.

2. Most manufactured drug solutions, such as injections, have their pH adjusted (e.g., with buffers) to a value for maximum solubility and/or stability of the drug.

Examples:

   Cimetidine Injection USP, which is Cimetidine Hydrochloride in Water for Injection, has a pH of 3.8 to 6.0; Cimetidine is a neutral weak base.

   Glycopyrrolate Injection USP has a pH between 2.0 and 3.0; Glycopyrrolate is neither an acid nor a base, it is a quaternary ammonium compound.

   Pentobarbital Sodium Injection USP has a pH between 9.0 and 10.5; Pentobarbital is a neutral weak acid.

Misconception #2:   If a drug has a reported pK_a, it must be a neutral weak acid because pK_b's are reported for neutral weak bases.

Fact: The pK values for both neutral weak acids and neutral weak bases are generally reported as pK_a's. The pK_a value reported for a neutral weak base is actually the pK value for the conjugate acid form of the base. For conjugate acid–base pairs the relationship is:

$$pK_w = pK_a + pK_b$$

Furthermore, one cannot tell from the numerical value of the pK_a whether the compound is a neutral weak acid or a neutral weak base. The following is true:

1. For neutral weak acids, as pK_a decreases, acid strength increases.

2. For neutral weak bases, as the pK_b decreases (and the pK_a of the conjugate acid form increases), base strength increases.

Examples:

Neutral weak acids: Carboxylic acids have pK_a's in the range of 2–6 and are relatively stronger acids than are phenols with pK_a's in the range of 7–11 and thiols with pK_a's in the range of 7–10.

Neutral weak bases: Aliphatic amines have pK_a's in the range of 8–11 (that is, the pK_a of their conjugate acid form) and are relatively stronger bases than are aromatic amines with pK_a's in the range of 4–7.

You cannot tell anything from a numerical value of a pK_a unless you know, using other evidence (such as chemical structure), that the compound in question is a neutral weak acid or is a neutral weak base.

FIGURE 37.1. HOW TO DETERMINE WHETHER A DRUG IS A NEUTRAL WEAK ACID OR A NEUTRAL WEAK BASE.

Misconception #3:   Since HCl, H_2SO_4, HNO_3, acetic acid, etc., are all acids, therefore, salts that are hydrochlorides, sulfates, nitrates, acetates, etc. must be salts of neutral weak acids.

Fact: The opposite is generally true; compounds that are hydrochlorides, sulfates, nitrates, etc. are usually the salts of neutral weak bases, because salts are formed from the reaction of an acid and a base.

How then can you tell if a compound is a neutral weak acid or a neutral weak base?

1. There are some functional groups that we readily recognize as having essentially neither acidic nor basic properties when in aqueous solution. Examples include, alcohols (R-OH) and polyols (e.g., sugars), ethers (ROR′), esters (RCOOR′), aldehydes (RCHO), ketones (RCOR′), and amides ($RCONH_2$).

2. There are other functional groups that we recognize are acids or have some acidic character. Examples include carboxylic acids (RCOOH), sulfonic acids (RSO_3H), phenols (ArOH), thiols (RSH), and imides (RCONHCOR′).

3. There are some functional groups that we recognize as bases or have some basic character. Examples include aliphatic amines ($R\text{-}NH_2$) and aromatic amines (either $ArNH_2$ or nitrogen as part of an aromatic ring structure).

4. Still, because drug molecules are complex structures, it is often difficult to look at the structure of a drug molecule and decide if it is a weak acid, a weak base, or neither. When this is true, a handy trick is to take note of the name of its salt form and use this information in making a determination.

Recall that in forming a salt, we combine an acid and a base; so consider the following:

Acid	+	Base	=	Salt
Mineral Acids	+	**Neutral Weak Bases**	=	Salt of the neutral weak base
HCl		Ranitidine		Ranitidine HCl
HBr		Homatropine		Homatropine HBr
H_2SO_4		Morphine		Morphine Sulfate
HNO_3		Pilocarpine		Pilocarpine Nitrate
H_3PO_4		Codeine		Codeine Phosphate
Organic Acids				
Malic Acid		Chlorpheniramine		Chlorpheniramine Maleate
Citric Acid		Clomiphene		Clomiphene Citrate
Neutral Weak Acids	+	Hydroxide Bases	=	Salt of the neutral weak acid
Phenobarbital		NaOH		Sodium Phenobarbital
Clavulanic Acid		KOH		Potassium Clavulenate
Saccharic Acid		$Ca(OH)_2$		Calcium Saccharate

It can be observed from the above that for the salts of the mineral and organic acids, the parent drug compound is a neutral weak base, and for salts of the hydroxide bases, the parent drug compound is a neutral weak acid. Therefore, when you encounter a drug that has as its salt form a sodium, potassium, calcium, or magnesium salt, the drug itself is most likely a neutral weak acid. Similarly for a salt that is a hydrochloride, sulfate, phosphate, maleate, tartarate, etc., the parent compound is likely a neutral weak base. There are 3 notable exceptions, so when making a final determination, the chemical structure of the drug must be known. In each of the following cases, the drugs are neither neutral weak acids nor neutral weak bases, and they are not subject to precipitation of a neutral form by a change in pH.

1. In some cases, an active drug compound is combined with an organic acid to give an ester rather than a salt. Examples would be desoxycortisone acetate, clobetasol proprionate, and erythromycin stearate.

2. For some halides, the resulting compound is a quaternary ammonium compound; that is nitrogen covalently bonded to four -R groups with no dissociable proton. Two examples are benzalkonium chloride and demecarium bromide.

3. Some compounds, such as sodium lauryl sulfate, are salts of strong acids and strong bases, and they are not sensitive to pH changes.

FIGURE 37.1. HOW TO DETERMINE WHETHER A DRUG IS A NEUTRAL WEAK ACID OR A NEUTRAL WEAK BASE. (*Continued*)

(1) For salts of weak bases use:

$$pK_a = pH - log\left(\frac{S_o}{S_T - S_o}\right)$$

(2) For salts of weak acids use:

$$pK_a = pH - log\left(\frac{S_T - S_o}{S_o}\right)$$

where:

pK_a = the pK_a of the drug (conjugate acid form)
S_T = the final total concentration of the drug in solution
S_o = the solubility of the neutral free form of the drug
pH = the limit of pH beyond which precipitation will occur at the given value of S_T (i.e., precipitation occurs at pH values lower than this limit for weak acids, but at pH values above this limit for weak bases)

(3) In using these equations, note that while technically the foregoing concentrations should be expressed in molar units, for the purposes of estimation used in compounding, a weight basis such as mg/mL or w/v% is often used. If more exact estimations are desired, molar quantities should be employed.

(4) Note also that while the pH of precipitation depends on three factors, two of them, the pK_a of the drug and the solubility of the free form (S_o), are properties of the drug and cannot be changed (in a given solvent).

(5) The third factor, the desired final drug concentration (S_T), varies with the situation. It is important to be aware of this when using references such as the *Handbook of Injectable Drugs*. Notice that the C/I (compatibility/incompatibility) rating in this reference is given for a particular drug concentration and for a particular vehicle. If these conditions are changed, there may or may not be a problem. Furthermore, in using these ratings, one may think that if a high concentration, such as 500 mg/L, shows compatibility, then surely a lower, more dilute concentration should be acceptable. This is usually but not always true. Injections usually contain buffers, and sometimes smaller volumes of drug solutions do not have sufficient buffer capacity to maintain the pH at the desired level for solubility when another drug or solution is added.

Example 37.4

In what pH range is it possible to prepare an aqueous solution of chlordiazepoxide having a concentration of 10 mg/5 mL?

1. The solubility of chlordiazepoxide (free base) is 1 g in >10,000 mL of water; this is, S_o. Chlordiazepoxide HCl is very soluble in water—1 g/10 mL.
2. Chlordiazepoxide has the chemical structure given here:

This drug is a neutral weak base. The water-soluble salt form of chlordiazepoxide is Chlordiazepoxide HCl, with an extra proton on the amine nitrogen.

3. From literature sources, $pK_a = 4.6$.
4. Express the total desired solubility (S_T) and the limiting solubility of the free base (S_o) in common terms (e.g., in percent):

$$S_T = 10 \text{ mg/5 mL} = 200 \text{ mg/100 mL} = 0.2 \text{ g/100 mL} = 0.2\%$$

$$S_o = 1 \text{ g/10,000 mL} = 0.01 \text{ g/100 mL} = 0.01\%$$

5. Using the equation for neutral weak bases, calculate the pH of precipitation:

$$pK_a = pH - log\left(\frac{S_o}{S_T - S_o}\right)$$

$$pH = 4.6 + log\left(\frac{0.01}{0.2 - 0.01}\right) = 4.6 + log\left(\frac{0.01}{0.19}\right)$$

$$pH = 4.6 + log\, 0.0526$$

$$pH = 4.6 - 1.279 = 3.3$$

Therefore, the drug is soluble at this desired concentration at any pH **below** 3.3; above this pH, precipitation will occur.

You can confirm that this is a reasonable solution by consulting the monograph for Chlordiazepoxide HCl Injection in the *Handbook of Injectable Drugs*. Here the desired concentration of the drug is higher (5%), and the formulators of the injectable product use both low pH (2.5–3.5) and a cosolvent system of water and propylene glycol to solubilize the drug (15).

---

   e. Possible strategies for handling solutions of weak electrolytes
   (1) If possible, control the pH at a desirable level. Though this sounds simple, in practice it may be more difficult. For example, most of the vehicles for oral solutions have pH's in the acid range, so if you want to make an oral solution of a drug that is a neutral weak acid (e.g., phenobarbital), this could be a problem. One possibility is to add a pH adjusting agent or a buffer. This is discussed in Chapter 18, Buffers and pH Adjusting Agents.
   (2) Keep drug solutions with incompatible pH's separate.
      (a) For IM injections, draw the drug solutions in separate syringes and give in different sites.
      (b) For IV injections, give at different times and flush the IV line between additions of the incompatible drug solutions. In some cases, multiple-lumen tubing may be used.
   (3) With oral or topical solutions, a cosolvent may be used if a suitable one that is available will keep the free form of the drug in solution.

Example 37.5   As shown in Example 37.3, the sodium salt of phenobarbital is soluble in water, but the neutral free acid is poorly soluble in water. If you were to dissolve the salt form in water and then add a liquid vehicle that has a low pH, the neutral free acid form would precipitate. This is the case with many oral flavored syrups because their pH's are in the range of 2.5 to 4.5. Alcohol can be added as a cosolvent to keep the free acid in solution. Table 37.6 show the percentage of alcohol needed to maintain the solubility of varying concentrations of phenobarbital at various pH ranges (16). Consider the following prescription order:

   Phenobarbital   15 mg/5mL

   Flavored Elixir   qs ad   100 mL

The pharmacy has available Alcohol USP and flavored, sweetened orange syrup, which contains no alcohol and has a pH of 3. Using the information in Table 37.6, calculate the amount of Alcohol USP that will be needed in this formulation to keep the phenobarbital in solution.

1. Note that the concentrations of phenobarbital in the table are given as a w/v%, so first convert the concentration of phenobarbital from 15 mg/5 mL to w/v%:

$$\frac{0.015\ g\ phenobarbital}{5\ mL\ solution} = \frac{x\ g\ phenobarbital}{100\ mL\ solution};\, x = 0.3\ g/100\ mL = 0.3\ \%$$

2. In Table 37.6, look in pH column 2 to 6 (the pH of our vehicle is 3) and find the concentration closest to 0.3%. The chart shows that at pH = 2 to 6; a 0.27% phenobarbital solution requires 20% alcohol to maintain a solution, so approximately 20% alcohol is needed to maintain the solubility of our 0.3% phenobaribital solution.

3. Calculate the amount of alcohol (that is, C_2H_5OH) that is needed for this preparation:

$$20\% \times 100\ mL = 20\ mL$$

Table 37.6	SOLUBILITY[a] OF PHENOBARBITAL IN ALCOHOL-AQUEOUS SYSTEMS AT VARIOUS pH VALUES				
			PH		
ALCOHOL, % (v/v)	2–6	7	8	9	10
0	0.11[b]	0.17	0.41	1.40	2.90
5	0.12	0.18	0.41	1.19	2.71
10	0.16	0.22	0.41	1.01	2.53
15	0.20	0.26	0.41	0.94	2.53
20	0.27	0.33	0.49	0.94	2.15
25	0.40	0.47	0.63	1.01	1.99
30	0.61	0.70	0.85	1.15	1.98
35	0.94	1.03	1.16	1.40	2.07
40	1.46	1.45	1.60	1.80	2.28
45	1.94	2.10	2.20	2.36	2.64
50	2.68	2.84	3.02	3.20	3.49

[a]Solubility was determined at 25 ± 0.02°.
[b]Denotes % phenobarbital (w/v).
Reprinted with permission from Urdang A, Leuallen EE. The effect of pH upon the solubility of phenobarbital in alcohol-aqueous solutions. JAPhA Sci Ed 1956;45:526.

4. Alcohol USP contain 95% alcohol. Calculate the number of mL of Alcohol USP that will give 20 mL of C_2H_5OH:

$$\frac{95 \text{ mL } C_2H_5OH}{100 \text{ mL Alcohol USP}} = \frac{20 \text{ mL } C_2H_5OH}{x \text{ mL Alcohol USP}}; x = 21 \text{ mL Alcohol USP}$$

5. Dissolve the phenobarbital (300 mg for 100 mL of preparation) in 21 mL of Alcohol USP and qs ad 100 mL with orange syrup.

The amount of alcohol needed can often be reduced by the use of a third cosolvent such as glycerin or propylene glycol. Notice in Table 37.7 that the concentration of alcohol can be reduced to 10% by adding 20% glycerin (17). This is particularly useful when making solutions for pediatric patients for whom the alcohol content should be minimal. (**Note:** A similar but more complex example is given on the CD ROM in the section Practice Calculations, Special Calculations Involving Alcohol.)

Table 37.7	SOLUBILITY OF PHENOBARBITAL IN ALCOHOL-GLYCERIN-WATER SYSTEMS AT 25°C										
					GLYCERIN						
ALCOHOL	0%	10%	20%	30%	40%	50%	60%	70%	80%	90%	100%
0%	0.12	0.19	0.20	0.21	0.23	0.28	0.37	0.48	0.66	0.82	1.16
10%	0.19	0.22	0.30	0.37	0.50	0.64	0.84	1.14	1.59	2.25	
20%	0.30	0.42	0.57	0.83	1.13	1.54	2.11	2.77	4.13		
30%	0.64	0.93	1.35	1.89	2.67	3.45	4.45	6.79			
40%	1.46	2.16	2.87	4.09	5.37	6.83	9.40				
50%	3.21	4.26	5.57	7.18	9.29	12.01					
60%	5.33	7.47	9.19	11.23	14.25						
70%	8.53	10.73	12.75	15.74							
80%	11.56	13.58	16.27								
90%	13.38	15.30									
100%	12.30										

Note: Where the sum of the percentages of alcohol and glycerin mixtures does not equal 100, the difference is water. Where the sum equals 100, no water is present in such mixtures.
Reprinted with permission from Krause GM, Cross JM. Solubility of phenobarbital in alcohol-glycerin-water systems. JAPhA Sci Ed 1951;40:139.

(4) For oral or topical solutions, check on the possibility of making a suspension.

(5) Dilute the final solution so that the concentration of the drug is below the precipitation concentration of the neutral free form.

(6) For injectable drugs that are sensitive to pH changes caused by absorption of CO_2, use short expiration times. Examples include Phenytoin Sodium Injection and Aminophylline Injection.

4. Formation of sparingly soluble salts: When a drug is dissolved in a solvent and another drug that is added forms a sparingly soluble salt with the first drug, precipitation can occur. Precipitation of sparingly soluble salts is actually a chemical rather than a physical change because a new compound is formed, but this subject is included here for completeness in the area of drug precipitations.

a. Inorganic precipitates

(1) Remember the general solubility product equation for sparingly soluble salts:

$$A_nB_m \rightarrow nA^{+m} + mB^{+n}$$

$$K_{sp} = [A^{+m}]^n [B^{+n}]^m$$

where precipitation occurs when K_{sp} is exceeded.

(2) Some typical pharmacy examples are shown here (shown as associations rather than dissociations):

$$Ag^+ + Cl^- \rightarrow AgCl \downarrow$$

$$Ca(Gluconate)_2 + K_2HPO_4 \rightarrow CaHPO_4 \downarrow + 2K^+ + 2\,gluconate^{-1}$$

(3) The example given here with the calcium phosphate can be a serious problem with parenteral nutrition (PN) solutions. In spring 1994, the FDA issued an alert after deaths attributed to the administration of PN solutions containing precipitated calcium phosphate. (See Figure 35.1 in Chapter 35, Total Parenteral Nutrition. Note that it is an especially difficult problem to handle because precipitation in these situations depends on so many factors; the *Handbook of Injectable Drugs* lists nine contributing factors, including pH, order of mixing, temperature, calcium salt used, and other ingredients present (15). A more thorough description of the factors involved is given in Chapter 35.

(4) General solubilities for inorganic salts are given in Table 37.8.

Table 37.8   SOLUBILITIES OF INORGANIC SALTS

CATIONS	Na	K	NH₄	Mg	Ca	Sr	Ba	Al Mn²⁺	Cr³⁺ Cu²⁺	Fe³⁺ Bi³⁺	Zn²⁺ Hg²⁺	Co²⁺	Ni²⁺ Cd²⁺	Ag	Pb²⁺	Hg⁺
Anions-NO₂	S	S	S	S	S	S	S	S	S	S	S	S	S	S	S	S
—Ac	S	S	S	S	S	S	S	S	S	S	S	S	S	S	S	S
—Cl	S	S	S	S	S	S	S	S	S	S	S	S	I	I	I	I
—SO₄	S	S	S	S	I	I	I	S	S	S	S	S	I	I	I	I
—CO₃	S	S	S	I	I	I	I	I	I	I	I	I	I	I	I	I
—PO₄	S	S	S	I	I	I	I	I	I	I	I	I	I	I	I	I
—S	S	S	S	I	I	I	I	I	I	I	I	I	I	I	I	I
—OH	S	S	S	I	I	I	I	I	I	I	I	I	I	I	I	I

S, soluble. I, insoluble. Soluble in this table includes the *USP* designations of *very soluble* (1 part of solute in less than 1 part of solvent), *freely soluble* (1 in 1 to 10), *soluble* (1 in 10 to 30), and *sparingly soluble* (1 in 30 to 100). Insoluble includes the *USP* designations of *slightly soluble* (1 in 100 to 1,000), *very slightly soluble* (1 in 1000 to 10,000), and *practically insoluble*, or *insoluble* (1 in more than 10,000).

Reprinted from King RE, ed. Dispensing of medications, 9th ed. Easton, PA: Mack Publishing Co., 1984;335.

b. Precipitation of large cation/large anion compounds

(1) Examples include heparin sodium, large antibiotic molecules such as gentamicin sulfate and kanamycin sulfate, quaternary ammonium compounds such as benzalkonium chloride, phenylmercuric nitrate, and many others. For example:

$$\text{Heparin Na} + \text{Gentamicin SO}_4 \rightarrow \text{ppt} \downarrow$$

(2) Strategies for handling possible precipitation

(a) Check the drug product inserts and available literature. As discussed in the beginning of this section, pay attention to all the details of the test conditions in compatibility reports.

(b) If no information is available, make test solutions first. When combining solutions, carefully monitor for precipitation and observe for a sufficient length of time. Precipitation often is not immediately apparent.

(c) If there will be a change in temperature during storage or use, be sure to test under these conditions also.

(d) If there is any doubt about compatibility, keep the solutions separate. For IM injections, draw the drug solutions in separate syringes and give in different sites. For IV injections, give at different times and flush the IV line between additions of the incompatible drug solutions. In some cases, multiple-lumen tubing may be used. Be especially carefully with Heparin solutions; they are often used as IV flush solutions, and Heparin is incompatible with many other drugs.

c. Drugs with unusual counter ions

(1) Any time you have a drug that is an organic salt with a special or unusual counter ion, such as mesylate, lactate, succinate, and the like, be cautious when adding a solution of another salt. When a drug manufacturer uses a special salt form, there is a good reason for this, and one reason is that the hydrochloride, sulfate, or other more common salt form of the drug is less soluble. Precipitation is dependent on concentrations and may also vary with other factors, such as a pH. Very often such combinations are compatible, but it is wise to be cautious.

(2) One example of this phenomenon involves the drug dihydroergotamine (DHE) mesylate. There was a published formula for this drug in a nasal solution with sodium chloride as the tonicity adjustor, but when the formula was attempted, there was precipitation of the hydrochloride salt of DHE owing to the addition of the sodium chloride.

d. Alkaloidal precipitants

(1) Alkaloids include a wide variety of amine drugs of plant origin. Some of our older and more widely used drugs, such as atropine, cocaine, codeine, colchicine, morphine, and ephedrine, are alkaloids. Many are complex molecules that contain other functional groups. Many years ago, when there was a more limited knowledge of the chemistry of these compounds, pharmacists would memorize lists of compounds that would cause alkaloids to precipitate from solution. These included citrate salts, tannins from wild cherry syrup, iodide, and picric acid. Although some of these reactions are simply caused by precipitation of the neutral free base as a result of a change in pH of the solution, other precipitations result from unique reactions.

(2) Possible strategies for handling alkaloidal precipitants vary with the compounds involved. Some pharmaceutical reference books, especially older editions, can be helpful. Often the addition of alcohol or glycerin prevents precipitation.

5. Colloids and polymers

a. Solutions of hydrophilic polymers such as methylcellulose and acacia depend on hydration through hydrogen-bonding and ion-dipole interactions. These polymers may be dehydrated and precipitated by concentrated electrolyte solutions (especially polyvalent ions) or phenolic compounds. Strategies for handling this type of problem include decreasing the concentration of the electrolyte and/or substituting another polymer gum that is not as easily dehydrated. This subject is discussed in Chapter 19, Viscosity-Inducing Agents.

b. For some viscosity-increasing polymers, interactions are required to form the desired gel. For example, sodium alginate is gelled with calcium ions, and carbomer is gelled by the addition of an inorganic (e.g., NaOH) or organic (e.g., triethanolamine) base. These gels are sensitive to the addition of some other additives or to changes in pH.

c. Regular amphotericin B forms a colloidal dispersion when reconstituted as directed. Preservative-free Sterile Water for Injection is required. The dispersion may then be diluted with Dextrose 5% in Water (D5W). The colloidal dispersion is very sensitive to pH, so the added

D5W must have a pH of at least 4.2. Buffers are present in the amphotericin B formulation to raise the pH of the final solution above 5.0 if the D5W has a pH of at least 4.2; if not, a sterile buffer must be added. The formula for a suitable phosphate buffer is given in the amphotericin B monograph in the *Handbook of Injectable Drugs* (15).

   d. Erythromycin lactobionate IV has restrictions similar to those of amphotericin B. The solubility and stability of the reconstituted erythromycin lactobionate IV solution are concentration-dependent; this is why different reconstitution instructions are given for the vial (in which a 5% solution results) and the piggyback (in which 0.5% solution is made).

  6. Effect of temperature

   a. The solubility of most drugs decreases as the temperature of the solution decreases.

    (1) Refrigeration is often recommended for solutions of drugs to increase their chemical stability or retard microbial growth, but this may cause problems with precipitation.

    (2) Parenteral drugs for which refrigeration is not recommended because of problems with precipitation include fluorouracil (5-FU), cisplatin, cotrimoxazole, metronidazole, and some brands of aminophylline.

   b. The opposite, though uncommon, can also be true. One example is the precipitation of dibasic calcium phosphate in parenteral nutrition solutions. Calcium phosphate and dibasic calcium phosphate are equilibrium products that result when calcium gluconate and potassium phosphate are added to PN solutions. Although at room temperature these products may be below the critical concentration for precipitation, if the PN solution is placed in a warm environment, such as a neonate crib, the insoluble dibasic calcium phosphate may precipitate from the solution. This unusual phenomenon is due to the fact that the calcium gluconate is more completely dissociated at higher temperatures, and this increases the concentration of calcium ion present in solution and leads to precipitation with the phosphate.

   c. Strategies for preventing precipitation of drug solutions sensitive to temperature changes

    (1) For injectable solutions, check the product package insert or a reference such as the *Handbook on Injectable Drugs*. Warnings concerning temperature effects on precipitation are found in these references. If an extemporaneously prepared sterile product cannot be refrigerated, the beyond-use date often needs adjustment.

    (2) For oral or topical solutions, be aware of possible problems when handling solutions at or near the saturation point. If such a solution must be stored or used at a temperature different from that at which it is made, appropriate steps to prevent or handle precipitation may be necessary. Patients should be alerted to this possibility and counseled about observing preparations that are refrigerated.

E. Sorption and leaching

  1. Sorption

   a. Sorption of drugs to containers, closures, IV tubing, bacterial filters, and administration devices can be a problem. Because this reaction cannot be seen, it was not originally recognized. Even now, this reaction cannot be detected by visual examination.

   b. Adsorption versus absorption: **Adsorption** is solely a surface phenomenon; molecules are concentrating at the interface between phases (liquid-liquid, liquid-solid, gas-solid). In contrast, with **absorption,** the molecules being absorbed are penetrating into the capillary spaces of the absorbing phase (6). Often we do not know whether absorption or adsorption is occurring, so the more general term, *sorption*, is used. In most instances, whether absorption or adsorption is occurring is inconsequential.

   c. Drugs may react with either glass or plastic, though generally there are fewer problems with glass.

    (1) With glass, the problems can be minimized by coating the glass surface (the process is called *silanization*) to decrease the number of sites for hydrophilic bonding. Silanization converts the -OH groups on the glass surface to silyl ethers, Si-O-Si.

    (2) With plastics, the most serious problems occur with materials that contain plasticizers. Polyvinyl chloride (PVC) is the plastic that most frequently gives problems. PVC is innately a rigid plastic that is made flexible by the addition of plasticizers such as Di(2-ethylhexyl)phthalate (DEHP) or dioctylphthalate. Certain drugs partition out of solution and into the liquid plasticizer.

   d. Logically, sorption is dependent on the hydrophilic/lipophilic nature of the drug and the binding site or the material in the capillary space of the interface.

    (1) A drug's **partition coefficient**, or its relative oil and water solubilities, is sometimes used to predict sorption tendencies.

     (a) Drugs that are poorly water-soluble or lipophilic have a greater tendency to sorb to PVC or dissolve in its plasticizer.

(b) For example, several of the benzodiazepines, beginning with diazepam, have been studied quite extensively. Lorazepam, with a water solubility of 0.08 mg/mL, has significant sorption problems both with PVC bags and some other plastics, whereas another benzodiazepine, midazolam HCl, which is water-soluble, does not have this difficulty (15,18–20).

(2) Sorption and binding are often **pH-dependent**.

(a) It is easy to see why the amount of binding or partitioning can be pH-dependent in the case of ionizable drugs. Depending on the hydrophilic/lipophilic nature of the binding site or plasticizer, either a ionized or neutral species will be attracted.

(b) For example, a chlorpromazine HCl solution with a pH = 5 (at this pH, this drug is present primarily in the hydrochloride salt form) and stored in PVC bags had only 5% sorption in 1 week at room temperature, but when the pH was adjusted upward to 7.4 (at this pH, the drug is largely in the neutral free-base form), approximately 86% was lost to sorption in the same period. The same behavior has been noted with midazolam HCl (15,20).

e. Examples of drugs that sorb to glass or plastic surfaces

(1) The first documented cases of sorption involved insulin, nitroglycerin, and diazepam. It is now recognized to be a problem with a wide variety of drugs.

(2) An article published in the *International Journal of Pharmaceutical Compounding* in March 2002 listed the following drugs with significant problems due to sorption to PVC containers and administration sets: amiodarone, calcitriol, diazepam, isosorbide dinitrate, lorazepam, nicardipine, nitroglycerin, propofol, quinidine gluconate, tacrolimus, and vitamin A. The authors stated that insulin is not listed because it sorbs to both PVC plastics and to glass and is titrated to the proper dose (21).

(3) Other drugs, including chlorpromazine HCl, thiopental Na, bleomycin, and many more, also pose problems in this regard. The *Handbook of Injectable Drugs* has a special section in each drug monograph devoted to the drug's sorption potential.

(4) Compatibility problems due to sorption will potentially become increasingly problematic with the development of protein and peptide drugs, many of which may sorb to surfaces.

f. Strategies for handling drugs that sorb to surfaces

(1) Check product package inserts and other references. As previously stated, the drug monographs in the *Handbook of Injectable Drugs* each have a section on sorption.

(2) Be suspicious of new drugs from an existing class where sorption problems with other members of that class have been documented.

(3) Special tubing or containers may be used. Consult the product package insert for recommendations. Because these special tubings and containers are expensive, be sure the problem is clinically significant and that it cannot be handled in another way. For example, insulin and nitroglycerin are two drugs with significant sorption problems, but both have their dosages titrated to patient response, so potentially either sorbing or nonsorbing materials could be used (22). There are two situations that require careful consideration:

(a) When using recommended doses for drugs with sorbing problems, be sure to either use the same type of tubing and containers or be prepared to make dosage adjustments. For example, product package inserts for Nitroglycerin Injection state that the usual starting doses that have been reported in clinical studies used PVC administration sets; the use of nonabsorbing tubing will result in the need for reduced doses.

(b) Furthermore, be exceedingly careful if it is necessary to switch container or tubing types for a patient stabilized with a drug that has a potential sorption problem.

(4) Because the degree of sorption increases with the length of contact time, the following strategies offer possibilities:

(a) Use short run-times for IVs containing drugs with potential sorption problems.

(b) Add the drug just before the time of administration.

(c) Consider giving the drug by IV push if possible.

(5) The number of binding sites is also a factor, so the use of short administration-set tubing can sometimes be helpful. One study with quinidine gluconate Injection showed a decrease in sorption from 30% to 3% by using shorter IV tubing (23).

(6) Temperature is another variable that can affect sorption, with sorption increasing with increasing temperature. Temperature can often be controlled to some degree by storing the product in the refrigerator until administration.

2. Leaching

   a. In recent years, there has been increasing concern about leaching of plasticizers from plastics such as PVC. Of particular concern is DEHP, because it has been classified by the federal Environmental Protection Agency as a probable human carcinogen based on studies performed in rodents (24).

   b. Drug solutions that contain surfactants or cosolvents are most at risk, because some of these have been found to extract plasticizer from the plastic and contaminate the drug solution.

      (1) For example, the approved labeling for paclitaxel, which uses a dehydrated alcohol-polyoxyethylated castor oil solvent system, requires use of non-PVC containers and administration sets. The manufacturer of paclitaxel gives a list of compatible administration sets, tubing, and infusion device components. There is a good discussion of the leaching studies done with this drug in *Trissel's Handbook of Injectable Drugs* (15).

      (2) Other drugs or drug products with potential problems include IV lipid emulsion, vitamin A, cyclosporine, docetaxel, propofol, tacrolimus, and teniposide and any others containing surfactants or cosolvents (21,24).

   c. The situation with DEHP has been clarified somewhat with a "Dear Colleague" letter sent from the Public Health Service in July 2002. The letter identified the two factors that determine the potential degree of risk to patients exposed to DEHP: (i) patient sensitivity and (ii) dose of DEHP received.

      (1) The patients listed at greatest risk are male fetuses and neonatal and peripubertal males. These have been identified because the animal (not human) studies have shown effects on the development of male reproductive systems and the production of normal sperm in young animals. Individuals in this group, as well as pregnant women carrying a male fetus or lactating women nursing a male infant, are considered in the at-risk group.

      (2) The letter also identified procedures that pose the greatest risk of delivering exposure to DEHP from PVC administration materials. They included such things as enteral nutrition, parenteral nutrition with IV lipid emulsion in PVC bags, multiple procedures, exchange transfusions, hemodialysis, and several others.

      (3) The letter stated that there is minimal or no risk of DEHP exposure when using PVC bags and tubing with crystalloid fluids (D5W, normal saline, lactated Ringer's injection, etc.).

      (4) The complete document, "Safety Assessment of Di(2-ethylhexyl)phthalate (DEHP) Released from PVC Medical Devices," is available on the FDA Center for Devices and Radiological Health (CDRH) Web site at http://www.fda.gov/cdrh/ost/dehp-pvc.pdf, accessed January 2008 (25).

   d. Strategies for handling situations where leaching may be a problem

      (1) Containers, administration sets, and device components that do not contain DEHP-plasticized materials can be substituted when there is concern about leaching.

      (2) Examples of such materials include glass, polyolefin, ethylene vinyl acetate, silicone, polyethylene, and polyurethane (21,25).

      (3) These materials are usually more costly, so the cost:benefit ratio (or risk) should be considered.

IV. CHEMICAL CHANGES

A. The *USP* Chapter ⟨1191⟩ states that in dosage forms, the following reactions usually cause loss of active drug content, and they usually do not provide obvious visual or olfactory evidence of their occurrence: oxidation, hydrolysis, epimerization, decarboxylation, dehydration, and photochemical decomposition (1). These reactions are enhanced by factors such as adverse temperatures, light, humidity, oxygen, and carbon dioxide.

Note: A review of basic chemical kinetics and equations useful in predicting rate of drug degradation is given in Figure 37.2.

B. Oxidation

   1. Drug classes susceptible to oxidation include the following:

      a. Catecholamines (compounds with $-OH$ groups present on adjacent carbon atoms on an aromatic ring; e.g., epinephrine)

      b. Phenolics (e.g., phenylephrine, morphine)

      c. Phenothiazines (e.g., chlorpromazine, promethazine)

      d. Olefins (alkenes; i.e., aliphatic compounds with double bonds)

      e. Steroids

      f. Tricyclics

1. **General equation:**

$$\text{Drug } [D] + \text{Reactant } [R] \rightarrow \text{Product } [P]$$

Since the rate of this reaction is dependent on the concentration of 2 components, the drug and the reactant, this is called a 2nd order reaction. The rate equation for this reaction is given by:

$$-\frac{dD}{dt} \propto [D][R] \quad or \quad -\frac{dD}{dt} = K_2[D][R]$$

where K_2 is the 2nd order rate constant

While we try to avoid adding to drug products any reactants that will cause drug degradation, sometimes this is unavoidable. For example, dosage forms, such as solutions, suspensions, and emulsions, require the presence of water, and water is a reactant for hydrolysis reactions; oxygen, a reactant in oxidation reactions, is present in the atmosphere.

2. **Apparent 1st order reactions**

In aqueous drug products and preparations, water is present in large excess so that its concentration is essentially constant. In this case we have kinetics that behave like a 1st order reaction in which, at any given temperature, the rate of reaction is dependent on the concentration of the drug in solution.

The apparent 1st order rate constant is given by:

$$K_1 = K_2[H_2O] \quad \text{where } [H_2O] \text{ is constant}$$

The rate equation for this reaction is then given by:

$$-\frac{dD}{dt} = K_2[D][H_2O] = K_1[D]$$

When we rearrange this equation and integrate over the interval $D_0 \rightarrow D_t$, we get the following equation for apparent 1st order reactions like hydrolysis:

$$\ln\frac{D}{D_0} = -K_1t \quad or \quad \ln[D] = \ln[D_0] - K_1t$$

When we solve this equation for t (that is, time) when D/D_0 is 0.5 (that is, the half-life of the drug product), we get:

$$t_{\frac{1}{2}} = \frac{0.693}{K_1}$$

When we solve this equation for t when D/D_0 is 0.9 (that is, the shelf-life of the drug product), we get:

$$t_{0.9} = \frac{0.105}{K_1}$$

These are important equations, since we can obtain the apparent 1st order rate constant, K_1, from either the half-life or shelf-life of the drug in this product.

3. **Apparent zero order reactions**

When the drug is present as a suspension, the concentration of drug in solution, $[D]$, is its solubility. The drug concentration is held essentially constant, because as the drug degrades and therefore is removed from solution, additional drug dissolves from the suspension particles to maintain a saturated solution. Products like this follow apparent zero order kinetics with a rate constant given by:

$$K_0 = K_1[D]$$

where $[D]$ is constant and is equal to the solubility of the drug in solution

The rate equation for an apparent zero order reaction is then given by:

$$-\frac{dD}{dt} = K_0$$

FIGURE 37.2. REVIEW OF CHEMICAL KINETICS: EQUATIONS FOR DRUG DEGRADATION.

In this case, at a given temperature, the rate is constant and is dependent on the rate constant for the reaction. The drug concentration at any time t is given by:

$$[D] = [D_0] - K_0 t$$

When we solve this equation for t when D/D₀ is 0.5 (that is, the half-life of the drug product) we get:

$$t_{\frac{1}{2}} = \frac{0.5[D_0]}{K_0}$$

When we solve this equation for t when D/D₀ is 0.9 (that is, the shelf-life of the drug product) we get:

$$t_{0.9} = \frac{0.1[D_0]}{K_0}$$

FIGURE 37.2 REVIEW OF CHEMICAL KINETICS: EQUATIONS FOR DRUG DEGRADATION. (*Continued*)

    g. Thiols [i.e., sulfhydryl compounds, R–SH (e.g., captopril)]
    h. Miscellaneous (e.g., amphotericin B, sodium nitroprusside, nitrofurantoin, tetracycline, furosemide, ergotamine, sulfacetamide)
  2. Factors that may affect the rate of oxidation
    a. Presence of oxygen
    b. Light
    c. Heavy metal ions
    d. Temperature
    e. pH
    f. Presence of other drugs or chemicals that can act as oxidizing agents
  3. Possible strategies for handling drugs that are subject to oxidation
    a. Protect from oxygen.
      (1) Manufacturers can seal vulnerable drug solutions under nitrogen gas.
      (2) The pharmacist can limit the effect of atmospheric oxygen by using tight containers and by limiting storage time through use of conservative beyond-use dates.
    b. Protect from light (3).
      (1) Use light-resistant containers or syringes.
      (2) Wrap drug containers, IV bags, and syringes with opaque or light-resistant wrappings. Examples of some light-sensitive injectable drug products that may be dispensed in this way include sodium nitroprusside, chlorpromazine HCl, amphotericin B, and doxycycline.
    c. Add a metal-chelating agent such as edetate disodium. This ties up heavy metal ions as chelates, which render the metal ions ineffective as oxidation catalysts (see Chapter 17, Antioxidants). For example, oral liquid preparations of captopril have been shown to be stabilized using edetate disodium (26). Sample Prescription 28.6 in Chapter 28 illustrates the use of edetate disodium in a compounded captopril suspension and Sample Prescription 33.1 in Chapter 33 uses it in a sulfite-free compounded epinephrine ophthalmic solution. This strategy is not usually used for IV admixtures.
    d. Add an antioxidant. Caution should be exercised when doing this because some antioxidants can cause other problems. For example, sodium bisulfite is a useful antioxidant, but it is also a strong nucleophile that initiates other undesirable degradative reactions (see Chapter 17, Antioxidants). This strategy is also not commonly used for IV admixtures.
    e. Control storage temperature. Usually the rate of oxidation is more rapid at elevated temperatures and can be retarded by storage of the sensitive product under refrigeration.
    f. Control pH. Be careful about mixing drug solutions or adding drugs to a solution when any component is subject to oxidation. Oxidation is most often favored by alkaline pH. For example, when sodium bicarbonate (pH = 7–8.5) is added to the oxidation-sensitive drug norepinephrine, rapid degradation of the norepinephrine results.
    g. Separate drugs that are easily oxidized from those that are easily reduced. Commercial preparations of parenteral multivitamin preparations illustrate this principle: Folic acid is incompatible with oxidizing agents, reducing agents, and metal ions; cyanocobalamin has

limited compatibility with ascorbic acid (about 24 hours), thiamine, and niacinamide. Therefore, injectable multivitamin products are either manufactured as lyophilized powder for
injection or are packaged as two separate solutions so the incompatible vitamins can be kept
separate until the time of administration.

C. Hydrolysis

1. Drug classes susceptible to hydrolysis include the following:
   a. Esters, R–CO–O–R (e.g., the local anesthetic "caines" such as procaine and tetracaine,
      aspirin, belladonna alkaloids, and especially strained ring-systems such as the lactones)
   b. Amides, R–CO–NH$_2$, and especially the strained ring-system amides such as the lactams
      (e.g., penicillins)
   c. Imides, R–CO–NH–CO–R′ (e.g., barbiturates)
   d. Thiolesters, R–CO–S–R′
2. Factors that affect the rate of hydrolysis
   a. Presence of water
   b. pH
   c. Presence of general acids and bases (citrate, acetate, phosphate), which are often used as
      buffers
   d. Concentration of the drug
   e. Temperature
   f. Presence of other components that may catalyze hydrolysis. Dextrose is reported to be a
      common offender.
3. Strategies for handling drugs subject to hydrolysis
   a. For solid drugs, control exposure to moisture by using tight containers and desiccants.
   b. Control the pH of aqueous formulations. Check the pH of all drug solutions that are to be
      combined and the usual pH generated by drugs that are to be added. The final pH of a solu-
      tion can be checked using pH paper or strips or a pH meter. This is illustrated with the
      applicable aqueous preparations that are given in sample prescriptions found in Part V, Non-
      sterile Dosage Forms and Their Preparation.
   c. Check appropriate references for possible negative effects of general acids or bases. If this
      can be a factor in accelerating hydrolysis, avoid adding these compounds as buffers or limit
      the amounts used, because this effect is concentration-dependent. Also avoid adding other
      drug solutions that contain these compounds.
   d. Consider drug concentration when this is a factor. Information on this is available in prod-
      uct package inserts and in references such as The *Handbook of Injectable Drugs*. Expiration
      times may be reduced greatly with concentrated solutions for some drugs subject to hydrol-
      ysis. The concentration-dependent rate of hydrolysis of Ampicillin Na is a classic example
      of this factor (27).
   e. Control storage temperature. The rate of hydrolysis is more rapid at elevated temperatures
      and can be retarded by storage of the sensitive product under refrigeration. You may need
      to limit or alter beyond-use dates for drugs subject to hydrolysis, depending on storage con-
      ditions.
      (1) The Arrhenius equation is a useful tool for estimating the effect of temperature on the
          rate of hydrolysis.

$$ ln\left(\frac{k_2}{k_1}\right) = \frac{E_a\,(T_2 - T_1)}{R\,T_2\,T_1} $$

where:

k_2 = rate constant for hydrolysis at T_2
k_1 = rate constant for hydrolysis at T_1
E_a = energy of activation for the reaction at the given conditions (concentrations,
     pH, solvent), in cal-mol^{-1}
R = the gas constant, 1.987 cal/deg-mole
T_1 = temperature in degrees K for rate constant k_1
T_2 = temperature in degrees K for rate constant k_2

      (2) Values for energies of activation (E_a) and half-lives for many common drugs can be found
          in *Chemical Stability of Pharmaceuticals* (28). An analysis of the energies of activation for
          drugs listed in *Chemical Stability of Pharmaceuticals* was done by author K. A. Connors. A
          normal-type distribution curve was found, with the lowest E_a at 4,000 cal/mol, the high-
          est at 44,000 cal/mol, and the majority clustered between 17,000 and 26,000 cal/mol.

(3) In a practical sense, this is useful information. Consider the following: In pharmacy practice, the situations in which we need to make predictions about changes in stability on the basis of influence of temperature are often in the area of reconstituted medications, antibiotics, and other drugs of limited stability. Most often, it concerns storage under refrigeration versus at room temperature. We can get an approximate quantitative determination of change in shelf life with these changes in storage temperature by solving the Arrhenius equation for the ratio of the rate constants, k_2/k_1, at the two temperatures.

Example 37.7

Set the following parameters in the Arrhenius equation:

$T_1 = 278$ K ($5°C$ or $41°F$, an average refrigerator temperature)

$T_2 = 295$ K ($22°C$ or $72°F$, an average room temperature)

$R = 1.987$ cal/deg-mol

$E_a = 22,000$ cal/mol—An average Ea for drugs

$$\ln\left(\frac{k_2}{k_1}\right) = \frac{22,000 \ (295 - 278)}{1.987 \ (295) \ (278)}$$

$$k_2/k_1 = 9.9 \approx 10$$

From this, it can be seen that for the "average" drug under "average" conditions, the rate of degradation reactions (such as hydrolysis) is approximately 10 times faster at room temperature than at refrigerator temperatures.

---

(4) A similar concept known as Q_{10} has been developed.
   (a) This is defined as the ratio of the rate constants, k_2/k_1, when the difference in temperature is $10°$.
   (b) Values of Q_{10} have been calculated for various energies of activation (E_a) between the normal ambient temperatures of $20°$ to $30°C$ ($68°$ to $86°F$). A list of these values and the development of Q_{10} from the Arrhenius equation is shown in Figure 37.3.
   (c) An equation using Q_{10}, also given at the bottom of Figure 37.3, calculates an estimate of the ratio of the rate constants for any temperature change, $Q_{\Delta T}$. Using the same data as was used in Example 37.7, a k_2/k_1 value of 8.3 is calculated, very close to the 9.9 value calculated using the Arrhenius equation. Either of these methods can be used to get an estimate of the change in rate of a reaction with a change in temperature.
(5) It is extremely important to remember that the energy of activation, E_a, varies with both the drug and the conditions.
   (a) For example, the Ea for the hydrolysis of ampicillin is 16,400 at pH 1.35, 18,300 at pH 4.93, and 22,300 at pH 9.78 (27), which correspond to rate constant ratios (k_2/k_1) of 5.5, 6.8, and 10.2 when going from $5°$ to $22°C$.
   (b) When the true energy of activation for the reaction is known, this should be used.
   (c) Even without known values of energy of activation, it is helpful to have some knowledge of the magnitude of the change of rate of reaction at temperatures of interest; for example, changes in the range of 5 to 15 times for most drugs when going from storage in the refrigerator to room temperature.
(6) Storage temperatures for drug products and preparations are defined in the General Notices of the *USP* and are discussed in section III of Chapter 13, Selection, Storage, and Handling Compounding Equipment and Ingredients. These define the allowable tolerance in storage circumstances at any location (e.g., pharmacies, hospitals, and warehouses). This terminology also allows patients or consumers to be counseled as to appropriate storage for the product. The *USP* also defines a Mean Kinetic Temperature (MKT) as the single calculated temperature at which the total amount of degradation over a specific time is equal to the sum of the individual degradations that would occur at various temperatures. This means that the MKT is an isothermal storage temperature that simulates the non-isothermal effects of storage temperature variation. It is not a simple arithmetic mean, but rather is based on the Arrhenius equation shown earlier. It is calculated from temperatures

Arrhenius Equation: $\ln \dfrac{k_2}{k_1} = \dfrac{E_a(T_2 - T_1)}{R\,T_2\,T_1}$ where temperature is in degrees K

Q_{10} is defined as the ratio of k_2/k_1 when the difference in temperature is 10°:

$$Q_{10} = \frac{k_{(T+10)}}{k_T}$$

Substituting this in the Arrhenius equation, we get:

$$\ln Q_{10} = \frac{E_a(T + 10 - T)}{R(T+10)(T)} = \frac{E_a}{R(T+10)T}\frac{10}{}$$

or $\qquad Q_{10} = e^{\frac{E_a}{R(T+10)T}\,10}$

Using one of these equations you can calculate the Q_{10} Values for the 10° interval about room temperature (25°C) for various E_a Values:

E_a (cal/mol)	Q_{10} (30 to 20°C)
10,000	1.76
12,200	2.0
15,000	2.34
19,400	3.0
20,000	3.11
22,000	3.48
24,500	4.0
25,000	4.12
30,000	5.48

These values can be used with the equation given below to obtain an approximation of the change of rate (k_2/k_1) for various temperature changes.

$$Q_{\Delta T} = Q_{10}^{(\Delta T/10)}$$

For example in going from 278 K (5°C, refrigerator temperature) to 295 K (22°C, room temperature), a ΔT of 17°, for a reaction with E_a of 22,000 cal/mol, we have

$$Q_{\Delta T} = Q_{10}^{(\Delta T/10)} = 3.48^{17/10} = 3.48^{1.7} = 8.33$$

Note: for more detailed treatment of this subject, see Connors KA, Amidon GL, Stella VJ, *Chemical stability of pharmaceuticals, 2nd ed.*, John Wiley & Sons, 1986.

FIGURE 37.3. Q10 VALUES AND CALCULATIONS.

measured over time in a storage facility (29). Methods for collecting temperature data in the pharmacy and calculation of MKT are discussed and illustrated in section III of Chapter 7, Systems of Measurement and Introduction to Pharmaceutical Calculations and in *USP* Chapters ⟨1150⟩ Pharmaceutical Stability and ⟨1160⟩ Pharmaceutical Calculations.

D. Evolution of gas (usually CO_2)
  1. Drugs that have problems
    a. Sodium bicarbonate and carbonate buffers are the most common offenders.
    b. Decarboxylation of *o*- and *p*-substituted benzoic acids (the antituberculosis drug *p*-aminosalicylic acid is an example) to give carbon dioxide can also occur.

   c. Note that this effect is actually desired in some preparations, such as effervescent powders and tablets (e.g., Alka Seltzer).

  2. Strategies for handling this problem

    a. Do not combine drug products that generate acid pH with sodium bicarbonate or drug products that contain carbonate buffers.

$$NaHCO_3 + H^+ \rightarrow H_2CO_3 \rightarrow H_2O + CO_2 \uparrow$$

    b. For vulnerable solid dosage forms, store and dispense in tight containers.

E. Displacement

  1. Cisplatin is the best-known example. The chemical structures given here show the active cisplatin molecule (center) and some displacement products that lack therapeutic activity.

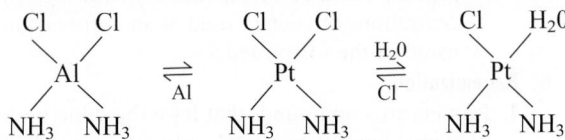

  2. After administration of cisplatin, one of the chloride ligands in the cisplatin molecule is slowly displaced by water (an aqua ligand), in a process termed *aquation*. The aqua ligand in the resulting $[PtCl(H_2O)(NH_3)_2]^+$ is then displaced, allowing cisplatin to coordinate to a basic site in DNA. Then the platinum cross-links two bases via displacement of the other chloride ligand.

  3. When cisplatin is diluted (such as in preparing an admixture in an LVP), the solution must have a sodium chloride concentration of at least 0.2% to maintain the chloride ions on the cisplatin molecule (15). These ions are essential to the activity of the cisplatin. Tests have found that 0.45% NaCl or 0.9% NaCl are satisfactory but not Sterile Water for Injection or D5W. Note that this is a reversible reaction.

  4. Because aluminum displaces the platinum when aluminum needles are used, stainless-steel needles must be used for drawing and administering this drug (15).

F. Complexation

  1. Tetracycline is the classic example of a drug that is inactivated by complexation.

    a. This reaction occurs with multivalent ions such as calcium, magnesium, iron, and aluminum.

    b. The usual strategy is to keep the drug separate from the offending ions. Tetracyclines should not be mixed with other drug products containing multivalent ions. Furthermore, patients taking tetracyclines (except some synthetic versions) should be counseled to avoid taking the drug with foods or drugs containing multivalent ions, including milk, most breads, iron-containing foods and drugs, and antacids.

  2. Aminophylline is an example of a drug that is a complex.

    a. In this case, theophylline, the active principle, is complexed in a 2:1 ratio with ethylenediamine. This is done to solubilize the theophylline because this drug has limited water solubility and does not form soluble salts.

    b. The complexation is a reversible reaction, and aminophylline may liberate the ethylenediamine. This is especially problematic when the drug is in solution because the theophylline then precipitates out of solution. Injectable solutions of aminophylline contain excess ethylenediamine to ensure that this does not happen, but these solutions should always be inspected for the presence of crystals and should not be used if any are present.

    c. The complexation is also pH-dependent.

      (1) King's *Dispensing of Medication* reports that Sorenson's phosphate buffer has been used to help maintain the stability of oral solutions of aminophylline (30).

      (2) The pH of Aminophylline Injection is maintained with the presence of excess ethylenediamine. The USP gives the pH range of injectable solutions of aminophylline as 8.6 to 9. The monograph states that excess ethylenediamine may be added but that no other substance may be added for the purpose of pH adjustment. It also notes that the injection should not be used if crystals are present (31).

  3. A third example of a drug that forms complexes is edetic acid, also known as *ethylenediaminetetraacetic acid* or *EDTA*. Various forms of edetic acid are used therapeutically and as stabilizing agents because of the ability of this compound to form complexes with various cations.

    a. There are two official injectable products: Edetate Disodium Injection and Edetate Calcium Disodium Injection. The disodium complex is used in emergency situations to treat hypercalcemia because the drug has a complexation site available to complex with and remove the excess calcium in the blood. The calcium disodium complex is used primarily to treat lead poisoning. In this case, the calcium disodium complex is used so that the drug will not remove calcium from the body.

b. Edetate disodium is also used in products subject to oxidation in which metal cations act as catalysts for the oxidation process. This is discussed in more detail in Chapter 17, Antioxidants.

c. The abbreviation EDTA has been used in the past for edetate; however, in January 2008, the FDA issued a public health advisory stating that the full product name edetate disodium (brand name, Endrate) or edetate calcium disodium (brand name, Calcium Disodium Versenate) should be used when prescribing or dispensing either of these drugs (32). The reason for the advisory is that there have been cases of death and injury when the wrong drug product was used therapeutically. Although this danger does not apply to the very small concentrations of edetate used as an antioxidant, it is important to use the appropriate specific name of the form used.

G. Racemization

1. Isomers are compounds that have the same molecular formula (i.e., the same number and kind of atoms) but different molecular structures. Enantiomers are isomers that are mirror images of each other. Enantiomers have identical chemical properties except toward optically active reagents and, more importantly in medicine, toward many enzymes, biologic receptors, and membranes. A mixture of equal parts of enantiomers is called a racemate, and the conversion of one enantiomer to a racemate is known as *racemization*.

2. Examples of drugs that undergo racemization include the following:

a. Epinephrine: The l-enantiomer has approximately 15 to 20 times the physiologic activity as the d-enantiomer (33).

b. Some local anesthetics, such as mepivacaine and bupivacaine, undergo racemization (33).

c. Other well-known drugs are available as both the racemic mixture and as the single enantiomer; examples include amphetamine and dextroamphetamine, albuterol and levalbuterol, and omeprazole and esomeprazole.

3. Problems exist only when one enantiomer is much more physiologically active than the other **and** when racemization easily takes place. The pharmacist should be aware of this and investigate the literature when handling any drugs that have this potential. In the future, more chiral drugs will be available as pure enantiomers than as racemates.

H. Epimerization

1. Optical isomers that are not superimposable and are not mirror images are called *diastereomers*. They have different physical properties: different melting points, boiling points, solubilities, and densities. They have the same functional groups and show similar chemical properties but exhibit different rates of reaction. A pair of diastereomers that differ only in the configuration about one carbon atom are called *epimers*.

2. One example of a drug that undergoes epimerization is tetracycline. It undergoes reversible epimerization to epitetracycline, a form that has little antibacterial activity. The chemical structures of tetracycline and epitetracycline differ only in the rotation of the $-N(CH_3)_2$ group on the C-4 atom.

a. Epimerization occurs to an appreciable extent only when tetracycline is in solution. The reaction rate is pH-dependent and is greatest at pH = 3. The rate also depends on temperature and the presence of citrate and phosphate ions. Solutions of Tetracycline Hydrochloride Injection are reported to lose 8–12% of their potency in 24 hours when stored at room temperature (34).

b. Because epimerization happens only to drug molecules in solution, suspensions of tetracycline are much more stable. Stable oral suspensions can be made by adding a buffer to maintain the pH at a level where the soluble form of tetracycline is minimized. Suspensions of tetracycline at pH 4 to 7 are reported to be stable for 3 months (34). One recommendation is to use a phosphate buffer with the pH adjusted to approximately 6.

c. In commercial solutions of tetracycline prescribed for the treatment of acne, the epimerization reaction is controlled by the addition of citric acid for buffering and excess 4-epitetracycline HCl. Because epimerization is a reversible reaction, the excess 4-epitetracycline shifts the equilibrium to prevent the active tetracycline from transforming to the inactive epi form. Extemporaneous topical solutions of tetracycline HCl should probably not be made extemporaneously unless the formulation is known to have ingredients that will control epimerization.

3. Pilocarpine is another example of a drug that may epimerize with loss of therapeutic activity.

REFERENCES

1. The United States Pharmacopeial Convention, Inc. Chapter ⟨1191⟩ 2008 USP 31/NF 26. Rockville, MD: Author 2007; 656–659.

2. ICH Guidance: Q1A(R2): Stability Testing of New Drug Substances and Products (Second Revision). Published in the Federal Register, Vol. 68, No. 225, November 21, 2003; pages 65717–65718.

3. ICH Guidance: Q1B: Photostability Testing of New Drug Substances and Products. Published in the Federal Register, Vol. 62, No. 95, May 16, 1997, pages 27115–27122.

4. ICH Guidance: Q1C: Stability Testing for New Dosage Forms. Published in the Federal Register, Vol. 62, No. 90, May 9, 1997, pages 25634–25635.

5. Dittert LW, ed. Sprowls' American pharmacy, 7th ed. Philadelphia: JB Lippincott, 1974; 333–334.

6. Sinko PJ. Martin's physical pharmacy and pharmaceutical sciences, 5th ed. Baltimore: Lippincott Williams & Wilkins, 2006.

7. Ecanow B, Sadik F. Powders. In: King RE, ed. Dispensing of medications, 9th ed. Easton, PA: Mack Publishing Co., 1984; 40.

8. Guillory JK. Generation of polymorphs, hydrates, solvates, and amorphous solids. In: Brittain HG, ed. Polymorphism in pharmaceutical solids. New York: Marcel Dekker, 1999; 183–226.

9. Griesser UJ. The importance of solvates. In: Hilfiker R, ed. Polymorphism in the pharmaceutical industry. Weinheim, Germany: Wiley-VCH, 2006; 211–257.

10. Kohut J III, Trissel LA, Leissing NC. Don't ignore details in drug-compatibility reports. Am J Health-Syst Pharm 1986; 53: 2339.

11. Oskroba DM, Leissing NC, Trissel LA. An automated process for determining the physical compatibility of drugs. Hosp Pharm 1997; 32: 1013–1020.

12. Stella VJ, Roberts RD. Unpublished results. In: Trissel LA, ed. Handbook of injectable drugs, 4th ed. Bethesda, MD: American Society of Hospital Pharmacists, 1986; XVII.

13. Raffa RB. Analgesic, antipyretic, and anti-inflammatory drugs. In: University of the Sciences in Philadelphia, ed. Remington: The science and practice of pharmacy, 21st ed. Baltimore: Lippincott Williams & Wilkins, 2005; 1524–1542.

14. Connors KA. Thermodynamics of pharmaceutical systems: An introduction for students of pharmacy. New York: John Wiley & Sons, Inc., 2002; 193–202.

15. Trissel LA, ed. Handbook of injectable drugs, 12th ed. Bethesda: American Society of Health-System Pharmacists, 2003.

16. Urdang A, Leuallen EE. The effect of pH upon the solubility of phenobarbital in alcohol-aqueous solutions. JAPhA Sci Ed 1956; 45: 526.

17. Krause GM, Cross JM. Solubility of phenobarbital in alcohol-glycerin-water systems. JAPhA Sci Ed 1951; 40: 139.

18. Trissel LA, Pearson SD. Storage of lorazepam in three injectable solutions in polyvinyl chloride and polyolefin bags. Am J Hosp Pharm 1994; 51: 368–372.

19. Stiles ML, Allen LV Jr, Prince SJ, Holland JS. Stability of dexamethasone sodium phosphate, diphenhydramine hydrochloride, lorazepam, and metoclopramide hydrochloride in portable infusion-pump reservoirs. Am J Hosp Pharm 1994; 51: 514–517.

20. Stiles ML, Allen LV Jr, Prince SJ. Stability of deferoxamine mesylate, floxuridine, fluorouracil, hydromorphone hydrochloride, lorazepam, and midazolam hydrochloride in polypropylene infusion-pump syringes. Am J Health-Syst Pharm 1996; 53: 1583–1588.

21. Rice SP, Markel JA. A review of parenteral admixtures requiring select containers and administration sets. IJPC 2002; 6: 120–122.

22. Altavela JL, Haas CE, Nowak DR, et al. Clinical response to intravenous nitroglycerin infused through polyethylene or polyvinyl chloride tubing. Am J Hosp Pharm 1994; 51: 490–494.

23. Darbar D, Dell'Orto S, Wilkinson GR, Roden DM. Loss of quinidine gluconate injection in a polyvinyl chloride infusion system. Am J Health-Syst Pharm 1996; 53: 655–658.

24. Landis NT. Advocacy group targets PVC i.v. equipment. Am J Health-Syst Pharm 1999; 56: 937–938.

25. Public Health Service, Center for Devices and Radiological Health, Food and Drug Administration. Public health notification: PVC devices containing the plasticizer DEHP. Rockville, MD: Author, July 12, 2002.

26. Lye MYE, Yow KL, et al. Effects of ingredients on stability of captopril in extemporaneously prepared oral liquids. Am J Health-Syst Pharm 1997; 54: 2483–2487.

27. Connors KA, Amidon GL, Stella VJ. Chemical stability of pharmaceuticals, 2nd ed. New York: John Wiley & Sons, 1986; 198–207.

28. Connors KA, Amidon GL, Stella VJ. Chemical stability of pharmaceuticals, 2nd ed. New York: John Wiley & Sons, 1986.

29. The United States Pharmacopeial Convention Inc. Chapter ⟨1150⟩ 2008 USP 31/NF 26. Rockville, MD: Author, 2007; 613–614.

30. Booth RE, Dale JK. Compounding and dispensing information. In: King RE, ed. Dispensing of medications, 9th ed. Easton, PA: Mack Publishing Co., 1984; 408.

31. The United States Pharmacopeial Convention Inc. USP Monographs 2008 USP 31/NF 26. Rockville, MD: Author, 2007.

32. Food and Drug Administration. FDA Public Health Advisory: Edetate Disodium (marketed as Endrate and generic products). Rockville, MD: Author, January 16, 2008, http://www.fda.gov/cder/drug/advisory/edetate_disodium.htm. Accessed February 2008.

33. Alexander KS. Appraisal of product quality. In: King RE, ed. Dispensing of medications, 9th ed. Easton, PA: Mack Publishing Co., 1984; 231.

34. Reynolds JEF, ed. Martindale: the extra pharmacopoeia, 30th ed. London: The Pharmaceutical Press, 1993; 212–213.

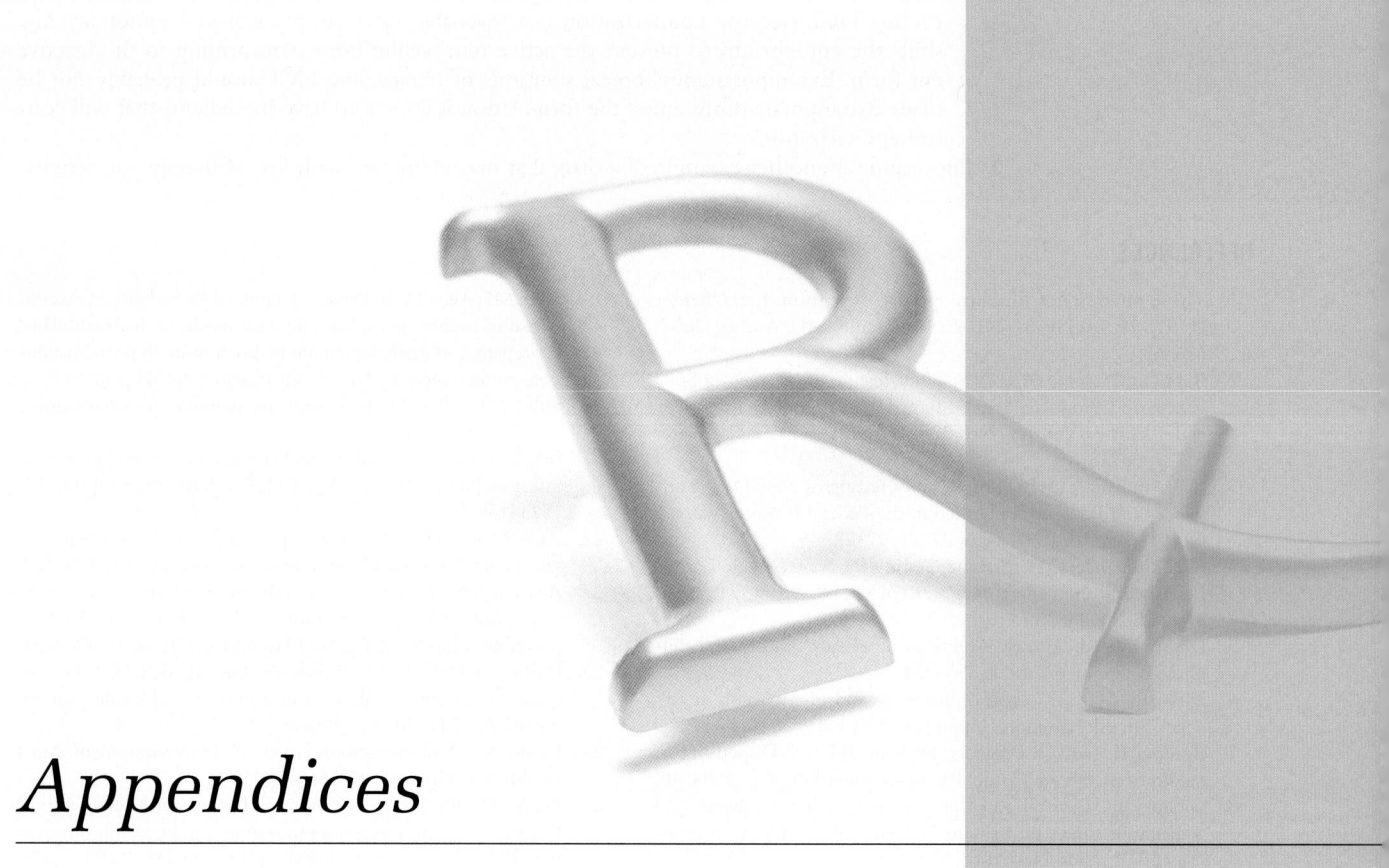

Appendices

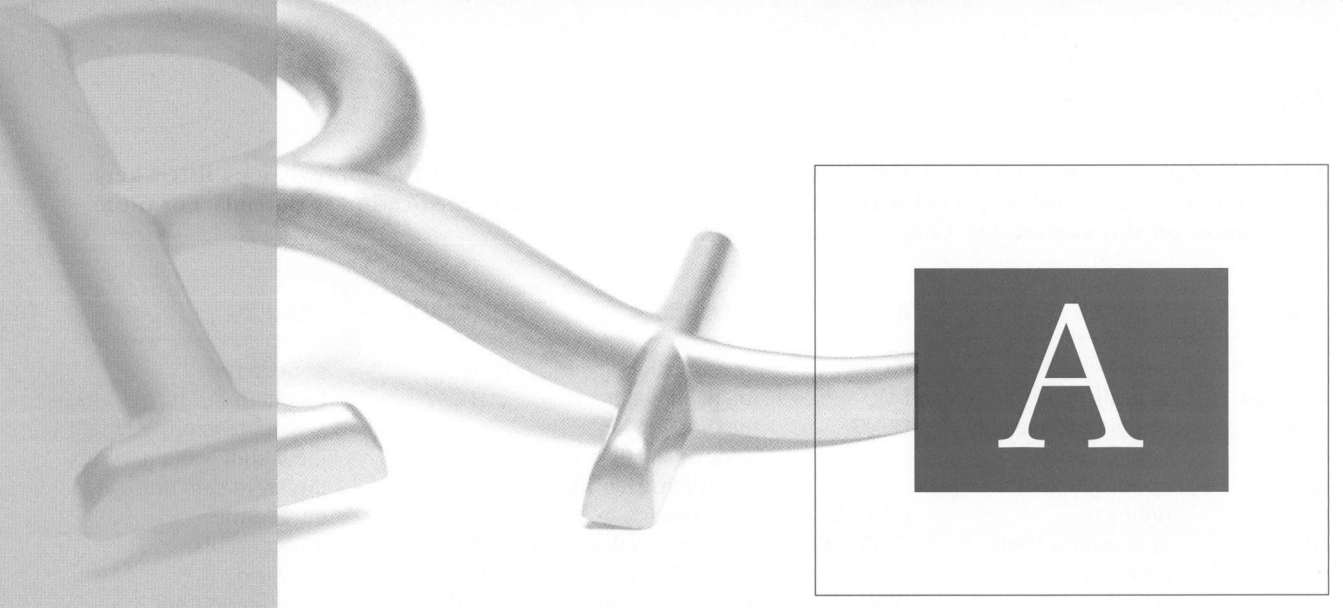

Abbreviations Commonly Used in Prescriptions and Medication Orders

These abbreviations are for informational purposes only; the use of some of the abbreviations listed here have been misread or misinterpreted with resulting errors when furnishing medication to patients. For more information on this subject, see Chapter 1 and Table 1.1.

ABBREV.	MEANING	ABBREV.	MEANING	ABBREV.	MEANING
a	before	d.t.d.	give of such doses	hs	at bedtime
aa. or $\overline{aa}$	of each	DW	distilled water	HT	height or
ABW	actual body weight	D5NS	dextrose 5% in		hypertension
a.c.	before meals		normal saline (0.9%	IBW	ideal body weight
ad	up to		sodium chloride)	ICU	intensive care unit
a.d.	right ear	D5½NS or	dextrose 5% in ½	ID	intradermal
ad lib.	at pleasure, freely	D5-0.45	normal saline	IM	intramuscular
a.m.	morning		(0.45% NaCl)	INH	isoniazid
amp.	ampul	D5W	dextrose 5% in water	I&O	input and output
APAP	acetaminophen	DX	diagnosis	inj.	injection
aq.	water	EC	enteric coated	IPPD	intermittent positive-
aq.dist.	distilled water	ECG or EKG	electrocardiogram		pressure breathing
a.s.	left ear	EDTA	edetate	IU or iu	international units
ASA	aspirin	EENT	eyes, ears, nose,	IV	intravenous
ASAP	as soon as possible		throat	IVP	intravenous push or
ATC	around the clock	EES	erythromycin		IV pyelogram
a.u.	each ear		ethylsuccinate	IVPB	intravenous
bid	twice a day	EFAD	essential fatty acid		piggyback
biw	twice a week		deficiency	L	liter
BM	bowel movement	elix.	elixir	LCD	coal tar solution
BP	blood pressure	e.m.p.	as directed	LR	lactated Ringer's
BS	blood sugar	EPI	epinephrine		injection
BSA	body surface area	EPO	erythropoietin	M.	mix
BUN	blood urea nitrogen	ER	emergency room	m^2 or M^2	square meter
BW	body weight	et	and	mcg or µg	microgram
C	centigrade	f. or ft.	make	MDI	metered-dose inhaler
c. or $\overline{c}$	with	F	Fahrenheit	mEq	milliequivalent
CA	cancer or cardiac	FBS	fasting blood sugar	mg	milligram
	arrest	FFA	free fatty acid	MI	myocardial infarction
cap	capsule	fl or fld	fluid	min	minute (s)
CBC	complete blood count	ft.	make	ml or mL	milliliter
cc	cubic centimeter	FU or 5-FU	fluorouracil	MMR	measles, mumps,
CCT	crude coal tar	g	gram		rubella
chart or	powder or powder	GI	gastrointestinal	MO	mineral oil
chartulate	paper	GFR	glomerular filtration	MOM	milk of magnesia
CHF	congestive heart		rate	mOsm or	milliosmoles
	failure	gr	grain	mOsmol	
CNS	central nervous	gtt, gtts	drop, drops	MR	may repeat
	system	GYN	gynecology	MRX_	may repeat_times
comp.	compound	GU	genitourinary	MS	morphine sulfate or
COPD	chronic obstructive	H	hypodermic		multiple sclerosis
	pulmonary disease	h or hr	hour	MVI	multivitamin
CPZ	chlorpromazine	HA	headache	n	nostril
crm	cream	Hb	hemoglobin	N&V	nausea and vomiting
C&S	culture and sensitivity	HBP	high blood pressure	NG	nasogastric
d	day	HC	hydrocortisone	NK	none known
disc or D.C.	discontinue	HCT	hematocrit	no. or No.	number
disp.	dispense	HCTZ	hydrochlorothiazide	noct.	night
div.	divide	HEPA	high-efficiency	non rep. or	do not repeat or no
DOB	date of birth		particulate air	N.R.	refills
DPT	diphtheria, pertussis,	HR	heart rate	NPO	nothing by mouth
	tetanus	HRT	hormone replacement	NS	normal saline
DS	double strength		therapy		

ABBREV.	MEANING	ABBREV.	MEANING	ABBREV.	MEANING
$^1/_2$NS	half-strength normal saline	pv	vaginally	tal.	such
		$\overline{q}$ or q	every	tal. dos.	such doses
NTG	nitroglycerin	qd	every day	tbsp.	tablespoonful
NVD	nausea, vomiting & diarrhea	qh	every hour	TCA	tricyclic antidepressant
		qid	four times a day		
O.	pint	qod	every other day	TCN	tetracycline
OB-GYN	obstetrics-gynecology	qs	a sufficient quantity	temp	temperature
OC	oral contraceptive	qs ad	a sufficient quantity to make	tid	three times a day
OD	overdose			tiw	three times a week
o.d.	right eye	r or R	rectal	TMP/SMX	trimethoprim– sulfamethoxizole
oint.	ointment	R.L. or R/L	Ringer's lactate		
o.l.	left eye	℞	prescription symbol (recipe or take thou)	top	topically
o.s.	left eye			TPN	total parenteral nutrition
OR	operating room	s or s	without		
OT	occupational therapy	sat.	saturated	tr.	tincture
OTC	over-the-counter	sid	once a day	tsp.	teaspoonful
o.u.	each eye	Sig.	write on label	U or u	unit(s)
o$_2$	both eyes	SL	sublingual	UA	urinalysis
oz	ounce (avoirdupois)	SOB	shortness of breath	u.d. or ut dict	as directed
p or per	by	sol.	solution		
Pb	phenobarbital	s.o.s.	if there is need	ung.	ointment
p.c.	after meals	SS	saturated solution	URI	upper respiratory infection
PCN	penicillin	ss. or $\overline{\overline{ss}}$	one-half		
p.m.	afternoon; evening	SSKI	saturated solution of potassium iodide	USP	United States Pharmacopeia
PO	by mouth				
post	after	stat.	immediately	UTI	urinary tract infection
post-op	after surgery	subc, subq, subcut, SC, or SQ	subcutaneously	UUN	urine urea nitrogen
PPD	purified protein derivative (tuberculin)			UV	ultraviolet
		supp.	suppository	vol.	volume
PPI	patient package insert	susp.	suspension	VS	vital signs
		SVR	alcohol	w/	with
PPM	parts per million	syr.	syrup	w.a. or WA	while awake
pr	rectally	SZ	seizure	WBC	white blood cell count
pre-op	before surgery	T&C	type and crossmatch		
p.r.n.	when required or as needed			wk.	week
		tab	tablet	w/o	without
PT	physical therapy	TAC	tetracaine, adrenalin, and cocaine	X	times
pulv.	powder			y.o.	year old
				ZnO	zinc oxide

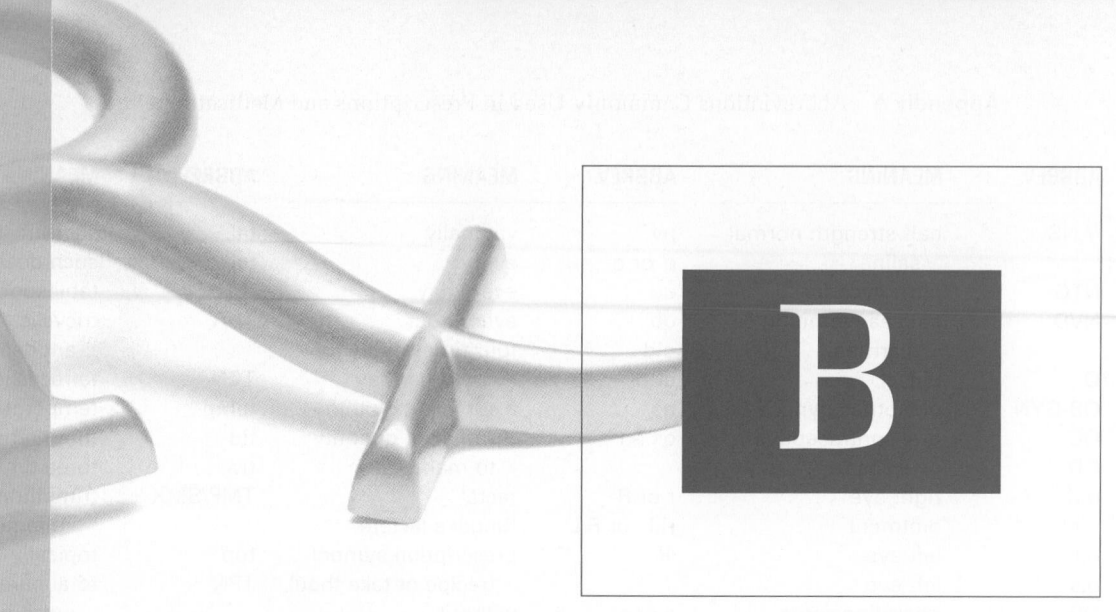

B

Nomograms for Determination of Body Surface Area from Height and Weight

Nomogram for Determination of Body Surface Area From Height and Weight

For Children

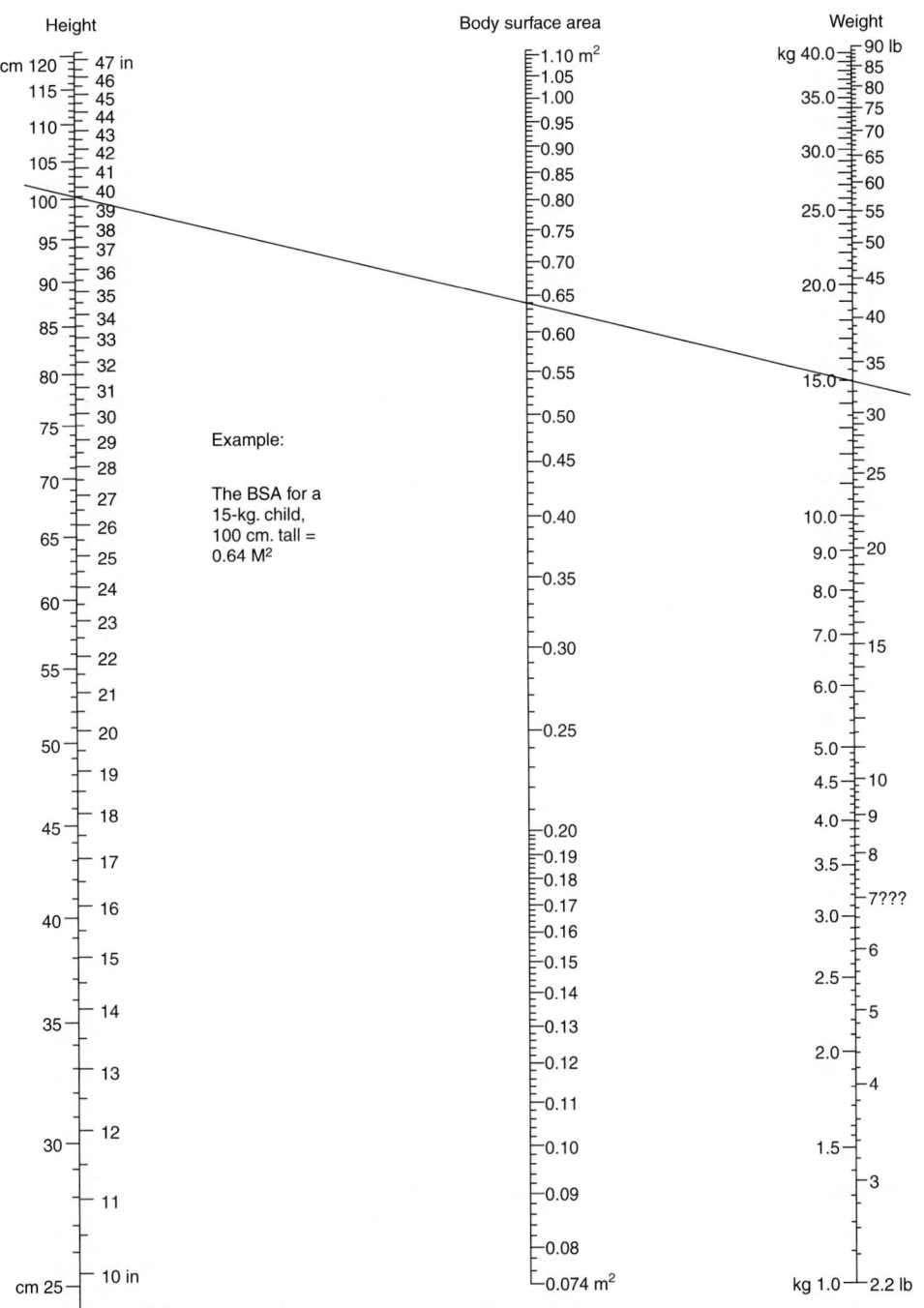

Example:

The BSA for a
15-kg. child,
100 cm. tall =
0.64 M²

From the formula of Du Bots and Du Bots, *Arch. intern. Med.*, 17, 863 (1916): $S = W^{0.425} \times H^{0.725} \times 71.84$, or
$\log S = \log W \times 0.425 + \log H \times 0.725 + 1.8564$ (S = body surface in cm², W = weight in kg, H = height in cm).

From Diem K, Lentner C, Geigy JR. Scientific tables. 7th ed. Basel, Switzerland: JR Geigy, 1970; 538.

Nomogram for Determination of Body Surface Area From Height and Weight

For Adults

Height	Body surface area	Weight

```
cm 200 ┬ 79 in                    ┬ 2.80 m²          kg 150 ╤ 330 lb
       ├ 78                                            145 ╪ 320
   195 ┼ 77                        ├ 2.70             140 ╪ 310
       ├ 76                                            135 ╪ 300
   190 ┼ 75                        ├ 2.60             130 ╪ 290
       ├ 74                                            125 ╪ 280
   185 ┼ 73                        ├ 2.50                 ╪ 270
       ├ 72                        ├ 2.40             120 ╪ 260
   180 ┼ 71                                            115 ╪ 250
       ├ 70                        ├ 2.30             110 ╪ 240
   175 ┼ 69                        ├ 2.20             105 ╪ 230
       ├ 68                                            100 ╪ 220
   170 ┼ 67                        ├ 2.10
       ├ 66                                             95 ╪ 210
   165 ┼ 65                        ├ 2.00              90 ╪ 200
       ├ 64                        ├ 1.95
   160 ┼ 63                        ├ 1.90              85 ╪ 190
       ├ 62                        ├ 1.85
   155 ┼ 61                        ├ 1.80              80 ╪ 180
       ├ 60                        ├ 1.75
   150 ┼ 59                        ├ 1.70              75 ╪ 170
       ├ 58                        ├ 1.65
   145 ┼ 57                        ├ 1.60              70 ╪ 160
       ├ 56                        ├ 1.55                 ╪ 150
   140 ┼ 55                        ├ 1.50              65 ╪
       ├ 54                        ├ 1.45                 ╪ 140
   135 ┼ 53                        ├ 1.40              60 ╪ 130
       ├ 52                        ├ 1.35
   130 ┼ 51                        ├ 1.30              55 ╪ 120
       ├ 50
   125 ┼ 49                        ├ 1.25              50 ╪ 110
       ├ 48                        ├ 1.20                 ╪ 105
   120 ┼ 47                        ├ 1.15              45 ╪ 100
       ├ 46                        ├ 1.10                 ╪ 95
   115 ┼ 45                                                ╪ 90
       ├ 44                        ├ 1.05              40 ╪ 85
   110 ┼ 43                        ├ 1.00                 ╪ 80
       ├ 42                        ├ 0.95              35 ╪ 75
   105 ┼ 41                        ├ 0.90                 ╪ 70
       ├ 40                                          kg 30 ╧ 66 lb
cm 100 ┴ 39 in                    ┴ 0.86 m²
```

From the formula of Du Bots and Du Bots, *Arch. intern. Med*, 17, 863 (1916): $S = W^{0.425} \times H^{0.725} \cdot 71.84$, or log S = log $W \times 0.425$ + log $H \times 0.725$ + 1.8564 (S = body surface in cm², W = weight in kg, H = height in cm).

From Diem K, Lentner C, Geigy JR. Scientific tables. 7th ed. Basel, Switzerland: JR Geigy, 1970; 538.

C

National Center for Health Statistics Growth Charts

Birth to 36 months: Boys
Length-for-age and Weight-for-age percentiles

NAME _____

RECORD # _____

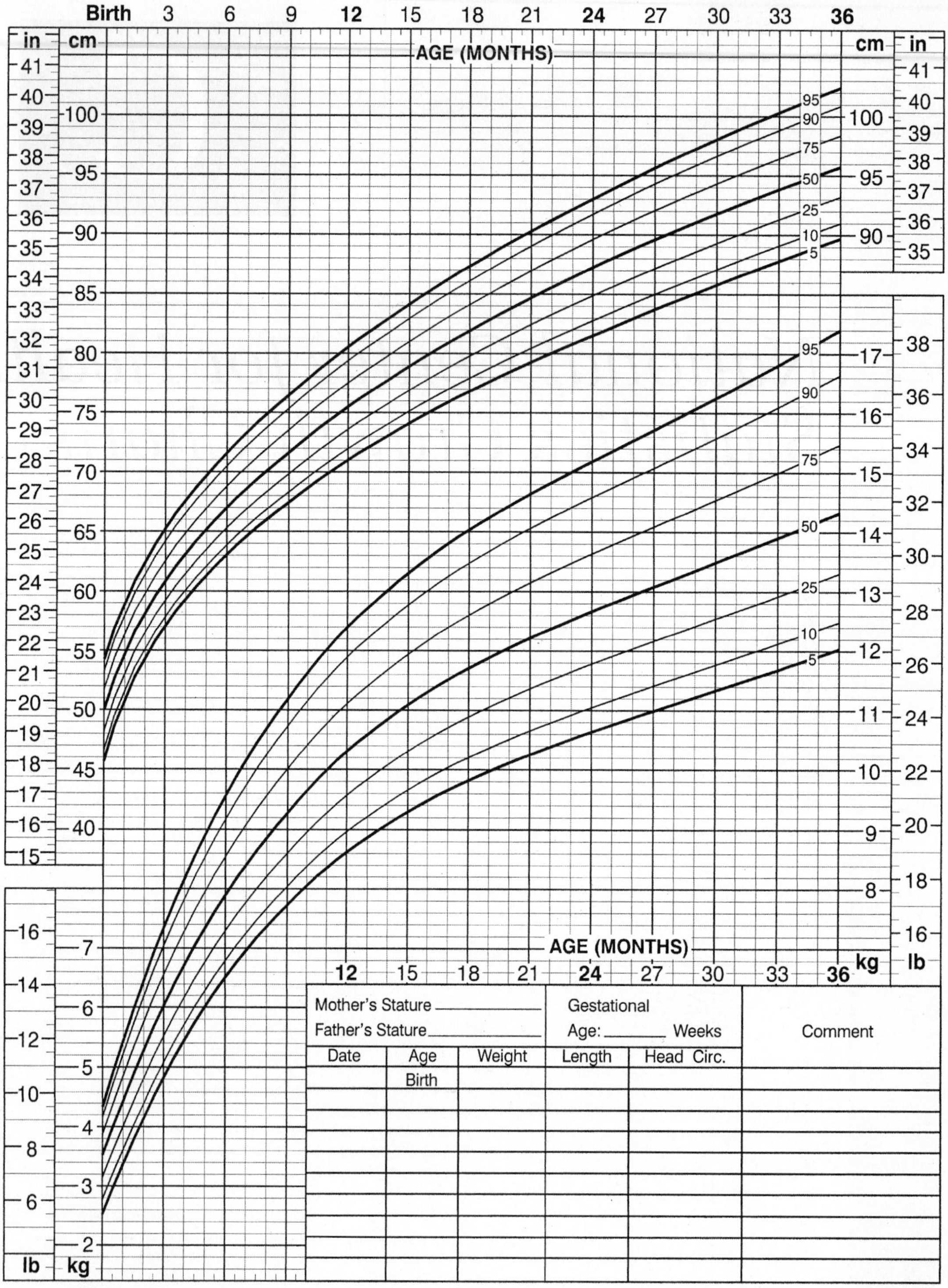

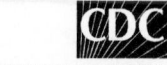

Published May 30, 2000 (modified 4/20/01).
SOURCE: Developed by the National Center for Health Statistics in collaboration with
the National Center for Chronic Disease Prevention and Health Promotion (2000).
http://www.cdc.gov/growthcharts

SAFER · HEALTHIER · PEOPLE™

Birth to 36 months: Girls
Length-for-age and Weight-for-age percentiles

NAME _____

RECORD # _____

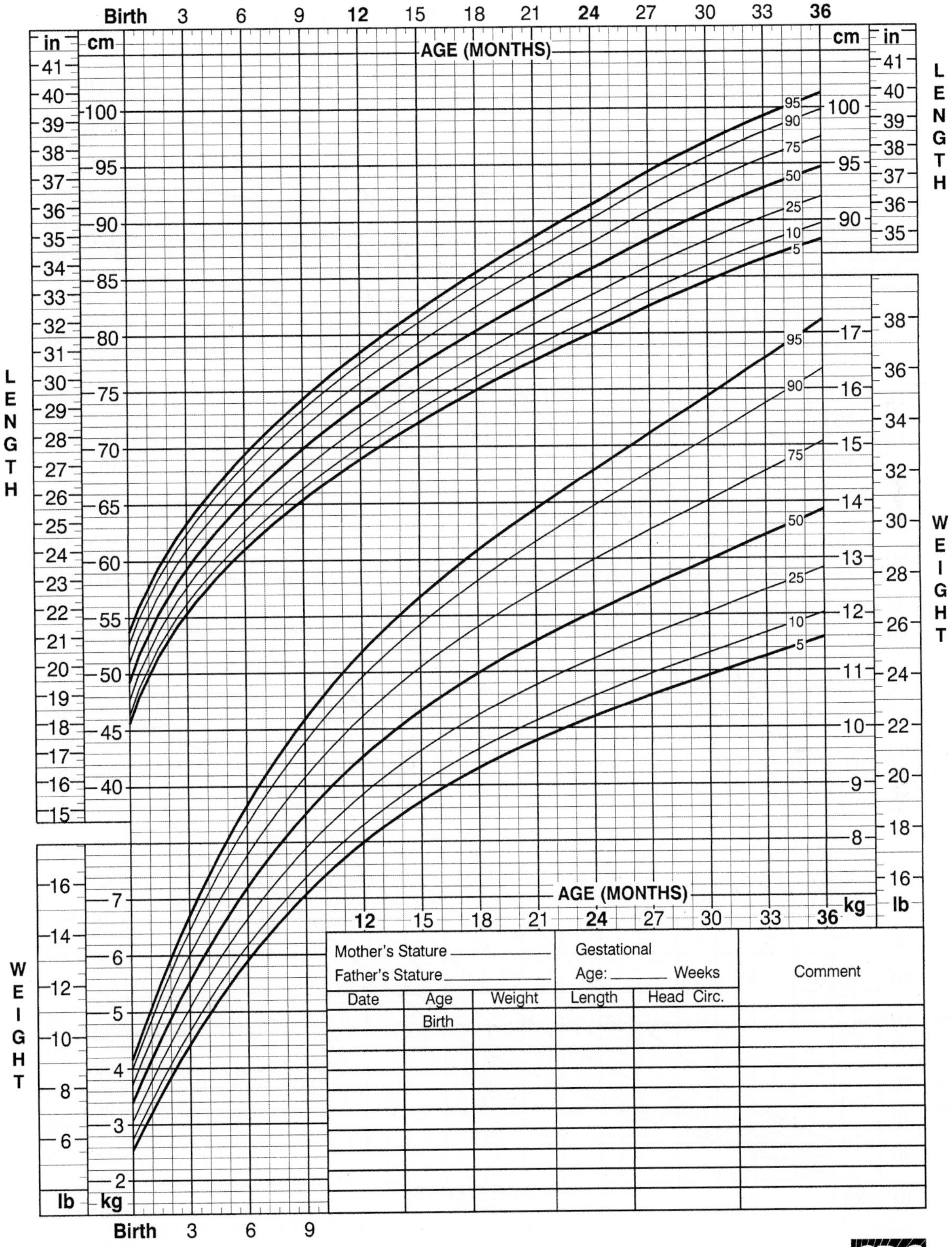

AGE (MONTHS)

Birth 3 6 9 **12** 15 18 21 **24** 27 30 33 **36**

LENGTH

WEIGHT

Mother's Stature _____	Gestational	
Father's Stature _____	Age: _____ Weeks	Comment

Date	Age	Weight	Length	Head Circ.	
	Birth				

Published May 30, 2000 (modified 4/20/01).
SOURCE: Developed by the National Center for Health Statistics in collaboration with
the National Center for Chronic Disease Prevention and Health Promotion (2000).
http://www.cdc.gov/growthcharts

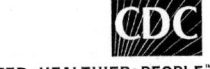

SAFER · HEALTHIER · PEOPLE™

2 to 20 years: Boys
Stature-for-age and Weight-for-age percentiles

NAME _____

RECORD # _____

Mother's Stature _____		Father's Stature _____		
Date	Age	Weight	Stature	BMI*

*To Calculate BMI: Weight (kg) ÷ Stature (cm) ÷ Stature (cm) x 10,000
or Weight (lb) ÷ Stature (in) ÷ Stature (in) x 703

AGE (YEARS)

STATURE

WEIGHT

Published May 30, 2000 (modified 11/21/00).
SOURCE: Developed by the National Center for Health Statistics in collaboration with
the National Center for Chronic Disease Prevention and Health Promotion (2000).
http://www.cdc.gov/growthcharts

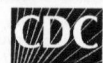

SAFER · HEALTHIER · PEOPLE™

CDC Growth Charts: United States

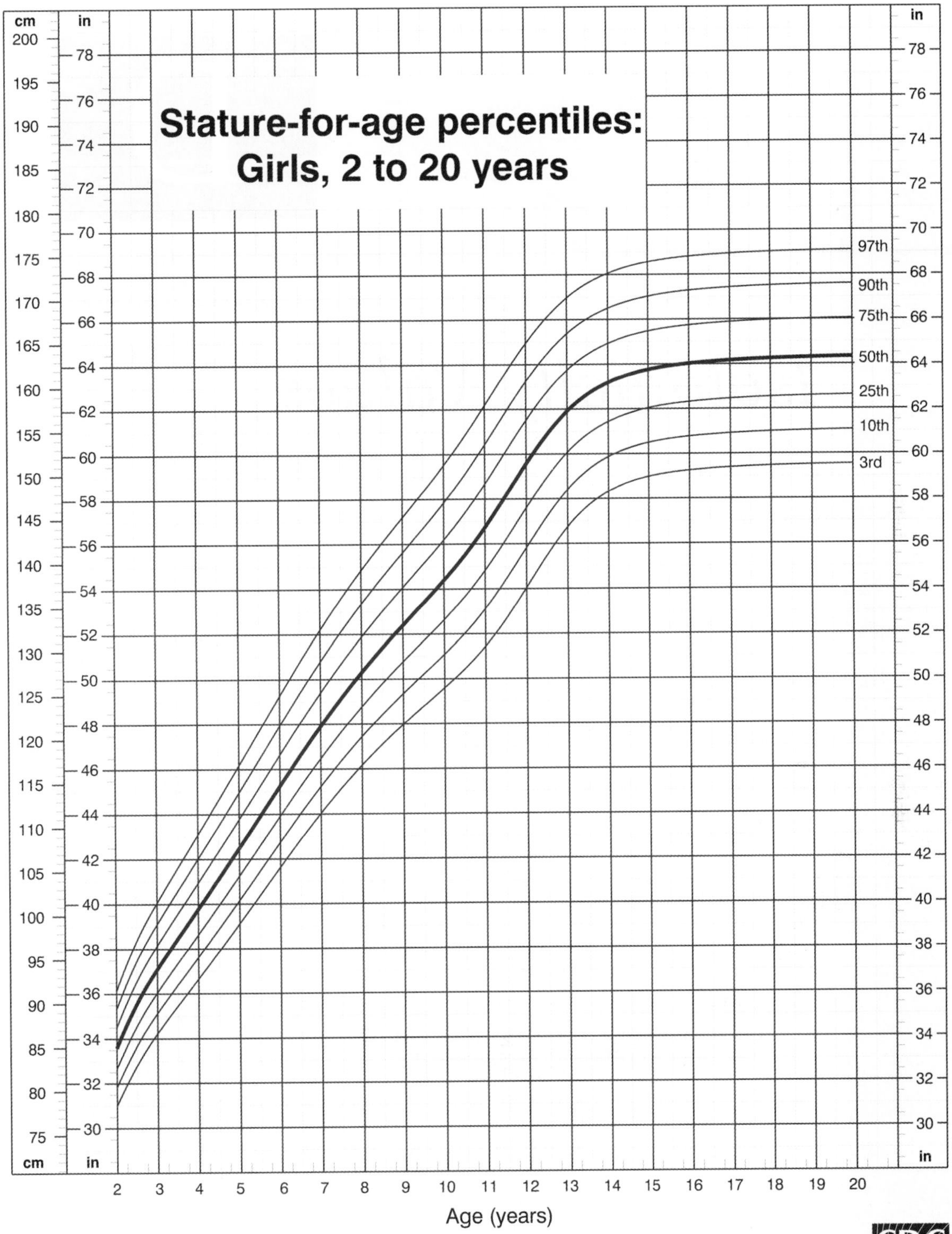

Stature-for-age percentiles:
Girls, 2 to 20 years

97th
90th
75th
50th
25th
10th
3rd

Age (years)

Published May 30, 2000.
SOURCE: Developed by the National Center for Health Statistics in collaboration with
the National Center for Chronic Disease Prevention and Health Promotion (2000).

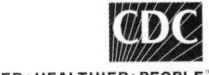

SAFER · HEALTHIER · PEOPLE™

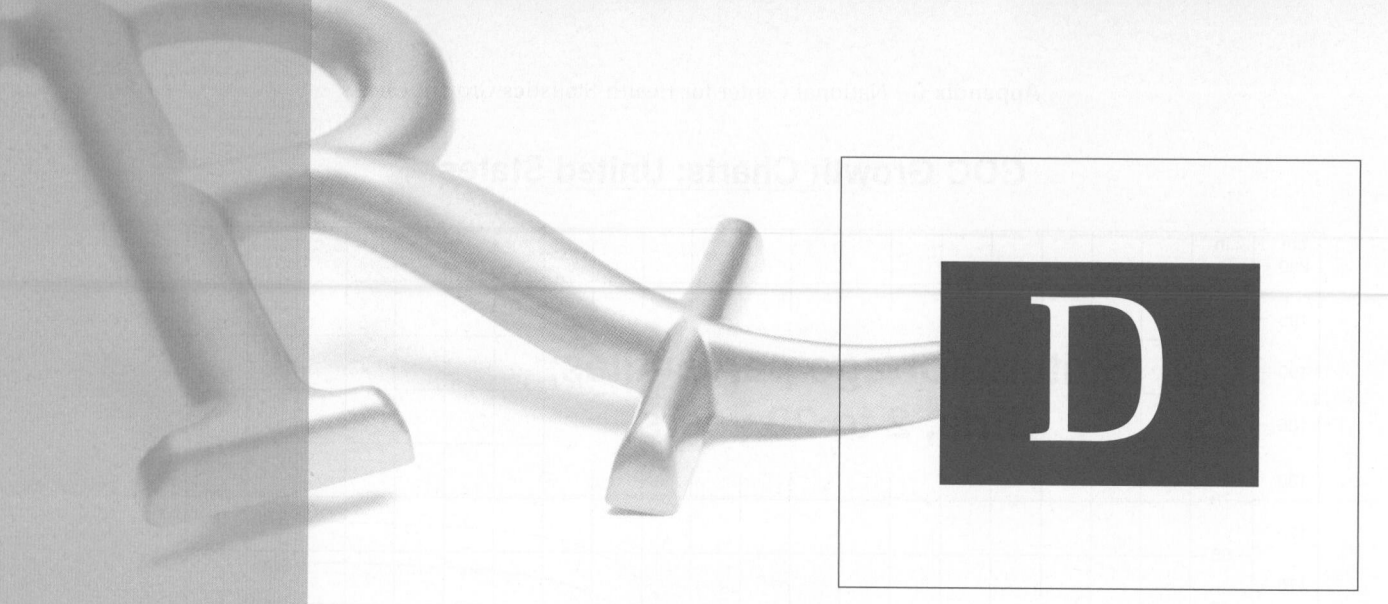

D

Isotonicity Values

CHEMICAL	MW	E$^{1\%}_{NaCl}$	V^{1g}	$\Delta T_f^{1\%}$	% ISO-OSMOTIC CONCENTRATION
Acetylcysteine	163.20	0.20	22.2	0.11	4.58
Alcohol USP (95%)	46.07	0.65	72.2	0.37	1.39
Alcohol, dehydrate	46.07	0.70	77.8	0.40	1.28
Alum, potassium	474.39	0.18	20.0	0.10	6.35
Amantadine hydrochloride	187.71	0.31	34.4	0.18	2.95
Aminoacetic acid (glycine)	75.07	0.41	45.6	0.23	2.20
Aminocaproic acid	131.18	0.26	28.9	0.14	3.52
p-Aminohippuric acid	194.19	0.13	14.4	0.07	
Aminophylline dihydrate	456.46	0.17	19.0	0.10	
p-Aminosalicylate sodium	153.14	0.29	32.2	0.16	3.27
Amitriptyline hydrochloride	313.87	0.18	20.0	0.10	
Ammonium chloride	53.50	1.08	120.0	0.64	
Ammonium phosphate, dibasic	132.06	0.55	61.1	0.31	1.76
Amobarbital sodium	248.26	0.25	27.8	0.14	3.6
Amphetamine sulfate	368.50	0.22	24.3	0.12	4.23
Ampicillin sodium	371.39	0.16	17.8	0.09	5.78
Anileridine hydrochloride	425.40	0.19	21.1	0.10	5.13
Antazoline phosphate	363.36	0.20	22.2	0.11	
Antimony potassium tartrate	333.93	0.18	20.0	0.10	
Antipyrine	188.23	0.17	19.0	0.09	6.81
Antistine hydrochloride	301.81	0.18	20.0	0.11	
Apomorphine hydrochloride	312.79	0.14	15.7	0.08	
L-Arginine hydrochloride	210.66	0.30	33.3	0.17	3.43
Ascorbic acid	176.12	0.18	20.0	0.11	5.94
Atropine sulfate	694.85	0.13	14.3	0.07	8.85
Bacitracin	NA	0.05	5.6	0.02	
Barbital sodium	206.18	0.30	33.3	0.17	3.12
Benoxinate hydrochloride	344.88	0.18	20.0	0.10	
Benzalkonium chloride	360(ave)	0.16	17.8	0.09	
Benzethonium chloride	448.09	0.05	5.6	0.02	
Benztropine mesylate	403.54	0.21	23.3	0.11	
Benzyl alcohol	108.14	0.17	18.9	0.09	
Betazole hydrochloride	184.07	0.51	56.7	0.29	1.91
Bethanechol chloride	196.68	0.39	43.3	0.22	3.05
Boric acid	61.84	0.50	55.7	0.29	1.9
Bretylium tosylate	414.36	0.14	15.6	0.08	
Bromodiphenhydramine hydrochloride	370.72	0.17	18.9	0.10	
Brompheniramine maleate	435.32	0.09	10.0	0.05	
Bupivacaine hydrochloride	342.90	0.17	18.9	0.09	5.38
Butabarbital sodium	234.23	0.27	30.0	0.15	3.33
Butacaine sulfate	710.95	0.20	22.3	0.12	
Caffeine	194.19	0.08	9.0	0.05	
Caffeine and sodium benzoate	NA	0.25	29.0	0.28	
Calcium chloride, anhydrous	110.99	0.70	77.8	0.40	1.29
Calcium chloride · 2H$_2$O	147.02	0.51	56.7	0.29	1.70
Calcium gluconate · H$_2$O	448.39	0.16	17.7	0.09	
Calcium lactate · 5H$_2$O	308.30	0.23	25.7	0.14	4.5
Calcium levulinate · 2H$_2$O	306.32	0.27	30.0	0.15	
Calcium pantothenate	476.54	0.19	21.1	0.10	5.6
Camphor	152.23	0.20	22.3	0.12	
Capreomycin sulfate	NA	0.04	4.4	0.02	
Carbachol	182.65	0.36	40.0	0.20	2.82
Carbenicillin disodium	422.36	0.20	22.2	0.11	4.40
Cefamandole nafate	512.50	0.14	15.6	0.07	
Cefazolin sodium	476.49	0.13	14.4	0.07	
Ceforanide	519.56	0.12	13.3	0.06	
Cefotaxime sodium	477.45	0.15	16.7	0.08	

CHEMICAL	MW	$E^{1\%}_{NaCl}$	V^{1g}	$\Delta T_f^{1\%}$	% ISO-OSMOTIC CONCENTRATION
Cefoxitin sodium	449.44	0.16	17.8	0.09	
Ceftazidime · 5H$_2$O	636.65	0.09	10.0	0.04	
Ceftizoxime sodium	405.39	0.15	16.7	0.08	
Ceftriaxone sodium	661.60	0.13	14.4	0.07	
Cefuroxime sodium	446.37	0.13	14.4	0.07	
Cephalothin sodium	418.42	0.17	18.9	0.09	6.80
Cephapirin sodium	445.45	0.13	14.4	0.07	7.80
Chloramphenicol	323.14	0.10	11.0	0.06	
Chloramphenicol sodium succinate	445.19	0.14	15.6	0.07	6.38
Chlordiazepoxide hydrochloride	336.22	0.22	24.4	0.12	5.50
Chlorobutanol, hydrated	177.47	0.24	26.7	0.14	
Chloroprocaine hydrochloride	307.22	0.20	22.2	0.10	
Chloroquine phosphate	515.87	0.14	15.6	0.08	7.15
Chlorpheniramine maleate	390.87	0.17	18.9	0.08	
Chlorpromazine hydrochloride	355.33	0.10	11.1	0.05	
Chlortetracycline hydrochloride	515.35	0.10	11.1	0.06	
Citric acid	192.13	0.18	20.0	0.09	5.52
Clindamycin phosphate	504.97	0.08	8.9	0.04	10.73
Cocaine hydrochloride	339.82	0.16	17.7	0.09	6.33
Codeine phosphate	406.38	0.14	15.6	0.07	7.29
Colistimethate sodium	1749.82	0.15	16.7	0.08	6.73
Cromolyn sodium	512.34	0.14	15.6	0.08	
Cupric sulfate · 5H$_2$O	249.69	0.18	20.0	0.09	6.85
Cupric sulfate, anhydrous	159.61	0.27	30.0	0.15	4.09
Cyclizine hydrochloride	302.85	0.20	22.2	0.12	
Cyclopentolate hydrochloride	327.85	0.20	22.2	0.11	5.30
Cyclophosphamide	279.10	0.10	11.1	0.06	
Cytarabine	243.22	0.11	12.2	0.06	8.92
Deferoxamine mesylate	656.79	0.09	10.0	0.04	
Demecarium bromide	716.61	0.12	13.3	0.06	
Dexamethasone sodium phosphate	516.42	0.17	18.9	0.09	6.75
Dexchlorpheniramine maleate	390.87	0.15	16.7	0.08	
Dexpanthenol	205.25	0.18	20.0	0.10	5.60
Dextroamphetamine sulfate	368.50	0.23	25.6	0.13	4.16
Dextrose, anhydrous	180.16	0.18	20.0	0.10	5.05
Dextrose, monohydrate	198.17	0.16	17.7	0.09	5.51
Diatrizoate sodium	635.90	0.09	10.0	0.04	10.55
Dibucaine hydrochloride	379.92	0.13	14.3	0.08	
Dicloxacillin sodium monohydrate	510.32	0.10	11.1	0.06	
Dicyclomine hydrochloride	345.96	0.18	20.0	0.10	
Diethanolamine	105.14	0.31	34.4	0.17	2.90
Diethylcarbamazine citrate	391.42	0.14	15.6	0.08	6.29
Dihydrostreptomycin sulfate	1461.43	0.06	6.7	0.03	21.4
Dimethyl sulfoxide	78.13	0.42	46.7	0.24	2.16
Diphenhydramine hydrochloride	291.81	0.27	22.0	0.15	
Dipivefrin hydrochloride	387.90	0.17	18.9	0.09	
Dobutamine hydrochloride	337.84	0.18	20.0	0.10	
Dopamine hydrochloride	189.64	0.30	33.3	0.17	3.11
Doxapram hydrochloride monohydrate	432.98	0.12	13.3	0.07	
Doxycycline hyclate	1025.89	0.12	13.3	0.07	
Dyclonine hydrochloride	325.88	0.24	26.7	0.13	
Dyphylline	254.24	0.10	11.1	0.05	
Echothiopate iodide	383.23	0.16	17.8	0.09	
Edetate disodium	372.24	0.23	25.6	0.13	4.44
Edetate calcium disodium	374.28	0.21	23.3	0.12	4.50
Edrophonium chloride	201.70	0.31	34.4	0.17	3.36
Emetine hydrochloride	553.56	0.10	11.0	0.06	

CHEMICAL	MW	$E^{1\%}_{NaCl}$	V^{1g}	$\Delta T_f^{1\%}$	% ISO-OSMOTIC CONCENTRATION
Ephedrine hydrochloride	201.69	0.30	33.3	0.18	3.2
Ephedrine sulfate	428.54	0.23	25.7	0.13	4.54
Epinephrine bitartrate	333.29	0.18	20.0	0.09	5.7
Epinephrine hydrochloride	219.66	0.29	32.3	0.16	3.47
Ergonovine maleate	441.49	0.16	17.8	0.08	
Erythromycin lactobionate	1092.25	0.07	7.8	0.04	
Ethylenediamine	60.10	0.44	48.9	0.25	
Ethylhydrocupreine hydrochloride	376.92	0.17	19.0	0.09	
Ethylmorphine hydrochloride	385.88	0.16	17.7	0.08	6.18
Eucatropine hydrochloride	327.84	0.18	20.0	0.11	
Ferrous gluconate	482.18	0.15	16.7	0.08	
Fluorescein sodium	376	0.31	34.3	0.18	3.34
Fluorouracil	130.08	0.13	14.4	0.07	
Fluphenazine dihydrochloride	622.63	0.14	15.6	0.08	
D-Fructose	180.16	0.18	20.0	0.10	5.05
Gallamine triethiodide	891.54	0.08	8.9	0.04	
Gentamycin sulfate	NA	0.05	5.6	0.03	
L-Glutamic acid	147.13	0.25	27.8	0.14	
Glycerin	92.09	0.35	37.7	0.20	
Glycine (also Aminocetic acid)	75.07	0.41	45.6	0.23	2.19
Glycopyrrolate	398.34	0.15	16.7	0.08	7.22
Heparin sodium	NA	0.07	7.8	0.04	12.2
Histamine phosphate	307.14	0.25	27.8	0.14	4.1
Homatropine hydrobromide	356.26	0.17	19.0	0.09	5.67
Homatropine methylbromide	370.29	0.19	21.1	0.10	
Hydralazine hydrochloride	196.64	0.37	41.1	0.21	
Hydromorphone hydrochloride	321.81	0.22	24.4	0.12	6.39
Hydroxyamphetamine hydrobromide	232.12	0.26	28.9	0.15	3.71
8-Hydroxyquinoline sulfate	388.40	0.21	23.3	0.11	9.75
Hydroxyzine hydrochloride	447.84	0.25	27.8	0.13	6.32
Hyoscyamine hydrobromide	370.29	0.19	21.1	0.10	
Hyoscyamine sulfate	712.86	0.15	16.7	0.08	
Imipramine hydrochloride	316.88	0.20	22.2	0.11	
Indigotindisulfonate sodium (indigo carmine)	466.36	0.30	33.3	0.17	
Iopamidol	777.09	0.03	3.3	0.01	
Isoetharine hydrochloride	275.77	0.23	25.6	0.13	4.27
Isometheptene mucate	492.65	0.18	20.0	0.09	4.95
Isoniazid	137.14	0.25	27.8	0.14	4.35
Isopropyl alcohol	60.10	0.53	58.9	0.30	1.71
Isoproterenol sulfate	556.63	0.14	15.6	0.07	6.65
Kanamycin sulfate	582.59	0.07	7.8	0.04	
Ketamine hydrochloride	274.19	0.21	23.3	0.12	4.29
Labetalol hydrochloride	364.87	0.19	21.1	0.10	
Lactic acid	90.08	0.41	45.6	0.23	2.3
Lactose monohydrate	360.31	0.07	7.7	0.04	9.75
Levobunolol hydrochloride	327.85	0.12	13.3	0.07	
Levorphanol tartrate	443.50	0.12	13.3	0.06	
Lidocaine hydrochloride	288.82	0.22	24.4	0.12	4.42
Lincomycin hydrochloride	443.01	0.16	17.8	0.09	6.60
Lithium carbonate	73.89	1.06	117.8	0.6	0.92
Mafenide hydrochloride	222.72	0.27	30.0	0.15	3.55
Magnesium chloride · 6 H_2O	203.30	0.45	50.0	0.26	2.02
Magnesium sulfate · 7H_2O	246.47	0.17	19.0	0.09	6.3
Magnesium sulfate, anhydrous	120.37	0.32	35.6	0.18	3.18

CHEMICAL	MW	$E^{1\%}_{NaCl}$	V^{1g}	$\Delta T_f^{1\%}$	% ISO-OSMOTIC CONCENTRATION
Mannitol	182.17	0.17	18.9	0.09	5.07
Menadiol sodium diphosphate	530.18	0.25	27.8	0.14	
Menthol	156.26	0.20	22.3	0.12	
Meperidine hydrochloride	283.79	0.22	24.3	0.12	4.8
Mepivacaine hydrochloride	282.82	0.21	23.3	0.11	4.6
Mercury bichloride	271.50	0.13	14.3	0.07	
Mesoridazine besylate	544.75	0.07	7.8	0.04	
Metaraminol bitartrate	317.30	0.20	22.2	0.11	5.17
Methacholine chloride	195.69	0.32	35.7	0.18	3.21
Methadone hydrochloride	345.92	0.18	20.0	0.10	8.59
Methamphetamine hydrochloride	185.69	0.37	41.0	0.20	2.75
Methanamine	140.19	0.23	25.6	0.12	3.68
Methicillin sodium	420.42	0.18	20.0	0.09	6.00
Methionine	149.21	0.28	31.1	0.16	
Methocarbamol	241.25	0.10	11.1	0.06	
Methotrimeprazine hydrochloride	364.94	0.10	11.1	0.06	
Methyldopa ethyl ester hydrochloride	275.73	0.21	23.3	0.12	4.28
Methylergonovine maleate	455.52	0.10	11.1	0.05	
Methylphenidate hydrochloride	269.77	0.22	24.4	0.12	4.07
Methylprednisolone sodium succinate	496.54	0.09	10.0	0.05	
Metoclopramide hydrochloride	354.27	0.15	16.7	0.08	
Metycaine hydrochloride	292.82	0.20	22.3	0.12	
Mezlocillin sodium	561.57	0.11	12.2	0.06	
Mild silver protein	—	0.17	20.0	0.09	
Minocycline hydrochloride	493.95	0.10	11.1	0.05	
Monoethanolamine	61.08	0.53	58.9	0.30	1.70
Morphine hydrochloride	375.84	0.15	16.7	0.08	
Morphine sulfate	758.82	0.14	15.6	0.07	
Nafcillin sodium	436.47	0.14	15.6	0.07	
Naloxone hydrochloride	363.84	0.14	15.6	0.08	8.07
Naphazoline hydrochloride	246.73	0.27	25.7	0.15	3.99
Neomycin sulfate	NA	0.12	12.3	0.06	
Neostigmine bromide	303.20	0.22	20.0	0.12	
Neostigmine methyl sulfate	334.39	0.20	22.2	0.10	5.22
Netilmicin sulfate	1441.56	0.07	7.8	0.04	
Nicotinamide	122.13	0.26	29.0	0.14	4.49
Nicotinic acid	123.11	0.25	27.8	0.14	
Novobiocin sodium	634.62	0.08	8.9	0.04	
Orphenadrine citrate	461.50	0.13	14.4	0.07	
Oxacillin sodium	441.44	0.17	18.9	0.09	6.64
Oxycodone hydrochloride	351.82	0.14	15.6	0.08	7.4
Oxymetazoline hydrochloride	296.84	0.22	24.4	0.12	4.92
Oxymorphone hydrochloride	337.81	0.16	17.8	0.08	
Oxytetracycline hydrochloride	496.91	0.14	15.6	0.08	
Papaverine hydrochloride	375.86	0.10	11.1	0.06	
Paraldehyde	132.16	0.25	27.8	0.14	3.65
Pentazocine lactate	375.51	0.15	16.7	0.08	
Pentobarbital sodium	248.26	0.25	27.8	0.14	
Penicillin G sodium	356.38	0.18	20.0	0.11	
Penicillin G procaine	588.71	0.10	11.0	0.06	
Penicillin G potassium	372.47	0.18	20.0	0.11	
Phenacaine hydrochloride	352.85	0.20	17.7	0.10	
Pheniramine maleate	356.42	0.16	17.8	0.09	
Phenobarbital sodium	254.22	0.24	26.7	0.13	
Phenol	94.11	0.35	39.0	0.19	2.8
Phentolamine mesylate	377.47	0.17	18.9	0.09	8.23

CHEMICAL	MW	$E^{1\%}_{NaCl}$	V^{1g}	$\Delta T_f^{1\%}$	% ISO-OSMOTIC CONCENTRATION
Phenylephrine hydrochloride	203.67	0.32	32.3	0.18	3.0
Phenylethyl alcohol	122.17	0.25	27.8	0.14	
Phenylpropanolamine hydrochloride	187.67	0.38	42.2	0.21	2.6
Physostigmine salicylate	413.46	0.16	17.7	0.09	
Physostigmine sulfate	648.45	0.13	14.3	0.07	7.74
Pilocarpine hydrochloride	244.72	0.24	26.7	0.13	4.08
Pilocarpine nitrate	271.27	0.23	25.7	0.13	
Piperacillin sodium	539.54	0.11	12.2	0.06	
Piperocaine hydrochloride	297.82	0.21	23.3	0.12	
Polyethylene glycol 300	NA	0.12	13.3	0.06	6.73
Polyethylene glycol 400	NA	0.08	8.9	0.04	8.50
Polyethylene glycol 1500	NA	0.06	6.7	0.03	10.00
Polyethylene glycol 1540	NA	0.02	2.2	0.01	
Polyethylene glycol 4000	NA	0.02	2.2	0.00	
Polymyxin B sulfate	NA	0.09	10.0	0.04	
Polysorbate 80	NA	0.02	2.2	0.01	
Polyvinly alcohol (99% hydrolyzed)	NA	0.02	2.2	0.00	
Potassium acetate	98.15	0.59	65.5	0.34	1.53
Potassium chloride	74.55	0.76	84.3	0.43	1.19
Potassium iodide	166.02	0.34	37.7	0.20	2.59
Potassium nitrate	85.11	0.56	62.2	0.32	1.62
Potassium permanganate	158.04	0.39	43.3	0.22	
Potassium phosphate, dibasic anhydrous	174.18	0.46	51.1	0.26	2.11
Potassium phosphate, monobasic	136.09	0.44	48.9	0.25	2.18
Potassium sorbate	150.22	0.41	45.6	0.23	2.23
Potassium sulfate	174.27	0.44	48.9	0.25	2.11
Potassium thiocyanate	97.18	0.59	65.5	0.34	1.52
Povidone	NA	0.01	1.11	0.00	
Pralidoxime chloride	172.62	0.32	35.6	0.18	2.87
Pramoxine hydrochloride	329.87	0.18	20.0	0.10	
Prilocaine hydrochloride	256.78	0.22	24.4	0.12	4.18
Procainamide hydrochloride	271.79	0.22	24.4	0.12	
Procaine hydrochloride	272.77	0.21	23.3	0.12	5.05
Prochlorperazine edisylate	564.15	0.06	6.7	0.03	
Promazine hydrochloride	320.89	0.13	14.4	0.07	
Promethazine hydrochloride	320.89	0.18	20.0	0.11	
Propantheline bromide	448.40	0.11	12.2	0.06	
Proparacaine hydrochloride	330.85	0.15	16.7	0.08	7.46
Propoxycaine hydrochloride	330.86	0.19	21.1	0.11	
Propranolol hydrochloride	295.80	0.20	22.2	0.12	
Propylene glycol	76.10	0.43	47.8	0.25	2.10
Pyridostigmine bromide	261.12	0.22	24.4	0.12	4.13
Pyridoxine hydrochloride	205.64	0.36	40.0	0.20	
Pyrilamine maleate	401.47	0.18	20.0	0.10	
Quinidine gluconate	520.58	0.12	13.3	0.06	
Quinidine sulfate	782.96	0.10	11.1	0.06	
Quinine bisulfate	422.50	0.09	10.0	0.05	
Quinine hydrochloride	396.91	0.14	15.7	0.07	
Ranitidine hydrochloride	350.87	0.18	20.0	0.10	
Resorcinol	110.11	0.28	31.1	0.16	3.3
Riboflavin phosphate (sodium)	514.36	0.08	8.9	0.04	
Ritodrine hydrochloride	323.81	0.20	22.2	0.11	
Scopolamine hydrobromide	438.32	0.12	13.3	0.06	7.85
Secobarbital sodium	260.27	0.24	26.7	0.13	3.9
Silver nitrate	169.89	0.33	36.7	0.19	2.74
Sodium acetate	136.08	0.46	51.1	0.26	2.03

CHEMICAL	MW	$E^{1\%}_{NaCl}$	V^{1g}	$\Delta T_f^{1\%}$	% ISO-OSMOTIC CONCENTRATION
Sodium acetate, anhydrous	82.03	0.77	85.5	0.44	1.18
Sodium ascorbate	198.11	0.32	35.6	0.18	2.99
Sodium benzoate	144.11	0.40	44.3	0.23	2.25
Sodium bicarbonate	84.00	0.65	72.3	0.38	1.39
Sodium bisulfite	104.06	0.61	67.7	0.35	1.5
Sodium borate · $10H_2O$	381.37	0.42	46.7	0.24	2.6
Sodium carbonate, anhydrous	105.99	0.70	77.8	0.40	1.32
Sodium carbonate, monohydrated	124.00	0.60	66.7	0.34	1.56
Sodium carboxymethylcellulose	NA	0.03	3.3	0.01	
Sodium chloride	58.45	1.00	111.0	0.58	0.9
Sodium citrate	294.10	0.31	34.4	0.17	3.02
Sodium iodide	149.89	0.39	43.3	0.22	2.37
Sodium lactate	112.06	0.55	61.1	0.31	1.72
Sodium lauryl sulfate	288.38	0.08	8.9	0.04	
Sodium metabisulfite	190.10	0.67	74.4	0.38	1.38
Sodium nitrate	84.99	0.68	75.7	0.39	1.36
Sodium nitrite	69.00	0.84	93.3	0.48	1.08
Sodium phosphate, dibasic anhydrous	141.98	0.53	59.0	0.30	1.75
Sodium phosphate, dibasic · $2H_2O$	178.05	0.42	46.7	0.24	2.23
Sodium phosphate, dibasic · $7H_2O$	268.08	0.29	32.3	0.16	3.33
Sodium phosphate, dibasic · $12H_2O$	358.21	0.22	24.3	0.12	4.45
Sodium phosphate, monobasic anhydrous	119.98	0.46	51.1	0.26	2.1
Sodium phosphate, monobasic ($NaH_2PO_4 · H_2O$)	138.00	0.43	44.3	0.24	2.21
Sodium phosphate, monobasic dihydrate	156.01	0.36	40.0	0.20	2.77
Sodium propionate	96.07	0.61	67.7	0.35	1.47
Sodium salicylate	160.11	0.36	40.0	0.20	2.53
Sodium succinate	162.05	0.32	35.6	0.18	2.90
Sodium sulfate · $10H_2O$	322.19	0.26	28.9	0.14	3.95
Sodium sulfate, anhydrous	142.04	0.54	60.0	0.30	1.78
Sodium sulfite, exsiccated	126.04	0.65	72.3	0.37	
Sodium tartrate · $2H_2O$	230.08	0.33	36.7	0.19	2.72
Sodium thiosulfate · $5H_2O$	248.18	0.31	34.4	0.18	2.98
Spectinomycin hydrochloride	495.35	0.16	17.8	0.09	5.66
Streptomycin sulfate	1457.40	0.07	7.7	0.03	
Strong silver protein	NA	0.08	9.0	0.04	
Succinylcholine chloride · $2H_2O$	397.34	0.20	22.2	0.11	4.48
Sucrose	342.30	0.08	9.0	0.04	9.25
Sulbactam sodium	255.22	0.24	26.7	0.14	3.75
Sulfacetamide sodium	254.24	0.23	25.7	0.14	
Sulfadiazine sodium	272.26	0.24	26.7	0.13	4.24
Sulfamerazine sodium	286.29	0.23	25.7	0.13	4.53
Sulfamethazine sodium	300.31	0.21	23.3	0.12	
Sulfanilamide	172.21	0.22	24.3	0.13	
Sulfapyridine sodium	271.27	0.23	25.6	0.13	4.55
Sulfathiazole sodium	304.33	0.22	24.3	0.12	4.82
Tannic acid	NA	0.03	3.3	0.01	
Tartaric acid	150.09	0.25	27.8	0.14	3.9
Terbutaline sulfate	548.65	0.14	15.6	0.08	6.75
Tetracaine hydrochloride	300.82	0.18	20.0	0.11	
Tetracycline hydrochloride	480.91	0.14	15.7	0.07	
Tetrahydrozoline hydrochloride	236.75	0.28	31.1	0.16	
Theophylline · H_2O	198.18	0.10	11.1	0.05	
Theophylline sodium glycinate	NA	0.31	34.4	0.18	2.94
Thiamine hydrochloride	337.27	0.25	27.8	0.13	4.24
Thiethylperazine maleate	631.77	0.09	10.0	0.05	
Thiopental sodium	264.32	0.27	30.0	0.15	3.5

CHEMICAL	MW	$E^{1\%}_{NaCl}$	V^{1g}	$\Delta T_f^{1\%}$	% ISO-OSMOTIC CONCENTRATION
Thioridazine hydrochloride	407.04	0.05	5.6	0.02	
Thiotepa	189.22	0.16	17.8	0.09	5.67
Ticarcillin disodium	428.40	0.20	22.2	0.11	4.62
Timolol maleate	432.49	0.13	14.4	0.07	
Tobramycin	467.52	0.07	7.8	0.03	
Tolazoline hydrochloride	196.68	0.34	37.8	0.19	3.05
Trifluoperazine dihydrochloride	480.43	0.18	20.0	0.10	
Triflupromazine hydrochloride	388.89	0.09	10.0	0.05	
Trimeprazine tartrate	747.00	0.06	6.7	0.03	
Trimethobenzamide hydrochloride	424.93	0.10	11.1	0.06	
Tripelennamine hydrochloride	291.83	0.30	24.3	0.17	
Tromethamine	121.14	0.26	28.9	0.15	3.41
Tropicamide	284.36	0.09	10.0	0.05	
Tubocurarine chloride · 5H$_2$O	785.77	0.13	14.4	0.07	
Urea	60.06	0.52	57.8	0.30	1.73
Vancomycin hydrochloride	1485.71	0.05	5.6	0.02	
Verapamil hydrochloride	491.06	0.13	14.4	0.07	
Warfarin sodium	330.31	0.17	18.9	0.09	6.10
Xylometazoline hydrochloride	280.84	0.21	23.3	0.12	4.68
Zinc chloride	136.30	0.61	67.8	0.35	
Zinc phenolsulfonate	555.84	0.18	20.0	0.11	
Zinc sulfate · 7H$_2$O	287.56	0.15	16.7	0.08	7.65
Zinc sulfate, dried	161.46	0.23	25.6	0.13	4.52

MW, molecular weight of the drug; $E^{1\%}_{NaCl}$, sodium chloride equivalent of the drug at 1% concentration (values may vary slightly with concentration); V^{1g}, volume in milliliters of isotonic solution that can be prepared by adding water to 1.0 g of the drug; $\Delta T_f^{1\%}$, freezing point depression of a 1% solution of the drug.
Sources (including but not limited to the following):

1. Hammarlund ER, Pedersen-Bjergaard K. New isotonic solution values J Am Pharm Assoc Pract Ed 1958; 19: 39.
2. Hammarlund ER, Pedersen-Bjergaard K. A simplified graphic method for the preparation of isotonic solutions J Am Pharm Assoc Sci Ed 1958; 47: 107–114.
3. Hammarlund ER, Pedersen-Bjergaard K. Hemolysis of erythrocytes in various iso-osmotic solutions J Pharm Sci 1961; 50: 24–30.
4. Hammarlund ER, Deming JD, Pedersen-Bjergaard K. Additional sodium chloride equivalents and freezing point depressions for various medicinal solutions J Pharm Sci 1965; 54: 160–162.
5. Hammarlund ER, Van Pevenage GL. Sodium chloride equivalents, cryoscopic properties and hemolytic effects of certain medicinals in aqueous solution J Pharm Sci 1966; 55: 1448–1451.
6. Fassett WE, Fuller TS, Hammarlund ER. Sodium chloride equivalents, cryoscapic properties and hemolytic effects of certain medicinals in aqueous solution II: Supplemental Values J Pharm Sci 1969; 58: 1540–1542.
7. Sapp C, Lord M, Hammarlund ER. Sodium chloride equivalents, cryoscopic properties, and hemolytic effects of certain medicinals in aqueous solution III: Supplemental Values J Pharm Sci 1975; 64: 1884–1886.
8. Hammarlund ER. Sodium chloride equivalents, cryoscopic properties and hemolytic effects of certain medicinals in aqueous solution IV: Supplemental Values J Pharm Sci 1981; 70: 1161–1163.
9. Hammarlund ER. Sodium chloride equivalents, cryoscopic properties and hemolytic effects of certain medicinals in aqueous solution section V: Supplemental Values J Pharm Sci 1989; 78: 519–520.
10. Budavari S., ed. The Merck index, 11th ed. Rahway, NJ: Merck, 1989; MISC 79–MISC 103.

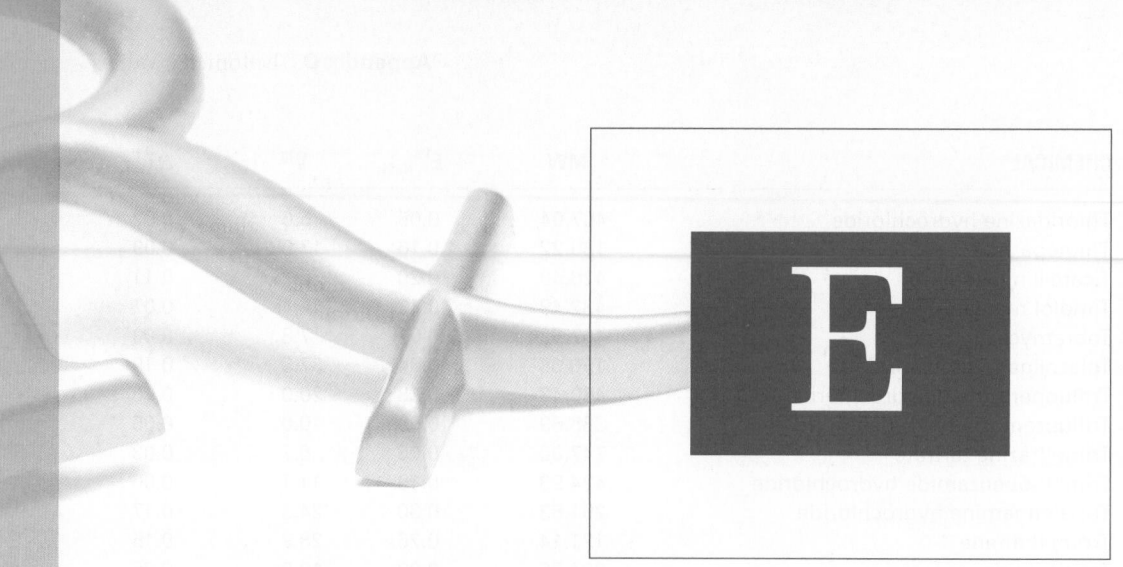

Code of Ethics for Pharmacists

PREAMBLE

Pharmacists are health professionals who assist individuals in making the best use of medications. This Code, prepared and supported by pharmacists, is intended to state publicly the principles that form the fundamental basis of the roles and responsibilities of pharmacists. These principles, based on moral obligations and virtues, are established to guide pharmacists in relationships with patients, health professionals, and society.

I. A pharmacist respects the covenantal relationship between the patient and pharmacist.
Considering the patient–pharmacist relationship as a covenant means that a pharmacist has moral obligations in response to the gift of trust received from society. In return for this gift, a pharmacist promises to help individuals achieve optimum benefit from their medications, to be committed to their welfare, and to maintain their trust.

II. A pharmacist promotes the good of every patient in a caring, compassionate, and confidential manner.
A pharmacist places concern for the well-being of the patient at the center of professional practice. In doing so, a pharmacist considers needs stated by the patient as well as those defined by health science. A pharmacist is dedicated to protecting the dignity of the patient. With a caring attitude and a compassionate spirit, a pharmacist focuses on serving the patient in a private and confidential manner.

III. A pharmacist respects the autonomy and dignity of each patient.
A pharmacist promotes the right of self-determination and recognizes individual self-worth by encouraging patients to participate in decisions about their health. A pharmacist communicates with patients in terms that are understandable. In all cases, a pharmacist respects personal and cultural differences among patients.

IV. A pharmacist acts with honesty and integrity in professional relationships.
A pharmacist has a duty to tell the truth and to act with conviction of conscience. A pharmacist avoids discriminatory practices, behavior or work conditions that impair professional judgment, and actions that compromise dedication to the best interests of patients.

V. A pharmacist maintains professional competence.
A pharmacist has a duty to maintain knowledge and abilities as new medications, devices, and technologies become available and as health information advances.

VI. A pharmacist respects the values and abilities of colleagues and other health professionals.
When appropriate, a pharmacist asks for the consultation of colleagues or other health professionals or refers the patient. A pharmacist acknowledges that colleagues and other health professionals may differ in the beliefs and values they apply to the care of the patient.

VII. A pharmacist serves individual, community, and societal needs.
The primary obligation of a pharmacist is to individual patients. However, the obligations of a pharmacist may at times extend beyond the individual to the community and society. In these situations, the pharmacist recognizes the responsibilities that accompany these obligations and acts accordingly.

VIII. A pharmacist seeks justice in the distribution of health resources.
When health resources are allocated, a pharmacist is fair and equitable, balancing the needs of patients and society.

Adopted by the membership of the American Pharmaceutical Association, October 27, 1994. Reprinted with permission.

Index

Page numbers in *italics* denote figures; those followed by a "t" denote tables.

725

Cómo establecer algunas metas

A la mayoría de las personas les parece muy iluminante saber cuánto necesitan ahorrar para lograr objetivos específicos. El querer jubilarse algún día es un objetivo muy común. El reto es que cuando usted tiene veinte o treinta y tantos años, es difícil tener objetivos más claramente definidos —tales como, saber que se quiere jubilar a la edad de 58 años y mudarse a Nuevo Méjico, dónde vivirá en una comunidad de viviendas compartidas y va a comprar una casa que cuesta $200.000. Pues no se preocupe —usted no necesita saber exactamente cuándo, dónde y cómo quiere jubilarse.

Lo que si quiere evitar son sorpresas desagradables. Cuando Pedro y Nancy llegaron a sus 40 años, dolorosamente se dieron cuenta que su jubilación se encontraba bien lejos en el tiempo porque todavía estaban tratando de pagar sus deudas y de establecer en forma regular un programa de ahorros. Ahora tienen que enfrentarse a una elección: tener que trabajar hasta los 70 años para alcanzar sus metas de jubilación o conformarse con un estilo de vida más modesto en su vida de jubilados.

Si la jubilación no es una de sus metas, ¡magnifico! Si usted quiere (y tiene capacidad) para continuar trabajando durante los 60, 70 y 80 años de edad, usted no necesitará acumular los grandes ahorros que otros necesitan para poder relajarse durante esos años dorados. Pero contar con tener la capacidad de trabajar durante toda su vida es riesgoso —usted no sabe cómo el mercado de trabajo y su salud podrían estar más adelante en su vida.

El dilema de los planes de ahorro para la jubilación

Las reformas impositivas de años anteriores eliminaron muchas de las deducciones de impuestos disponibles que existían hasta entonces, excepto por una de las mejores y con más deducciones asequibles: los aportes a los planes o cuentas de jubilación. El dinero que usted contribuye a una cuenta o plan de jubilación que tiene con un empleador —tales como un 401(k) o un 403(b)—, o a un plan para trabajadores independientes —tales como un SEP-IRA o un Keogh— es generalmente deducible del impuesto. Esto le ahorra tanto impuestos federales como estatales en el año en el cual se hace la contribución. Además, todo el dinero en estas cuentas se capitaliza con el tiempo sin el efecto de los impuestos. (***Nota:*** Los relativamente nuevos planes de ahorro para jubilación Roth IRA son diferentes porque aunque no ofrecen una deducción inmediata de los impuestos, permiten retirar el dinero de la cuenta sin pagar impuestos, siempre y cuando satisfaga ciertos requisitos que debe reunir.) Estos planes o cuentas de jubilación que reducen impuestos son unas de las mejores formas de ahorrar su dinero y de incrementarlo.

El reto para la mayor parte de las personas es mantener sus gastos bajos, en un nivel que les permita ahorrar lo suficiente para contribuir a estos beneficiosos planes que reducen impuestos. Supóngase que actualmente está gastando todo su ingreso (cosa que típicamente hacen los norteamericanos) y que usted quiere ser capaz de ahorrar un 10 por ciento del mismo. Gracias a los ahorros impositivos que usted obtendría por contribuir a su cuenta de jubilación, si usted puede reducir sus gastos en tan solo 7,5 por ciento y colocar esos ahorros en una de estas cuentas de jubilación deducibles de impuestos, usted será capaz de alcanzar su meta del 10 por ciento.

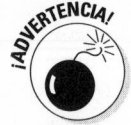

Hablando en forma general, cuando usted contribuye a un plan de pensión, no tiene acceso al dinero a menos que pague una multa o penalización. Así que si usted está guardando dinero para el pago inicial de una casa, el colocarlo en una cuenta de jubilación es generalmente una mala idea. ¿Por qué? Porque cuando usted retira dinero de una cuenta de fondos para la jubilación, usted no solamente debe impuestos sobre la renta, sino que también debe una penalización considerable (el 10 por ciento del monto que se retira debe ir a Internal Revenue Services [IRS, por sus siglas en inglés] y, además, debe pagar también cualquier penalización que establezca el estado donde usted reside).

De modo que el dilema es que usted puede ahorrar en otras cuentas que no sean las de jubilación y tener acceso al dinero del pago inicial, pero tiene entonces que pagar mucho más impuestos. O, usted puede contribuir a su cuenta de jubilación y obtener los beneficios impositivos, pero no tener acceso al dinero para la compra de su casa.

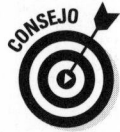

Existen dos maneras de eludir este dilema. Averigüe si su empleador le permite hacer préstamos contra los saldos del plan de jubilación. Y si usted tiene una Cuenta de Jubilación Personal (IRA, por sus siglas en inglés), ya sea una estándar IRA o la más reciente Roth IRA, usted puede retirar hasta $10.000 (como máximo en su vida) para la compra de una casa, siempre y cuando usted no haya sido propietario de una vivienda en los últimos dos años. La cuenta Roth IRA es una mejor inversión porque no se pagan impuestos por retirar dinero siempre que la cuenta tenga un mínimo de 5 años de haber sido abierta. Aunque una cuenta estándar IRA no tiene esa restricción relativa al tiempo, los retiros de esta cuenta son considerados ingresos para efectos impositivos; usted obtendrá, para el pago inicial de la casa, sólo el monto resultante después que los impuestos sean deducidos.

Ya que la mayoría de nosotros disponemos de una restringida cantidad de dinero que podemos gastar en lo que queramos, debemos decidir cuáles son nuestras prioridades. Ahorrar para la jubilación y reducir el impuesto que se paga es importante, pero cuando usted está intentando ahorrar para comprarse una casa, alguno de sus ahorros o la mayoría necesitan estar fuera de la cuenta de jubilación que está protegida de los impuestos. Está bien dejar de ahorrar para su jubilación y ahorrar para acumular una cantidad para el pago inicial, siempre y cuando sea por corto tiempo. Sin embargo, sea cuidadoso y compre una casa que le permita suficiente flexibilidad en el presupuesto, como para contribuir a su cuenta de jubilación después de la compra. ¡Haga el ejercicio de presupuesto de la Tabla 2-1 que presentamos al principio de este capítulo!

Otras razones para ahorrar

Casi nunca, la única razón para ahorrar es el querer tener los recursos financieros para dejar de trabajar algún día. La mayoría de las personas tienen otras razones, que son igualmente importantes, para ahorrar dinero. Aquí presentamos otros objetivos financieros típicos que motivan a las personas (o que deberían estar motivándolas) a ahorrar dinero. También le decimos cómo hacer que cada meta encaje con su deseo de comprar una casa y con su situación financiera en general.

✔ **Reserva para emergencias:** El problema no es que cosas malas pasan al azar, sino *cuándo* pasan. Simplemente usted no puede predecir qué impacto podrán tener sobre usted y su familia la pérdida del trabajo o la muerte de un familiar, un accidente o un gasto muy grande e inesperado. Por eso es una buena idea tener una reserva de dinero segura y de fácil acceso que usted pueda usar en caso que la necesite.

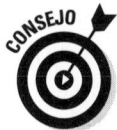

Asegúrese que tiene acceso a por lo menos, un mínimo equivalente a tres meses de gastos (si usted tiene un trabajo muy inestable y un ingreso volátil, quizás sean necesarios seis meses). Idealmente, usted debería mantener su dinero en un fondo de mercado monetario, porque tales fondos le ofrecen alto rendimiento y liquidez. Las principales compañías de fondos mutuales (tales como Vanguard, Fidelity y T. Rowe Price) ofrecen fondos monetarios con rendimientos competitivos, facilidades para emitir cheques y acceso a otras buenas inversiones. (Vea el Capítulo 3 para conocer más acerca de estos fondos y cómo usted puede usarlos para invertir su dinero del pago inicial.) Alternativamente, una cuenta de ahorros en un banco puede funcionar también para estos propósitos, pero probablemente le ofrezca un rendimiento menor. Si usted tiene unos familiares benevolentes que estén dispuestos a darle dinero rápidamente, también ellos le pueden servir de reserva para emergencias.

✔ **Gastos educativos:** Si usted tiene unos pequeños querubines en su casa, seguramente quiere lo mejor para ellos, y eso típicamente incluye una buena educación universitaria. Así que cuando los primeros regalos en efectivo comienzan a llegar desde la casa de los abuelos, muchos padres establecen una cuenta de inversión en nombre del niño.

Sus mejores intenciones podrían volverse en contra suya cuando su hijo solicite inscripción en la universidad. Si todo sigue como hasta ahora, cuanto más dinero tenga usted disponible en cuentas distintas a las de jubilación y, en nombre de su hijo, menos dinero podrá solicitar él como ayuda financiera para sus estudios. (Por ayuda financiera queremos decir todo tipo de ayuda, incluyendo becas y préstamos que no están basados en el criterio de necesidad). A menos que usted sea rico o que esté seguro que puede pagar por el costo completo de la educación universitaria de sus hijos, piénselo bastante antes de poner dinero a nombre de ellos. Aunque esto puede parecer egoísta, usted les hace a su familia y a sí mismo un favor al aprovechar todas las oportunidades que tenga de contribuir a sus cuentas de jubilación. Recuerde también que una de las ventajas de ser propietario es que usted puede pedir prestado contra la ganancia de capital de la vivienda para ayudar a pagar los gastos de universidad de sus hijos.

✔ **Fondos para comenzar un negocio:** Otra razón para ahorrar dinero es si usted espera tener o comprar un negocio algún día. Cuando usted tenga suficiente ganancia de capital acumulada en su casa, usted puede hacer un préstamo contra esa ganancia para ser usado en el negocio. O, quizás, desee acumular el dinero en otras inversiones por separado para este propósito.

No importa cuáles son sus objetivos financieros y personales, usted probablemente va a necesitar un monto decente de dinero para alcanzarlos. Piense en cuáles son sus metas y cuánto necesita ahorrar para lograrlas, especialmente la jubilación. Ponga sus finanzas en orden antes de decidir cuánto realmente usted puede pagar por una casa. De otra manera, usted puede terminar siendo un prisionero de su vivienda.

Cómo Proteger a Sus Dependientes, a Sí Mismo y a Sus Bienes

No tener una cobertura de seguros apropiada es potencialmente desastroso — tanto para usted como para sus dependientes. No estamos hablando en este caso del seguro de la propiedad. (¡Caramba, ni siquiera hemos explicado cómo encontrar una casa u obtener un préstamo todavía! Explicaremos el seguro de propiedad en el Capítulo 13.)

Personalmente, usted, necesita una protección de seguros adecuada para sí mismo y para sus bienes. Claro que usted puede arriesgarse y tener la esperanza de que nunca va a contraer una enfermedad grave, o que tenga un accidente de tránsito horrible o sufra cualquier otra desgracia o mala suerte. Pero, generalmente, la desgracia y la mala suerte llegan sin avisar.

Créanos cuando le decimos que somos unas personas optimistas y positivas. Sin embargo —y este es un gran *sin embargo*—, conocemos muchas personas que se metieron o metieron a sus familias (o ambos casos) en dificultades financieras después de comprar una casa porque por descuido no se aseguraron apropiadamente.

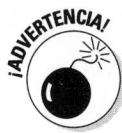

Aquí le presentamos algunos casos que lo ayudarán a ser cauteloso:

- ✔ Steve compró una casa y luego se enteró que tenía esclerosis múltiple. Tuvo que cortar dramáticamente las horas de trabajo, y como no tenía un seguro de incapacidad de largo plazo adecuado y estaba ganando mucho menos dinero, se vio forzado a vender su casa con pérdida porque el mercado inmobiliario en su zona estaba deprimido.

- ✔ María era dueña de una casa en California y a pesar del riesgo conocido de terremotos en la zona, María no había comprado seguro con cobertura para eventos sísmicos. Ella decía: "Es tan costoso y, además, las compañías de seguro no podrán hacerle frente a todos los reclamos en caso de un terremoto grande. El gobierno nos podrá ayudar." Más adelante, después de un terremoto, la casa de María fue una pérdida total, y aunque el gobierno le hizo un préstamo, *no pagó* por la pérdida y, en última instancia, el dinero tuvo que salir del bolsillo de ella.

- ✔ Maggie y Donald vivían una vida encantadora en el área campestre de Nueva Inglaterra con sus dos hijos, una casa en la granja, un perro y un gato — hasta que Maggie se enfermó con cáncer. Maggie tuvo que dejar su trabajo, y esto puso un poco de presión en las finanzas familiares. Después de muchos tratamientos, Maggie falleció y Donald y los niños se vieron forzados a salir de la casa porque Maggie no tenía un seguro de vida que los cubriera.

- ✔ Michelle tenía la acera de su casa rota. Desafortunadamente, un día un señor mayor tropezó y se hirió seriamente. Para hacer de esta larga historia una corta, después de largos trámites legales, el veredicto fue a favor del señor, y el pago que se le hizo fue lo suficientemente grande como para forzar a Michelle a vender su casa. Una buena parte del acuerdo legal salió del bolsillo de Michelle porque ella no tenía suficiente seguro de responsabilidad civil (para daños a terceros).

Ahora bien, no estamos tratando de decirle que tener seguro hubiera hecho que esas situaciones terminaran bien. Generalmente, estar asegurado no puede prevenir problemas médicos grandes, hacer que una persona no fallezca, o detener la demanda de alguien contra usted. Sin embargo, un seguro apropiado puede protegerlo a usted y su familia de las adversas y serias consecuencias financieras de problemas de esta magnitud. El tipo correcto de cobertura de seguro puede establecer la diferencia entre mantener o perder su casa, y puede ayudarlo a su familia y a usted a mantener su estándar de vida.

Hacer caso omiso de la necesidad de asegurarse es tentador y es una tendencia natural de los humanos. Después de todo, el seguro le cuesta el dinero que ha ganado con tanto esfuerzo, después de impuestos, y asegurarse no tiene un beneficio tangible e inmediato (a diferencia de una comida fuera de casa, unas vacaciones o un nuevo equipo de sonido).

Usted tiene la esperanza de no tener que usar su seguro, pero si llegara a necesitarlo, estará contento de tenerlo disponible para su protección, y en algunos casos, la de su familia. Si ocurre una verdadera catástrofe y usted tiene una cobertura muy baja, esto no lo protegerá a usted y a los suyos. De modo que usted necesita el monto correcto de cobertura que logre un buen balance de costos y una adecuada protección.

Cómo protegerse a sí mismo

Antes de que usted compre una casa, ponga en orden todo lo relacionado a la cobertura de seguros (para usted y para sus bienes más valiosos). Fallar en hacer esto es, financieramente, el equivalente de conducir un carro muy pequeño por la autopista a 90 millas por hora sin tener el cinturón de seguridad puesto. Usted debería comprar suficiente cobertura para prevenir una catástrofe financiera.

Seguro de incapacidad

Su habilidad para producir ingresos debería estar asegurada. Durante los años que usted puede trabajar, su habilidad para generar ingresos en el futuro es probablemente su activo más valioso —mucho más valioso que un carro o aun su casa.

El seguro de incapacidad a largo plazo reemplaza la mayor parte de los ingresos no percibidos en el evento que una invalidez le impida trabajar. Los casos de invalidez mayor son el resultado de accidentes o problemas médicos —cosas que por supuesto no se pueden predecir. Aun si usted no tiene personas que dependan financieramente de usted, probablemente necesita tener cobertura por incapacidad. A menos que sea bastante rico y ya no necesite trabajar para obtener ingresos, ¿no es *usted* financieramente hablando dependiente de su cheque de pago? Aunque muchas compañías grandes ofrecen seguro de incapacidad a largo plazo, muchos empleados de compañías pequeñas y personas que trabajan por su cuenta no tienen esta cobertura —ésta es una situación riesgosa.

Seguro de vida

Cuando usted tiene personas que dependen de usted, también puede necesitar la protección de un seguro de vida. La pregunta que debe hacerse a sí mismo y a su familia es cómo se mantendrían financieramente si usted falleciera y ellos no tuvieran los ingresos que usted produce. Si su familia depende de su ingreso, y usted quiere que ellos mantengan su estándar de vida actual en su ausencia, usted necesita la cobertura de un seguro de vida.

El seguro de vida a término, como la mayoría de otros tipos de seguro, es la protección de seguro en su forma pura y es el mejor tipo de protección para la gran mayoría de las personas. El monto de cobertura que usted compre debe estar basado en el *valor* de cuántos años de sus ingresos usted quiere proveerle a su familia en caso de su muerte.

A los agentes de seguro les encanta vender el seguro de vida con valor en efectivo (también se le conoce como seguro de vida total o universal) por la comisión tan considerable que pueden ganar vendiendo este tipo de seguro. (Estas comisiones por supuesto salen de su bolsillo.) Algunas entidades hipotecarias tratan de presionarlo para que compre el seguro de vida hipotecario que ellos venden. Evite la compra de cualquiera de estas opciones. El seguro de vida hipotecario es simplemente un seguro a término más costoso, y el seguro de vida con valor en efectivo generalmente es una combinación de un seguro de vida costoso y una cuenta de inversión con rendimientos relativamente bajos.

Seguro de enfermedad

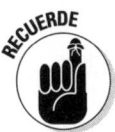

Además del seguro de incapacidad y el de vida, todas las personas deberían tener una póliza de seguro de enfermedad a todo riesgo. Aún si usted goza de buena salud, usted nunca sabe cuándo una enfermedad o un accidente pueden ocurrir. Los gastos médicos pueden crecer vertiginosamente de mil a cientos de miles de dólares en poco tiempo. No deje de tener un seguro de enfermedad a todo riesgo.

Cómo asegurar sus bienes

A medida en que su riqueza se vaya acumulando con los años (idealmente, y al menos en parte, debido al aumento del valor de la casa que le estamos ayudando a comprar), en esa misma medida aumenta el riesgo de perder sus valiosos bienes o de enfrentar una demanda que proviene de ellos. Por ejemplo, usted debe tener un seguro contra todo riesgo de su casa y de su(s) carro(s). Si su casa se destruye en un incendio, una póliza de seguro de propietario a todo riesgo pagaría por el costo de reconstruir la casa. Igualmente, si su carro es destruido en un accidente, el seguro del carro debe pagar para reemplazarlo.

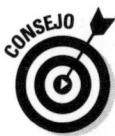

En todos los tipos de seguro que usted compre, escoja el deducible más alto que usted pueda pagar cómodamente. El *deducible* es una cantidad de dinero que usted debe pagar de su bolsillo cuando tiene una pérdida por la cual usted hace un reclamo. Cuando los deducibles son altos, esto le ayuda a mantener bajo el costo del seguro y a eliminar las molestias relacionadas con el sometimiento de reclamos pequeños.

Testamentos, fideicomisos activos, y planificación del patrimonio

Aunque a ninguno de nosotros nos guste admitirlo, o siquiera pensar en eso, todos vamos a morir. Debido a la forma como nuestro sistema legal y de impuestos trabaja, a menudo es beneficioso tener en orden ciertos documentos legales que especifiquen detalles importantes tales como lo que debería hacerse con sus bienes (incluyendo su casa) cuando usted fallezca.

El *testamento* es el más básico de esos documentos. Para la mayoría de las personas y, particularmente para aquellos que son jóvenes y que no tienen gran cantidad de bienes, es el único y más importante documento a tener. A través de un testamento, usted puede indicar a qué personas les serán entregados sus bienes en caso de su muerte y quién va a tener custodia de sus hijos menores. En ausencia de un testamento, las leyes estatales deciden sobre estos asuntos importantes.

Además de su testamento, piense también en tener un *testamento en vida* y un *poder para decisiones médicas.* Estos documentos ayudan a su doctor y miembros de la familia a tomar decisiones importantes relacionadas con su salud, en caso de que usted esté incapacitado para tomar esas decisiones por usted mismo.

Un testamento y otros documentos médicos y legales de apoyo, puede que todavía no sean suficientes para hacerles llegar sus bienes a los herederos elegidos por usted, ni para minimizar los impuestos y los gastos legales. En la mayoría de los estados, cuando usted tiene una cantidad de bienes considerable (tales como una casa y un negocio), que no forman parte de las cuentas de jubilación exentas de impuestos, esos bienes deben ser *validados o legalizados* —esto se refiere al proceso que es administrado por un tribunal para implementar su testamento. Los honorarios que cobran los abogados por este servicio pueden llegar a ser bastante altos— hasta un 5 por ciento del valor de los bienes legalizados. El preparar y poner su casa y otros bienes en un *fideicomiso activo,* puede eliminar muchas de estas dificultades y eliminar el costo de legalización del testamento ante el tribunal.

Finalmente, si su patrimonio (activos menos pasivos) excede los $2 millones al momento de su muerte, el gobierno federal (y quizás también el estatal) le impondrá unos impuestos considerablemente altos. (Para el año 2009, el monto que usted puede pasar a sus herederos, libres de impuestos sobre transmisiones patrimoniales, aumentará a $3,5 millones.) La planificación del patrimonio puede ayudar a minimizar la porción del mismo que está sujeta a los impuestos. Una estrategia de planificación simple, pero poderosa, es repartir el dinero entre los herederos designados por usted para reducir el patrimonio gravable. (Si sus familiares se encuentran en posesión de una gran riqueza, ellos pueden dar hasta $11.000 anuales libres de impuestos a tantos beneficiarios como ellos quieran. Si le dan a usted $11.000, usted puede usar este dinero para el pago inicial de su casa.)

Los testamentos, fideicomisos en vida y la planificación del patrimonio son solamente formas de asegurarse. Recuerde que toma tiempo y dinero generar estos documentos, y los beneficios están lejos en el futuro, así que no exagere haciendo muchas de estas cosas ahora, sino hasta que sea mayor y tenga un monto de activos importantes. Lea la última edición de *Taxes For Dummies* (Wiley), de la cual Eric es coautor, para aprender más acerca de la planificación del patrimonio.

Junto con la compra de seguros para cubrir los costos de reemplazo por la pérdida o daño de sus bienes, usted puede (y debe) comprar un seguro de responsabilidad civil adecuado para esos bienes. Los seguros de propiedad y de automóviles incluyen coberturas para daños a terceros. Asegúrese que tiene cobertura de responsabilidad civil de por lo menos el doble del valor de su *patrimonio* (activos menos pasivos).

Además de la cobertura de responsabilidad civil que viene con el seguro de automóviles y el de propiedad, usted puede comprar una póliza de responsabilidad complementaria conocida como *seguro de cobertura general o de responsabilidad excedente*. Este seguro es comprado en incrementos de $1.000.000,00, y esta cobertura puede proteger a personas que tengan patrimonios más grandes. Recuerde que esta cobertura no protege contra demandas que provienen de su trabajo.

Invierta en Sí Mismo

Por último, pero no por eso menos importante, en su entusiasmo por construir su imperio financiero y comprar viviendas más grandes y más costosas cada vez, no olvide cuál es su mejor inversión: usted. No lleve su vida y su cuerpo a la ruina trabajando largas horas solo para poder pagar la casa de sus sueños.

Además de invertir en su salud, su familia y sus amigos, invierta en aprender más y en hacerse cargo de sus asuntos financieros. Si necesita más ayuda para evaluar su salud financiera, para reducir sus gastos, sus impuestos y deudas, y elaborar un plan financiero (incluso manejar sus inversiones y seguros), actúe inteligentemente y busque una copia de la edición más reciente de *Personal Finance For Dummies* de Eric (Wiley).

Capítulo 3

¿Cuánto Puede Pagar por Su Vivienda?

En Este Capítulo

▶ Cómo determinar los costos de la propiedad

▶ Cómo entender los beneficios impositivos de ser propietario

▶ Cómo reunir e invertir el pago inicial

Cuando usted entra en un negocio de venta de automóviles, una de las primeras preguntas que los vendedores le hacen (después que usted se los quita de encima) es: ¿Cuál es su presupuesto? O, ¿cuánto puede usted pagar por un carro? Por supuesto que ellos esperan que el número que salga de su boca sea grande. Y si usted es como muchos compradores de automóviles, probablemente diga algo así como: "Bueno, realmente no estoy seguro".

Hoy en día, muchos compradores de carros financian su compra —de modo que dejan que un banco u otra entidad crediticia decida qué automóvil se pueden comprar. Tales decisiones están basadas en los ingresos del comprador y en sus otras obligaciones de deuda.

Pero aquí es donde la mayoría de las personas se confunden. Cuando una entidad de préstamo dice que usted reúne los requisitos para pedir prestado, digamos, $30.000 para la compra de un carro, esto no quiere decir que usted *puede* pagar esa cantidad en un automóvil. Lo que la entidad crediticia realmente está diciéndole es "basado en lo poco que sé de su situación y en el hecho de que yo no puedo controlar su conducta futura, éste es el monto máximo que nuestra organización puede prestarle tomando un riesgo prudente".

La entidad crediticia normalmente requiere una cuota o pago inicial para protegerse contra la posibilidad de que usted no pague el préstamo. Si usted no paga y cae en mora, por ejemplo, la entidad de préstamo tiene que enviar al agente de recobros de posesiones para quitarle su carro y venderlo. Este proceso toma tiempo y dinero y el banco, con seguridad, obtiene menos por el carro que la suma que usted pagó por él.

Las Entidades de Préstamo No Pueden Decirle lo que Usted Puede Pagar

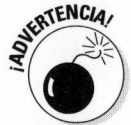

En última instancia, a su banco o entidad financiera no le importan su situación económica ni sus otras necesidades ni usted, siempre y cuando ellos tengan protegidos sus propios intereses financieros. Esta es la realidad, bien sea que usted esté pidiendo prestado para comprar un carro o una casa. La entidad de préstamo no sabe ni le importa si, por ejemplo, usted:

✔ No ha ahorrado lo suficiente para la jubilación.

✔ Quiere ahorrar dinero para otras metas financieras importantes, tales como empezar o comprar su propio negocio.

✔ Tiene un pequeño pelotón de niños (o espera aumentos en los costos de la educación privada).

✔ No tiene una cobertura de seguro adecuada.

Allí es donde está el problema de tomar la decisión sobre cuánto puede usted pagar por una casa (o un carro) basado en cuánto dinero la entidad de préstamo está dispuesta a prestarle. Y, eso es lo que Walter y Susana hicieron. La pareja se dispuso a comprar la casa cuando el negocio de Walter estaba prosperando y estaban ganando más de $200.000 al año.

Walter y Susana realmente querían comprar la casa más grande y mejor que pudieran pagar. Cuando se reunieron con el banco de su comunidad, éste estaba más que dispuesto a mostrarles cómo podían prestar $900.000 a través de una hipoteca con tasa ajustable. (Usted puede leer todo lo relacionado a estas hipotecas en el Capítulo 6. Aquí le diremos simplemente que algunas hipotecas con tasa ajustable o variable, empiezan con una tasa artificialmente baja que "engancha" al deudor, y que le permite reunir las condiciones para prestar mucho más de lo que podrían hacerlo con una hipoteca tradicional de interés fijo.)

Walter y Susana compraron la casa de sus sueños con una hipoteca de $900.000 con tasa de interés ajustable. A los pocos años, esta casa de sus sueños se transformó en una pesadilla. La hipoteca era como una soga alrededor de sus cuellos.

Ahora que Walter y Susana disfrutaban la bendición de tener niños pequeños, no querían trabajar largas horas; pero se vieron forzados a hacerlo para poder cumplir con los gigantescos pagos de la hipoteca. Los primeros pagos de la hipoteca de tasa ajustable ya eran altos, pero se dispararon vertiginosamente cuando la tasa de interés del préstamo aumentó. El estrés financiero conllevó a Walter y a Susana al estrés personal, ya que tenían discusiones frecuentes acerca del dinero, y del cuidado de los niños.

Sabemos de otras personas que se comprometieron financieramente más allá de lo que podían, de la misma manera que Walter y Susana lo hicieron. Muchos de ellos continuaron esclavizados trabajando largas horas en trabajos que no les gustaban y haciendo otros sacrificios innecesarios, tales como limitar el tiempo que le dedicaban a la familia para poder hacer los pagos de la vivienda. Algunos terminaron divorciándose debido, en parte, a la tensión financiera. Otros quedaron en mora con sus deudas y perdieron sus casas y su buen crédito.

Personas de todos los niveles de ingresos, incluso los adinerados, pueden meterse en problemas y sobre extenderse al comprar una casa más cara que la que pueden pagar, y al adquirir más deudas que las que pueden cómodamente amortizar. Sólo porque un banco o un agente de bienes raíces le dice que usted cumple y reúne los requisitos para un cierto monto de dinero, no quiere decir que eso es lo que usted puede pagar dada su situación financiera personal. Las entidades de préstamo *no* pueden decirle lo que usted puede pagar. Ellos *sólo* pueden decirle el máximo que están dispuestos a darle prestado.

El Costo de Comprar y de Ser Propietario de una Vivienda

Antes que usted emprenda la búsqueda de la casa de sus sueños, una de las preguntas más sencillas e importantes que usted debe hacerse es, ¿cuánto puedo pagar por una casa? Para poder responder esta pregunta inteligentemente, primero, necesita saber cuáles son sus metas financieras, qué va a necesitar para alcanzarlas, y en qué situación se encuentra usted hoy en día. Si usted no ha leído todavía el Capítulo 2, ahora es el momento de hacerlo (a menos que esté 100 por ciento seguro que sus finanzas están en excelentes condiciones).

En las siguientes secciones, profundizamos en los costos de compra y los costos de ser propietario de una vivienda.

Los pagos de la hipoteca

En el Capítulo 6, presentamos cómo seleccionar el mejor tipo de hipoteca que se ajusta a sus circunstancias particulares. Mientras tanto, usted todavía tiene que afrontar las hipotecas (con nuestra ayuda), porque indudablemente las hipotecas constituyen el componente más grande del costo total de ser dueño de una casa.

Empecemos por lo más sencillo: una *hipoteca* es un préstamo que usted obtiene para comprar una vivienda. Una hipoteca le permite comprar una casa de $150.000 aun cuando usted tiene muchísimo menos de esa cantidad para darla para la compra.

Con muy pocas excepciones, los préstamos hipotecarios en los Estados Unidos de América se pagan típicamente en un período de 15 a 30 años y casi todos requieren pagos mensuales. Una hipoteca funciona de la siguiente manera: imagínese que usted compra una casa de $150.000, y para ello (siguiendo nuestro sabio consejo, el cual se encuentra más adelante en este capítulo) usted ha ahorrado con esmero un 20 por ciento ($30.000, en este ejemplo) para el pago inicial. De esta manera, usted termina con un préstamo hipotecario de $120.000.

Usted va a una entidad hipotecaria y le piden que complete una montaña de papeles (nosotros lo acompañamos a lo largo de este pantanoso camino en el Capítulo 7) que hace parecer diminuta la montaña de papeles de su declaración de impuestos sobre la renta. Justo cuando usted cree que lo peor ha terminado (después que el torbellino de papeles pasa), la entidad le da un dolor de cabeza todavía más grande al decirle (así como suena) de las miles de opciones y variaciones de la hipoteca.

¡Pero no se preocupe —nosotros podemos ayudarlo a cortar camino en esa multitud de opciones! Imagine, por un momento, un mundo sencillo donde las entidades crediticias le ofrecen sólo dos opciones de hipoteca: una hipoteca de tasa fija por 15 años y una hipoteca de tasa fija por 30 años (*tasa fija* significa simplemente que la tasa de interés sobre el préstamo no cambia, y permanece igual durante el período del préstamo). Estos serían los pagos mensuales para cada una de las opciones:

$120.000, hipoteca de 15 años @ 7,00 por ciento = $1.079 por mes

$120.000, hipoteca de 30 años @ 7,25 por ciento = $819 por mes

Como explicamos en el Capítulo 6, típicamente la tasa de interés de una hipoteca de 15 años es un poco más baja que la de una de 30 años, porque los préstamos a corto plazo son un poco menos riesgosos para las entidades hipotecarias. Fíjese que el pago mensual del préstamo a 15 años es mucho más alto que el pago a 30 años. Estos pagos de una hipoteca de 15 años tienen que ser más altos, porque usted está pagando un préstamo del mismo monto 15 años antes.

Pero no deje que los montos mensuales más altos de su hipoteca de 15 años lo hagan olvidar que al final de ese período, ya no tiene que hacer más pagos, mientras que con la hipoteca de 30 años, usted todavía tiene 15 años más de pagos mensuales por hacer. Así pues, usted tiene desembolsos mensuales más altos con la hipoteca de 15 años, pero observe la diferencia en los pagos totales y en los intereses de las dos opciones de préstamo:

Tipo de Hipoteca	Total de Pagos	Total de Intereses
Hipoteca de 15 años (180 meses)	$194.147	$74.147
Hipoteca de 30 años (360 meses)	$294.700	$174.700

Nota: En caso de que usted esté curioso por saber cómo obtuvimos el monto total de interés, simplemente restamos el monto de préstamo que ya se ha pagado ($120.000), del "Total de pagos". Los montos mensuales de los pagos que mencionamos antes, así como los montos del total de pagos y total de intereses, están redondeados, de modo que si usted intenta multiplicar 180 ó 360 por los montos de pagos mensuales, no obtendrá respuestas idénticas a las de arriba.

En el caso de la hipoteca de 30 años, debido a que usted está pidiendo prestado el dinero por 15 años adicionales (comparada con la hipoteca de 15 años), no debería ser una sorpresa que (con una hipoteca de un monto moderado como ésta), usted termine pagando más de $100.000 adicionales de intereses. El préstamo de 30 años no es necesariamente malo; por ejemplo, los pagos más bajos le pueden permitir alcanzar sus otros objetivos financieros importantes, tales como ahorrar en una cuenta de jubilación deducible del impuesto. (Vea el Capítulo 6 para más información sobre la comparación de la hipoteca de 15 años y la hipoteca de 30 años.)

En los primeros años durante los cuales está pagando su hipoteca, casi todo el pago que se hace se destina a cubrir los intereses sobre el dinero que usted prestó. No es sino hasta años más adelante en su hipoteca, que usted comienza a pagar rápidamente el saldo del préstamo, como se muestra en la Figura 3-1.

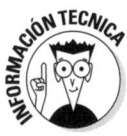

En la medida en que las tasas de interés aumentan, también aumenta el tiempo necesario para pagar la mitad del préstamo. Por ejemplo, a una tasa de interés del 10 por ciento, pagar la mitad del préstamo toma casi 24 años de los 30 años del tiempo total de la hipoteca, mientras que a una tasa del 14 por ciento, toma más de 25 años del tiempo total.

Los límites de las entidades hipotecarias

Hemos visto personalmente las consecuencias financieras que han afrontado personas que prestan más allá de sus posibilidades (aún dentro de los límites establecidos por las entidades crediticias) y, por eso, usted no nos escuchará decir en esta sección que las entidades hipotecarias le pueden decir el monto que usted puede pagar por una casa. Las entidades no tienen la capacidad para hacer esto. Todo lo que las entidades crediticias pueden hacer es decirle los criterios que emplean para aprobar o negar las solicitudes de préstamos y para calcular el máximo monto que le pueden prestar. (Para tener una idea más completa de cómo funcionan las entidades hipotecarias, y los límites que emplean, por favor vea la primera sección de este capítulo.)

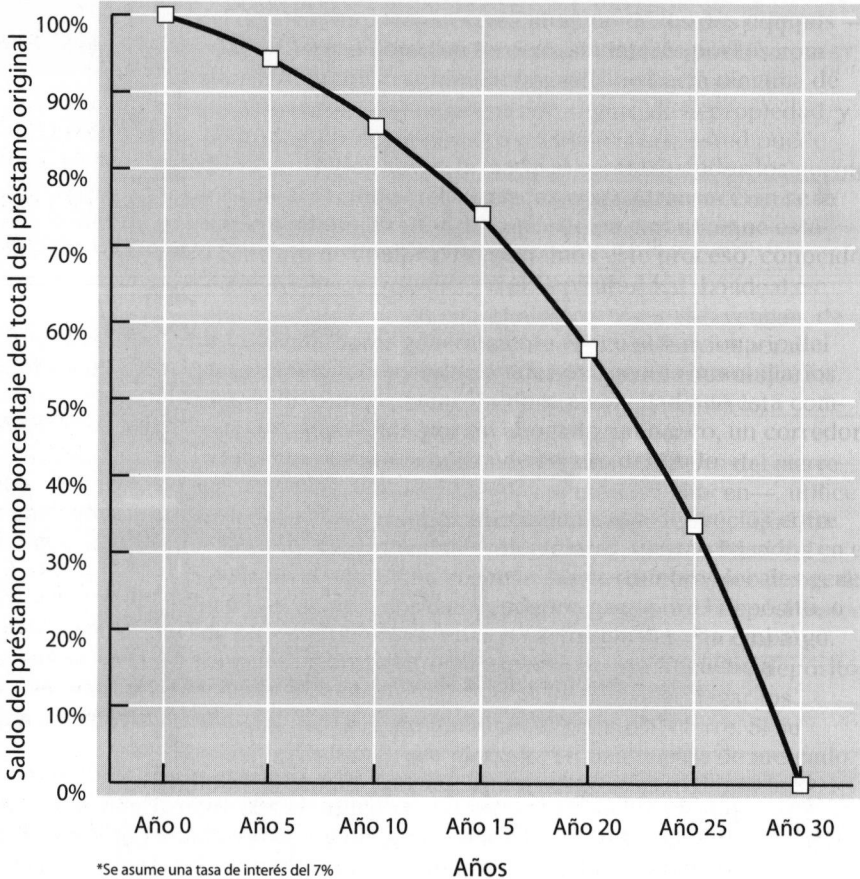

Pago de un préstamo de 30 años*

Saldo del préstamo como porcentaje del total del préstamo original

100% · 90% · 80% · 70% · 60% · 50% · 40% · 30% · 20% · 10% · 0%

Año 0 · Año 5 · Año 10 · Año 15 · Año 20 · Año 25 · Año 30

Años

*Se asume una tasa de interés del 7%

Figura 3-1: Toma muchos años del tiempo de la hipoteca para empezar a amortizar el capital del préstamo. En este caso, pagar la mitad del capital toma cerca de 22 años.

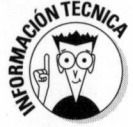

La mayoría de las entidades hipotecarias, pero no todas, emplean criterios muy parecidos para la evaluación de préstamos, porque ellas en realidad venden los préstamos hipotecarios que hacen en los mercados financieros, a inversionistas exigentes. Las agencias del gobierno —tales como *Fannie Mae* (Asociación Hipotecaria Nacional Federal), FNMA por sus siglas en inglés, y *Ginnie Mae* (Asociación Hipotecaria Nacional del Gobierno), GNMA por sus siglas en inglés— garantizan el pago del capital y los intereses en tales préstamos, siempre y cuando la entidad financiera que hace la hipoteca siga ciertos criterios específicos para aceptar o rechazar la solicitud del préstamo hipotecario. Quizás, en el mundo tan confuso de las inversiones, usted haya escuchado el término *Ginnie Maes*. Pues bien, cuando usted invierte en valores respaldados por hipotecas, lo que usted está básicamente comprando son bonos que son hipotecas y, ¡quizás hasta compre la suya sin saberlo!

Una entidad hipotecaria lleva la cuenta de su *gasto mensual de vivienda*, cuyos componentes ellos consideran que son los siguientes:

	Pago de la hipoteca	(capital e intereses; ***PI***, por sus siglas en inglés)
+	Impuestos de la Propiedad	(***T***, por su sigla en inglés)
+	Seguro	(***I***, por su sigla en inglés)
=	Lo que la entidad crediticia define como *gasto de la vivienda* (**PITI**, por sus siglas en inglés, se refiere al *capital*, *interés*, *impuestos*, y *seguro*)

Para una propiedad determinada que usted esté pesando comprar, la entidad hipotecaria estima el gasto de la vivienda, y normalmente requiere que éste no exceda un cierto porcentaje (generalmente alrededor del 35 por ciento) de su ingreso mensual antes de impuestos (bruto). (Algunas entidades crediticias permiten que este porcentaje sea un poco más alto.) De modo que, por ejemplo, si su ingreso bruto mensual es de $6.000, la entidad crediticia no permitirá que su gasto mensual de la vivienda sea mayor que $2.100 (si ella está usando el 35 por ciento). Cuando usted trabaja por su cuenta, y hace su declaración de impuestos, *Formulario 1040, Anexo C (Schedule C) del IRS,* las entidades financieras usan sus ingresos después de los gastos (*netos*), que se encuentra en la última línea de dicho anexo.

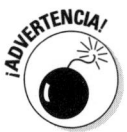

Ahora bien, si usted ha estado prestando atención a este capítulo, hasta este momento, debe haberse dado cuenta que es erróneo usar este enfoque tan simplista que recoge todo en un solo número. Este porcentaje del gasto de la vivienda ignora por completo casi todas las otras metas, sus necesidades y sus obligaciones financieras. También omite los gastos de mantenimiento y remodelación de la vivienda, los cuales pueden comerse gran parte del dinerito del propietario.

Los únicos otros elementos (además de sus ingresos) que la entidad de préstamo toma en consideración son sus otras deudas. Ella analiza, específicamente, los pagos mensuales de préstamos educativos, préstamos para automóviles, las cuentas de las tarjetas de crédito y otras deudas. Además del porcentaje de sus ingresos que las entidades de préstamo permiten para gastos de la vivienda, también, usualmente, establecen que un 5 por ciento adicional de su ingreso mensual se destine al pago de otras deudas. De modo que su gasto mensual por vivienda y el pago mensual de otras deudas pueden llegar hasta el 40 por ciento de su ingreso, pero nunca excederlo.

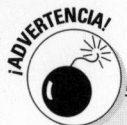

Comprometerse financieramente más allá de lo que las entidades hipotecarias le permitirían

Algunas veces, los compradores potenciales de vivienda creen que ellos pueden hacerle frente a una mayor deuda que la que las instituciones financieras le permitirían. Estos compradores probablemente busquen pedir prestado más dinero de la familia, o piensan mentir sobre sus ingresos en la solicitud de hipoteca. (Los trabajadores por cuenta propia tienen mayores oportunidades para hacer esto.) Esta manera de actuar no es nada diferente de la mala conducta de algunos jóvenes, que conducen por encima del límite de velocidad, beben y fuman cosas prohibidas, o se pasan de la hora de permiso y entran por la puerta de atrás de la casa.

Aunque algunos de esos jóvenes se salen con la suya con esta conducta tan riesgosa, otros terminan metidos en problemas académicos o sicológicos (u otros peores). Lo mismo les ocurre a propietarios que se comprometen demasiado, financieramente hablando, para comprar una propiedad más cara. Algunos sobreviven sin problemas, pero otros terminan con problemas financieros y emocionales.

Cada vez más están apresando a compradores que mienten en sus solicitudes de hipotecas. ¿Y cómo hacen esto? Cuando usted está listo para hacer el cierre del préstamo, la entidad crediticia puede (y generalmente lo hace) pedirle que firme una planilla autorizándolos a solicitar una copia de su declaración de impuestos al *IRS*. Esto le permite a la entidad crediticia verificar su ingreso. (Vea el Capítulo 7 para más detalles).

Así que, aunque hemos dicho que la palabra de la entidad crediticia no es la última en términos de establecer cuánto puede usted pagar por una casa, tenemos que dejar claro que decir la verdad en su solicitud de hipoteca es la única manera de hacer las cosas (esto le evita cometer el delito de perjurio y fraude). Decir la verdad no es sólo lo correcto, sino que evita que usted se zambulla de cabeza y se comprometa más allá de sus posibilidades con estas obligaciones. Los bancos no quieren que usted incumpla en los pagos de su préstamo y usted tampoco debería querer tomar ese riesgo.

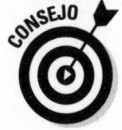

Si tiene deuda de consumidor, asegúrese de leer el Capítulo 2. Debe bastarle con que le digamos aquí que usted debe liberarse (y mantenerse libre) de esas deudas. La deuda de consumidor tiene un costo alto, y a diferencia de un préstamo hipotecario, el interés que se paga sobre este tipo de deuda no es deducible de los impuestos. La deuda de consumidor limita la posibilidad de que le aprueben, y de que pueda pagar su hipoteca. *La deuda de consumidor es un cáncer financiero.*

Cómo calcular los pagos de la hipoteca

Calcular el monto del pago de la hipoteca, después que usted sabe el monto que quiere prestar, es muy simple. La parte difícil para la mayoría de las personas es determinar cuánto pueden pedir prestado. Si usted ya sabe cuánto es la cantidad mensual que usted puede pagar, ¡excelente! ¡Siéntese en la primera fila! Suponga que usted trabajó en su presupuesto en el Capítulo 2, y calculó que usted puede pagar $1.500 mensuales por la vivienda. Determinar el monto exacto de la hipoteca que le permite mantenerse dentro de este límite es bastante difícil, porque el costo mensual de vivienda que usted calculó que podía pagar ($1.500, en nuestro ejemplo) está formado por varios componentes. Por suerte para usted, nosotros cubrimos cada uno de esos componentes en este capítulo, entre ellos el pago de la hipoteca, los impuestos a la propiedad, el seguro y el mantenimiento. (Fíjese que aunque las entidades crediticias no toman en cuenta los gastos de mantenimiento cuando calculan lo que usted puede pagar por una casa, usted no debería obviar este gasto tan real e importante).

En la medida en que usted cambia el monto que está dispuesto a pagar por una casa, el tamaño o monto de la hipoteca con el que usted se va a comprometer, usualmente cambia, y de la misma manera cambian los otros elementos del costo de propiedad. De modo que usted tiene que jugar con los números un poco, hasta que éstos sean los que usted quiere. Usted puede escoger una casa de cierto precio y calcular los impuestos a la propiedad, seguro, mantenimiento y otros factores. Cuando usted suma todo, probablemente se dé cuenta que el total está por encima o por debajo de la meta que usted se ha propuesto ($1.500, en nuestro ejemplo). Obviamente, si se pasa un poco, usted necesita revisar el monto de la vivienda y escoger una propiedad un poquito menos costosa o con una hipoteca más pequeña.

Si usa la Tabla 3-1, usted puede calcular los pagos de la hipoteca basados en el monto que usted quiere pedir prestado, en la tasa de interés del préstamo y en el número de años que van a durar los pagos del préstamo. Para calcular los pagos mensuales de la hipoteca, simplemente multiplique el número que corresponda de la Tabla 3-1 por el monto de la hipoteca expresado en (dividido por) miles de dólares. Por ejemplo, si usted va a solicitar una hipoteca de $150.000 a 30 años, a una tasa de interés del 7,5 por ciento, multiplique 150 por 7 (de la Tabla 3-1) para llegar al pago mensual de $1.050,00.

Tabla 3-1	Cálculo del Pago Mensual de la Hipoteca	
Tasa de Interés	*Hipoteca de 15 Años*	*Hipoteca de 30 Años*
4	7,40	4,77
4⅛	7,46	4,85
4¼	7,52	4,92
4⅜	7,59	4,99
4½	7,65	5,07
4⅝	7,71	5,14
4¾	7,78	5,22

(continúa)

Tabla 3-1 *(continuación)*

Tasa de Interés	Hipoteca de 15 Años	Hipoteca de 30 Años
$4\frac{7}{8}$	7,84	5,29
5	7,91	5,37
$5\frac{1}{8}$	7,98	5,45
$5\frac{1}{4}$	8,04	5,53
$5\frac{3}{8}$	8,11	5,60
$5\frac{1}{2}$	8,18	5,68
$5\frac{5}{8}$	8,24	5,76
$5\frac{3}{4}$	8,31	5,84
$5\frac{7}{8}$	8,38	5,92
6	8,44	6,00
$6\frac{1}{8}$	8,51	6,08
$6\frac{1}{4}$	8,58	6,16
$6\frac{3}{8}$	8,65	6,24
$6\frac{1}{2}$	8,72	6,33
$6\frac{5}{8}$	8,78	6,41
$6\frac{3}{4}$	8,85	6,49
$6\frac{7}{8}$	8,92	6,57
7	8,99	6,66
$7\frac{1}{8}$	9,06	6,74
$7\frac{1}{4}$	9,13	6,83
$7\frac{3}{8}$	9,20	6,91
$7\frac{1}{2}$	9,28	7,00
$7\frac{5}{8}$	9,35	7,08
$7\frac{3}{4}$	9,42	7,17
$7\frac{7}{8}$	9,49	7,26
8	9,56	7,34
$8\frac{1}{8}$	9,63	7,43
$8\frac{1}{4}$	9,71	7,52

Tasa de Interés	Hipoteca de 15 Años	Hipoteca de 30 Años
8⅜	9,78	7,61
8½	9,85	7,69
8⅝	9,93	7,78
8¾	10,00	7,87
8⅞	10,07	7,96
9	10,15	8,05
9⅛	10,22	8,14
9¼	10,30	8,23
9⅜	10,37	8,32
9½	10,45	8,41
9⅝	10,52	8,50
9¾	10,60	8,60
9⅞	10,67	8,69
10	10,75	8,78
10⅛	10,83	8,87
10¼	10,90	8,97
10⅜	10,98	9,06
10½	11,06	9,15
10⅝	11,14	9,25
10¾	11,21	9,34
10⅞	11,29	9,43
11	11,37	9,53
11¼	11,53	9,72
11½	11,69	9,91
11¾	11,85	10.10
12	12,01	10,29
12¼	12,17	10,48
12½	12.17	10,48

Use este espacio genial de trabajo (que se presenta a través de este capítulo) para ver sus gastos estimados de la propiedad, empezando con el pago de la hipoteca:

Concepto	Gasto Mensual Estimado
Pago de la hipoteca	$_____
Impuestos a la propiedad	+ $_____
Seguro	+ $_____
Mejoras, mantenimiento y otros	+ $_____
Gastos de la propiedad (antes de los impuestos)	= $_____
Ahorros Impositivos	– $_____
Gastos de la propiedad (después de ahorros impositivos)	= $_____

Impuestos a la propiedad

Si usted vive y respira, ya sabe que escaparse de pagar impuestos es casi imposible. Cuando usted compra y es propietario de una vivienda, su gobierno local (típicamente a través de la llamada Oficina de Recaudación de Impuestos del Condado (*County Tax Collector's Office*) le envía la cuenta de sus impuestos de propiedad, expresada en un monto anual único. Nunca es divertido recibir y pagar esta cuenta porque la mayoría de las comunidades envían esta cuenta sólo una o dos veces al año. A algunos propietarios de viviendas, les parece una molestia estar pagando tantos impuestos de propiedad además de los impuestos federales, estatales y los impuestos a las ventas que ya pagan. En caso que usted se lo esté preguntando, los impuestos a la propiedad sirven para pagar los gastos de la comunidad, tales como las escuelas públicas y el paleado de la nieve (para aquellos de nosotros lo suficientemente tontos como para vivir donde el invierno es muy frío). Especialmente en zonas de costos más altos, por ejemplo: con pocos establecimientos comerciales o pocas empresas que pagan impuestos, los impuestos a la propiedad residencial pueden ser bastante altos.

Si usted va a hacer un pago inicial (típicamente definido como menos del 20 por ciento del precio de compra), muchas entidades de préstamos insisten en que usted tenga unas *cuentas de depósitos en garantía* para pagar los impuestos a la propiedad y los seguros. Estas cuentas requieren que usted pague esos conceptos junto con el pago mensual de la hipoteca.

Normalmente, los impuestos a la propiedad están basados en el valor de la misma. Aunque una tasa de impuesto promedio es alrededor del 1,5 por ciento del precio de compra de la propiedad, por año, usted debe saber cuál es la tasa exacta en su zona. Llame a la Oficina del Recaudador de Impuestos de la ciudad donde usted está pensando comprar la vivienda, e indague cuál es la tasa de impuesto de la propiedad y cuáles cargos adicionales y gravámenes se emplearían en su caso. Puede encontrar ese número de teléfono en la sección de páginas del gobierno del directorio local de teléfonos y busque "Recaudador de Impuestos", "Tesorero" o "Asesor de Impuestos".

Tenga cuidado de que está comparando peras con peras cuando analice las comunidades y los impuestos a la propiedad. Por ejemplo, algunas ciudades pueden sacarle hasta el último centavo en gravámenes extras, por servicios que, en otras comunidades, están incluidos en las cuentas estándar de impuestos a la propiedad.

Los listados de viviendas a la venta, los cuales generalmente son elaborados por los agentes inmobiliarios, pueden indicar lo que el dueño actual de la vivienda está pagando en impuestos. Pero basarse en esta información para saber cuáles van a ser sus impuestos a la propiedad si usted comprara dicha vivienda, puede ser una acción financieramente riesgosa. Los impuestos que paga el dueño actual pueden estar basados en una valoración de la propiedad más baja o que no está actualizada. Así como es peligroso manejar hacia adelante mirando por el espejo retrovisor de su coche, usted no debería comprar una propiedad y presupuestar los impuestos de la misma, sólo basado en los impuestos que paga el dueño actual. Sus impuestos a la propiedad (si usted compra la casa) serán probablemente recalculados basados en el precio que usted paga por la vivienda.

Concepto	*Gasto Mensual Estimado*
Pago de la hipoteca	$_____
Impuestos a la propiedad	+ $_____
Seguro	+ $_____
Mejoras, mantenimiento y otros	+ $_____
Gastos de la propiedad (antes de los impuestos)	= $_____
Ahorros Impositivos	– $_____
Gastos de la propiedad (después de ahorros impositivos)	= $_____

El seguro

Cuando usted compra una casa, es casi seguro que la entidad hipotecaria no le permitirá cerrar la compra hasta que usted haya demostrado que tiene el seguro de la propiedad requerido. Las entidades crediticias no están siendo paternalistas en este caso, si no que están velando por sus propios intereses. ¿Cómo es esto? Si usted compra la casa y hace un pago inicial, digamos del

20 por ciento del precio de compra, la entidad crediticia está poniendo el otro 80 por ciento del precio. Si una vivienda se incendia y resulta una pérdida total, esto puede importarle más a la entidad, al menos financieramente hablando, que a usted. En la mayoría de los estados, la vivienda es la garantía del préstamo para las entidades hipotecarias.

En años pasados, algunas entidades financieras aprendieron de la manera más difícil, que a algunos dueños de vivienda puede que no les importe perder sus propiedades. En algunos casos, en los cuales las viviendas fueron una pérdida total, los propietarios que tenían, financieramente hablando, poco que perder en la propiedad e insuficiente cobertura de seguro, simplemente se fueron y dejaron a la entidad con el problema financiero. Debido a casos como ésos, hoy en día, casi todas las entidades hipotecarias requieren que usted compre un *seguro de hipoteca privado* (*PMI,* por sus siglas en inglés) si usted aporta menos del 20 por ciento del precio de compra. (Mas adelante en este capitulo, hablamos del *PMI* con más detalle, en la sección titulada "La solución del 20 por ciento").

Cuando compra una casa, usted debería proteger su inversión en la propiedad (así como tener cobertura para los costos importantes de reemplazo de la propiedad, en caso de que ésta sea dañada o robada). Reemplazar su ropa, los muebles, artefactos eléctricos de la cocina y su colección de latas de cervezas puede acumular rápidamente un monto notable de dinero.

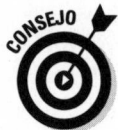

Cuando compre el seguro de propietario, debe comprar la cobertura más completa que usted pueda, y tener el deducible más alto que pueda pagar, para ayudar así a disminuir el costo. En el Capítulo 13, le explicamos cómo hacer todo esto. Para poder estimar cuánto va a costarle el seguro de la propiedad, le sugerimos que contacte algunas de las compañías aseguradoras que recomendamos en el Capítulo 13. Explíqueles qué tipo de propiedad usted está considerando comprar, las categorías de precios y en cuáles localidades (indique los códigos postales), y ellos deberían poder darle un estimado del costo mensual del seguro. El llamar a los agentes de seguro ahora, le permitirá comenzar a evaluar cuáles aseguradoras ofrecen este servicio y la cobertura que usted desea, y estar preparado para cuando llegue el momento justo de comprar la casa de sus sueños.

Del mismo modo como usted debe hacer cuando compra un carro, asimismo, debe buscar cotizaciones de seguros de propiedad mientras los evalúa, o pregúnteles a los dueños lo que ellos pagan por su cobertura. (Solo acuérdese que algunos propietarios pagan demás o no compran el tipo de cobertura correcto, así que no tome lo que ellos paguen como la verdad absoluta). Si usted obvia los costos de seguro hasta después que haya acordado comprar una propiedad, está exponiéndose a una sorpresa no muy agradable.

Concepto	*Gasto Mensual Estimado*
Pago de la hipoteca	$_____
Impuestos a la propiedad	+ $_____
Seguro	+ $_____
Mejoras, mantenimiento y otros	+ $_____
Gastos de la propiedad (antes de los impuestos)	= $_____
Ahorros Impositivos	− $_____
Gastos de la propiedad (después de ahorros impositivos)	= $_____

La diferencia entre el mantenimiento y las mejoras desde el punto de vista de los impuestos

Mientras sea dueño de su vivienda, a usted le conviene llevar un control del dinero que gasta en mejoras. ¿Por qué? Porque cuando usted vaya a vender su casa en algún momento, el *IRS* le permite deducir de sus impuestos esa porción de sus ganancias que fue producto de las mejoras de capital. (Como explicamos en el Capítulo 15, las normas impositivas del *IRS* que rigen la venta de propiedades también le permiten, a las personas que pagan impuestos y que cumplen los requisitos, deducir de los impuestos federales un monto considerable de beneficios —hasta $250.000 para quienes declaran como solteros, y $500.000 para parejas de casados que declaran conjuntamente.)

Para efecto de los impuestos, el *IRS* le permite agregar el costo de las *mejoras,* pero no el dinero gastado en mantenimiento, a su precio original de compra. ¿Cuál es la diferencia? Bueno, *hay* una diferencia, pero así como en todos los asuntos donde el *IRS* tiene una opinión, esta diferencia no está demarcada muy claramente.

✔ Las *mejoras de capital* son cosas que usted le hace a su vivienda que aumentan su valor en forma permanente y que alargan su duración. Las mejoras de capital incluyen conceptos tales como diseños de jardinería en su patio, agregar una cubierta con piso, comprar nuevos artefactos eléctricos (siempre y cuando usted los deje en la casa cuando la venda), instalar un nuevo sistema de calefacción o techo, remodelar y agregar habitaciones y otras cosas más.

✔ Los *gastos de mantenimiento y reparación* incluyen solamente esos tipos de arreglos que necesitan hacerse alrededor de la casa de vez en cuando. Mantenimiento y reparación incluyen cosas tales como arreglar una tubería rota o un baño que gotea, pintar, pagarle a alguien para que corte su césped y saque la mala hierba, y otras similares.

Así que cuando compre una vivienda, mantenga a mano un archivo en el cual pueda poner todos los recibos de los gastos de mejoras. Si tiene duda de si un gasto determinado es de mantenimiento o mejora del capital, guarde el recibo y decida sobre el asunto cuando llegue el momento de vender su casa.

Costos de mantenimiento y otros costos

Como propietario, usted *tiene* que pagar su hipoteca y su seguro de propiedad. Si no lo hace, eventualmente perderá su casa. Además, las viviendas también necesitan mantenimiento a lo largo de los años y usted tendrá que hacer ciertos tipos de mantenimiento (reparaciones, por ejemplo) en un momento determinado. Usted nunca sabe precisamente cuándo puede necesitar arreglar un problema eléctrico, reparar el techo, o reemplazar la lavadora y secadora —hasta que el problema asoma su nariz—, por lo cual el mantenimiento es algo difícil de presupuestar. (El pintar y otras mejoras optativas pueden hacerse a su discreción.)

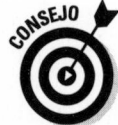

Como regla general, espere gastar cerca del 1 por ciento del precio de compra de su vivienda, en mantenimiento cada año. Entonces, por ejemplo, si usted gasta $150.000 en una casa, usted debe presupuestar cerca de $1.500 por año (o alrededor de $125 mensuales) para mantenimiento. Aunque en algunos años usted podría gastar menos, en otros años usted podría gastar más. Cuando se daña su techo, por ejemplo, reemplazarlo puede costarle el valor de varios años de sus gastos presupuestados de mantenimiento. En ciertos tipos de viviendas, tales como condominios, usted realmente paga un monto mensual a una asociación de propietarios, que cuida del mantenimiento del complejo residencial. En este caso, usted es sólo responsable del mantenimiento del interior de su propiedad. Antes que usted compre dicha propiedad, verifique con la asociación para ver cuánto es la cuota, y si ellos están planificando algún otro pago para reparaciones futuras. (Vea el Capítulo 8 para más información.)

Además del mantenimiento necesario, usted debe estar consciente (y tener cuidado) de lo que puede gastar en mejoras no esenciales para la vivienda. La categoría de *Otros* puede meterlo realmente en problemas. Las propagandas, sus vecinos y sus compañeros de trabajo, pueden inducirlo a gastar grandes cantidades de dinero en muebles nuevos, proyectos permanentes de remodelación, en diseños del jardín y muchos otros.

¿Debe usted incluir esos elementos no esenciales en su presupuesto? En general, la respuesta es sí. El problema potencial es que su casa se puede convertir en un foso de dinero al hacer que usted gaste demasiado y no ahorre lo suficiente y, posiblemente, se endeude a través de las tarjetas de crédito y otros medios. (Cubrimos el tema de los peligros de excederse en las mejoras en el Capítulo 8.) A menos que usted sea un excelente ahorrador y logre sus metas de ahorro, y tenga mucha flexibilidad en su presupuesto, asegúrese de no pasar por alto esta parte en su presupuesto de gastos del hogar.

El monto que usted espera gastar en mejoras es sólo un estimado. Éste depende de cuán *terminada* esté la casa que usted compre, y de sus deseos y gustos personales. Tome en cuenta su conducta de gasto y los tipos de proyectos que usted espera hacer, cuando esté considerando viviendas potenciales para la compra.

Concepto	*Gasto Mensual Estimado*
Pago de la hipoteca	$_____
Impuestos a la propiedad	+ $_____
Seguro	+ $_____
Mejoras, mantenimiento y otros	+ $_____
Gastos de la propiedad (antes de los impuestos)	= $_____
Ahorros Impositivos	– $_____
Gastos de la propiedad (después de ahorros impositivos)	= $_____

Los beneficios impositivos de ser propietario

Uno de los beneficios de ser propietario es que el *IRS* y la mayoría de los gobiernos estatales le permiten deducir dentro de ciertos límites los intereses de la hipoteca y los impuestos de la propiedad, cuando usted hace su declaración anual de impuestos sobre la renta. Cuando hace la declaración en el *Formulario 1040,* los intereses de la hipoteca y los impuestos a la propiedad de su vivienda son desgravámenes o deducciones detalladas en el Anexo A (*Schedule A*) (vea la Figura 3-2). En los préstamos hipotecarios de hoy en día, usted puede deducir el interés del primer millón ($1.000.000) de dólares de deuda, así como también todos los impuestos de la propiedad. Los buenos amigos del *IRS* también le permiten deducir los intereses que paga por un préstamo hipotecario sobre el *capital de la propiedad* (segunda hipoteca) hasta un máximo de $100.000 de préstamo.

Pero sólo porque los intereses de la hipoteca y los impuestos de la propiedad son deducciones permitidas en su declaración de impuestos sobre la renta, no piense que el gobierno está, literalmente, pagando por ellos por usted. Tome en cuenta que cuando usted se gana un dólar de ingreso y tiene que pagar impuestos sobre ese dólar, usted no paga el dólar completo al gobierno en impuestos. Su categoría impositiva (vea Tabla 3-2) determina el monto de impuestos que usted paga sobre ese dólar.

SCHEDULES A&B (Form 1040)
Department of the Treasury Internal Revenue Service (99)

Schedule A—Itemized Deductions

(Schedule B is on back)

▶ Attach to Form 1040. ▶ See Instructions for Schedules A&B (Form 1040).

OMB No. 1545-0074 | 2006 | Attachment Sequence No. 07

Name(s) shown on Form 1040 | Your social security number

Section	Line	Description	Box
Medical and Dental Expenses		**Caution.** Do not include expenses reimbursed or paid by others.	
	1	Medical and dental expenses (see page A-1)	1
	2	Enter amount from Form 1040, line 38 [2]	
	3	Multiply line 2 by 7.5% (.075)	3
	4	Subtract line 3 from line 1. If line 3 is more than line 1, enter -0-	4
Taxes You Paid (See page A-3.)	5	State and local income taxes	5
	6	Real estate taxes (see page A-3)	6
	7	Personal property taxes	7
	8	Other taxes. List type and amount ▶	8
	9	Add lines 5 through 8	9
Interest You Paid (See page A-3.)	10	Home mortgage interest and points reported to you on Form 1098	10
	11	Home mortgage interest not reported to you on Form 1098. If paid to the person from whom you bought the home, see page A-3 and show that person's name, identifying no., and address ▶	11
Note. Personal interest is not deductible.	12	Points not reported to you on Form 1098. See page A-4 for special rules	12
	13	Investment interest. Attach Form 4952 if required. (See page A-4.)	13
	14	Add lines 10 through 13	14
Gifts to Charity If you made a gift and got a benefit for it, see page A-4.	15	Gifts by cash or check. If you made any gift of $250 or more, see page A-5	15
	16	Other than by cash or check. If any gift of $250 or more, see page A-5. You **must** attach Form 8283 if over $500	16
	17	Carryover from prior year	17
	18	Add lines 15 through 17	18
Casualty and Theft Losses	19	Casualty or theft loss(es). Attach Form 4684. (See page A-6.)	19
Job Expenses and Certain Miscellaneous Deductions (See page A-6.)	20	Unreimbursed employee expenses—job travel, union dues, job education, etc. Attach Form 2106 or 2106-EZ if required. (See page A-6.) ▶	20
	21	Tax preparation fees	21
	22	Other expenses—investment, safe deposit box, etc. List type and amount ▶	22
	23	Add lines 20 through 22	23
	24	Enter amount from Form 1040, line 38 [24]	
	25	Multiply line 24 by 2% (.02)	25
	26	Subtract line 25 from line 23. If line 25 is more than line 23, enter -0-	26
Other Miscellaneous Deductions	27	Other—from list on page A-7. List type and amount ▶	27
Total Itemized Deductions	28	Is Form 1040, line 38, over $150,500 (over $75,250 if married filing separately)? ☐ **No.** Your deduction is not limited. Add the amounts in the far right column for lines 4 through 27. Also, enter this amount on Form 1040, line 40. ☐ **Yes.** Your deduction may be limited. See page A-7 for the amount to enter. ▶	28
	29	If you elect to itemize deductions even though they are less than your standard deduction, check here ▶ ☐	

For Paperwork Reduction Act Notice, see Form 1040 instructions. Cat. No. 11330X **Schedule A (Form 1040) 2006**

Figura 3-2: Detalle de las deducciones de los intereses sobre hipoteca e impuestos a la propiedad en el Anexo A del Formulario 1040.

Tabla 3-2	Categorías Impositivas y Tasas del Impuesto sobre la Renta 2006	
Ingreso Gravable para Solteros	*Ingreso Gravable para Casados Que Declaran Conjuntamente*	*Tasa de Impuestos sobre la Renta*
Menor que $7.550	Menor que $15.100	10%
Desde $7.550 hasta $30.650	$15.100 a $61.300	15%
Desde $30.650 hasta $74.200	$61.300 a $123.700	25%
Desde $74.200 hasta $154.800	$123.700 a $188.450	28%
Desde $154.800 hasta $336.550	$188.450 a $336.550	33%
Mayor que $336.550	Mayor que $336.550	35%

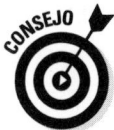

Técnicamente hablando, usted paga impuestos federales y estatales, así que usted también debe tomar en cuenta las deducciones o ahorros impositivos estatales cuando calcule sus ahorros impositivos como propietario. Sin embargo, para simplificar, y aun lograr obtener un estimado confiable de estos beneficios impositivos, simplemente multiplique el pago de la hipoteca y de los impuestos a la propiedad por su tasa *federal* de impuestos sobre la renta. Este atajo funciona bien porque la pequeña porción de su pago de la hipoteca que no es deducible (porque es para amortizar el capital) compensa aproximadamente los ahorros impositivos estatales que se hayan pasado por alto.

Concepto	*Gasto Mensual Estimado*
Pago de la hipoteca	$_____
Impuestos a la propiedad	+ $_____
Seguro	+ $_____
Mejoras, mantenimiento y otros	+ $_____
Gastos de la propiedad (antes de los impuestos)	= $_____
Ahorros Impositivos	– $_____
Gastos de la propiedad (después de ahorros impositivos)	= $_____

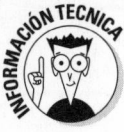

Usted podría estar interesado también en saber —pero muy probablemente no le importe— que la posibilidad de deducir los intereses de una hipoteca de hasta $1.000.000 de préstamo como máximo, cubre la deuda de su residencia principal y de su residencia secundaria. (Comprar y mantener dos viviendas es una tarea costosa, y la cual pocas personas pueden hacerlo, ¡así que no agarre ninguna idea loca porque nosotros mencionamos este bocadito deducible!)

¡Felicitaciones! Usted ha calculado lo que la casa de sus sueños debería costarle mensualmente, después de incluir los beneficios impositivos de ser propietario. No se olvide de tomar en cuenta, dentro de sus planes de gastos mensuales presentes, estos costos de propietario que se esperan (vea el Capitulo 2), para así asegurarse de que pueda pagar esa cantidad en una vivienda y también alcanzar sus metas financieras.

Los Costos de Cierre

El día cuando la casa sea suya oficialmente (conocido éste como *día del cierre*), muchas personas (además del vendedor) tendrán las manos en su billetera. Numerosos costos de cierre pueden dejarlo pobre y arruinado, o enviarlo corriendo a buscar ayuda financiera de sus padres o familiares.

No queremos que no pueda cerrar la compra de su casa, o que se vea forzado a arrodillarse ante su suegra y rogarle por dinero. (Esa humillación no sólo le afecta su ego, sino que también su suegra probablemente le cobre un 25 por ciento de interés en el dinero prestado y, por si fuera poco, espere tres nietos en los próximos cinco años). El prepararse con antelación para los costos de cierre lo ayudará a mantener su cordura y sus finanzas.

A continuación presentamos algunos costos de cierre comunes (presentados de los más grandes a los más pequeños), y cuánto debe usted presupuestar para cada uno (los valores exactos varían de acuerdo a los costos de la propiedad y la zona):

- **Costos de tramitación (puntos) y otros cargos relacionados con el préstamo:** Estos cargos pueden estar entre cero y el 3 por ciento del monto prestado. Las entidades crediticias generalmente cobran toda clase de tarifas o cargos por conceptos tales como valuación de la propiedad, obtención de su puntuación crediticia, preparación de los documentos del préstamo y procesamiento de su solicitud, así como también por tramitación del préstamo, el cual puede ser el 1 o 2 por ciento del monto del mismo. Si no dispone del dinero, puede buscar un préstamo que tenga menos gastos para su tramitación o, quizás, ninguno; sin embargo, tales préstamos tienen tasas de interés típicamente más altas durante su periodo de vigencia. Como se explica en el Capítulo 12, quizás usted pueda llegar a un acuerdo con el vendedor para que él pague esos costos de cierre del préstamo.

✔ **Gastos de depósitos en garantía:** estos costos oscilan entre cientos de dólares hasta más de mil dólares, y están basados en el precio de compra de la vivienda. Estos cargos cubren el costo de manejar los documentos y fondos relacionados con la compra. Explicamos estos costos con mucho más detalle en los Capítulos 9 y 14.

✔ **Seguro de propietario:** este seguro normalmente cuesta entre cientos de dólares hasta más de mil dólares por año, dependiendo del valor de su vivienda y cuánta cobertura quiere. Como explicamos al principio de este capítulo, usted no puede obtener un préstamo a menos que pueda demostrarle a la entidad hipotecaria, que tiene una cobertura adecuada de seguro de propietario. Prometerle a la entidad crediticia que va a obtener esta cobertura no es suficiente; las entidades generalmente insisten en que usted pague la prima del primer año de la póliza de seguro al momento del cierre.

✔ **Seguro del título de propiedad:** este seguro generalmente oscila entre cientos de dólares hasta mil dólares, dependiendo del precio de compra de la vivienda. Las entidades crediticias exigen que usted compre un seguro del título de propiedad cuando compra la vivienda, para asegurarse de que usted tenga un título limpio de problemas y que pueda venderse. Entre otras cosas, el *seguro de título de propiedad* lo protege a usted y a la entidad hipotecaria, de la posibilidad remota de que la persona que le esté vendiendo la vivienda no sea la dueña legal de la misma. Explicamos con más detalle el seguro del título de propiedad en el Capítulo 13.

✔ **Impuestos a la propiedad:** el costo de estos impuestos oscila entre cientos de dólares hasta dos mil dólares, y depende del precio de compra de la casa y de la fecha de cierre. Al momento del cierre, usted puede que tenga que rembolsarles a los vendedores algún impuesto a la propiedad que ellos hayan pagado por adelantado. Por ejemplo, suponga que (antes de que ellos le vendieran la casa a usted) los vendedores de la vivienda ya habían pagado sus impuestos de la propiedad hasta el 30 de junio. Si la venta ocurre el 30 de abril, usted le debe a los vendedores dos meses de impuestos a la propiedad — el recaudador de impuestos no va a rembolsarles los impuestos a la propiedad que ya se han pagado correspondientes a los meses de mayo y junio.

✔ **Gastos legales:** estos costos van desde cero hasta cientos de dólares. En algunos estados del este de los Estados Unidos, los abogados siempre están involucrados en las compras de bienes inmobiliarios. Sin embargo, en la mayoría de los estados, los abogados no son necesarios para realizar la transacción de compra y venta, siempre y cuando los agentes de bienes raíces utilicen contratos preestablecidos y estándar. Tales contratos tienen el aporte legal y la bendición de los leguleyos.

✔ **Inspecciones:** estos costos pueden ir desde $200 hasta $1.000 (dependiendo del tamaño de la propiedad y de la eficacia de la inspección). Como explicamos en el Capítulo 13, nunca debe pensar en comprar una casa sin haberla inspeccionado antes. Como probablemente usted no es muy experto en inspecciones de viviendas, usted se beneficiará al contratar a alguien que sea un experto en las mismas. Algunas veces, usted simplemente paga estos costos directamente; otras veces usted los paga al momento del cierre.

- **Seguro de hipoteca privado (PMI, por sus siglas en inglés):** si llegara a necesitarlo, este seguro puede costarle cientos de dólares, o más, por año. Como se describe en la siguiente sección de este capítulo, si usted pagó menos del 20 por ciento de pago inicial en la vivienda, muchas entidades crediticias van a exigirle que compre un seguro de hipoteca privado. Este tipo de seguro protege a la entidad crediticia en caso de que usted incumpla con sus pagos hipotecarios. Al momento del cierre, usted necesita pagar por adelantado cualquier suma, que puede estar entre un par de primas mensuales hasta más de la prima total de un año. Si usted puede, evite este costo poniendo un 20 por ciento de pago inicial, o buscando un financiamiento 80-10-10, el cual explicamos en la sección "Cómo comprar una casa poniendo menos dinero de inicial", más adelante en este capítulo.

- **Intereses prepagados del préstamo:** las entidades pueden cobrarle hasta 30 días de interés sobre su préstamo para cubrir los intereses que se acumulan desde el día en que los fondos del préstamo están disponibles (generalmente un día laborable antes del cierre) hasta 30 días antes de su primer pago de hipoteca ya programado. La cantidad exacta que usted tenga que pagar depende de la fecha de su primer pago mensual. Si usted es inteligente, y sabemos que lo es, debe hablar sobre esto con la entidad crediticia de modo que no tenga que pagar por adelantado ningún interés por el préstamo.

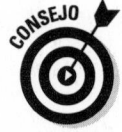

Para evitar pagar inútilmente tres días de intereses, *nunca programe el cierre para el día lunes.* Si usted hace el cierre un lunes, la entidad hipotecaria tiene que colocar los fondos de su hipoteca en reserva el viernes anterior. Como resultado de esto, a usted le cobran intereses sobre el préstamo por los días viernes, sábado y domingo, aun cuando usted no es el dueño de la casa sino hasta el cierre el día lunes. (Este pequeño consejo paga en su totalidad, y tal vez más, el costo de este libro. ¿No se siente más inteligente ahora?).

- **Registro:** el gasto para registrar el documento de propiedad y la hipoteca es alrededor de $50.

- **Costos de envío:** usualmente estos gastos son menos de $50. ¿Recuerda cuando usted envió algo a través del correo postal de los Estados Unidos, a una dirección a la cuál usted pudo haber conducido y llegado en unas pocas horas, pero que les tomó a ellos la mayor parte de la semana llevarlo hasta allá (o quizás lo perdieron)? Bien, las entidades crediticias y otras personas que participan en los negocios de bienes raíces saben que estos inconvenientes pueden ocurrir sin aviso, y como no quieren entorpecer su transacción o tener que pagar dinero, a menudo envían los documentos por el medio más rápido que pueden. ¿Y por qué no hacerlo? ¡Después de todo, es su dinero el que están gastando y no el de ellos!

- **Notaría:** las tarifas del notario van desde $10 hasta $20 *por firma por comprador.* Al momento del cierre, usted firma toda clase de documentos importantes con los cuales compromete todas las posesiones que tiene en este mundo, y hasta su hijo primogénito, en caso que usted incumpla con las obligaciones de la hipoteca. Por lo tanto, usted necesita tener su firma autenticada por un notario de modo que todos en la transacción sepan que usted realmente es quien dice ser.

Como puede ver, los costos de cierre se acumulan rápidamente. En una transacción típica de bienes raíces, estos gastos representan entre el 2 y el 5 por ciento del precio de compra de la propiedad. Así que no debería pasarlos por alto cuando esté calculando el monto de dinero que necesita para cerrar la compra. Tener suficiente dinero para cubrir el pago inicial de su préstamo, simplemente, no es suficiente.

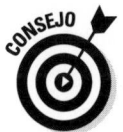

Si no tiene suficiente dinero ahorrado y está ansioso por comprar una casa lo antes posible, usted puede obtener una hipoteca que no tenga estos costos inmediatos ni puntos (vea el Capítulo 6). Puede tratar de negociar con el vendedor de la propiedad, para que él pague otros costos del cierre (vea el Capítulo 12). En este caso, anticipe que deberá pagar una tasa de interés más alta en la hipoteca por un préstamo con gastos o costos iniciales bajos. De acuerdo a estas condiciones, proyecte también pagar un precio de compra más alto (con el correspondiente aumento de la hipoteca) para convencer al vendedor que le pague esos otros gastos de cierre. Igualmente, no acepte ciegamente todos los costos de cierre que llegan al momento del mismo. En el Capítulo 14, le explicamos la importancia de revisar los documentos de cierre.

Cómo Ahorrar Dinero para el Pago Inicial

Jeremías salió a ver casas y, rápidamente, se enamoró de una de ellas. Desafortunadamente, después que encontró la casa de sus sueños, se dio cuenta de toda la documentación que se requería para el préstamo, de los honorarios extras y de las penalizaciones que tendría que pagar por tener una cuota inicial tan baja. Al final, Jeremías no pudo comprar la casa que quería porque no había ahorrado lo suficiente. "Si yo hubiera sabido, hubiera comenzado a ahorrar mucho antes —pensaba que ahorrar para el futuro era algo que uno hacía cuando uno está en la edad madura", le dijo a Eric.

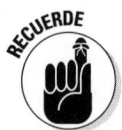

No queremos que se lleve una mala sorpresa cuando salga finalmente a comprar una vivienda. Por eso es que ahora, en la comodidad de su vivienda alquilada, en el tren o en el bus (o donde sea que usted esté leyendo este libro), nos gustaría que considerara lo siguiente:

- Cuánto dinero tiene que ahorrar para el pago inicial y para los costos de cierre de la compra de su casa
- De dónde va a provenir el dinero de su pago inicial
- Cómo debería invertir ese dinero mientras está esperando por la compra y el cierre

La solución del 20 por ciento

Idealmente, usted debería comprar una casa y tener suficiente dinero acumulado para el pago inicial, de tal manera que éste represente el 20 por ciento del precio de compra de la propiedad. ¿Por qué 20 por ciento y no 10 ó 15 ó 25 ó 30 por ciento? El 20 por ciento de pago inicial es el número mágico, porque es un colchón lo suficientemente grande como para proteger a las entidades crediticias contra incumplimiento de los pagos. Suponga, por ejemplo, que un comprador pone solo un 10 por ciento de inicial, y el valor de la propiedad baja un 5 por ciento y, además, el comprador no paga la deuda. Cuando la entidad crediticia ejecute la hipoteca —*después* de pagar una comisión de bienes raíces, impuesto de transferencia y otros gastos de la venta — la misma estará en serios aprietos. A las entidades hipotecarias no les gusta perder dinero. Ellos saben que tienen menos probabilidades de perder dinero en hipotecas, cuando el prestatario ha puesto un pago inicial de por lo menos un 20 por ciento del valor de la propiedad.

Si usted planifica prestar dinero de un banco, como lo hacen la mayoría de las personas, o de otra entidad financiera, esté consciente que casi todos requieren que usted obtenga (y pague) un seguro de hipoteca privado (PMI) si su pago inicial es menor del 20 por ciento del precio de compra. Aunque el PMI generalmente aumenta el costo de su préstamo en cientos de dólares anualmente, este seguro protege financieramente a la entidad crediticia en caso que usted no cumple sus obligaciones de la hipoteca. Si usted comprara una casa costosa —de cien mil dólares o más— el PMI puede agregarle $1.000 o más, anualmente, a su cuenta de la hipoteca. (Cuando hace un pago inicial menor del 20 por ciento, debe anticipar términos menos favorables en su préstamo, tales como pagos iniciales más altos o una tasa de interés más alta en el préstamo.)

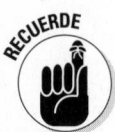

El PMI no es un costo permanente. Su necesidad del PMI se termina cuando usted demuestra que tiene al menos el 20 por ciento de *ganancia de capital* (el valor de la vivienda menos el saldo pendiente por pagar del préstamo) en la propiedad. El 20 por ciento puede venir por haber pagado el préstamo, de una revalorización de la vivienda, de mejoras hechas a la misma o por una combinación de estas tres condiciones. También, tome en cuenta que para eliminar el PMI, la mayoría de las entidades crediticias requerirán que se haga una valoración de la propiedad —a costa suya.

Nota: Si usted tiene (o espera tener) el 20 por ciento del dinero y, también, suficiente dinero para los costos de cierre, pase por alto la siguiente sección y vaya a la sección "Cómo invertir su pago inicial".

Cómo comprar una casa poniendo menos dinero de inicial

Especialmente si usted está empezando a ahorrar o está todavía pagando préstamos educativos o algo peor —saliendo de la duda de consumidor—, ahorrar el 20 por ciento del precio de compra de una casa más los costos de cierre, puede parecer una montaña muy difícil de escalar.

No se asuste y no se dé por vencido. A continuación le presentamos un grupo de alternativas que no han fallado a través del tiempo, y de las cuales puede escoger, para sobrepasar este obstáculo aparentemente gigante:

✔ **Aumente su tasa de ahorros.** Digamos que quiere acumular $30.000 para la compra de su casa y que está ahorrando sólo $100 mensuales. A ese paso, ¡le tomará cerca de dos décadas alcanzar su meta! Sin embargo, si usted puede aumentar su tasa de ahorros a $300 por mes, usted debería alcanzar el objetivo en aproximadamente 5 años.

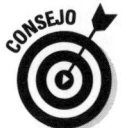

Ser eficiente con sus gastos es un buen hábito financiero, pero ahorrar más rápido es una *necesidad* para casi la mayoría de los compradores de vivienda. Si usted no tiene familiares benevolentes ni llenos de dinero, ni otras fuentes que lo provean con una ganancia inesperada, va a tener que acumular dinero de la forma antigua como millones de otros compradores de vivienda lo hicieron en el pasado: ahorrándolo gradualmente. La mayoría de las personas tienen "excesitos" en sus presupuestos. Comience por leer el Capítulo 2 para buscar maneras de evaluar sus gastos presentes y aumentar su tasa de ahorros.

✔ **Baje un poco sus aspiraciones.** El veinte por ciento de un número grande, es un número grande, de modo que podemos decir con seguridad que el 20 por ciento de un número más pequeño, es un número más pequeño. Si el pago inicial y los costos de cierre necesarios para comprar una vivienda de $300.000 están por encima de sus posibilidades presentes, recorte su objetivo a una vivienda de $240.000 ó $200.000, lo cuál debería reducir sus requerimientos de efectivo para la compra, entre un 20 y un 33 por ciento.

✔ **Verifique los programas de préstamos con bajo pago inicial.** Algunas entidades crediticias ofrecen programas de préstamos hipotecarios con bajo pago inicial, donde usted puede poner de inicial entre un 3 y un 10 por ciento del precio de compra. Para reunir los requisitos para tales hipotecas, generalmente usted debe tener un crédito excelente y comprar un seguro de hipoteca privado (PMI). Con estos préstamos de bajo pago inicial, además del gasto extra del PMI, proyecte que va a obtener peores condiciones para el préstamo — tasa de interés más alta y más costos de cierre. Para explorar esta alternativa, consulte con las entidades crediticias locales y con agentes de bienes raíces en su zona.

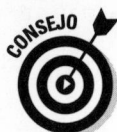

A menos que usted esté demasiado ansioso por comprar una casa, tómese más tiempo y trate de ahorrar para un pago inicial más grande. Sin embargo, si usted es del tipo de personas que tiene problemas ahorrando y puede que nunca acumule un pago inicial del 20 por ciento, comprar con menos pago inicial puede ser su mejor opción. En este caso, asegúrese de buscar los préstamos con las mejores condiciones.

✔ **Saque dinero de las cuentas de jubilación.** Algunos empleadores le permiten prestar dinero de su plan de ahorros para la jubilación. Sólo asegúrese de que entiende las reglas para pagar y devolver ese dinero, de tal manera que no se equivoque y tenga que considerar el préstamo que realice como un ingreso gravable. Usted puede hacer retiros libre de penalizaciones de las Cuentas de Jubilación Individual cuando compra casa por primera vez (vea el Capítulo 2).

✔ **Busque ayuda de la familia.** A sus padres o abuelos les podrían gustar, o quizás encantar, poder ayudarlo con el pago inicial y los costos de cierre de la casa de sus sueños. ¿Y por qué harían eso? Bueno, quizás ellos tuvieron la ayuda financiera de su familia cuando compraron una casa por primera vez en aquel entonces. Otra posibilidad es que ellos tienen más dinero ahorrado para su futuro y jubilación del que puedan necesitar. Si ellos tienen activos importantes, mantener todos estos activos hasta el momento de su muerte, podría dar origen a innecesarios impuestos a la propiedad. Una última razón por la cuál ellos estarían dispuestos a prestarle dinero, es que ellos sean del tipo de inversionistas conservadores que invierten en bancos y bonos, y estén obteniendo unos rendimientos irrisorios.

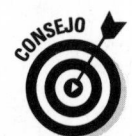

Si sus padres o abuelos (u otros familiares) abordan el tema de darle o prestarle dinero para la compra de su casa, siga adelante y converse sobre el asunto. Pero en muchas situaciones, usted (como comprador de vivienda potencial) probablemente sea quien necesite mencionar el tema primero. Algunos padres simplemente no se sienten cómodos hablando acerca de dinero o pueden preocuparse de que usted tome su oferta de una manera equivocada.

✔ **Examine un posible financiamiento por parte del vendedor.** Algunos vendedores no necesitan todo el dinero de la propiedad cuando cierran la venta. Estos vendedores pueden estar dispuestos a ofrecerle una segunda hipoteca para ayudarlo a comprar la propiedad. De hecho, a menudo anuncian que están dispuestos a ayudar con el financiamiento. El financiamiento del vendedor tiene un plazo de cinco a diez años. Esto le da a usted tiempo para acumular ganancia de capital o para ahorrar lo suficiente y refinanciar con una nueva, más grande y convencional hipoteca del 80 por ciento, antes de que se venza el préstamo del vendedor.

Sea cauteloso con el financiamiento del vendedor. Algunos vendedores que ofrecen propiedades con financiamiento incluido están tratando de salir de una casa que tiene defectos grandes. También es posible que el precio de la vivienda esté por encima del valor justo de mercado. Antes de aceptar el financiamiento del vendedor, asegúrese de que la propiedad

no tenga problemas graves (lleve a cabo una inspección profesional pro-
funda, como explicamos en el Capítulo 13), y de que su precio es com-
petitivo. También asegúrese de que la tasa de interés del vendedor sea
igual o más baja que la tasa que usted puede obtener a través de una
entidad hipotecaria tradicional.

✔ **Averigüe acerca del financiamiento 80-10-10.** Este financiamiento es llamado 80-10-10 porque un banco, una asociación de ahorro y préstamo ú
otra entidad crediticia, otorgan una primera hipoteca tradicional del 80
por ciento, usted obtiene una segunda hipoteca del 10 por ciento y hace
un pago inicial igual al 10 por ciento del precio de compra de la vivienda.
Usted puede obtener la segunda hipoteca ya sea de la entidad crediticia
que le dio la primera hipoteca o del vendedor que mencionamos previamente. Desde el punto de vista de la entidad financiera, el financiamiento
80-10-10 es tan bueno como el 20 por ciento de pago inicial.

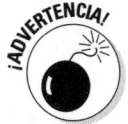

No se preocupe por el nombre. Solo porque este financiamiento es conocido como financiamiento 80-10-10, no significa que usted tiene que
aportar el 10 por ciento en efectivo. El mismo principio se usa si, por
ejemplo, usted puede disponer solamente del 5 por ciento de inicial —
un financiamiento 80-15-5 también es posible. Sin embargo, dado que un
pago inicial menor aumenta el riesgo de incumplimiento para la entidad
hipotecaria, usted sin duda tendrá que pagar gastos de préstamos más
altos y una tasa de interés más alta por el financiamiento 80-15-5, que el
que pagaría por el 80-10-10. El libro *Mortgages For Dummies* (Wiley), el
cuál escribimos nosotros también, profundiza en los detalles de préstamos especiales como éste.

✔ **Busque un socio.** Como en muchas otras situaciones de la vida, en la
unión está la fuerza. Usted puede obtener más por su dinero, y puede
necesitar reunir menos dinero inicialmente para gastos, si encuentra
socios para la compra de una propiedad multifamiliar. Por ejemplo,
usted puede encontrar uno o dos socios, e ir juntos a comprar una
vivienda o un edificio de apartamentos para dos familias o tres.

Involucrarse en un negocio en bienes raíces en donde se piensa que con
el "doble o triple de participantes, mejor es el negocio" (esto es, con dos
o más personas), no está libre de riesgo. Antes de que vaya a formar una
sociedad para comprar una propiedad, asegúrese de que ha contemplado
todas las posibilidades del juego "¿qué pasa si...?". (¿Qué pasa si uno de
ustedes se quiere salir de la sociedad después de un año? ¿Qué pasa si
uno de ustedes no paga la cuota que le corresponde de gastos? ¿Qué
pasa si uno de ustedes quiere remodelar y el otro no? Y así sucesiva-
mente.) Haga que un abogado prepare un acuerdo para los socios, deli-
neando específicamente cómo estos asuntos van a ser resueltos. De lo
contrario, más adelante en el camino, usted podría encontrar grandes
desacuerdos, aun si usted pacta el negocio con unos amigos o con personas que cree que conoce muy bien. Nosotros explicamos las ventajas
y desventajas de estas sociedades en el Capítulo 8.

Cómo invertir su pago inicial

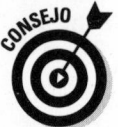

Como con todas las decisiones de inversión bien analizadas, las inversiones que usted considere en dónde poner su dinero del pago inicial, deben estar determinadas por cuan pronto usted va a necesitar nuevamente ese dinero. Mientras más largo sea el tiempo durante el cual usted puede invertir, más orientada al crecimiento y más riesgosa (esto es, más *volátil*) puede ser la inversión. Y a la inversa, cuando el tiempo que tiene para invertir es muy corto —cinco años o meno — escoger inversiones volátiles es peligroso.

Cómo comprar una casa "sin inicial"

Unos cuantos libros escritos por "expertos" en negocios de bienes raíces (y una serie de conferencias costosas conducidas por los mismos) afirman que usted puede no solamente comprar una propiedad sin aportar el pago inicial, sino también que usted puede obtener montones de dinero si lo hace. Hace una generación, esta forma de pensar fue popularizada por Robert Allen en su libro *Nothing Down.*

Allen dice que la clave para comprar una propiedad sin inicial, es encontrar un vendedor desesperado del tipo "por lo que sea se la vendo" —esto es, alguien que "haría cualquier cosa por deshacerse de su propiedad". ¿Por qué alguien estaría así de desesperado? Bueno, quizás la persona se encuentre en dificultades financieras por la pérdida de su trabajo, por haberse extendido en su crédito o por una enfermedad grave.

Quizás, antes, cuando más personas estaban acostumbradas a vivir en comunidades más pequeñas e integradas, dónde todas las personas se ayudaban unas a otras, este tipo de capitalismo salvaje no hubiera prosperado. Pero en estos tiempos, Allen dice, un "por lo que sea se la vendo" puede ofrecerle a usted hipotecas con las mejores condiciones, tales como un pago inicial bajo y una tasa de interés baja.

¿Cómo encuentra usted esas almas oprimidas que están esperándolo sólo para que usted se aproveche de ellas? De acuerdo a los estimados de Allen, el 10 por ciento de los vendedores en el mercado de bienes raíces son del tipo "por lo que sea se la vendo". Sencillamente, llame a la gente que tiene propiedades listadas para la venta en el periódico, o ponga usted mismo unos anuncios diciendo que comprará de inmediato.

En nuestra experiencia, encontrar casas que pueden ser compradas sin dar una inicial, no es algo fácil de hacer. Si usted puede encontrar ese vendedor desesperado, esté consciente de que la propiedad puede tener problemas o fallas grandes. Si la propiedad fuera una buena propiedad, la lógica nos dice que el vendedor no tendría que venderla con condiciones tan desfavorables para él. Si usted tiene la paciencia de ir de caza, y de escudriñar quizás cientos de propiedades para encontrar una buena que esté disponible con financiamiento del vendedor sin pago inicial, pues le invitamos a que lo haga. Pero, no espere a que la tarea sea fácil o muy lucrativa. Es mejor buscar buenas propiedades y financiamiento de entidades financieras, con bajo pago inicial, y empezar a ahorrar para un pago inicial considerable que le permita reunir los requisitos para optar a un mejor préstamo.

Cuando el mercado de valores está subiendo, como ocurrió muy a menudo durante la década de los noventa, usted puede estar tentado a dejar el dinero de su pago inicial invertido en acciones. Después de todo, cuando está obteniendo rendimientos del 20 por ciento o más anual, usted va a alcanzar su objetivo de ahorrar el pago inicial más rápidamente. Inversionistas más avariciosos, que codician las acciones de alta tecnología e Internet, las cuales parecen duplicarse en valor cada 90 días, esperan transformar rápidamente sus pequeños ahorros para una casita, a una montaña de dinero para una mansión.

Invertir el dinero del pago inicial en acciones es una estrategia riesgosa. La compra de su vivienda podría ser pospuesta por años debido a portafolios de inversión que bajan precipitadamente de precio. Generalmente, las acciones son inversiones inadecuadas para el dinero del pago inicial, cuando usted espera utilizarlo en los próximos cinco años. La inversión en acciones específicas es más peligrosa aun y, debe tener un plazo de tiempo más largo —idealmente de siete a diez años o más. Recuerde lo que le pasó a los sueños de aquellos amigos que querían comprar una propiedad, pero que tontamente invirtieron sus ahorros, para el pago inicial de su vivienda, en el mercado de valores, antes y durante la terrible baja del mercado a principios de la década del dos mil.

Inversiones por cinco años o menos

La mayoría de los futuros compradores de vivienda no están en posición de tomar muchos riesgos con su dinero del pago inicial. Mientras más pronto espera comprar, menos riesgo debería tomar. A menos que usted anticipe comprar después de cinco años, usted ni siquiera debería considerar invertir en esas inversiones más orientadas al crecimiento, tales como en acciones.

Aunque pueda parecerle aburrido, el primer (y posiblemente el mejor) lugar para acumular su pago inicial, es en un fondo mutual. Así como ocurre con las cuentas de ahorros de los bancos, los fondos de inversión en activos del mercado monetario no arriesgan su capital —el valor de su inversión original (capital) no fluctúa. En lugar de eso, usted simplemente gana intereses sobre el dinero que ha invertido. Los fondos de mercado monetario invierten en inversiones súper seguras, tales como en pagarés o letras del Tesoro de los Estados Unidos, certificados bancarios de depósito, y *pagarés financieros* (o sea, pagarés a corto plazo emitidos por las corporaciones financieramente más firmes y que se conocen como *IOUs*).

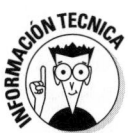

Los fondos de inversión en activos del mercado son uno de los tres grupos más grande de fondos mutuales —los otros dos son aquéllos que se concentran en bonos (fondos de bonos) y aquéllos que se concentran en acciones (fondos de inversión en acciones o capital). Muchas personas creen que los fondos mutuales son inversiones riesgosas, en parte porque ellos asemejan las inversiones de los fondos, con el invertir en el mercado de valores. Sin embargo, la realidad es que según las normas de la Comisión de la Bolsa de

Valores (*SEC*, por sus siglas en inglés), los fondos de mercado monetario sólo pueden invertir en acciones seguras, y las inversiones en estos fondos deben tener una madurez máxima promedio de 90 días. El hecho de ser a corto plazo, elimina el riesgo de que los fondos de mercado monetario sean inestables porque no están sujetos a cambios de las tasas de interés, como lo están los bonos y los fondos de bonos.

Aunque las cuentas de ahorro de algunos bancos pagan tasas de interés moderadas, casi todas pagan menos intereses que los mejores fondos de mercado monetario. ¿Por qué es esto? Porque los bancos no son tan eficientes y bajos en costos, como lo son los fondos del mercado monetario. Por cierto, ¿quién cree usted que está pagando por los alquileres de todas esas sucursales de bancos?

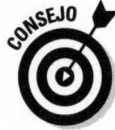

Si usted realmente quiere ahorrar a través de un banco, busque, busque y busque. Las cooperativas de ahorro y préstamo pequeñas, y las de crédito, generalmente ofrecen rendimientos más competitivos que los bancos más grandes que gastan grandes cantidades de dinero en publicidad y que tienen sucursales en casi cada esquina. Recuerde, más gastos generales significan rendimientos más bajos para su dinero.

Además de rendimientos más altos, los mejores fondos de mercado monetario ofrecen servicios de cuentas de cheques (de modo que usted tiene fácil acceso a sus fondos) y vienen en versiones libre de impuestos. Si usted está en una categoría impositiva alta, un fondo de mercado monetario libre de impuestos, puede permitirle ganar un rendimiento efectivo más alto que un fondo monetario que paga intereses gravables. (***Nota:*** Usted paga impuestos sólo en el dinero invertido fuera de las cuentas de jubilación libre de impuestos.) Cuando usted está en una categoría impositiva alta (vaya a la Tabla 3-2 al principio de este capítulo), usted debería invertir en fondos de mercado monetario libres de impuestos. Si usted vive en un estado con altos impuestos, considere un fondo de mercado monetario estatal, el cual paga intereses libres de impuestos estatales y federales.

Los mejores fondos de mercado monetario también ofrecen servicios de transferencias y cancelaciones a través del teléfono y, de servicios automatizados de transferencia de su cuenta bancaria a otras o viceversa. Las inversiones automáticas son muy útiles para ahorrar el pago inicial de una vivienda. Una vez al mes, por ejemplo, usted puede hacer que le transfieran dinero de su cuenta bancaria a su fondo de mercado monetario.

Debido a que un tipo particular de fondo de mercado monetario (general, Tesoro, o bonos municipales libre de impuestos) está básicamente invirtiendo en los mismos valores que sus competidores, opte por un fondo que mantenga los gastos bajos. Los gastos operativos de un fondo de mercado monetario, los cuales son deducidos antes del pago de dividendos, son un factor muy importante en la determinación del rendimiento del fondo. De la misma manera como ocurre con los gastos generales de los bancos, mientras más altos son los gastos operativos de los fondos monetarios, más bajo es su rendimiento. Los excelentes fondos monetarios de las mejores compañías de fondos mutuales, están a su disposición sólo por el pago de unos gastos operativos anuales de 0,5 por ciento o menos. Recomendamos unos fondos muy buenos en esta sección.

Cuando usted no está en una categoría impositiva federal alta y tampoco en una categoría impositiva estatal alta (esto es, paga menos del 5 por ciento en sus impuestos estatales), tome en cuenta los siguientes fondos de mercado monetario gravables, para invertir el dinero del pago inicial de la compra de su casa:

- ✔ Fidelity Cash Reserves (requiere un mínimo de $2.500 para abrir)
- ✔ Fidelity's Spartan Money Market (tiene rendimientos más altos si usted tiene $20.000 para invertir)
- ✔ T. Rowe Price Summit Cash Reserves (requiere un mínimo de $25.000 para abrir)
- ✔ Vanguard's Prime Money Market (requiere un mínimo de $3.000 para abrir)

Si usted duerme mejor de noche después de prestarle su dinero a una organización con más de $7 billones en deuda pendiente, usted puede invertir en un fondo de mercado monetario que invierte en fondos de bonos del Tesoro de los Estados Unidos, los cuáles tienen el respaldo del gobierno federal.

Desde el punto de vista impositivo, y debido a que los títulos de deuda emitidos por el Tesoro de los Estados Unidos están libres de impuestos estatales, pero son gravables a nivel federal, estos bonos del Tesoro son buenos cuando usted no está en una categoría impositiva federal alta, pero está en una categoría impositiva estatal alta (5 por ciento o más). Si usted decide invertir en un fondo de mercado monetario que invierte en fondos del Tesoro de los Estados Unidos, tome en cuenta los siguientes fondos:

- ✔ Fidelity's Spartan U.S. Treasury Money Market (requiere un mínimo de $20.000 para abrir)
- ✔ USAA's Treasury Money Market (requiere un mínimo de $3.000 para abrir)
- ✔ Vanguard Treasury Money Market (requiere un mínimo de $3.000 para abrir)
- ✔ Vanguard's Admiral Treasury Money Market (tiene rendimientos más altos si usted tiene $50.000 para invertir)

Cómo comunicarse con las empresas de fondos mutuales

La mayoría de las compañías de fondos mutuales no tienen muchas (o tal vez ninguna) oficinas locales. Generalmente, este hecho ayuda a estas compañías a mantener sus gastos bajos de modo que pueden pagarle a usted rendimientos más altos en un fondo de mercado monetario.

Entonces, ¿cómo hace para relacionarse con una compañía de inversiones sin una oficina cerca de usted? Pues es muy simple: usted abre y mantiene su cuenta de fondo mutual por la línea telefónica gratis de la compañía, por correo y por el Internet. Algunos proveedores de fondos mutuales también tienen sucursales.

Aquí le presentamos cómo contactar, por teléfono o por Internet, a las compañías más grandes de fondos que recomendamos en esta sección:

- Fidelity: 800-544-8888; `www.fidelity.com`
- T. Rowe Price: 800-638-5660; `www.troweprice.com`
- USAA: 800-382-8722; `www.usaa.com`
- Vanguard: 800-662-7447; `www.vanguard.com`

Los fondos monetarios *municipales* (también conocidos como *muni*) invierten en deudas a corto plazo emitidas por los gobiernos estatales y locales. Un fondo de mercado monetario municipal, el cual paga dividendos libres del impuesto federal, invierte en esos fondos "munis" emitidos por los gobiernos estatales y locales de todo el país. Un fondo municipal de un estado específico invierte en "munis" emitidos por el gobierno estatal y local de ese estado, tal como Nueva York. De modo que si usted vive en Nueva York y compra del fondo municipal de ese estado, los dividendos de ese fondo están, generalmente, libres de impuestos federales y de impuestos del estado de Nueva York.

Entonces, ¿cómo decide usted si comprar un fondo municipal de escala nacional o un fondo de un estado específico? Los fondos monetarios libres de impuestos federales son apropiados cuando usted está en una categoría impositiva federal alta, y en una categoría impositiva estatal baja (esto es, menos del 5 por ciento). Puede ser que el estado donde vive no tenga un fondo de mercado monetario libre de impuestos estatales, o no son buenos. Si vive en unos de esos estados, posiblemente sería mejor invertir en uno de los siguientes fondos monetarios nacionales:

- T. Rowe Price Summit Municipal Money Market (requiere un mínimo de $25.000 para abrir)
- USAA Tax-Exempt Money Market (requiere un mínimo de $3.000 para abrir)
- Vanguard Tax-Exempt Money Market (requiere un mínimo de $3.000 para abrir)

Bonos a corto plazo y fondos de bonos

Usted puede estar pensando, "de tres a cinco años es un tiempo muy largo para mantener mi dinero, sin hacer nada, en un fondo de mercado monetario".

A eso podemos responder, sí y no. Durante ciertos períodos, inversionistas que compraron bonos que maduraban en cinco años obtuvieron muy poco en términos de rendimientos extras, comparados con lo que pudieron haber obtenido en un buen fondo de mercado monetario. Durante otros periodos, bonos de tres a cinco años ganaron mucho más intereses que los que ganaron los fondos monetarios.

En cualquier momento que usted invierte en bonos que no maduran en un tiempo corto, usted está tomando riesgos. Primero, tiene el riesgo de que quien emite el bono pueda caer en problemas financieros, y este riesgo comienza desde el momento en que usted compra el bono hasta el momento en que el mismo vence. Segundo, tiene el riesgo de que las tasas de interés en general puedan aumentar considerablemente. Si esto último ocurre, debido generalmente al efecto de la inflación, usted puede terminar quedándose con un bono que le paga menos que la tasa de inflación.

La mayoría de las veces, los bonos que vencen en unos pocos años deberían producir una tasa de retorno un poco más alta que las cuentas de ahorro y de mercado monetario. Sin embargo, si usted invierte en esos bonos, recuerde que puede terminar ganando lo mismo (o quizás menos) que lo que usted hubiera ganado si se hubiera quedado con el fondo de mercado monetario. Las tasas de interés que están en aumento pueden hacer disminuir el valor de la inversión en los bonos.

Invierta en bonos solamente si usted anticipa retenerlos por un periodo de tres a cinco años. Si quiere invertir en ciertos bonos en particular, y no se encuentra en una categoría impositiva alta, piense en bonos del Tesoro, cuyo riesgo crediticio no requiere ser monitoreado — esto es, ¡a menos que el gobierno de los Estados Unidos caiga en mora! Además, fíjese en los rendimientos de los certificados de depósitos de los bancos. Usted también puede considerar algunos fondos mutuales de bonos a corto plazo y de alta calidad que invierten —¡ya lo adivinó!—, en bonos a corto plazo. Uno de estos fondos buenos es el Vanguard's Short-Term Investment Grade Portfolio.

Si usted se encuentra en una categoría impositiva alta, es difícil ganarle a un fondo mutual monetario libre de impuestos como alternativa de inversión. Algunos fondos de bonos libres de impuesto federal que se pueden investigar son el bono a corto plazo Vanguard's Short-Term Tax-Exempt y los de tiempo limitado Vanguard's Limited-Term Tax-Exempt. Buenos fondos de bonos a corto plazo y que sean deducibles de ambos gravámenes, federales y estatales, al mismo tiempo, simplemente no existen.

Los fondos monetarios libres de impuestos estatales son apropiados cuando usted está ubicado en una categoría impositiva federal alta y también en una categoría impositiva estatal alta (5 por ciento o más). Contacte las compañías de fondos mutuales que hemos mencionado en la sección "Cómo comunicarse con las empresas de fondos mutuales" para verificar si ellos ofrecen un fondo monetario de su estado.

Inversiones de más de cinco años

Si está anticipando que va a mantener el dinero del pago inicial de su casa por más de cinco años, usted puede pensar tranquilamente en inversiones un poco más riesgosas, como bonos de largo plazo, y en acciones más conservadoras. Eric cubre esos tipos de inversiones y muchas otras más en sus libros *Investing For Dummies* y *Mutual Funds For Dummies* (Wiley).

Capítulo 4

¿Por Qué los Precios de la Vivienda Suben y Bajan?

En Este Capítulo

▶ Cómo determinar el valor actual de la vivienda y su valor en el futuro

▶ Cómo estimar la tendencia del cambio de precios de la vivienda en su localidad

▶ Estrategias de compra para hacer una buena inversión en cualquier mercado

Si usted está considerando comprar una vivienda, puede que le preocupe la tendencia futura de los precios de las mismas. Después de todo, ¿quién quiere comprar una casa justo antes de que los precios bajen precipitadamente? O, por el contrario, ¿a quién, en su buen juicio, no le encantaría entrar en el mercado de bienes raíces antes de que los precios suban al cielo? Para entender cuáles son los factores que afectan los precios de compra y venta de las casas, usted debe examinar a qué se debe la fluctuación de la demanda y la oferta de viviendas.

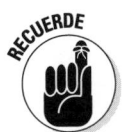

RECUERDE

A medida que presentamos en este capítulo las causas de la subida y bajada de los precios, por favor, tenga en cuenta lo siguiente: cuando se trata de comprar una vivienda y convertirse en propietario, no se preocupe demasiado por el estado actual del mercado de bienes raíces en su localidad. Si usted cree que cuando compre una casa es posible que sea su dueño por muchas décadas, entonces el preocuparse por escoger el momento oportuno para comprarla, no vale la pena. *El momento oportuno* —esto es, comprar cuando los precios están bajísimos y vender cuando los precios de bienes raíces están muy altos— es muy difícil de predecir. Conocemos a personas que comenzaron a esperar, desde hace una generación, por una baja de precios de las viviendas, y ¡todavía están esperando!

No es fácil pronosticar lo que va a ocurrir con los precios de bienes raíces en un determinado vecindario o ciudad, región o estado, el próximo año o en los subsiguientes años. En última instancia, la demanda y los precios de las viviendas en una zona dependen en gran parte de la salud de la economía en esa zona y de su vitalidad. Con el aumento de fuentes de trabajo, especialmente de los que ofrecen buenos salarios, surge una mayor demanda de viviendas.

Si usted compra su primera casa durante sus 20, 30 o 40 años de edad, probablemente terminará siendo propietario por varias décadas. Con seguridad, en
ese largo lapso de tiempo, el mercado de bienes raíces en el que usted invirtió su dinero pasará por algunos altos y bajos. La historia muestra que los
precios de los bienes raíces experimentan más y grandes subidas que bajadas
durante un período largo de tiempo; por eso, si consulta con un adivino y ve
nubarrones en la bola de cristal, no se preocupe.

Es decir, puede ser que tenga dudas acerca de comprar una vivienda en diferentes etapas de su vida. Y, puede ser que no esté seguro si va a quedarse en
esa localidad por un período de tres a cinco años. Cuanto más corto sea el
período de tiempo que espera quedarse en la misma localidad, mucho más
importante es el considerar cuidadosamente cuándo comprar. Entonces,
parte de su decisión en el proceso de adquisición de una casa, puede depender de si los precios actuales de viviendas en su localidad están ofreciéndole
una buena compra. Aun si decide permanecer a la espera por cierto tiempo,
el entender las causas de las subidas y bajadas de los precios, y el conocer
las maneras de maximizar las oportunidades de hacer una buena compra,
pueden justificar la espera. Este capítulo le ayudará a entender estos puntos.

¿Qué Factores Influyen en el Mercado de Bienes Raíces y en Sus Precios?

Si va a comprar una casa, usted va a hacer una gran inversión —quizás, la
única inversión más grande de las que ha hecho en su vida. Por lo que seguramente usted hará una extensa investigación para decidir qué comprar, y
dónde y cuándo hacer la compra.

En el resto de este capítulo le explicaremos qué debe buscar en una localidad
y en la propiedad que vaya a comprar, desde el punto de vista de un inversionista. En algunos casos, la información que le ofrecemos requiere que usted
piense como un inversionista. Por supuesto, para mucha gente, la decisión de
la compra de una casa en la que vivirá con su familia, es distinta a la de una
casa como inversión en bienes raíces, con el fin de alquilar la propiedad.

Nota: En el Capítulo 8 presentamos los diferentes tipos de propiedades (residencias unifamiliares, condominios y otras construcciones como ésas), y sus
atractivos como inversión.

Empleos, maravillosos empleos

Una vivienda provee refugio del clima y de cambios atmosféricos, y provee
también un lugar para guardar y mantener las posesiones que adquiere
como consumidor. Como las viviendas cuestan dinero para adquirirlas y

mantenerlas, y como lo más probable es que usted no sea un descendiente de los Rockefeller, los Getty o de Bill Gates, necesitará una fuente de ingresos constante para poder ser propietario de una de ellas. ¿De dónde sale ese dinero? De un trabajo.

Bueno, usted puede llamarlo *una carrera* o, mejor aún, una de sus pasiones. Pero si usted es como la mayoría de la gente, usted trabaja para pagar sus cuentas. Y una casa y los gastos que ella ocasiona son una de las mayores fuentes de gastos que la gente tiene (y es una de las razones por la que trabajamos muchas décadas en nuestra edad madura).

Ésa es la razón por lo que la demanda de viviendas y la habilidad de pagar por ellas, están directamente relacionadas con el número de empleos y calidad de los mismos en una comunidad o zona. Desde la perspectiva de una inversión, una zona ideal en donde las viviendas aumentan de valor rápidamente, tiene las siguientes características:

✔ **El crecimiento del mercado de trabajo:** entonces, ¿qué ocurre si una región tiene miles o millones de empleos pero está perdiendo muchos de ellos? La zona metropolitana de la Ciudad de Nueva York tenía millones de empleos pero sin embargo sufrió una caída en los precios de bienes raíces al principio de la década de los noventa debido a una disminución de empleos. La creación de empleos es un factor vital para que exista un mercado local de bienes raíces atrayentes. Investigue cómo están las condiciones de empleo en la zona que le interesa y examine cómo ha cambiado la tasa de desempleo en los últimos años. Las señales positivas son una declinación de la tasa de desempleo y un crecimiento en el número de empleos.

✔ **La diversificación del mercado de trabajo:** no, no estamos hablando aquí de lo que se llama "políticamente correcto". Si una comunidad depende de una fábrica de papel y de un fabricante de ropa interior, y ambos representan la mitad de las fuentes de trabajo, usted no debería confiar en comprar una casa allí. Porque si ambas compañías cerraran sus puertas, el mercado de bienes raíces sufriría una declinación segura. Este tipo de escenario se ha visto en comunidades más pequeñas que fueron seriamente perjudicadas cuando grandes fábricas de materiales para la industria de defensa, y bases militares, perdieron muchos empleados debido a una reducción en la inversión de ese tipo de industria.

✔ **Calidad del empleo:** no todos los empleos son iguales. ¿Cuál zona cree usted que tiene bienes raíces con un aumento de valor más rápido? ¿Una zona con más empleos que pagan altos salarios en industrias en crecimiento (como la industria tecnológica) o una zona donde la mayoría de los empleos requieren un nivel bajo en destrezas, y ofrecen salarios bajos (por ejemplo, los trabajos en los restaurantes de comida rápida)? Al igual que la comida, las diversiones y el sexo, la calidad es tan importante como la cantidad, o talvez más. Cuando la mayoría de los trabajos en una comunidad provienen de sectores de empleo de bajo crecimiento o que están reduciéndose (como la industria agrícola, las pequeñas tiendas, los fabricantes de zapatos y ropa, y empleos en el gobierno), los precios de bienes raíces probablemente no van a aumentar su valor rápidamente en el futuro. Por otra parte, las áreas con una mayor cantidad de industrias de alto crecimiento (como la tecnológica) van a tener más oportunidades de notar un incremento más rápido en el valor de los bienes raíces.

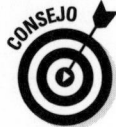

¿Dónde puede usted obtener información que le presente este tipo de perspectiva? *The U.S. Bureau of Labor Statistics* (El Departamento de Estadísticas Laborales de los Estados Unidos) compila datos de empleo y desempleo para las zonas metropolitanas y los condados. Usted puede encontrar el gran tesoro de estadísticas de esa entidad, a través de la Internet, en el sitio Web www.bls.gov o puede visitar una buena biblioteca o la cámara de comercio local. También, un agente de bienes raíces puede ayudarlo a encontrar la información deseada.

Disponibilidad de viviendas

Aunque los empleos crean una demanda de viviendas, la cantidad de viviendas disponibles —tanto las existentes como las nuevas— representan la oferta, en la ecuación de oferta y demanda. Aún cuando se están creando empleos nuevos, los precios de la vivienda pueden mantenerse sin cambio alguno si hay una disponibilidad abundante de viviendas. Por otro lado, una tasa de empleo relativamente baja en un área con escasez de viviendas, puede provocar un aumento significativo en los precios de los bienes raíces.

Comience por examinar cómo la oferta de viviendas existentes está siendo utilizada. Las tasas de vacantes son un indicador útil en el proceso de investigación. Ellas indican cuán alta o baja es la demanda por viviendas o unidades existentes para alquilar. *La tasa de vacantes* se calcula fácilmente dividiendo el número de unidades desocupadas (no alquiladas) por el número total de unidades de alquiler disponibles. Así, por ejemplo, si 50 unidades de alquiler están desocupadas en Happy Valley, Tennessee, y hay un total de 1.000 unidades disponibles, la tasa de vacantes es del 5 por ciento (50 dividido por 1.000).

Una tasa de vacantes baja (por debajo del 5 por ciento) es un buen indicador de la futura apreciación de los bienes raíces. Cuando la tasa de vacantes es baja y su valor continúa disminuyendo, existe más competencia por las pocas unidades de alquiler existentes (o surgirá una competencia pronto). Esta competencia tiende a aumentar los precios del alquiler, haciendo que el alquilar se vuelva más caro y menos deseable.

Por otra parte, una tasa de vacantes alta, indica que hay una oferta abundante de unidades de alquiler, lo que baja los costos de los alquileres porque los propietarios tienen que competir por atraer inquilinos. Las tasas de vacantes altas (entre un 7 y 10 por ciento) y el incremento progresivo de ellas son generalmente una señal: una señal mala para los vendedores de bienes raíces y para los precios, pero buena para los compradores potenciales de vivienda.

Además de examinar la tasa de vacantes, que le va decir si la cantidad de viviendas existentes están habitadas, los inversionistas astutos en bienes raíces también observan lo que está ocurriendo con los permisos de construcción. Para construir nuevas casas es necesario obtener un permiso de construcción. La tendencia ascendente o descendente del número de permisos de construcción, pueden revelarle con qué rapidez o lentitud la oferta de propiedades de bienes raíces puede ir cambiando en el futuro.

Un aumento significativo del número de permisos que se emiten, puede ser una señal importante pues puede indicar una saturación del mercado de viviendas en el futuro. Tales aumentos, frecuentemente ocurren después de un tiempo prolongado de aumento de precios de las viviendas en una zona. A medida que los precios alcanzan un nivel muy alto, los constructores se apresuran a construir y ofrecer nuevas viviendas para capitalizarse con los precios altos.

Por el contrario, precios bajos o una construcción a alto costo pueden dar como resultado un escaso desarrollo de nuevas viviendas. Con el tiempo, esta tendencia puede favorecer los precios de los bienes raíces locales.

La cantidad de viviendas disponibles está también determinada, en parte, por la cantidad de tierra disponible para el desarrollo. A menos que usted piense que las casas flotantes o los basureros sean la tendencia del futuro, debe aceptar que se necesita tierra para construir viviendas. Una cantidad limitada de tierra, generalmente favorece el aumento del precio de bienes raíces a largo plazo en una zona. Por eso, los bienes raíces han ido aumentando de valor por décadas en áreas como Manhattan, San Francisco, Hawai, Hong Kong y Tokio (que son muy caros hoy en día), y que se encuentran localizadas alrededor de lagos y océanos. Por otra parte, los precios de la vivienda tienden a subir lentamente cuando existen grandes extensiones de tierra para desarrollar.

Inventario de viviendas en venta y ventas finalizadas

Así como extensiones grandes de tierra disponible y una excesiva cantidad de edificios nuevos frenan el aumento potencial de los precios de bienes raíces en el futuro, de ese mismo modo lo frenan un número creciente de listados de propiedades en venta. Las asociaciones locales de agentes de bienes raíces, mediante sus "Servicios de listado múltiple" *(Multiple Listing Service* [MLS, por sus siglas en inglés]), típicamente consultan continuamente el número total de los *listados* (contratos de trabajo entre un agente de bienes raíces y el dueño de la propiedad). Las propiedades que son "vendidas directamente por el propietario" (es decir, sin la ayuda de un agente), no están incluidas en esos listados. Pero dichas ventas no registradas en el MLS tienden a seguir las mismas tendencias que las propiedades registradas por los agentes. (No sabemos de nadie que lleve un control del número de propiedades vendidas directamente por el propietario).

En un mercado de bienes raíces normal, la cantidad de viviendas en venta incluidas en la lista permanece a un nivel relativamente constante, ya que nuevas viviendas entran en el mercado continuamente, mientras que otras se venden. Sin embargo, cuando el precio de las propiedades comienza a alcanzar un nivel alto, y algunos propietarios e inversionistas de bienes raíces tratan de sacarle provecho y hacen nuevas inversiones, el *inventario del listado* (el número de viviendas registradas para la venta) puede aumentar significativamente. Un número creciente de compradores potenciales optan por alquilar cuando los precios de las viviendas alcanzan valores altos comparados con el precio del alquiler (vea la sección siguiente). El interés de los compradores también puede disminuir como consecuencia de un enfriamiento de la actividad económica.

Un aumento en el número de casas registradas para la venta, y un alto inventario de casas sin vender, son dos señales de que probablemente los precios de las viviendas van a bajar en el futuro. Al tener muchas opciones para elegir, los compradores potenciales pueden ser más exigentes antes de comprar. Esta competencia entre muchos vendedores por los pocos compradores existentes es lo que comienza a forzar una baja de precios en el mercado, y puede crear un *mercado de compradores,* o sea, un mercado preferido por los compradores porque los precios son bajos debido a que la oferta excede ampliamente la demanda.

Un número decreciente de nuevos registros en los listados y un inventario bajo de propiedades registradas para la venta, favorecen la subida de los precios de las mismas. Las ventas rápidas, pocas viviendas a la venta y numerosas ofertas de compra indican que la demanda de los compradores excede la oferta de propiedades en venta —es *un mercado para el vendedor.*

Cuando la economía local es fuerte y la vivienda no es cara, comparada con los precios de los alquileres, un mayor número de inquilinos elige comprar (o tiene los medios financieros para hacerlo), lo que resulta en un aumento en las actividades de ventas. Si usted es un vendedor, se siente como en las nubes. Como comprador, puede sentirse frustrado por los precios en constante ascenso, o por perder la oportunidad de compra debido a múltiples peticiones o porque otros compradores interesados le han ganado la carrera hacia la nueva casa puesta en venta.

Tasas de interés y precios de la vivienda

Generalmente, el gasto mayor que tiene un propietario de vivienda es el pago mensual de la hipoteca; por lo tanto, el nivel de las tasas de interés de las hipotecas debiera tener un impacto importante en los precios de las viviendas. A medida que bajan las tasas de interés, las mensualidades de hipoteca de un cierto monto pueden bajar también.

Piense en una hipoteca de $100.000 con una tasa de interés fija, a pagar en 30 años. Si la tasa de interés es del 6 por ciento, la mensualidad de la hipoteca es de $600. Si la tasa de interés es un 10 por ciento, la mensualidad de la hipoteca sube drásticamente a $878.

Es cierto que tasas de interés bajas permiten a más inquilinos ser propietarios. Por lo que usted puede pensar que una disminución de las tasas de interés podría producir un alza de los precios de las viviendas y, viceversa, que el aumento de las tasas de interés podría acarrear una caída de los precios de las mismas. Pero ésta no es la manera en que el mundo trabaja, y esto está probado por el hecho de que al final de la década de los ochenta y al principio de la década de los noventa, en muchas partes de los Estados Unidos los precios de la vivienda disminuyeron al mismo tiempo que las tasas de interés estaban bajando. Aún cuando las tasas de interés tendían a subir al final de la década de la década de los noventa, los precios de las viviendas subieron rápidamente en muchas comunidades en toda la nación.

Claramente, hay otros factores que influyen en los precios de la vivienda, especialmente el estado de la economía local y nacional y la confianza del consumidor. Y aunque las tasas de interés bajas ponen la vivienda al alcance de muchos, ellas también permiten construir más viviendas a un costo más bajo. Un gran inventario de viviendas tiende a desalentar el aumento de los precios.

¿Qué nos enseña esta historia? Nos enseña que no debe decidir cuándo comprar una vivienda basándose en lo que está ocurriendo, o en lo que usted espera que vaya a suceder con las tasas de interés. En verdad, los cambios futuros del valor de su casa pueden sorprenderlo.

El mercado de viviendas de alquiler

Los precios de los alquilares son un indicador útil de la demanda de vivienda. Cuando la demanda de viviendas de alquiler excede la oferta, y la economía local continúa creciendo, el costo del alquiler también aumenta. Esta situación favorece el aumento de los futuros precios de la vivienda. Cuando el costo del alquiler aumenta, la compra de una vivienda es mucho más deseada por los inquilinos que estudian el mercado de bienes raíces y están considerando la posibilidad de comprar.

Pero, la tendencia de los alquileres y el nivel absoluto de los mismos, no le dicen todo lo que usted necesita saber. Suponga que una casa de 1.100 pies cuadrados, con dos habitaciones y un baño, en un vecindario de su ciudad, se alquila por $1.200 mensuales. ¿Y qué? Lo que usted también necesita saber es cómo el costo del alquiler de esa casa se compara con el costo de comprarla y ser el dueño de ella.

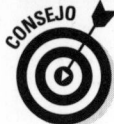

Compare el costo del alquiler de una vivienda determinada con el costo de si usted la comprara. En realidad, ésta es la comparación que hacen los inquilinos cuando sopesan los costos de la compra y de salirse de la vivienda alquilada. La comparación entre el costo de ser el dueño de una vivienda con el costo de alquilarla, sirve para conocer la realidad de los precios de las viviendas.

A fin de hacer una comparación justa entre alquilar y comprar, usted debe comparar el costo mensual de una vivienda alquilada con el costo de la misma si usted es el propietario. Pero si compara el costo de alquilar una vivienda por $1.200 mensuales, con el precio de compra de la misma por $250.000, usted está comparando peras con manzanas. Esos $250.000 son el costo total de la compra de la vivienda, pero no es su costo mensual si fuese su dueño.

Cuando usted calcule los costos de ser propietario, debe también incluir los beneficios de las deducciones impositivas permitidas. Sus mayores gastos como dueño de una propiedad —los intereses de la hipoteca e impuestos a la propiedad— son generalmente deducibles de su declaración de impuestos (vea el Capítulo 3).

¿Son los precios de bienes raíces una burbuja a punto de romperse?

Aún durante la gran baja del mercado de valores al principio del 2000, los precios de las viviendas en la mayoría de las comunidades continuaron la marcha ascendente, que habían comenzado a mediados de la década de los noventa. Los comentaristas y expertos se asombraban y predecían más y más, que los precios estaban en camino hacia una caída de gran magnitud.

En uno de esos artículos, titulado *That Sinking Feeling* (Ese sentimiento deprimente), el autor opinaba que los precios de los bienes raíces eran la próxima inversión a punto de sufrir una crisis. Desafortunadamente, el autor pasó completamente por alto el indicador más útil de todos, para los compradores potenciales, cuando ellos están tratando de decidir si es bueno comprar o alquilar. Se puede conocer este indicador comparando el costo mensual de ser propietario de una vivienda, después de haber deducido los impuestos, con el costo del alquiler de la misma. Si el costo de ser propietario es considerablemente mayor, esa es una señal de alarma que advierte que los precios de la vivienda están aumentados o inflados. Como decimos en otra parte en este capítulo, quien esté preocupado por los precios de las viviendas en un lugar determinado porque los precios son muy altos, debería hacer este sencillo análisis antes de comprometerse a comprar.

Pensamos que el análisis del autor es muy simplista. Básicamente, lo que él argumenta es que los precios de las viviendas son muy altos porque la rapidez de la apreciación ha sobrepasado el ritmo de crecimiento de los ingresos. Esto casi siempre es verdad a largo plazo, especialmente durante los períodos cuando las tasas de interés están bajando.

Los compradores potenciales tienen la opción de alquilar, por lo que el análisis de "alquilar versus comprar" es una herramienta increíblemente simple pero poderosa para discernir si los precios de la vivienda son demasiado altos, demasiado bajos, o simplemente los apropiados.

Las viviendas nunca han perdido repentinamente su atractivo para los propietarios, como les ha pasado a los inversionistas con sus acciones. ¿Recuerda cuando las acciones de Enron se fueron en picada después de publicarse la noticia de los hechos delictivos de la corporación? La caída fue de $49 por acción, en septiembre del 2001, a 25 centavos por acción, a finales de noviembre de ese mismo año. ¿Y qué decir del doble golpetazo del llamado "Black Friday" y del "Meltdown Monday", un lunes en octubre de 1987, cuando el promedio del Dow Jones perdió alrededor del 25 por ciento de su valor en dos días?

Aún en las épocas más difíciles, los precios de la vivienda nunca han bajado de precio precipitadamente. Ciertamente, los precios decayeron de vez en cuando, pero nunca bajaron precipitadamente. No hay que confundir la forma en que opera el mercado de valores con la forma en que opera el mercado de bienes raíces residenciales.

Los propietarios de vivienda no tienen la mentalidad gregaria de los accionistas. Suponga que las tasas de interés de las hipotecas repentinamente subieran a dos dígitos, como ocurrió en la década de los ochenta. ¿Cree usted que todos los propietarios pondrían sus viviendas en venta simultáneamente? Por supuesto que no. Las tasas altas de los préstamos nuevos no afectarían a millones de las hipotecas existentes. Y la vida continuaría como si nada.

Por supuesto, los precios de la vivienda sufrirían una baja por algún tiempo. Pero tarde o temprano, como suele suceder, las tasas de interés se normalizarían de nuevo. Y lo mismo pasaría con los valores de los inmuebles.

Si usted no vende cuando los precios están bajos, no pierde dinero. Sin embargo, si usted tiene que vender en un mercado deprimido, debido a un divorcio, jubilación u otro cambio importante en su vida, descubrirá que los dioses de los bienes raíces son meticulosamente justos. Cualquier cosa que pierda cuando vende, generalmente lo recuperará cuando compre su nueva vivienda. Los precios de los inmuebles son como los corchos flotantes en una laguna: todos tienden a subir y a bajar al mismo tiempo.

Ser propietario no es sólo una inversión. También ofrece una gama de beneficios: un refugio físico, una ventaja contra la inflación y deducciones de los intereses de la hipoteca y de los impuestos a la propiedad cuando paga sus impuestos. Según la actual legislación impositiva, los vendedores de viviendas pueden deducir de los impuestos una cantidad considerable de sus ganancias (en el Capítulo 17 hay más información sobre esta maravillosa deducción). Las viviendas son excelentes inversiones *a largo plazo*.

El siguiente ejemplo de la vida real muestra cómo comparar los costos de alquilar con los de ser propietario. A mediados de la década de los ochenta, viviendas de tres dormitorios, en lotes medianos, en comunidades populares de la península de San Francisco, se vendían por alrededor de $250.000. Esas mismas casas se podían alquilar por unos $1.200 mensuales. El costo de ser propietario de esa casa (suponiendo un pago del 20 por ciento del valor de la casa como pago inicial) llegaba aproximadamente a $1.300 mensuales. Esta cantidad incluye el interés de la hipoteca y los gravámenes a la propiedad que se pueden deducir de los impuestos.

Entonces, en ese momento, usted podría haber comprado una casa en esa magnífica zona, económicamente fuerte y diversificada, y haber tenido los mismos costos que hubiera tenido si la alquilaba. Y no se olvide que con el correr del tiempo, el costo del alquiler estaría sujeto a la inflación, mientras que si usted hubiera comprado su casa con una hipoteca de interés fija, los costos como propietario se hubieran mantenido en gran parte constantes (vea el Capítulo 3). La compra de una casa en ese momento hubiera sido un buen negocio, teniendo en cuenta estos hechos.

Ahora, vamos al año 1990. En el lapso de apenas unos pocos años, los precios de las viviendas en esa zona subieron como un cohete al espacio. Y esas viviendas de $250.000 se vendían a $400.000. Los alquileres habían subido más lentamente. Así, el costo de ser propietario de esa casa ascendió a más de $2.400 mensuales, a pesar de que el costo de alquilarla permaneció en $1.300. Entonces en 1990, los compradores de viviendas en esa zona estaban pagando una diferencia considerable para comprar (versus alquilar) una vivienda similar.

Abundaban señales de que el mercado de compra de viviendas estaba sobrevaluado, pero el mayor factor a considerar era que el pago mensual del propietario sobrepasaba enormemente la mensualidad del alquiler de una propiedad. ¿Adivina lo qué pasó después? Pues, menos inquilinos tenían los medios económicos para comprar porque los precios eran demasiado altos. Y muy pocos inquilinos querían comprar porque, por comparación, el alquilar era mucho más barato. Por eso, disminuyó la demanda de viviendas en venta, lo que provocó una disminución de los precios de las mismas. Y aumentó la demanda de viviendas de alquiler, lo que causó un aumento sorprendente de los alquileres. Las leyes de la oferta y la demanda corrigieron un sistema que estaba desequilibrado. Cuando la economía comenzó a disminuir su ritmo de crecimiento, como lo hace eventualmente, los compradores potenciales se paralizaron, y no quisieron gastar tanto dinero en una casa, ni comprometerse a pagar una hipoteca tan grande.

Ahora, avancemos rápidamente unos cinco años. Y, ¡oh, sorpresa!, el mercado corrigió su desequilibrio. Esas viviendas de $400.000 bajaron de valor hasta unos $350.000 en 1995. Mientras tanto, los alquileres aumentaron a medida que el número de viviendas de alquiler se redujo. Así, el costo de comprar esa vivienda en 1995 era de $1.790 mensuales (versus $1.600 mensuales por el alquiler). En otras palabras, usted podía ser propietario por un monto escasamente más alto que el del alquiler —¡exactamente como era a mediados de la década de los ochenta! (En este mismo período, las tasas de interés bajaron, ayudando a reducir también los costos de propiedad.)

Desde 1995, los precios de la vivienda en la zona de San Francisco Bay han subido otra vez como un cohete espacial —ellas han duplicado su valor, en la mayoría de las comunidades—, y los alquileres también subieron de la misma manera.

La salud total de la economía de la región en la que usted vive, sin duda tiene también un impacto directo sobre los precios de la vivienda. Si las compañías en su zona tienen que reducir la fuerza laboral, y la compensación de los empleados está estancada, o quizás decrece, los consumidores tendrán menos dinero disponible para gastar en vivienda, y los precios de éstas sentirán las consecuencias.

Una corrección (reducción) del 20 por ciento de los precios de la vivienda es muy posible ante estas circunstancias. Aquellos que piensan que la lentitud en el aumento de los precios o que un periodo de precios estable es lo peor que podría suceder serían muy inocentes en sus pensamientos.

Cómo enriquecerse en bienes raíces con sólo un suspiro

Se han escrito y ofrecido muchos libros y seminarios caros que afirman tener el enfoque de inversiones en bienes raíces que pueden "ganarle al sistema." A menudo estos promotores le dicen que usted puede convertirse en multimillonario mediante la compra de propiedades *con problemas* —propiedades con problemas financieros, legales o físicos. Una estrategia sugerida es comprar propiedades en las cuales el vendedor no ha cumplido con sus obligaciones financieras o está a punto de no hacerlo. ¿Y si se compra una propiedad que está en el testamento de otra persona a través del tribunal de sucesiones? ¡O quizás le gustaría probar su suerte como inversionista en una propiedad que ha sido expropiada o que está contaminada con deshechos tóxicos!

Es posible hacer un "buen negocio" al comprar una propiedad con problemas con un descuento más grande que el costo de repararla. Pero no es fácil encontrar esas oportunidades, y los vendedores de tales inmuebles generalmente no quieren vender con un descuento lo suficientemente grande como para dejarle a usted una ganancia aceptable. Si usted no sabe cómo evaluar completa y correctamente los problemas de la propiedad, puede terminar pagando demás. Es posible que usted se tenga que quedar con una propiedad que tiene defectos irremediables tales como una mala ubicación, ruido excesivo o sin terreno al fondo. (En el Capítulo 8 le indicamos cómo separar las piedras de los "diamantes en bruto", que se pueden pulir.)

En algunos casos, las estrategias que estos gurúes o especialistas de bienes raíces recomiendan, es aprovecharse de la falta de conocimiento de la gente. Por ejemplo, algunas personas no saben que pueden proteger la participación en el capital invertido en su casa declarándose en quiebra. Cuando encuentre vendedores que estén en una desesperada situación financiera, es probable que pueda negociar la compra de sus viviendas.

Otros métodos de obtener buenas propiedades de este tipo demandan mucho tiempo e investigación. Algunos serían hacer llamadas al azar, así por así, a los dueños de las propiedades para ver si ellos están interesados en vender. Si usted llama a miles de personas de esta forma, eventualmente, podría encontrar a un buen candidato. Sin embargo, cuando toma en cuenta el valor de su tiempo, estos métodos raramente se consideran buenos.

El comparar el costo de ser dueño de una vivienda con el costo del alquiler de la misma, es un sencillo pero poderoso indicador de si los bienes raíces en la región tienen un precio excesivamente alto, demasiado bajo o el precio adecuado. El comprar es generalmente más seguro (y una buena inversión) cuando cuesta casi lo mismo que alquilar la vivienda. Sin embargo, en algunas comunidades especialmente atractivas y en demanda, ser propietario cuesta casi siempre más que alquilar. ¿Cuál sería una prima asequible? No hay una respuesta sencilla, pero si el costo mensual de ser propietario es mayor que el costo mensual de alquilar la vivienda en un 20 al 30 por ciento, tenga cuidado.

Después que compre una casa, probablemente será su propietario por muchas décadas. Por lo tanto, no se preocupe acerca de cuándo es el mejor momento para comprar una vivienda. El buscar el mejor momento para comprar tiene más importancia si piensa mudarse antes de los cinco años. En ese caso, trate de no comprar en un mercado sobrevaluado. El nivel de los precios de bienes raíces comparado con los alquileres, el estado del mercado laboral y el número de viviendas en los listados de propiedades en venta, son indicadores útiles para conocer el estado del mercado de la vivienda.

Cómo Hacer un Buen Negocio en Cualquier Mercado

Bien, ¿qué pasa si usted tiene que (o quiere) comprar cuando el mercado beneficia a los vendedores? ¿O si simplemente tiene miedo de pagar demasiado en cualquier mercado, porque usted es un novato en este tipo de transacción? A nadie le gusta que lo engañen, y a la mayoría de la gente le gusta sentir o creer que está haciendo una buena compra.

Muchas veces, cuando usted contrata servicios y compra productos de compañías (especialmente de vendedores al por menor), le dicen qué descuento o rebaja le están ofreciendo:

¡UN 60 POR CIENTO DE DESCUENTO!

LIQUIDACIÓN POR CIERRE — ¡DEBE VENDERSE TODO!

¡AHORRE HASTA $3 POR LIBRA!

¡LIQUIDACIÓN DE PRIMAVERA!

A algunos vendedores de vivienda y, con más frecuencia, a sus agentes, les gusta usar el mismo tipo de publicidad. Los siguientes ejemplos se han tomado de los avisos comerciales de viviendas en venta:

¡GRAN REDUCCIÓN DE PRECIO!

¡$20.000 DE DESCUENTO!

¡PRECIO REDUCIDO! ¡OTRA VEZ EN EL MERCADO! ¡EL DUEÑO TIENE QUE VENDER!

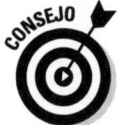

Cuando vea este tipo de avisos, en vez de pensar: "¡Increíble, esto es un excelente negocio!", usted debería pensar: esa propiedad debe haber estado sobrevaluada o es probable que tenga un defecto grande.

No le estamos diciendo que no puede conseguir y hacer un *buen negocio* (en otras palabras, comprar una vivienda a un precio menor a su *precio de mercado)*. Pero no es fácil hacerlo, y el encontrar justamente la oportunidad perfecta requiere mucho trabajo. Para la mayoría de la gente el no pagar más del valor real —en otras palabras, pagar el valor justo del mercado (que no es necesariamente el precio pedido)— es un buen objetivo. Vea el Capítulo 10 para obtener más información acerca de cómo determinar del valor de la vivienda.

Lea nuestras sugerencias para conseguir una buena compra, aún cuando esté dispuesto a pagar el precio justo de mercado. Estas ideas pueden ayudarlo a evitar pagar un precio excesivo.

Busque oportunidades escondidas para aumentar el valor

Los problemas más fáciles de corregir en una propiedad son los estéticos. Algunos vendedores y sus agentes son tan perezosos que ni siquiera se preocupan por limpiar la propiedad. Pintar, sacar la alfombra sucia, renovar los pisos de madera, reemplazar gabinetes y aparatos electrodomésticos fuera de moda, y cambiar el diseño del jardín, no son necesariamente proyectos difíciles de hacer. Y esos cambios pueden transformar la apariencia de la vivienda y hacer que luzca mucho mejor.

Una manera un poco más complicada para aumentar el valor es identificar propiedades que no están totalmente en uso o desarrolladas, según las ordenanzas locales de zonificación de propiedades. A veces, usted puede darle un uso más productivo a una propiedad. Por ejemplo, quizá pueda convertir una propiedad de dos viviendas adyacentes en dos condominios. A algunas residencias para una familia se les podría agregar una vivienda para alquilar si las ordenanzas de zonificación local así lo permitieran. Quizás usted pueda agregar otro piso para crear una vista panorámica. Un buen agente de bienes raíces, un contratista, y la oficina local de planeamiento del pueblo o ciudad en la que está buscando propiedades, podrían ayudarlo a identificar inmuebles cuyo uso actual puede cambiarse.

Identificar, evaluar, comprar y reparar una propiedad toma un tiempo precioso y mucha energía. Si usted tiene el talento de ver esas oportunidades escondidas y está dispuesto a invertir el tiempo necesario para coordinar las reparaciones, sin lugar a dudas, invierta su talento y su dinero en ellas. Pero asegúrese de ser realista cuando haga la evaluación, y vea si los defectos pueden corregirse, cuánto dinero va a necesitar para mejorar la propiedad y cuánto valor pueden las mejoras realmente agregarle a la vivienda. También, cerciórese de emplear a un inspector de propiedades bien competente. (Vea el Capítulo 13.)

Compre cuando otros teman hacerlo

El número de viviendas vendidas generalmente decrece cuando la economía se desequilibra y el desempleo aumenta, y el ambiente se siente sombrío y desalentador. De igual forma, los precios tienden a bajar. Esta situación puede señalar un momento muy bueno para adelantarse y comprar. Compre cuando las casas "estén rebajadas" y cuando no tenga que competir con otros compradores. Compre cuando pueda elegir entre muchas ofertas en un listado extenso de viviendas en venta.

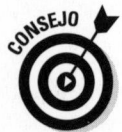

Muy poca gente se siente segura cuando hace una inversión en algo que se ha devaluado, especialmente cuando las cosas parecen tener un futuro incierto. (Pero por alguna razón psicológica inexplicable, a muchos de nosotros nos encanta comprar gangas en una tienda de venta al por menor). He aquí varios signos de que un mercado flojo de bienes raíces que se está fortaleciendo:

✔ El costo mensual de ser propietario de una vivienda es casi el mismo al costo mensual del alquiler de una vivienda similar. Uno de los atractivos de una reducción de los precios de bienes raíces es que puede poner nuevamente los costos de comprar una casa al mismo nivel que los costos de alquilarla.

✔ El inventario de viviendas en venta, incluidas en los listados, comienza a bajar de las nubes cuando las ventas comienzan a subir.

✔ El mercado de alquiler se reduce (como se puede ver, por el aumento de los alquileres y la disminución de vacantes). Otra buena señal es la escasa construcción de nuevas viviendas.

✔ El mercado de trabajo mejora. Recuerde que los empleos aumentan la demanda de viviendas. Los precios de las viviendas se recuperan cuando el índice de empleo aumenta. Esté pendiente de una disminución de la tasa de desempleo en su región.

A pesar de los precios bajos de la vivienda, de que la economía esté mejorando y de los inventarios mostrando una reducción de viviendas de alquiler y en venta, los compradores potenciales generalmente muestran mucho menos interés en comprar una vivienda cuando las cosas todavía parecen inciertas o inseguras. Es necesario tener valor para comprar durante esas épocas, cuando los titulares de los periódicos y las noticias de la televisión pregonan a los cuatro vientos las últimas cifras de los recientes despidos. No pierda la cabeza, y aproveche las oportunidades de comprar cuando ellas aparecen. Con el correr de los años, usted se alegrará de haberlo hecho.

Consiga un vendedor entusiasta

Una vez que haya dedicado tiempo a examinar un número suficiente de propiedades, eventualmente conocerá a un dueño de propiedad que realmente necesita vender o que desea vender. Puede ser que el dueño necesite trasladarse a otra parte del país por su trabajo, o quizás, se está mudando a una vivienda más grande y necesita el dinero de la venta de la propiedad actual a fin de comprar su nueva vivienda. A veces ocurre que el dueño de una propiedad no tiene los medios económicos para mantener por más tiempo la vivienda debido a sus problemas financieros.

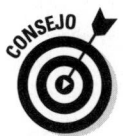

De cualquier manera, la compra de una vivienda al precio justo de mercado o por debajo de él, es mucho más fácil si el vendedor tiene un *motivo* por el cual tiene que vender. Nosotros lo llamamos un vendedor *motivado*. ¿Cómo consigue un vendedor *motivado*? Es muy sencillo: ¡Haga preguntas y más preguntas! Es sorprendente el número de compradores potenciales que son muy tímidos como para preguntarle al vendedor por qué es un vendedor, o no creen que es importante. Muchos vendedores serán sinceros con usted. Y, a un buen número de agentes de bienes raíces (especialmente a aquellos que les gusta hablar) les gusta contar sus historias y dan un montón de detalles. ¡Pero usted tiene que preguntar!

Compre en períodos de poca actividad

La mayoría de los mercados de bienes raíces locales pasan con regularidad por períodos predecibles, como un reloj, de mucha y poca actividad. Así como tiene sentido comprar cuando todo el mercado de bienes raíces en una región está deprimido, también puede ser beneficio comprar durante esos períodos típicamente lentos.

Por ejemplo, muy pocos compradores potenciales tienden a buscar vivienda durante la temporada de las fiestas en el invierno. En la mayoría de los mercados, el período entre el Día de Gracias hasta enero o febrero, tiende a ser muy tranquilo. Cuanto más fría sea la región donde usted vive, más largo será este período invernal. En las regiones más septentrionales de los Estados Unidos, donde el tiempo es tempestuoso y nieva con frecuencia, el mercado de bienes raíces no comienza realmente a activarse sino hasta abril. Pero en lugares soleados y con temperaturas más altas todo el año, como Florida y el sur de California, las ventas de viviendas comienzan a iniciarse desde el comienzo de febrero.

Otro período típicamente lento es durante los meses de verano, o sea de julio a agosto. Mucha gente se va de vacaciones, y aquellas familias que querían comprar antes del inicio del nuevo año escolar, probablemente ya han comprado para esas fechas. El calor asfixiante de las regiones del sur también mantiene a la gente dentro de sus casas, con el aire acondicionado prendido y tomando té helado.

La ventaja de buscar durante los períodos sin mucha actividad es que tiene mucho menos competencia con otros compradores potenciales. Si usted puede encontrar un vendedor *motivado*, podrá negociar una buena compra sin la intromisión de otros posibles interesados.

Sin embargo, no le estamos diciendo que solamente busque en los períodos lentos del año o que, sin lugar a dudas, va a hacer un buen negocio durante esos períodos. Tiene que ser realista. Casi siempre, en la mayoría de los mercados, hay menos propiedades en venta durante el tiempo de menor actividad. Los vendedores con experiencia venden sus propiedades durante los períodos más activos, en la primavera y el otoño. Comprenda también que una buena porción de las propiedades en el mercado durante períodos lentos pueden ser viviendas que nadie quiso.

Conviértase en un gran negociador

Conseguir una buena compra puede ser tan sencillo como ser un buen negociador. Las buenas habilidades para negociar lo capacitarán para comprar una propiedad a un precio menor del precio justo del mercado, especialmente si usted encuentra a un vendedor que necesita cerrar la venta rápidamente.

Su posición para negociar es también mejor si actúa como si *no tiene* que comprar. Si tiene mucha paciencia y está dispuesto a dejar todo si no logra lo que quiere, tendrá más posibilidades para negociar un buen precio. El tener otra propiedad como una segunda opción o el recordar que hay muchas otras propiedades en venta a su alrededor, también ayuda. Vea el Capítulo 12 para descubrir cómo ser un negociador de primera clase.

Compre en un buen vecindario

Si compra una vivienda en una zona atrayente, usted tiene una mayor probabilidad de hacer una buena inversión. En el Capítulo 8 le explicamos cómo analizar si un vecindario es bueno o no.

Cuando usted compra una buena propiedad y la mantiene por un período largo, podrá obtener un rendimiento mejor en su inversión. Al paso de los años, el haber comprado una propiedad con un pequeño descuento pasa a ser algo insignificante. Usted ganará dinero por el hecho de ser propietario de una vivienda (y quizás de otras inversiones en bienes raíces) a medida que el mercado de bienes raíces, como un todo, incrementa su valor.

Parte II
Finanzas 101

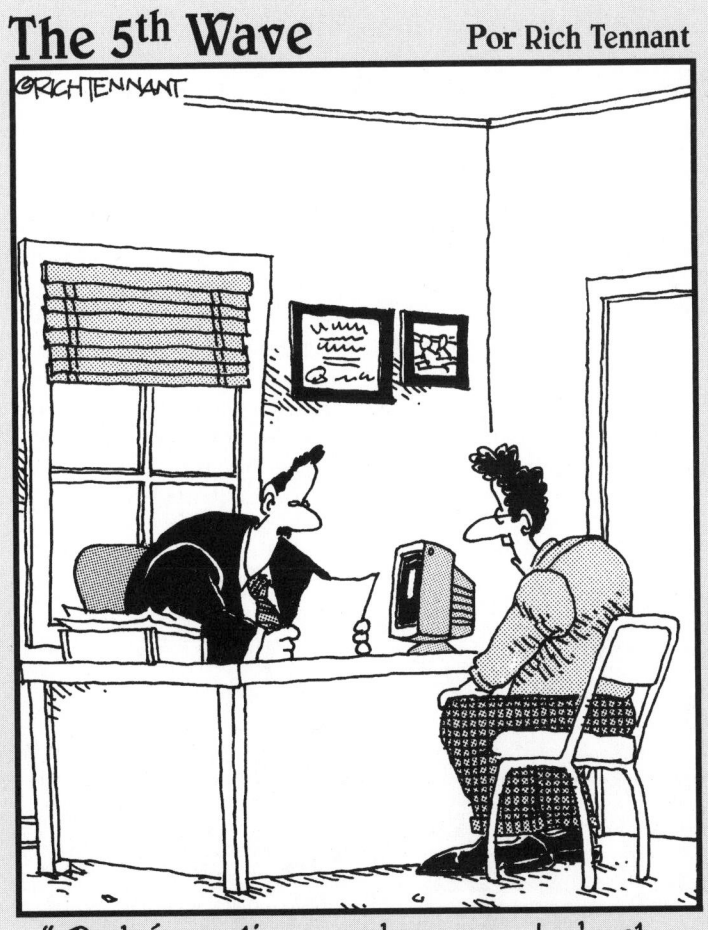

"¿Podría explicarme de nuevo, todo el programa de préstamos, pero esta vez sin usar las palabras bla, bla, bla, bla, bla?"

En esta parte . . .

A algunas personas la palabra *hipoteca* les da inmediatamente dolor de cabeza. No se ponga nervioso. Lea los siguientes capítulos y estará al corriente de los diferentes tipos de hipotecas que hay y de toda esa jerga técnica que se usa. También aprenderá cómo seleccionar una hipoteca que se ajuste a su situación financiera. Además, le explicamos cómo conseguir la mejor hipoteca posible, y lo guiamos a través de la montaña de papeles que tiene que llenar cuando hace su solicitud. Asimismo, le explicamos cómo funciona el reporte de crédito y, lo que es mejor aún, le decimos cómo mejorarlo.

Capítulo 5

Entienda y Mejore Su Puntuación de Crédito

Debe comprender que la compra de una vivienda no es un juego ya que puede perder el partido si no tiene cómo pagarla. Y la mayoría de las personas no pueden pagar una vivienda sin un préstamo hipotecario.

Cuando solicita un préstamo, las entidades crediticias tratan de determinar el nivel de riesgo de su crédito. Si ellas deciden darle el préstamo, ¿cuál es la probabilidad de que usted cumpla con sus pagos a tiempo?

Para saber el riesgo de su crédito, la mayoría de las entidades crediticias, miran su puntuación de crédito. Esta puntuación influye en el crédito que se le ofrecerá y en las condiciones de cualquier préstamo hipotecario que se le conceda.

La mayoría de las entidades crediticias también consideran otros factores para tomar la decisión de prestarle o no. Ellas miran el monto de su deuda y sus ingresos, y consideran lo que sensatamente usted podría pagar y, además, examinan su historial laboral y su historial crediticio. Basadas en la interpretación de toda esa información, así como también en sus propias pólizas del seguro de garantía, las entidades crediticias pueden darle crédito aunque su puntuación sea baja, o pueden negarle su solicitud aunque su puntuación sea alta. Pero sus posibilidades de que le aprueben el crédito y de recibir un préstamo con las mejores condiciones posibles, son mejores cuando usted tiene una puntuación de crédito alta.

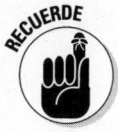

El entender la importancia de la puntuación de su crédito puede ayudarlo a administrar el estado de su crédito. Al saber cómo los prestamistas evalúan el riesgo de prestarle dinero, usted puede hacer algo para disminuir ese riesgo —y así, mejorar su puntuación— con el paso del tiempo. Una buena puntuación puede significar mejores opciones y condiciones de préstamos para usted.

Siga los consejos prácticos de este capítulo para saber cómo manejar eficientemente la puntuación de su crédito. El mejorar su puntuación puede ayudarle a:

- Obtener mejores ofertas de crédito
- Bajar sus tasas de interés
- Una rápida aprobación del crédito

El Documento que No Puede Ignorar: El Reporte de Su Historial Crediticio

Probablemente ha escuchado algo sobre los reportes de antecedentes crediticios y se ha dado cuenta de que ellos pueden causar la aprobación o rechazo de su solicitud de crédito. Sin embargo, estos reportes son un misterio para la mayoría de nosotros porque no sabemos qué se incluye en ellos ni tampoco lo que podemos hacer para mejorar nuestra puntuación de crédito. ¡No más dudas . . . !

La información que contiene su historial crediticio

Los reportes de crédito le dicen a la entidad crediticia cómo usted administra sus finanzas y, detalla su historial crediticio según fue reportado a las agencias de reportes de crédito nacionales por las compañías o entidades crediticias que le han dado crédito. Su reporte crediticio contiene:

- El tipo de crédito que usa
- El tiempo que ha tenido con esas cuentas
- Si ha pagado sus cuentas a tiempo

El reporte le dice a los prestamistas la cantidad de crédito que ha usado y si está buscando nuevas fuentes de crédito. Además, les ofrece una visión más amplia de su historial crediticio que la que se obtiene de su banco personal (a menos que todos sus créditos anteriores hayan sido concedidos por ese banco).

La información que incluye su reporte crediticio

Aunque cada una de las agencias de reportes de crédito nacionales tiene su manera particular de presentar y reportar la información, todos los reportes de crédito contienen básicamente el mismo tipo de información:

- **Datos de identificación:** para identificarlo se usa su nombre, dirección, número de Seguro Social, fecha de nacimiento e información de empleo. Sin embargo, estos factores no se incluyen en el cálculo de su puntuación. La actualización de esta información es la que usted provee a los prestamistas.

- **Renglones incluidos:** éstas son sus cuentas de crédito. Las entidades crediticias reportan información sobre cada cuenta que usted haya establecido con ellas. Ellas reportan el tipo de cuenta (tarjeta de crédito, préstamo para la compra de un automóvil, hipoteca, etc.), la fecha en la que usted abrió la cuenta, la cantidad límite del crédito o monto total al que tiene acceso, el balance de la cuenta, su historia de pagos y cuándo cerró la cuenta.

- **Copias del reporte:** cuando usted solicita un préstamo, usted está autorizando a su prestamista a que pida una copia del reporte de su crédito. Así es como aparecen las indagaciones hechas de su reporte de crédito. La parte de solicitud de información contiene una lista de todas las personas que han pedido acceso a su información de crédito en los últimos dos años. El reporte que usted ve, contiene las solicitudes *voluntarias*, que surgen cada vez que usted presenta una solicitud de crédito y, también, las solicitudes *involuntarias* que son las que hacen otros prestamistas para poder hacerle una oferta que ellos le envían por correo, pero que han aprobado previamente.

- **Información de registro público y cobro de deudas:** las agencias nacionales de reportes de crédito también obtienen información de los tribunales del estado y del condado, e información sobre deudas morosas de las agencias de cobranza. La información de registro público incluye bancarrotas, embargos hipotecarios, demandas, retenciones del sueldo para satisfacer una deuda, gravámenes y dictámenes judiciales.

Junto con el reporte del historial crediticio, las entidades crediticias pueden también comprar su puntuación crediticia basándose en la información de este reporte.

Por qué debe verificar su reporte de crédito

Debe verificar su reporte de crédito para saber si éste contiene errores o está incompleto, o contiene información de otra persona. Esto ocurre típicamente porque:

- ✔ Usted solicitó créditos bajo nombres algo diferentes (Robert Jones o Bob Jones, etc.).

- ✔ Alguien cometió un error en la oficina al leer o anotar su nombre o domicilio incorrectamente, cuando los copió de una solicitud manuscrita.

- ✔ Alguien dio un número de Seguro Social incorrecto, o el prestamista leyó mal el número.

- ✔ Los pagos de una tarjeta de crédito o de un préstamo fueron acreditados erróneamente a otra cuenta.

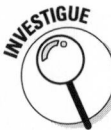

Información peyorativa en su reporte crediticio puede forzarlo a una hipoteca con una tasa de interés más alta y con cargos, o causar que la solicitud de su préstamo hipotecario sea negada. Si encuentra un error, las agencias nacionales de reportes de crédito deben investigar, y responderle en un plazo no mayor de 30 días. Si está en el proceso de solicitar un préstamo, notifique de inmediato a su entidad crediticia de cualquier información incorrecta en su reporte. Para obtener su reporte crediticio, vea la última sección de este capítulo, donde encontrará la información sobre cómo contactar las agencias nacionales de reportes de crédito.

La Puntuación Más Popular de Todas: La Puntuación FICO

La puntuación de crédito que los prestamistas usan con más frecuencia en la actualidad, fue desarrollada por la Corporación Fair Isaac y se llama "puntuación FICO" (*FICO score,* en inglés). Las puntuaciones de FICO van de 300 puntos a un máximo de 850 puntos. Cuanta más alta es su puntuación, más bajo es el riesgo que usted representa para los prestamistas. Los prestamistas reciben estas puntuaciones de las tres agencias de reportes de crédito nacionales: Equifax, Experian y TransUnion.

Aunque la puntuación de FICO es la más usada para determinar los riesgos de prestarle dinero, los prestamistas pueden usar otras puntuaciones para evaluar lo mismo. Éstas incluyen lo siguiente:

✔ **Uso de la puntuación de riesgo:** muchos prestamistas usan sistemas de puntuación que incluye la puntuación de FICO pero también consideran la información contenida en su solicitud de préstamo.

✔ **La puntuación de riesgo del solicitante:** un prestamista puede usar estas puntuaciones para tomar las decisiones de crédito sobre sus clientes actuales. Estas puntuaciones, conocidas también como *puntuación del comportamiento*, consideran la puntuación de FICO y, además, la información de cómo ha pagado sus deudas a ese acreedor en el pasado.

✔ **Otras puntuaciones del registro de crédito:** estas puntuaciones pueden evaluar su reporte de crédito de manera diferente al de la puntuación FICO y, en algunos casos, una puntuación más alta puede significar más riesgo y no menos, como lo es con la puntuación FICO.

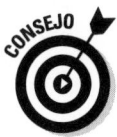

Si a usted le niegan un crédito, la Ley de Igualdad de Oportunidades de Crédito (*Equal Credit Opportunity Act, ECOA*) le da el derecho a saber el porqué se le ha negado el crédito, en un período no mayor de 30 días. También tiene derecho a recibir una copia gratis de su reporte, en un período no mayor de 60 días, la cual puede solicitar a las agencias de reportes de crédito. Si la puntuación de su crédito fue el motivo principal de la decisión del prestamista, éste usará las puntuaciones para explicar por qué no le fue aprobado el crédito.

Cómo funcionan las puntuaciones: La versión corta

Cada puntuación de crédito se calcula usando una ecuación matemática que evalúa muchos tipos de datos de la información de su crédito en esa agencia. Al comparar esta información con los patrones de cientos de miles de información de créditos previos, la puntuación refleja un nivel estimado del riesgo de crédito en el futuro.

A fin de calcular su puntuación FICO, el reporte debe contener por lo menos una cuenta que se haya abierto en los previos seis meses o antes. Además, el reporte crediticio debe incluir por lo menos una cuenta que haya sido actualizada en los últimos seis meses. De esta forma se asegura que hay suficiente información reciente en su reporte para calcular la puntuación.

Su puntuación puede cambiar cuando cambia su información crediticia. Pero su puntuación probablemente no cambiará mucho de un mes para otro.

Aunque una bancarrota o pago atrasado pueden bajar su puntuación rápidamente, el mejorarla lleva tiempo. Por eso es una buena idea verificar su puntuación (especialmente si tiene motivos para preocuparse por su historial crediticio), al menos seis meses antes de solicitar un préstamo hipotecario. Esto le da tiempo para tomar una acción correctiva si es necesario. Si usted está tratando conscientemente de mejorar su puntuación, debería verificarla trimestralmente o, mejor aún, mensualmente, para estar al tanto de los cambios.

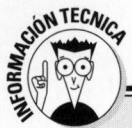

Las agencias de registro de crédito pueden presentar puntuaciones diferentes

La Corporación Fair Isaac hace las puntuaciones de FICO tan consistentes como le es posible, entre las tres agencias de reportes de crédito. Si su información fuera exactamente igual en las tres agencias, las puntuaciones de las tres agencias deberían tener una diferencia de muy pocos puntos entre ellas.

Sin embargo, a veces su puntuación de FICO puede ser muy diferente en cada una de estas agencias. La manera en que los prestamistas y otros negocios envían la información a las agencias que registran el crédito, hace que existan, a veces, datos diferentes en su información en las diferentes agencias. Las agencias de reportes de crédito también presentan la información de manera diferente. Lo que es más, las pequeñas diferencias de la información en las tres agencias de reportes pueden influir en su puntuación.

Dado que los prestamistas pueden obtener su puntuación de cualquiera de las tres agencias de registro de crédito, es mejor que usted verifique su información crediticia en las tres, para asegurarse de que es correcta (la última sección de este capítulo le dirá cómo hacerlo).

Pero ninguna puntuación, aunque sea alta o baja, indica si usted será un cliente "bueno" o "malo". Aunque muchos prestamistas usan las puntuaciones de FICO para tomar sus decisiones de otorgar crédito, cada uno de ellos tiene también sus propias estrategias, incluso el nivel de riesgo que les parece aceptable para un cierto tipo de préstamos. No hay una puntuación mínima única que sea usada por todas las entidades crediticias.

Cómo la puntuación de FICO evalúa su historial crediticio: La versión larga

La puntuación de FICO evalúa varias categorías de información: su historia de pagos, el monto de su deuda, cuántos años están representados en su historia crediticia, nuevos y recientes créditos, tipo de crédito que usa y el número de solicitudes de información de su crédito. Como puede imaginar, algunos son más importantes que otros. Por eso es importante notar que:

- ✔ **Una puntuación incluye todas esas categorías de información, y no solamente una o dos.** Ninguna categoría en particular ni ningún factor individual determinan su puntuación.

- ✔ **La importancia de cualquier factor depende de la información total que aparece en su historial crediticio.** Un factor en particular puede ser más importante que otros para algunas personas que tienen otra historia de crédito. Además, a medida que cambia la información en su historial crediticio, también cambia la importancia de cualquier factor en la determinación de su puntuación. Por eso es imposible decir exactamente cuál es la importancia de un factor determinado en el resultado de su puntuación — incluso, la importancia relativa de un factor mostrada en las siguientes secciones, es para la población en general y varía para los distintos perfiles de crédito.

✔ **Su puntuación de FICO solamente está basada en la información de su historial crediticio.** Los prestamistas también tienen en cuenta otras cosas cuando toman una decisión sobre crédito, como sus ingresos, el tiempo que ha trabajado en su empleo actual y el tipo de crédito que está solicitando.

✔ **Su puntuación considera tanto lo positivo como lo negativo de su información de crédito.** Los pagos atrasados bajan su puntuación, pero al establecer o restablecer una buena trayectoria haciendo sus pagos a tiempo suben su puntuación.

✔ **El aumentar su puntuación es un poco como ponerse físicamente en forma.** Lleva tiempo y no hay una solución inmediata. De hecho, los esfuerzos para lograr soluciones rápidas, pueden fracasar. El mejor consejo es que maneje su crédito responsablemente todo el tiempo.

Estos porcentajes están basados en la importancia de las cinco categorías estudiadas en la población total. Para grupos específicos —por ejemplo, gente que no ha usado su crédito por mucho tiempo— la importancia de estas categorías puede ser diferente.

Las secciones siguientes ofrecen una visión completa de la información que está incluida en la puntuación de FICO. Para una representación gráfica de lo que contribuye a su puntuación crediticia, por favor, vea la Figura 5-1.

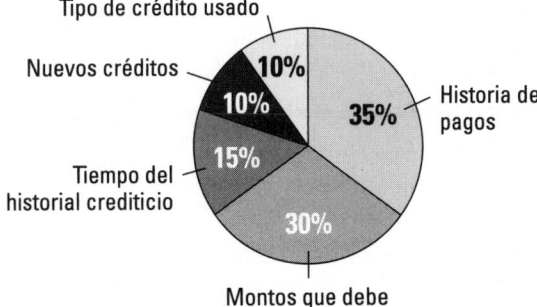

Figura 5-1:
Composición de la puntuación de crédito.

Tipo de crédito usado — 10%
Nuevos créditos — 10%
Tiempo del historial crediticio — 15%
Montos que debe — 30%
Historia de pagos — 35%

Su historia de pagos

Lo primero que un prestamista quiere saber es si usted ha pagado otros créditos a tiempo. Su historia de pagos de deudas saldadas a sus acreedores influye aproximadamente un 35 por ciento de su puntuación.

Los pagos atrasados no "matan" automáticamente la posibilidad de crédito. Sin embargo, la presentación de un crédito bueno en su totalidad puede tener más peso que quizás una o dos instancias de pagos atrasados de tarjetas de crédito. Por otro lado, el no tener pagos atrasados en su información crediticia tampoco garantiza que automáticamente va a tener una puntuación alta. Entre un 60 a un 65 por ciento de los historiales crediticios no muestran pagos atrasados. La historia de su crédito es solamente una parte de la información que se usa para calcular su puntuación.

En cuanto a los pagos, su puntuación toma en cuenta lo siguiente:

- **La información de pagos de muchos tipos de cuentas:** estos incluyen tarjetas de crédito como Visa, Master Card, American Express y Discover; tarjetas de crédito de negocios en donde usted compra; *préstamos reembolsables a plazos* (como los hipotecarios, en los que usted hace regularmente pagos) y cuentas de compañías financieras.

- **Información de registro público y cobro de deudas:** esta documentación incluye los reportes sobre bancarrotas, embargos hipotecarios, demandas, retenciones del sueldo para satisfacer una deuda, gravámenes y dictámenes judiciales. Estos datos son considerados muy importantes, aunque los más antiguos y los de montos pequeños cuentan menos que los más recientes o aquéllos de un monto mayor. Las bancarrotas permanecen en su reporte de crédito de siete a diez años, según el tipo.

- **Detalles sobre pagos atrasados u omitidos *(morosos)*, los reportes de registro público y las facturas a cobrar:** la puntuación de FICO considera la duración del retraso de los pagos, el monto de lo que debe, cuándo ocurrieron los pagos atrasados y cuántos hay. Como regla general, un pago atrasado 60 días no es tan malo como un pago atrasado 90 días. Sin embargo, un pago atrasado 60 días que fue pagado justo hace un mes, es más perjudicial que uno atrasado 90 días hace cinco años.

- **Cuántas cuentas no tienen pagos atrasados:** una buena trayectoria de pagos en la mayoría de sus cuentas de crédito aumenta su puntuación de crédito.

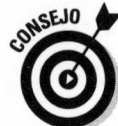

Cómo mejorar su puntuación de FICO:

- **Pague sus cuentas a tiempo.** Pagos morosos y cobranzas de facturas no saldadas pueden tener un mayor impacto negativo en su puntuación.

- **Si usted omite algún pago, actualice su cuenta y manténgala actualizada.** Su puntuación será mejor si siempre hace los pagos de las cuentas a tiempo.

✔ **Saldar una cuenta o cerrarla no la elimina de su historial crediticio.** La puntuación seguirá considerando la información porque refleja su patrón de pagos en el pasado.

✔ **Si tiene problema en cumplir con sus obligaciones financieras, busque ayuda.** Esto no mejora de inmediato su puntuación, pero si puede comenzar a manejar su crédito y a pagar a tiempo, su puntuación mejorará con el paso del tiempo. Por favor, vea en el Capítulo 2 nuestros consejos relacionados con las estrategias para solucionar problemas de crédito.

La cantidad que debe

Alrededor del 30 por ciento de su puntuación está basado en su deuda actual. El tener cuentas de crédito, y con un balance, no significa que usted sea un prestatario de gran riesgo, ni que va a recibir una puntuación baja. Sin embargo, el tener deudas de mucho monto en muchas cuentas puede indicar que la persona ha adquirido obligaciones en exceso a sus ingresos, y es más probable que haga algunos pagos atrasados o los omita por completo. Parte de la ciencia de asignar puntuación es determinar qué monto es demasiado grande para cierto tipo de prestatario.

En cuanto a las deudas, su puntuación toma en cuenta:

✔ **El monto total adeudado de todas las cuentas.** Note que aunque pague mensualmente el balance total de sus tarjetas de crédito, su reporte de crédito puede mostrar un balance en esas tarjetas. Generalmente, ese reporte mostrará el monto total correspondiente al balance de su último estado de cuenta.

✔ **La cantidad adeudada en todas las cuentas y en diferentes tipos de cuentas.** Además del total de su deuda, la puntuación considera el monto que debe en tipos específicos de cuentas, como tarjetas de crédito y préstamos hipotecarios.

✔ **Si muestra balances en cierto tipo de cuentas.** En algunos casos, tener un pequeño balance sin ningún pago atrasado indica que usted maneja responsablemente su crédito. Por otro lado, cerrar cuentas de crédito en desuso que muestran un balance de cero y que tienen buenos antecedentes no aumenta su puntuación.

✔ **Cuántas cuentas tienen balances.** Un gran número de cuentas con balances indica un mayor riesgo de sobre extenderse.

✔ **Cuánto del monto límite del crédito permitido está usado en tarjetas de crédito y en otras cuentas de *crédito rotativo* (que mantienen un balance de mes a mes).** Alguien que está cerca de "llegar a su máximo límite" en muchas tarjetas de crédito puede tener problemas para hacer pagos en el futuro.

✔ **Cuánto es el total que debe todavía en un crédito de reembolso a plazos comparado con el monto total del préstamo original**. Por ejemplo, si usted recibió un préstamo de $10.000 para la compra de un automóvil, y ha pagado $2.000, debe aún (con los intereses) más del 80 por ciento del monto del préstamo original. Disminuir la deuda de los préstamos de reembolso a plazos es una buena señal de que usted es capaz y, además, desea administrar bien su dinero y saldar la deuda.

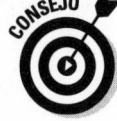

Cómo mejorar su puntuación de FICO:

✔ **Mantenga bajos los balances de las tarjetas de crédito y de otros créditos rotativos.** Una gran deuda pendiente puede influir negativamente en su puntuación.

✔ **Cancele la deuda.** La manera más efectiva de mejorar su puntuación en este renglón es disminuir su deuda de crédito rotativo.

✔ **No cierre cuentas de tarjetas de crédito en desuso como estrategia a corto plazo para aumentar su puntuación.** Generalmente, esto no tiene ese efecto. De hecho, puede bajar su puntuación. Los pagos atrasados asociados con cuentas viejas no desaparecen de su historial crediticio si usted cierra la cuenta. Cuentas establecidas por mucho tiempo muestran que tiene una larga historia de administrar su crédito, y eso es algo positivo. Y tener crédito disponible que usted no usa no disminuye su puntuación. Puede ser que usted tenga otras razones que no tienen nada que ver con la puntuación cuando cierre cuentas de tarjetas de crédito viejas y en desuso, pero no lo haga con la esperanza de lograr una puntuación mejor.

✔ **No abra nuevas tarjetas de crédito que no necesite, solamente para aumentar su disponibilidad de crédito.** Este enfoque puede perjudicarlo y, en realidad, disminuir su puntuación.

El tiempo que cubre su historial crediticio

¿Está bien establecida su historia de crédito? Alrededor del 15 por ciento de su puntuación está basado en esa información. En general, una larga historia crediticia aumentará su puntuación. Sin embargo, aún la gente que no ha usado crédito por mucho tiempo, puede lograr puntuaciones altas, pues depende de lo que muestra el resto de su historial crediticio.

En este aspecto, su puntuación toma en cuenta:

✔ **Cuánto tiempo hace que tiene establecidas sus cuentas de crédito, en general.** La puntuación considera dos: el tiempo de su cuenta más vieja y un promedio del tiempo de todas sus cuentas.

✔ **Por cuánto tiempo han estado establecidas cuentas específicas de crédito.**

✔ **Cuánto tiempo ha pasado desde que usted usó ciertas cuentas.**

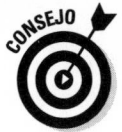

Cómo mejorar su puntuación de FICO:

✔ **Si usted ha administrado su crédito por poco tiempo, no abra nuevas cuentas demasiado rápido.** Las nuevas cuentas bajan el promedio del tiempo de las cuentas, lo cual tiene una gran influencia en su puntuación si no tiene mucha información crediticia de otro tipo. También, la creación rápida de nuevas cuentas puede parecer riesgosa si usted es un usuario nuevo.

Su crédito nuevo

La introducción de nuevas deudas también cambia su puntuación. Aproximadamente el 10 por ciento de su puntuación está basado en créditos nuevos y en las solicitudes de crédito.

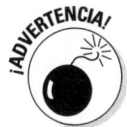

Hoy en día, la gente desea tener más crédito y desea comprar a crédito más que en cualquier otra época —usando la Internet y otros medios—, y las puntuaciones de crédito reflejan esta realidad. Sin embargo, las investigaciones muestran que la apertura de varias cuentas de crédito en un corto período de tiempo, representa más riesgo, especialmente para aquellas personas que no tienen un historial crediticio largo y bien establecido.

El solicitar varias tarjetas de crédito nuevas también representa más riesgo. Pero, las puntuaciones de FICO son tan buenas que distinguen entre las solicitudes de información hechas por *muchas* cuentas de crédito nuevas y la de *una* sola cuenta nueva con una tasa de interés más baja.

En cuanto al crédito nuevo, su puntuación toma en cuenta:

✔ **Cuántas cuentas nuevas tiene usted.** La puntuación considera, por tipo de cuenta, cuántas cuentas nuevas tiene (por ejemplo, cuántas cuentas de tarjetas de crédito abrió recientemente). Asimismo, puede considerar cuántas de sus cuentas son nuevas.

✔ **Cuánto tiempo hace desde que usted abrió una cuenta nueva.** De nuevo, la puntuación considera esto de acuerdo al tipo de cuenta.

✔ **Cuántas solicitudes de crédito ha hecho usted recientemente.** Esto está indicado por el número de solicitudes hechas de su información crediticia, a las agencias de reportes de crédito. La cantidad de solicitudes permanece en su historial de crédito por dos años, aunque la puntuación de FICO considera solamente las solicitudes hechas durante los últimos 12 meses. También, las puntuaciones han sido cuidadosamente diseñadas para contar únicamente las solicitudes que verdaderamente impactan el riesgo del crédito.

✔ **El período de tiempo desde que los prestamistas han indagado sobre el reporte crediticio.** Cuánto más viejas sean estas solicitudes de información, mucho mejor es. No se toman en cuenta las solicitudes hechas hace más de un año. En este caso, es bueno que las ignoren.

✔ **Si usted tiene una buena historia de crédito reciente, después de problemas pasados.** El restablecimiento de su crédito y el hacer los pagos a tiempo, después de un período de pagos atrasados, contribuyen con el paso del tiempo, a subir la puntuación.

Cómo mejorar su puntuación de FICO:

✔ **Busque la mejor tasa de interés para un préstamo determinado dentro de un período de tiempo específico.** Las puntuaciones de FICO distinguen entre una solicitud para un préstamo solamente, y la solicitud para muchas nuevas tarjetas de crédito, en parte, por el período de tiempo en que ocurrieron cada una de esas solicitudes. Para más información sobre este tema, vea la sección "El número de solicitudes en su historial crediticio", más adelante en este capítulo.

✔ **Restablezca su historial crediticio si ha tenido problemas.** El abrir nuevas cuentas conscientemente y pagarlas a tiempo, subirá su puntuación a lo largo del tiempo.

✔ **Está bien que pida y verifique su propia información de crédito y la puntuación de FICO.** Esto no cambia su puntuación, siempre que haga la solicitud de su información crediticia directamente a las agencias nacionales de reportes de crédito, o por medio de una organización autorizada para proveer esta información a los consumidores, por ejemplo, www.myfico.com.

Tipos de crédito que está usando

Una variedad de créditos no es un factor de importancia en la determinación de su puntuación — pero se le da más peso si su historial crediticio no tiene otro tipo de información que se pueda considerar para la puntuación. Alrededor del 10 por ciento de su puntuación está basado en esta categoría.

En este aspecto, su puntuación toma en cuenta:

✔ **Los tipos de cuentas de crédito que usted tiene.** Su puntuación considera la mezcla de cuentas, tales como: sus tarjetas de crédito, cuentas de minoristas, préstamos rotativos, cuentas de compañías de financiamiento y préstamos hipotecarios. No se sienta obligado a tener una de cada clase.

✔ **Cuántas cuentas de crédito de cada tipo tiene.** La puntuación considera el número total de cuentas que usted tiene. Un número considerado demasiado alto varía según el tipo de crédito. No necesita tener una cuenta de cada tipo y, no abra cuentas de crédito que no intenta usar, solamente para subir la puntuación.

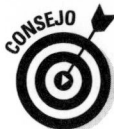

Cómo mejorar su puntuación de FICO:

- ✔ **Solicite y abra nuevas cuentas de crédito solamente cuando sea necesario.** No abra cuentas sólo para tener una mayor variedad —esto probablemente no subirá su puntuación.

- ✔ **Tenga tarjetas de crédito —pero manéjelas responsablemente.** En general, tener tarjetas de crédito y préstamos de reembolsos a plazos (y pagarlos a tiempo) sube su puntuación.

- ✔ **Tome nota: cerrar una cuenta no la elimina de su historial crediticio.** Una cuenta cerrada todavía aparece en su reporte de crédito, y puede incluirse en su puntuación.

El número de solicitudes en su historial crediticio

Una búsqueda de crédito nuevo puede significar un riesgo mayor. Por eso, la puntuación de FICO cuenta el número de indagaciones hechas —esas solicitudes de información que hacen los prestamistas sobre su historial crediticio o de su puntuación cuando usted solicita crédito.

Las puntuaciones de FICO toman seriamente en consideración el número de solicitudes hechas porque no todas están vinculadas al riesgo del crédito. Debe poner atención a tres cosas acerca de las solicitudes de su historial crediticio:

- ✔ **Las solicitudes no influyen mucho en las puntuaciones.** Para la mayoría de la gente, una solicitud más acerca de su crédito le disminuirá la puntuación de FICO en menos de 5 puntos. Sin embargo, las solicitudes pueden causar un impacto mayor si usted tiene pocas cuentas o una historia de crédito corta. Un gran número de solicitudes también significa un mayor riesgo: la gente con seis solicitudes o más en su reporte crediticio sugiere que hay un mayor riesgo de que se declare en bancarrota en comparación con la gente que no tiene solicitudes en su reporte crediticio.

- ✔ **Muchos tipos de solicitudes no se toman en cuenta.** La puntuación no toma en cuenta cuando usted solicita su propio historial crediticio o su puntuación de una agencia de reportes de crédito. Tampoco toma en cuenta las solicitudes que hacen los prestamistas —para enviarle ofertas de crédito aprobadas por adelantado o para examinar su cuenta con ellos—, aun cuando estas solicitudes aparezcan en su historial crediticio. Tampoco toma en cuenta las solicitudes hechas por los empleadores.

- ✔ **La puntuación verifica si buscó una mejor tasa de interés.** La búsqueda de un préstamo, bien sea hipotecario o para la compra de un vehículo, puede originar muchas solicitudes sobre su historial crediticio hechas por diferentes prestamistas, aún cuando usted está buscando solamente *un* préstamo. Para compensar por esas solicitudes, la puntuación considera todas esas solicitudes que se han hecho en un período de 15 días como si fueran una sola. Además, ignora *todas* las solicitudes hechas en los últimos 30 días antes de hacer el cálculo. Entonces, si usted encuentra un préstamo en esos 30 días, las solicitudes hechas no influyen en su puntuación mientras usted está buscando una mejor tasa de interés.

Lo que la puntuación de FICO ignora

Las puntuaciones de FICO consideran una amplia variedad de información en su reporte de crédito. Sin embargo, no consideran:

- ✔ Su raza, color, religión, origen, sexo y estado civil

  Las leyes de los Estados Unidos prohíben que esos factores se incluyan en el cálculo de la puntuación del crédito, así como también recibos de asistencia social y cualquier información que se encuentre protegida por "Ley de Protección al Crédito del Consumidor" *(Consumer Credit Protection Act).*

- ✔ Su edad
- ✔ Sus ingresos, ocupación, título, empleador, fecha de empleo o antecedentes de trabajo

Sin embargo, los prestamistas pueden tener en cuenta la siguiente información:

- ✔ Dónde vive
- ✔ Cualquier tasa de interés en una tarjeta de crédito en particular u otra cuenta
- ✔ Cualquier información relacionada con pensión para el sustento de los hijos o alimenticia, y contratos de alquiler
- ✔ Cierto tipo de solicitud del historial crediticio (solicitud de su información crediticia o de su puntuación)

  La puntuación *no* toma en cuenta ninguna solicitud hecha por usted mismo ni por los empleadores, ni tampoco las hechas por prestamistas sin su previa autorización

- ✔ Cualquier información que no se encuentra en su historial crediticio
- ✔ Cualquier información que no sea útil para predecir el comportamiento futuro del manejo de su crédito

Por qué su puntuación es como es

Cuando un prestamista recibe su puntuación de FICO, también recibe hasta *cuatro razones* que la explican. Ésas son las cuatro razones principales por las que su puntuación no es más alta. Si el prestamista le niega su solicitud de crédito, y su puntuación de FICO fue en parte la razón, estas razones pueden ayudar al prestamista a explicarle a usted el porqué de la negativa.

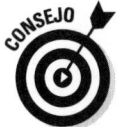

Para usted, estas razones pueden serle más útiles que la misma puntuación. Ellas le ayudan a determinar si hay errores en su historial crediticio, y cómo puede mejorar su puntuación de crédito. Sin embargo, si usted ya tiene una puntuación de FICO alta (por ejemplo, unos setecientos puntos o más) algunas razones pueden no ser útiles porque pueden referirse a factores secundarios relacionados con categorías menos importantes, como su extenso historial crediticio, nuevos créditos o tipos de crédito en uso.

Cómo Obtener Su Reporte Crediticio y Su Puntuación

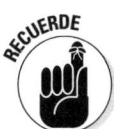

Es una buena idea, obtener y guardar una copia de su reporte de crédito personal. Como su propio reporte crediticio contiene una historia de su uso (¡y abusos!) de crédito, es importante que esté consciente de lo que contiene y de verificar si la información es correcta.

Si usted está solicitando un préstamo hipotecario, puede entonces pedir una copia de su reporte crediticio —después de todo, ¡usted está pagando por él! También es bueno que sepa que los prestamistas deben mandarle a usted una copia de su informe crediticio gratis si le niegan un préstamo.

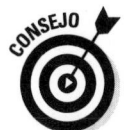

El Congreso de los Estados Unidos nos ha dado el derecho a obtener un reporte de crédito gratis de cada una de las tres mayores agencias nacionales de reportes de crédito —Experian (888-397-3742; www.experian.com), Equifax (800-685-1111; www.equifax.com) y Trans Union (800-888-4213; www.transunion.com)—, una vez al año. Generalmente, otras oficinas de crédito también deben proveerle una copia gratis de su reporte si le han negado un crédito, un empleo, vivienda, o seguro, en los últimos 60 días, a causa de la información en su reporte de crédito. También puede comprar una copia de su reporte crediticio de cualquiera de las tres agencias nacionales (generalmente cuestan menos de $10 cada una). Le recomendamos que por lo menos obtenga anualmente sus copias gratis. Sin embargo, solamente el reporte es gratis. Si desea saber cuál es su puntuación de crédito, tiene que pagar por él.

Es fácil verificar su puntuación de FICO y descubrir qué medidas específicas puede tomar para mejorarla. Hay sitios en la Web de muchos bancos, de instituciones financieras y de agencias de reportes de crédito que ofrecen la puntuación de FICO por un precio, al igual que el enlace Web myFICO, `www.myfico.com`, de Fair Isaac.

La información que usted recibe incluye:

✔ Su puntuación de FICO actual

✔ Su reporte de crédito en el que la puntuación de FICO está basada

✔ Una explicación de su puntuación, los factores positivos y negativos del mismo y cómo los prestamistas ven el riesgo de su crédito

✔ Un simulador de la puntuación de FICO que puede usar para ver los diferentes resultados en que acciones específicas, tales como pagar los balances de sus tarjetas, afectarían su puntuación

✔ Consejos específicos de lo que puede hacer para mejorar su puntuación de FICO con el tiempo

Además, usted puede ver información vigente de las tasas de interés para los préstamos de vivienda que corresponden a los diferentes niveles de la puntuación de FICO.

Capítulo 6

Cómo Seleccionar
un Préstamo Hipotecario

*L*a mayoría de nosotros necesitamos conseguir una hipoteca para comprar una vivienda por la sencilla razón de que es la única forma en que podemos pagar por una propiedad que es apropiada a nuestras necesidades. Este capítulo ayuda a todas aquellas personas, que no tienen suficiente dinero, a entender los tipos de hipotecas y a escoger una apropiada para ellos. (Si usted *es* rico y tiene mucho dinero como para invertirlo en una propiedad, este capítulo también puede ayudarlo a decidir cuánto de su dinero debe invertir o destinar para la compra de su vivienda).

Empecemos por lo más básico. ¿Qué es una hipoteca? Una hipoteca no es nada más que un préstamo que usted obtiene para cubrir la diferencia entre el dinero en efectivo que usted tiene para el pago inicial de la vivienda y el precio de la vivienda que está comprando. Las viviendas en la zona dónde vive pueden costar $70.000, $170.000 ó $770.000. Pero esto carece de importancia —la mayoría de las personas no tienen esa cantidad de dinero disponible en el banco.

Generalmente, las hipotecas requieren que usted haga pagos mensuales para bajar la deuda. Los pagos de la hipoteca están compuestos por el *interés,* que es lo que la entidad crediticia le cobra a usted por el uso del dinero que le ha prestado, y el *capital,* que es el pago o amortización del monto original del préstamo.

El seleccionar una hipoteca que sea apropiada para sus necesidades, le asegura felicidad por muchos años como propietario. Usted también necesita entender cómo hacer un buen negocio cuando esté buscando la hipoteca porque ese es, generalmente, el gasto mensual más alto relacionado con su propiedad (y quizás también, del total de su presupuesto del hogar). Es común que usted pague más por cargos totales de intereses durante el plazo de su hipoteca, que el monto que usted pagó inicialmente por su humilde morada.

Suponga que el palacio de sus sueños cuesta $180.000. Usted contribuye $36.000 de sus ahorros como pago inicial y pide prestada la diferencia, $144.000. Si usted obtiene esos $144.000 con una hipoteca de interés fijo a 30 años al 7 por ciento de interés, usted termina pagando la increíble suma de $200.892, solamente en intereses durante el plazo de su préstamo. Esta última cifra no es sólo un monto muy grande de interés, ¡sino que además es mayor que el precio de compra de la vivienda y del monto que usted originalmente tomó prestado!

De manera que para que no gaste más de lo necesario en su hipoteca y para que consiga la más apropiada para usted, ha llegado el momento de ocuparse de la tarea de entender las opciones o tipos de hipotecas que tiene a su disposición.

¿Interés de Tasa Fija o de Tasa Variable? Ésta Es una Pregunta Interés(ante)

Quizás usted recuerde la escena del programa *Saturday Night Live* en la cual los actores Dan Aykroyd y John Belushi trabajaban en un restaurante que sólo servía hamburguesas con queso, papitas y Pepsi. Los clientes que trataban de ordenar una hamburguesa, papas fritas y Coca Cola, no corrían con la suerte de ser atendidos. No hay hamburguesa, solo hamburguesa con queso; no hay papitas, sólo papas fritas; y no hay Coca Cola, sólo Pepsi. En ese restaurante, sus alternativas ya estaban definidas. ¡Si tan sólo corriéramos con la misma suerte con las hipotecas!

Como en el caso de otros productos financieros y de inversión, existen diferentes opciones de hipotecas entre las cuales usted puede escoger. Las variaciones entre ellas pueden ser importantes o triviales, costosas o menos costosas.

Usted se dará cuenta a través de este capítulo que existen fundamentalmente dos tipos de hipotecas. Ellas se diferencian en la forma en que la tasa de interés se calcula. Estos dos tipos de hipotecas son la hipoteca con tasa de interés fija y la hipoteca con tasa de interés variable o ajustable.

Cómo distinguir las hipotecas de tasas fijas de las de tasas ajustables

Antes que existieran las hipotecas con tasa de interés variable, solo había disponible las hipotecas con tasa de interés fija. Generalmente otorgadas por plazos de 15 o de 30 años, las *hipotecas con tasa de interés fija* (como su nombre lo indica) tienen tasas de interés que son *fijas* (invariables) durante el plazo del préstamo.

Con una hipoteca de este tipo, la tasa de interés se mantiene fija y su pago mensual del préstamo es siempre el mismo. No hay sorpresas, no hay incertidumbre y no hay ansiedad acerca de cambios en la tasa de interés ni cómo eso afectaría su pago mensual. Si a usted le gusta poder predecir que su programa favorito de televisión lo presentan a la misma hora todos los días, a usted probablemente le gustarán las hipotecas con tasas de interés fijas.

Por el contrario, las *hipotecas con tasas de interés ajustables o variables* (*ARM,* por sus siglas en inglés), tienen una tasa de interés que cambia (o se *ajusta*). La tasa de interés de una hipoteca *ARM* generalmente se ajusta cada 6 a 12 meses, pero puede llegar a cambiar hasta una vez por mes.

Como presentamos más adelante en este capítulo, la tasa de interés de una hipoteca ajustable está determinada principalmente por lo que esté pasando con las tasas de interés en el mercado. Generalmente, cuando las tasas de interés aumentan, entonces la tasa de su hipoteca *ARM* también aumenta y, por lo tanto, incrementa el monto mensual del pago de su hipoteca. Lo opuesto también ocurre, cuando las tasas de interés bajan, también disminuyen las tasas de la hipoteca ajustable y los pagos.

Si a usted le gusta el cambio, usted puede pensar que las hipotecas de tasa ajustable son apropiadas y quizás opine que el cambio es lo que hace la vida más interesante. Por favor, siga leyendo, porque aún si usted piensa que en la variedad está el gusto, ¡a usted podría no gustarle la variedad y el gusto de las tasas ajustables!

Los préstamos híbridos

Si tan solo el mundo fuera más simple, y sólo existieran los préstamos puros de tasa de interés fija y los de tasa de interés variable. Pero una de las ventajas de vivir en una sociedad capitalista es que, a menudo, un individuo tiene una amplia gama de opciones para todo. Un ejemplo son los *préstamos híbridos,* o los que las entidades hipotecarias llaman a veces, préstamos ajustables intermedios (*intermediate ARM*). Estos préstamos comienzan como préstamos con tasas de interés fija —la tasa inicial puede ser constante por tres, cinco, siete y hasta diez años— y luego se convierte en una hipoteca ajustable, generalmente ajustando la tasa cada 6 a 12 meses a partir de ese momento (aunque algunas hipotecas tienen solamente un ajuste en la tasa).

Un comienzo riesgoso: Hipotecas de sólo interés

Como los precios de las viviendas, ya bastantes altos, aumentaban rápidamente en zonas urbanas y en las ciudades circunvecinas, las entidades crediticias respondieron con aún otra opción, y comenzaron a promocionar préstamos de *sólo interés*. A diferencia de las hipotecas tradicionales, las *hipotecas de sólo interés* atraen a los prestatarios ofreciéndoles pagos artificialmente bajos en los primeros años del préstamo. Esto es posible porque los primeros pagos sólo incluyen los intereses (sin que se amortice el capital), y de allí el nombre del préstamo.

Posteriormente, en un tiempo predeterminado del plazo (tres, cinco, siete o diez años), comienza la amortización del capital, y el monto mensual del préstamo da un salto notable de un 20, 30 ó 40 por ciento o más. Y allí es donde radica el problema principal con estos préstamos, ya que algunos prestatarios pueden no estar financieramente preparados para estos pagos mucho más altos. En el peor de los casos, estos préstamos son generalmente préstamos disfrazados porque son préstamos con un pago final global, o sea, reembolsables al vencimiento y tienen todas las desventajas de préstamos reembolsables (vea las notas identificadas por la barra vertical gris más adelante en este capítulo).

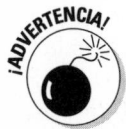

Como ya puede haberse dado cuenta, no somos grandes aficionados de las hipotecas de *sólo interés*. Lo instamos a que examine completamente todos los términos y condiciones que rigen el préstamo, antes que decida aceptar un préstamo de este tipo.

La decisión de tasas fijas o tasas ajustables

Entonces, ¿cómo escoge usted entre un préstamo de tasa fija y uno de tasa ajustable? ¿Es esta decisión tan sencilla como una prueba de personalidad?

En esta sección, le vamos a presentar las ventajas y desventajas de las diferentes alternativas en hipotecas, pero le pedimos por favor que tenga en mente un factor muy importante: al final del análisis, la hipoteca que es mejor para usted es aquélla que encaja perfectamente en su situación personal y financiera. *Usted* es quién está en la mejor posición para decidir si un préstamo de tasa fija o uno de tasa variable es el que se ajusta mejor a su situación y sus deseos.

Hipotecas con tasa de interés fija

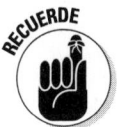

Es lógico pensar que dado que la tasa de interés no cambia en una hipoteca de tasa fija, la ventaja de este tipo de hipoteca es que usted sabe con seguridad cuál va a ser el pago mensual de la misma y, de esta manera, el presupuestar y planificar es más fácil.

Para que la entidad crediticia se comprometa a prestarle dinero durante todos esos años a una tasa fija, usted tendrá que pagar algo por ese beneficio y, generalmente, es en forma de una tasa de interés más alta. Cuanto más largo sea el tiempo del préstamo que la entidad financiera le da con una tasa de interés fija, más riesgo está asumiendo la misma. Una entidad hipotecaria que acuerda prestarle el dinero, por ejemplo, durante 30 años a un 8 por ciento, se lamentará si las tasas de interés suben a un nivel del 15 por ciento o más (como ocurrió al principio de los años ochenta). (Con el aumento de las tasas de interés e inflación en aquel entonces, las entidades hipotecarias estaban pagando tasas de interés sobre depósitos que eran casi el doble del nivel de las tasas que estaban cargando por hipotecas que habían comenzado hacía una década antes. ¡Ésta, obviamente, no es la manera más rentable de administrar un banco!)

Otra desventaja potencial de los préstamos a tasa fija, además de pagar una tasa de interés más alta cuando usted saca el préstamo, es que si las tasas de interés bajan significativamente después que usted saca la hipoteca, usted tiene el riesgo de quedarse varado con su costosa hipoteca. Esto podría pasar si usted no reúne los requisitos (debido a un deterioro en su situación financiera o a una disminución del valor de su propiedad) para *refinanciar* (sacar un préstamo nuevo que reemplace el viejo). Aún si usted reúne las condiciones para obtener un refinanciamiento, hacerlo toma tiempo, y además hay que gastar dinero en la nueva evaluación crediticia, en los gastos de tramitación del préstamo y en el seguro de título.

Otras dos posibles desventajas, de menor importancia, que tienen las hipotecas de tasa de interés fija, son las siguientes:

✔ Si usted vende su casa antes de pagar totalmente la hipoteca, probablemente los compradores de su propiedad no podrán adquirir ese mismo préstamo. La posibilidad de traspasar el préstamo al próximo comprador (dicho en el lenguaje de bienes raíces: el nuevo comprador compra su préstamo) puede ser útil si usted se ve forzado a vender durante un período poco común de tasas de interés ultra altas, tal como ocurrió a principios de la década de los ochenta.

✔ Algunas veces, las hipotecas con tasa de interés fija tienen penalizaciones si usted paga el préstamo antes del plazo programado (éstas se explican en la sección "Evite los préstamos con penalizaciones por pago adelantado").

Préstamos reembolsables al vencimiento o balón

Un tipo de hipoteca conocido como *préstamo reembolsable al vencimiento* (también llamado *préstamo con cuota balón* [*balloon loan*]), parece ser, a primera vista, un préstamo híbrido. La tasa de interés es fija, por ejemplo, por cinco, siete, o diez años. Sin embargo, y éste es un *sin embargo* muy grande, al final del plazo del préstamo, el balance o saldo total del mismo vence. En otras palabras, usted tiene que pagar el total de la cantidad o deuda pendiente.

Los prestatarios se sienten atraídos a estos tipos de préstamos por la misma razón que se sienten atraídos por los préstamos híbridos o por los préstamos de tasa ajustable: porque comienzan con una tasa de interés más baja que las hipotecas con tasas de interés fija. Se sienten inclinados a tomar este tipo de préstamo durante períodos de tasas de interés altas o cuando no reúnen los requisitos necesarios, o no pueden pagar las mensualidades de una hipoteca tradicional.

Nosotros no le recomendamos los préstamos reembolsables al vencimiento porque pueden ser bastante riesgosos. Por ejemplo, usted puede quedarse sin una hipoteca si no tiene la opción de *refinanciar* (o sea, de obtener un nuevo préstamo para reemplazar el viejo) cuando se venza el plazo del préstamo. Puede tener dificultades para refinanciar si, por ejemplo, usted pierde su trabajo o sus ingresos bajan, el valor de la propiedad declina o su evaluación crediticia resulta muy baja como para optar a un nuevo préstamo, o si las tasas de interés aumentan y usted no reúne las condiciones para un préstamo a esas tasas más altas.

En el negocio de bienes raíces, los préstamos reembolsables al vencimiento también son llamados "préstamos metralla" (*bullet loans*). ¿Y porqué los llaman así? Porque las personas en la industria opinan que si el préstamo se vence durante un período de tasas altas, ese momento es como ser alcanzado por una metralla.

Recuerde que refinanciar una hipoteca *no es* una cosa segura. Tomar un préstamo reembolsable al vencimiento, puede ser una solución financieramente muy riesgosa. Más aún, es una solución de corto plazo para sus necesidades financieras de largo plazo.

La única circunstancia bajo la cual nosotros pensamos que está bien *considerar* tener un préstamo de este tipo es, si absolutamente, usted tiene que tener esa propiedad en particular, y el préstamo amortizable al vencimiento es su única alternativa de hipoteca. Si éste es su caso, usted debería asegurarse tanto como pueda, de que podrá refinanciar cuando el préstamo se venza. Si usted tiene familiares que puedan ayudarlo con el refinanciamiento, ya sea sirviendo de aval o prestándole directamente el dinero, ése es un buen respaldo. Ah, y si usted *tiene* que tomar uno de estos préstamos, consiga el plazo más largo que le sea posible, idealmente, no menos de siete años y, preferiblemente, por diez años.

Hipotecas de tasa de interés ajustable o variable

Las hipotecas de tasas de interés fijas no son su única opción. Las entidades hipotecarias fueron lo suficientemente inteligentes como para darse cuenta que ellos no podían prever si las tasas de interés aumentarían o disminuirían en el futuro; por esta razón, surgieron las hipotecas con tasas de interés ajustables (o simplemente, préstamos *ajustables*).

Aunque algunos préstamos ajustables son más volátiles que otros, todos son similares en el hecho de que *fluctúan* (o varían) de acuerdo al nivel de las tasas de interés en el mercado. Si la tasa de interés varía, también varía el pago mensual. Y en esto radica el riesgo: como el pago de la hipoteca es posiblemente el gasto mensual más grande para usted, una hipoteca de tasa de interés ajustable que aumente, puede ocasionar un desastre en su presupuesto.

Dados todos los problemas, reveses y retos de la vida, como lo sabemos, usted podría preguntarse —y con toda razón—, ¿por qué entonces alguien aceptaría una hipoteca con tasa de interés variable? Pues bien, personas que están tratando de comprar más allá de sus posibilidades —tales como quienes compran por primera vez o aquéllos que están tratando de *mudarse a una propiedad más costosa*— pueden verse forzados financieramente a aceptar una hipoteca con tasa variable. Como esta hipoteca ajustable empieza con una tasa de interés más baja, la misma le permite al prestatario, *reunir los requisitos* para prestar más. Y como lo dijimos en el Capítulo 2, sólo porque usted reúne tales requisitos para prestar, no significa que usted *puede pagar* toda esa cantidad de dinero, dadas sus otras metas y necesidades financieras.

Evite los préstamos con penalizaciones por pago adelantado

Algunas hipotecas vienen con una condición que penaliza al prestatario por pagar el balance del préstamo antes del plazo de su vencimiento. Estas penalizaciones pueden llegar a representar varios puntos porcentuales del saldo del préstamo que se va a pagar anticipadamente.

Cuando usted paga una hipoteca antes del plazo establecido, ya sea porque usted vendió la propiedad o porque quiere refinanciar el préstamo para aprovechar tasas de interés más bajas, algunas entidades hipotecarias no imponen penalizaciones mientras usted haga la nueva hipoteca con ellos. Aún así, financieramente usted está atado de manos, a menos que solicite refinanciar con la misma entidad acreedora.

Muchos estados establecen límites en el monto y la duración de la penalización que los prestamistas pueden cobrar por hipotecas sobre propiedades residenciales habitadas por el propietario. La única manera de saber si un préstamo tiene penalización es preguntar y revisar cuidadosamente la declaración de veracidad y el pagaré que el prestamista hipotecario le provee. Nosotros pensamos que debe evitar este tipo de préstamos. (Muchos de los llamados préstamos *sin puntos* tienen este tipo de penalización).

Algunos compradores que reúnen los requisitos ya sea para una hipoteca de interés ajustable o una de interés fijo, por el mismo monto, escogen la hipoteca con tasa de interés ajustable. ¿Por qué hacen esto? Probablemente porque pueden ahorrarse dinero, en forma de cargos de intereses totales más bajos, que con un préstamo de tasa fija.

Puesto que usted acepta el riesgo de un posible aumento de la tasa de interés, las entidades crediticias le hacen ciertas concesiones. La *tasa de interés inicial* en una hipoteca ajustable (llamada algunas veces "tasa tentadora" [*teaser rate*]), debería ser menor que la tasa de interés inicial de un préstamo a tasa fija por el mismo monto. De hecho, la tasa de interés de una hipoteca ajustable para el primer o segundo año del préstamo es generalmente más baja que la tasa de una hipoteca fija.

Otra ventaja de una hipoteca ajustable es que si usted compra su vivienda durante un período de altas tasas de interés, usted puede empezar a pagar su hipoteca con una tasa inicial artificialmente baja. Si las tasas disminuyen más adelante, usted puede disfrutar los beneficios de tasas más bajas sin necesidad de refinanciar.

Cuándo considerar un préstamo híbrido

Si desea tener una mayor estabilidad en sus pagos mensuales que la que puede lograr con una hipoteca ajustable y, además, anticipa tener su préstamo por un período entre 5 a 10 años, un préstamo *híbrido*, el cual explicamos anteriormente en este capítulo, puede ser el mejor préstamo para usted.

Sabemos que mientras más largo sea el tiempo que esté asegurada o fija la tasa de interés inicial, más alta ésta será. La tasa inicial de un préstamo híbrido es casi siempre más baja que la tasa de una hipoteca fija a 30 años. Comparadas con una hipoteca ajustable, las hipotecas híbridas tienen una tasa de interés más alta; esto se debe a que la tasa de interés inicial de una hipoteca híbrida está asegurada por un período de tiempo más largo que el período típico de seis meses o un año de las hipotecas ajustables regulares.

En épocas cuando existía poca diferencia entre las tasas de interés de corto plazo y las de largo plazo, los ahorros por tasa de interés con un préstamo híbrido o uno regular ajustable (comparados con un préstamo de tasa fija) eran mínimos (menos del 1 por ciento). De hecho, por cierto tiempo, la tasa de interés inicial en un híbrido de 7 a 10 años de plazo, era exactamente igual que la de un préstamo con tasa fija a 30 años. En circunstancias como ésas, los préstamos de tasa fija son en general la mejor alternativa.

Para evaluar los préstamos híbridos, usted debe sopesar la probabilidad de que usted venda la propiedad antes que la tasa de interés inicial del préstamo venza. Tomemos como ejemplo, un préstamo híbrido a 7 años en el que usted está ahorrando, digamos, un 0,5 por ciento por año comparado con una hipoteca de tasa fija a 30 años. Si usted está bastante seguro que se va a mudar antes de los siete años, el híbrido probablemente le ahorre dinero. Por el contrario, si usted piensa que existe una probabilidad moderada de quedarse en la misma propiedad por más de ese tiempo, entonces usted debería optar por la hipoteca de tasa fija a 30 años.

Una situación en la cuál los préstamos con tasa variable tienen otra ventaja sobre sus hermanos de tasa fija es cuando las tasas de interés declinan, y usted no reúne los requisitos para refinanciar su hipoteca y aprovechar esta ventaja del mercado. La buena nueva para los propietarios que no pueden refinanciar y tienen una hipoteca ajustable es que usualmente reciben los beneficios de tasas más bajas. Con un préstamo de tasa fija, usted tendría que refinanciar para beneficiarse de la baja de las tasas.

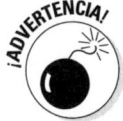

La desventaja de un préstamo con tasa ajustable es que, si en general las tasas de interés aumentan, los intereses de su préstamo y los pagos mensuales posiblemente aumenten también. Generalmente, si las tasas aumentan más del 1 ó 2 por ciento y se mantienen altas, el préstamo de tasa ajustable es probable que le cueste más que un préstamo de tasa fija.

Antes que usted haga la elección final entre una hipoteca de tasa fija y una de tasa ajustable, lea las siguientes dos secciones.

¿Qué efecto tiene el aumento de las tasas de interés en sus finanzas?

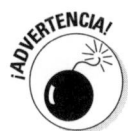

Muchísimos compradores de vivienda, especialmente los que compran por primera vez, toman una hipoteca de tasa ajustable porque les permite prestar más y comprar una casa más cara. Aunque esta decisión de prestar demás, es causada por esta moderna actitud norteamericana de despilfarro: ¡Me muero si no lo tengo ahora!, excederse en el monto a prestar, es también propiciado por algunos vendedores de bienes raíces e hipotecas. Después de todo, los ingresos de estos vendedores, en forma de comisión, dependen del costo de la casa que usted compre y del monto de la hipoteca que acepte.

Si no los ha leído aún, regrésese a los Capítulos 2 y 3. Léalos con detenimiento y estúdielos cabalmente para que pueda entender mucho mejor cuánto realmente puede usted pagar por una casa, dadas sus otras necesidades, compromisos y metas.

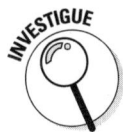

Si está considerando una hipoteca ajustable, usted debe entender absolutamente y sin ninguna duda, el efecto que el aumento de las tasas de interés (y, por consiguiente, un pago mensual de hipoteca mayor) tendría sobre sus finanzas personales. Examine la posibilidad de tomar una hipoteca de este tipo, sólo si puede responder afirmativamente a las siguientes preguntas:

✔ ¿Su presupuesto mensual es tal que le permitirá hacer pagos más altos de la hipoteca y todavía lograr otras metas financieras importantes, tales como ahorrar para la jubilación?

✔ ¿Tiene usted una reserva de dinero para emergencias (equivalente a seis meses mínimos de gastos mensuales) a la cuál usted puede recurrir para hacer unos pagos de hipoteca mensuales potencialmente más altos?

✔ ¿Puede usted pagar el pago más alto previsto en la hipoteca de tasa ajustable?

La entidad hipotecaria puede decirle el máximo pago mensual posible, el cual usted tendría que pagar si la tasa de interés de su hipoteca ajustable llegara al límite máximo permitido en el plazo del préstamo.

✔ Si se está extendiendo financieramente más allá de sus límites, prestando cerca de la cantidad máxima que la entidad crediticia está dispuesta a otorgarle, o un monto que llevaría su presupuesto al límite, ¿son su trabajo y sus ingresos estables?

✔ Si usted anticipa que va a tener niños en el futuro, ¿ha usted considerado que los gastos de su hogar aumentarán y su ingreso disminuirá con la llegada de sus pequeños polluelos?

✔ ¿Puede usted manejar el estrés psicológico de tasas de interés y pagos de hipoteca variables?

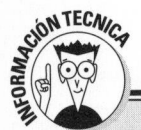

Tasas de interés a corto plazo y tasas a largo plazo

Cuando están decidiendo entre una hipoteca de tasa ajustable y una de tasa fija, muchas personas no se dan cuenta que están haciendo una elección entre hipotecas, en las cuales la tasa de interés está determinada ya sea por las tasas de interés de largo plazo o por las de corto plazo.

Usted se preguntará: ¿Qué es una tasa de interés a corto plazo y en qué se diferencia de una a largo plazo?" Cuando una entidad crediticia le cotiza una tasa de interés para un tipo de préstamo en particular, ellos deberían especificarle el plazo del préstamo en términos de cuántos años van a pasar hasta que el préstamo se pague completamente.

La mayoría de las veces, los prestatarios tienen que pagar una tasa de interés más alta para prestar dinero por un período de tiempo más largo. Y a la inversa, los prestatarios generalmente pagan una tasa de interés más baja por préstamos de plazos más cortos. ¿Y?

Bueno, las tasas que se usan para determinar la mayoría de las hipotecas ajustables son *tasas de interés a corto plazo*, mientras que las tasas de interés de hipotecas de tasa fija están determinadas por las *tasas de interés a largo plazo*. Durante la mayoría del tiempo, las tasas de interés a largo plazo son más altas que las de corto plazo, debido al mayor riesgo que la entidad acreedora acepta al comprometerse con una tasa a largo plazo.

Por consiguiente, parece razonable, que cuando existen diferencias pequeñas en el nivel de mercado de las tasas de interés de corto plazo y las de largo plazo, las tasas de las hipotecas fijas no deberían ser tan diferentes de las tasas de hipotecas ajustables. Por este motivo, las hipotecas ajustables parecen menos atrayentes mientras que las fijas sí lo son.

Por otra parte, cuando las tasas de interés a corto plazo, son significativamente más bajas que las de largo plazo, las hipotecas de tasa ajustable deberían estar disponibles a unas tasas mucho más bajas que las tasas para préstamos con tasa fija. Si las demás condiciones son las mismas, entonces, las hipotecas ajustables se ven más atractivas durante estos períodos, y le ahorrarán más dinero durante los primeros años de su préstamo.

Si usted tiene una situación económica que le permite tomar el riesgo financiero de una hipoteca de tasa ajustable, entonces considere tomarla —nosotros no estamos tratando de convencerlo de que se decida por un préstamo de tasa fija. Usted tiene todas las posibilidades de ahorrar dinero, en la forma de intereses y pagos más bajos, con una hipoteca ajustable. Su tasa de interés al comienzo es baja y generalmente se mantiene baja, si el nivel gene-ral de las tasas de interés no cambia. Y aún si las tasas aumentaran, como a veces tienden a hacerlo, seguramente bajarán de nuevo. Así que, si puede tener la hipoteca ajustable en tiempos de tasas de interés altas y bajas, usted todavía puede salir ganando.

También tiene que saber que aunque las hipotecas ajustables llevan consigo el riesgo de una tasa de interés fluctuante, casi todos esos préstamos limitan, o ponen un *tope,* al aumento permitido en la tasa de interés. Ciertamente, nosotros no recomendaríamos que usted tome una hipoteca de tasa ajustable sin topes. Comúnmente, los topes son del 2 por ciento por año y del 6 por ciento durante el plazo total del préstamo. (Más adelante en este capítulo, explicamos los topes de las tasas de interés de una hipoteca ajustable.)

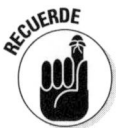

Piense en una hipoteca con tasa ajustable sólo si usted está financiera y emo-cionalmente seguro de poder hacerle frente a los máximos pagos posibles durante un período largo de tiempo. Las hipotecas ajustables son más apro-piadas para prestatarios que toman préstamos más bajos que la cantidad para la cual reúnen los requisitos, o para quiénes sistemáticamente ahorran más del 10 por ciento de sus ingresos mensuales. Si usted se decide por una hipoteca ajustable, asegúrese de que tiene suficiente dinero en reserva y a la que tiene acceso fácilmente en caso de que las tasas aumenten. No se decida por una ajustable sólo porque las tasas de interés más bajas al principio del período le permiten comprar inicialmente una vivienda más costosa. Es mejor comprar una casa que usted pueda pagar con una hipoteca a tasa fija. (Y no se olvide de los préstamos híbridos si usted quiere un préstamo con más estabilidad en los pagos, pero no está dispuesto a pagar extra por el interés fijo de una hipoteca a largo plazo).

¿Por cuánto tiempo piensa usted permanecer en su vivienda y tener su hipoteca?

Como explicamos anteriormente en este capítulo, una entidad hipotecaria toma más riesgo cuando presta dinero a una tasa de interés fija por muchos años (15 o 30). Por ese riesgo extra, las entidades le cobran algo, general-mente, en forma de una tasa de interés más alta que la tasa inicial de una hipoteca ajustable.

Si no planifica permanecer en la casa por un tiempo largo, debería considerar la hipoteca con tasa ajustable. En la mayoría de estos préstamos, el ahorro por cargos de interés está generalmente garantizado en los primeros dos a tres años. Esto es posible porque una hipoteca ajustable comienza con una tasa de interés más baja que una hipoteca fija. Si usted está bastante seguro de que va a vivir en esta vivienda por menos de cinco años, debería entonces escoger una hipoteca ajustable. Sin embargo, también debería preguntarse por qué está pasando por toda esta molestia, e incurriendo en más gastos, si piensa vender tan pronto.

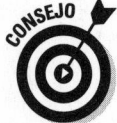

Si usted anticipa que va a tener la vivienda por un tiempo largo —de cinco a siete años— un préstamo de tasa fija puede tener más sentido, especialmente cuando no está en posición de afrontar los cambios de los pagos mensuales que una hipoteca de tasa ajustable tiene.

Cuando usted está considerando un período intermedio (es decir, anticipando que va a quedarse en la vivienda entre siete a diez años, por ejemplo), considere los préstamos híbridos que explicamos anteriormente en este capítulo.

Si está todavía indeciso, tome un préstamo de tasa fija. Una hipoteca fija es financieramente más segura que una hipoteca de tasa variable —y es más fácil de obtener.

Cómo decidir el plazo del préstamo: ¿A 15 ó a 30 años?

Usted podría pensar que después que ha decidido qué tipo de hipoteca va a obtener —fija o ajustable— ya dejó atrás sus dilemas hipotecarios. Desafortunadamente no es así. Usted todavía tiene que tomar otra decisión importante —escoger entre una hipoteca a 15 años o una a 30 años. (No todas las hipotecas vienen solamente para 15 o 30 años. Usted puede encontrar algunas versiones de 20 y 40 años, pero eso no va a cambiar los temas que vamos a abordar a continuación).

Cuando usted se está extendiendo financieramente más allá de lo que puede para comprar la casa que quiere, usted quizás está obligándose, a sí mismo, a tomar la hipoteca de 30 años. Hacer esto no es necesariamente malo y, de hecho, tiene sus ventajas.

La principal ventaja que tiene una hipoteca de 30 años sobre una de 15 años, es que la primera tiene pagos mensuales más bajos, dejando así libre más de su ingreso mensual para otros propósitos como ahorrar para objetivos importantes, tales como la jubilación. También, quizás usted quiera tener más dinero disponible de modo de no ser un prisionero financiero de su casa y ¡poder vivir su vida! Una hipoteca de 30 años tiene pagos mensuales más bajos porque tiene un período más largo para pagarla (lo que se transfiere a más pagos). Por ejemplo, una hipoteca con tasa fija a 30 años y a una tasa de interés del 7 por ciento, tiene pagos que son aproximadamente un 25 por ciento más bajos que aquéllos de una hipoteca a 15 años.

Nadie puede predecir el futuro de las tasas de interés

Probablemente todos los expertos en lógica están comentando que la elección entre una hipoteca de tasa ajustable y una de tasa fija es muy simple de hacer. Todo lo que usted necesita saber para tomar una buena decisión es qué va a pasar con las tasas de interés. Es lo más lógico. Si las tasas de interés están a punto de aumentar, una hipoteca con tasa fija sería favorable. Asegure una tasa baja y sonría satisfecho cuando las tasas de interés aumenten vertiginosamente.

Ahora, si pensó que las tasas de interés se iban a mantener igual o a bajar, usted querría una hipoteca con tasa ajustable. Algunos libros de bienes raíces que hemos leído, llegan a atreverse a decir que su ¡pronóstico personal de las tasas de interés debería determinar si optar por una hipoteca con tasa variable o una hipoteca con tasa fija! "Los pronósticos de las tasas de interés deberían ser el factor más importante en la decisión de tomar o no una hipoteca con tasa ajustable", señala uno de esos libros.

Ahora bien, nosotros no creemos que usted sea tonto, pero usted *no* va a poder determinar qué va a pasar con las tasas de interés. El movimiento de las tasas de interés no obedece a la lógica y, ciertamente, usted no puede predecirlo. Si pudiera hacerlo, haría una fortuna invirtiendo en bonos, en futuras tasas de interés y sus opciones.

Aún los profesionales que trabajan todo el tiempo con tasas de interés y bonos, no pueden predecir con regularidad las tasas de interés. Fíjese en el hecho de que los gerentes de fondos de bonos en las compañías de fondos mutuales tienen dificultad para adelantarse a los índices de acumulación del mercado de bonos. Si estos gerentes de fondos pudieran predecir el comportamiento de las tasas de interés, fácilmente podrían superar los promedios al vender y comprar bonos en el momento que anticiparan cambios en las mismas.

¿Qué pasaría si usted pudiera hacer pagos más altos que los que requiere una hipoteca de 15 años? Bueno, esto no significa necesariamente que usted debe tomarla. ¿Qué pasaría si en lugar de hacer pagos altos en la hipoteca a 15 años, usted hace pagos más bajos en la hipoteca a 30 años y pone ese dinero a producir más dinero para usted?

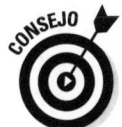

Si usted, realmente, hace algo productivo con ese dinero extra, la hipoteca de 30 años es para usted. Un excelente uso para esa plata extra, es contribuir en una cuenta de jubilación, deducible del impuesto, y a la que usted tenga acceso con facilidad. Las contribuciones que usted hace a su plan de jubilación 401(k) y 403(b) con un empleador (y las cuentas SEP-IRA o Keoghs para quienes trabajan por cuenta propia), no sólo le dan a usted una reducción inmediata de sus impuestos, sino que permiten que su inversión se capitalice, con impuestos diferidos, a los años futuros. Todas las personas con ingresos provenientes de un empleo pueden también contribuir a una cuenta de jubilación individual (*IRA*). Sin embargo, las contribuciones a esta cuenta pueden no ser deducibles del impuesto inmediatamente, si su empleador (o el de su cónyuge) ofrece una cuenta de jubilación o un plan de pensión.

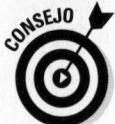

Si usted ha agotado todas sus opciones para contribuir a todas las cuentas de jubilación lo más que pueda, pero aún le es difícil tener su propio plan de ahorros, la hipoteca de 15 años le ofrece entonces un buen programa de ahorros forzados.

Cuando usted elige una hipoteca a 30 años, usted tiene la flexibilidad de pagarla más rápido si usted quiere. (Sólo esté seguro de evitar esas hipotecas que penalizan por pagar antes del plazo.) Pero obligarse a sí mismo a hacer unos pagos mensuales más altos con la hipoteca de 15 años tiene un riesgo. Si usted llega a enfrentar tiempos difíciles financieramente hablando, quizás no pueda realizar los pagos de la hipoteca que se requieren.

Cómo Encontrar una Hipoteca de Tasa Fija

Si usted decide, basado en nuestros consejos y criterios de selección, optar por un préstamo de tasa fija, pues ¡excelente! Usted no va a decepcionarse. En lugar de eso, tendrá la tranquilidad que proveen hipotecas con pagos estables. Y como los préstamos de tasa fija tienen menos opciones, son mucho más fáciles de comparar que los préstamos de tasa ajustable.

Sin embargo, no queremos darle la falsa impresión de que los préstamos de tasa fija son tan fáciles de encontrar como las gaseosas. Desafortunadamente, debido a las numerosas entidades crediticias que ofrecen tales préstamos, y al número aparentemente interminable de pagos extras y gastos que las entidades le añaden a los préstamos, usted necesita ponerse su saco y pantalones de consumidor inteligente y prepararse con su lapicero número 2.

Asegúrese de entender las siguientes secciones antes de intentar escoger el mejor préstamo con tasa fija que se ajuste a sus necesidades.

La importancia de la tasa de interés

Si usted alguna vez ha prestado dinero, sabe que las entidades crediticias no son organizaciones de beneficencia. Las entidades hipotecarias ganan dinero al cobrarle a usted, en forma de interés, por el uso de su dinero. Por lo general, las entidades le cotizan la *tasa de interés* como un porcentaje por año del monto prestado. Usted quizás esté familiarizado con las tasas de interés si alguna vez ha tomado prestado dinero para préstamos educativos, préstamos para automóviles o las tarjetas de crédito. En estos casos, las entidades crediticias pueden haberle cobrado un 8, 10, 12 o, quizás, hasta un 18 por ciento o más por el privilegio de usar esos recursos monetarios. Igualmente, las entidades hipotecarias también le cotizan una tasa de interés anual.

Usted ha comprado otros productos y servicios por vía telefónica, así que puede hacer lo mismo con los préstamos y llamar a diferentes entidades hipotecarias. Quizás la primera que usted llame le cotice un préstamo de tasa fija al 7,5 por ciento, pero luego llama a una segunda entidad financiera para tratar de mejorar esa tasa, y la entidad le dice, "Claro que sí, nosotros podemos ofrecerle un préstamo a tasa fija al 7,25 por ciento".

Los puntos más importantes de los puntos

Si usted escoge ciegamente el préstamo al 7,25 por ciento, usted puede estar cometiendo un error muy caro. Puede tener una idea de lo que queremos decir si ha escuchado la frase "No juzgue al pasajero sólo por la maleta". Bien, usted tampoco debería juzgar una hipoteca únicamente por su tasa de interés, sino que también debe entender los puntos y otros gastos de tramitación del préstamo que la entidad hipotecaria carga.

Así como Abbott y Costello, Laurel y Hardy, y Calvin y Hobbes, no pueden separarse en su mente, asimismo la tasa de interés va unida a los puntos del préstamo. No estamos hablando de los puntos que un jugador de básquetbol acumula durante un juego por cada canasta que logra. Los puntos en una hipoteca le cuestan a usted dinero.

Los *puntos* son intereses anticipados. Las entidades crediticias los cobran para compensar el trabajo y los gastos de procesar su préstamo. Cuando usted compra una casa, los puntos son deducibles del impuesto —usted puede declararlos como un gasto deducible en el Anexo A (*Schedule A*) de su formulario 1040 (vea el Capítulo 3). Pero, cuando usted refinancia, para efectos del impuesto sobre la renta, los puntos deben ser repartidos y deducidos sobre el plazo del nuevo préstamo.

Las entidades hipotecarias cotizan los puntos como un porcentaje del monto de la hipoteca y requieren que usted los pague al momento del cierre de la compra de la vivienda y al comienzo del largo curso de pagar su préstamo. Un *punto* es igual al 1 por ciento del monto que usted está pidiendo prestado. Por ejemplo, si una entidad dice que el préstamo que le están proponiendo tiene dos puntos, eso simplemente significa que usted debe pagar el 2 por ciento del monto del préstamo por ese concepto. En un préstamo de $120.000, por ejemplo, dos puntos le cuestan $2.400. ¡Ésos no son centavitos de cambio!

La tasa de interés en un préstamo de tasa fija tiene una relación inversa con los puntos de ese préstamo. Cuando usted puede (o desea) pagar más puntos en una hipoteca, la entidad hipotecaria debería reducir la tasa de interés del préstamo. Esta reducción puede ser beneficiosa para usted, si tiene el efectivo para pagar más puntos y quiere disminuir la tasa de interés que pagará año tras año. Si anticipa que va a tener la casa y la hipoteca por muchos años, mientras más baja sea la tasa de interés que acuerden, mucho mejor es.

Y a la inversa, si usted quiere (o necesita) pagar menos puntos (quizás porque esté limitado por dinero cuando vaya a comprar la vivienda), puede pagar una tasa de interés más alta. Mientras más corto sea el tiempo que usted piensa tener la hipoteca, más sentido tiene esta estrategia de pagar menos dinero al comenzar.

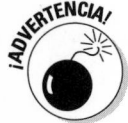

No pase por tonto, creyendo que los préstamos "sin puntos" son un buen negocio ya que nada es gratis en el mundo de bienes raíces. Recuerde la relación entre puntos y tasas de interés: si usted paga menos en puntos, la tasa de interés es más alta. De modo que si un préstamo tiene cero puntos, éste debe tener una tasa de interés más alta. Esto no significa necesariamente que el préstamo es mejor o peor que préstamos similares de otras entidades hipotecarias. Sin embargo, nuestra experiencia ha sido que las entidades hipotecarias que presionan fuertemente para otorgar préstamos sin puntos, no son las entidades hipotecarias más competitivas en términos de precios. Los préstamos sin puntos tienen sentido cuando usted no dispone de dinero en el momento de la compra de su vivienda, y cuando anticipa que no va a tener la casa y la hipoteca por un largo plazo.

Fíjese en las siguientes opciones de hipoteca para entender la relación entre puntos y la tasa de interés. Suponga que usted quiere pedir prestado $150.000. Una entidad hipotecaria le cotiza 7,25 por ciento en un préstamo de 30 años de tasa fija y le cobra 1 punto (1 por ciento). Otra entidad le cotiza 7,75 por ciento y no le cobra puntos. ¿Cuál oferta es mejor? La respuesta depende principalmente de cuánto tiempo piensa usted tener el préstamo.

El préstamo al 7,25 por ciento, le cuesta $1.024 por mes, comparado con $1.075 por mes de la hipoteca al 7,75 por ciento. Usted puede ahorrar $51 mensuales con el préstamo al 7,25 por ciento, pero tiene que pagar $1.500 en puntos para obtenerlo.

Para saber cuál préstamo es mejor, divida el costo de los puntos entre los ahorros mensuales ($1.500 dividido por $51 es igual a 29,4). Este resultado es el número de meses que le tomará recuperar el costo de los puntos (en este caso 29,4 meses). El préstamo al 7,25 por ciento cuesta 0,5 por ciento menos en intereses anualmente que el préstamo al 7,75 por ciento. Año tras año, el préstamo de 7,25 por ciento le ahorra 0,5 por ciento. Pero como usted tiene que pagar un punto por adelantado en la hipoteca a 7,25 por ciento, a usted le tomará cerca de 30 meses (dos años y medio) ganar esos ahorros para cubrir el costo de ese punto. Así que si usted anticipa tener el préstamo por más de 30 meses, acepte la opción de 7,25 por ciento y un punto. Si usted no espera tener la hipoteca por más de ese tiempo, escoja el préstamo sin puntos.

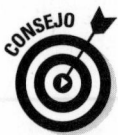

Para hacer una comparación justa de hipotecas de diferentes entidades crediticias, solicite a las entidades que le coticen tasas de interés al *mismo* nivel de puntos. Pídales a las entidades, por ejemplo, que le digan cuál sería la tasa de interés de una hipoteca de tasa fija con un punto. También, asegúrese que los préstamos tienen el mismo plazo —por ejemplo, que ambos son de 30 años.

Otros cargos de las entidades hipotecarias

Usted puede pensar que como está pagando puntos con su hipoteca, usted no tendrá que pagar otros costos iniciales. Pues bien, piénselo de nuevo. Existen tantos gastos iniciales y de procesamiento del préstamo, que usted debe investigarlos cuando esté comparando las diferentes hipotecas. Si usted no entiende la estructura de los costos iniciales, puede terminar con un préstamo costoso o quedar corto de dinero cuando venga el momento de cerrar la compra de la vivienda.

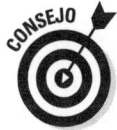

Pídales a cada entidad hipotecaria cuyos servicios usted está considerando seriamente, que le den un desglose, por escrito, de todos estos "otros" cargos. Para reducir sus posibilidades de desperdiciar dinero en una hipoteca para la cual usted probablemente no reúne los requisitos, pregúntele a la entidad crediticia si su solicitud puede ser rechazada por alguna razón. Por ejemplo, mencione cualquier problema potencial de la propiedad que haya sido descubierto durante las inspecciones de la misma.

De igual manera, así como algunas entidades acreedoras tienen hipotecas sin puntos, algunas entidades tienen *hipotecas sin costos iniciales.* Si una entidad está ofreciendo un préstamo libre de estos costos, lo más probable es que le vaya a cobrar más en otras formas o conceptos, especialmente, en la tasa de interés de su préstamo.

Gastos de tramitación y solicitud del préstamo

Las entidades hipotecarias generalmente cobran de $200 a $300 por adelantado por *gastos de tramitación o por la solicitud.* Este cargo es, principalmente, para asegurarse que usted realmente tiene la intención de obtener un préstamo de ellos, y para compensación en el caso de que su préstamo sea rechazado. Las entidades hipotecarias quieren evitar perder dinero en tramitar solicitudes de préstamos que finalmente no se materialicen en un préstamo. Muy pocas entidades hipotecarias no cobran este cargo, pero si lo hacen, le devuelven su dinero si acepta el préstamo.

Reporte crediticio

Su reporte de crédito le dice a una entidad hipotecaria cuán responsable usted ha sido con sus préstamos anteriores. ¿Pagó usted la totalidad de sus préstamos anteriores (y a tiempo)? Los reportes crediticios no cuestan mucho, pero usted puede pagar alrededor de $50 para que la entidad obtenga una copia actualizada del suyo.

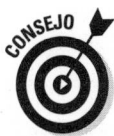

Si sabe que tiene problemas en su reporte de crédito, resuelva esos problemas *antes* de solicitar la hipoteca. Si no lo hace, va a perder tiempo y dinero. No solicite un préstamo que usted ya sabe le será negado.

Avalúo o tasación de la propiedad

Las entidades hipotecarias quieren que la propiedad sea valuada por una entidad independiente, para asegurarse que la vivienda que está comprando, vale lo que usted acordó pagar por ella —éste es el trabajo de un perito o tasador. ¿Por qué es esto tan importante para la entidad hipotecaria? Muy sencillo— porque seguramente la entidad le está prestando una gran parte del precio de compra de la propiedad. Si usted paga un precio mayor que el valor real de la vivienda y ese valor baja, o usted termina en dificultades financieras, usted podría estar dispuesto a abandonar la propiedad y dejar a la entidad crediticia con todo el problema.

El costo de un avalúo varía de acuerdo al tamaño, la complejidad y el valor de la propiedad. Por una valuación de propiedades de precio módico, promedio, anticipe pagar unos cientos de dólares.

Cómo Obtener la Mejor Tasa de Interés Ajustable

Si usted es del tipo de persona que es calmada, serena y que no es propensa al pánico, y que puede resistir la volatilidad de las tasas de interés y ha decidido, gracias a nuestro sabio consejo, a optar por una hipoteca de tasa ajustable, necesitará saber algo más para poder escoger una buena hipoteca. Las hipotecas ajustables son más complicadas de evaluar y seleccionar que las de tasa fija.

Además de tener que aprender sobre los puntos y otros gastos asociados al préstamo —que explicamos en la sección anterior sobre préstamos con tasas de interés fijas—, usted va a ser bombardeado con una jerga como *márgenes, topes e índices*. Los maniáticos de números pueden pasar fácilmente cientos de horas comparando diferentes permutaciones de hipotecas de tasa ajustable, y determinando cómo pueden comportarse éstas en diferentes escenarios de tasas de interés.

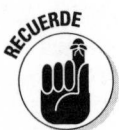

A diferencia de una hipoteca de tasa fija, en una hipoteca de tasa ajustable no es posible determinar en forma exacta el monto del dinero que va a costarle. Ese mismo cuidado que tuvo para escoger una casa, debe ser usado para seleccionar una hipoteca de tasa ajustable que se ajuste a su presupuesto y necesidades. Esto involucra llegar a un acuerdo y decidir qué es importante para usted. Así que aquí tiene un curso acelerado para entender las hipotecas de tasa de interés ajustable.

De dónde proviene la tasa de interés de una hipoteca ajustable

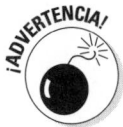

La mayoría de las hipotecas con tasa de interés ajustable comienzan con una tasa artificialmente baja. La selección de una hipoteca ajustable basada solamente en la baja tasa de interés inicial, probablemente es un gran error porque usted no estará pagando esa tasa baja por mucho tiempo. Quizás sólo la tendrá por 6 ó 12 meses o, tal vez, ¡por sólo un mes! Las entidades hipotecarias y los agentes de hipotecas son como muchos otros vendedores: les gusta promocionar algo que capturará su atención y que lo haga pensar que usted va a realizar un excelente negocio. Probablemente, ésa sea la razón por la cuál las entidades y agentes hipotecarios mencionan, primero que otra cosa, la tasa inicial baja.

La tasa inicial de una hipoteca ajustable, no es tan importante como lo es la tasa de interés del préstamo en el futuro. El factor más importante que usted debe entender al momento de evaluar la hipoteca ajustable, es cómo se calcula la futura tasa de interés de la hipoteca.

Todas las hipotecas de tasas ajustables que nosotros hemos visto están siempre basadas en una ecuación que incluye un índice y un margen. Estos dos elementos se suman para calcular y establecer la tasa de interés futura del préstamo. Antes de continuar, por favor, asegúrese de entender los siguientes conceptos:

- ✔ **Índice:** el índice es una medida de las tasas de interés que la entidad crediticia usa como referencia. Por ejemplo, el índice bancario de depósitos a plazo fijo de seis meses, se utiliza como referencia para muchas hipotecas. Suponga que la tasa actual en depósitos a plazo fijo de seis meses es aproximadamente el 5 por ciento. Teóricamente, este índice indica cuánto le cuesta al banco obtener fondos para luego prestarlos.

- ✔ **Margen:** el margen es la ganancia de la entidad hipotecaria (o margen de utilidad) sobre el dinero que ellos piensan prestar. La mayoría de los préstamos tienen márgenes de alrededor del 2,5 por ciento, pero el margen exacto depende de cada entidad crediticia y del índice que la misma esté usando. Cuando usted compara préstamos que están relacionados con el mismo índice y el resto de las características son las mismas, el préstamo con el margen más bajo es el mejor para usted, porque representa la alternativa con el costo más bajo.

- ✔ **Tasa de interés:** la tasa de interés es la suma del índice y del margen. Es lo que usted pagará (sujeto a ciertas limitaciones) por su préstamo.

Poniendo todos estos conceptos juntos en nuestro ejemplo —el índice de depósito a plazo fijo de seis meses del 5 por ciento, más el margen del 2,5 por ciento—, da como resultado una tasa de interés del 7,5 por ciento. Esta cifra es conocida como *tasa de interés indexada completa*. Si este préstamo comienza con el 5 por ciento, por ejemplo, la tasa indexada le dice a usted a qué tasa aumentaría la hipoteca, si el nivel de las tasas de interés en el mercado — medido con el índice de depósitos a plazo fijo—, permanece constante. Nunca acepte una hipoteca de tasa ajustable a menos que comprenda este concepto tan importante de la tasa indexada:

> Índice + margen = tasa de interés

Muchas entidades hipotecarias saben que un gran número de prestatarios prestan atención solamente a la tasa inicial de la hipoteca ajustable y pasan por alto el margen y el índice que determinan la tasa del préstamo. Escuche nuestro consejo y fíjese, en la tasa inicial de la hipoteca ajustable, *de último*. Cuando evalúe una hipoteca de tasa variable, comience por ver con cuál índice está relacionada y qué margen tiene. Las siguientes secciones explican los índices más comunes de las hipotecas con tasa ajustable.

Letras del Tesoro

El gobierno federal de los Estados Unidos es el mayor prestatario en el mundo al momento, de modo que no debe sorprendernos que al menos un índice de la hipoteca de tasa ajustable esté basado en la tasa de interés que el gobierno paga sobre algún tipo de deudas de las muchas que tiene. Los índices de tasas de interés del gobierno más comúnmente utilizados para hipotecas ajustables, son los de las Letras del Tesoro a 6 y a 12 meses.

Estos índices tienden a estar entre los índices que más cambian, o sea, que responden más rápidamente a los cambios del mercado de tasa de interés.

Depósitos a plazo fijo

Los *depósitos a plazo fijo* (*CDs*) son inversiones bancarias que devengan intereses por un período de tiempo determinado. Las hipotecas ajustables están generalmente vinculadas a la tasa de interés promedio que los bancos pagan en los depósitos a plazo fijo de seis meses.

Así como las letras del Tesoro, los depósitos a plazo fijo tienden a cambiar rápidamente con los cambios generales de las tasas de interés. Sin embargo, las tasas de interés de estos depósitos tienden a aumentar más lentamente cuando se producen aumentos de las tasas en general. Esto sucede porque los bancos, enfocados siempre en sus ganancias, prefieren ser lentos cuando tienen que pagar más intereses a los ahorristas. Y, a la inversa, las tasas de los depósitos a plazo fijo tienden a bajar rápidamente cuando las tasas bajan, de modo que los banqueros puedan mantener sus ganancias.

Índice de Costo de Fondos del Distrito 11

El índice de Costo de Fondos del Distrito 11 (también conocido como *COFI*, por sus siglas en inglés, el cual se pronuncia como la bebida con cafeína que algunas personas toman por la mañana), es publicado mensualmente por el Directorio del Banco Federal de Préstamos para Viviendas (*Federal Home Loan Bank Board*). Este índice muestra el costo promedio ponderado de los ahorros, préstamos y anticipos de los bancos miembros localizados en los estados de California, Arizona y Nevada (el Distrito 11). Debido a que este índice *COFI* es un promedio que cambia mensualmente porque se basa en las tasas que los banqueros han pagado a los ahorristas durante los meses más recientes, tiende a ser un índice relativamente estable.

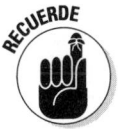

Una hipoteca de tasa ajustable que está vinculada a un índice más lento, tal como el índice *COFI*, tiene la ventaja de aumentar más lentamente cuando las tasas de interés están subiendo. Por otro lado, usted tiene que ser paciente para beneficiarse de tasas de interés en descenso cuando las tasas están bajando. El índice del Distrito 11 baja muy despacio cuando las tasas de interés, en general, bajan.

Debido a que las hipotecas de tasa ajustable vinculadas al índice *COFI* aumentan más lentamente cuando las tasas en general aumentan, ellas generalmente comienzan a una tasa de interés más alta que las hipotecas ajustables vinculadas a índices que cambian más rápido.

Índice de tasa LIBOR

Bueno, aquí vamos a explicar un índice más raro que los anteriores. El índice *London Interbank Offered Rate Index* (*LIBOR,* por sus siglas en inglés), es un promedio de las tasas de interés que los bancos internacionales más grandes se cobran entre ellos por prestarse dólares estadounidenses en el mercado interbancario de Londres. Tal como los índices del Tesoro de los Estados Unidos y los de depósitos a plazo fijo (*CD*), la tasa LIBOR tiende a moverse y a ajustarse rápidamente a los cambios de las tasas de interés.

¿Por qué necesitamos un índice internacional de tasas de interés? Porque inversionistas extranjeros compran hipotecas estadounidenses como inversiones, y no debe sorprendernos que estos inversionistas prefieran que las hipotecas de tasas ajustables estén vinculadas a un índice que ellos entienden y con el cuál están más familiarizados.

¿Con qué frecuencia se ajusta la tasa de interés?

Las entidades hipotecarias generalmente ajustan las tasas sobre sus hipotecas cada 6 ó 12 meses y usan para ello la fórmula hipoteca-tasa que presentamos al principio de esta sección. Sin embargo, hay préstamos que se ajustan mensualmente. (Generalmente, estos ajustes mensuales son avisos para reconocer préstamos de amortización negativa. En la sección "Evite las hipotecas de tasa ajustable con amortización negativa" explicamos cómo mantenerse alejado de estos préstamos.) Antes de cada ajuste, la entidad hipotecaria debe enviarle un aviso explicando en detalle cómo han calculado la nueva tasa, de acuerdo a las condiciones establecidas en su préstamo de tasa ajustable.

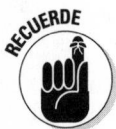

Mientras menos frecuente sea el ajuste de su préstamo, menos riesgo financiero está usted aceptando. A cambio de tomar menos riesgo, la entidad hipotecaria normalmente espera que usted pague una tasa de interés inicial más elevada.

Límites a los ajustes de la tasa de interés

A pesar del hecho de que una hipoteca de tasa ajustable tiene un sistema para calcular la tasa de interés futura (sumando el margen y el índice del préstamo), los bancos limitan la dimensión de los cambios que pueden ocurrir en la tasa real que usted paga. Estos límites, también conocidos como *topes de las tasas,* influencian cada futuro ajuste de la tasa de la hipoteca ajustable al terminarse el período de vigencia de la tasa inicial.

Los *topes de ajuste periódico* establecen lo máximo que puede cambiar la tasa, hacia arriba o hacia abajo, permitida para cada ajuste. Para hipotecas que se ajustan cada seis meses, el tope de ajuste es generalmente el 1 por ciento. Las hipotecas que se ajustan más de una vez al año, también restringen el máximo cambio de tasa permitido durante el año. Este tope anual es, por lo general, el 2 por ciento.

Finalmente, casi todas las hipotecas ajustables vienen con *topes* máximos a usar durante la vigencia del préstamo. Por eso, usted nunca debe aceptar una hipoteca ajustable que no indique el tope máximo de ajuste. Estos topes limitan la tasa máxima permitida durante la vigencia del préstamo. Las hipotecas de tasas ajustables generalmente tienen un tope máximo permitido de un 5 ó 6 por ciento más alto que la tasa inicial.

Cuando usted se decida por una hipoteca de tasa variable, asegúrese de que puede amortizar el máximo pago posible permitido, en caso de que la tasa de interés de la hipoteca ajustable llegue al tope máximo permitido durante la vigencia del préstamo.

Cómo Encontrar las Mejores Entidades Hipotecarias y el Más Bajo Interés

Para aquellos de ustedes que detestan ir de compras, tenemos malas noticias: a menos que disfruten tirar por la ventana miles de dólares, necesitan buscar las mejores condiciones para su hipoteca. Piensen en esto como si estuvieran "pescando por dólares" (o, "navegando en busca de dólares", para ésos que son usuarios de la Web).

No importa si usted decide hacerlo por sus propios medios o contratar a alguien competente para que lo ayude. Lo importante es que se asegure que esta comparación se haga.

Suponga que usted está buscando una hipoteca de $100.000 a 30 años. Si al hacerlo en forma persistente y juiciosa, usted es capaz de obtener una hipoteca que es, por ejemplo, 0,5 por ciento más baja por año que la que usted hubiera obtenido de cualquier otra manera, usted ahorrará aproximadamente en intereses $14.000 durante la existencia de su préstamo (dadas las tasas aproximadas de interés actuales). Estos ahorros se duplican si la hipoteca es de $200.000.

Aunque nosotros lo animamos a que encuentre las entidades crediticias con más bajos costos, debemos primero hacerle una advertencia: si alguien le ofrece a usted unas condiciones que son muchísimo mejores que las de cualquier otra entidad hipotecaria, no lo crea a primeras y dude un poco. Esa entidad crediticia le puede estar lanzando un anzuelo con un préstamo que no existe o con uno para el cual usted no reúne los requisitos y, como consecuencia, usted se puede quedar atrapado en un préstamo costoso si no tiene tiempo de solicitar otra hipoteca en alguna otra parte.

Cómo buscar cotizaciones de tasas de interés por usted mismo

En la mayoría de las comunidades, hay un gran número de entidades crediticias. Aunque tener innumerables opciones entre las cuales escoger es bueno por la competencia, muchas alternativas pueden darle dolor de cabeza cuando salga de compras.

Muchos tipos de compañías ofrecen hipotecas hoy en día. Las empresas de hipotecas más comunes, los *originadores* (como se conocen en el ambiente de los negocios) son los bancos, las entidades de ahorro y préstamo y los banqueros hipotecarios.

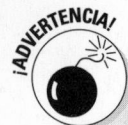

Evite las hipotecas de tasa ajustable con amortización negativa

Algunas hipotecas de tasa ajustable ponen un tope al aumento de su pago mensual, pero no al aumento de la tasa de interés y, por consecuencia, el monto de su pago mensual podría no reflejar todos los intereses que usted realmente debe de su préstamo. De modo que, en lugar de pagar el interés que usted debe y amortizar parte del saldo de su préstamo cada mes, usted puede terminar pagando algo, pero no todo, del interés que debe. Así que el interés extra no pagado mensualmente, se lo suman a su saldo pendiente de deuda.

A medida que paga su hipoteca, con el transcurso del tiempo, el saldo del préstamo que usted todavía debe se reduce gradualmente en un proceso llamado *amortización de la deuda*. Lo contrario de este proceso (es decir, el aumento del saldo de su préstamo) es llamado *amortización negativa*.

La amortización negativa es como realizar sólo el pago mínimo requerido en una cuenta de la tarjeta de crédito. Usted continúa acumulando intereses adicionales en el saldo si solamente paga el monto mensual mínimo. Sin embargo, hacer esto con una hipoteca aminora

el propósito de prestar un monto que se ajuste a sus objetivos financieros en general (vea el Capítulo 3).

Algunos bancos tratan de ocultar el hecho de que una hipoteca de tasa ajustable que ellos le están proponiendo tiene una amortización negativa. ¿Cómo puede usted evitar un préstamo de este tipo? ¡Pregunte, pregunte y pregunte!

Sepa también que la amortización negativa aparece más frecuentemente en aquellas hipotecas que las entidades acreedoras consideran riesgosas. Si usted tiene problemas para encontrar entidades crediticias dispuestas a ofrecerle una hipoteca, entonces sea más cauteloso.

Por último, pero no por eso menos importante, sepa que muchas entidades crediticias no proveerán financiamiento adicional en forma de hipotecas secundarias o préstamos con líneas de crédito, sobre el capital en la propiedad, para respaldar un préstamo de amortización negativa. Ellos temen que si el préstamo de amortización negativa se hace muy grande, puede agotar todo el capital de la propiedad.

Usted se puede preguntar, ¿y porqué es importante saber eso? Pues bien, los banqueros hipotecarios solamente tramitan hipotecas, y los mejores de ellos ofrecen tasas muy competidoras. Los bancos más pequeños y las entidades de ahorro y préstamo también pueden darle una buena oferta. Pero en cambio, los bancos grandes, cuyos nombres están fijos en su cabeza como producto de la propaganda, generalmente no ofrecen las mejores tasas.

Cuando usted comience su expedición en búsqueda de la hipoteca, no tiene que hacerlo completamente solo. Si ha escogido un buen agente de bienes raíces para ayudarlo en la compra de la vivienda, por ejemplo, el agente debe estar en capacidad de ofrecerle una lista corta de buenas entidades crediticias y de agentes hipotecarios en su zona (vea la siguiente sección). Sólo recuerde y compare los préstamos de estas entidades con los ofrecidos por las entidades hipotecarias que usted mismo encuentra.

Algunos agentes de bienes raíces, que en general son buenos, pueden recomendarle entidades crediticias que no necesariamente ofrecen las mejores tasas de interés para hipotecas. Algunos puede que no estén actualizados en quién tiene los mejores préstamos o no se preocupan en buscar quién los ofrece. Otros puede que se sienten cómodos trabajando con ciertas entidades crediticias o han obtenido clientes enviados por esas entidades.

Como usted seguramente sabe, el Internet ofrece aún otro método para llegar a compañías específicas. En el Capítulo 11, le damos muchos consejos y recomendaciones de páginas Web que pueden ayudarlo en la búsqueda de hipotecas.

Otra manera de encontrar entidades crediticias es mirar las tablas con las tasas de interés que se publican los domingos en la sección de bienes raíces de los periódicos más grandes. Sin embargo, no crea que dichas tablas contengan las mejores entidades crediticias en su zona. De hecho, muchas de esas tablas son enviadas gratis a los periódicos por compañías que distribuyen información de agentes hipotecarios. No obstante, usted puede usar las tablas como un punto de partida para llamar a las organizaciones financieras que ofrecen las mejores tasas (sepa, por supuesto, que estas tasas pueden cambiar diariamente, y las que ve en el periódico pueden no reflejar lo que está disponible en ese momento).

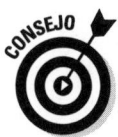

Si usted es un "busca datos", la compañía *HSH Associates* (800-873-2837; www.hsh.com) publica semanalmente las listas de docenas de cotizaciones de tasas de interés de entidades crediticias, para la mayoría de las zonas metropolitanas. El paquete inicial, el cual viene con panfletos detallados, cuesta $20. Si usted desea comprar los fascículos que siguen, ésos cuestan $10 cada uno.

Cómo trabajar con un agente hipotecario

Los *agentes o corredores hipotecarios* son intermediarios, independientes de los bancos y de otras instituciones financieras, que tienen dinero para prestar. Estos agentes pueden hacer la búsqueda por usted.

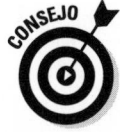

Si su historial crediticio y su posibilidad de reunir los requisitos para una hipoteca son dudosos, un buen agente hipotecario puede ayudarlo a pulir y reunir todo los requisitos necesarios para su solicitud, y guiarlo hacia aquellas entidades hipotecarias que podrían darle un préstamo. Los agentes también

pueden ayudarlo si las entidades financieras no quieren hacer préstamos para propiedades poco comunes en las cuales usted podría estar
interesado en comprar. A muchas entidades no les gusta vincularse con
negocios de cooperativas y viviendas multifamiliares con áreas comunes
(vea el Capítulo 8), con prestatarios con problemas de créditos o con
compradores que solicitan en préstamo casi todo el valor de la
propiedad (el 90 por ciento o más).

Características de las entidades crediticias eficientes

Es cierto que existen miles de entidades hipotecarias por allí. Sin embargo, muy pocas son
buenas entidades hipotecarias. Los agentes de
bienes raíces y otros en el mismo negocio, así
como otros prestatarios que usted conoce,
pueden ser útiles para encaminarlo hacia las
entidades hipotecarias de primera categoría y
alejarlo de las malas. (Para estar seguro de que
las recomendaciones que usted está recibiendo
son objetivas, pregúntele a su agente si le pagan
un honorario por esas recomendaciones que
da.) A medida que usted pide información y
comienza a visitar las entidades crediticias,
trate de encontrar las que reúnen las siguientes
características:

✔ **Son directas:** los agentes de préstamo eficientes, explican sus diferentes programas
de préstamos en un lenguaje sencillo, sin
usar ambigüedades o jerga, y lo ayudan
a comparar su préstamo con los de la competencia. Aléjese tan rápido como pueda
de aquellos agentes de hipoteca que lo
tratan como si usted no pudiera entender
los programas e intentan confundirlo con
un lenguaje complicado.

✔ **Aprueban los préstamos localmente:** las
entidades crediticias buenas aprueban su
préstamo localmente. No tienen que enviar
su solicitud a un comité de préstamo fuera

de la ciudad, donde lo convierten de un
humano que respira y vive a un número sin
vida. Las buenas entidades usan tasadores
que están familiarizados con el mercado de
bienes raíces local y tienen experiencia valuando los tipos de propiedades que son
vendidas comúnmente en la localidad.
Igualmente, estas organizaciones trabajan
activamente con usted y su agente para
obtener la aprobación de su préstamo.

✔ **Conocen el mercado:** las buenas entidades
conocen el tipo de propiedad que usted
quiere comprar. Y aquí radica otra gran ventaja de la aprobación local del préstamo: no
ocurren cancelaciones inesperadas de
préstamos o de última hora, porque usted,
sin darse cuenta, se metió en problemas
con alguna norma institucional poco clara.

Este tipo de obstáculo generalmente ocurre
cuando un agente hipotecario intenta conseguir un préstamo con la tasa de interés
más baja que la que está siendo ofrecida en
ese momento en cualquier lugar del uni-
verso. Encontrar un préstamo es relativamente fácil, pero obtener el dinero es otra
cosa, y es casi imposible porque usted no
sabe qué extrañas peculiaridades yacen en
las profundidades de las letras pequeñitas
del documento del préstamo.

Estos préstamos tan particulares generalmente se otorgan a propiedades prístinas. Por ejemplo, una vez una entidad crediticia ubicada fuera del estado aprobó un préstamo bajo la condición de que todos los trabajos pendientes de reparación debieran estar listos y la vivienda pintada por dentro y por fuera, antes del cierre de la garantía. Dado que el préstamo fue aprobado un lunes y la compra estaba programada para cerrar el viernes, no había forma de que el trabajo fuese hecho en cuatro días.

✔ **Son competitivas:** las entidades buenas son competitivas en precios. No tenga miedo de pedirle a la entidad crediticia de su preferencia si puede darle la misma tasa de interés que encontró en otra entidad y que es una tasa más baja. Lo peor que podría pasar es que la entidad le niegue su requerimiento; y, lo mejor, es que usted podría terminar haciendo el negocio con la organización que desea y con las condiciones del préstamo que quiere. Las tasas y los gastos de los préstamos *son* negociables.

✔ **Prestan atención a los mínimos detalles:** las entidades crediticias buenas cumplen con las fechas del contrato y aprueban y dan los fondos del préstamo a tiempo. Su agente conoce cuáles entidades cumplen con sus promesas y cuáles no. Hablar es fácil, pero usted necesita hechos, no promesas falsas. Acuérdese que incumplir con las fechas establecidas puede echar a perder su compra.

Los agentes hipotecarios generalmente le dicen que pueden conseguirle las mejores condiciones de préstamo porque salen a solicitar cotizaciones entre las entidades hipotecarias. Ellos hasta podrían decirle que otro beneficio de usar sus servicios es que pueden explicarle el sinnúmero de opciones de préstamos que hay disponibles, que lo ayudan a seleccionar el préstamo y lo guían a través de la montaña de papeles que, desafortunadamente, es necesario llenar para obtener la hipoteca.

Estos agentes, cuando son eficientes, pueden cumplir la mayoría de estas promesas y, por este servicio, reciben una parte del monto que usted está prestando —típicamente, desde un 0,5 por ciento hasta un 2 por ciento en préstamos pequeños. No es barato, pero dado que encontrar una buena hipoteca y cerrar la compra son dolores de cabeza, contratar un agente hipotecario puede ser exactamente lo que le recomendó su doctor financiero.

Si usted va a trabajar con un agente hipotecario, por favor recuerde que el negocio de estos agentes es la "venta" de las hipotecas, y que obtienen una comisión por este trabajo, tal como lo hacen los corredores de bolsa que venden acciones y los vendedores de automóviles que venden carros. Una diferencia, sin embargo, es que la tasa de interés y los puntos que usted paga por obtener la hipoteca a través de un agente son los mismos que los que usted hubiera pagado a una entidad hipotecaria directamente. Las entidades hipotecarias piensan que ellas pueden compartir sus honorarios normales con un agente hipotecario que no es un empleado del banco. Después de todo, si usted obtuviera el préstamo directamente del banco, usted tendría que trabajar y utilizar más el tiempo de uno de los empleados del banco.

Sin embargo, algunas entidades crediticias, incluso aquéllas que tienen las tasas más bajas, no venden a través de agentes hipotecarios. Y algunas veces un préstamo que se obtiene a través de un agente puede terminar costándole más que si usted lo hubiese solicitado directamente de la entidad —por ejemplo, si el agente hipotecario está quedándose con una comisión grande para él.

La comisión que el agente hipotecario recibe no es fija y es totalmente negociable, especialmente para préstamos grandes. En un préstamo de $100.000, el 1 por ciento de comisión es $1.000. La misma comisión en un préstamo de $300.000 resulta en un monto de $3.000 para el agente, aun cuando este préstamo, tres veces más grande que el primero, no toma tres veces más del tiempo que el agente usa. Usted tiene todo el derecho de preguntarle al agente cuál es su tarifa. No sienta vergüenza y recuerde: es su dinero, ¡y usted tiene derecho de conocer esta información! Pregunte y no dude en negociar.

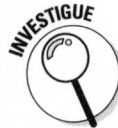

Además de conocer y negociar la comisión del agente hipotecario, cuando realiza su proceso de selección, haga las siguientes preguntas:

✔ **¿Con cuántas entidades hipotecarias hace negocios el agente? ¿Qué hace para estar actualizado con respecto a nuevas entidades y préstamos que puedan ser mejores?** Algunos agentes hipotecarios, ya sea por hábito o flojera, mantienen relaciones comerciales con sólo unas pocas entidades y no le pueden conseguir un préstamo con mejores condiciones. Pregúnteles a los agentes cuáles entidades los han autorizado para representarlas a ellas.

✔ **¿Cuánto sabe el agente sobre los diferentes programas de préstamo? ¿Tiene el agente hipotecario paciencia para explicarle todas las características importantes de los mismos?** Mientras más entidades hipotecarias un agente represente, menos probable es que el agente conozca los detalles y matices de todos y cada uno de los préstamos. Sea especialmente cauteloso con un vendedor que trata de venderle a todo costo cierto tipo de préstamo y pasa por alto o ignora explicarle los puntos importantes que discutimos en este capítulo para evaluar ciertas hipotecas en particular.

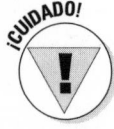

Todos los consejos que le dimos para seleccionar una buena entidad hipotecaria, también pueden usarse para escoger un buen agente hipotecario. Se sabe que algunos agentes, por ejemplo, tratan de convencer al prestatario de programas con altísimas tasas de interés y puntos; esto no debería sorprenderlo porque les genera una mayor comisión a ellos. Este problema ocurre más frecuentemente con prestatarios que tienen un crédito dudoso u otros problemas para reunir los requisitos para un préstamo.

Estudio preliminar y aprobación previa de un préstamo

Cuando usted ya tiene un contrato para comprar una vivienda y ha gastado cientos de dólares en gastos de procesamiento e inspección de la misma, el rechazo de su solicitud (después de esperar varias semanas) puede causarle la pérdida de la propiedad. Lo que es peor, usted puede perder la vivienda en la cual probablemente invirtió innumerables horas de búsqueda y mucho trabajo para asegurarla. Algunos vendedores de vivienda puede que no estén dispuestos a esperar o quizás necesiten vender rápidamente. Asimismo, si los vendedores tienen otros compradores esperando por la propiedad, es probable que usted la pierda.

¿Cómo pudo haber evitado esta molestia? Bueno, puede que haya escuchado a algunas personas en el negocio de bienes raíces, tales como los agentes inmobiliarios e hipotecarios, recomendarle que haga un estudio preliminar y obtenga una aprobación previa para determinar si usted reúne los requisitos para el préstamo o hipoteca.

El estudio preliminar (*prequalification*) es una discusión informal entre el prestatario y la entidad crediticia. Esta última emite una opinión acerca del monto del préstamo que usted puede solicitar basado únicamente en lo que usted, el prestatario, le dice a dicha entidad. La entidad no verifica ninguna información que usted haya dado y no está obligada a darle el préstamo cuando usted esté listo para comprar.

La aprobación previa es un proceso mucho más riguroso, por lo que nosotros lo preferimos, si usted tiene alguna razón para pensar que tendrá dificultades en reunir las condiciones del préstamo que desea. La aprobación previa del préstamo está basada en información que ha sido verificada y documentada en relación a la probabilidad de que usted tenga su empleo, en sus ingresos, sus obligaciones o deudas y en el dinero que usted tenga disponible para cerrar la compra de la casa. El único aspecto que la entidad crediticia no puede aprobar previamente, es la propiedad que usted tiene intención de comprar porque, por supuesto, usted no la ha encontrado todavía.

Pasar por todo este proceso es una muestra para los vendedores de viviendas de cuán decidido usted está de comprar una casa —esto es como un sello de calidad de buen prestatario. La carta de aprobación previa de la entidad crediticia es mucho más importante que una carta de estudio preliminar. En una situación en la cual existen varias ofertas realizadas por compradores potenciales por una misma propiedad, aquellos compradores que han sido previamente aprobados para un préstamo tienen una ventaja con respecto a otros compradores cuya situación crediticia no ha sido verificada.

Las entidades hipotecarias no cobran por hacer un estudio preliminar. Pero dado el trabajo que la aprobación previa requiere, algunas entidades sí cobran por ella (quizás unos cientos de dólares). Otros bancos, sin embargo, ofrecen hacer la aprobación previa gratis para ganar la lealtad del prestatario. No escoja una entidad financiera sólo porque no cobre por la tramitación previa del préstamo, ya que ella podría no ofrecerle las mejores condiciones para el mismo.

Si usted decide obtener la aprobación previa de una entidad hipotecaria que cobra por el proceso, asegúrese que usted va a realizar pronto la compra de la casa. De otra manera, usted habrá tirado el dinero por la ventana.

Asimismo, protéjase si su agente hipotecario lo insta a tomar un préstamo reembolsable al vencimiento o uno de amortización negativa (presentados anteriormente en este capítulo). Los préstamos reembolsables al vencimiento —los cuáles son pagaderos en su totalidad cuando se vencen después de varios años que usted lo ha obtenido— son peligrosos porque usted puede tener dificultades en conseguir un nuevo financiamiento y podría verse forzado a vender la propiedad.

Si usted está indeciso acerca de si contratar un agente hipotecario o no, haga esta sencilla prueba: si usted es del tipo de persona que detesta salir de compras y espera hasta el último momento para comprar un regalo, entonces un buen agente hipotecario probablemente puede ayudarlo a ahorrar dinero. Un agente competente puede ser de gran beneficio para aquéllos que no se molestan en buscar los préstamos con mejores condiciones o que puedan ser rechazados por la mayoría de las entidades hipotecarias.

Aún si usted planifica buscar el préstamo usted mismo, hablar con un agente hipotecario puede valer la pena. Al menos, usted puede comparar lo que usted encuentre, con lo que los agentes dicen que pueden conseguirle.

Sepa que algunos agentes solamente le dicen lo que usted quiere escuchar, o sea, que ellos pueden ofrecerle algo mejor de lo que usted encontró por sí mismo. Más adelante, podría descubrir que el agente no es capaz de cumplir con su promesa. Si usted encuentra un buen préstamo por sí mismo y quiere comprobar con un agente hipotecario para ver lo que él o ella pueden ofrecerle, sería prudente no decirle las condiciones del préstamo que usted consiguió. Si usted lo hace, a muchos agentes siempre se les ocurrirá algo que pueden decirle que es mejor de lo que ya usted tiene en las manos.

Cuando un agente hipotecario le cotiza una buena tasa y buenas condiciones para un préstamo (usted sabrá cuáles son si ya ha salido en busca de una hipoteca), pregunte quién es la entidad hipotecaria. La mayoría de los agentes se niegan a revelar esta información hasta que usted pague unos cuantos dólares para cubrir los costos de valuación de la propiedad y del reporte crediticio. En la mayoría de los casos, usted puede consultar con la misma entidad para corroborar la tasa de interés y los puntos que el agente le cotizó, y asegurarse que usted reúne las condiciones necesarias para que le sea aprobado el crédito. Algunos bancos no venden préstamos directamente al público.

Si usted descubre, al llamar a la entidad crediticia directamente, que ésta no ofrece dichas condiciones tan buenas a sus clientes, no llegue a la conclusión de que el agente hipotecario le mintió. En ciertos casos, un agente hipotecario puede ofrecerle unas condiciones un poquito mejor que las que usted hubiese podido conseguir por sí mismo.

¿Debería usted solicitar más de una hipoteca?

Cuando usted solicitó inscripción en la universidad o solicitó trabajo, probablemente no lo hizo solamente en la institución que consideraba su primera opción. Quizás, usted tenía otra opción como respaldo, o dos, o tres. De modo que cuando llegue el momento de solicitar una hipoteca, puede sentirse tentado a solicitar un préstamo en más de una entidad hipotecaria. A lo mejor piensa que es una ventaja, que si una entidad crediticia le niega el préstamo, tiene como respaldo a la otra, o sea, alguien más a quien recurrir.

Sin embargo, nosotros creemos que si usted hace bien lo que tiene que hacer y escoge una buena entidad hipotecaria con una reputación de tener tasas bajas, buena calidad de servicio, de ser responsable y de satisfacer las expectativas de los clientes, solicitar más de una hipoteca no es necesario en la mayoría de los casos. Cuando usted solicita un segundo préstamo, usted tiene que pagar gastos adicionales por la solicitud y gastar más tiempo y esfuerzo en completar el papeleo de nuevo.

El hacer solicitudes a más de una institución hipotecaria tiene sentido en situaciones especiales, en las cuales usted corre un mayor riesgo de que le nieguen su petición. El primer caso es cuando usted tiene problemas de crédito. En relación a esto, lea el Capítulo 2 para poner sus finanzas en orden antes de emprender la expedición de compra de una vivienda; asimismo, lea el Capítulo 7 para enterarse de algunos consejos de cómo hacer más interesante su solicitud de préstamo al banco.

El segundo caso en el cual tendría sentido solicitar un préstamo a más de una entidad hipotecaria, es cuando usted quiere comprar una propiedad con problemas estructurales o legales "difíciles". Es imposible, por supuesto, saber anticipadamente todos los tipos de propiedades que por sus características particulares puedan no gustarle a una entidad específica. De hecho, a nosotros dos, hace cierto tiempo, nos negaron los préstamos porque nuestras viviendas potenciales tenían unas cosas con las que una entidad hipotecaria en particular no estaba de acuerdo. Por eso, disminuya las probabilidades de una sorpresa negativa preguntándoles a su agente y al inspector de la propiedad, si algún aspecto de la misma puede representar una preocupación para la entidad hipotecaria.

Si usted solicita dos préstamos, dígale a cada entidad crediticia que usted está solicitando un préstamo en las dos. Esto es importante porque cuando la segunda entidad solicite su reporte de crédito la indagación de la primera entidad aparecerá registrada en el sistema. (Prestatarios cuya característica no es precisamente la franqueza casi siempre quedan en evidencia de esta manera). También, dígale a ambas entidades acreedoras que usted está verdaderamente interesado —así como le diría a cualquier compañía que pueda potencialmente ofrecerle trabajo.

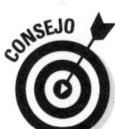

Si el agente estaba tratando de confundirlo para poder hacer trato con usted, el pagar la comisión del agente hipotecario con su tarjeta de crédito le da la oportunidad de hacer un reclamo por este cargo y recobrar su dinero.

Capítulo 7

Dilemas, Interrogantes y Papeleo de Hipotecas

*N*o es un proyecto tan difícil el entender los diferentes tipos de présta- mos hipotecarios y el seleccionar uno (el tema del Capítulo 6) después de interpretar el palabrerío técnico, y de conocer bien su situación financiera y sus metas.

Desgraciadamente, cuando solicita una hipoteca pueden interponerse obstáculos. En este capítulo le enseñamos cómo movilizarse ante estos retos molestosos y, en ocasiones, no exactamente triviales. También contestamos sus preguntas en relación a otras alternativas confusas (y en algunos casos, deseables) que pueda tener.

En la última sección de este capítulo le explicamos cómo llenar esas temidas solicitudes para tramitar un préstamo hipotecario.

Superación de Problemas Comunes de Hipotecas

Pocas cosas en la vida son más frustrantes que no poder obtener algo que realmente se quiere, especialmente si percibe, correcta o incorrectamente, que la mayoría de la gente que usted conoce sí lo tiene. Si quiere comprar una casa y no logra financiar la compra, lo más seguro es que su sueño tendrá que pasar a un segundo plano.

No pierda las esperanzas si se interponen obstáculos en su camino. Es posible que tenga que tener más paciencia de lo normal, pero jamás hemos conocido a alguien que estuviera determinado a comprar una casa y que no haya podido superar problemas de crédito o de otro tipo. Este capítulo le enseña cómo obtener el financiamiento que necesita y ¡merece!

Ingresos insuficientes

Es posible que su entidad crediticia deseada rechace su solicitud si parece que usted se está sobre extendiéndose económicamente. Aunque enojarse y clavarle alfileres en un muñeco vudú del banquero es una reacción inicial natural, la realidad es que debería estar agradecido. ¿Por qué? Porque es posible que el banquero le esté haciendo un favor enorme al prevenir que compre una casa que no le permitirá ahorrar y lograr otras metas financieras que puedan ser importantes para usted a lo largo del tiempo. (Para más sobre este tema, lea los Capítulos 2 y 3 sobre cómo poner en orden su economía doméstica y determinar, de acuerdo a sus finanzas, qué cantidad puede pagar realmente por su vivienda).

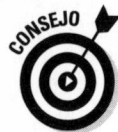

Si *sabe* que puede pagar una casa que ya tiene en mente, aquí están algunas claves para lograr que aprueben su préstamo:

✔ **Tenga paciencia.** Cuando tiene ingresos bajos (por ejemplo, si trabaja por sí mismo y ha estado deduciendo como gasto empresarial todo menos el aire que respira), es posible que necesite esperar un año o dos para que pueda demostrar ingresos más altos.

✔ **Incremente su cuota o pago inicial.** Si da una cuota inicial del 25 al 30 por ciento o más, algunos prestamistas hipotecarios pueden aprobarlo para un préstamo hipotecario que no requiere verificación de ingresos (en casos especiales lo dan con un 20 por ciento de inicial). Por lo general, tales hipotecas tienen tasas de interés más altas que los préstamos convencionales, por lo cual tendrá que reconocer que va a pagar más por este tipo de préstamo.

✔ **Consiga un aval.** Siempre supo que molestaría nuevamente a sus padres algún día, pidiéndoles ayuda y favores. Si sus padres están económicamente bien, es posible que puedan firmar su préstamo como aval para ayudarle a reunir los requisitos. Un hermano económicamente solvente, una tía rica o un amigo adinerado también pueden hacerlo.

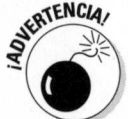

Asegúrese de considerar las ramificaciones económicas y no económicas de pedirle a algún familiar o amigo que firmen de aval en su préstamo. El impago de la hipoteca o pagos atrasados mancharán no solamente su historial crediticio sino también el de su aval. Por lo menos hable francamente sobre estas cuestiones antes de comprometerse a tal arreglo y asegúrese de redactar un acuerdo para el préstamo junto con su aval.

Deudas y problemas de crédito

Cuando solicita un préstamo hipotecario, los prestamistas examinan su historial crediticio, el cual detalla su crédito personal en un reporte. Los prestamistas también analizan sus deudas y responsabilidades actuales, las cuales usted proporciona en su solicitud para la hipoteca. Sus deudas actuales e historial crediticio pueden producir varias advertencias que hagan que los prestamistas vacilen en cuanto a darle el préstamo. Esta sección le dice cómo enfrentarse con los problemas típicos que les preocupan a los prestamistas.

Errores tontos en el reporte de créditos

Como seguramente ya sabe, los acreedores pueden reportar sus incumplimientos e impagos de los préstamos a las agencias de crédito. Estas manchas aparecerán en su reporte de créditos.

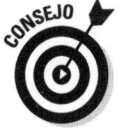

Este es el plan de ataque que sugerimos para resolver esos problemas:

- **Sea competente y hágale frente.** Si usted sabe que su crédito incluye defectos e imperfectos, escriba una carta concisa al prestamista explicando el porqué de las imperfecciones. Por ejemplo, quizás hizo varios pagos a su préstamo tarde en una ocasión porque estaba fuera del país y no procesó sus cuentas a tiempo. O, quizás, perdió su trabajo inesperadamente y se atrasó en sus pagos hasta que encontró otro trabajo.

- **Compare servicios en la búsqueda de prestamistas comprensivos y flexibles.** Algunos prestamistas son más comprensivos al hecho de que usted es un ser humano y que ha cometido algunos errores. Al entrevistar prestamistas, pregunte si las manchas crediticias que tenga representarán un problema. También puede considerar contratar los servicios de un agente hipotecario que pueda estar más acostumbrado a enfrentar problemas de préstamos.

- **Hable con el vendedor cuando busque un préstamo.** Vendedores de propiedad que están interesados en ser prestamistas, también pueden ser flexibles. Como cosa sorprendente, algunos ni siquiera revisan su reporte crediticio. Aquellos que sí revisan su reporte crediticio puede que estén más dispuestos a perdonar problemas anteriores que los bancos, especialmente si hoy por hoy usted está económicamente bien y estable.

- **Pelee y corrija errores.** Las agencias de reportes de crédito y los acreedores que reportan información a ellas cometen errores. Desgraciadamente, en el mundo de las finanzas, usted es culpable hasta que convenza a las agencias de crédito que es inocente. Empiece por identificar la información equivocada en su reporte de crédito. Si la información equivocada se relaciona con una cuenta que usted nunca tuvo, comuníqueselo a la agencia de crédito para ver la posibilidad de que esa información perjudicial pertenezca al reporte de otra persona.

Si la información negativa *sí es* de una de sus cuentas, pero un acreedor (por ejemplo, el "Banco Usura", del que obtuvo un préstamo para automóvil) ha cometido un error, lo más seguro es que tenga que fastidiar al acreedor hasta que éste le comunique a la agencia de crédito que corrija el error. Para arreglar este tipo de errores, tiene que ser persistente y paciente. Por ley, las agencias de crédito tienen que responder a su petición en un periodo no mayor de 30 días. Si recibe puras evasivas de los representantes de servicio al cliente con los que habla al principio, pídales hablar con un supervisor o gerente hasta que quede satisfecho. Si esa técnica no funciona, encuentre el *Better Business Bureau* de su localidad (consulte la guía telefónica local), y someta una queja. También puede someter una declaración de desacuerdo o disconformidad en su reporte crediticio para que los posibles acreedores, tales como los prestamistas hipotecarios, puedan ver su versión de lo sucedido al solicitar su reporte de crédito. Pero, su mejor estrategia es hacer que eliminen la mala información de su reporte.

✔ **Consiga un aval.** Tal como sugerimos anteriormente, un aval, como un familiar, también puede ayudar con los problemas crediticios que estén impidiendo la aprobación de su solicitud para el préstamo.

✔ **Ahorre más y establezca un historial mejor.** Si puede continuar rentando, quizás lo mejor que puede hacer es esperarse un poco. ¿Qué caso tiene apurarse a comprar si los prestamistas le huyen como de una plaga, y lo rechazan o sólo le ofrecen préstamos con intereses altísimos? Dedíquese un par de años a ahorrar dinero y a mantener su crédito limpio, ¡y a la larga tendrá a los prestamistas tras de usted rogándole para hacer negocios!

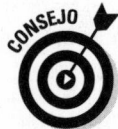

Si tiene problemas para lograr que le aprueben el crédito, hable con su agente de préstamos y haga una lista de los elementos que tiene que corregir para que se lo puedan dar. Así, en vez de tratar de adivinar qué es lo que está mal, tendrá una lista de todo lo que necesita corregir.

Deuda excesiva

Si le niegan la hipoteca a causa de deuda excesiva (como tarjetas de crédito y préstamos para autos), sea agradecido. ¡El prestamista de hecho le está haciendo un favor! A largo plazo, tal deuda es un obstáculo serio en relación a su capacidad para ahorrar dinero y vivir según sus ingresos.

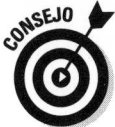

Si tiene dinero disponible para poder liquidar parte o toda su deuda, le recomendamos muchísimo hacerlo. Los prestamistas de hipotecas con frecuencia piden esto como condición para financiar una hipoteca, especialmente cuando tiene deudas grandes o cuando está en el límite para ver si puede ser aprobado para el préstamo que está pidiendo. Si no tiene suficiente dinero para pagar y disminuir su deuda, ni tampoco para comprar la casa que desea, escoja entre las siguientes opciones:

- ✔ **Propóngase metas más realistas.** Compre una casa menos costosa con un préstamo hipotecario para el cual usted reúne los requisitos.

- ✔ **Póngase a dieta económicamente.** La mejor manera de deshacerse de deudas de consumo es analizando detenidamente sus costumbres en cuanto a gastos (consulte el Capítulo 2) e identifique qué cosas puede recortar. Use sus ahorros para pagar y disminuir su deuda. También vea cómo incrementar sus ingresos.

- ✔ **Consiga ayuda de su familia.** Otra posible opción es pedirle ayuda a su familia ya sea con una firma de aval o con dinero prestado o regalado para pagar parte de su deuda de alto interés.

Puntuación de crédito (FICO)

Los prestamistas normalmente usan un sistema de puntuación para hacer más eficiente el procesamiento de solicitudes de crédito. El sistema de puntuación de crédito más usado por prestamistas hipotecarios es la puntuación FICO. FICO es abreviatura del nombre de la compañía que desarrolló este sistema: Fair Isaac Corporation.

Puntuaciones más altas significan que el prestatario tiene mucha más probabilidad de hacer pagos a tiempo y completos al tomar prestado el dinero. En otras palabras, tales prestatarios son del tipo que los prestamistas prefieren al dar préstamos y por lo general se consideran de "bajo riesgo".

Las puntuaciones de crédito como las de FICO se determinan usando información de su reporte de crédito. Como hay tres agencias de crédito principales (Equifax, Experian y TransUnion), usted puede tener una puntuación de cada uno de sus reportes FICO. (Hablamos sobre los reportes de crédito y cómo obtenerlos en el Capítulo 5.)

Si es que lo rechazan para un préstamo hipotecario o de otro tipo, pida una copia de su reporte de crédito y una explicación de su prestamista dando la razón específica por la cual se le negó el crédito. Usted puede mejorar su puntuación de crédito a través del tiempo resolviendo las preocupaciones de los prestamistas y usando las soluciones que le presentamos en otras partes de este capítulo para enfrentarse a los problemas comunes relacionados con la solicitud para una hipoteca.

La mejor defensa para no ser rechazado es examinar, entender y mejorar su puntuación de crédito *antes* de solicitar una hipoteca. Por favor, consulte el Capítulo 5 para todos los detalles.

Falta de dinero para el pago inicial

Ahorrar dinero en los Estados Unidos, en donde de un momento a otro *todo* se considera una necesidad, puede ser un gran reto. Si le falta dinero para el pago inicial, consulte las sugerencias en el Capítulo 3 de cómo conseguir financiamiento.

Cómo Enfrentar Sus Problemas de Avalúo

Puede ser que su solicitud para préstamo vaya viento en popa por los canales de aprobación de préstamos —gracias a su impecable (o al menos aceptable) situación económica— y luego, de repente, como en un episodio de Batman y Robin:

¡¡¡PUF!!! ¡¡¡PAF!!! ¡¡¡PUM!!! ¡¡¡ZAS!!!

La propiedad de la que se ha enamorado no vale lo que usted se comprometió a pagar por ella, al menos no según el *valuador* —la persona que valúa la propiedad para los prestamistas. Es posible que usted quede pasmado, desilusionado o hasta espantado porque el valuador haya dado una valuación muy baja. El plan de acción que debe de tomar depende de cual de los siguientes tres problemas causaron la baja valuación.

Usted ha pagado por demás

Generalmente, las valuaciones no resultan más bajas que el precio de compra en el contrato. Pero cuando esto sucede, casi siempre es porque usted (y quizás su agente de bienes raíces) sobreestimó el valor de la casa. Si éste es el caso, agradezca que el valuador le ha proporcionado una enorme advertencia de que está a punto de tirar su dinero (quizás miles de dólares) a la basura si decide llevar a cabo el pago del precio especificado en su contrato de compra. También es posible que la valuación haya sido baja porque la casa necesita un techo nuevo, cimientos nuevos o alguna otra reparación estructural importante. (Cubrimos la inspección de propiedades en el Capítulo 13).

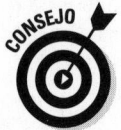

Como obviamente le gusta la propiedad (después de todo, ya hizo una oferta para comprarla) use la valuación como herramienta ya sea para renegociar un precio más bajo con el vendedor o para obtener un descuento del vendedor para hacer las reparaciones necesarias. Si el vendedor no está dispuesto a hacer eso, busque otra propiedad. También evalúe nuevamente el conocimiento de su agente de inmuebles acerca del valor de las propiedades y sus motivos —considere buscar un nuevo agente si el agente actual lo incitó a pagar demás.

El valuador no conoce su zona

Si usted y su agente conocen el valor de las propiedades locales y han visto casas comparables que justifican por completo el precio que se comprometió a pagar, es posible que el valuador simplemente no conozca el valor de las propiedades en esa zona. Un indicio de que éste pueda ser el caso es si el valuador no valúa viviendas en su zona normalmente. Otro indicio sería si las propiedades que escogió para la comparación no son similares ni representativas de la zona. Hablamos detalladamente sobre lo que es y no es una propiedad comparativamente similar en el Capítulo 10.

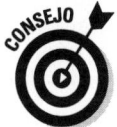

Si tiene motivo para creer que el valuador puede estar equivocado, exprese sus preocupaciones al prestamista de la hipoteca con el que está trabajando. Pida también una copia del avalúo, esto es algo a lo que tiene derecho. El prestamista puede darle más información sobre los antecedentes y la experiencia del valuador en la valuación de casas en su localidad. Algunas veces puede pedir un nuevo avalúo sin cargo adicional.

El valuador o el prestamista están frustrando sus esfuerzos

La explicación menos probable del porqué de una valuación baja es que su prestamista hipotecario pudo haber registrado un avalúo bajo para liberarse de darle un préstamo que considera poco deseable. Dentro de la industria, a este tipo de engaño se le conoce como *sandbagging*.

Las entidades crediticias que usan valuadores internos son los que mejor pueden deshacerse de un préstamo que no quieren dar. Quizás se pregunte, ¿por qué lo engañaría de esta manera un prestamista con un préstamo para el cual ha aceptado tan de buena gana su solicitud? Recuerde que lo más seguro que pasó es que el empleado entusiasta en el banco hipotecario o el agente hipotecario que asignó su préstamo a la entidad, trabajan a comisión y no son las personas que toman las decisiones dentro de la compañía para aprobar una hipoteca.

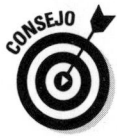

Si sospecha que su préstamo está siendo valuado por debajo del precio real (*sandbagging*), pida una copia del avalúo. Si los datos de ventas de viviendas similares muestran que la valuación está baja, plantéele a su entidad crediticia este problema y vea qué le responde al respecto. Si le da la vuelta y usted no está satisfecho, pida un reembolso completo del dinero de su solicitud para el préstamo y del gasto por el avalúo, y haga su negociación con otra entidad hipotecaria. También puede considerar el someter una queja al organismo estatal que rige a los prestamistas hipotecarios en su localidad.

Esa Montaña de Papeles para Préstamos Hipotecarios

Cuando finalmente llegue a la parte de la compra de la vivienda en la que está solicitando la hipoteca, es factible que se canse de tanto papeleo que soñará con una sociedad en donde todo se realice sin papel. Quizás le interese saber que algunos prestamistas (especialmente los prestamistas que están usando los servicios de la Internet, sobre los cuales hablaremos detalladamente en el Capítulo 11) están cambiando hacia procesos basados en programas de computación (y menos basados en papel y tinta) para sus solicitudes. Eso no importa ahora porque de cualquier manera tendrá que proporcionar mucha información personal y financiera.

En esta sección veremos los documentos que normalmente se le pedirán que llene en el proceso para la solicitud de una hipoteca. Si está trabajando con una persona con experiencia en la compañía hipotecaria o ha escogido un agente hipotecario, estas personas le pueden ayudar a navegar a través de la mayor parte de esta montaña de papeles.

Pero sabemos que probablemente tiene preguntas sobre el tipo de información que tiene que proporcionar y la información que no tiene que proporcionar. También es posible que no esté a gusto revelando ciertos datos, digamos poco favorables, sobre su situación, datos que quizás crea que puedan poner en peligro la aprobación de su préstamo. Finalmente, no importa qué tan buena sea la persona con la que esté trabajando para sacar el préstamo, la responsabilidad de acumular los datos, los montos y documentos sigue siendo suya. Así que aquí estamos junto con usted para guiarlo y persuadirlo todo el camino.

Lista de quehaceres relacionados con los documentos requeridos

Muchas compañías hipotecarias le proporcionan una lista increíblemente larga de información que requieren junto con la solicitud para la hipoteca (vea la Figura 7-1). ¡Un vistazo rápido a la lista es suficiente como para hacer que la mayoría de posibles compradores opten por seguir alquilando!

Pero no pierda las esperanzas. Esta lista tiene que cubrir todas las posibles situaciones, así que puede que algunas de las preguntas o datos pedidos no le conciernen a usted. Esperamos que, por ejemplo, no esté recibiendo un diploma ni divorciándose, o mudándose por su trabajo o llenando papeles para declararse en bancarrota, ¡todo al mismo tiempo!

La mayoría de la información de esta lista se requiere para comprobar y corroborar su estado financiero actual ante la compañía hipotecaria y, subsecuentemente, ante otras organizaciones que pudieran comprar su préstamo en un futuro. Los recibos de pago, las declaraciones de impuestos y los estados de cuentas bancarios y de inversiones ayudan a documentar sus ingresos y bienes. Los prestamistas evalúan el riesgo de prestarle dinero y determinan cuánto pueden prestarle basándose en esa lista.

Si se está preguntando por qué los prestamistas no pueden confiar en su palabra en cuanto a hechos y cifras financieras, personales y confidenciales, recuerde que hay personas que no dicen la verdad. A pesar de que sabemos que usted es una persona sincera, los prestamistas no tienen forma de saber quién es sincero y quién no lo es. Las consecuencias, desafortunadamente, son que los prestamistas tienen que tratar a todos los solicitantes como si no lo fueran.

LO QUE DEBE LLEVAR AL SOLICITAR SU PRÉSTAMO

Use la siguiente lista para verificar que lleva consigo todos los documentos requeridos para que la experiencia de solicitar su préstamo sea fácil y sin problemas. <u>SE REQUIEREN LOS ORIGINALES A MENOS QUE SE INDIQUE LO CONTRARIO.</u>

_____ **El contrato de compra y venta** (la compra de la nueva casa)

_____ **Recibos originales de sueldos o salarios de los últimos 30 días** (que reflejen sus ingresos del año en curso hasta el presente, su nombre y número de seguro social)

_____ **Documentos originales de los formularios W-2 de los últimos 2 años más recientes**

_____ **Declaraciones de impuestos Federales de los últimos 2 años más recientes** (con todos los anexos y firmados con tinta azul)

_____ **Estados de Pérdidas y Ganancias del año en curso y Balances de cuentas bancarias vigentes** (si es trabajador independiente únicamente)

_____ **Información sobre su historial residencial** (de los últimos 2 años, direcciones y fechas)

_____ **Talón de pagos o estados de cuentas más recientes de cualquier préstamo y de las tarjetas de crédito**

_____ **Estados de cuenta de todas sus cuentas bancarias de los últimos 3 meses** (en caso de cuentas abiertas recientemente o de depósitos considerables, traer documentación para probar el origen de esos fondos)

_____ **Estados de cuenta de su plan de jubilación IRA/Keogh/401K/Participaciones de los últimos 3 meses**

_____ **Certificado de estudios o diploma** (si ha sido estudiante en los últimos 2 años)

_____ **Información sobre préstamos y rentas de inmuebles que le pertenecen y sus direcciones** (si aplican)

_____ **Nombre, teléfono y dirección de su arrendador actual o cheques cancelados de los últimos 12 meses**

_____ **Copia del contrato de venta** (si está vendiendo su casa actual)

_____ **Papeles de divorcio o de acuerdo de separación legal completos** (si paga o recibe manutención de menores o pensión alimenticia)

_____ **Acuerdo de traslado** (si lo están trasladando a esta localidad)

_____ **Documentos de bancarrota, incluyendo plan de pagos a acreedores y documentos de descarga** (si aplica)

_____ **Carta de indemnización y copia del cheque más reciente** (si recibe beneficios del seguro social, de jubilación o incapacidad)

_____ **Comprobante de pago de sus coches** (si los coches tienen 5 años o menos)

_____ **Copia de la licencia para conducir y del seguro social** (préstamos FHA únicamente)

_____ **Certificado original de elegibilidad y el DD214** (si solicita un préstamo VA únicamente)

_____ $_____ **Cheque para el Avalúo y el Reporte de Crédito**

Figura 7-1: Éste es un ejemplo de los muchísimos documentos que su entidad crediticia le pedirá que le entregue.

A pesar de que los prestamistas requieren toda esta documentación, aún así algunos compradores falsifican información. Peor aún, algunos agentes hipotecarios animan a los compradores a mentir para poder llenar los requisitos para el préstamo, con el fin de ellos poder cerrar más préstamos y ganar más en comisiones. Un ejemplo de cómo algunas personas hacen trampas: algunas personas que trabajan independientemente inventan declaraciones de impuestos falsas con ingresos exagerados. A pesar de que algunas personas se han salido con la suya con tales engaños, le recomendamos mucho que no siga este camino impredecible —es un fraude.

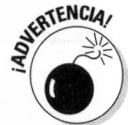

La falsificación de un documento para un préstamo es perjurio y fraude y no es de beneficio para usted. Aparte de las repercusiones legales obvias, puede acabar con más deuda hipotecaria de la que realmente puede pagar. Además, los prestamistas hipotecarios pueden darse cuenta de sus mentiras. ¿Cómo? Bueno, muchos de los prestamistas le piden que firme un contrato (al cerrar el contrato de la casa o durante el proceso de compra o al solicitar el préstamo) que les permite a ellos pedir directamente al *IRS* una copia de la declaración de impuestos que usted presentó. El *Formulario 4506* le da permiso al prestamista a obtener copia de su declaración de impuestos. Otro documento con el que lo puede sorprender el prestamista es el *Formulario 8821,* que los prestamistas le dan a prestatarios que no tienen un buen reporte. Este formulario le pide al *IRS* que confirme específica información y, lo más probable es que el prestatario es quien lo solicite para verificar su información financiera tal y como usted la reportó por motivos de impuestos (vea la Figura 7-2). Típicamente recibirá todos estos documentos al cerrar la compra, y usted puede rehusarse a firmarlos, pero claro, ¡el prestamista puede entonces negarse a darle el préstamo!

Cuando no reúne los requisitos para una hipoteca, sin tener que recurrir a engaños, el rechazo es por su propio bien. Los prestamistas tienen criterios para asegurarse de que usted va a poder pagar el dinero que toma prestado y de que usted no se sobre extienda.

Permisos para inspeccionar sus finanzas

Para que un prestamista hipotecario realice una evaluación apropiada de su situación financiera presente, el prestamista necesita pedir una detallada documentación. Por lo tanto, los prestamistas hipotecarios o los agentes de bienes raíces piden que firme una autorización (como la de la Figura 7-3) que los autoriza y les permite pedir tal documentación de su empleador y de las instituciones financieras con las que usted tiene relaciones comerciales, y también de otras instituciones.

Tal y como lo recomendamos en varias partes de este libro, antes de hacer un negocio con una compañía de préstamos hipotecarios, usted debe obtener *por escrito* un estimado de cuáles serán sus gastos extras para poder efectuar la compra. La buena nueva para usted es que al prestamista se le requiere, por ley, que le proporcione a usted un *Cálculo aproximado de buena fe* de los costos de cierre, en un período no mayor de tres días, después de haber iniciado el proceso de compra con ellos.

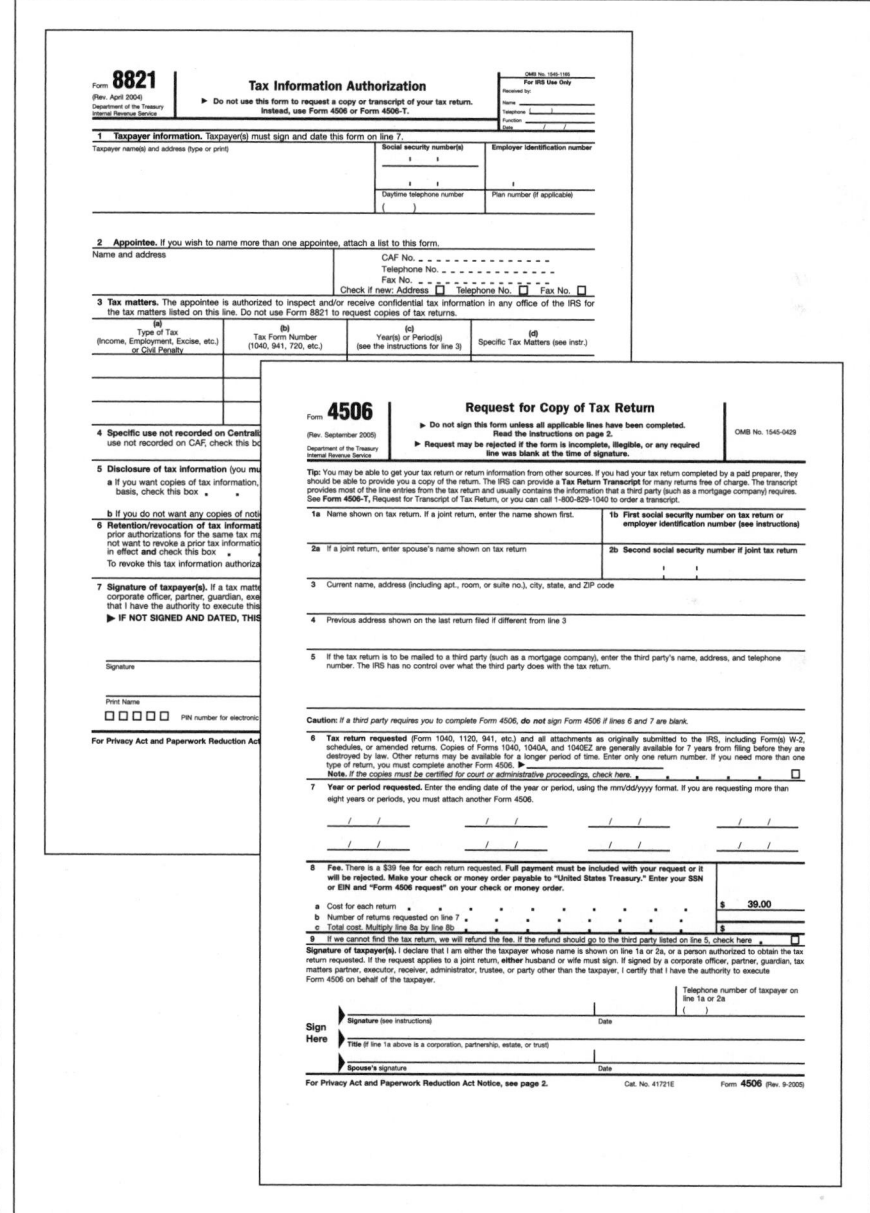

Figura 7-2:
Estos documentos pueden sorprenderlo entre los papeles de cierre que la entidad crediticia le entregue.

AUTORIZACIÓN

Por medio de la presente yo (nosotros) autorizo (autorizamos) a ComUnity Lending para verificar la información necesaria en relación a la solicitud de un préstamo hipotecario *F.H.A., V.A.* o Conventional o Second Trust Deed/Equity Line. Dicha información incluye, pero no está limitada a lo siguiente:

1. *Historial crediticio*
2. *Historial laboral*
3. *Cuentas bancarias*
4. *Historial hipotecario*

Además, esta autorización le da el derecho a ComUnity Lending a usar una copia fotostática de mi (nuestras) firma(s) abajo, con el objeto de obtener información relacionada en cualquiera de los puntos anteriormente mencionados.

_____
SOLICITANTE (Prestatario)

_____
NÚMERO DE SEGURO SOCIAL

_____
SOLICITANTE (Prestatario)

_____
NÚMERO DE SEGURO SOCIAL

CLU/CR

Figura 7-3: Este tipo de documento le da permiso a su entidad hipotecaria o agente a verificar y documentar los datos financieros de su vida.

Solicitud para préstamo hipotecario residencial uniforme

Este es el pez gordo, toda la enchilada o como lo quiera llamar. Los prestamistas y los agentes hipotecarios a lo largo de este vasto país usan la "Solicitud para Préstamo Hipotecario Residencial Uniforme" (*The Uniform Residencial Loan Application*) para obtener datos esenciales sobre compras de casas y de préstamos propuestos. Muchas entidades crediticias usan este documento estándar, conocido como el *Formulario 1003* dentro de la industria hipotecaria, porque venden sus hipotecas a inversionistas. Cuando los préstamos hipotecarios se venden, las organizaciones gubernamentales llamadas Fannie Mae y Freddie Mac aceptan garantizar (si es que los préstamos hipotecarios cumplen con los requisitos estándares federales) el pago del capital y de los intereses, lo cual hace más fácil para los prestamistas vender sus préstamos y para los inversionistas el querer comprarlos.

Algunos prestamistas hipotecarios quizás le den el *Formulario 1003* y esperarán que lo llene y lo entregue. Otros prestamistas y agentes lo ayudarán a llenarlo y, algunas veces, hasta lo llenan por usted.

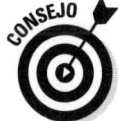

Si usted le permite a alguien llenar la solicitud de su préstamo hipotecario residencial uniforme por usted, sepa que usted sigue siendo responsable de que la información en el formulario sea correcta y verdadera. También esté consciente de que en sus esfuerzos por vender, algunas entidades hipotecarias y agentes puede que lo inviten a sus oficinas o se invitan a sí mismos a su casa u oficina para completar este formulario por usted o con usted. Aunque el buen servicio no lo vemos como problema, sí queremos que tenga en mente que usted no tiene ningún compromiso ni obligación para con los prestamistas o agentes, ¡aunque se ofrezcan ir a su casa a lavarle el carro y a darle un "pedicure"! El dinero es suyo y es su compra, así que compare préstamos o agentes hipotecarios. (También guarde una copia de todos los formularios que haya llenado para un prestamista hipotecario para ahorrar tiempo en caso de que quiera solicitar el préstamo con otro prestamista.)

Si usted hace el primer intento de llenar el formulario sólo, como la mayoría de la gente, nos parece que las siguientes secciones (en las que le explicamos paso a paso las partes más importantes de esta solicitud) le serán útiles.

1. Tipo de hipoteca y condiciones del préstamo

Los puntos principales que le conciernen en la primera sección de la solicitud (vea la Figura 7-4) son el monto del préstamo (*cantidad*), la *tasa de interés,* la duración del préstamo (*Nº de meses*) y el tipo de préstamo (tasa de interés fija o ajustable [*ARM*, por sus siglas en inglés]). Si al momento de estar solicitando su hipoteca, no está seguro de algunas de estas opciones o de lo que va a escoger, simplemente deje las casillas en blanco.

Su entidad crediticia o agente hipotecario llenarán las casillas, en esta sección, que no tienen sentido para usted — *Número de préstamo de la agencia* y *Número de préstamo del prestamista.* ¡No llene estas casillas!

11. Información de la propiedad y propósito del préstamo

Su entidad hipotecaria o prestador tiene curiosidad por saber por qué quiere pedir prestado esa enorme cantidad de dinero que puso en la parte I —por consiguiente, le pide que llene la parte II (vea la Figura 7-5). Además de querer saber la dirección de la propiedad, también quiere saber la descripción legal de la propiedad. La *Descripción legal de la propiedad* en cuestión se refiere simplemente al número de la cuadra y del lote de la propiedad que se obtiene del reporte titular preliminar. Tanto su agente como su entidad hipotecaria y usted deben tener copias de este reporte después de haber firmado el acuerdo de compra.

Figura 7-4:
En la Parte I
de la
Solicitud
para
Préstamo
Hipotecario
Residencial
Uniforme,
usted
explica en
detalle el
tipo de
préstamo
que quiere
y las
condiciones.

I. TYPE OF MORTGAGE AND TERMS OF LOAN/*TIPO DE HIPOTECA Y CONDICIONES DEL PRÉSTAMO*				
Mortgage Applied for/ *Préstamo Hipotecario Solicitado:*	☐ VA/*VA* ☐ FHA/*FHA*	☐ Conventional/*Convencional* ☐ USDA/Rural Housing Service *USDA/Servicio Rural de Vivienda*	☐ Other (explain)/ *Otro (explique)*:	Agency Case Number/ *Nº de Préstamo de la Agencia*	Lender Case Number/ *Nº de Préstamo del Prestador*
Amount/*Cantidad Total del Préstamo* $	Interest Rate/ *Tasa de Interés* %	No. of Months/ *Plazo (Meses)*	Amortization Type/ *Tipo de Amortización:*	☐ Fixed Rate/ *Tasa Fija* ☐ GPM/*GPM*	☐ Other (explain)/ *Otro (explique)*/ ☐ ARM (type)/ *ARM (tipo)*:

La información que usted incluya en la sección *Propósito del préstamo* le dice al prestamista si piensa usar la hipoteca para comprar una casa, refinanciar un préstamo existente o construir una casa nueva (Construcción). El prestamista también quiere saber si la propiedad va a ser su residencia principal o secundaria o una propiedad para inversión. Sus respuestas a estas preguntas determinarán qué tipo de préstamo su propiedad puede tener y las condiciones del mismo. Desde el punto de vista del prestamista, los préstamos de construcción y préstamos de propiedades para inversión son más riesgosos que otros préstamos y, por lo general, tienen tasas de interés más altas.

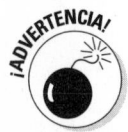

Quizás usted esté tentado (como también lo han estado algunos agentes hipotecarios) a mentir en esta parte de la solicitud hipotecaria para obtener condiciones más favorables para el préstamo. Esté consciente de que las entidades hipotecarias pueden —y a veces deciden— exigirle que compruebe que va a estar viviendo en la propiedad si sospechan lo contrario. Aún después de cerrar la compra y su préstamo, se ha visto que los prestamistas piden pruebas de que el prestatario está viviendo en la propiedad. Es posible que le pidan facturas de servicios públicos (para ver si las facturas están a su nombre) y ¡hasta se ha visto que algunas entidades crediticias mandan a un representante a que toque a las puertas de sus prestatarios para ver quién está viviendo en la vivienda!

Al momento en que usted solicita su hipoteca, tiene que declarar cómo va a registrar el título de la propiedad —en pocas palabras, cómo se estructurará la posesión de la casa para propósitos legales. Cubrimos esta importante decisión en el Capítulo 14.

II. PROPERTY INFORMATION AND PURPOSE OF LOAN/*INFORMACIÓN SOBRE LA PROPIEDAD Y PROPÓSITO DEL PRÉSTAMO*

Subject Property Address (street, city, state & ZIP)/ *Dirección de la Propiedad (calle, ciudad, estado y código postal)* — No. of Units/ *Nº de Unidades*

Legal Description of Subject Property (attach description if necessary)/ *Descripción Legal de la Propiedad (adjunte descripción si es necesario)* — Year Built/ *Año de Construcción*

Purpose of Loan/ *Propósito del Préstamo*
☐ Purchase/*Compra* ☐ Construction/*Construcción* ☐ Other (explain)/ *Otro (explique)*
☐ Refinance/ *Refinanciamiento* ☐ Construction-Permanent/ *Financiamiento Permanente de Construcción*

Property will be/*La propiedad será:*
☐ Primary Residence/ *Residencia Principal* ☐ Secondary Residence/ *Residencia Secundaria* ☐ Investment/ *Inversión*

Complete this line if construction or construction-permanent loan./ *Complete esta línea si es un préstamo para construcción o financiamiento permanente de construcción.*

Year Lot Acquired/ *Año en que se Adquirió el Lote*	Original Cost/ *Costo Original*	Amount Existing Liens/ *Monto de los Gravámenes Actuales*	(a) Present Value of Lot/ *Valor Actual del Lote*	(b) Cost of Improvements/ *Costo de las Mejoras*	Total (a + b)/ *Total (a + b)*
	$	$	$	$	$

Complete this line if this is a refinance loan./ *Complete esta línea si es un préstamo de refinanciamiento.*

Year Acquired/ *Año en que se Adquirió*	Original Cost/ *Costo Original*	Amount Existing Liens/ *Monto de los Gravámenes Actuales*	Purpose of Refinance/ *Propósito del Refinanciamiento*	Describe Improvements/ *Descripción de las Mejoras*	☐ made/ *realizadas* ☐ to be made/ *por realizarse*
	$	$		Cost/*Costo:* $	

Title will be held in what Name(s) /*Nombre(s) que se Registrará(n) en el Título*

Manner in which Title will be held/ *Manera en que se Registrará el Título*

Estate will be held in/ *La propiedad se mantendrá en:*
☐ Fee Simple/ *Pleno Dominio*
☐ Leasehold (show expiration date)/ *Arrendamiento (indique fecha de vencimiento)*

Source of Down Payment, Settlement Charges, and/or Subordinate Financing (explain)/ *Origen de Pago Inicial, Costos de Cierre y/o Financiamiento Subordinado (explique)*

Figura 7-5: La descripción legal de la propiedad y lo que va a hacer con el préstamo.

A las entidades hipotecarias también les gusta saber de dónde proviene su pago inicial y el pago de los costos de cierre para asegurarse de que el dinero no es de otro préstamo adicional que pueda ser un problema en cuanto a su capacidad para pagar el dinero que ellas le están prestando. Lo ideal para los prestamistas es ver que el pago inicial y el dinero para los costos del cierre vengan de sus cuentas de ahorros. Diga la verdad —los prestamistas tienen muchas maneras de hacerlo caer en sus propias trampas aquí. Por ejemplo, pueden pedir ver los estados de cuenta de su cuenta bancaria o de inversión de los últimos meses para verificar que, por ejemplo, un familiar no le haya dado el dinero recientemente.

III. Información del prestatario

En la tercera parte de la *Solicitud para préstamo hipotecario residencial uniforme* (vea la Figura 7-6) es donde a usted le toca escribir su nombre, años de educación y número de serie. Si está comprando la propiedad con alguien más, como su cónyuge, tiene el privilegio adicional de proporcionar la información de la otra persona también.

Años de educación simplemente se refiere al número total de años de estudios formales que ha estudiado. Si se graduó de la secundaria o preparatoria, tiene 12 años de escuela. Las universidades de dos y cuatro años agregan ese número de años a los 12 anteriores. Si se aventó a estudiar el postgrado, agregue el número de años que se dedicó a la lucha por esos pedacitos de papeles adicionales que colgó en la pared de su oficina o sala.

Borrower/*Prestatario*				III. BORROWER INFORMATION/ *INFORMACIÓN SOBRE EL PRESTATARIO*	Co-Borrower/*Co-Prestatario*			

Figura 7-6: Parte III dice, "Ahora, cuéntenos sobre usted. . ."

III. BORROWER INFORMATION/ *INFORMACIÓN SOBRE EL PRESTATARIO*

Borrower's Name (include Jr. or Sr. if applicable)/ *Nombre del Prestatario (indique Jr., o Sr. si aplica)*

Co-Borrower's Name (include Jr. or Sr. if applicable)/ *Nombre del Co-Prestatario (indique Jr., o Sr. si aplica)*

Social Security Number/ *Número de Seguro Social*	Home Phone (incl. area code)/ *Teléfono de la Casa (incluya código de área)*	DOB (mm/dd/yyyy)/ *Fecha de nacimiento (mm/dd/aaaa)*	Yrs. School/ *Años de Educación*	Social Security Number/ *Número de Seguro Social*	Home Phone (incl. area code)/ *Teléfono de la Casa (incluya código de área)*	DOB (mm/dd/yyyy)/ *Fecha de nacimiento (mm/dd/aaaa)*	Yrs. School/ *Años de Educación*

☐ Married *Casado* ☐ Unmarried (include single, divorced, widowed)/ *No está casado (incluye soltero, divorciado, viudo)* ☐ Separated *Separado*

Dependents (not listed by Co-Borrower)/ *Dependientes (no incluidos por el Co-Prestatario)*   No./*Nº*   Ages/*Edades*

☐ Married *Casado* ☐ Unmarried (include single, divorced, widowed)/ *No está casado (incluye soltero, divorciado, viudo)* ☐ Separated *Separado*

Dependents (not listed by Borrower)/ *Dependientes (no incluidos por el Prestatario)*   No./*Nº*   Ages/*Edades*

Present Address (street, city, state, ZIP)/ *Dirección Actual (calle, ciudad, estado, código postal)*   ☐ Own *Propietario* ☐ Rent *Inquilino* ___ No. Yrs./ *Nº de Años*

Present Address (street, city, state, ZIP)/ *Dirección Actual (calle, ciudad, estado, código postal)*   ☐ Own *Propietario* ☐ Rent *Inquilino* ___ No. Yrs./ *Nº de Años*

Mailing Address, if different from Present Address/ *Dirección donde recibe su correspondencia, si es diferente de su dirección actual*

Mailing Address, if different from Present Address/ *Dirección donde recibe su correspondencia, si es diferente de su dirección actual*

If residing at present address for less than two years, complete the following:/Si habita en dicha dirección hace menos de dos años, por favor complete:

Former Address (street, city, state, ZIP)/ *Dirección Anterior (calle, ciudad, estado, código postal)*   ☐ Own *Propietario* ☐ Rent *Inquilino* ___ No. Yrs./ *Nº de Años*

Former Address (street, city, state, ZIP)/ *Dirección Anterior (calle, ciudad, estado, código postal)*   ☐ Own *Propietario* ☐ Rent *Inquilino* ___ No. Yrs./ *Nº de Años*

La entidad crediticia también quiere saber dónde ha estado viviendo recientemente. (Además, la compañía necesita saber si la dirección donde recibe su correspondencia es diferente de la de su domicilio).

Los prestatarios están buscando estabilidad en esto. La mayoría de ellos también piden una carta de su arrendador para verificar que usted paga su renta a tiempo. Si se ha mudado frecuentemente en los últimos años, la mayoría de los prestamistas verificarán la información con otros arrendadores además de su último arrendador. Si su solicitud está en el límite de no ser aceptada, buenas referencias pueden darle un empujoncillo a su favor. Si ha pagado lo que debe y lo ha pagado a tiempo, no tiene nada de qué preocuparse. Pero, si no lo ha hecho, debería de explicarlo ya sea por medio de una carta aparte al prestamista o en el espacio en blanco en la página 8 de la solicitud.

IV. Información sobre el empleo

Tal como los prestamistas quieren saber sobre sus residencias recientes, también quieren saber sobre su historia laboral reciente. (Vea la Figura 7-7). Si ha estado en un empleo menos de dos años, ése es el único empleo que tiene que listar. De otra manera, necesita poner sus empleos anteriores hasta cubrir los últimos dos años. Nuevamente, el prestamista está buscando ver estabilidad, la cual puede ayudar a avanzar una solicitud marginal por los canales de la aprobación de su préstamo.

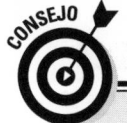

CONSEJO

¿Debería de excluir ciertos empleos y residencias de su solicitud para hipoteca?

Muchas personas que preparan un currículum vitae deciden omitir información sobre trabajos en los que estuvieron solamente por poco tiempo o residencias en donde vivieron por poco tiempo. Las razones varían al hacerlo, pero la mayoría de las personas lo hacen para que su currículum vitae se vea más completo y para evitar ser percibidos como pájaros saltarines.

Cuando hay intervalos de tiempo vacíos en su historia laboral, es mejor incluir el intervalo a que lo pillen con las manos en la masa — frecuentemente los prestamistas piden las fechas de sus empleos. No mienta; los prestamistas que se dan cuenta que ha mentido en una

cosa, examinan doblemente con cuidado su solicitud en busca de más fallas. A los prestamistas no les importan los cambios de empleos.

Otra sección de la verificación de empleo que recibe su empleador del prestamista, pregunta acerca de cuáles son sus prospectos en cuanto a continuar en ese empleo. La respuesta a esa pregunta también es importante.

De cierta manera, una solicitud para una hipoteca es como un currículum vitae. Necesita presentar su información de la mejor manera posible, pero siempre con la verdad.

Si usted es una persona que se fija en detalles, quizás se pregunte por qué la solicitud le pide su ingreso mensual de trabajos anteriores, pero no el del actual. La razón es que usted proporciona un ingreso para su posición presente en la siguiente sección de la solicitud (parte V).

Quizás también se pregunte (y le preocupe) por qué quiere el prestamista el teléfono de su jefe actual y de los anteriores. Es posible que el prestamista llame a su jefe, poco antes de que cierre la compra, para verificar si aún tiene trabajo; esta verificación normalmente se hace por correo. Es poco probable que el prestamista llame a sus jefes anteriores.

V. Ingresos mensuales y proyecciones de costos de vivienda

La parte V (vea la Figura 7-8) decide para bien o para mal el camino de muchas de las solicitudes. Aquí, usted da sus ingresos actuales, incluyendo lo que reciba de inversiones de cuentas bancarias, de corretaje y de fondos mutuales. Para la mayoría de las personas, sus sueldos son los que los ayuda a que les presten el dinero para la compra. Si sus ingresos fluctúan de un mes a otro, simplemente escriba el promedio de sus ingresos mensuales de los últimos 12 meses. (Algunos prestamistas usan el promedio de los últimos 24 meses si trabaja independientemente).

Borrower/*Prestatario*			IV. EMPLOYMENT INFORMATION/ *INFORMACIÓN SOBRE EL EMPLEO*	Co-Borrower/*Co-Prestatario*	
Name & Address of Employer/ *Nombre y Dirección del Empleador*	☐ Self Employed/ *Empleado por Cuenta Propia*	Yrs. on this job/ *Años en este trabajo* Yrs. employed in this line of work/profession/ *Años de empleo en este tipo de trabajo/profesión*		Name & Address of Employer/ *Nombre y Dirección del Empleador*	☐ SelfEmployed/ *Empleado por Cuenta Propia*	Yrs. on this job/ *Años en este trabajo* Yrs. employed in this line of work/profession/ *Años de empleo en este tipo de trabajo/profesión*
Position/Title/Type of Business/ *Posición/Título/Tipo de Negocio*		Business Phone (incl. area code)/*Teléfono en el lugar de trabajo (incluya código de área)*		Position/Title/Type of Business/ *Posición/Título/Tipo de Negocio*	Business Phone (incl. area code)/*Teléfono en el lugar de trabajo (incluya código de área)*

If employed in current position for less than two years or if currently employed in more than one position, complete the following:/
Si ha estado trabajando en la posición actual menos de dos años o si actualmente está empleado en más de una posición, complete lo siguiente:

Name & Address of Employer/ *Nombre y Dirección del Empleador*	☐ Self Employed/ *Empleado por Cuenta Propia*	Dates (from – to)/ *Fechas de empleo (desde – hasta)* Monthly Income/ *Ingreso Mensual* $	Name & Address of Employer/ *Nombre y Dirección del Empleador*	☐ Self Employed/ *Empleado por Cuenta Propia*	Dates (from – to)/ *Fechas de empleo (desde – hasta)* Monthly Income/ *Ingreso Mensual* $
Position/Title/Type of Business/ *Posición/Título/Tipo de Negocio*		Business Phone (incl. area code)/ *Teléfono en el lugar de trabajo (incluya código de área)*	Position/Title/Type of Business/ *Posición/Título/Tipo de Negocio*		Business Phone (incl. area code)/ *Teléfono en el lugar de trabajo (incluya código de área)*
Name & Address of Employer/ *Nombre y Dirección del Empleador*	☐ Self Employed/ *Empleado por Cuenta Propia*	Dates (from – to)/ *Fechas de empleo (desde – hasta)* Monthly Income/ *Ingreso Mensual* $	Name & Address of Employer/ *Nombre y Dirección del Empleador*	☐ Self Employed/ *Empleado por Cuenta Propia*	Dates (from – to)/ *Fechas de empleo (desde – hasta)* Monthly Income/ *Ingreso Mensual* $
Position/Title/Type of Business/ *Posición/Título/Tipo de Negocio*		Business Phone (incl. area code)/ *Teléfono en el lugar de trabajo (incluya código de área)*	Position/Title/Type of Business/ *Posición/Título/Tipo de Negocio*		Business Phone (incl. area code)/ *Teléfono en el lugar de trabajo (incluya código de área)*

Figura 7-7: En la parte IV, el prestamista quiere saber si su trabajo es estable.

V. MONTHLY INCOME AND COMBINED HOUSING EXPENSE INFORMATION/ *INFORMACIÓN SOBRE EL INGRESO Y LOS GASTOS MENSUALES COMBINADOS DE VIVIENDA*

Gross Monthly Income *Ingreso Bruto Mensual*	Borrower *Prestatario*	Co-Borrower *Co-Prestatario*	Total	Combined Monthly Housing Expense/*Gastos Mensuales Combinados de Vivienda*	Present *Actual*	Proposed *Propuesto*
Base Empl. Income* *Ingreso Básico del Empleado**	$	$		Rent *Alquiler*	$	
Overtime *Horas extra*				First Mortgage (P&I) *Hipoteca Principal (Principal e Interés)*		$
Bonuses *Pagas Extras*				Other Financing (P&I) *Otro Financiamiento (Principal e Interés)*		
Commissions *Comisiones*				Hazard Insurance *Seguro Contra Riesgos*		
Dividends/Interest *Dividendos/Intereses*				Real Estate Taxes *Impuestos Sobre Bienes Raíces*		
Net Rental Income *Ingreso Neto por Alquiler*				Mortgage Insurance *Seguro de Hipoteca*		
Other (before completing, see the notice in "describe other income", below) *Otros (antes de llenar, vea el aviso en "describa otros ingresos", a continuación)*				Homeowner Assn. Dues *Cuotas de la Asociación de Propietarios* Other: *Otro:*		
Total	$	$	$	Total	$	$

* Self Employed Borrower(s) may be required to provide additional documentation such as tax returns and financial statements.

* *Se podrá requerir al Prestatario o Prestatarios que trabajan por cuenta propia que proporcionen documentos adicionales, tales como
declaraciones y planillas de impuestos y estados financieros.*

Describe Other Income/ *Describa Otros Ingresos*

Notice: Alimony, child support, or separate maintenance income need not be revealed
if the Borrower (B) or Co-Borrower (C) does not choose to have it considered
for repaying this loan.

Aviso: *La pensión conyugal, pensión para el sustento de los hijos o ingreso de
mantenimiento por separación, no tienen que declararse si el Prestatario
(B) o Co-Prestatario (C) no desea que se considere para el pago de este Préstamo.*

B/C		Monthly Amount *Cantidad Mensual* $

Figura 7-8: ¿Cuánto gana y cuánto gastará?

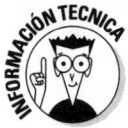

La propiedad rentada es propiedad que compró con el propósito de alquilarla. El *Ingreso neto por alquiler* se refiere a la diferencia entre las rentas mensuales recibidas por sus inmuebles alquilados y los gastos (excluyendo la depreciación). Por lo tanto, el *ingreso neto por alquiler* es la ganancia o pérdida que tiene cada mes por las propiedades alquiladas que le pertenecen (excluyendo la depreciación). Si ha comprado recientemente la propiedad para alquilar, el prestamista toma en cuenta solamente el 75 por ciento de la renta actual que está cobrando. Cuando haya tenido su propiedad para alquilar por suficiente tiempo y puede suministrar una declaración de impuestos, la mayoría de los prestamistas usan las ganancias o pérdidas reportadas en su declaración de impuestos (excluyendo la depreciación).

Si tiene otras fuentes de ingreso, tales como pensión para el sustento de los hijos o pensión alimenticia, detállelas en el renglón marcado *Otros*, y descríbalas en la última porción de esta sección. Cuantos más ingresos pueda poner, mejor preparado estará para ser aprobado para una hipoteca con condiciones más favorables para usted.

El renglón de *Gastos mensuales combinados de vivienda*, al lado derecho de esta sección, le permite calcular sus gastos caseros de hoy en día y los que propone que va a tener. Si está alquilando al presente, simplemente escriba el monto de su alquiler en la casilla que corresponde. Los gastos que propone tener se refieren a los gastos que calcula que tendrá después de que compre la casa. Su prestamista o agente hipotecario le pueden ayudar a llenar esta sección tan importante.

Si está estirando el dinero para comprar una vivienda, asegúrese de que los cálculos que su prestamista o agente inserten en la sección de gastos mensuales propuestos sean moderados y que no estén aumentados. Algunos prestamistas hipotecarios hacen cálculos demasiado altos porque están tratando de proteger sus espaldas y asegurándose de que usted no se sobre extienda. Si, por ejemplo, el prestamista hipotecario calcula que el seguro de propietario le costará $100 dólares al mes, pero usted ya tiene en la mano una buena cobertura por $80 dólares al mes, indíqueles la diferencia.

Si se da el caso en que usted está justo en el límite entre si le dan o no el préstamo, los prestamistas estarán menos dispuestos a dárselo si hay una diferencia grande entre sus gastos de vivienda actuales y los gastos que propone como propietario. Los prestamistas y agentes hipotecarios se refieren a personas en esta situación como personas que se exponen a sí mismas a un *susto de pago*. Si usted está en esta situación, debería de evaluar si realmente puede vivir con este aumento tan considerable en sus gastos de vivienda mensuales (consulte los Capítulos 2 y 3).

VI. Bienes y pasivos

En la parte VI (vea la Figura 7-9) usted presenta su balance general, el cual resume sus bienes (activos) y pasivos (responsabilidades). Sus bienes se dividen en activos líquidos (por ejemplo, cuentas que no son de jubilación) y activos que no son líquidos (tales como inmuebles). *Líquido*, en este ejemplo, significa simplemente los bienes que puede vender rápidamente para tener dinero constante y sonante en las manos para la compra de una casa o algún otro propósito.

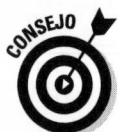

Nos confunde el porqué hay tantos espacios para las cuentas corrientes y de ahorros. Si no logra que quepan sus otros bienes de cuentas de corretaje o fondos mutuos de inversión (no asignados para su jubilación), en el pequeño espacio asignado para *Acciones y Bonos,* use los renglones vacíos designados para las cuentas bancarias y explique lo que está enumerando allí.

Los *Pasivos* son cualquier préstamo o deuda que tenga pendiente. Cuantas más obligaciones de éstas tenga, más resistirá el prestamista hipotecario en prestarle una cantidad grande de dinero.

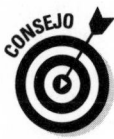

Cuando tenga el dinero disponible para poder pagar préstamos de consumo de alto costo, tales como préstamos de tarjetas de crédito y de automóvil, considere hacerlo sin demora. (Si escogió la opción de satisfacer los requisitos antes de hacer el préstamo o su aprobación previa, como lo presentamos en el Capítulo 6, lo más seguro es que el prestamista le recomendó que se deshiciera de las deudas en ese momento). Tales deudas por lo general tienen un interés alto que no es deducible de los impuestos y disminuyen sus posibilidades de obtener un préstamo hipotecario (consulte el Capítulo 3 para una explicación sobre este tema).

Figura 7-9:
¿Cuánto dinero y cuántos bienes tiene reservados para el pago inicial y para el cierre? ¿Y cuánto debe?

VI. ASSETS AND LIABILITIES/*BIENES Y PASIVOS*

This Statement and any applicable supporting schedules may be completed jointly by both married and unmarried Co-Borrowers if their assets and liabilities are sufficiently joined so that the Statement can be meaningfully and fairly presented on a combined basis; otherwise, separate Statements and Schedules are required. If the Co-Borrower section was completed about a non-applicant spouse or other person, this Statement and supporting schedules must be completed about that spouse or other person also.

Esta Declaración y cualquier anexo respaldatorio pertinente pueden llenarse conjuntamente tanto por Co-Prestatarios casados como no casados si sus bienes y deudas están suficientemente unidos de manera que la Declaración pueda presentarse con sentido sobre una base combinada y de una forma fiel; o de lo contrario, se requieren Declaraciones y Anexos por separado. Si en la sección del Co-Prestatario se completó la parte sobre el cónyuge, no solicitante u otra persona, esta Declaración y los anexos respaldatorios también deben completarse para dicho cónyuge u otra persona.

Completed/*Se completó* ☐ Jointly/*En Conjunto* ☐ Not Jointly/*Por Separado* ☐

ASSETS/*BIENES* Description/*Descripción*	Cash or Market Value/ *Valor en Efectivo o* *Valor en el Mercado*	Liabilities and Pledged Assets. List the creditor's name, address, and account number for all outstanding debts, including automobile loans, revolving charge accounts, real estate loans, alimony, child support, stock pledges, etc. Use continuation sheet, if necessary. Indicate by (*) those liabilities, which will be satisfied upon sale of real estate owned or upon refinancing of the subject property.
Cash deposit toward purchase held by:/ *Depósito en efectivo para* *la compra en poder de:*	$	*Deudas y Bienes Gravados.* *Indique al nombre, la dirección y el número de cuenta de todas las deudas pendientes, incluyendo préstamos para autos, cuentas de poder de: crédito rotativo, préstamos de bienes raíces, pensión conyugal, pensión para el sustento de hijos, valores gravados, etc. Si es necesario, use una hoja adicional. Indique con un (*) aquellas deudas que se satisfarán al venderse o refinanciarse la propiedad inmobiliaria en cuestión.*

		LIABILITIES/*PASIVOS*	Monthly Payment & Months Left to Pay/ *Pago Mensual y N° de Pagos Mensuales que quedan por pagar*	Unpaid Balance/ *Balance Pendiente*
List checking and savings accounts below/ *Indique abajo las cuentas de cheques y de ahorros*		Name and address of Company/ *Nombre y dirección de la Compañía*	$ Payment/Months *$ Pagos Meses*	$
Name and address of Bank, S&L, or Credit Union/ *Nombre y dirección del Banco, Asociación de Ahorro y Préstamo o* *Cooperativa de Crédito*				
		Acct. no./*N° de Cuenta*		
Acct. no./*N° de Cuenta*	$	Name and address of Company/ *Nombre y dirección de la Compañía*	$ Payment/Months *$ Pagos Meses*	$
Name and address of Bank, S&L, or Credit Union/ *Nombre y dirección del Banco, Asociación de Ahorro y Préstamo o* *Cooperativa de Crédito*				
		Acct. no./*N° de Cuenta/*		
Acct. no./*N° de Cuenta*	$	Name and address of Company/ *Nombre y dirección de la Compañía*	$ Payment/Months *$ Pagos Meses*	$
Name and address of Bank, S&L, or Credit Union/ *Nombre y dirección del Banco, Asociación de Ahorro y Préstamo o* *Cooperativa de Crédito*				
		Acct. no./*N° de Cuenta*		
Acct. no./*N° de Cuenta*	$	Name and address of Company/ *Nombre y dirección de la Compañía* creditor	$ Payment/Months *$ Pagos/Meses*	$
Name and address of Bank, S&L, or Credit Union/ *Nombre y dirección del Banco, Asociación de Ahorro y Préstamo o* *Cooperativa de Crédito*				
		Acct. no./*N° de Cuenta*		
Acct. no./*N° de Cuenta*	$	Name and address of Company/ *Nombre y dirección de la Compañía*	$ Payment/Months *$ Pagos/Meses*	$
Stocks & Bonds (Company name/number and description)/ *Acciones y Bonos (Nombre de la compañía número y descripción de los valores y bonos)*	$	Acct. no./*N° de Cuenta*		
Life insurance net cash value/ *Valor en efectivo neto del seguro de vida*	$	Name and address of Company/ *Nombre y dirección de la Compañía*	$ Payment/Months *$ Pagos/Meses*	$
Face amount: *Monto de la póliza:* $				
Subtotal Liquid Assets/ ***Subtotal de los Bienes Líquidos***	$			
Real estate owned (enter market value from schedule of real estate owned)/ *Propiedad inmobiliaria de la cual es dueño (indique el valor en el mercado según el anexo de la propiedad inmobiliaria)*	$			
Vested interest in retirement fund/ *Intereses adquiridos en el fondo de retiro*	$			
Net worth of business(es) owned (attach financial statement)/ *Valor neto de negocio(s) propio(s) (incluya estados financieros)*	$	Acct. no./*N° de Cuenta*		
Automobiles owned (make and year)/ *Automóviles de los cuales es dueño (marca y año)*	$	Alimony/Child Support/Separate Maintenance Payments Owed to:/ *Pensión Alimenticia Pensión Para el Sustento de los Hijos/Manutención por Separación:*	$	
Other Assets (itemize)/ *Otros Bienes (detalle)*	$	Job-Related Expense (child care, union dues, etc.)/ *Gastos Relacionados con el Empleo(cuidado de los hijos, cuotas de sindicatos, etc.)*	$	
		Total Monthly Payments/ ***Total de Pagos Mensuales***	$	
Total Assets a./ *Total de Bienes a.*	$	Net Worth (a minus b) ► *Valor Neto (a menos b)* $	Total Liabilities b. *Total de Pasivos b.* $	

Figura 7-9: *(continuado)*

Schedule of Real Estate Owned (If additional properties are owned, use continuation sheet.) *Anexo de Propiedades Inmobiliarias (Si es dueño de más propiedades, use la hoja a continuación.)*							
Property Address (enter S if sold, PS if pending sale or R if rental being held for income)/ *Dirección de la Propiedad (ponga una S por vendida, una PS por venta pendiente o una R si recibe ingreso por alquiler)* ▼	Type of Property/ *Tipo de Propiedad*	Present Market Value/ *Valor Actual en el Mercado*	Amount of Mortgages & Liens/ *Cantidad de Hipotecas y Gravámenes*	Gross Rental Income/ *Ingreso Bruto por Alquiler*	Mortgage Payments/ *Pagos Hipotecarios*	Insurance, Maintenance, Taxes & Misc./ *Seguro, Mantenimiento, Impuestos y Otros*	Net Rental Income/ *Ingreso Neto por Alquiler*
		$	$	$	$	$	$
	Totals/ *Totales*	$	$	$	$	$	$

List any additional names under which credit has previously been received and indicate appropriate creditor name(s) and account number(s):/ *Indique otros nombres bajo los cuales ha recibido crédito anteriormente, así como los nombres de los acreedores y el número de las cuentas.*

Alternate Name/*Otro Nombre*   Creditor Name/*Nombre del Acreedor*   Account Number/*Número de Cuenta*

Figura 7-9: *(continuado)*

Fíjese (al final de la columna de pasivos) que tiene que poner la manutención de menores y los pagos de manutención por separación que hace, y también de los gastos que tenga que se relacionen con su trabajo, si no trabaja independientemente. Tales gastos mensuales son como deudas en el sentido de que hay que pagarlos mensualmente.

La parte VI continúa en las páginas 4 y 5 e incluye renglones para los detalles de bienes raíces o inmuebles que ya tenga. Si obtiene ganancias de tales propiedades, las ganancias pueden ayudarlo a mejorar sus probabilidades de llenar los requisitos para otras hipotecas. Pero, un *flujo de efectivo negativo* (los gastos de propiedad son mayores que sus ingresos) de propiedades que tiene en alquiler reduce la cantidad que un prestamista hipotecario le prestará. La mayoría de los prestamistas hipotecarios quieren una copia de su declaración de impuestos (y posiblemente de sus contratos de arrendamiento de sus inquilinos) para verificar la información que puso en este espacio.

VII. Detalles de la transacción

En la parte VII (vea la Figura 7-10) usted detalla las condiciones de compra de la vivienda que desea comprar. El propósito de la primera parte de esta sección es calcular el costo total de la vivienda, incluyendo los costos de cierre. Después de restar el monto solicitado del préstamo, esta columna da la cantidad de dinero que necesita conseguir para cerrar el negocio de la compra de la casa. Algunos posibles compradores descubren que después de llenar esta sección, tienen que ir a suplicarles a sus familiares por dinero o pedir más dinero prestado para cerrar la compra.

VIII. Declaraciones

La parte VIII (vea la Figura 7-11) no debería llamarse *Declaraciones;* debería llamarse: *¡Interrogatorio personal!*

Las preguntas de la *a* a la *i* (arriba de la línea quebrada) son posibles advertencias para los prestamistas. Si contesta sí a cualquiera de estas preguntas, explique la razón en una página aparte o en el espacio en blanco en la página 8 de la solicitud.

VII. DETAILS OF TRANSACTION/ *DETALLES DE LA TRANSACCIÓN*		
a.	Purchase price/*Precio de compra*	$
b.	Alterations, improvements, repairs/ *Remodelaciones, mejoras, reparaciones*	
c.	Land (if acquired separately)/ *Terreno (si fue adquirido por separado)*	
d.	Refinance (incl. debts to be paid off)/ *Refinanciamiento (incluya deudas que se pagarán)*	
e.	Estimated prepaid items/ *Estimado de partidas prepagadas*	
f.	Estimated closing costs/ *Estimado de los costos de cierre*	
g.	PMI, MIP, Funding Fee/ *Seguro de hipoteca privado (PMI), Primas de seguro de hipoteca (MIP), Costos de Financiamiento*	
h.	Discount (if Borrower will pay)/ *Descuento (si el Prestatario lo pagará)*	
i.	Total costs (add items a through h)/ **Total de costos (sume las líneas "a" hasta la "h")**	
j.	Subordinate financing/ *Financiamiento subordinado*	
k.	Borrower's closing costs paid by Seller/ *Costos de cierre del Prestatario pagados por el Vendedor*	
l.	Other Credits (explain)/ *Otros Créditos (explique)*	
m.	Loan amount (exclude PMI, MIP, Funding Fee financed)/ *Cantidad del Préstamo (excluya PMI, MIP, Costos de Financiamiento financiados)*	
n.	PMI, MIP, Funding Fee financed/ *Seguro de hipoteca privado (PMI), Primas de seguro de hipoteca (MIP), Costos de Financiamiento financiados*	
o.	Loan amount (add m & n) / *Cantidad del Préstamo (sume líneas "m" y "n")*	
p.	Cash from/to Borrower (subtract j, k, l & o from i)/ *Dinero del / para el Prestatario (reste j, k, l & o de i)*	

Figura 7-10: Es hora de calcular sus costos de cierre.

Las demás preguntas son detalles importantes que los prestamistas necesitan saber, pero no se preocupe porque un sí aquí no eliminará su solicitud para el préstamo.

VIII. DECLARATIONS/ *DECLARACIONES*				
If you answer "Yes" to any questions a through i, please use continuation sheet for explanation. / *Si responde "Sí" a cualquier de las preguntas de la "a" a la "i", debe utilizar una hoja adicional para dar una explicación.*	**Borrower/** *Prestatario*		**Co-Borrower/** *Co-Prestatario*	
	Yes/*Sí*	No	Yes/*Sí*	No
a. Are there any outstanding judgments against you? *¿Existe alguna sentencia o fallo judicial pendiente en contra suya?*	☐	☐	☐	☐
b. Have you been declared bankrupt within the past 7 years? *¿Se ha declarado en bancarrota durante los últimos 7 años?*	☐	☐	☐	☐
c. Have you had property foreclosed upon or given title or deed in lieu thereof in the last 7 years? *¿Se le ha entablado una ejecución hipotecaria o ha transferido el título de propiedad en sustitución de una ejecución hipotecaria en los últimos 7 años?*	☐	☐	☐	☐
d. Are you a party to a lawsuit? *¿Es usted parte en una demanda judicial?*	☐	☐	☐	☐
e. Have you directly or indirectly been obligated on any loan which resulted in foreclosure, transfer of title in lieu of foreclosure, or judgment? *¿Ha estado usted obligado, directa o indirectamente, en algún préstamo que provocó una ejecución hipotecaria, transferencia de título en sustitución de una ejecución hipotecaria, o alguna sentencia, o fallo en su contra?*	☐	☐	☐	☐
(This would include such loans as home mortgage loans, SBA loans, home improvement loans, educational loans, manufactured (mobile) home loans, any mortgage, financial obligation, bond, or loan guarantee. If "Yes," provide details, including date, name, and address of Lender, FHA or VA case number, if any, and reasons for the action.) *(Esto incluye préstamos tales como préstamos hipotecarios para vivienda, préstamos SBA, préstamos para mejoras en la casa, préstamos educacionales, préstamos para casa móviles, cualquier hipoteca, obligación financiera, bono o préstamo garantizado. Si la respuesta es "Sí", incluya la fecha, el nombre y la dirección del Prestador, o el número de caso de FHA o VA, si lo hubiera, y las razones de la acción.)*				
f. Are you presently delinquent or in default on any Federal debt or any other loan, mortgage, financial obligation, bond, or loan guarantee? If "Yes," give details as described in the preceding question. *¿Se encuentra atrasado, moroso o en incumplimiento con alguna deuda federal o cualquier otro préstamos, hipoteca, obligación financiera, bono o garantía de préstamos? Si la respuesta es "Sí", provea detalles según se describe en la pregunta anterior.*	☐	☐	☐	☐
g. Are you obligated to pay alimony, child support, or separate maintenance? *¿Está obligado a pagar por pensión alimenticia, pensión para el sustento de los hijos, o manutención por separación?*	☐	☐	☐	☐
h. Is any part of the down payment borrowed? *¿Le prestaron alguna parte del pago inicial?*	☐	☐	☐	☐
i. Are you a co-maker or endorser on a note? *¿Es usted co-prestatario o fiador de un pagaré?*	☐	☐	☐	☐
---				
j. Are you a U.S. citizen? *¿Es usted ciudadano de los Estados Unidos?*	☐	☐	☐	☐
k. Are you a permanent resident alien? *¿Es usted un residente extranjero permanente de los Estados Unidos?*	☐	☐	☐	☐
l. Do you intend to occupy the property as your primary residence? If "Yes," complete question m below. *¿Tiene usted la intención de ocupar la propiedad como su residencia principal? Si la respuesta es "Sí" conteste la pregunta "m".*	☐	☐	☐	☐
m. Have you had an ownership interest in a property in the last three years? *¿Ha tenido usted participación como dueño en una propiedad en los últimos 3 años?* (1) What type of property did you own—principal residence (PR), second home (SH), or investment property (IP)? *¿De qué tipo de propiedad era usted dueño—residencia principal (PR), reisdencia secundaria (SH) o propiedad de inversión (IP)?* (2) How did you hold title to the home—solely by yourself (S), jointly with your spouse (SP), or jointly with another person (O)? *¿Cómo estaba registrado el título—a nombre suyo solamente (S), conjuntamente con su cónyuge (SP), o conjuntamente con otra persona (O)?*	☐ _____ _____	☐	☐ _____ _____	☐

Figura 7-11:
Es hora de
confesarlo
todo.

IX. Reconocimiento y acuerdo

Si no ha sido sincero en este formulario, considere la parte IX su oportunidad para cometer un perjurio (Figura 7-12).

Si algún agente hipotecario u otra persona le han ayudado a llenar esta solicitud, usted no se ha librado de su responsabilidad. Repase las respuestas que ellos proporcionaron antes de firmar el acuerdo. Éste es el momento de hacerse preguntas (y de verificar sus respuestas) para asegurarse de que está presentando su información de una manera positiva y verdadera.

X. Información para fines de verificación por parte del gobierno

Puede saltarse esta parte X (Figura 7-13) si quiere. El Gobierno Federal lleva cuenta del origen y sexo de los compradores para ver si los prestamistas están discriminando contra ciertas personas (entre otras cosas).

Hoja de continuación

Vaya a la página 8 de la *Solicitud para Préstamo Hipotecario Residencial Uniforme* y va a ver una hoja casi en blanco. Este espacio es para aquellas respuestas que no caben fácilmente en ninguna otra parte de la solicitud. Aquí, por ejemplo, puede explicar brevemente por qué se ha cambiado tanto de empleo, puede justificar sus problemas de crédito, registrar sus bienes y pasivos adicionales o explicar por qué lo arrestaron corriendo desnudo en la ciudad universitaria cuando estudiaba allí. Si no tiene nada importante que revelar, ¡puede escoger por decorar el espacio con garabatos usando sus creyones favoritos! Quizás hasta pueda esbozar los detalles de su primer proyecto de renovación de su casa.

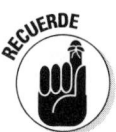

Si no tiene nada que poner en la página 8, lo que debe hacer es dibujar una línea diagonal dividiendo la hoja para que el prestamista sepa que la vio y que no tiene nada más que añadir. Asegúrese de firmar al final de la página también, aunque no escriba nada en ella. Muchas personas no firman, ¡lo cual no es de sorprenderse con el Gran Cañón de espacio que hay entre el encabezado de la página y la línea donde debe firmar al pie de ella!

Otros documentos típicos

Todos los prestamistas y agentes tienen su propio paquete, individualizado, de documentos para que usted los llene. Algunos documentos son estándares porque son por mandato federal. El presentar todos estos formularios no está dentro del ámbito de este libro —ni dentro de los límites de la capacidad de atención de la mayoría de la gente. A continuación hay algunos de los otros documentos que su prestamista o agente hipotecario pueden probablemente presentarle.

IX. ACKNOWLEDGEMENT AND AGREEMENT/*RECONOCIMIENTO Y ACUERDO*

Each of the undersigned specifically represents to Lender and to Lender's actual or potential agents, brokers, processors, attorneys, insurers, servicers, successors and assigns and agrees and acknowledges that: (1) the information provided in this application is true and correct as of the date set forth opposite my signature and that any intentional or negligent misrepresentation of this information contained in this application may result in civil liability, including monetary damages, to any person who may suffer any loss due to reliance upon any misrepresentation that I have made on this application, and/or in criminal penalties including, but not limited to, fine or imprisonment or both under the provisions of Title 18, United States Code, Sec. 1001, et seq.; (2) the loan requested pursuant to this application (the "Loan") will be secured by a mortgage or deed of trust on the property described in this application; (3) the property will not be used for any illegal or prohibited purpose or use; (4) all statements made in this application are made for the purpose of obtaining a residential mortgage loan; (5) the property will be occupied as indicated in this application; (6) the Lender, its servicers, successors or assigns may continuously rely on the information contained in the application, and I am obligated to amend and/or supplement the information provided in this application if any of the material facts that I have represented herein should change prior to closing of the Loan; (8) in the event that my payments on the Loan become delinquent, the Lender, its servicers, successors or assigns may, in addition to any other rights and remedies that it may have relating to such delinquency, report my name and account information to one or more consumer reporting agencies; (9) ownership of the Loan and/or administration of the Loan account may be transferred with such notice as may be required by law; (10) neither Lender nor its agents, brokers, insurers, servicers, successors or assigns has made any representation or warranty, express or implied, to me regarding the property or the condition or value of the property; and (11) my transmission of this application as an "electronic record" containing my "electronic signature," as those terms are defined in applicable federal and/or state laws (excluding audio and video recordings), or my facsimile transmission of this application containing a facsimile of my signature, shall be as effective, enforceable and valid as if a paper version of this application were delivered containing my original written signature.

Cada uno de los suscritos representa específicamente al Prestamista y a los verdaderos o posibles agentes, corredores, procesadores, abogados, aseguradores, administradores, sucesores y cesionarios del Prestamista, y está de acuerdo y acepta que: (1) la información que se proporciona en esta solicitud es exacta y correcta a partir de la fecha expuesta en la línea opuesta a mi firma, y que toda distorsión, intencional o negligente, de esta información contenida en esta solicitud pudiera resultar en una penalidad civil, incluyendo daños monetarios, hacia cualquier persona que sufra alguna pérdida debido a la toma de decisiones hecha en base a cualquier declaración falsa que yo haya hecho en esta solicitud, o en castigos penales, incluyendo, pero sin limitar a, multa o arresto o ambos, de acuerdo con las disposiciones del Título 18, del Código de los Estados Unidos, Sec. 1001, et seq.; (2) el préstamo solicitado de acuerdo a esta solicitud (el "Préstamo") estará asegurado por una hipoteca o escritura de fideicomiso sobre la propiedad descrita en la presente solicitud; (3) la propiedad no se utilizará para ningún propósito o uso ilegal o prohibido; (4) todas las declaraciones realizadas en esta solicitud se hacen con el fin de obtener un préstamo hipotecario residencial; (5) la propiedad se ocupará de acuerdo con lo indicado en la presente solicitud; (6) el Prestamista, sus administradores, sucesores o cesionarios pudieran retener los registros originales o electrónicos contenidos en esta solicitud, se apruebe o no el Préstamo; (7) el Prestamista y sus agentes, corredores, aseguradores, administradores, sucesores y cesionarios, pueden tomar decisiones constantemente en base a la información contenida en esta solicitud, y yo estoy obligado a corregir y complementar la información proporcionada en esta solicitud si alguno de los hechos significativos que he declarado en la presente solicitud cambia antes del cierre del Préstamo; (8) en el caso de que mis pagos al Préstamo se atrasen, el Prestamista, sus administradores, sucesores o cesionarios pudiera, además de cualquier otro derecho y recurso que pueda tener relacionado a dicho atraso, reportar mi nombre e información de cuenta a una o más agencias de información de crédito del consumidor; (9) la propiedad del Préstamo o la administración de la cuenta del Préstamo pudiera transferirse otorgando la notificación que requiera la ley; (10) ningún Prestamista ni sus agentes, corredores, aseguradores, administradores, sucesores o cesionarios me han hecho alguna manifestación o garantía, expresa o implícita, respecto a la propiedad, o la condición o el valor de la propiedad; (11) mi transmisión de esta solicitud como un "registro electrónico" que contenga mi "firma electrónica", como se definen esos términos en las leyes federales y estatales correspondientes (excluyendo grabaciones de audio y video), o mi transmisión de facsímil de esta solicitud que contenga un facsímil de mi firma, deberá ser tan eficaz, acatable y válida como si se hubiera entregado una versión en papel de esta solicitud que contenga mi firma escrita original.

Acknowledgement. Each of the undersigned hereby acknowledges that any owner of the Loan, its servicers, successors and assigns, may verify or reverify any information contained in this application or obtain any information or data relating to the Loan, for any legitimate business purpose through any source, including a source named in this application or a consumer reporting agency.

Reconocimiento. Cada uno de los abajo firmantes reconocen por la presente que el titular del Préstamo, sus administradores, sucesores y cesionarios pueden verificar y reverificar cualquier información incluida en esta solicitud u obtener cualquier información o datos relacionados con el Préstamo, para cualquier propósito comercial legítimo, a través de cualquier fuente, incluida una fuente mencionada en esta solicitud o una agencia de crédito del consumidor.

THE SPANISH TRANSLATION IS FOR CONVENIENCE PURPOSES ONLY. IN THE EVENT OF AN INCONSISTENCY BETWEEN THE ENGLISH AND SPANISH LANGUAGE VERSIONS OF THIS FORM, THE ENGLISH LANGUAGE VERSION SHALL PREVAIL.
LA TRADUCCIÓN AL ESPAÑOL ES PARA SU CONVENIENCIA ÚNICAMENTE. EN CASO DE QUE EXISTA UNA INCONSISTENCIA ENTRE LA VERSIÓN EN INGLÉS Y LA VERSIÓN EN ESPAÑOL DE ESTE FORMULARIO, PREVALECERÁ LA VERSIÓN EN INGLÉS.

LEA ESTO PRIMERO: Este documento contiene una traducción al español de su texto en inglés.

Borrower's Signature/*Firma del Prestatario*	Date/*Fecha*	Co-Borrower's Signature/*Firma del Co-Prestatario*	Date/*Fecha*
X		X	

Figura 7-12: Firme aquí.

X. INFORMATION FOR GOVERNMENT MONITORING PURPOSES/*INFORMACIÓN PARA FINES DE VERIFICACIÓN POR EL GOBIERNO*

The following information is requested by the Federal Government for certain types of loans related to a dwelling in order to monitor the lender's compliance with equal credit opportunity, fair housing and home mortgage disclosure laws. You are not required to furnish this information, but are encouraged to do so. The law provides that a lender may not discriminate either on the basis of this information, or on whether you choose to furnish it. If you furnish the information, please provide both ethnicity and race. For race, you may check more than one designation. If you do not furnish ethnicity, race, or sex, under Federal regulations, this lender is required to note the information on the basis of visual observation and surname if you have made this application in person. If you do not wish to furnish the information, please check the box below. (Lender must review the above material to assure that the disclosures satisfy all requirements to which the lender is subject under applicable state law for the particular type of loan applied for.)

La siguiente información la solicita el gobierno Federal para ciertos tipos de préstamos relacionados con una vivienda, con el fin de verificar el cumplimiento del Prestador con las leyes de igualdad de Oportunidades de Crédito, "fair housing" y las leyes de divulgación de hipotecas para viviendas. Usted no está obligado a proporcionar esta información, pero le instamos a hacerlo. La ley dispone que un Prestador no puede discriminar en base a esta información ni por el hecho de que decida o no proporcionarla. Si usted decide proporcionarla debe indicar grupo étnico y raza. Usted puede indicar más de una raza. Si usted no desea suministrar la información, de acuerdo a las reglamentaciones federales, el Prestador debe anotar la raza y el sexo basado en una observación visual y de acuerdo a su apellido si usted preparó esta solicitud en persona. Si usted no desea proporcionar la información, sírvase marcar en el cuadro ubicado en la parte inferior. (El Prestador debe evaluar el material arriba mencionado para asegurarse de que la información proporcionada cumple con todos los requisitos a los que está sujeto el Prestador bajo la ley estatal pertinente para el tipo de préstamo en particular que se ha solicitado.)

BORROWER/*PRESTATARIO* ☐ I do not wish to furnish this information / *No deseo proporcionar esta información*	CO-BORROWER/*CO-PRESTATARIO* ☐ I do not wish to furnish this information / *No deseo proporcionar esta información*
Ethnicity: ☐ Hispanic or Latino/ ☐ Not Hispanic or Latino/ *Grupo étnico Hispano o Latino No Hispano o Latino*	**Ethnicity:** ☐ Hispanic or Latino/ ☐ Not Hispanic or Latino/ *Grupo étnico Hispano o Latino No Hispano o Latino*
Race/*Raza*: ☐ American Indian or Alaska Native/ *Indio Americano o Nativo de Alaska* ☐ Asian/ *Asiático* ☐ Black or African American/ *Negro o Afroamericano* ☐ Native Hawaiian or Other Pacific Islander/ *Nativo de Hawai o de otra isla del Pacífico* ☐ White/*Blanco*	**Race/*Raza*:** ☐ American Indian or Alaska Native/ *Indio Americano o Nativo de Alaska* ☐ Asian/ *Asiático* ☐ Black or African American/ *Negro o Afroamericano* ☐ Native Hawaiian or Other Pacific Islander/ *Nativo de Hawai o de otra isla del Pacífico* ☐ White/*Blanco*
Sex/*Sexo*: ☐ Female/*Femenino* ☐ Male/*Masculino*	**Sex/*Sexo*:** ☐ Female/*Femenino* ☐ Male/*Masculino*

To be Completed by Interviewer *A COMPLETARSE POR EL ENTREVISTADOR* This application was taken by: *Esta solicitud se obtuvo por:* ☐ Face-to-face interview/*Entrevista en persona* ☐ Mail/*correo* ☐ Telephone/*teléfono* ☐ Internet/*Internet*	Interviewer's Name (print or type) *Nombre del Entrevistador (use en letra de imprenta o a máquina)* Interviewer's Signature Date/*Fecha* *Firma del Entrevistador* Interviewer's Phone Number (incl. area code) *Nº de Teléfono del Entrevistador (inc. código de área)*	Name and Address of Interviewer's Employer *Nombre y Dirección del Empleador del Entrevistador*

Figura 7-13: El Gran Hermano omnipresente quiere saber.

Su derecho a recibir una copia del avalúo

Ahora usted tiene derecho a recibir copia del reporte de valuación, pero no siempre fue así. El hecho de que el prestatario no siempre tuviera este derecho es algo absurdo —después de todo, ¡usted es el que está pagando por la valuación!

Para asegurarse de que sabe que tiene este derecho, el gobierno exige que las entidades hipotecarias y los agentes hipotecarios le presenten el documento mostrado en la Figura 7-14.

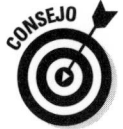

A pesar de que la notificación le dice que haga su petición por escrito, intente hacerlo verbalmente para ahorrarse tiempo. Luego, si su petición es ignorada, tómese la molestia de escribir una petición (en un período no mayor de 90 días después de que se haya tomado la decisión de aprobar o rechazar su préstamo). Es bueno tener los avalúos en su expediente —nunca sabe cuándo una le será útil. Al menos puede ver cuáles propiedades se usaron como propiedades similares a la suya, para saber qué tan buena o mala es la valuación.

La Ley de Igualdad para la Oportunidad al Crédito
(ECOA, por sus siglas en inglés)
(Reglamento B)

Derecho a recibir copia del avalúo

Usted tiene el derecho a recibir una copia del reporte de valuación usado en relación a su solicitud para crédito. Si desea una copia, por favor escríbanos a la dirección proporcionada. Tenemos que recibir su petición por escrito, en un período no mayor de 90 días, después que le notifiquemos sobre la acción tomada en cuanto a su solicitud de crédito, o si usted retira su solicitud. En su carta nos tiene que proporcionar su nombre, la dirección de la propiedad deseada, su dirección actual y el número del préstamo asignado a su solicitud.

Yo (nosotros) he (hemos) leído y entendido las condiciones anteriormente mencionadas con respecto a mi (nuestro) derecho a recibir una copia de mi (nuestra) valuación y certifico (certificamos) haber recibido una copia de esta información.

_____   _____
           Solicitante   Fecha

_____   _____
           Solicitante   Fecha

Figura 7-14: Ejerza su derecho a tener el reporte de valuación de su propiedad —pida una copia.

Ley de igualdad para la oportunidad al crédito

Otra planilla que probablemente verá es una que declara que la ley federal prohíbe al prestamista hipotecario rechazar su solicitud de préstamo por causas personales como: su raza, sexo, estado civil, edad u otras más. Usted tampoco tiene que revelar ingresos que recibe como resultado de estar divorciado (aunque nosotros consideramos que es de su beneficio hacerlo porque ese ingreso puede ayudarlo a conseguir que aprueben su préstamo).

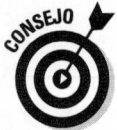

Si tiene motivos para creer que la entidad hipotecaria está discriminándolo, contacte con el Departamento de Bienes Raíces (*Department of Real Estate*) o con el departamento gubernamental que regula a las entidades hipotecarias en su estado, y presente una queja. Ahora, emprenda la búsqueda por un prestamista mejor y más ético.

Parte III
Propiedades, Participantes y Precios

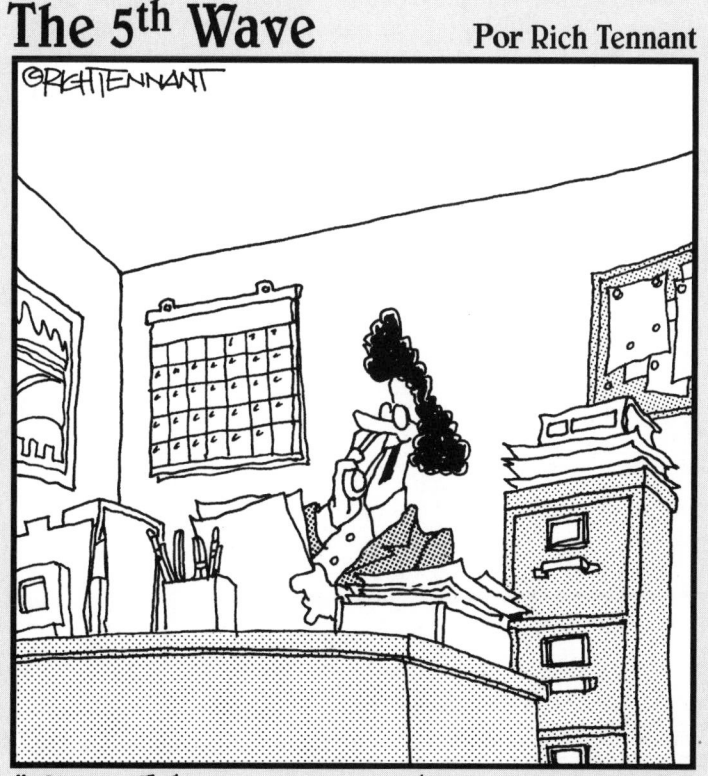

"¡Señor Johnson, creo que hemos encontrado la casa de sus sueños! Y de paso, ¿me puede decir qué piensa de los fantasmas, cementerios y hechizos?"

En esta parte . . .

*E*s el momento de presentarle los diferentes tipos de viviendas que puede considerar al comprar y las personas que puede contratar para ayudarlo en la compra de la suya.

Además de guiarlo hacia estrategias exitosas y excelentes profesionales, también lo ayudamos a evitar propiedades con problemas y, en general, a evitar las desilusiones. En esta parte le damos un curso intensivo en cómo distinguir una buena compra de una súper cara para que no tenga que pagar demás cuando esté comprando la casa de sus sueños y, de hecho, poder lograr hacer un buen negocio.

Para cerrar esta sección, le explicamos cómo usar el potencial de la Internet cuando esté haciendo la investigación para la compra de su casa.

Capítulo 8

Dónde y Qué Comprar

· ·

En Este Capítulo

▶ Sitio, valor y buenos vecindarios

▶ Cómo maximizar su inversión

▶ Casas unifamiliares separadas y casas adyacentes (condominios y apartamentos cooperativos)

▶ Premios y riesgos de casas con necesidad de reparación y embargos hipotecarios

▶ Ventajas y desventajas de sociedades residenciales

· ·

¿**O**ué se imagina al pensar en el coche perfecto, en el trabajo perfecto y la manera perfecta de pasar el día? ¿Hubiera dicho lo mismo hace diez años? Probablemente no, ¿verdad? La perfección es un blanco que cambia frecuentemente —cambia a medida que usted cambia.

¿La casa *perfecta*? No existe tal cosa. Para empezar, pocas personas tienen los recursos económicos para comprar lo que consideran "la casa perfecta". Aunque usted sea uno de los pocos suertudos con suficiente dinero para tirar, aún así es muy poco probable que encuentre una casa perfecta de arriba a abajo. La casa que parece perfecta a los veintitantos años, cuando está libre y sin compromisos, seguramente no lo será a los cuarenta y tantos, si está casado y con hijos. Adelántese otros veinte años más hacia la edad en que esté por jubilarse, y es posible que quiera o necesite mudarse a una casa más pequeña que le sea más fácil de mantener.

No se apure. Aunque no haya una casa que sea perfecta para siempre, este capítulo le enseñará cómo lograr perfección en la secuencia de la adquisición de sus casas, de una manera lucrativa; y, puesto que es caro mudarse, también le enseñamos cómo minimizar el número de veces que usted compra y vende.

Es probable que conozca a alguien que perdió dinero en la venta de su casa. Estamos seguros de que no está en sus planes ser la próxima víctima de un mercado de bienes raíces caprichoso. Conseguir una ganga al comprar su casa es un buen objetivo, pero no se quede ahí. ¿Es qué no quiere que el valor de su casa también aumente mientras sea suya?

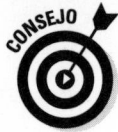

El mejor momento para pensar sobre cuánto quiere por su casa al venderla, es antes de comprarla. Nunca permita que su entusiasmo por una casa lo ciegue y no vea los defectos de la misma. Antes de comprar, trate de ver la propiedad a través de los ojos del *próximo* posible comprador. Lo más seguro es que cualquier cosa que a usted le moleste de la casa o del vecindario, también le molestará al próximo comprador.

No estamos sugiriendo que planee vender su casa inmediatamente después de comprarla. Quién sabe, pero quizás viva feliz para siempre en la casa que está a punto de comprar; por otra parte, un cambio de vida inesperado, como un traslado a otra ciudad o el crecimiento de su familia, puede forzarlo a vender. Si eso sucede, una buena ganancia puede aliviar un poco el estrés de la mudanza.

El aumento de valor es bueno para mucho más que incrementar su valor neto. Dado que el valor de su casa incrementa a través del tiempo, es posible que un día usted concluya que *el valor líquido de la vivienda* (la diferencia entre el valor en el mercado y la hipoteca que usted debe) le puede ayudar a lograr una multitud de metas financieras y personales. Puede usar el dinero como guste —aumentar los ahorros para su jubilación, ayudar a pagar la educación universitaria de sus hijos, empezar su propio negocio o viajar en el Expreso de Oriente de Londres a Venecia para celebrar su vigésimo quinto aniversario de bodas. Los ahorros son herramientas financieras muy versátiles y, ¡no tienen polillas!

En un mundo lleno de incertidumbre, nadie le puede garantizar que el valor de su casa aumentará. Sin embargo, comprar una buena casa en una urbanización codiciada incrementa sus probabilidades de ganar mucho dinero. Este principio es cierto ya sea en un mercado de bienes raíces fuerte o débil, a la hora de vender.

Los precios de los inmuebles no son fijos; ellos suben y bajan por factores tales como el mercado laboral local, la oferta y la demanda de viviendas disponibles y de viviendas para alquilar, tasas de interés y ciclos anuales de actividad alta o baja en el mercado. (Para más información sobre este tema, consulte el Capítulo 4.) La mayoría de esos factores están fuera de sus manos y de su capacidad para predecirlos, pero eso no significa que su realidad económica como propietario de su vivienda sea el resultado de un capricho del destino. Al contrario, usted controla tres factores importantes que afectan el valor de su casa:

✔ Cuánto paga por su casa.

✔ Dónde está situada su casa.

✔ Qué tipo de casa compra.

El factor controlable principal es cuánto paga por su casa. Si paga por demás al comprarla, tendrá que correr con mucha suerte para poder sacarle ganancias al venderla. Es por eso que dedicamos el Capítulo 10 a identificar propiedades a buen precio y a evitar precios sobre valorados, y así asegurarnos de que usted sabe exactamente qué comprar.

Este capítulo se enfoca en los otros dos factores importantes bajo su control: dónde y qué comprar.

Ubicación, Más Ubicación y Valor

Si es extravagantemente rico, usted puede pagar para vivir en donde mejor le plazca. El resto de nosotros, sin embargo, tenemos presupuestos un poco más limitados. Aún así, a menos de que esté rebuscando en el último eslabón de la cadena alimenticia en el mundo de las viviendas, usted tendrá muchas opciones al decidir en qué gastar su dinero. Dónde decida comprar, será finalmente, su decisión.

Lo más seguro es que ya ha oído que las tres cosas más importantes que debe buscar al comprar una vivienda son "la ubicación, la ubicación y la ubicación". Este axioma es bastante cierto, porque cuando la gente compra, compra tanto el vecindario como la casa. En buenos y malos tiempos, la gente paga por vivir en vecindarios mejores. En cambio, vecindarios o urbanizaciones pésimas destrozan el valor de las viviendas. Hasta el Taj Mahal tendría problemas de venderse si estuviera rodeado de pocilgas y gallineros.

El decir simplemente que el secreto de hacer dinero en bienes raíces es "la ubicación, la ubicación y la ubicación", es equivalente a decir que se hará millonario con la bolsa de valores si compra a precios bajos y vende a precios altos. Toma más que generalidades para hacer dinero. Necesita acciones específicas.

Primeramente, no estamos de acuerdo en que los tres factores más importantes al comprar una vivienda sean la ubicación, la ubicación y la ubicación. Además, no vemos el caso de estarnos repitiendo tres veces —¡usted no está sordo! El *valor* —lo que recibe a cambio de su dinero— también es importante.

Si, por ejemplo, todo el mundo sabe que la Colonia Selecta es la *mejor* urbanización, entonces usted pagará una cantidad considerable para vivir ahí; y a pesar de que la Colonia Selecta es en estos momentos la urbanización más admirada de todas, y probablemente vaya a seguir siéndolo, también es cierto que esta ubicación no tiene más remedio que bajar de precio.

Otros vecindarios, que hoy por hoy no se consideran tan preferidos, a la larga pueden mejorar lo que tienen que ofrecerle al propietario y, finalmente, tener un aumento en su valor mucho mayor. El comprar una vivienda con una buena ubicación, aunque importante, no debe ser su único criterio para comprar. Si quiere comprar una casa que sea una buena inversión, tiene que encontrar algo de buen valor. Explicaremos cómo hacer esto en este capítulo.

Las características de un buen vecindario

Los buenos vecindarios, como la belleza, son según el cristal con que se miren. Por ejemplo, la proximidad a buenas escuelas es importante para usted si tiene niños pequeños. Al contrario, si está listo para jubilarse, quizás le llame la atención mudarse a un lugar tranquilo con actividades al aire libre; y, el vivir al lado de una secundaria ruidosa talvez le parezca una pesadilla. Si es una persona libre y sin compromiso, es posible que ninguna de las dos opciones anteriores le convenga. Su vecindario ideal probablemente es un complejo de condominios de gente soltera, en el centro, para poder estar cerca de donde está la acción, día y noche.

Si dejamos a un lado las preferencias personales, todos los buenos vecindarios tienen las siguientes características:

✔ **El estado económico:** nada mata el valor de las propiedades más rápido que un bosque de letreros anunciando casas "En venta", ocasionado por despidos corporativos. Consulte el Capítulo 4 para ver las maneras de evaluar compañías y mercados laborales de las comunidades en las que esté contemplando comprar casa.

✔ **El esparcimiento:** los medios de esparcimiento son características especiales de una localidad que hacen de ella un lugar atractivo y deseable para vivir. Ejemplos perfectos de los servicios que le agregan valor serían calles amplias, flanqueadas por robles majestuosos, parques verdes exuberantes, vistas al mar, tranquilidad, estacionamiento y cercanía a escuelas, iglesias, centros comerciales y restaurantes, transporte, patios con juegos infantiles, canchas de tenis y playas. Claro, poca gente tiene la posibilidad económica para comprar en una zona con todas estas comodidades, pero entre más beneficios de éstos tenga, mejor es.

✔ **Escuelas de buena calidad:** quizás no le importe qué tan buenas o malas sean las escuelas si no tiene niños en edad escolar. Sin embargo, a menos que esté comprando dentro de una comunidad remota para jubilados o de tipo vacacional, mejor crea que cuando esté listo para vender su casa, la mayoría de los compradores potenciales con niños van a estar profundamente preocupados por el sistema escolar. Pero, también le debería importar la calidad de las escuelas cercanas por motivos más allá del valor de la casa: las escuelas buenas producen niños mejores y esto indudablemente afecta la calidad de vida en la comunidad. No dependa de las calificaciones de los exámenes ni de la opinión de alguien al evaluar la calidad de las escuelas; hable con los padres y maestros para tener una idea de cómo son las escuelas de la localidad.

✔ **Baja incidencia de criminalidad:** la mayoría de las personas hoy en día están preocupadas por la delincuencia —y deberían de estarlo, ya que la incidencia de criminalidad en muchas partes de los Estados Unidos está demasiado elevada. Así como con las escuelas, no dependa de la opinión de terceros o de reportes aislados para saber esto. Las comunidades normalmente recopilan estadísticas de delincuencia por zonas. Llame a la estación de policía local, visite su sitio Web o la biblioteca pública del vecindario para confirmar los datos.

✔ **Estabilidad:** algunas comunidades están en un estado constante de movimiento. Su lema es "adiós a lo pasado y bienvenido a lo nuevo". Imagínese lo que le pasaría al valor de las propiedades si se reemplazara un basurero con un parque hermoso. ¿Qué tal la situación inversa: aparece un edificio feo para estacionamiento, de concreto y de varios pisos, donde había un parque hermoso? Verifique con el apartamento de planificación local y con un buen agente de bienes raíces para ver los desarrollos propuestos en las zonas que está considerando.

✔ **Orgullo de propietario:** el costo de una casa no influye en la intensidad del orgullo del propietario al tenerla. Dé una vuelta por cualquier vecindario, elegante o modesto, y verá al instante si las personas que viven ahí se enorgullecen de sus casas o no. Un vecindario lleno de casas bien cuidadas y jardines bien cortados expresa a gritos el orgullo de los propietarios.

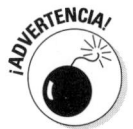

El valor de las propiedades baja cuando los propietarios ya no se enorgullecen de sus propiedades. Evite vecindarios en decadencia, donde encuentra señales de propietarios que han perdido el interés: casas mal cuidadas, jardines llenos de basura, carros abandonados en la calle, muchos propietarios ausentes rentando la propiedad, altos niveles de vandalismo a la propiedad y de delincuencia y otros más. El deterioro de un vecindario es como una plaga que se contagia de una casa a otra.

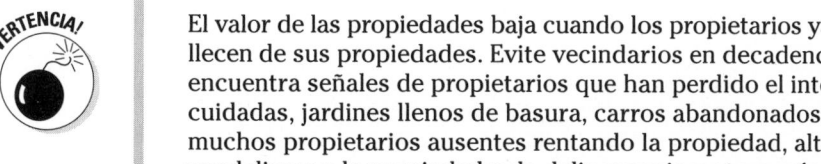

Cómo seleccionar el mejor vecindario

Es posible que corra con suerte y encuentre el vecindario de sus sueños rápidamente. Sin embargo, es mucho más factible que acabe evaluando el lado bueno y el lado malo de varios vecindarios al tratar de decidir en cuál comprar. Si tiene un presupuesto —y la mayoría de las personas lo tienen— tiene que tolerar y cambiar unas cosas por otras.

Supongamos que un vecindario tiene escuelas que le gustan, pero otro es más cercano a su oficina (lo que le ahorraría una hora de transporte todos los días) y el último está en un pueblo con una playa encantadora. Todos son buenos vecindarios. ¿Cuál escoger? Ésta es una decisión muy difícil de tomar.

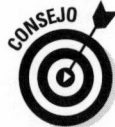

A continuación presentamos diferentes maneras de investigar y seleccionar el mejor vecindario *para usted*.

Déle prioridad a sus necesidades

Comprar una casa cuando tiene limitaciones económicas significa cambiar unas cosas por otras. Por ejemplo, si quiere vivir en el pueblo con las escuelas buenas y los parques, lo más probable es que tenga que conformarse con una casa más pequeña que la que podría tener en una comunidad de precios asequibles. A la hora de la verdad, cuando ya tiene que escoger dónde vivir, tiene que decidir qué es lo más importante para usted.

Investigación

Tal y como lo indicamos anteriormente en este capítulo, en la sección de "Las características de un buen vecindario", debe examinar el estado de la economía local, los servicios de esparcimiento, tales como parques y entretenimiento, la calidad de las escuelas y el nivel de criminalidad antes de comprar una casa. Y bien, ¿dónde puede encontrar toda esta información?

✔ **Aproveche los recursos locales.** Consulte las bibliotecas de la localidad. La cámara de comercio local también es una fuente de información excelente.

✔ **Hable con la gente que vive en el vecindario.** ¿Quién sabe más sobre un vecindario que la misma gente que vive en él? Además de preguntarles qué opinan sobre el vecindario, pídales opiniones sobre los otros vecindarios que usted está considerando. Si puede inspirar algo de rivalidad entre los vecindarios, podrá enterarse de los detalles de otros vecindarios, como su clima espantoso, sus problemas de estacionamiento, los residentes antipáticos o arrogantes y otras cosas más. Los inquilinos también son una excelente fuente de información. Como no tienen un montón de billetes invertido en una casa, los inquilinos normalmente son francos al hablar sobre los problemas de un vecindario. Finalmente, pero no por eso menos importante, conduzca o camine por el vecindario a diferentes horas del día y de la noche para asegurarse de que su encanto perdura las 24 horas del día.

✔ **Obtenga de su agente de bienes raíces las estadísticas sobre los días en el mercado** (*Days On the Market*, [DOM, por sus siglas en inglés]). Las estadísticas *DOM* indican el tiempo promedio que tarda en venderse una vivienda de la zona después de ponerla en el mercado. Por lo general, entre más rápido se vende una propiedad, más probable es que cierre cerca del precio que se pidió originalmente. Ventas rápidas indican una fuerte demanda por parte de los compradores, lo cual es buenísimo cuando está usted listo para vender.

✔ **Obtenga ayuda de un profesional.** Pídale a una entidad hipotecaria, a un agente de bienes raíces o valuador que comparen el potencial positivo del valor de las casas en cada vecindario. Así como lo explicamos en el Capítulo 9, el comprar una casa es un esfuerzo de equipo. Consiga un análisis de los valores presentes y futuros de cada vecindario con los agentes de bienes raíces que trabajan a tiempo completo.

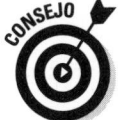

Ni los agentes de bienes raíces ni las entidades prestamistas cobran por opiniones sobre los valores. Sin embargo, ellos tienen un interés personal en venderle algo. Por otra parte, los valuadores no tienen un interés personal que proteger. Es cierto que los tasadores cobran por analizar valores de propiedad y las tendencias de los precios de los vecindarios, pero si va a gastar miles y miles de dólares en una casa, pagar unos cientos de dólares más para obtener un análisis neutral y profesional de los valores de las propiedades de un vecindario puede ser una buena inversión.

✔ **Métase en línea.** Varios sitios Web de bienes raíces proporcionan datos e información de la comunidad local. Consulte el Capítulo 11 para sitios recomendados y estrategias de búsquedas por el Internet.

Principios Fundamentales para Escoger una Casa

¡Buenas noticias! No importa si compra una cabaña o una casa estilo Cape Cod colonial, o francesa provincial, victoriana estilo Queen Victoria o californiana tipo rancho, usted puede hacer dinero con cualquier propiedad siguiendo tres principios fundamentales al escoger la casa que va a comprar. A medida que lea las siguientes pautas, recuerde que no son reglas estrictas y que existen excepciones.

Los principios de progresión: Motivo para comprar una de las casas más baratas de la cuadra

Un valuador le dirá que el *principio de progresión* indica que la propiedad de menor valor aumenta en valor por su cercanía a mejores propiedades. ¿En español, por favor? Compre una de las casas más baratas de la cuadra, porque las casas más caras que la rodean aumentarán el valor de la suya.

Por ejemplo, digamos que un agente le muestra una casa que acaba de salir al mercado en un vecindario y que le gusta. A $175.000 es una de las casas menos costosas que ha visto en la zona. El agente le dice que las demás casas alrededor probablemente se venderán entre $225.000 y $275.000. A usted se le cae la barbilla.

No saque su chequera todavía. Infórmese y averigüe por qué está tan barata esa casa. Si los defectos son aceptables, haga la oferta. Si los defectos no son aceptables, continúe viendo otras propiedades.

Defectos corregibles

Si una casa es una ganga porque tiene defectos que no son difíciles o caros de arreglar, cómprela. Por ejemplo, quizás la casa sea como el patito feo y sólo necesite un poco de pintura, jardinería ornamental u otros toques estéticos pequeños para transformarse en un bello cisne. Quizás es la única casa en la cuadra con dos dormitorios, pero tiene un área de almacenaje que puede convertir en una tercera habitación por menos de $15.000. Por $190.000 ($175.000 por la casa más $15.000 para construir la habitación), puede estar viviendo en un vecindario con valores entre $225.000 y $275.000. ¡Una ganga!

Problemas como ésos son *defectos corregibles,* o sea, defectos de la propiedad que pueden arreglarse por medio de una mejora o reparación y que se hacen con relativamente poco dinero. Pintar, modernizar un baño, instalar mostradores y gabinetes nuevos en la cocina y actualizar el sistema eléctrico son ejemplos de defectos corregibles.

Defectos incorregibles

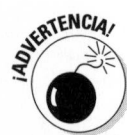

Si una casa tiene problemas graves, no es una ganga a ningún precio. ¿Quién quiere vivir al lado de un basurero? ¿O que tal si es una casa muy fea? Solo porque el vendedor se haya hecho millonario en la industria del chorizo no significa que usted (ni nadie más) quiera vivir en una casa en forma de un "perro caliente" gigantesco. Puede ser que una casa esté barata porque el contratista dice que está a punto de derrumbarse y tendrá que gastar al menos $125.000 en un techo y cimientos nuevos, plomería nueva y cableado nuevo en toda la casa.

Defectos enormes como ésos se llaman *defectos incorregibles* ya que no es económicamente viable repararlos. Tampoco hay nada que pueda hacer si la casa está mal situada. Ni tiene sentido, normalmente, pagar $175.000 por la casa en forma de "perro caliente" sólo para derrumbarla y construir una nueva (a menos que los lotes vacíos similares se vendan a esos precios). Por otro lado, si paga $175.000 por aquella ruina y luego le invierte $125.000 más para arreglarla, tendrá el honor dudoso de ser el propietario de la casa más cara del vecindario.

No nos interprete mal, no todas las casas para renovar son malas inversiones. Entramos en detalles sobre las casas que necesitan arreglo más adelante en este capítulo.

Los beneficios de renovar casas más económicas

Las casas más económicas de la cuadra también son las menos riesgosas para renovar, gracias al principio de progresión. Por ejemplo, digamos que acaba de pagar $175.000 por una casa que necesita mucho trabajo de reparación, pero que está situada justamente en medio de un vecindario de casas de $250.000.

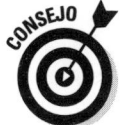

La diferencia entre su precio de compra y el valor de las casas alrededor determina aproximadamente lo máximo que debería considerar gastar en la renovación.

En el ejemplo anterior, usted no debería gastar más de $75.000 para llevar su casa a los estándares de las demás casas. Claro, suponiendo que usted puede gastar esa cantidad (consulte el Capítulo 2) y que tiene el tiempo y la paciencia para coordinar el trabajo o hacerlo usted mismo. Siempre y cuando mejore la propiedad de manera eficaz, y respete su presupuesto, lo más probable es que recupere la mayor parte del dinero invertido, o todo, en las mejoras al vender la propiedad.

Use el principio de progresión junto con el de ubicación, ubicación y valor. El comprar una de las casas menos caras en un vecindario bueno aumenta la probabilidad de que la propiedad se aprecie en el futuro.

El principio de regresión: Motivo para no comprar la casa más cara de la cuadra

¡Lo adivinó! El *principio de regresión* es económicamente lo opuesto al principio de progresión.

Si compra la vivienda más cara de la cuadra, el principio de regresión lo castigará al venderla. Cuanto más bajo sea el valor de todas las demás casas, más disminuirá el valor de la suya.

Si un espíritu diabólico le susurra al oído que debería de comprar la casa más cara de la cuadra para lucir su gran estatus en la vida, consulte con un exorcista inmediatamente. No tiene que ceder ante los encantos del espíritu diabólico, a menos que le cause gran regocijo la idea de perder dinero al vender. Satisfaga su ego —y haga una inversión más inteligente— comprando una de esas casas menos costosas en vecindarios mejores.

La vivienda más cara de la cuadra también es la peor candidata para una renovación. Digamos que compra una casa a $250.000 en un vecindario de casas de $150.000. Desde la perspectiva de un tasador, la casa ya resalta como una mosca en un vaso de leche. Gastarse otros $50.000 para agregarle una nueva cocina lujosa a la que ya es la casa más cara de la cuadra, solo agrave su problema más. Es casi seguro que la cocina nueva no incrementará el valor de su casa a $300.000. Nadie puede negarle el hecho de que haya gastado $50.000 en la cocina si tiene los recibos para comprobar lo que gastó, pero la gente que compra casas a $300.000 normalmente quiere estar rodeada de casas que valgan lo mismo o más, que la que están comprando.

Las casas son como los vasos, cuando los llena demasiado se derraman. De la misma manera, cuando hace reparaciones excesivas a su casa (en base al precio de venta de casas similares del vecindario), el dinero que gasta en las mejoras se va por la borda. Este fenómeno se llama *mejora excesiva de la propiedad.*

Aunque compre la casa menos costosa del vecindario, puede arreglarla demasiado si gasta mucho más al mejorarla. El mejor momento para cuidarse de no hacer mejoras excesivas es antes de comenzar el trabajo.

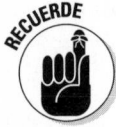

Si va a acabar con la casa más cara de la cuadra al terminar un proyecto, no lleve a cabo el proyecto.

El principio de similitud: Motivo por el cual lo diferente es normalmente costoso

Los principios de progresión y regresión están relacionados con la similitud económica. Si quiere maximizar la probabilidad de la valorización de la casa que va a comprar, su casa también tiene que ser similar a las demás casas del vecindario o urbanización en cuanto a tamaño, edad, condición y estilo. Este es el *principio de similitud.*

Este principio no quiere decir que su casa tiene que ser un clon idéntico de todas las casas de la cuadra. Sin embargo, sí debe estar dentro de los estándares predominantes de su vecindario. Por ejemplo:

- **Tamaño:** su casa no debe sobrepasar a las demás casas de la cuadra haciéndolas ver como miniaturas, ni viceversa. Si su casa es más pequeña que las demás, use el principio de progresión como guía, para que se vea como las demás y así aumentará su valor. En cambio, si tiene una casa de tres dormitorios en una urbanización con casas de dos y tres dormitorios, el agregarle una cuarta quebrantaría el principio de regresión.

✔ **Edad:** casi nunca se ve una casa más vieja en una cuadra de casas nuevas y modernas. Sin embargo, de vez en cuando se ve una casa nueva insertada ilógicamente entre casas más viejas. Una casa moderna típicamente se ve fuera de lugar en un vecindario de elegantes casas más antiguas. Aunque le ofrezcan una súper ganga, la falta de semejanza a las demás casas de la cuadra vendrá a causarle dolores de cabeza al tratar de venderla.

✔ **Condición:** la condición estética de su casa tiene un impacto tremendo en su valor. No es de sorprenderse que su casa pierda valor si es una casa dilapidada comparada con el resto de las casas de la cuadra.

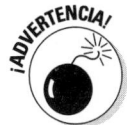

Paradójicamente, no es bueno tener su casa en condiciones demasiado superiores a las de las demás del vecindario. Aunque su casa sea similar a todas las demás casas en cuanto al tamaño, edad y estilo, usted podría mejorar excesivamente su casa si la calidad de los materiales, de la fabricación y de los aparatos en su casa excede mucho más los estándares de calidad predominantes en el vecindario.

✔ **Estilo:** la arquitectura de la casa que compre no es tan importante — mientras sea similar al estilo arquitectónico predominante en la urbanización. Desde el punto de vista de una inversión, por ejemplo, no es prudente comprar la única casa victoriana "Queen Anne" en una cuadra llena de casas coloniales estilo "Menonita" o viceversa. Tampoco debe comprar una casa de tres pisos cuando todas las casas alrededor son de un piso.

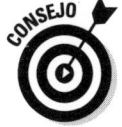

Su casa no tiene que ser una aburrida réplica, sin gracia, de todas las demás casas de la cuadra. Puede seguir el principio de similitud y aún así expresar su individualismo por medio de un jardín ornamental, la pintura y los muebles de la casa. Sabe que lo ha hecho bien cuando la gente usa palabras como, "de buen gusto" y "exquisita" para describir su casa. Por otra parte, el estilo de su casa es problemático si la gente se refiere a su casa como, algo "extraña" o "excéntrica".

Cómo Se Define Hogar, Dulce Hogar

¿Qué es exactamente un hogar? Si nos vamos a lo más elemental, un hogar, en sí, es un concepto impreciso. Todo el mundo sabe, por ejemplo, que el hogar es donde reside nuestro corazón. Esto está bien para el que es romántico, pero no es muy útil para el que está comprando una casa.

Hasta ahora, hemos usado los términos "hogar" y "casa" en forma casual para indicar un lugar donde quiere vivir. Bajo esa definición, desde un estudio en Manhattan hasta una choza de paja en una playa hawaiana se pueden considerar como hogar. Sin embargo, ahora es el momento de ser más precisos porque estamos a punto de enfocarnos en tipos de propiedades específicos o que probablemente usted compre: viviendas unifamiliares separadas, condominios y apartamentos cooperativos. Cada una de estas opciones ofrece a los propietarios ventajas y desventajas económicas y personales, que necesitan entender para poder tomar una decisión de compra inteligente.

Viviendas unifamiliares separadas

Si creció en una ciudad grande, la imagen mental que tiene de un hogar probablemente es la de un apartamento en un edificio de concreto y metal, de varios pisos, o una casa adyacente tipo "brownstone" o algún otro tipo de casa en hilera. Por otra parte, si creció en un pueblo pequeño, cuando alguien dice "hogar" lo más seguro es que se imagine una vivienda de ladrillos o con marco de madera, con una cerca blanca, un jardín y columpios en el patio.

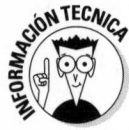

Para distinguir el tipo de casa que ve en zonas donde los terrenos baratos abundan (y en programas de la TV como *Leave It to Beaver*) como condominios, cooperativas u otro tipo de viviendas que les sirven de hogar a muchas personas, la terminología correcta para propiedades del tipo de la cerca blanca es *vivienda unifamiliar separada*. La palabra clave es "separada" porque tales casas no están adyacentes a ninguna otra propiedad. Ahora que ya lo hemos impresionado con la profundidad de nuestro conocimiento, podemos llamarlos simplemente "hogares" o "casas" como lo hacen todos los demás.

Las viviendas unifamiliares separadas, como los carros, son de dos tipos: *nuevas* y *usadas*.

Viviendas nuevas

Si usted es del tipo de persona que nunca considera comprar coches usados porque le gusta el olor a coche nuevo y no le gusta comprar los problemas ajenos, es posible que piense de la misma manera en cuanto a casas. Esto tiene ventajas muy atrayentes:

✔ **Una casa nueva construida correctamente se construye para satisfacer al comprador de hoy.** El escoger una casa nueva hecha por una conocida constructora por su alta calidad le da la tranquilidad de saber que su casa no contiene asbestos, pinturas con plomo, formaldehído, ni ninguna otra sustancia peligrosa ni tóxica. Además, puede estar seguro de que su casa nueva cumple con los vigentes (y más estrictos) códigos federales, estatales y locales de construcción, de incendios y seguridad, y del medio ambiente. ¡Claro, no hay garantía que en el futuro no se descubran más peligros!

✔ **Una casa nueva construida correctamente debe tener un gasto de administración y mantenimiento más económico.** Los gastos de administración se minimizan porque una casa nueva debe tener la tecnología más reciente en sistemas más eficientes de calefacción y aire acondicionado energéticamente, en plomería y servicios eléctricos modernos, en aparatos electrodomésticos energéticamente eficientes y en niveles de aislamiento apropiados. Con una casa nueva, sus gastos iniciales de mantenimiento casi ni existen porque todo es nuevo — el techo, los aparatos electrodomésticos, la pintura interior y exterior, las alfombras y otras cosas más. Aparte de cambiar las bombillas de luz, ¿qué más puede necesitar reparación?

✔ **Una casa nueva correctamente diseñada no lo obligará a ajustar su modo de vida a las limitaciones de ella.** Al contrario, casas nuevas tienen suficientes enchufes en las paredes y en los pisos para todos sus juguetes de alta tecnología — el horno de microondas; la cafetera de café expreso, las conexiones para el satélite y el cable de la tele; videograbadoras y tocadores de CD y DVD; secadoras de pelo, máquinas de afeitar eléctricas y cepillos de dientes eléctricos; equipo para oficinas en la casa como computadoras, monitores, impresoras, conexiones de Internet de banda ancha, faxes, etc. Usted no sufrirá los peligrosos y antiestéticos nidos de cables enredados.

Las casas nuevas sólo pueden ser tan buenas como lo son las constructoras que las edifican. Visite varios de los proyectos hechos por el constructor. Vea con sus propios ojos qué tan bien han aguantado los años esas construcciones. Pregúnteles a los propietarios en vecindarios más viejos si comprarían otra casa nueva de la misma constructora. Vea qué tipo de problemas han tenido a través de los años, si es que los han tenido, y pregunte si la constructora cerró el trato a tiempo y si cumplió con todos los compromisos del contrato a tiempo, incluso los de completar trabajos de construcción no terminados. También averigüe si la constructora arregló de buena gana los defectos que hayan tenido las viviendas o si los propietarios tuvieron que iniciar alguna acción legal para que se corrigieran los problemas. Pregúnteles a los agentes en cuánto han aumentado de valor las casas en esos vecindarios a través del tiempo, y cómo se comparan, en general, con las otras casas de la zona.

Como es de esperarse, las casas nuevas también tienen desventajas. Por ejemplo:

✔ **Lo que normalmente ve, no es lo que recibe.** Usted ve una casa modelo profesionalmente decorada, amueblada de modo exquisito y con jardinería preciosa. Usted, por el contrario, compra una casa vacía, sin muebles, donde casi todo — aparatos eléctricos, alfombras, cortinas, pintura, acabados de la chimenea, jardinería, etcétera — es adicional y no está incluido en el precio básico. Los constructores gastan, con frecuencia, miles y miles de dólares decorando sus casas modelos extravagantemente. Los propietarios nuevos e inexpertos pueden gastar pequeñas fortunas tratando de duplicar el estilo de la casa modelo. Al ver una casa modelo, pregúntele al vendedor lo qué está y no está incluido exactamente en el precio básico, sin nada más agregado.

✔ **Los precios son menos negociables.** Los constructores mantienen el precio original a fin de proteger el valor de las casas no vendidas y para mantener los valores de los avalúos para propósito de los préstamos. Es más, el constructor que recorta precios le está indicando que el proyecto está fracasando. En vez de reducir el precio que están pidiendo, los constructores negocian con usted dándole cosas adicionales gratis o le dan mejoras (por ejemplo, alfombras de mejor calidad, mejores aparatos eléctricos, mostradores de granito en la cocina en vez de Formica).

Algunos constructores atraen compradores a una casa básica y vacía ofreciendo un precio que está muy cerca al del costo real de ellos. Luego, ellos generan sus ganancias por medio de las mejoras y cosas extras que ofrecen. Si al comparar precios se da cuenta de que estas mejoras están exageradamente valoradas, no se las compre a la constructora. En su lugar, compre la casa vacía y compre las cosas adicionales de otros proveedores.

✔ **Basándose en un precio por pie cuadrado, las casas nuevas normalmente son más caras que las usadas.** Es obvio. El costo del terreno, la mano de obra y el material son hoy en día más caros de lo que fueron hace unos años cuando se construyeron las casas; y no se olvide que está comprando una casa sin el desgaste del uso cotidiano.

✔ **Las casas nuevas en zonas de más desarrollo están construidas normalmente en sitios que anteriormente se consideraban poco deseables o inutilizables para la construcción.** Es el viejo principio de "recibir por orden de llegada". Los constructores que llegan primero reciben los mejores sitios. Los constructores de hoy en día toman cualquier terreno disponible —laderas empinadas, llanos inundados y terrenos situados muy lejos del centro del área comercial. En diez o veinte años, los sitios que hoy se consideran pésimos serán considerados de primera para las nuevas construcciones —todo es relativo.

✔ **Las casas nuevas pueden tener costos de administración que no se ven a simple vista.** Los vecindarios que ofrecen muchas amenidades normalmente les cobran cuotas a los propietarios para cubrir los costos de administración y mantenimiento de áreas comunes como piscinas, canchas de tenis, instalaciones para ejercicios, casa club y cosas por el estilo. Algunas asociaciones de propietarios le cobran la misma cuota anual a cada propietario. Otras, prorratean las cuotas en base al tamaño de la casa o al precio de compra — cuanto más grande o más cara su casa, más alta será su cuota. Si el vecindario tiene una asociación de propietarios, averigüe cómo están estructuradas las cuotas y cuánto sería la suya. También averigüe qué reglas (llamadas convenios) controlan lo que puede hacerle a su casa como parte del vecindario. Algunos convenios limitan los colores que puede usar al pintar la casa, los anexos que le puede hacer a la propiedad y si puede o no rentar la propiedad, entre otros. A pesar de que la intención es mantener en alto el valor de las propiedades, algunas de las reglas pueden crearle problemas a la hora de tratar de adaptar su propiedad a su estilo de vida. Para más información detallada sobre los documentos y convenios importantes relacionados con las asociaciones de propietarios, asegúrese de consultar la sección "Residencias adyacentes" posteriormente en este capítulo.

A veces, las cuotas de las asociaciones de propietarios son establecidas artificialmente bajas para camuflar el costo real del vecindario. Cuando sucede esto, tarde o temprano le llegan a los propietarios con ajustes especiales para volver a pintar la casa club, recubrir las canchas de tenis y otras cosas más. Asegúrese de que la asociación de propietarios del vecindario que está considerando tiene reservas adecuadas y que sus cuotas reflejan costos de administración y mantenimiento con precisión. También revise y verifique si la regularidad del aumento de las cuotas ha sido justificada y van de acuerdo a la tasa general de inflación vigente. Eso es algo que probablemente puede determinar preguntándole a su prestamista.

✔ **Es posible que tenga que usar como representante suyo al agente de bienes raíces del constructor.** Los constructores siempre tienen su propio personal de ventas y sus propios contratos de compra. Sin embargo, algunos constructores le permitirán tener un agente de bienes raíces que no trabaja para ellos. Otros insisten en que use el agente de ellos y no es un asunto negociable. Si no está de acuerdo, tiene la opción de no comprarles la casa.

Si se ha enamorado de una casa nueva, pero el constructor no acepta agentes externos, le recomendamos que pague por una valuación independiente para obtener una opinión imparcial sobre el valor de la casa. También es prudente que usted elija un abogado especializado en bienes raíces para que revise su contrato. (Consulte el Capítulo 9 sobre cómo encontrar un agente y lo que puede hacer por usted.)

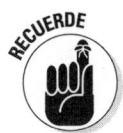

Sólo porque la casa sea completamente nueva no significa que esté libre de defectos. Las casas son construidas por personas y las personas son humanas. Errar es humano — y de ahí la expresión *error humano*. Además, las constructoras trabajan para generar ganancias, sin mencionar que algunas constructoras simplemente no son muy buenas. Por lo tanto, una casa *nueva en la que nadie ha vivido* debe ser inspeccionada *minuciosamente* desde los cimientos al techo por un inspector profesional de propiedades con el fin de descubrir los errores antes de comprarla. Cubrimos el tema de inspección de propiedades, a nuestra manera meticulosa, en el Capítulo 13.

Casas usadas

Quizás se pregunte por qué clasificamos todas las casas como nuevas o usadas. ¿Por qué no usar "nuevas" y "viejas" en vez de "nuevas" y "usadas?" Porque "viejo" no es un término preciso. ¿Qué tan viejo es viejo? ¿Se considera vieja una casa de más de 25 años? ¿O, se debe definir el límite a partir de casas construidas hace más de 50 años? Si las casas construidas hace más de 50 años se consideran viejas, ¿cómo denominamos las casas construidas hace 100 o 200 años? ¿Decrépitas? Por otra parte, *usado* simplemente significa que alguien ha sido dueño de esa casa antes que usted. (Considerando lo caras que son las viviendas, quizás prefiera referirse a la que compre usted como "vivienda con propietario anterior". Si esto lo hace sentirse mejor, adelante.)

Llámelas como las llame, las casas usadas tienen muchas características recomendables:

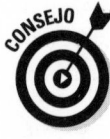

- ✔ **Las casas usadas normalmente son más económicas que las nuevas.** Por lo general, la gente que compró casa hace varios años pagó menos por sus casas de lo que cobran los constructores por construir una casa similar hoy. Además, siempre hay más casas usadas en el mercado que casas nuevas. La siempre fiable competencia mantiene bajo el precio de las casas usadas.

- ✔ **Los precios de venta de las casas usadas son por lo general mucho más negociables que los precios de venta de las casas nuevas.** Los vendedores de casas usadas no tienen que proteger el valor de todo un nuevo vecindario. Típicamente solo quieren cobrar su dinero y continuar con la próxima gran aventura de sus vidas.

- ✔ **Las casas usadas están normalmente situadas en vecindarios bien conocidos y establecidos.** Con una vivienda usada, no tiene que preguntarse cómo acabará siendo el vecindario en algunos años cuando esté completamente establecido. Simplemente vea a su alrededor y podrá ver exactamente qué tipo de escuelas, transporte, comercios, entretenimientos y otros servicios tienen.

- ✔ **Las casas usadas han sido aprobadas con el tiempo.** Para cuando compre la casa usada, sus dueños anteriores normalmente han descubierto los problemas que se ven con el tiempo como: asentamientos, defectos estructurales y defectos de construcción. No tendrá que adivinar qué tan bien envejecerá la casa a través de los años. Puede verlo con sus propios ojos.

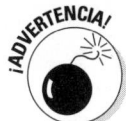

No importa qué tan bien envejezca una casa, de todas maneras un profesional capacitado tiene que inspeccionarla minuciosamente (por dentro y por fuera) antes de que usted la compre. Es posible que los propietarios anteriores no hayan tenido tiempo, dinero o deseos de arreglar los problemas. También puede ser que no hayan estado conscientes de los problemas que no se ven a simple vista. Asegúrese de que la casa cumple con los códigos de construcción vigentes; que no tiene peligros ambientales, para la salud o de seguridad; y que tenga buen material aislante. Nunca trate de ahorrar en inspecciones sólo porque ve bien la casa. La única excepción a esta estricta regla es si sucede que usted es un profesional en inspección de propiedades. (Consulte el Capítulo 13 para más información sobre inspección de viviendas e inspectores).

✔ **Las casas usadas son propiedades "terminadas".** Cuando compra una casa, por lo general no tiene que tomarse la molestia de gastar en comprar e instalar alfombras, cortinas y artefactos de iluminación; poner acabados para la chimenea; sembrar césped; poner un jardín ornamental; construir cercas y patios; instalar sistemas de riego, y otros. El trabajo ya está hecho (a menos que la casa sea un proyecto de remodelación grande) y normalmente todo está incluido en el precio de compra.

✔ **Comprar una casa usada quizás sea la única manera de conseguir el estilo arquitectónico, artesanía o material de construcción que quiere.** ¿Qué tal si lo que quiere es una casa tipo granja de Nueva Inglaterra del siglo diecinueve o una victoriana tipo "Queen Anne"? Quizás quiera paredes con enlucido, pisos de parqué, vitrales, o algún otro tipo de material o artesanía que es carísimo o imposible de conseguir en una casa nueva. Si éste es el caso, compre una casa usada.

Así como las casas nuevas tienen algunas desventajas, las casas usadas también:

✔ **Las casas usadas normalmente son más caras que las nuevas en cuanto a su administración y mantenimiento.** Algunas casas usadas han sido modernizadas con sistemas energéticamente más eficientes de calefacción y aire acondicionado. Aún así, en una casa usada con techos a una altura de 12 pies, la calefacción siempre será más cara que en una con techos a 9 pies. De la misma manera, entre más viejos sean el techo, los desagües, la plomería, el horno, el calentador de agua, y los aparatos eléctricos, más pronto tendrá que repararlos o reemplazarlos.

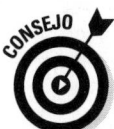

Antes de comprar una casa, pídale al vendedor copias de las facturas de los servicios públicos de los últimos 2 años (gas, electricidad, agua y aguas servidas) para que pueda ver por sí mismo exactamente cuánto le costará el mantenimiento de la casa. Si las facturas de los servicios son muy altas, pregúntele al inspector de la propiedad sobre el costo de hacer la casa energéticamente más eficiente.

El valor de la inversión en una casa unifamiliar separada

Los norteamericanos siempre han tenido un afecto profundamente arraigado por las casas unifamiliares separadas. Como salmones regresando a reproducirse al río donde nacieron, a la hora de comprar casa, mucha gente se ve inexorablemente atraída por el tipo de casa en la que crecieron. Aunque usted no haya crecido en una casa unifamiliar, quizás codicie una porque los programas de televisión y los comerciales le han insistido mucho que estas casas son deseables y que son símbolos de éxito.

La demanda por las casas unifamiliares separadas hace que éstas sean una buena inversión.

Comparadas con residencias adyacentes, como condominios y apartamentos cooperativos, las casas unifamiliares separadas tienden a conservar mejor su valor en mercados bajos y aumentan su valor más rápido en mercados altos. Pídales a los agentes de bienes raíces locales un cotejo del aumento del valor de propiedades de residencias adyacentes, comparadas con residencias unifamiliares separadas y verá a lo que nos estamos refiriendo.

✔ **Las casas usadas, normalmente, son hasta cierto punto funcionalmente anticuadas.** Ejemplos de casas obsoletas funcionalmente, son un diseño y distribución en donde falta una habitación principal, hay un solo baño en una casa de tres dormitorios, falta de cochera, servicio eléctrico inadecuado y falta de calefacción o aire acondicionado central. ¿Cuánta obsolescencia funcional es demasiada? Eso depende de usted. Lo que a nosotros nos parece encantador, a usted le puede parecer un desastre inhabitable. Hablamos sobre casas funcionalmente obsoletas en la sección de reparación de viviendas.

✔ **Las casas usadas maravillosas a veces se encuentran en vecindarios no tan maravillosos.** Es posible que le atraiga una casa antigua y encantadora en un vecindario espantoso. A pesar de lo mucho que cree que le encantaría vivir en ella, no se olvide que tendrá que pasar por la parte indeseable cada vez que quiera salir o llegar a la casa de sus sueños.

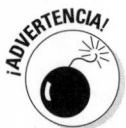

A pesar de que usted puede ignorar guerras entre pandillas y graffiti en todas las paredes, ¿podrán hacerlo los posibles compradores futuros cuando esté listo para vender? Recuerde: "ubicación, ubicación y valor". No importa qué tan despampanante sea la propiedad ni qué tan bueno sea el precio que le ofrezcan, no compre los problemas de alguien más.

Residencias adyacentes

Si no puede aceptar las reglas y normas que por necesidad se le impondrían en viviendas comunales, no lea más. Usted es de espíritu demasiado libre para poder ser feliz en una residencia adyacente.

Pero si está dispuesto a tolerar las limitaciones de una vida comunal para gozar de sus ventajas económicas y del estilo de vida asociado con ella, continúe leyendo. Puede descubrir sorpresas agradables.

Condominios (propiedad horizontal)

¿Qué tipo de propiedad les ofrece a los compradores novatos la opción más económica de vivienda y también les da a personas mayores propietarias de una casa unifamiliar, una alternativa ideal de estilo de vida para la tercera edad? Si dijo "los condominios", le toca una estrellita en la frente.

Algunas personas creen que un *condominio* o propiedad horizontal es un tipo de edificio. Están equivocados. El tipo de edificio en el que se encuentra un condominio no importa. Los condominios pueden ser apartamentos en un edificio de varios pisos en Chicago o una "townhouse" de dos pisos en Dallas o un piso victoriano en San Francisco. Lo que lo hace un condominio es la estructura del *título*.

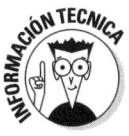

Primero, tomemos un breve descanso para la clase de idiomas de hoy. En Latín, *con* significa "con" y *dominium* significa "dominio". Junte las dos palabras y tenemos *condominio,* que se traduce como "dominio o titularidad con otros" (propiedad con dominio). Definitivamente impresionará a sus colegas con este bocadito de conocimiento etimológico.

Digamos que compra un condominio en un edificio de varios pisos de Chicago. Tiene una hipoteca, impuestos sobre la propiedad y un título de propiedad tan elegante que hasta lo podría enmarcar con lo que puede comprobar que usted es el dueño de la unidad 603, uno de los 100 condominios de ese edificio. Hasta este punto, tener un condominio es más o menos lo mismo que tener una casa unifamiliar pero que flota en el cielo.

Cuando compra una casa unifamiliar aislada, una línea invisible corre alrededor de los límites de su propiedad para separar lo que le pertenece a usted y lo que es de su vecino. Pero, cuando usted compra un condominio los bordes limítrofes de la propiedad son la superficie interior (paredes, piso, techo, ventanas y puertas) de su unidad. En otras palabras, con un condominio, usted tiene derecho o título al aire dentro de su unidad y todo lo que en él está —alfombras, cortinas y lo demás. El mejoramiento del aire y del interior es todo lo que usted posee.

Usted y los demás propietarios en un complejo de condominios comparten la titularidad del *terreno* sobre el cual está situado el proyecto y *edificio* de varios pisos que contiene sus unidades individuales. Por lo tanto, todos ustedes son dueños de parte del techo, de las paredes exteriores del edificio, los cimientos —y también de un trozo del estacionamiento, de los ascensores, la planta baja, los pasillos, la piscina, las canchas de tenis, las instalaciones del gimnasio, etcétera. Todas las partes del complejo que estén más allá de las unidades individuales se conocen como *áreas comunes* porque usted es dueño de ellas junto con los otros dueños de los condominios *en común*. No son cosas suyas nada más.

Si compra un condominio, usted se convierte en miembro de la asociación de propietarios automáticamente. No tiene que asistir a las juntas a menos que quiera, pero tiene que pagar las cuotas de la asociación de propietarios. Las cuotas cubren los gastos de operación y mantenimiento de las áreas comunes, desde sueldos para personal, cloro para la piscina y alumbramiento de la planta baja, hasta colección de basura y seguro contra incendios para el edificio. Una porción de las cuotas va a un fondo de reservas para cubrir reparaciones inevitables, como pintar el edificio de vez en cuando y reemplazar el techo.

Antes de comprar un condominio, averigüe exactamente qué porcentaje tendría de la titularidad común en todo el complejo de condominios. Esto establece cuánto se le cobrará mensualmente para la asociación de propietarios y qué porcentaje pagará de un cobro especial que se puede imponer a los propietarios para cubrir gastos imprevistos de las áreas comunes. Eso también determinará cuántos votos le corresponderán en casos "catastróficos" que afecten al complejo, como decidir si el color del exterior se debiese cambiar a turquesa o mandarina, o si es mejor reparar la caminadora del gimnasio o comprar una nueva, etcétera.

Los condominios usan varios métodos diferentes para establecer los porcentajes de propiedad o titularidad. El método más sencillo es dar a cada propietario una porción igual por todo el complejo. Por lo tanto, a cada dueño le corresponde un voto por la misma cantidad mensual y cualquier otro cobro especial.

Si el porcentaje de titularidad se basa en el tamaño o valor en el mercado del condominio, las personas que tengan las unidades más grandes o caras tienen mayor influencia sobre lo que sucede con el complejo que los dueños de los condominios más pequeños o económicos. Sin embargo, estas personas de influencia también tienen las cuotas más altas para la asociación de propietarios correspondientes y pagan un porcentaje más alto de los cobros especiales.

¿Por qué un condominio?

Tomando en cuanta la complejidad de un condominio, ¿por qué compra la gente condominios? ¿Por qué todos, simplemente, no comprar casas unifamiliares separadas? Por lo siguiente:

- **Las residencias adyacentes aumentan su poder de compra.** Compare el precio de un condominio de dos dormitorios con el de una vivienda unifamiliar separada, de dos dormitorios, en el mismo vecindario. Basándose en pies cuadrados habitables, los condominios normalmente se venden por lo menos en un 20 o 30 por ciento menos que las casas unifamiliares similares. El tener su propio techo, cimientos y terreno es mucho más caro que compartir estos gastos con muchos otros propietarios.

  Para algunos compradores potenciales, la opinión es: comprar un condominio que cumple con sus necesidades de espacio o continuar alquilando. La necesidad económica explica porqué el camino que conduce al sueño americano —para cada casi uno de cinco compradores novatos— es la titularidad de un condominio. La unión hace la fuerza... en la compra.

✔ **El mantenimiento de residencias adyacentes normalmente cuesta menos que el de una casa unifamiliar separada.** Digamos que usted es uno de los 100 propietarios de los condominios en un edificio de varios pisos en Chicago. A diferencia del propietario de una casa unifamiliar separada que tiene que pagar todos los costos de mantenimiento —tales como la instalación de un techo nuevo o pintura exterior—, usted puede compartir estos gastos de mantenimiento con los otros 99 propietarios. A pesar de que en términos absolutos, reemplazar el techo del edificio de varios pisos, por ejemplo, cuesta mucho más que reemplazar el techo de una casa unifamiliar separada, el costo por propietario debe ser mucho menos. La unión hace la fuerza... en el ahorro.

✔ **Las residencias adyacentes tienen servicios que de otra manera no podrían pagar.** ¿Cuántas personas conoce usted que tengan una casa unifamiliar separada con canchas de tenis, piscinas y gimnasios lujosos? Muchos propietarios no pueden pagar lujos como éstos; pero cuando el costo se comparte con los demás propietarios en un complejo de condominios grande, ese sueño imposible de repente se vuelve su realidad hedonística. La unión hace la fuerza... en el lujo.

✔ **Las residencias adyacentes son los hogares ideales para algunas personas de la tercera edad.** A medida que se acerca su jubilación, es posible que se sienta como un cascabelito en una sonajera enorme en una casa unifamiliar separada. Quizás, un condominio de dos dormitorios en un edificio sin problemas de mantenimiento y, un portero que remite su correspondencia mientras usted anda en una de sus muchas vacaciones, podría solucionar todos sus problemas. La unión hace la fuerza... en el estilo de vida.

Desventajas de los condominios

Al igual que las casas unifamiliares separadas, los condominios no son para todos. Juzgue por sí mismo cuánto le pueden afectar las siguientes desventajas a usted:

✔ **Los condominios ofrecen menos privacidad.** Paredes compartidas significa que puede oír a los demás más fácilmente. La contaminación del ruido es uno de los problemas más grandes de tener un condominio y el aspecto que la mayoría de los posibles compradores pasan por alto. Visite la unidad a diferentes horas y días para observar el nivel de ruido. Hable con los dueños de los condominios en el complejo y vea si les molesta la contaminación del ruido. De ser posible, pase unas horas o una tarde en una unidad. Asegúrese de apagar la música suave que tenía en el fondo el agente de bienes raíces cuando le mostró la unidad.

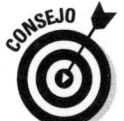

Por lo general, entre menos paredes comparta con un vecino, más privacidad tendrá dentro de su unidad. Ése es uno de los motivos por los cuales las unidades de las esquinas se venden a precios más altos; y si su unidad está en el último piso, no tendrá a nadie caminando en su techo (a menos que haya acceso a la azotea, claro). Si tiene el dinero, en cuanto a privacidad en un condominio, lo mejor es una unidad en esquina en el último piso y no en planta baja.

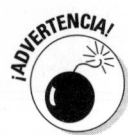

✔ **Los condominios son legalmente complejos.** Antes de comprar su condominio, debe recibir copias de tres documentos sumamente importantes: el título de propiedad principal o declaración de convenios, condiciones y restricciones (*Declaration of Covenants, Conditions and Restrictions,* [*CC&Rs,* por sus siglas en inglés]); las reglas internas de la asociación de propietarios y el presupuesto de la asociación de propietarios. (Consulte las notas "Documentos de condominios" resaltadas en color gris.) Por favor, lea estos documentos de pe a pa.

Los *CC&R,* las reglas internas y el presupuesto comprometen legalmente a todos los propietarios del condominio. A pesar de que hacen mucho bulto y son numerosos y aburridos, tiene que leerlos con muchísimo cuidado. Si tiene preguntas sobre lo que significan estos documentos o si no entiende su importancia, asesórese con un abogado de bienes raíces. Ya que estamos hablando de cosas legales, averigüe con su agente o con la asociación de propietarios si el condominio está implicado en un litigio o va a estarlo en un futuro cercano. Las demandas son caras.

✔ **Los condominios son financieramente complicados.** Como posible propietario, repase el presupuesto de administración actual. Asegúrese de que cubra en forma realista los costos de mantenimiento, personal, servicios, recolección de basura, primas de seguro y otros gastos operativos normales. Si el presupuesto está demasiado bajo, prepárese para que, tarde o temprano, le vengan con aumentos masivos. De la misma manera, asegúrese de que el presupuesto incluye fondos de reservas adecuadas para cubrir gastos importantes previsibles, tales como retoques a la pintura exterior de vez en cuando y techos nuevos. ¿Cuánto es adecuado? Normalmente, del tres al cinco por ciento del presupuesto bruto de administración se considera una reserva mínima aceptable. Si los fondos reservados están muy bajos, hay peligro de que le hagan un cobro especial en caso de una emergencia económica.

Recomendamos que revise los presupuestos de mantenimiento y los estados de cuenta de los últimos años para ver si hay indicaciones de mala gestión fiscal. Las siguientes son alertas de mala administración de las que se tiene que cuidar:

- **Aumentos frecuentes y grandes de las cuotas de la asociación de propietarios.** Las cuotas no deben de subir anualmente a un ritmo más acelerado del ritmo de la inflación vigente.

- **Cobros especiales que no hubieran sido necesarios si la asociación hubiera tenido una reserva adecuada.** Al hablar sobre el presupuesto y el fondo de reservas, averigüe si se anticipan aumentos en las cuotas o si hay cobros especiales en un futuro cercano para compensar el déficit de administración o cubrir el costo de proyectos grandes.

- **Hay demasiados propietarios con cuotas impagadas.** Los costos administrativos continúan paguen o no las cuotas todos los propietarios.

✔ **Algunos reglamentos de condominios son excesivamente restrictivos.**
Las personas que viven cerca unos con otros necesitan algunas reglas
para mantener orden y conservar la armonía. Sin embargo, demasiadas
reglas pueden convertir su condominio en una prisión. Por ejemplo, los
condominios pueden tener reglas especificando qué tipo de piso y cortinas tiene que tener en su unidad, y el tamaño y número de mascotas que
puede tener en su unidad; reglas limitando su capacidad para alquilar
su unidad a alguien más o prohibiéndole hacer cambios o mejoras a su
unidad; reglas limitando cuándo o qué tan seguido puede tener invitados en su apartamento, y otras más. Antes de comprar, lea los *CC&R* y
las reglas internas cuidadosamente para averiguar exactamente qué tipo
de restricciones de uso contienen. Algunas de estas restricciones también pueden verse en nuevos proyectos de casas unifamiliares separadas, como se mencionó anteriormente.

Si descubre que el condominio (o proyecto nuevo de viviendas) tiene
restricciones que no le gustan, no compre la unidad. El tratar de modificar los *CC&R* o las reglas internas para eliminar restricciones después
de haber comprado la unidad es, generalmente, una práctica en el arte
de lo inútil y frustrante. Sabemos que usted tiene mejores cosas que
hacer que desperdiciar una gran parte de su tiempo regateando con
asociaciones de condominios y sus abogados.

Las restricciones prudentes sobre arrendamientos son un tesoro. Lo ideal
es que todas las unidades estén ocupadas por sus dueños. Si algunos
dueños *a veces* le permiten a sus amigos usar sus unidades, o rentan sus
unidades por una o dos semanas cuando están de vacaciones, no hay
problema. Sin embargo, si la mayoría de las unidades les pertenecen a
inversionistas ausentes que las rentan a un desfile de desconocidos fies-
teros, es malo, y especialmente si a usted le cuesta trabajo dormir con
música a todo volumen durante la noche. También puede ser difícil
conseguir un préstamo hipotecario en un complejo con demasiados
inquilinos.

✔ **Condominios completamente nuevos tienen las mismas ventajas y
desventajas que las casas unifamiliares separadas nuevas, pero son
más complicados por la complejidad legal y económica que tienen.** Si
no ha leído la sección anterior en este capítulo sobre casas unifamiliares
separadas nuevas, ahora es el momento de hacerlo. Todos los avisos de
precaución que dimos para esas casas también son pertinentes a condominios nuevos. Así como con las casas nuevas, los nuevos proyectos de
condominios son tan buenos o malos como lo sean los constructores que
los construyeron y los abogados que los crearon. Ya que ningún proyecto
nuevo por definición tiene historial, deberá visitar proyectos hechos
anteriormente por el mismo constructor para ver qué tan bien han enve-
jecido los condominios y cuán satisfechos están los dueños de ellos.

Algunos constructores de condominios nuevos, sin escrúpulos, calculan
a propósito un costo mensual de administración demasiado bajo con el
fin de engañar a posibles compradores para que éstos piensen que es
menos costoso vivir ahí de lo que realmente es. Esos constructores

pagan una porción de los gastos mensuales, de sus propios bolsillos, para mantener el costo del proyecto artificialmente bajo. La guillotina económica cae cuando la compañía entrega el proyecto a la asociación de propietarios, que pronto se ve forzada a subir las cuotas para cubrir los gastos administrativos verdaderos. Cuando el costo de administración proyectado se ve demasiado bueno como para ser verdad, lo más seguro es que no lo es. Compare los gastos administrativos proyectados con los gastos administrativos de otros proyectos similares ya establecidos.

✔ **En cuanto al estacionamiento y almacenaje en condominios, lo que parece ser obvio, no lo es.** Por ejemplo, ¿su título de propiedad incluye una cochera o espacio titulado que solamente usted puede usar, o se usan los espacios "por orden de llegada?" ¿Hay cobros adicionales para estacionarse o están incluidos en las cuotas mensuales? ¿Hay disponibilidad de espacios para invitados? ¿Hay estacionamiento para lanchas o remolques? ¿Tiene un área de almacenaje de su propiedad que esté situada fuera de su unidad? Si la tiene, ¿dónde está? Si necesita aún más almacenaje, ¿hay disponible y cuánto cuesta? Le conviene mucho más obtener respuestas a estas preguntas antes y no después de comprar.

✔ **Algunos edificios de apartamentos que han sido adaptados a condominios pero tienen problemas obsoletos de funcionamiento.** Con frecuencia los edificios más viejos tienen detalles y artesanía excelente. Sin embargo, con frecuencia también tienen sistemas de calefacción y aire acondicionado anticuados; y es posible que les falten elevadores, que son bastante útiles si, por ejemplo, está cargando el mandado o maletas y tiene que subir varios pisos. Si está comprando un condominio en un edificio más viejo, averigüe si los servicios se calculan por unidad o si están incluidos en la cuota mensual de la asociación de propietarios. ¿Su unidad tiene termostato para controlar la calefacción o el aire acondicionado, o tienen un control centralizado?

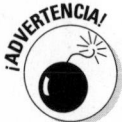

Si se incluyen los servicios públicos en las cuotas mensuales, los demás propietarios de los condominios no tienen incentivos para economizar por medio del uso moderado de la calefacción o del aire acondicionado. Si usted es una persona ahorrativa, simplemente acabará subsidiando a los propietarios que no lo son. Al mismo tiempo, en un edificio con calefacción y aire acondicionado centrales, es posible que sus opciones climáticas se limiten a estarse asando en el inverno y a congelarse en el verano. Aunque usted pueda vivir con esos sobrecargos de servicios o la incomodidad personal, estos factores pueden ahuyentar a futuros compradores cuando trate de vender su unidad.

✔ **El tamaño puede ser un problema.** Los complejos de condominios grandes, con frecuencia, tienen un aspecto impersonal y similar a un hotel. Por lo general, las personas que viven en complejos grandes tienden a no prestar atención a las finanzas y a los detalles diarios de administración porque la asociación de propietarios contrata una compañía administradora de propiedades para que manejen todo en nombre de los propietarios. Sin embargo, tener un condominio en un complejo grande tiene una que otra ventaja que recompensa. Si, por ejemplo, varios propietarios de un complejo de 100 dueños no cumplen con el pago de su cuota mensual, no es el fin del mundo económicamente. Lo que es más, socialmente hablando, la probabilidad de toparse con un propietario que no le guste mucho disminuye en un complejo residencial grande.

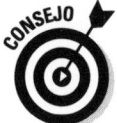

No compre en un complejo de condominios pequeño a menos que disfrute de la amistad personal con sus vecinos. Evalúe a los demás dueños cuidadosamente y asegúrese de que sean del tipo de personas de las que puede estar seguro que cumplirán su parte con sus obligaciones económicas y administrativas. En un complejo pequeño, usted participa en forma activa en la asociación de propietarios porque tiene que hacerlo. Cada voto tiene un impacto inmediato en sus finanzas y en la calidad de vida. No tiene que adorar a los demás propietarios, PERO si algunos de ellos, o todos, son personas con las que usted no se va a poder llevar bien, no compre la unidad.

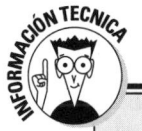

Documentos del condominio

Si usted es del tipo de persona que sólo le interesa saber la hora, sáltese esta parte. Si, por otra parte, le intriga saber cómo se fabrican los relojes, le encantará esta sección porque le explica las menudencias de cómo se crean y administran los condominios.

Un proyecto de condominios nace cuando una compañía registra el Título de propiedad principal o la Declaración de convenios, condiciones y restricciones (*CC&R*) en la oficina de registros del condado, lo que hace que esta información sea de conocimiento público, a la vista de todo el mundo. Los *CC&R* establecen el condominio al crear una asociación de propietarios, al estipular cómo se manejarán el mantenimiento y las reparaciones, y al establecer control de lo que se puede o no hacer en las unidades individuales y en las áreas comunes del condominio. En nuevos desarrollos planificados de casas unifamiliares separadas algunas veces usan un procedimiento similar.

Las reglas internas permiten el buen funcionamiento de los condominios. Ellas también describen con mucho detalle los poderes legales administrativos, las responsabilidades y el manejo de la asociación de propietarios. Estas reglas internas también cubren elementos esenciales de cómo se eligen los miembros de la directiva de la asociación de propietarios y el poder que se le otorga para imponer cargos a los propietarios de las unidades del condominio.

Finalmente, el planificador de la construcción crea un presupuesto. A diferencia de nuestro gobierno, el presupuesto de los condominios no puede (en teoría, al menos) operar en números rojos. El presupuesto actual establece lo que el condominio espera gastar este año en administración y mantenimiento. Los propietarios de los condominios también reciben anualmente un estado de cuenta de ingresos y gastos, indicando específicamente cómo se gastaron las cuotas del año anterior y detallando la situación financiera presente de los condominios.

Después de leer las desventajas de ser dueño de un condominio, quizás piense que sólo un tonto compraría un condominio. ¡No es verdad! Nosotros conocemos a muchos propietarios de condominios que están muy contentos y que nunca considerarían comprar una vivienda unifamiliar separada. En nuestro afán por protegerlo, muchas veces, se nos pasa la mano con las precauciones. Lo hacemos con su bienestar en mente.

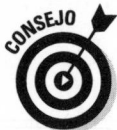

Los condominios tienen más sentido para las personas que no quieren molestias de administración y mantenimiento (recuerde que aún así, tendrá el *gasto*), y que quieren maximizar el valor de su dinero en cuanto a gastos de espacio y que no necesitan un jardín privado. Comprar un condominio por unos años, mientras ahorra dinero para comprarse una casa unifamiliar separada, no tiene mucho sentido financieramente. Dados los gastos de compra y venta de un condominio, combinados con el hecho de que lo más probable es que no se valorice mucho, lo más seguro es que le convenga más esperar y comprar una casa unifamiliar si cree que lo hará en unos cinco años o menos.

Apartamentos cooperativos

Los dos tipos de residencias adyacentes más comunes son los condominios y los apartamentos cooperativos, normalmente llamados cooperativas. No puede distinguir cuál es cuál con sólo ver el edificio o las unidades individuales. Al igual que los condominios, lo que crea una cooperativa es su estatus legal.

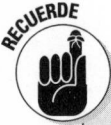

También hay que inspeccionar los condominios

Cuando compre un condominio, tiene que inspeccionar el edificio entero —no sólo su unidad. Como se explica en los Capítulos 9 y 13, necesita un inspector profesional porque la condición estructural y mecánica de la propiedad afecta enormemente el valor. ¿En qué condiciones están los componentes caros de las áreas comunes, tales como el techo, los sistemas de calefacción y aire acondicionado, los sistemas de plomería y eléctricos, los elevadores y los cimientos? ¿Están en buenas condiciones las áreas de recreación como las canchas de tenis, la piscina y el gimnasio? Puesto que está comprando parte de todas las áreas comunes junto con su unidad individual, necesita la opinión de un profesional sobre las condiciones de todo el complejo.

Revise el aislamiento para el ruido preguntándoles a otros propietarios si les molestan los ruidos de las unidades que rodean su unidad. El edificio tiene problemas de ventilación si usted puede oler dentro de su unidad o en el pasillo comida cocinándose en otras unidades. Si descubre que hacen falta reparaciones o mantenimientos caros, y las reservas de los condominios no tienen, ni por asomo, la cantidad de dinero necesaria para cubrir los costos anticipados, no compre una unidad en este complejo. Tarde o temprano, a los dueños les llegará un cobro especial o un incremento enorme en sus cuotas.

Le encantará saber que la mayoría de las ventajas y desventajas de tener un condominio también son iguales a las de una cooperativa, así que no tiene que leer un montón de cosas nuevas. (Si no leyó las secciones anteriores sobre condominios, léalas ahora). En las siguientes secciones nos enfocaremos en las tres maneras en que los condominios y las cooperativas se diferencian: la definición del título de propiedad, la administración y sus opciones financieras.

Definición de propiedad: título o acciones

Cuando compra un condominio, le dan el título de propiedad de su unidad. Cuando compra una cooperativa, le dan un certificado de acciones (que comprueba que usted es dueño de cierta cantidad de acciones en la corporación cooperativa) y un *arrendamiento de propiedad* que le da derecho a vivir en el apartamento que compró. La corporación es propietaria del edificio y tiene el título de propiedad a su nombre como, por ejemplo, "Corporación 10 West 86th Street". Por lo tanto, usted es copropietario del edificio y, simultáneamente, inquilino del mismo.

En la mayoría de las cooperativas, las acciones se destinan en base al tamaño de la unidad y en qué piso está. Por lo tanto, un apartamento en el último piso normalmente tiene más acciones que una unidad del mismo tamaño en planta baja. Entre más acciones tenga, mayor será su influencia sobre la cooperativa, porque cada acción le da un voto. Desgraciadamente, el poder tiene su precio. Su parte prorrateada de los gastos de mantenimiento total también se basa en la cantidad de votos que tenga en la cooperativa. Si tiene muchas acciones, sus gastos mensuales serán proporcionalmente más altos; cuando esté listo para vender su apartamento, los gastos mensuales que son proporcionalmente más altos pueden reducir su valor.

Gestión: asociación de propietarios o mesa directiva

Si alguna vez ha soñado con ser el director de una mesa directiva, aquí está su oportunidad: compre apartamento en una cooperativa y ascienda en la organización. Como su unidad está en un edificio que es de una corporación, lo rige una mesa directiva elegida por usted y por los demás propietarios. Aparte del nombre, así como la asociación de propietarios en un condominio, una mesa directiva es responsable de la administración y finanzas de la cooperativa.

Financiamiento de su compra

Puede que sea difícil conseguir un préstamo para financiar su vivienda cooperativa. Muchos prestamistas se rehúsan rotundamente a aceptar acciones de una corporación cooperativa como garantía de la hipoteca. Del mismo modo, algunas cooperativas se rehúsan rotundamente a un financiamiento personal por encima del valor de la hipoteca que tiene todo el edificio o cooperativa. Estas cooperativas creen que una prueba de su solvencia de crédito es su capacidad para pagar su unidad en efectivo.

Comprar y vender una cooperativa es frecuentemente un reto

El comprar y vender una cooperativa normalmente es mucho más difícil que comprar y vender condominios. La mayoría de las cooperativas estipulan que los propietarios no pueden vender o transferir sus acciones o los arrendamientos de la propiedad sin el consentimiento expreso de la mesa directiva o de la mayoría de los propietarios.

Los compradores potenciales por lo general tienen que proporcionar varias cartas de referencia sobre su excelente carácter y calidad de persona con alta solvencia crediticia. Además, es posible que tengan que someterse a toda una inquisición por parte de la mesa directiva. Dado que los propietarios viven tan cerca y dependen económicamente el uno del otro, tener la posibilidad de eliminar parranderos, desobligados y otros seres similares, es prudente, con tal de que este poder no se abuse para discriminar injustamente contra los compradores.

Aún así, algunos compradores sienten que el proceso de aprobación es extremadamente revelador y se oponen completamente a entregar sus estados financieros a desconocidos. El proceso de aprobación también tiende a demorar la venta de unidades de una cooperativa.

Ser dueño de una cooperativa es un arma de dos filos. Como dueño de una cooperativa, tendrá muchísimo más control sobre quiénes son (o no son) sus vecinos comparado con un condominio. Desgraciadamente, ese control tiene dos desventajas. Cuando trate de vender su unidad, las personas que usted considere compradores perfectos pueden ser rechazadas por la cooperativa porque sus vecinos creen que los posibles compradores tendrían demasiados invitados o no pueden con la carga económica. Renunciar al hecho de vender su cooperativa al mejor comprador, puede ser un precio demasiado caro por el derecho de escoger sus vecinos.

A menos que sea más rico que Midas, no compre en una cooperativa si solamente uno o dos prestamistas en su área dan préstamos para apartamentos en cooperativas. Lo más probable es que tenga que pagar un interés más alto por falta de competencia entre las entidades prestamistas y por la preocupación de los prestamistas sobre el alto riesgo que conllevan las cooperativas. Peor aún, ¿qué sucede si estas entidades dejan de ofrecer hipotecas para cooperativas y ningún otro prestamista toma su lugar? Usted no podrá vender su apartamento hasta que no encuentre a alguien que lo compre al contado (y de esos hay muy pocos) o hasta tener los recursos económicos para prestarle el dinero al posible comprador usted mismo.

Cómo Encontrar una Ganga

Si es como la mayoría de las personas, tiene la desdicha de tener gustos de magnate y bolsillo de bolero. Las casas que tanto desea cuestan mucho más de lo que puede pagar. Para comprar estas casas tendría que encontrar una ganga increíble o ganarse la lotería.

Las gangas increíbles *sí* existen. El truco es saber dónde encontrarlas y cómo evaluarlas. No pierda el tiempo buscando casas perfectas si busca una buena ganga. La gente paga precios de lujo por la perfección. Las casas que se encuentran a precios increíbles son las propiedades imperfectas —casas con problemas estructurales o económicos. La oferta que se le ofrece es un incentivo para que usted enfrente el problema. La pregunta es si la oferta le conviene más a usted o al vendedor.

En el Capítulo 4 hablamos sobre las estrategias para una buena compra en cualquier tipo de mercado. En el resto de este capítulo cubrimos situaciones especiales de propiedades que pueden ser buenas ofertas o gato por liebre.

Cómo encontrar viviendas para reparar

Las viviendas para reparación son casas destartaladas con problemas estructurales. Los agentes de bienes raíces normalmente se refieren a este tipo de casas con eufemismos como casas que "necesitan trabajo" o que "tienen gran potencial".

Las viviendas para reparación no son muy populares en un mercado de bienes raíces lento. La mayoría de los compradores en tales mercados no quieren molestarse con los problemas e incertidumbres de financiamiento relacionados con una casa con reparaciones complicadas. Prefieren comprar casas en condiciones habitables. Estas casas son seguras, pero son inversiones pasivas. Como su valor potencial se ha logrado completamente, el nuevo propietario no puede hacerle mucho para aumentar su valor.

Por otra parte, una casa en pésimas condiciones, ofrece posibles recompensas más grandes para personas que tienen la visión de ver más allá del desastre presente y "ver" la casa maravillosa que puede ser. El comprador de una casa en necesidad de reparaciones también tiene que tener los recursos económicos y el valor para llevar a cabo las reparaciones. Si usted es de este tipo de personas, éste puede ser el futuro que gozará después de haber transformado su patito feo en un bello cisne:

- ✔ Estará viviendo en una casa más bonita y en un vecindario mejor al que normalmente podría pagar.

- ✔ En vez de comprar una casa decorada con lo que alguien más considera buen gusto, su casa estará como a usted le gusta.

- ✔ Es posible que haya aumentado el valor justo del mercado de su casa mucho más que los gastos que tuvo que hacer para mejorarla.

Por ejemplo, si es muy hábil y diestro, puede aumentar el valor de su casa en miles de dólares si hace usted mismo los trabajos laboriosos como pintar, empapelar y la jardinería. La participación en forma del sudor de su frente puede pagar dividendos muy grandes.

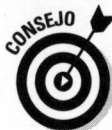

Si es como nosotros, con pocas destrezas, olvídese de hacer estas labores. A la larga, es menos frustrante y más económico ganarse la vida haciendo lo que sabe hacer y usar parte de ese dinero para contratar a personas competentes para que hagan lo que *ellos* saben hacer. El trabajo mal hecho es un ahorro falso: se ve horrible y disminuye el valor de la propiedad. Es mucho más fácil y rápido hacer el proyecto bien la primera vez. Además, es mucho más económico, que hacerlo mal usted mismo y luego tener que pagarle a alguien más para que arregle su desastre. Si usted es una de esas raras personas que puede hacer un buen trabajo, entonces, adelante. Inténtelo —sólo sea realista con el tiempo y el costo requerido.

Algunas viviendas en malas condiciones son fáciles de identificar; parecen casas de espanto y brinco como para celebrar el día de las brujas —la pintura se está pelando, las contraventanas se están cayendo, el césped parece bosque y otras cosas más. Por supuesto, las cosas en su interior no son mejores. Es posible que estas casas necesiten todo, desde una buena limpieza hasta cambios totales del sistema eléctrico y de la plomería.

Sin embargo, otras viviendas que necesitan reparación son mucho más engañosas. Algunas casas, condominios y cooperativas más viejas, por ejemplo, pueden verse bien al principio, pero tienen un funcionamiento obsoleto. Son aptas para vivir, pero necesitan mejoramientos, tales como una habitación principal, baños o garajes, y la modernización de sus sistemas eléctricos para que cumplan con los estándares más rigurosos de hoy en día.

Cómo encontrar un diamante en el pedregal

Encontrar una vivienda en pésimas condiciones, pero adecuada, no es cuestión de suerte; al contrario, requiere de mucha persistencia, habilidad y tenacidad. Usted invierte mucho tiempo examinando propiedades e invierte mucho más tiempo — de su precioso tiempo — evaluando promesas que a fin de cuentas económicamente no tienen sentido; pero, de pronto, cuando ya está a punto de darse por vencido, descubre finalmente el diamante en bruto y lo compra.

Esta es la manera de separar los diamantes de las piedrecillas:

✔ **Lea este libro.** Todo lo que necesita saber está aquí. Preste atención en especial a los temas que se cubren en este capítulo (buenos vecindarios; principios de progresión, regresión y similitud; casas y condominios usados). También el Capítulo 10 (cómo determinar el valor justo del mercado con precisión para que no pague demás) y el Capítulo 13 (inspecciones a la propiedad). También asegúrese de que puede sobrellevar el desembolso económico para arreglar la casa después de la compra (consulte el Capítulo 2).

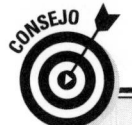

Reparaciones estructurales y mejoras

El trabajo que se le hace a una vivienda en necesidad de reparación cabe en dos categorías amplias: reparaciones estructurales y renovaciones o mejoras. *Las reparaciones estructurales* son cambios que le hace a la propiedad para que ésta cumpla con los estándares de sanidad y seguridad. Este trabajo puede incluir reparaciones a los cimientos, reemplazo del techo, instalación de nuevos sistemas de electricidad y plomería nueva, entre otros — cosas que cuestan mucho dinero pero que agregan relativamente poco valor a la propiedad. Lo ideal es conseguir un descuento del vendedor para hacer parte, si no todas, las reparaciones estructurales necesarias. Entre menos tenga que desembolsar para hacer reparaciones, más puede gastar en mejoras o renovaciones.

Las renovaciones aumentan el valor de la casa al modernizarla. Algunos ejemplos de renovaciones importantes que hacen que la casa sea más funcional, agradable y valiosa al venderla incluyen la remodelación de una cocina vieja, la instalación de un segundo baño y agregar una cochera.

Las renovaciones estéticas (pintura, alfombras, jardinería ornamental y cosas similares) también aumentan el valor con mucho menos gasto y problemas. Las casas en necesidad de reparación que son ideales para comprar son las que se ven espantosas pero que sólo necesitan arreglos estéticos para verse de lo mejor.

✔ **Inspeccione de arriba a abajo la vivienda que necesita reparación antes de comprarla.** La propiedad debe de inspeccionarse cuidadosamente antes de comprarse (consulte el Capítulo 13.) Una vivienda en estas condiciones necesita un examen aún más profundo para que usted sepa exactamente en qué se está metiendo. Su oferta de compra debe estar sujeta a las condiciones de la inspección de la propiedad y de la resolución satisfactoria de los problemas que descubran. Puede encontrar estas cláusulas en el Capítulo 12.

✔ **Obtenga presupuestos de contratistas para las reparaciones estructurales y las renovaciones.** Puede usar los diferentes presupuestos de constructores como herramientas de negociación, para obtener un abono para pagar por los daños o puede obtener un precio más bajo de compra por parte del vendedor para las reparaciones estructurales — como daños por termitas y un techo nuevo. También debe conseguir presupuestos para renovaciones tales como la modernización de un baño, una cocina y gabinetes nuevos, calefacción central y cualquier otra cosa que se requiera para modernizar la propiedad.

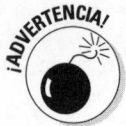

Si los presupuestos que recibe indican que acabará con la casa más cara de la cuadra, no haga el proyecto. El trabajo de reparación tiene tres reglas que nunca fallan:

- Siempre es más trabajo del que se esperaba.

- Siempre toma más tiempo del que se planeaba.

- Siempre cuesta más de lo que se calculaba.

Por lo tanto, si los costos de reparación hacen que la propiedad sea la más cara de la cuadra, para cuando el trabajo termine, ¡el costo real hará que la casa sea la más cara del estado!

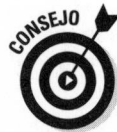

Normalmente conseguir un préstamo es difícil si el costo anticipado de las reparaciones excede el 3 por ciento del valor de la propiedad, que casi siempre es el caso de casas con problemas mayores. Sin embargo, un buen agente de bienes raíces debe saber cuáles entidades prestamistas en su zona se especializan en préstamos para casas que necesitan reparaciones grandes. Si ese prestamista lo considera digno de crédito y ve factible su proyecto, es posible que le dé un préstamo hipotecario para comprar la propiedad *y* un préstamo de construcción para llevar a cabo las mejoras.

Comentario final sobre viviendas en necesidad de reparación

Es normal sentirse abrumado por los riesgos relacionados con una vivienda que necesita reparación. Ahora usted entiende por qué muchos de los compradores normalmente las evitan. Temen caer en un pozo sin fondo que interrumpa sus vidas por completo y se trague todos sus ahorros. Alquile las películas *Mr. Blandings Builds His Dream House* y *The Money Pit* en su tienda de videos para que tenga una idea de lo que podría ser su futuro en bienes raíces.

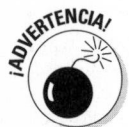

Desgraciadamente, la mayoría de los compradores novatos subestiman el tiempo y costo requerido para las casas que necesitan reparaciones. A fin de cuentas, casi todas las personas descubren que les hubiera costado lo mismo, o menos, comprar una casa terminada y evitar los dolores de cabeza de hacer o coordinar las renovaciones. Algunas personas han acabado en la ruina y hasta se han divorciado por el estrés causado por tales renovaciones.

Si disfruta de los retos y está dispuesto a investigar mucho, recuerde los siguientes consejos para maximizar sus posibilidades de éxito en una vivienda que necesita reparación:

- ✔ Compre en el mejor vecindario que pueda pagar.

- ✔ Compre una de las casas más económicas de la cuadra.

- ✔ Asegúrese de que los trabajos de renovación compensen la inversión y generen plusvalía.

- ✔ Asegúrese de que el precio de la casa sea lo suficientemente bajo como para permitirle hacer las reparaciones y renovaciones sin convertir su propiedad en la casa más cara de la cuadra.

Si los dioses de bienes raíces jugaran limpio, quien comprara la casa exquisitamente *terminada* que usted transformó de un patito feo a un cisne hermoso, debiera pagar un bono por su visión, por reconocer el potencial de esa casa, por su audacia al enfrentarse al riesgo económico y por su paciencia al aguantar el caos y el polvo de la remodelación. Si (y solamente si) elige inteligentemente y negocia el precio inteligentemente, y hace las renovaciones inteligentemente, podrá disfrutar de años felices viviendo en la casa maravillosa que ha creado — y además tener una ganancia muy buena al venderla.

Adquisición de un embargo hipotecario

Para conseguir una hipoteca, usted le da a la entidad hipotecaria el derecho a quitarle su casa y venderla para pagar el saldo pendiente si:

- ✔ No hace los pagos mensuales del préstamo.

- ✔ No paga los impuestos sobre la propiedad.

- ✔ Deja vencer la póliza del seguro de propiedad.

- ✔ Hace cualquier cosa que ponga en peligro su casa económicamente.

La acción legal para embargar una casa y venderla es un *embargo hipotecario o ejecución hipotecaria.*

Cada año, cientos y miles de casas terminan con un embargo hipotecario. Estos embargos hipotecarios con frecuencia son el resultado del uso indebido del crédito. Sin embargo, en otros casos hay gente que simplemente pasa por malas rachas: pierden su trabajo, tienen gastos médicos inesperados, sufren una muerte en la familia o se divorcian.

Es posible que haya oído historias sobre personas que consiguieron buenas ofertas al comprar casas embargadas a un precio muy por debajo del valor del avalúo de la casa. De hecho, algunas personas que compran propiedades embargadas corren con suerte, pero por cada ganador con suerte hay muchos más que no ganan nada o que, de hecho, pierden dinero al comprar una propiedad embargada.

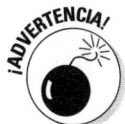

Por favor, tenga cuidado — las propiedades embargadas normalmente son un infierno legal y económico. A menos que tenga un experto con usted que lo guíe a través del proceso completo del embargo hipotecario, de principio a fin, ni siquiera piense en comprar una propiedad embargada.

Si compra una casa embargada, lo más seguro es que también compre los problemas del propietario anterior. A continuación tiene una lista de los riesgos que debe considerar:

- ✔ **Estéticos:** algunos propietarios reaccionan ante la desgracia emocional de un embargo hipotecario con una actitud de "si no puede ser nuestra, nos aseguraremos de que nadie la quiera". Antes de irse, se llevan los aparatos electrodomésticos, los artefactos de iluminación, los gabinetes, los lavabos, los escusados y otras cosas de valor. En casos extremos, rompen las ventanas, tiran concreto por el drenaje de la cocina y del baño, arrancan el cableado eléctrico de las paredes, desentierran los arbustos, cortan los árboles y hacen cualquier otra cosa que se les ocurre para destrozar la propiedad. ¿Qué tal si usted es el ganador de una casa saboteada vendida en una subasta de propiedades embargadas? ¡Qué golpe de suerte, ¿no?!

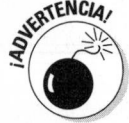

Normalmente los prestamistas no le permitirán inspeccionar la casa antes de la subasta. Tampoco puede hacer una oferta de compra con la condición de obtener el préstamo. El riesgo de comprar una propiedad que no puede inspeccionar primero es muchísimo mayor que una posible recompensa.

✔ **Económicos:** dependiendo del estado en el que esté la casa, la ejecución hipotecaria puede tardar entre cuatro meses y un año para llevarse acabo. Supongamos que consigue lo que parece ser una ganga, personas que de hecho están vendiendo en medio del proceso del embargo. ¿Qué pasa si estas personas están mintiendo sobre cuánto deben de la hipoteca y de los impuestos sobre la propiedad? ¿Qué tal si no lo dicen sobre hipotecas no registradas, juicios legales o gravámenes federales y estatales (cuotas tributarias pendientes) de la casa? Adivine quién es responsable por las deudas de la propiedad. ¡Qué golpe de suerte, ¿verdad?!

✔ **De posesión:** supongamos que después de comprar una casa embargada en una subasta, visita su nueva casa y descubre que los dueños anteriores aún están habitándola con la última posesión que les queda —un rifle—, y no tiene la menor intención de irse por las buenas. ¿A quién cree que le toca el placer de desalojarlos? ¡Qué golpe de suerte!

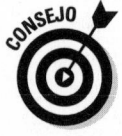

La compra de una casa embargada nunca es *completamente* segura debido a la posibilidad de un sabotaje por parte de los dueños anteriores. La manera menos arriesgada de comprar una, es comprando directamente de una entidad prestamista la cual tiene el título de propiedad porque nadie la compró en la subasta. Éstas son las razones:

✔ Cualquier hipoteca que la casa tenga, registrada o no publicada, o juicios legales o gravámenes son eliminados de la propiedad o al menos le son revelados antes de la compra.

✔ Usted puede —y de hecho, debe— tener la casa inspeccionada profesionalmente por un inspector de propiedades de la manera más minuciosa posible. Si ha sido una propiedad embargada, tiene que averiguar si los dueños anteriores le dejaron sorpresas escondidas.

✔ El precio y los términos de venta son negociables. Aunque los embargos normalmente están publicados según su avalúo, los prestamistas pueden hacer concesiones para trabajos de reparación, bien sea reduciendo el precio de la casa o dándole un crédito para realizar el trabajo. Generalmente, ofrecen también buenos términos para el préstamo (baja cuota inicial, no cargos por el préstamo, tasa de interés por debajo del mercado) para deshacerse rápidamente de estas propiedades con problemas. Después de todo, ellos están en el negocio de dar préstamos y no en el de vender propiedades.

Piénselo bien antes de comprar una casa embargada. Aunque compre directamente de un prestamista, puede estar comprando una casa empapada de techo a cimientos por las lágrimas de sueños destrozados. Una casa así probablemente no ha recibido el mejor cuidado. Investigue cuidadosamente, inspeccione la casa a fondo y entienda *perfectamente* en lo que se está metiendo antes de comprar.

Propiedades otra vez en el mercado

Cuando una casa registrada para la venta recibe una oferta aceptable, los vendedores normalmente le dicen a su agente que no promueva activamente la propiedad ni acepten nuevas ofertas, mientras trabajan con el comprador para satisfacer los términos y condiciones del contrato de venta — como inspecciones a la propiedad y financiamiento. Si esa propiedad se pone a la venta nuevamente (*BOM,* o "back on the market" en inglés, según la jerga de bienes raíces), esto significa que el trato no se cerró.

Las propiedades se vuelven a poner a la venta por muchos motivos: quizás los compradores no reunieron los requisitos para el préstamo o talvez cambiaron de opinión. O, quizás el prestamista pensó que la casa no valía la cantidad de dinero que los compradores estaban dispuestos a pagar por ella, y no aprobaron la solicitud del préstamo. Sin embargo, la razón más común, casi siempre, por la que no se cierran los contratos es que los compradores y vendedores no se pudieron poner de acuerdo sobre cómo resolver los problemas estructurales y estéticos descubiertos durante la inspección.

Lo irónico es que el castillo codiciado por todos los compradores cuando era una nueva casa en el listado ahora se convierte en "esa vieja casucha" al ponerla otra vez de venta en el mercado. Los compradores desconfiados se preguntan qué defectos tendría la casa. De repente, el estigma, real o imaginario, de ser una posible propiedad problemática ahuyenta a mucha gente. Casi nadie quiere comprar una casa rechazada por alguien más. Como resultado de la pérdida de entusiasmo por parte de los compradores, las casas que están de vuelta en el mercado (*BOM*), con frecuencia se venden por menos la segunda vez.

No rechace inmediatamente una vivienda porque la ponen de nuevo en el mercado. Averigüe por qué está otra vez en venta. Si el problema se relaciona con defectos de la propiedad, pídales a los vendedores que le muestren copias de los reportes de inspección. Si los problemas son corregibles y puede negociar un buen trato, la mala suerte del vendedor puede ser la buena suerte de usted. A los vendedores que les ha tocado un trato no realizado, con frecuencia, están más dispuestos a negociar el precio y los términos con el siguiente comprador. Si utiliza los principios que cubrimos en la sección de casas que necesitan reparaciones en este capítulo, usted puede conseguir una ganga con una casa que es puesta otra vez a la venta.

Junte Sus Recursos: Sociedades Especiales

Así como han aumentado los precios de las viviendas en muchas partes densamente pobladas del país, también ha aumentado la frecuencia de personas sin relación personal que forman sociedades especiales para comprar casas. Estas personas no están necesariamente involucradas emocionalmente. Al contrario, generalmente son personas que decidieron que una buena manera de hacer realidad su sueño americano de comprar una casa era uniendo sus recursos como socios.

Tipos de sociedades residenciales

Un tipo de sociedad especial conocida como *coparticipación de propiedad,* incluye a inversionistas que no viven en la propiedad. El inversionista proporciona el dinero en efectivo para comprar la casa en la que vive su socio mientras el valor de la propiedad (en el mejor de los casos) se incrementa. Después de un periodo de tiempo específico —digamos cinco años— el socio que vive en la casa tiene la opción de comprar la parte de la propiedad del inversionista o vender la casa y compartir la ganancia.

En *sociedades de convivencia,* el otro tipo de sociedad especial, todos los socios viven en la propiedad comprada en común. Al juntar su dinero y sus ingresos para una cuota inicial, con su pareja o un amigo o un familiar, estas personas compran su propia casa; ésta es un refugio fiscal y, si los dioses de bienes raíces son generosos, es también una ganancia cuando la vendan y cada quién sigue su propio camino.

Sociedades de convivencia son una versión de los gemelos Siameses en bienes raíces. Las personas que conviven todos los días cerca a su pareja tienen una relación personal que es mucho más intensa que el de una sociedad de coparticipación de propiedad.

Hemos visto sociedades de convivencia que han funcionado perfectamente bien. Con el paso del tiempo, los socios se convirtieron en mejores amigos de lo que eran antes de comprar la casa. Sin embargo, la mayoría de estas sociedades no son más que matrimonios de conveniencia que los socios deben sobrellevar para poder cosechar los beneficios económicos. Las discusiones sobre cosas como, si se debe arreglar un techo que gotea o reemplazarlo, sobre quién dejó los platos sucios en el fregadero (¡otra vez!), si se debe pintar de morado o de dorado la sala o a quien le toca usar el jardín para su fiesta el próximo sábado, pueden estresar hasta la mejor de las relaciones.

Cómo estructurar una sociedad exitosa

Muchas son las sociedades que acaban mal innecesariamente. ¿Por qué? Porque los socios no anticipan los problemas que puedan surgir relacionados con la convivencia. Lo irónico es que la mayoría de los problemas se pueden prevenir y evitar. Un planeamiento adecuado previene los problemas.

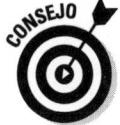

Antes de formar una sociedad residencial, puede hacer dos cosas para aumentar más las probabilidades de tener éxito:

- **Póngala a prueba.** Si está considerando una sociedad de convivencia, recomendamos que viva con su posible socio por lo menos seis meses antes de comprar una casa juntos. Quizás descubra que tiene un problema de compatibilidad muy serio —por ejemplo, que usted se va a la cama a las nueve de la noche y a su compañero le encanta parrandear hasta la madrugada. O, si usted, Maestro Limpio, insiste en que todo debe estar en su lugar y su posible socio es un demonio de Tasmania que considera que el suelo también puede servir de closet. Imagínese los placeres de la convivencia si usted siempre paga sus cuentas para el día primero del mes y el deporte favorito de su socio es jugar a las escondidas con los cobradores.

- **Póngalo por escrito.** También recomendamos que un abogado, con experiencia en sociedades residenciales de bienes raíces, prepare un documento de asociación cuanto antes. No busque inventar el hilo negro; deje que un abogado con experiencia lo guíe a usted y a su posible socio por los posibles problemas de una sociedad.

Lo ideal es redactar un contrato antes de hacer la oferta de compra. ¿Cuál es la prisa? Tiene que asegurarse de que usted y su socio entienden precisamente cómo funciona la sociedad y qué responsabilidades tienen el uno con el otro. El acuerdo debe cubrir cuestiones importantes tales como las siguientes:

- **Acuerdos económicos:** esta sección del contrato es sobre las finanzas de la compra, el mantenimiento y la venta de la propiedad. También especifica, para cada socio, cómo se pueden deducir de los impuestos los intereses de la hipoteca y los impuestos sobre la propiedad, si es que las contribuciones a la sociedad son desiguales.

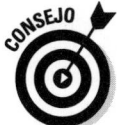

¿Qué sucede si, por ejemplo, su socio se muere de repente o se declara en bancarrota? La manera en la que el título está descrito es importante. (Cubrimos este importante tema en el Capítulo 14). En el caso de una sociedad de convivencia, ¿debería tener el socio la primera opción a compra antes de que se pueda vender a un tercero? Planear para lo inesperado es mucho mejor que reaccionar ante una crisis. Su acuerdo también debe tener cláusulas para disolver la sociedad.

✔ **Resolución de conflictos:** ¿Qué pasa si su socio y usted acaban peleándose por cuestiones de "importancia", como si se deben plantar margaritas o rosas al lado de la casa? Si sólo dos socios están involucrados, ¿cómo se rompe el empate? Anticipe los conflictos. Muchas veces hasta los mejores amigos no están de acuerdo y esto es una realidad de la vida. Proporcione un método (como la mediación o el arbitraje) para resolver los problemas que no logren resolver entre ustedes.

✔ **Plan de ataque:** si usted y su socio tienen la intención de mejorar la propiedad que van a comprar, por ejemplo, remodelando la cocina o convirtiendo dos apartamentos en un condominio, el contrato de su sociedad debe ser lo más específico posible en cuanto al tipo de trabajo, el tiempo y costo del proyecto, etcétera. Planee ahora para evitar conflictos después.

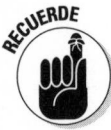

Nunca se apresure a formar una sociedad —las consecuencias económicas de un error pueden ser catastróficas. Sopese cuidadosamente las ventajas y desventajas. Y, luego, ponga todo por escrito con la ayuda de un abogado con experiencia para cubrir todos los posibles problemas, en caso de que no todo vaya tan maravillosamente como usted espera.

Una sociedad infernal

Desafortunadamente, algunas veces una sociedad se convierte en un desastre infernal. La historia trágica de Irv ilustra algunos de los obstáculos de las sociedades residenciales.

Irv y Sid eran buenos amigos desde hacía 25 años y compraron juntos un condominio. Irv usó el dinero que heredó de su madre para la cuota inicial del condominio y los costos de cierre. Sid, que tenía un sueldo muy superior al de Irv, pero que no tenía dinero disponible, tenía el condominio como residencia principal. Sid pagaba las mensualidades de la hipoteca, los impuestos sobre la propiedad y las cuotas de la asociación de propietarios, y también le pagaba alquiler a Irv.

Era una sociedad perfecta. Sid tenía las deducciones de impuestos que necesitaba y además un 25 por ciento del aumento del valor del condominio al venderlo. Los pagos de alquiler de Sid a Irv le daban a éste una buena ganancia sobre la inversión que hizo, y le tocaba la porción más grande del valor del condominio al venderlo. Irv y Sid estaban fascinados con el arreglo.

Todo funcionó bien por casi un año. Luego, sin aviso, Sid se declaró en bancarrota.

Los pagos del alquiler a Irv pararon, por supuesto. Lo que es más, el tribunal a cargo de la bancarrota puso un gravamen sobre el condominio congelando los bienes de Sid —y sin querer, congeló todo el dinero de Irv también. Lo peor de todo es que Irv y Sid no tenían un contrato de sociedad, por escrito, describiendo la división de la participación en un 75 y 25 por ciento. Sin documentos escritos, Irv no pudo comprobar este hecho satisfactoriamente ante el tribunal.

Cómo Armar el Mejor Equipo de Trabajo en Bienes Raíces

*W*inston Churchill caracterizó a la anterior Unión Soviética como "un enigma envuelto en un misterio dentro del enigma". La apropiada descripción de Churchill es también acertada al hablar del proceso de compra de una vivienda. Si usted es como la mayoría de las personas que están buscando una vivienda, usted no es un experto en el valor de propiedades, en el financiamiento, o en la legislación impositiva o de bienes raíces. Y cuando sus ahorros de toda la vida están en juego, la ignorancia no es una ventaja. El no entender lo que involucra el proceso de comprar una vivienda puede costarle mucho más dinero y no sentirse feliz con la vivienda que finalmente compre.

¿Cómo se puede ver el camino en medio del intricado laberinto de constantes cambios de las condiciones de los bienes raíces, de las ordenanzas locales, de los reglamentos y de los códigos impositivos? ¿Dónde puede usted inscribirse en un curso intensivo de valores de las viviendas? Y aún, si tiene la aptitud, ¿cómo va a encontrar el tiempo para convertirse en un experto en tantos campos de conocimiento?

Una manera de resolver esto es no hacer nada. No puede meterse en problemas si se queda acurrucado en un rincón, doblado en una posición fetal. Por supuesto, la desventaja de no hacer nada es que nada pasa sin su participación activa. Nunca llegará a comprar una vivienda usando este método.

El leer este libro *"La compra de una vivienda para Dummies"*, tercera edición, pone en sus manos un método mucho más dinámico. Este libro le muestra cómo puede convertirse en un comprador inteligente, sin embargo, no puede hacer todo por usted.

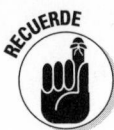

El entender la teoría del valor de la propiedad y el saber cuál es el valor real de la casa de sus sueños son dos cosas diferentes. Igualmente, leer acerca de cómo comprar una vivienda no le asegura que va a acertar todo justo en el blanco, ni le garantiza que será un comprador experto —porque no existe ningún substituto para los años de experiencia en este campo. También necesitará algunos expertos a su lado. Pero no se preocupe, nosotros le explicaremos cómo encontrar expertos competentes que pueden ayudarle a comprar una vivienda y no le cobrarán un ojo de la cara para ayudarlo.

El Concepto de Equipo

Una y otra vez, hemos visto gente inteligente meter la pata y acabar en situaciones horribles durante el proceso de compra de una vivienda. Y, más de lo que cree, lo que los puso en situaciones difíciles fue el desconocimiento de algo que ellos (o sus agentes) debían saber, pero que ignoraban.

Aunque le parezca mentira no es importante que usted mismo sepa todo. Lo que es importante es tener buena gente en su equipo —gente que sabe lo que usted necesita saber, para que ellos puedan ayudarlo a resolver los problemas que invariablemente aparecen.

Como alinear a los participantes

Usted no tiene que convertirse instantáneamente en un experto en el valor de las propiedades, hipotecas, legislación de bienes raíces y de impuestos, seguros de propiedad, depósitos garantizados, control de pestes y técnicas de construcción, a fin de participar correctamente en el juego de compra de una vivienda. Puede contratar a personas que dominan las habilidades que le faltan a usted. La compra de una vivienda es un trabajo de equipo, y como en un equipo deportivo, su responsabilidad es dirigir y entrenar al equipo, y no en todas las posiciones. Después de que usted haya armado un equipo ganador, sus participantes deberían darle consejos bien fundamentados para que usted pueda tomar brillantes decisiones.

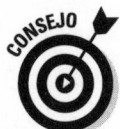

Si el dinero no fuera problema, usted elegiría a todos los expertos que pudiera. Pero, como probablemente no tiene un presupuesto ilimitado, necesita determinar qué expertos son absolutamente necesarios, y cuáles tareas puede hacer usted mismo. En este capítulo, explicamos cuáles son los expertos que es bueno contratar, y cuáles puede pasar por alto. En última instancia, lógicamente usted debe determinar sus propias destrezas o la carencia de ellas en los varios aspectos del proceso de compra de la vivienda.

Aquí tiene una pequeña reseña de los posibles participantes de su equipo:

✔ **Usted:** recuerde siempre que usted es el participante más importante de su equipo. En casi todas las compras de vivienda, algo puede salir mal — uno de sus jugadores pierde la pelota o no satisface sus necesidades. Usted tiene el derecho absoluto de, diplomáticamente, pero con energía, insistir en que se corrijan los errores. Recuerde que usted contrata (y paga) a los jugadores de su equipo. Ellos trabajan para usted. Los malos jugadores pueden ver la relación al revés —les gustaría pensar, (y quieren creer) que ellos son los que tienen el poder de decisión. Pueden tratar de manipularlo para que actúe a favor de los intereses de ellos, y no de los suyos. No tolere esta situación. Usted es el jefe —y puede despedir tanto como contratar.

✔ **Agente de bienes raíces:** como la casa que está por comprar probablemente será la mayor inversión de su vida, debe tener a alguien en su equipo que conozca los valores de la propiedad. La misión principal de su agente es ayudarle a encontrar la vivienda de sus sueños, decirle cuál es el valor de la propiedad y negociarla en su favor.

✔ **Corredor de bienes raíces:** todos los estados otorgan dos tipos de licencias de bienes raíces, la licencia de vendedor y la licencia de corredor. La gente con licencia de corredor debe completar una educación más avanzada y tener estándares de experiencia satisfactorios. Si su agente de bienes raíces no es un corredor inmobiliario independiente, o un corredor para una oficina de bienes raíces, él o ella, debe ser supervisado(a) por un corredor que sea responsable de lo que su agente hace o deja de hacer. Cuando se presentan problemas, el éxito de su transacción puede depender del apoyo que el corredor inmobiliario le brinda a su agente.

✔ **Entidad crediticia:** si no puede pagar, no puede comprar. Y como la mayoría de las personas no tienen para pagar por sus casas con dinero en efectivo, es posible que usted necesite un préstamo para comprar la vivienda de sus sueños. Un buen prestamista ofrece préstamos con precios competitivos y, quizás pueda ayudarle a seleccionar el mejor tipo de préstamo entre la multitud de programas crediticios de hoy en día.

✔ **Inspector de propiedades:** la condición estructural y estética de un inmueble influye enormemente en su valor. La casa de sus sueños tiene que ser inspeccionada minuciosamente desde los cimientos hasta el techo antes de que usted la compre, para asegurarse de que realmente está comprando lo que usted piensa que está comprando.

✔ **Oficial de custodia del depósito de garantía:** la desconfianza mutua es una regla que está presente en todas las transacciones en bienes raíces. Usted y el vendedor necesitan un tercer participante neutral, esto es un oficial de custodia de la garantía, para que maneje los fondos y el papeleo relacionado con la transacción sin tener ningún favoritismo. El oficial de custodia de la garantía es el árbitro en el juego de compra de una vivienda.

✔ **Asesores financieros e impositivos:** antes de comprar una vivienda debe comprender la manera en que la compra va a encajar en el plan total de su situación financiera. Usted debe considerar cuáles son las circunstancias de sus metas financieras y, de acuerdo a esas metas, determinar cuál es costo de vivienda que estaría a su alcance. En el Capítulo 2, le explicamos cómo hacerlo.

✔ **Abogado:** usted puede tener o no tener, un abogado en su equipo. Esto dependerá de la complejidad del contrato, de la ubicación de la vivienda de sus sueños, y de su propia idea de lo que es necesario para vivir confortablemente. Al firmar el contrato de compra cuando adquiere una casa, usted contrae una obligación legal. Si tiene algunas preguntas sobre la legalidad del contrato, incluya en su equipo a un abogado especializado en legislación de bienes raíces.

Es raro que gane un partido si no tiene un equipo ganador. Pero recuerde que sus jugadores son *consejeros* —y no les corresponde tomar decisiones. Usted es el jefe y es el que toma las decisiones. Usted es el que tiene la última palabra. Después de todo, es su dinero el que está en juego.

Ignore los consejos gratuitos

Lo repetimos otra vez: la compra de una vivienda es un trabajo de equipo. Las transacciones exitosas resultan de los esfuerzos coordinados de muchas personas —agentes, corredores, prestamistas, inspectores de propiedades, oficiales de custodia del depósito, asesores de impuestos y abogados. Cada jugador trae diferentes conocimientos y habilidades al juego y debería hacer contribuciones importantes al equipo.

Mientras los expertos hagan lo que saben hacer, todo funcionará sin complicaciones. Sin embargo, en cuanto uno de los expertos invade el campo de conocimiento del otro, la guerra estalla ruidosamente.

Las opiniones no solicitadas referentes a los valores de la propiedad son un ejemplo de un tipo de consejos gratuitos que pueden causar efectos devastadores. Generalmente, esas opiniones son dadas por los asesores de impuestos y los abogados durante la revisión de su transacción. Los abogados y los tasadores de impuestos no conocen los valores de la propiedad. Si se hace una mala jugada basada en sus malos consejos, aunque se hayan hecho con buena intención, puede detenerse a mitad del camino la compra de la casa de sus sueños.

Aunque parezca increíble, algunos compradores, tontamente, solicitan asesoramiento gratuito en un intento equivocado de ahorrar unos pocos dólares. "¿Por qué —se preguntan a sí mismos los compradores— emplear a un contador público para recibir asesoramiento de impuestos cuando podemos obtener consejos sobre impuestos gratis de nuestro agente?" "¿Por qué pagar por el asesoramiento legal de un abogado si el oficial de custodia del depósito nos va a dar opiniones, sin costo, sobre la mejor manera de obtener el título de propiedad con el nombre y datos personales, que deben ser los mismos que están en el seguro hipotecario de nuestra casa?"

¿Por qué? Porque si usted tiene suerte, el consejo gratuito de un experto de fuera de su equipo, vale exactamente lo que usted paga por él: cero. Cero. Nada. Absolutamente nada.

En cambio, si no tiene suerte, el consejo gratis puede salirle muy caro. El *IRS* no tiene misericordia si comete un error basado en un asesoramiento equivocado. Desgraciadamente, este tipo de error, por lo general, le sale mucho más caro que los honorarios de un abogado o asesor impositivo si ellos le hubieran dado el asesoramiento correcto.

Dadas las consecuencias adversas de un mal consejo, los *buenos* expertos no le dan consejos en asuntos para los que no están capacitados. Si usted les pide un consejo, se van a negar categóricamente a dárselo. En cambio, guiarán a sus clientes hacia los expertos apropiados. Los verdaderos expertos son lo suficientemente inteligentes como para saber lo que no saben, y son lo suficientemente humildes para admitirlo. Y en un tono más egoísta, ellos no quieren ser enjuiciados por sus clientes porque les dieron un asesoramiento equivocado.

Sea cauteloso y evite a los expertos que ofrecen consejo gratuito fuera de sus campos de estudio y experiencia.

Atraiga a un Agente de Bienes Raíces

¿Cuánto cuesta?

¡La respuesta incorrecta a esta pregunta puede costarle mucho dinero! Pero aún, no hay una respuesta fácil a esta pregunta que parece tan sencilla porque los precios de la vivienda no son exactos. Como lo explicamos en el Capítulo 10, los precios de las viviendas no pueden reducirse a un problema matemático donde 2 más 2 siempre son 4. Los precios de las viviendas no son fijos —por el contrario, ellos se mueven ampliamente de un lado para otro.

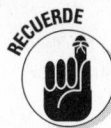

Las casas se venden por el precio justo del mercado, el cual es cualquier cantidad que ofrecen los compradores y que aceptan los vendedores. El precio justo del mercado no es un número específico, es una gama de precios.

Imagine que hace una oferta por una vivienda cuyo valor es de alrededor de $150.000. Si el vendedor tiene un agente mejor que el suyo, y usted está desesperado por comprar, puede acabar pagando $160.000. Por otro lado, si usted no tiene urgencia y su agente sabe cómo negociar, es posible que compre esa misma propiedad por $140.000. Los precios de las viviendas frecuentemente están directamente relacionados con ambos, con el conocimiento del agente acerca de los precios de propiedades similares que ya se vendieron y con las habilidades del agente como negociador. Por supuesto, otros factores (como la motivación del vendedor y del comprador, sus necesidades y conocimientos) son también importantes.

Un buen agente puede ser el pilar de su equipo de bienes raíces. Puede ayudarlo a encontrar la casa que satisfaga sus necesidades, negociar por esa vivienda en su nombre, supervisar las inspecciones de la propiedad y coordinar el cierre de la transacción. A menudo, los agentes lo pueden guiar con información útil para obtener préstamos hipotecarios. Las habilidades de negociador de un buen agente y su conocimiento de los valores de las propiedades pueden ahorrarle miles de dólares.

Algunas personas piensan que un "buen agente" es un contrasentido. Estos individuos le dirán que todos los agentes buscan siempre sus propios intereses y no los suyos. Por ejemplo, haciéndole comprar viviendas más caras de las que usted puede afrontar, con el solo fin de aumentar el monto del cheque de su comisión.

Algunos agentes pueden presionarlo para que compre más pronto (y tener que pagar más de lo que debería) a fin de aumentar sus propias comisiones. Asimismo, por desgracia, andan también por allí muchos agentes bien intencionados, pero incompetentes. En este capítulo le explicamos cómo evitar a los malos agentes —y cómo identificar entre la multitud de ellos a los mediocres— para reducir la lista de nombres y dejar en ella solamente los buenos agentes que merecen sus comisiones.

Tipos de relación con el agente

Digamos que usted ha estado trabajando con un agente llamado Al, quien le ha mostrado propiedades durante varios meses. Ayer, finalmente encontró la vivienda que le gustaba. La propiedad parece tener un precio apropiado, pero usted le dijo a Al que hiciera una oferta por un monto más bajo de todas maneras. (Todo el mundo sabe que los precios son negociables, ¿verdad? Si los vendedores no aceptan la oferta, déjenlos que presenten una contraoferta.) Pero, ¿qué pasa si su agente echa todo a perder? Suponga que Al le contó a los vendedores sus más íntimos secretos —por ejemplo, cuánto dinero tiene usted para un depósito de garantía, y cuánto, realmente, está dispuesto a pagar por la vivienda. Ahora el vendedor puede ganarle en su propio juego. Si usted descubre lo que Al hizo, (muchos compradores son víctimas pero no lo saben) seguramente se sentirá herido, traicionado y realmente furioso. Usted debería preguntarle a Al para qué lado del equipo está él.

La respuesta a esa pregunta ha cambiado un poco a través de los años. En décadas pasadas, tales compradores pensaban que tenían agentes que los representaban. Pero en realidad, no era cierto. En esa época, los agentes o subagentes tenían la obligación legal de representar a *los vendedores.*

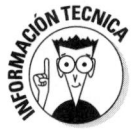

Agentes con una responsabilidad diferente, también llamados *agentes en relación cooperativa,* trabajan entre sí como miembros del *Servicio de listado múltiple (MLS,* por sus siglas en inglés). Los agentes usan los servicios de listado múltiple para promover sus propios listados de bienes raíces y ofrecen compartir sus comisiones con agentes de otras oficinas que son realmente los que venden las propiedades en las listas. Como agentes en relación cooperativa del vendedor, los participantes en los *MLS* están obligados a obtener el más alto precio posible para los vendedores de las propiedades.

Desgraciadamente, muchos compradores no sabían que los mismos agentes que trabajaban con ellos estaban en verdad representando los intereses de los vendedores. Y la ley no les exigía a los agentes que les notificaran a los compradores a quién verdaderamente representaban, antes de preparar las ofertas en nombre de sus compradores.

Sin embargo, los tiempos han cambiado. Algunos estados (como California) han aprobado leyes para mejorar la protección al consumidor. Estos estados aprobaron leyes que requieren que los agentes les den a ambos, a los compradores y a los vendedores, un documento de sus responsabilidades como agentes de ellos. Estas leyes les permiten a los compradores y a los vendedores seleccionar el tipo de relación que quieren tener con sus agentes.

Los compradores y los vendedores de vivienda pueden tener tres tipos diferentes de relación con los agentes de bienes raíces. Explicamos las *"agencias que representan a ambas partes y los conflictos de interés",* al representar a ambas partes, en los párrafos enmarcados con fondo gris.

Las otras relaciones posibles son de dos tipos de *agencias de servicio exclusivo,* es decir, donde los agentes representan solamente a una de las partes en la transacción.

> ✔ **Agente del vendedor:** En este tipo de agencia de servicio exclusivo, la agencia trabaja solamente para el vendedor.
>
> ✔ **Agente del comprador:** En este tipo de agencia de servicio exclusivo, la agencia trabaja solamente para el comprador. El agente de un comprador no puede ser el agente del vendedor, aún cuando el agente del comprador recibe una porción de la comisión pagada por el vendedor.

Aunque la agencia de servicio exclusivo mejoró el sistema viejo, los agentes del comprador todavía sufren un conflicto de interés el cual es inherente al recibo de una comisión, ya que esta comisión está determinada por un porcentaje que está directamente relacionado al precio final que paga el comprador por la propiedad.

En raros casos, los agentes del comprador no aceptan dinero de los vendedores. En cambio, un comprador firma un contrato de trabajo exclusivo con un agente, y el comprador le paga al agente un adelanto por su disponibilidad, que luego cuenta como parte del pago de honorarios correspondientes, cuando dicho agente encuentre una propiedad para el comprador. Según como sean las provisiones del contrato, el adelanto puede o no devolverse al comprador, si el agente no encuentra una propiedad que satisfaga a su cliente.

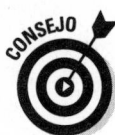

He aquí la forma de tener lo mejor de los dos mundos con el agente del comprador. Esta técnica elimina el incentivo de su agente de hacerle gastar más, y le permite a usted evitar pagar por un servicio que no se realizó. Ofrézcale a su agente una suma global de comisión, más una bonificación si, *y solo si,* el agente le consigue una compra mejor. Por ejemplo, si el agente normalmente recibe el 3 por ciento del precio de venta de una vivienda y usted espera comprar una propiedad de aproximadamente $200.000, ofrézcale al agente una cantidad fija de $5.000 de comisión y un bono adicional de $100 por cada $1.000 de reducción de los $200.000 que el agente consiga, hasta un máximo de $6.000 de bonificación.

¿Es su agente su aliado o su enemigo? Como las leyes de los diferentes estados les asignan diferentes responsabilidades legales a los agentes, es importante que usted conozca cómo se juega el juego en su estado. Asegúrese de determinar a quién representa su agente antes de comenzar a trabajar juntos.

Cómo se les paga a los agentes

Una compañía de corretaje en bienes raíces es un negocio de todo o de nada. Como regla, los agentes cobran una comisión solamente cuando se vende la propiedad. Si la propiedad no se vende, no se les paga a los agentes.

Agencia que representa a ambas partes y conflictos de interés

En ciertas transacciones un agente representa a ambos, al vendedor y al comprador. Este tipo de representación se llama de *agencia que representa a ambas partes*.

La agencia representante de ambas partes es el tipo más confuso. La mayoría de la gente piensa que esta agencia significa que el mismo agente representa a ambos, al comprador y al vendedor. Esa situación es posible, pero es muy poco común, y mucho menos recomendable. Es imposible que un mismo agente represente sus mejores intereses como comprador al mismo tiempo que represente los mejores intereses del vendedor.

En un tipo más común de agencia que representa a ambas partes, la venta de una propiedad específica involucra dos agentes diferentes, pero ambos trabajan para el mismo corredor de bienes raíces. Suponga que Sam Seller decide, en un domingo con mucho sol, incluir su vivienda en la lista de ventas con Sara, una agente de Acme Realty. Sara sonríe cuando firma el contrato para representar a Sam como su agente exclusiva.

Simultáneamente, Betty Compradora se encuentra casualmente con Bob, quien también es un agente de Acme Realty, el domingo, en una casa en exhibición para que la visiten los interesados potenciales. A Betty le gusta Bob y le pide que la represente a ella, exclusivamente como su agente para comprar una vivienda. Bob acepta representarla con mucha alegría.

Por ahora, todo marcha bien. Sam tiene a Sara como su agente exclusivo; Betty tiene a Bob como su agente exclusivo. Las cosas se complican más tarde ese mismo día cuando Bob le muestra a Betty la casa de Sam que Sara acaba de incluir en la lista. Betty está deslumbrada. Le encanta la casa y le dice a Bob que presente una oferta de inmediato.

Cuando Betty decide hacer una oferta para la casa de Sam, la relación que Betty y Sam tenían con sus respectivos agentes cambió. Le guste o no, repentinamente, Sarah se encontró representando a ambos, a Sam y a Betty. De la misma manera, Bob se convirtió en el representante de Betty y de Sam.

¿Por qué? Aún cuando hay dos agentes diferentes involucrados, ambos trabajan para el mismo corredor de bienes raíces, Acme Realty. Tan pronto como Bob comenzó a trabajar en la oferta de Betty, Acme Realty representaba al vendedor y al comprador de la misma propiedad. Esto es lo que significa una agencia que representa a ambas partes.

La agencia que representa a ambas partes no sería un problema si usted acaba trabajando con un agente de una oficina pequeña que tiene pocos agentes. La posibilidad de que compre una vivienda listada por otro agente en la agencia de su agente es mínima. Sin embargo, si el agente que usted selecciona trabaja para una gran operación de corretaje con oficinas múltiples y miles de agentes (como *Coldwell Banker*), la posibilidad de que tenga que trabajar con una agencia de representación doble aumenta astronómicamente.

Como comprador, debe cuidarse de dos problemas potenciales cuando se encuentre trabajando con una agencia de representación a ambas partes. Primero, asegúrese de que su agente no esté compartiendo información confidencial con los otros agentes de su compañía de bienes raíces. Segundo, tenga cuidado con los agentes que promueven las listas de su propia firma, porque el vender una vivienda de

(continúa)

(continuación)

su lista genera una comisión más grande para ellos.

La mayoría de los estados permiten las relaciones de agencias dobles siempre que el estatus de la agencia se les informe con anterioridad a ambos, compradores y vendedores, y ambas partes estén de acuerdo. Cuando una agencia de representación doble no revela su estatus, pueden existir condiciones que causen la anulación de un acuerdo de compra, y generalmente, le permite a las partes que son perjudicadas buscar indemnización por parte de los agentes de bienes raíces.

Este método de pago puede crear conflicto de interés entre usted y su agente. El método de pago no creará ningún conflicto de interés con los *buenos* agentes, porque los buenos agentes ponen sus intereses primero, y no su deseo de ser pagados. Sin embargo, usted sabe que está trabajando con un mal agente si éste está más interesado en cerrar la venta rápidamente y le hace pagar el precio de venta, en vez de educarlo diligentemente y conseguirle el mejor precio posible.

Permítanos contestar estas preguntas de vital importancia sobre las comisiones en bienes raíces.

✔ **¿Cuánto reciben en comisiones los agentes de bienes raíces?** Las comisiones se calculan como un porcentaje del precio de venta. Aunque dependen de costumbres locales, las comisiones sobre las viviendas varían entre el 4 y el 7 por ciento del precio de venta.

✔ **¿Quién paga la comisión?** Típicamente, los vendedores. Después de todo, los vendedores reciben el dinero cuando la propiedad se vende. Raramente los compradores tienen mucho dinero después de hacer el pago inicial por la vivienda de sus sueños, y de pagar el costo del préstamo, cargos por la inspección de la propiedad, la prima del seguro de propiedad, costos de la mudanza y otros gastos relacionados con la compra, según lo mencionamos en el Capítulo 3. Como la comisión es parte del precio de venta, sin embargo, el costo efectivo de la comisión sale de ambos, de los bolsillos del comprador y del vendedor.

✔ **¿Son negociables las comisiones?** Categóricamente, sí. Los acuerdos de listado (los contratos que los dueños de la propiedad firman con los corredores para vender el inmueble) y los acuerdos de compra, generalmente establecen que las comisiones no están establecidas por ley, y son negociables entre los vendedores y los corredores.

✔ **¿Cómo se distribuye la comisión?** Piense en una vivienda que se vende por un total de $200.000. Suponiendo una tasa del 6 por ciento de comisión, la venta genera una comisión de $12.000. Es un montón de dinero. Sería así si toda esa suma fuera para una sola persona, pero como regla general, las comisiones no se administran de esa manera.

Por lo general, la comisión se divide por la mitad cuando se cierra la venta. El corredor de la lista, que representa a los vendedores, recibe la mitad ($6.000, en nuestro ejemplo) de la comisión, y la otra mitad ($6.000) va al corredor de la venta, quien representa a los compradores.

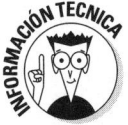

Si el agente del comprador o del vendedor trabajan para un corredor, éste, típicamente, recibe una porción de la comisión. La operación de corretaje típicamente toma del 30 al 50 por ciento de la comisión, lo que le deja al agente entre un 50 al 70 por ciento. En algunas firmas, tales como *RE/MAX*, los agentes pagan una cuota mensual a su firma de corretaje y acaban quedándose con un 80 al 90 por ciento de las comisiones que traen a la firma. Los agentes que trabajan por su cuenta como corredores independientes, por supuesto, no tienen que dividir sus comisiones con nadie.

Cómo comprar sin un agente

Es posible que usted vea un cartel o dos durante su búsqueda de vivienda que digan "Venta directa por el propietario", (*FSBO,* por sus siglas en inglés). Los vendedores quizás sean amigos, vecinos o colegas del trabajo. Como en la venta no intervienen agentes de bienes raíces, el propietario no tiene que pagar la comisión. Eso elimina el pago de un montón de dinero que se necesita en los otros casos.

Si la propiedad que está en venta directa por su propietario, la encontró usted mismo y satisface sus requisitos, se preguntará si necesita un agente para completar la compra. Después de todo, si los vendedores no tienen que pagarle comisión a su agente, ellos deberían estar dispuestos a rebajar el precio de la propiedad.

Algunos compradores de propiedades han hecho satisfactoriamente la compra de la vivienda de sus sueños, sin contratar a un agente. Otros han metido la pata con este método.

Si usted es novato, normalmente tiene sentido contratar a un agente. Tenga en cuenta el valor adicional que un agente contribuye a la transacción, además de encontrarle la propiedad —tal como la negociación, el estimado valor en el mercado, la coordinación de las inspecciones de la propiedad, la eliminación de condiciones para la venta, la información del vendedor, el financiamiento, el depósito de garantía, y muchísimos más detalles.

También puede considerar pedirle a su agente que acepte una comisión estándar o inferior al 3 por ciento ya que usted mismo encontró la propiedad. Si usted decide no contratar a un agente, le sugerimos que contrate los servicios de un abogado, pagándole sus honorarios por hora, a fin de que maneje los importantes detalles legales de la transacción.

Características de los buenos agentes

Los buenos agentes pueden ser hombres o mujeres, y los hay de diferentes razas, colores, experiencias y edades. Sin embargo, los buenos agentes reúnen las siguientes características que benefician a los compradores:

- ✔ **Un buen agente lo educa a usted.** Su agente conoce bien el proceso de la compra de una vivienda y le explica cada paso para que usted *siempre* comprenda lo que está pasando. Los agentes deben ser pacientes, sin presionar al cliente. Un buen agente *nunca* se aprovecha de su ignorancia para manipularlo.

- ✔ **Los buenos agentes no toman las decisiones por usted.** Su agente *siempre* le explica cuáles son sus opciones de manera que *usted* tome las decisiones correctas en relación al plan de acción.

- ✔ **Los buenos agentes le dicen cuándo piensan que es aconsejable incluir a otros expertos (inspectores, abogados, etc.) en su equipo.** Los expertos no intimidan a un buen agente. El amor propio del agente debería siempre ser secundario a su primera misión que es prestarle buenos servicios.

- ✔ **Los buenos agentes voluntariamente se restringen a una zona geográfica y a un tipo de propiedad.** Idealmente, su agente ya aprendió que no puede cubrir todos los aspectos del proceso de compra por sí mismo, pues esto invariablemente resulta en un servicio mediocre. Diferentes comunidades pueden tener condiciones de mercado, legislación y restricciones radicalmente diferentes. (Para obtener más información, vea la parte identificada con una barra gris vertical "Agentes que trabajan fuera de sus campos de experiencia son peligrosos".)

- ✔ **Los buenos agentes trabajan a tiempo completo, porque servirle a usted adecuadamente demanda una dedicación completa a esa actividad.** Para reducir el impacto financiero del cambio de trabajo, mucha gente comienza su carrera en bienes raíces trabajando a medio tiempo, y lo hacen después de sus horas de trabajo normales, y también en los fines de semana. Esto es bueno para esos agentes, pero no para usted.

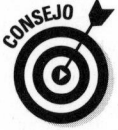

Una de las primeras preguntas que debe hacerle a cualquier agente con el que considere trabajar es: "¿Trabaja como agente a tiempo completo?" Así como usted no se arriesgaría a contratar los servicios de un abogado defensor que sólo trabaja a medio tiempo, no permite que lo represente un agente a medio tiempo tampoco.

- ✔ **Los buenos agentes tienen muchos contactos.** La gente prefiere trabajar con personas que conocen, respetan y son de su confianza. Usted puede usar las relaciones comerciales de su agente con entidades prestamistas locales, inspectores de propiedad, abogados, funcionarios de la oficina de títulos de propiedad, agentes de seguro, funcionarios del gobierno, y otros agentes de bienes raíces. Los buenos agentes les recomendarán a proveedores de servicios altamente calificados que ofrecen precios competitivos.

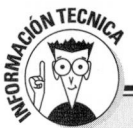

Dónde invierte su tiempo el agente

Algunas personas piensan que las comisiones de bienes raíces son exageradas teniendo en cuenta el tiempo del trabajo de los agentes: ésa es una forma diplomática de decir que su pago es extraordinariamente excesivo.

Es más fácil justificar la comisión de los agentes si se entiende lo que nosotros llamamos la Teoría del iceberg. Como probablemente ya sabe, el 90 por ciento del volumen del iceberg está escondido debajo del agua. Usted no puede determinar el tamaño de un iceberg por la porción que se ve flotando sobre el nivel del agua. Por otra parte, no puede decir por cuánto tiempo los agentes estuvieron trabajando para usted. Los buenos agentes pasan al menos nueve horas detrás del escenario por cada hora que están en contacto con el cliente.

Desgraciadamente, la mayoría de los compradores y vendedores no lo saben. Los compradores y los vendedores piensan que las comisiones son excesivas basándose en las pocas horas en las que ven personalmente a sus agentes.

A diferencia de los abogados y otros profesionales que le mandan la cuenta al cliente por horas de trabajo, los agentes de bienes raíces no detallan el tiempo que pasaron en una transacción desde el principio hasta el final. Si lo hicieran, usted tendría una mejor idea en dónde invierten su tiempo los agentes.

Típicamente, los buenos agentes invierten 20 horas por semana visitando propiedades nuevas y verificando inmuebles que han estado en el mercado por cierto tiempo, a fin de ver cuáles viviendas todavía están disponibles, y cuáles han recibido ofertas. Los agentes hacen este trabajo de campo semana tras semana, para mantenerse al día de lo que hay en el mercado y de cómo cambian los valores de la propiedad.

Después de que usted seleccione a un agente, ella o él comienzan a determinar cuáles viviendas pueden interesarle a usted. Los agentes con experiencia investigan varias propiedades por cada una de las que eventualmente le muestran, ahorrándole así a usted el tiempo de visitarlas todas. Su agente invierte tiempo en el teléfono hablando con agentes que tienen listas de inmuebles, tratando de obtener instrucciones acerca de cómo mostrar esas propiedades, y fijando la cita para mostrarlas. Entonces ella o él invierten más horas con usted, visitando las viviendas y en busca de esa vivienda maravillosa que ve en sus sueños.

Una vez que encuentra la propiedad de sus sueños, su agente necesita tiempo para preparar una oferta de compra, para presentarla, y para negociar ofertas diferentes que hace el agente del vendedor con respecto al precio y a las condiciones de la venta. Una vez que se acepta la oferta, un buen agente pasa más horas ayudándole a hacer cosas como asegurar un préstamo hipotecario; coordinar los detalles de la transacción con el agente del vendedor; proveer el papeleo y presentación del depósito de garantía al funcionario correspondiente; acompañar a los varios inspectores de propiedad, y verificar el cumplimiento de las declaraciones requeridas de los vendedores por la legislación local, estatal y federal.

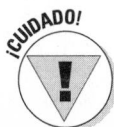

Tenga cuidado con los agentes malintencionados que tienen intereses escondidos. En vez de recomendarles a los mejores proveedores de servicios, estos agentes limitan sus recomendaciones a personas que les pasan transacciones a ellos o que les pagan una comisión.

✔ **Los buenos agentes tienen tiempo disponible.** Los agentes se ganan la vida vendiendo su tiempo, no las viviendas. El éxito es una espada de doble filo para los agentes muy ocupados. Un agente que esté ya trabajando con varios compradores y vendedores, probablemente no tiene suficiente tiempo para servirle adecuadamente. Algunos conflictos de horario son a veces inevitables. Pero si usted se da cuenta de que sus necesidades frecuentemente no son satisfechas porque su agente está involucrado en demasiados negocios, busque otro agente.

Los agentes que trabajan en campos fuera de su especialidad son peligrosos

A los compradores desprevenidos les esperan muchos riesgos cuando confían en agentes que trabajan en campos fuera de su especialidad. Aunque el siguiente ejemplo de la vida real es extraño, muestra el desastre causado por un agente especializado en la propiedad ubicada en Sonoma, una tranquila ciudad a 40 millas al norte de San Francisco.

La agente de Sonoma representaba a su amiga en la compra de un pequeño edificio de apartamentos ubicado en San Francisco. La compradora pensaba transformar los apartamentos en condominios y entonces venderlos individualmente y beneficiarse con una ganancia.

Desgraciadamente, la agente de Sonoma no sabía nada de las restricciones estrictas en San Francisco para las viviendas de alquiler y tampoco conocía las ordenanzas, igualmente estrictas, para la conversión de departamentos en condominios. El intento de estas leyes es desalentar a la gente de transformar apartamentos baratos en condominios de alta categoría.

Si el edificio hubiera sido convertido en condominios, el total de la venta de cada condominio hubiera sido menos que el precio pagado por el comprador originalmente por el edificio, debido a la naturaleza restrictiva de estas leyes. La negligencia de la agente resultó en la pérdida de $125.000 del comprador, cuando ella vendió el edificio más tarde.

Esta agente no sólo cometió el error de trabajar en "tierra extranjera", sino también omitió recomendarle a la compradora que incluyera a un abogado local de bienes raíces en su equipo para que la aconsejara sobre estos asuntos legales. La compradora pudo haber demandado a la agente por negligencia en el ejercicio de su responsabilidad, pero no lo hizo porque la agente era su amiga.

Con amigos como ésta, el comprador no necesita enemigos. Si la agente de Sonoma hubiera sido una amiga verdadera, le hubiera recomendado a la compradora un buen agente de San Francisco.

Los agentes que se apartan de su zona geográfica o del ámbito de sus conocimientos, lo hacen porque son avaros, o sencillamente incapaces porque son muy tontos al no conocer sus limitaciones. Cualquiera que sea la razón, evite a estos agentes como si fueran la plaga.

Cómo seleccionar a un agente

Ahora que ya conoce las cualidades generales y relucientes de un hipotético agente bueno, está preparado para ir al grano y considerar los detalles específicos para elegir a su propio agente. Le recomendamos con insistencia que entreviste por lo menos tres agentes antes de seleccionar el mejor para usted.

Cómo descubrir fuentes de referencia

Si tiene dificultad en encontrar tres buenos agentes para entrevistar, aquí le ofrecemos algunas fuentes de referencia:

- **Amigos, colegas de su negocio y miembros de organizaciones religiosas, profesionales y sociales a las que pertenece:** en resumen, cualquier persona que conozca, que esté buscando una vivienda o que sea propietaria de una en el vecindario donde quiere comprar, puede ser una buena fuente de recomendación de nombres de agentes. No pregunte solamente por los nombres, averigüe por qué a ellos le gustan sus agentes.

- **Su empleador:** la compañía en la que usted trabaja quizás tenga un servicio de traslados que puede consultar.

- **Los profesionales en campos relacionados:** son buenas fuentes de referencia de asesores financieros, impositivos y legales.

- **El agente que vendió su vivienda anterior:** si usted es propietario y se va a mudar a una nueva zona, pregúntele al agente que le vendió su casa si le puede recomendar a un buen agente en esa nueva zona. Los buenos agentes tienen redes de contacto con otros.

- **Viviendas abiertas al público los domingos:** mientras investiga las viviendas, ponga atención a los agentes. Estos agentes ya han probado (al ver la concurrencia a las viviendas abiertas al público) que trabajan en el vecindario en el que usted desea comprar.

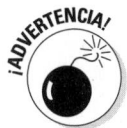

No acepte cualquier recomendación, aun si es del Papa, como si fuera el Evangelio. La mayoría de la gente que da recomendaciones tiene experiencia limitada o vieja con el agente que recomiendan. Además, la persona que da la recomendación probablemente no es un agente de bienes raíces.

Cómo pedir una lista de actividad

Después que ya haya identificado a tres buenos agentes que quiere entrevistar, comienza la parte más entretenida. Para evitar un malentendido, dígale a cada uno de los agentes que tiene planes de entrevistar a varios agentes antes de seleccionar al que va a trabajar con usted. Pídale a cada agente que traiga a la entrevista una lista de *cada* propiedad que listó o vendió durante los 12 meses anteriores. Esta lista, llamada *lista de actividad,* es una herramienta extremadamente poderosa y analítica.

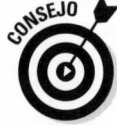

He aquí lo que debe incluir la lista de actividad y cómo debe usarla durante la entrevista.

- ✔ **Dirección de la propiedad:** las direcciones le ayudan a localizar cuál es la zona geográfica de operación del agente. Vea por sí mismo exactamente cuántas propiedades vendió el agente y las que listó en el vecindario que usted quiere. Elimine a los agentes cuya zona está fuera de la que usted quiere y los agentes que no tienen una zona geográfica.

- ✔ **El tipo de propiedad (casa, condominio, viviendas dúplex, etc.):** puede usar esta información para determinar si el agente tiene experiencia en el tipo de vivienda que usted intenta comprar. Si, por ejemplo, un agente se especializa en condominios, y usted quiere comprar una casa para una familia, puede tener problemas.

- ✔ **Precio de venta:** ¿Maneja el agente viviendas en el nivel de precios que está buscando? Un agente que trabaja con propiedades de precios *mucho* más altos o *mucho* más bajos de los que espera comprar, no es un buen agente para usted. Por ejemplo, si su plan es gastar $150.000, y la vivienda más barata que el agente vendió tenía un valor de $300.000, éste no será un buen miembro de su equipo. Tales agentes probablemente no invertirán mucho tiempo en usted porque tienen cosas más importantes que hacer.

- ✔ **Fecha de la venta:** las actividades de las ventas deberían estar distribuidas regularmente a lo largo del año. Si no es así, investigue por qué. La carencia de ventas recientes puede deberse a enfermedad o problemas familiares que pueden disminuir la capacidad del agente.

- ✔ **A quién representa el agente —al vendedor o al comprador:** los agentes con experiencia trabajan la mitad del tiempo con los compradores y la otra mitad con los vendedores. Los agentes más nuevos trabajan con los compradores. Evite a los agentes que trabajan casi siempre con los vendedores. Estos agentes, generalmente, carecen o de interés o de aptitud para trabajar exitosamente con los compradores.

- ✔ **El valor total en dólares vendido durante los 12 meses previos:** la comparación del total de las ventas de propiedades de los tres agentes inmobiliarios es una manera rápida de medir la actividad individual y el respectivo éxito de cada uno. Sin embargo, hay otros factores igualmente importantes a considerar cuando seleccione su agente. Usted no quiere necesariamente un "productor máximo". Estos agentes llegan a esa posición por medio de listados y gran cantidad de ventas de propiedades. Usualmente no tienen ni tiempo ni paciencia para tomarlo de la mano y educarlo si lo necesita, especialmente si es la primera vez que usted compra un inmueble.

✔ **El nombre y el número de teléfono actualizado de los vendedores y compradores:** usted usará esta información después para verificar las referencias.

Los hechos dicen más que las palabras. La lista de actividad transforma una charla trivial en hechos reales. Los buenos agentes dan amablemente sus listas y le animan a que verifique las referencias de sus clientes. Los malos agentes no quieren que usted hable con sus víctimas descontentas. Elimine tomar en consideración a cualquier agente que no quiera darle una lista de actividad completa —probablemente está tratando de esconder la falta de ventas, o los clientes descontentos.

Cómo entrevistar a los agentes

Comience cada entrevista dedicando unos pocos minutos al análisis de la lista de actividad del agente. Una vez que termine de revisar la lista y haya tenido tiempo de organizar sus pensamientos, obtenga respuestas a las siguientes preguntas:

✔ **¿Es usted un agente inmobiliario a tiempo completo?** Debería haber hecho esta pregunta antes de invitar al agente a la entrevista. Si se le olvidó, hágalo ahora. No trabaje con agentes que sólo dedican medio tiempo a este trabajo.

✔ **¿A quién representa?** Esto regresa a la pregunta fundamental de la agencia. ¿Es el agente exclusivamente su representante, o es un agente de representación a ambas partes, a usted y al vendedor? Asegúrese de saber exactamente a quién representa su agente en todo momento.

✔ **¿Qué puede decirme usted acerca de su oficina?** Hable del tamaño de la oficina, del personal auxiliar, de su especialización en el mercado, y de la reputación. Investigue si el corredor del agente tiene experiencia, si usted tendrá acceso a él en caso de ser necesario, y si tiene talento para resolver problemas. En un apuro, el éxito (o fracaso) de su transacción puede depender de la calidad de la ayuda que usted y su agente reciban.

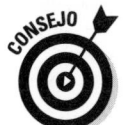

No le dé demasiado peso al tamaño de la oficina del agente. Algunos agente excelentes trabajan por su cuenta, y otros igualmente excelentes prefieren la energía y los servicios de apoyo que se encuentran en una oficina grande. Aunque las oficinas grandes tienden a tener más listados, ninguna oficina tiene un monopolio de los buenos listados de propiedades. La calidad del servicio es más importante que la cantidad de los listados o los agentes.

✔ **¿Cuánto tiempo hace que trabaja como agente inmobiliario?** Usted desea un agente que continúa aprendiendo y ganando experiencia. Después de cinco años en bienes raíces, un buen agente tiene 5 años de experiencia, mientras que una agente mediocre tiene un año de experiencia cinco veces. El tiempo en la montura no es muestra de que domina al caballo.

✔ **La licencia de vendedor o la licencia de corredor.** Un agente debe estudiar más tiempo y debe tener experiencia de campo para cumplir con los requisitos para obtener la licencia de corredor inmobiliario. Muchos agentes muy competentes tienen solamente la licencia de vendedor inmobiliario durante toda su carrera. Aunque la licencia de corredor no es garantía de excelencia, los buenos agentes a menudo obtienen una licencia de corredor para mejorar sus destrezas profesionales, y para acrecentar su ventaja en situaciones de selección de un agente.

✔ **¿Tiene usted alguna designación profesional? ¿Ha tomado recientemente algunas clases de bienes raíces? ¿Lee usted material publicado para mantenerse al día en su profesión?** La asistencia a cursos de educación continua, y la lectura de bibliografía pertinente a bienes raíces para actualizarse y conocer los cambios ocurridos en el mercado inmobiliario, son una buena señal. También lo es la obtención de certificaciones profesionales, como los de Estudios Superiores del *Graduate Realtor Institute* (*GRI,* por sus siglas en inglés) y el de Especialista residencial certificado (*Certified Residencial Specialist* [*CRS,* por sus siglas en inglés]) que se obtienen a través de los programas de estudio de la Asociación Nacional de Corredores de Bienes Raíces (*National Association of Realtors*). Sin embargo, las credenciales no son en sí mismas una garantía de aptitud o ética.

✔ **¿Comprende bien el agente lo que usted necesita para comprar una vivienda?** Probablemente usted ya le ha dicho al agente el tipo de propiedad que quiere comprar, el vecindario en el que desea vivir y cuánto puede gastar. Compruebe si el agente recuerda lo que usted dijo. Si el agente no lo recuerda, tenga cuidado. Usted necesita un agente que escucha atentamente lo que usted dice.

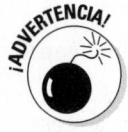

✔ **¿Qué piensa usted de los otros dos agentes (diga sus nombres) a quiénes estoy entrevistado?** Para estimular franqueza, asegure a los agentes que no va a repetir lo que ellos le dicen. Los buenos agentes no aprovechan la oportunidad para destruir la reputación de los otros. Si los tres agentes son buenos, no escuchará ningún comentario despectivo. Sin embargo, si uno de los agentes (o la firma del agente) tiene mala reputación en la comunidad inmobiliaria, los otros dos deberían decírselo. Sea buena o mala la reputación de su agente y la de la oficina del agente, ésta se le atribuirá a usted también.

✔ **¿Cuántos compradores y vendedores representa usted en estos momentos?** Si, por ejemplo, el agente tiene cada fin de semana tres viviendas abiertas al público y está trabajando con otros seis compradores, ¿cuándo le va a dar una cita a usted? Aunque algunos conflictos de horarios son inevitables, usted no debería tener que cambiar su vida para ajustarla al horario del agente. Un buen agente tiene tiempo para acomodarse a su horario.

✔ **¿Trabaja usted en asociación con otro agente o utiliza asistentes?** Algunos agentes trabajan en equipo con otros agentes para darles servicios a compradores y a vendedores entre los dos. Si éste es el caso, usted debe entrevistar a los dos agentes. Otros agentes delegan detalles que demandan mucho tiempo a sus asistentes para poder así dedicarse a los aspectos importantes de la transacción. Si el agente confía en sus asistentes, verifique si los asistentes son capaces y sepa exactamente cómo y cuándo, durante el proceso de compra, su agente trabajará directamente con usted. No quiere contratar a un agente y descubrir luego que va a terminar tratando casi todo el tiempo con su asistente — quien no le cae nada bien.

✔ **¿Hay algo que no le haya preguntado a usted o a su firma, y que usted piensa que debería saber?** Quizás el agente esté planeando cambiar de firma, o la próxima semana se va a hacer un viaje de 80 días alrededor del mundo. O, el corredor del agente está cerrando sus oficinas. *Esto es asegurarse de que sabe todo lo que necesita saber para tomar una buena decisión.*

Cómo verificar las referencias del agente

Aquí tiene la oportunidad de aprovecharse de los errores de otra gente, lo que es infinitamente mejor que cometerlos usted mismo. Usted debería tener las listas de actividad con los nombres y números de teléfono de cada comprador y vendedor que los agentes representaron durante los previos 12 meses. Puede seleccionar a las personas a las que quiere llamar, y no restringirse a la lista selectiva de referencias, cuyos miembros piensan que estos agentes son el regalo de Dios a la industria inmobiliaria.

¿Qué y quién le va a impedir a los agentes omitir selectivamente sus peores transacciones? Nada, ni nadie. Pero cuantas más transacciones omitan, mostrarán una actividad menor en su lista de actividad —y será peor aún cuando usted compare la actividad total de los agentes.

Suponga que cada agente le da una lista que incluye 50 transacciones. Si considera que hay un comprador o vendedor para cada transacción, 50 clientes por agente multiplicado por los tres entrevistados, es equivalente a 150 llamadas telefónicas. Usted estará llamando por teléfono toda una eternidad.

¡Buenas noticias! No tiene que llamar a cada uno ni a todos los clientes para verificar las referencias. Usted puede obtener una muy buena idea de cada agente, si hace, por decir, seis llamadas por agente.

He aquí una manera fácil y rápida para lograr una muestra representativa de las referencias de los clientes:

1. **Como usted es un comprador, ignore las referencias de los vendedores.**

   Si lo hace así, probablemente corta la lista por la mitad.

2. **Dedique su atención a las personas que compraron una propiedad similar en precio, ubicación y tipo de propiedad como la que usted quiere comprar.**

3. **Llame a dos de esos compradores que compraron hace alrededor de 12 meses, otros dos compradores que compraron hace seis meses, y los dos que hicieron más recientemente sus depósitos de garantía.**

   Al distribuir las referencias a lo largo del año pasado, puede descubrir si el tipo de servicio del agente ha sido regularmente bueno.

Ahora que ya ha identificado a los compradores que va a llamar, lo siguiente es lo que tiene que preguntarles cuando los tenga en el teléfono:

- ✔ **¿Es el agente digno de confianza? ¿Es sincero? ¿Cumplió con sus promesas?** Su agente no puede ser poco confiable o no siempre sincero, o poco cumplidor. Una respuesta negativa a cualquiera de estas preguntas es el beso de la muerte.

- ✔ **¿Tuvo el agente tiempo suficiente para servirlo adecuadamente? ¿Estuvo disponible el agente, como se requiere, acomodándose a su horario?** Ocasionalmente, los conflictos de horario son inevitables. Pero los conflictos frecuentes son absolutamente inaceptables.

- ✔ **¿Le explicó el agente todo lo que pasaba durante el procesos de compra, claramente y con detalles suficientes para satisfacerlo?** Lo que una persona piense de lo que son detalles suficientes, pueden no serlo para otros. Usted se conoce bien — haga las preguntas de verificación que considere necesarias.

- ✔ **¿Fijó el agente fechas límites realistas para el contrato y las cumplió o adelantó?** "El tiempo es oro" y es una condición de cada contrato en bienes raíces. El plazo para obtener un préstamo, completar las inspecciones de la propiedad, y otras cosas semejantes son extremadamente importantes y deben respetarse estrictamente o el negocio se pierde. Los buenos agentes preparan contratos bien escritos con plazos realistas, y luego se aseguran que se cumplan todas las fechas de vencimiento el día establecido o antes.

- ✔ **¿Las siguientes palabras describen al agente: iniciativa, dedicación, motivación?** A nadie le gustan los prepotentes. Pero si usted está bajo la presión de concretar la compra rápidamente, la última cosa que necesita es un agente súper lento. No debería tener que sacudir periódicamente a su agente con una descarga eléctrica para estar seguro de que todavía respira. Descubra cuánta energía tiene el agente que está considerando y si está preparado para trabajar.

✔ **¿Quién encontró la casa que compró —usted o el agente?** Esta pregunta es para verificar de nuevo si el agente conoce el mercado. Los buenos agentes no sólo saben lo que ya está en el mercado, sino también conocen las viviendas que van a estar pronto en el mercado. Usted no debería tener que encontrar el inmueble que va a comprar —ése es el trabajo del agente.

✔ **¿Negoció el agente un buen precio para su vivienda?** Vea si los compradores del agente *todavía* piensan que hicieron un buen negocio. Los buenos agentes son frugales cuando gastan el dinero del cliente. También usan el conocimiento del valor de la propiedad y sus habilidades de negociador para asegurarse que sus clientes pagan el precio justo del mercado, o menos, por las viviendas que compran. La gente que compró una propiedad hace un año o seis meses, puede decirle si su compra ha conservado el precio del mercado a través del tiempo.

✔ **¿Usaría usted al mismo agente otra vez?** Ésta es la última prueba para conocer la satisfacción del cliente. Si alguien dice "no", pregunte por qué no. La respuesta negativa puede resultar de un conflicto de personalidades entre el comprador y el agente, que no le importa a usted. Por otro lado, la respuesta negativa puede revelar un defecto serio del agente que usted aún no ha descubierto.

✔ **¿Hay algo que no le haya preguntado a usted, o acerca de la oficina del agente, que usted piensa que yo debería saber?** Nunca se sabe lo que descubrirá cuando hace la famosa pregunta que lo abarca todo.

Cómo tomar su decisión

Después de analizar la lista de actividad de los tres agentes, de entrevistarlos y de hablar con sus compradores, usted tiene los hechos que necesita para tomar una decisión bien fundada. A continuación hay tres consideraciones finales que le ayudarán a seleccionar el agente ejemplar y virtuoso que necesita para su equipo de bienes raíces.

✔ **¿Se sentirá orgulloso de que el agente lo represente?** La gente que entra en contacto con su agente forma opiniones de usted basadas en sus impresiones de su agente inmobiliario. No puede arriesgarse a tener a alguien en su equipo que no sea un profesional altamente calificado.

✔ **¿Tiene una buena comunicación con su agente?** Los buenos agentes quieren estar seguros de que usted comprende todo lo que le dicen. Si no puede entender a su agente, no es que usted sea tonto —el agente es un mal comunicador.

✔ **¿Le gusta la personalidad del agente?** Comprar una vivienda incluye el pasar por un proceso estresante, aun para los que son tan frescos como la lechuga. Compartirá situaciones extremadamente intensas con su agente. Si trabaja con un agente que le agrada, el proceso de compra de una vivienda, que puede ser una experiencia horrible, puede transformarse en una aventura emocionante.

Cómo lograr una buena relación con su agente

Después de haber trabajado tanto para seleccionar al mejor agente, sería una lástima que sin quererlo, se dañara la relación entre ustedes. La buena relación entre el comprador y el agente no es accidental. Tales relaciones están asentadas en los pilares de lealtad y confianza mutuas.

Por el contrario, las relaciones difíciles resultan de una idea falsa sobre cómo se juega el partido. Algunos compradores actúan de la forma que consideran mejor para sus intereses, pero acaban dañándose a sí mismos sin intentarlo.

Más no es siempre mejor

Es un error pensar que cinco agentes son cinco veces mejor que uno. ¡La teoría parece tan lógica! Si usted trabaja con agentes de diferentes oficinas, puede ganar una mayor presencia en el mercado y tener la primicia de los listados nuevos que cada oficina pone en el mercado. Cuantos más agentes trabajan con usted, son mejores las posibilidades de encontrar rápidamente la casa de sus sueños.

Pero las cosas no funcionan así en el mundo real. Cuando agentes veteranos lo conocen por primera vez, probablemente le preguntarán si está trabajando con otros agentes. Dichos agentes están tratando de saber cuánto conoce el mercado (así ellos evitan el riesgo de mostrarle propiedades que usted ya visitó) y para saber qué no le gustó de las propiedades que ya vio.

Un buen agente puede rápidamente mostrarle todas las propiedades en el mercado que cumplen con sus especificaciones de precio, vecindario, tamaño y condición. Si no le ha gustado ninguna propiedad, los agentes competentes continuarán buscando hasta que llegue al mercado la que usted busca. Los buenos agentes no limitan sus búsquedas a sólo las viviendas listadas en sus oficinas. Investigan todo lo que sea aun remotamente similar a lo que usted desea, sin importarles cuál oficina listó la propiedad. Si trabaja con un agente o con cien, usted verá las mismas viviendas.

Los agentes saben que no recibirán ningún pago si usted no compra. El riesgo de que eso ocurra es parte del trabajo. Lo que más odian los agentes es perder una venta después de meses de trabajo arduo, porque ellos lo llamaron a usted justo después que otro agente lo contactó en relación a la misma propiedad. Ése riesgo es innecesario. Por supuesto, usted es libre de trabajar con tantos agentes como quiera. De hecho, trabajar con más de un agente tiene sentido si usted está buscando una vivienda en más de una localidad geográfica, pero no se sorprenda, sin embargo, si buenos agentes en la misma zona abandonan la carrera. Las probabilidades de recibir una comisión aumentan notablemente cuando usan su tiempo con compradores que trabajan exclusivamente con ellos. La lealtad engendra lealtad.

El riesgo de tantear el terreno raramente vale la pena. Un agente leal, totalmente comprometido a encontrarle su vivienda, es infinitamente mejor que cinco agentes trabajando para usted sin mucho interés, solamente porque lo consideran a usted un poquitín mejor que el traidor norteamericano Benedict Arnold. Como en los matrimonios, la mejor relación entre el comprador y el agente es la monogamia.

Su agente no es su enemigo

Otro error es ver a su agente como si fuera su adversario. Es verdad, usted no le cuenta sus íntimos secretos a un hablador indiscreto que descuidadamente los ventilará al vendedor o al agente del vendedor. Algunos compradores piensan que cuanto menos sepa el agente de ellos, mejor es. Tales compradores creen que después de que los agentes sepan lo que ellos quieren comprar y cuánto dinero tienen, de alguna manera los agentes van a manipularlos para que gasten mucho más de lo que pueden por la vivienda, que eventualmente van a comprar.

Eso no es verdad. Los agentes con experiencia hacen preguntas porque necesitan asegurarse de que usted reúne los requisitos para obtener el financiamiento, a fin de evitar la pérdida de tiempo de ellos y la de usted, la cual finalmente será verdad si no tiene los medios para comprar las propiedades que le muestren. Si su agente sabe que usted está bajo presión para comprar dentro de un plazo determinado, le dará prioridad para buscar la vivienda.

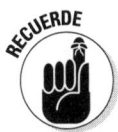

Los buenos agentes no traicionarán su confianza. Ellos saben que si cumplen con su responsabilidad, la comisión llegará completita al final. Si usted no confía en su agente, no finja su confianza ni esconda su disgusto, y busque a un nuevo agente.

Aunque parezca mentira, muchos agentes expertos le temen a usted tanto, o más, de lo que usted les teme a ellos. Saben que usted tiene el poder de afianzar o destruir sus carreras. Si lo hacen feliz, usted se convertirá en una fuente de elogios y de futuros clientes. Si no llenan sus expectativas, usted le dirá a todo el mundo que conoce que ellos hicieron un trabajo pésimo.

Aproveche el inmenso poder de las recomendaciones potenciales para manejar su relación con el agente. Si su agente hace un pobre trabajo, no se enoje — dígale al mundo entero cada detalle horrendo de su espantosa experiencia. No hay nada que arruine más rápido la carrera de un agente que sus clientes descontentos.

Cómo Cazar a un Corredor Inmobiliario

La selección de un corredor es fácil. Cuando usted elige a un agente, éste trae consigo al corredor con quien trabaja. Es el paquete completo; lo tiene todo.

Si su transacción se desliza sobre ruedas desde el momento en que aceptan su oferta hasta el cierre, probablemente nunca conocerá al corredor. Pero si el motor comienza a fallar y las ruedas empiezan a separarse del vehículo, es posible adivinar quién es el candidato para hacer un trabajo rápido de reparación. Los corredores inmobiliarios son el combustible invisible que mueve las transacciones problemáticas.

Todos los estados emiten dos tipos completamente diferentes de licencias de bienes raíces: una para los vendedores (los agentes) y una para los corredores inmobiliarios. Los agentes que tienen también la licencia de corredores deben satisfacer un nivel de educación mucho más riguroso y estándares de experiencia más altos que los agentes que tienen licencia de ventas solamente.

Su agente puede tener cualquiera de esos tipos de licencia. Los corredores licenciados tienen la opción de trabajar independientemente o, trabajar para otro corredor. Un agente con licencia inmobiliaria, por el contrario, *debe* trabajar bajo la supervisión directa de un corredor para que usted tenga acceso a un mayor grado de experiencia en caso de necesitarla.

Cuando Harry Truman era presidente, tenía un cartel en su escritorio que decía: "La responsabilidad final termina aquí". Como Truman, los corredores competentes no les pasan la responsabilidad a otros. Éstas son algunas de sus otras características:

- **Reputación excelente:** la imagen del corredor inmobiliario será obvia por los comentarios que escucha mientras verifica las referencias del agente. Usted quiere que el vendedor, el prestamista y otra gente involucrada en su transacción trabajen a su lado en virtud de la reputación del corredor, y no a pesar de ella. La compra de una vivienda es de por sí complicada como para agregarle el sentirse abrumado por su relación con los miembros de su equipo. Si las referencias del agente menosprecian al corredor del agente inmobiliario, no trabaje con él.

- **Múltiples relaciones comerciales:** los buenos corredores desarrollan y mantienen relaciones con la gente que tiene relaciones comerciales con su oficina —otros corredores inmobiliarios, funcionarios de la oficina de títulos, funcionarios del gobierno local y otros similares. Este conjunto preexistente de buenos contactos le será útil a usted cuando encuentre problemas durante el proceso. Los corredores con relaciones comerciales importantes pueden hacer cosas casi milagrosas para usted en una crisis.

- **Experto en la resolución de problemas:** los participantes en las relaciones comerciales inmobiliarias a veces se dejan llevar por la emoción.

Cuando su vida está en juego, en algunas ocasiones, es posible que usted ataque verbalmente a su agente y a otros miembros del equipo. Alguien tiene que resolver las peleas y malentendidos. Esa persona es el corredor.

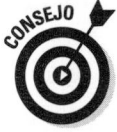

El trabajo del corredor inmobiliario es ayudarle a resolver sus problemas. Invite al corredor a unirse al equipo si su agente está paralizado por un problema serio, o si usted tiene problemas con su agente. Todo lo que su agente hace o deja de hacer es, en última instancia, responsabilidad del corredor inmobiliario.

Cómo Encontrar a un Prestamista

Todos piensan que la compra de una casa es probablemente la compra más cara de su vida. Excepto, si usted piensa comprar la vivienda con dinero en efectivo, todos los demás están equivocados. He aquí el porqué.

Vamos a suponer que el precio de compra de la vivienda de sus sueños es $250.000. Usted hace un depósito en garantía de $50.000 y obtiene un préstamo hipotecario con una tasa de interés fijo al 7,5 por ciento de su simpático prestamista. En los próximos 30 años, usted paga responsablemente su préstamo en cuotas mensuales de $1.400. (Le mostramos en el Capítulo 3 y en el 6, cómo puede analizar y calcular estos números usted.)

El monto total de sus 360 pagos mensuales del préstamo hipotecario será de $500.000. Si originalmente le concedieron un préstamo de $200.000, la diferencia de $300.000 que pagó equivale a los intereses de su préstamo. El total de los intereses fue *mayor* que el precio de compra de su propiedad.

Si no puede pagar, no puede jugar. Usted necesita un buen prestamista en su equipo para que lo convierta de buscador de vivienda a propietario de la misma. Si encuentra a un buen prestamista, se puede ahorrar un montón de dinero durante la vigencia del préstamo.

No existe un préstamo que sea bueno para todos. Una persona que recién se graduó de la universidad y que está luchando para comprar un condominio con un pago en garantía del 5 por ciento, tiene que cumplir con requisitos muy diferentes que una pareja más madura y rica que puso el 50 por ciento de depósito en garantía por una casita para vivir después de la jubilación, usando el capital de la venta de su vivienda anterior.

Para las generaciones anteriores fue fácil encontrar un préstamo adecuado. Podían obtener cualquier tipo de hipoteca que quisieran, siempre que el préstamo fuera para pagar en 30 años y tuviera un interés fijo. Todos los préstamos hipotecarios eran básicamente iguales, excepto por variaciones mínimas en las cuotas y en las tasas de interés.

Conocimiento por experiencia y conocimiento de los libros

La gente con conocimiento obtenido de los libros tiene un conocimiento teórico. Saben sólo lo que debiera ocurrir en un mundo perfecto, según lo que han leído. Usted está recibiendo en estos momentos el conocimiento que se adquiere de los libros.

Por el contrario, la gente que tiene el conocimiento por experiencia de la vida, sabe cómo son las cosas en la realidad del mundo. Ellos aprendieron de sus propios errores a lo largo de años de práctica y experiencia. Un buen corredor inmobiliario en su equipo es uno de los mejores conocedores por experiencias de la vida real.

La gente aprende muy poco de las cosas cuando todo sale bien y sin tropiezos, y las transacciones son rutinarias: es como si volaran en un avión con piloto automático. La experiencia de la vida es el conocimiento de un trabajo logrado con el sudor de la frente. Por fortuna, la mayoría de los agentes pasan anualmente sólo por uno o dos de estos problemas que les retuercen las entrañas. Cuando ocurren estas transacciones problemáticas, podemos decir que el corredor inmobiliario es el que asume el control del avión.

A raíz de que el corredor participa directa o indirectamente, en cada asunto que pasa por su oficina, su experiencia práctica tiene una relación directa con el número de agentes en la oficina. Un corredor inmobiliario que supervisa una oficina con 25 agentes, por ejemplo, adquiere una experiencia de 25 años en un año normal. Cualquier corredor inmobiliario que sobrevive cinco años administrando todas las transacciones verdaderamente horribles de la oficina se convierte en una persona con una magnífica habilidad para resolver problemas.

Esas épocas mejores y más simples son ahora una historia del pasado. Hoy día, usted se encuentra frente a una gama desconcertante de programas con tasas de interés fijo y con tasas de interés ajustable (*ARM*). En el Capítulo 6, revelamos el misterio de cómo asegurar un préstamo hipotecario y cómo seleccionar a un prestamista.

Cómo Conseguir a los Inspectores de Propiedades

El precio de un inmueble está directamente relacionado con la condición estructural y estética. Las viviendas en excelentes condiciones se venden por precios más altos. Las que necesitan renovación tienen precios más reducidos porque quienquiera que las compre tiene que gastar dinero en reparaciones para ponerlas nuevamente en mejores condiciones.

Aun si usted es un científico espacial, al ver la propiedad, no puede saber con exactitud cuánto va a costar la renovación que es necesaria. No puede ver si los techos van a gotear, si el sistema eléctrico es defectuoso, si la plomería es deficiente, si el intercambiador de calor de la calefacción está rajado, si la chimenea está floja, o si hay una infestación de termitas en las partes de madera. Defectos invisibles como éstos requieren reparaciones costosas.

Como usted no quiere convertirse, sin saberlo, en el propietario de una vivienda que tenga tantos problemas escondidos, necesita inspectores de propiedad en su equipo. Ninguno de los otros participantes de su equipo — incluyendo los agentes de bienes raíces, los prestamistas y los corredores inmobiliarios— tiene el conocimiento necesario para darle consejo sobre la condición estructural de la propiedad, o el costo del trabajo de renovación necesario. En el Capítulo 13, le damos información sobre todo lo que necesita saber acerca de las inspecciones de la vivienda y de la selección de los inspectores de propiedad.

Aunque una vivienda no es tan compleja como una nave espacial, tiene sin embargo, una buena cantidad de sistemas caros que pueden descomponerse. El ahorro de dinero por eliminación de las inspecciones, sólo porque el inmueble parece estar en buenas condiciones, es un ahorro falso. La gran mayoría de los problemas de una vivienda no son visibles. Nunca compre una casa que no haya sido detalladamente inspeccionada desde los cimientos hasta el techo por inspectores expertos elegidos por usted.

Cómo Seleccionar a un Administrador de Depósito en Garantía

Un denominador común aparece en casi todos los negocios de bienes raíces: la desconfianza mutua. Como comprador, ¿le daría usted al vendedor el dinero ganado con el sudor de su frente antes de estar satisfecho con todas las condiciones de la venta? Probablemente no. Si su posición fuera la opuesta, y usted fuera el vendedor, ¿le daría el *título* de la propiedad de su vivienda al comprador antes de recibir su dinero? Por supuesto que no.

Los negocios se paran en seco si no existe un puente de unión para saltar el abismo de desconfianza que hay entre el comprador y el vendedor. Aun la transacción más sencilla incluye una multitud de detalles que deben resolverse a satisfacción de las partes antes de que se complete la venta. Es por eso que en el juego de bienes raíces, como en cualquier otro juego, se necesita un árbitro.

El funcionario o administrador de depósito en garantía es el árbitro que mantiene civilizado el partido entre los equipos. Claramente hablando, los administradores del depósito no pertenecen a ninguno de los dos equipos — ellos son neutrales. Ellos actúan como un tercero, sin interés por los compradores o vendedores, y sin mostrar ningún favoritismo hacia ninguna de las partes.

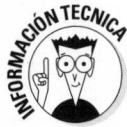

Después que usted y el vendedor hayan firmado el contrato, todos los documentos, fondos e instrucciones relacionadas con su transacción se le entregan al funcionario o administrador de depósito en garantía que está especificado en su contrato de compra. Presentamos este proceso, conocido como *apertura de un depósito en garantía,* en el Capítulo 14.

Los compradores y los vendedores generalmente eligen al funcionario del depósito en garantía según la recomendación de sus agentes inmobiliarios. La costumbre local dicta, según la ubicación de la propiedad que está comprando, si el depósito está manejado por un abogado, un banco, un corredor inmobiliario, o una firma que emite la póliza de seguro del título.

Los honorarios del depósito en garantía cubren una gama de precios entre unos cientos de dólares hasta algunos miles de dólares, y están basados en el precio de compra de la propiedad. Una vez más, las costumbres locales generalmente determinan si el comprador o el vendedor paga por el depósito, o si los honorarios de éste son divididos en dos partes iguales. Sin embargo, como lo explicamos en el Capítulo 12, este aspecto es con frecuencia negociable.

Cómo Encontrar (U Omitir) Asesores Financieros e Impositivos

El juego de bienes raíces requiere dinero real —su dinero, fruto de su trabajo. Es probable que usted haya escatimado, ahorrado y dejado de comprar cosas para reunir el dinero necesario para el pago inicial. Cuando algún día venda su casa, su capital en ella será probablemente una buena parte de su patrimonio. De cualquier manera, si compra o si vende, está en juego mucha plata.

La compra de una vivienda tiene una importancia enorme sobre sus finanzas personales. Antes de comprar una vivienda, necesita comprender qué papel jugará esa compra en el contexto de la totalidad de sus finanzas y de sus otras metas. No deje de leer los Capítulos 2 y 3, que tratan de estos asuntos importantes.

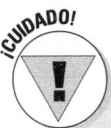

Algunos expertos dan asesoramiento equivocado

Ray no sabía mucho acerca de asesores impositivos cuando se mudó a San Francisco. Algunas personas con las que Ray trabajó le recomendaron que utilizara el asesor impositivo de ellos. Él lo seleccionó teniendo en cuenta esas recomendaciones (más el hecho de que su oficina estaba sólo a dos cuadras de la suya).

Ray se dio cuenta de que cometió un error cuando fue a su oficina para verificar la declaración de impuestos que ella le había preparado. Él le preguntó cómo había llegado a las deducciones detalladas de sus gastos de automóvil y de entrenamiento profesional. En ambos casos, eran mucho más altas que los totales de los recibos que Ray le había dado.

Ella le explicó que estas deducciones más altas reducían lo que tenía que pagar, y le dijo que nadie se daría cuenta, pues estaban dentro de los límites aceptables en las directivas del *IRS*. Ray aún así no comprendió el concepto de deducir más dinero del que había gastado.

La asesora de impuestos de Ray, con cierta impaciencia, le explicó nuevamente la declaración impositiva, más lentamente, y usando palabras más sencillas esta segunda vez. Terminó diciéndole que no debía preocuparse por lo que ella había hecho porque todo el mundo aumenta los gastos declarados.

Ray sabía que ella estaba hablando en inglés porque reconocía casi todas las palabras, pero ellas parecían rebotar de su cabeza, sin penetrar su cerebro. Comenzó a sentirse más y más frustrado, y su asesora impositiva estaba retrasándose para sus otras citas. Ella, desesperada, le dio a Ray la declaración de impuestos y lo mandó a su casa para que pensara, tratándolo como si él fuera un niño de edad escolar.

Y él lo pensó.

Ray decidió que el problema no era que él era estúpido. El problema era que le habían dado un consejo falto de ética profesional. En su celo por ahorrarle dinero a su cliente, la asesora impositiva había falsificado las deducciones de Ray. Esta falsificación era incorrecta y, lo que es peor, era ilegal. Ray resolvió el problema buscando a un nuevo asesor.

Nunca siga, a ciegas, el consejo de expertos solamente por el hecho de que usted admira sus conocimientos. Los expertos pueden estar tan equivocados como todos los demás mortales.

Usted puede optar por contratar a un asesor financiero, pero la mayoría de esos asesores no están preparados para responder con objetividad las preguntas sobre la compra de una vivienda. La razón es que los asesores financieros ganan dinero del asesoramiento que ofrecen. Muchos de los llamados consultores financieros reciben comisiones de las inversiones que le venden. Si éste es el caso, ¿la motivación del asesor lo llevará a aconsejarle a que use su dinero para comprar una vivienda, o a que, en cambio, haga una inversión para su portafolio? Los asesores que manejan dinero por un precio determinado (o por un porcentaje) tienen el mismo conflicto de intereses.

Si piensa contratar a un asesor, busque uno que cobre por hora de trabajo y que no tenga un interés personal en su decisión de comprar una vivienda. Muy pocos asesores financieros trabajan de esta manera. Y, aunque los asesores impositivos probablemente trabajan de esta forma, ellos tienden a tener una perspectiva financiera más reducida de lo que es necesario. Un asesor impositivo competente podría ayudarle a estructurar la compra de la propiedad al mismo tiempo que maximiza los beneficios en sus impuestos. Sin embargo, para la mayoría de las transacciones, un asesor impositivo es innecesario.

Si usted desea contratar a un asesor impositivo, entreviste a varios antes de seleccionar uno. Consulte con su agente, su banquero, su abogado, sus colegas en negocios, y con sus amigos para que le den los nombres de algunos de ellos. Así como lo hizo con la selección de su agente, aquí también debería obtener referencias de los clientes de asesores impositivos y verificar esas referencias.

Esto es lo que debe buscar en un buen asesor impositivo o financiero:

- ✔ **¿Dedica el asesor tiempo completo a este trabajo?** El ámbito del campo de finanzas personales y de impuestos es demasiado amplio para confiar en un asesor que trabaja a medio tiempo. Usted necesita los servicios de un profesional con dedicación a tiempo completo.

- ✔ **¿Es su lenguaje comprensible?** Los buenos asesores pueden explicar sus alternativas financieras en términos sencillos. Si usted no entiende exactamente lo que el asesor impositivo le dice, pídale una explicación mejor. Y, si todavía no entiende, busque otro asesor impositivo. (Vea el subtítulo: "Algunos expertos dan asesoramiento equivocado".)

- ✔ **¿Es objetivo el asesor?** Contrate a alguien que cobra solamente por hora y que no tiene un interés personal en el consejo que le está dando en relación a cuándo comprar y cuánto gastar.

- ✔ **¿Cuánto cobra por el asesoramiento?** Los honorarios por hora varían muchísimo. No elija a alguien solamente por lo que cobra por hora. Un asesor que recién comienza su carrera, por ejemplo, puede cobrar sólo la mitad comparado con otro que tiene 20 años de experiencia. Si el novato trabaja cuatro horas por lo que el asesor con experiencia hace en una hora, ¿cuál asesor es más caro al final? Además, la calidad del consejo del asesor con experiencia puede ser superior a la del novato.

- ✔ **¿Es el asesor impositivo un Contador Público certificado (*CPA*, por sus siglas en inglés) o un agente profesional (*Enrolled Agent* [*EA*, por sus siglas en inglés]) certificado por el gobierno de los EE.UU. para representar a los contribuyentes ante el *IRS?*** Estas designaciones profesionales indican que el asesor impositivo ha satisfecho requisitos de educación y experiencia y ha pasado un riguroso examen para obtener su licencia. Un Contador Público (*CPA*) practica contabilidad en general y prepara declaraciones de impuestos. Un *EA* trabaja específicamente con los impuestos. Sólo los *CPA*, *EA* y los abogados están autorizados a representarlo ante el *IRS* en el caso de una auditoría.

✔ **¿Tiene el asesor impositivo experiencia con transacciones de bienes raíces?** El ejercicio de la profesión en impuestos es como la abogacía y la medicina, es un campo extremadamente amplio. Los asesores impositivos que usa IBM (por ejemplo) son, sin duda, muy buenos, pero esos asesores impositivos no son necesariamente los más apropiados para usted. Usted necesita un asesor de impuestos cuyos clientes tienen problemas impositivos semejantes a los suyos.

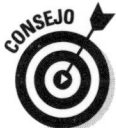

Los mejores asesores del mundo no pueden hacer mucho para cambiar las consecuencias financieras e impositivas de una transacción *después* del cierre de la misma. Si usted va a consultar a asesores, hágalo *antes* de tomar decisiones financieras de importancia. Planee su situación financiera e impositiva, en vez de reaccionar a las consecuencias después del hecho.

La Búsqueda de Abogados

Los abogados son como los cinturones de seguridad. Nunca se sabe cuándo los vamos a necesitar. Su proceso de compra se desliza plácidamente y sin tropiezos, cuando de pronto —¡puf, paf, zas!— usted tropieza con un bache legal y termina en la ciudad El Juicio Final.

Ese contrato de compra que usted firmó, terminó siendo un contrato con un vínculo legal entre usted y el vendedor. Si tiene alguna duda sobre la legalidad de su contrato, contrate a un abogado, y *muy pronto*. Nadie en el equipo está capacitado para darle consejo legal.

He aquí lo que determina si usted necesita un abogado:

✔ **La ubicación de la propiedad que compra:** en estados como California, los abogados raramente trabajan en asuntos que sólo requieren llenar los espacios en blanco de un contrato estándar, que está previamente impreso y aprobado por los miembros del colegio de abogados. En otros estados, como Nueva York, sin embargo, los abogados rutinariamente hacen todo, desde la preparación de los contratos de compra hasta el cierre del depósito en garantía. Su agente debe saber el papel que los abogados tienen en su localidad.

✔ **La complejidad de su transacción:** usted necesita un abogado en cualquier momento en que se encuentre en una situación que no está prevista en un contrato estándar. A menos de que su agente sea un abogado o abogada, él o ella no están capacitados para redactar un documento legal. Los casos complicados deben ser manejados por abogados, como lo son aquéllos en contratos de sociedad entre gente sin relación alguna de parentesco que compran juntos una propiedad, y las complejas ramificaciones de recibir el título de su vivienda, que ocurren con frecuencia. (Hablamos de los contratos de sociedades residenciales especiales en el Capítulo 8 y de la obtención del título en el Capítulo 14.)

✔ **Cuando no hay agente de por medio:** digamos que usted está comprando una casa que está en venta directa por el dueño. Si, ni usted ni el vendedor tienen un agente, contrate a un abogado para que prepare el contrato y para que haga las cosas que normalmente estarían a cargo del agente. El no tener un agente no elimina la necesidad de las declaraciones financieras, de las inspecciones, de las condiciones para la venta, y de una multitud de otros detalles incluidos en el proceso de compra de una vivienda.

✔ **Para dormir bien por la noche:** puede ser que usted tenga el caso más fácil del mundo; pero, si se siente mejor teniendo un abogado que revise el contrato, su tranquilidad ciertamente vale el costo de una hora o dos del tiempo de un abogado.

Cómo seleccionar a su abogado

Si por cualquier razón usted decide que necesita un abogado, entreviste a varios antes de tomar su decisión. La ley, lo mismo que la medicina, es un campo de conocimiento sumamente especializado. Un abogado corporativo o el que tuvo a su cargo el divorcio de su vecino, no son los mejores candidatos para su equipo de bienes raíces. Busque a un abogado especializado en transacciones inmobiliarias residenciales. Su agente y el corredor son excelentes fuentes de referencias porque ellos trabajan todo el tiempo con abogados de bienes raíces en sus transacciones.

Un buen abogado:

✔ **Es un abogado que trabaja a tiempo completo en su profesión y está licenciado para practicar en su estado:** ¡Por supuesto!

✔ **Es una persona de la región y con talento:** la legislación inmobiliaria, como el corretaje de bienes raíces, es extremadamente regional. La ley varía no solamente de estado a estado, sino también de una zona a otra dentro del mismo estado. Las leyes de control de los alquileres, los estatutos de conversión de los condominios, y los códigos de zonificación son generalmente aprobados por las agencias de gobierno de la ciudad o del condado. Un buen abogado local conoce las leyes y ha establecido relaciones personales con la gente que administra las leyes en su zona.

✔ **Tiene tarifas justas:** los honorarios por hora varían muchísimo. Un buen abogado calcula el monto aproximado de sus honorarios de acuerdo a su caso. Lo mismo que con los asesores financieros e impositivos, la experiencia del profesional es importante. Los abogados con experiencia generalmente cobran honorarios por hora más altos que un abogado novato, pero tienden a completar más trabajo por hora que abogados con poca experiencia. Un costo menor no es una ganga si el novato está aprendiendo mientras usted le paga.

✔ **Tiene una buena trayectoria profesional:** si su caso tiene que ir a un tribunal, verifique si el abogado tiene experiencia en los tribunales. Algunos abogados no trabajan con casos en litigación. Luego, pregunte acerca del récord del abogado en cuanto al número de juicios ganados y perdidos. ¿Cuál es el beneficio de tener a un abogado con una gran experiencia en litigación, si nunca ha ganado un juicio?

✔ **Puede cerrar un trato o puede encontrar una salida legal (según sea el caso):** algunos abogados son buenos en conectar todos los aspectos de una transacción. Otros se especializan en confundirlo y perderlo. Cada una de estas habilidades es importante. Los abogados buenos en cerrar los acuerdos, no siempre son igualmente buenos en romperlos y viceversa. Dependiendo de lo que usted necesite, el abogado para salir de un contrato o uno para hacerlo, asegúrese de que tiene el tipo de abogado apropiado para su situación.

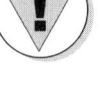

Si su abogado *solamente* piensa que la solución de todos los problemas es entablando un juicio e ir a tribunales, usted está en las garras de un abogado que quiere cobrarle altos honorarios legales. Busque otro abogado.

✔ **Habla su lenguaje:** los buenos abogados le explican sus opciones clara y concisamente sin usar la jerga legal incomprensible, y le dan la *evaluación del riesgo* de sus opciones a fin de ayudarle a tomar una buena decisión. Por ejemplo, el abogado puede decirle que su primer plan de acción llevará más tiempo, pero le ofrecerá un 90 por ciento de probabilidades de éxito; mientras que la opción más rápida le da solamente el 50 por ciento de probabilidades de ganar.

Obtenga el mejor servicio de su abogado

Quién haya dicho que más vale prevenir que curar, debe haber estado pensando en los abogados. Una consulta de dos horas con su abogado es muchísimo mejor que un juicio que dure dos meses, y que podría ocurrir sólo porque usted decidió "ahorrarse dinero" eliminando la consulta legal.

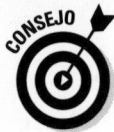

Si no está seguro de que necesitará un abogado, el Capítulo 12 contiene una cláusula que se puede incluir en su contrato para romper un acuerdo comercial que no haya sido aprobado por su abogado. No necesita realmente contratar los servicios de un abogado si usa esta cláusula; ella le da la opción de que el contrato sea revisado más tarde por un abogado de su elección, si usted así lo desea.

Los buenos abogados son estrategas. Si se les da tiempo al principio, pueden estructurar casi cualquier tipo de contrato para que lo beneficie. Al contrario, si usted incorpora a su equipo abogados fantásticos después de cerrar el negocio, lo único que le pueden ofrecer es controlar el daño ya hecho. La mejor defensa es una buena ofensiva.

Esté alerta del "factor de admiración" hacia el profesional legal. Algunas personas sienten admiración por los abogados porque consideran que su palabra es la ley. Ellos piensan que si usted desobedece a un abogado, acaba en la cárcel. Eso es mentira. No siga ciegamente el consejo de su abogado. Si no entiende el consejo, o si no está de acuerdo con él, dígaselo. Es posible que usted tenga razón, y que el abogado esté equivocado. Los abogados pueden equivocarse tanto como cualquier otra persona.

Capítulo 10

¿Cuánto Cuesta?

*U*sted ha recorrido una vivienda que está en venta. El precio es de $249.500. ¿Es esa encantadora casita una ganga o un robo disfrazado?

Si no tiene la menor idea, no se preocupe. Eso es normal. La mayoría de los compradores no conocen el valor de las propiedades cuando comienzan la búsqueda de una vivienda. Para convertirse en un *comprador instruido*, necesita tiempo para familiarizarse con el valor de las propiedades.

Cuando Ray comenzó su carrera inmobiliaria, pasó horas y horas cada semana mirando casas. Igual que muchos agentes novatos, su apetito por propiedades no tenía límites y era indiscriminado: casas grandes, condominios pequeñitos, propiedades viejas, y viviendas nuevas en condiciones inmaculadas, o en necesidad de renovación, en el distrito residencial, en el centro y alrededor del centro. Si tenía techo y un cartel de "En venta", Ray visitaba y revisaba la propiedad por dentro y por fuera.

¿Por qué? Porque la mejor manera de aprender el valor de las propiedades es darle una pasada a tantas viviendas como sea posible, y luego hacerles un seguimiento hasta que se vendan. Así es como los agentes aprenden por sí mismos.

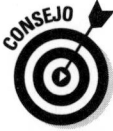

Usted no necesita ver todas las viviendas en la ciudad para aprender. Un buen agente puede acelerar su período de aprendizaje usando una versión del juego escolar de mostrar y describir las propiedades. Tendrá que visitar solamente las viviendas que reúnen los requisitos específicos que usted indicó en su lista de condiciones en cuanto a presupuesto, tamaño y vecindario. Después de ver más de una docena de viviendas semejantes a la vivienda de sus sueños, usted será un comprador instruido.

No se sorprenda si está completamente confundido después que ha pasado un día entero recorriendo propiedades en venta. Cuando ve seis o siete casas una tras otra, es un desafío recordar cuál tenía una cocina maravillosa y cuál el enorme patio con un juego de columpios. Para que la visita de las propiedades sea más productiva, siga los siguientes consejos:

- **Tome notas.** Probablemente recibirá una lista de propiedades (una página de avisos de viviendas en venta o avisos de mercadeo), folletos, o la hoja informativa de los Servicios de listado múltiple, que describen cada una de las propiedades que visita. Para ayudarle a recordar la vivienda, tome notas directamente en su hoja de información mencionando las características distintivas, por ejemplo, la sala a un nivel más bajo, un plano no común del interior de la propiedad, o la ubicación cerca de una parada del tren suburbano.

- **Examine sus notas sobre las propiedades.** Al terminar el día de visitas, comente con su agente las viviendas que vio (si tiene un agente). Si su memoria no es clara respecto a una o dos propiedades que visitó, posiblemente su agente podrá completarle los detalles.

- **Guarde las hojas informativas.** Como verá cuando lea la sección: "Cómo determinar el valor justo de mercado: Análisis comparativo del mercado", más adelante en este capítulo, los precios de venta son importantísimas herramientas de negociación. Pídale a su agente (o al agente del listado, si no tiene un agente) que le informe cuando se venda la casa que usted visitó, y a qué precio se vendió. Anote el precio y la fecha de la venta en su hoja informativa para referencia futura.

Los Tres Componentes Fugaces del Valor

Oscar Wilde dijo que un cínico es alguien que sabe el precio de todo y el valor de nada. En el juego de bienes raíces, *ni el costo ni el precio* son equivalentes al *valor*. Cuando comprenda el significado de estas palabras y sus diferencias, usted podrá reemplazar la emoción por la objetividad cuando mira las propiedades y durante las negociaciones del precio después de finalmente hacer una oferta. En una negociación, aquéllos que presentan hechos, en lugar de argumentos basados en emociones, casi siempre ganan.

El valor es un blanco en movimiento

El *valor* es su opinión personal de lo que vale una vivienda determinada, basado en el uso que usted piensa darle ahora y en el futuro. El valor no está esculpido en piedra, por el contrario, es algo muy difícil de captar.

Por un lado, las opiniones son subjetivas. Nosotros, sus humildes autores, podemos pensar que nos parecemos a Robert Redford y a Paul Newman. Usted, por otro lado, tiene la opinión que nos parecemos a Boris Karloff y a Bela Lugosi —con todo y el disfraz de monstruos. Eso no importa siempre que nos demos cuenta de que hay una gran diferencia entre las opiniones subjetivas y los hechos objetivos.

Además, *factores internos* —cosas relacionadas con su situación personal— tienen una forma astuta de cambiar con el paso del tiempo. Imagine que en la actualidad usted valora mucho una casa con cuatro dormitorios y un gran jardín o patio con cerca atrás. La casa debe estar ubicada en una ciudad con un buen distrito escolar. ¿Por qué estas preferencias? Porque tiene hijos menores.

Dentro de veinte años, cuando los niños hayan crecido y se hayan ido de la casa (¡su deseo!), es posible que decida vender la casa. ¿Por qué? Porque ya no necesita una casa tan grande. Ni la casa ni el distrito escolar han cambiado —lo que cambió fueron los factores internos relacionados con el uso de la propiedad y, así, el valor que tuvo antes para usted.

Los factores externos son aquellos que están fuera de su control y cambian el valor de las propiedades. Si el tiempo que le toma llegar a su trabajo se corta por la mitad, porque después que compró su vivienda el servicio de tren llegó a su vecindario, esto aumenta el valor de la propiedad. Si por el contrario, construyen un basurero al lado de su propiedad, tendrá un gran problema para obtener un buen precio por su casa cuando la venda.

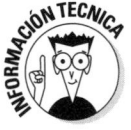

La ley de la oferta y la demanda es otro factor externo que influye en el valor. Si hay más gente que quiere comprar que vender, los compradores deben competir por las propiedades, y el precio subirá. Por el contrario, si hay más gente que quiere vender que comprar, los precios bajan. Vea el Capítulo 4 para una explicación completa de todos los factores que influyen en los precios.

El costo es de ayer

El *costo* mide gastos del pasado —por ejemplo, lo que los vendedores pagaron cuando compraron su vivienda. Lo que los vendedores pagaron originalmente, o cuánto gastaron en renovación de la vivienda después de comprarla, no significa mucho en cuanto al valor presente o futuro de la propiedad. Eso fue entonces, y esto es ahora.

Por ejemplo, cuando los precios de la vivienda subieron drásticamente en muchas partes de ambas costas, en la segunda mitad de la década de los 90 y en los años 2000, algunos compradores acusaron a los vendedores de avaricia. "Usted pagó $400.000 hace siete años. Ahora está pidiendo $850.000", decían ellos. "Si logra que le paguen su precio, tendrá una ganancia escandalosa".

"Así es, ¿no?" Responden los vendedores compasivamente. Si usted no quiere pagar nuestro modesto precio de venta, hágase a un lado, y deje que otros compradores que esperan detrás de usted, puedan presentar su oferta. En un mercado que favorece a los vendedores, la gente que hace una oferta basada en el precio pagado originalmente por la propiedad, hace perder el tiempo de todos.

Sin embargo, el mercado inmobiliario no permanece siempre en la misma dirección. Al principio de los 90, por ejemplo, los precios habían disminuido en muchas zonas. Los vendedores se hubieran sorprendido de encontrar compradores que quisieran pagarles lo que ellos habían pagado hacía cinco años, cuando los precios eran excesivos.

Los compradores sin conocimiento son mentirosos involuntarios

Ray sólo tiene que mirarse en un espejo para ver el prototipo perfecto de un comprador mentiroso y sin el conocimiento necesario. Como todos los compradores, Ray sinceramente creía que le estaba diciendo la verdad al agente cuando él y su dulce esposa, Annie B., comenzaron la búsqueda de una vivienda en la región de los viñedos, 50 millas al norte de San Francisco. Cuando se encontraron por primera vez con su agente, Beverly Mueller, Ray no malgastó ni un momento para establecer las reglas del juego de la búsqueda de la vivienda.

"No necesitamos el Taj Mahal", le dijo Ray a Beverly. "Soy miembro del ejército de bienes raíces, no un ciudadano como sus otros compradores. Créame cuando le digo que $300.000 es categórica y absolutamente la suma máxima que vamos a pagar".

"Lo entiendo, Ray. Solamente miraremos propiedades de un precio máximo de $300.000", le dijo Beverly.

Y realmente, así lo hicieron. Durante los meses siguientes, Beverly les mostró todas las casas en el mercado de Sonoma Valley en su nivel de precios. Ray y Annie rechazaron todas y cada una de las propiedades que vieron. O les gustaba el terreno pero odiaban la vivienda, o viceversa. Ya estaban a punto de abandonar la causa cuando tuvieron suerte.

Ray y Annie encontraron Woodpecker Haven, la vivienda que finalmente compraron en Glen Ellen, gracias a Karen y Herman Isman, amigos suyos que también estaban trabajando con Beverly. Karen and Annie manejaron de San Francisco a Glen Ellen juntas para ver una casa que Beverly pensó que les iba a gustar a los Isman. Fue amor a primera vista.

¿Por qué Beverly no les había mostrado la casa a Ray y a Annie? Porque el precio que pedían era de $390.000 —bastante más de lo que Ray había ordenado. El error de Beverly fue creer lo que le dijo Ray en su primer encuentro.

¿Por qué mintió Ray? No fue intencional. Si él y Annie hubieran encontrado lo que querían por menos de $300.000, Ray habría dicho la verdad. Solamente tres meses después de comenzar la búsqueda de la propiedad era claro que lo que Ray y Annie querían gastar y lo que querían para vivir estaba desconectado de la realidad del mercado.

Muchos compradores chocan con la misma pared tarde o temprano durante su proceso educativo. Ray y Annie se dieron cuenta tarde de que debían hacer algunas concesiones —ya sea reduciendo sus expectativas para ajustarlas a su presupuesto, o ampliando su presupuesto hasta que se satisficieran sus expectativas.

Entonces fue cuando se transformaron en compradores instruidos. Finalmente fueron lo suficientemente realistas para tomar decisiones difíciles.

Lo que le ocurrió a Ray y a Annie, le pasa a la mayoría de las personas. Por ejemplo, usted decide con pesadumbre abandonar o la idea de la piscina o de la sala para la familia, porque no tiene los medios para comprar una vivienda que tenga las dos cosas, si aún desea comprar en el vecindario que le gusta. O, quizás, decide optar por mantener su lista de requisitos, y comprar en un vecindario no tan maravilloso. Hay que ceder en algo cuando no tiene más remedio que enfrentar la realidad.

La otra alternativa es ampliar su poder adquisitivo. Su deseo es tener la seguridad de un préstamo hipotecario a pagar en 30 años con una tasa de interés fija, pero decide obtener una hipoteca con una tasa de interés ajustable (*ARM*) porque le permite cumplir con los requisitos de un préstamo más grande. Aunque de verdad le gustaría comprar sin la ayuda financiera de sus padres, se traga su orgullo y les pide un préstamo. Nuevamente, hay que hacer alguna concesión.

Groucho Marx dijo una vez que nunca pertenecería a ningún club que lo aceptara como miembro. Interpretando las palabras de Groucho, la mayoría de las personas más bien no se conformarían con la vivienda que pueden comprar, si con sólo estirarse financieramente un poco, pueden comprar la propiedad de sus sueños.

El precio es lo que vale hoy día

Los vendedores fijan el *precio de venta* de sus propiedades. Los compradores establecen una oferta o *precio de oferta* en sus contratos. Ambos negocian el precio subiéndolo o bajándolo hasta que establecen el *precio de compra* de la vivienda. El precio de compra de hoy es el costo de mañana. ¿Es el precio de compra un buen valor del mercado? Eso depende.

Es posible que usted consiga una buena ganga si encuentra una vivienda cuyos dueños no saben cuál es el valor de su propiedad, o que deben vender de inmediato debido a un cambio negativo en sus vidas como por ejemplo, divorcio, pérdida de empleo, o la muerte de un familiar. Las personas que no tienen tiempo para sentarse a esperar a compradores que quieran pagar un buen precio, usualmente sufren pérdidas cuando venden. El enemigo del vendedor es el tiempo, mientras que éste es un gran amigo del comprador.

Sin embargo, si usted debe reubicarse rápidamente porque tiene un trabajo nuevo, o para establecerse antes del comienzo del año escolar, tenga cuidado. Es probable que pague demás porque no tiene suficiente tiempo para buscar y hacer un buen negocio.

El costo es cosa del pasado, el precio es el presente, y el valor es algo subjetivo (como la belleza) y depende de quién lo evalúa. Lo que los vendedores pagaron por su vivienda hace años, o lo que desean obtener hoy, no tiene importancia. No derroche su dinero ganado con el sudor de su frente, en una propiedad con un precio excesivo, para satisfacer la fantasía irrealista del vendedor.

Valor Justo de Mercado

Dejando a un lado los desastres naturales, cada vivienda se venderá a un precio justo. Ese precio se define como el *valor justo de mercado* (*FMV,* por sus siglas en inglés) — el precio que un comprador pagará y un vendedor aceptará por la vivienda, cuando ni el vendedor, ni el comprador, están bajo *coerción*. La coerción puede resultar de cambios en la vida, como un problema de salud serio, divorcio, reubicación por trabajo, o repentina pérdida de empleo, los cuales ponen al comprador o al vendedor bajo la presión de concretar rápidamente el negocio. Si los tasadores saben que la venta se hizo bajo coerción, suben o bajan el precio de venta de la vivienda, a fin de que refleje más exactamente el verdadero y justo valor de mercado.

El valor justo de mercado es más poderoso que el *valor* pasado. Como comprador, usted tiene su opinión del valor de la casa. El vendedor tiene igualmente una opinión diferente del valor de su propiedad, que no es necesariamente igual (probablemente, es más alta). Estos valores son opiniones, no hechos, y las opiniones no tienen un valor económico.

A diferencia del valor, el precio justo de mercado es un hecho. Se convierte en un hecho cuando los compradores y vendedores acuerdan un *precio mutuamente aceptable*. Así como se necesitan dos para bailar un tango, es necesario un comprador y un vendedor para que exista un precio justo de mercado. Los hechos sí tienen un valor económico.

Cuando el precio justo del mercado no es justo —es necesario un precio base

Cuando el mercado de bienes raíces se torna débil y flojo, muchos vendedores potenciales sienten que el valor justo de mercado no es nada justo. "¿Por qué no se vende nuestra casa?" se preguntan. "¿Por qué no podemos venderla al precio que pedimos? No es justo."

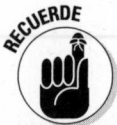

No permita que su sentido altamente desarrollado de lo que es justo, le haga una mala jugada. Los vendedores con frecuencia confunden "justo" con "imparcial." A pesar de su nombre amistoso, el valor justo de mercado no es como un hada madrina cariñosa y adorable. Por el contrario, puede ser descorazonado y cruel. La necesidad no es un componente del valor justo de mercado. Al valor justo de mercado no le importa ninguno de los siguientes elementos:

✔ Lo que necesitan recibir los vendedores porque pagaron un precio excesivo cuando compraron la propiedad.

✔ La cantidad que *necesitan* los vendedores para recobrar el dinero que gastaron renovando su vivienda después de comprarla.

✔ El dinero que *necesitan* los vendedores para pagar por completo sus préstamos.

✔ El dinero que *necesitan* obtener de la venta para comprar su próximo modesto hogar: el palacio Buckingham.

He aquí el porqué el *precio base necesario* del vendedor no es parte del valor justo de mercado. Imagine que hay dos casas idénticas, una al lado de la otra, que están en venta. Una casa fue comprada por $32.000 hace tres décadas. La otra casa se vendió hace un par de años por $320.000, inmediatamente después de que los precios alcanzaron su punto máximo en la zona. El préstamo de la primera vivienda está ya saldado. La otra todavía tiene una gran hipoteca.

"No puede vender" y "no va a vender"

Dos semanas de extraordinarias lluvias torrenciales dañaron la tierra de la subdivisión en la zona de Anaheim Hills, en los Ángeles. Después de que la tierra se empapó, las viviendas en las 25 acres de este desarrollo residencial comenzaron a deslizarse hacia abajo a un promedio de 1 pulgada por día.

Los cimientos y las piscinas se rajaron. Las calles y las veredas sufrieron daños. Las autoridades locales finalmente ordenaron a todos la evacuación de sus hogares, hasta que la tierra se estabilizara.

A diferencia de la mayoría de otros vendedores frustrados que conocemos, estas personas realmente *no podían* vender sus viviendas. Las fuerzas naturales fuera de su control redujeron a cero el valor de sus propiedades. Excepto por algún valor de salvamento que tuvieran, no existe un mercado para estas viviendas que, sin intención de nadie, se volvieron móviles.

Afortunadamente, la mayoría de los propietarios que se quejan de "no poder" vender sus viviendas, no tienen este problema. No son víctimas de desastres cuyos hogares de pronto pierden todo su valor por un acto de Dios. Por el contrario, tienen compradores en abundancia para sus casas, y también montones de entidades crediticias que otorgarían préstamos a esos compradores.

Si no hay nada negativo en sus casas, ¿cuál es entonces el problema? Los propietarios. El problema no es que *no pueden* vender, sino que estos propietarios *no quieren* vender.

Mientras haya propietarios que *eligen* no aceptar lo que los compradores quieren pagar por sus viviendas, ellos no venderán —y esas propiedades permanecerán en el mercado a sus precios excesivos. La profecía entonces se convierte en un hecho. Como comprador potencial de una vivienda, tenga cuidado de estos vendedores irrealistas y codiciosos.

Bill y Mary, dueños de la casa que compraron hace dos años, *necesitan* más dinero que Ed, dueño de la casa comprada hace 30 años. Después de todo, ellos pagaron diez veces más que Ed por su vivienda, y ahora le deben al banco un montón de dinero para pagar el total de su préstamo.

Como las casas son básicamente iguales en tamaño, edad, condición y ubicación, ellas tienen el mismo valor justo de mercado. No es una sorpresa que las dos se vendan por $275.000. Este monto le da a Ed un lindo nido para cuando se jubile, pero es apenas suficiente para saldar el préstamo hipotecario de Mary y Hill. ¿Es esto justo? Ed piensa que sí. Bill y Mary creen que no.

El valor justo de mercado es terriblemente imparcial. Es lo que es —no lo que vendedores o compradores quieren que sea.

La mediana de los precios y el valor justo de mercado

Algunas personas piensan que la mediana de los precios indica el valor justo de mercado, pero no es así.

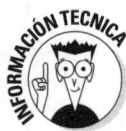

Organizaciones tales como la Asociación Nacional de Agentes de Bienes Raíces, la cámara de comercio, y firmas de investigación privadas, generan información sobre la *mediana de los precios de venta,* mediante la observación de las ventas de viviendas en una región geográfica específica, tal como una ciudad, un condado o un estado. Una función de estas organizaciones es la de reunir los datos de investigación de mercado acerca de la actividad de ventas de viviendas.

No hay nada mágico acerca de la *mediana de los precios de venta*. Sencillamente, es el punto medio en una distribución de todas las ventas de viviendas ocurridas durante un período determinado. La mitad de las ventas ocurridas durante el período de recolección de datos están arriba de la mediana, y la otra mitad, debajo de la misma. La mediana del precio de una vivienda, en otras palabras, es la que está exactamente en el medio de los precios de todas las propiedades vendidas.

Cuando este libro fue a la imprenta, la mediana de los precios de la vivienda en los Estados Unidos era de $220.000, lo cual nos dice que la mitad de las viviendas vendidas en el país se vendieron por más de $220.000, y la otra mitad por menos de esa cantidad. Desgraciadamente, lo único que se sabe sobre esta propiedad hipotética que se corresponde con la mediana de los precios, es su precio.

No se sabe cuántos dormitorios o baños tiene esta vivienda. Tampoco se sabe de cuántos pies cuadrados de espacio para vivir dispone, ni la edad de la propiedad, ni si tiene un garaje o un patio en el fondo. Ni siquiera se sabe la ubicación de esta vivienda que se corresponde con la mediana, excepto que está en algún lugar de los Estados Unidos.

Si la información sobre la mediana de los precios es tan vaga, ¿para qué sirve? Porque le dice dos cosas importantes:

- **La tendencia de los precios:** si la mediana de los precios de una vivienda en los Estados Unidos era de $140.000 hace cinco años, y es ahora de $220.000, usted sabe que, en general, los precios de las viviendas han aumentado. No se sabe por qué la mediana de los precios ha subido, sólo se sabe que ha ocurrido.

- **Relatividad del precio:** si la mediana de los precios de la vivienda en Yakima, Wahington, se vende por $185.000, mientras la mediana de una vivienda en Honolulu es de $550.000, usted sabe que su dólar le rendirá mucho más en Yakima. Honolulu tiene muchas características excelentes, pero la vivienda barata no es una de ellas.

Las estadísticas de la mediana de los precios de la vivienda son una información interesante, pero no son más exactas para determinar los valores específicos de una vivienda, que las estadísticas de la mediana de los ingresos para pronosticar cuánto va a ganar usted en su próximo empleo. Se necesita información mucho más precisa sobre el valor de la propiedad, antes de que invierta una porción grande de los ahorros de toda su vida en ella.

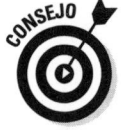

El Capítulo 3 puede ayudarle a determinar cuánto puede invertir en la compra de una vivienda. En el Capítulo 11 puede encontrar la dirección de algunos sitios de la Web, en los que puede localizar zonas con precios módicos al comparar la mediana de los precios de la vivienda, ciudad por ciudad, y vecindario por vecindario. Cuando la mediana de los precios indique que los mismos están subiendo o bajando bruscamente, investigue las razones leyendo y hablando con miembros de su equipo de bienes raíces, tal como su agente.

Cómo Determinar el Valor Justo de Mercado: Análisis Comparativo del Mercado

Créalo o no, las casas son como las manzanas rojas deliciosas. La mayoría de las casas son verdes y necesitan más tiempo en el árbol de bienes raíces antes de que estén listas para ser escogidas. Sólo unas pocas están maduras para ser escogidas ahora mismo. El truco es saber cuál es cuál, porque las casas no se vuelven rojas cuando maduran.

Ésa es una razón por la que usted debe entender el valor justo de mercado, y saber el precio inicial y los precios de ventas de casas similares a la que quiere comprar. Los compradores de vivienda instruidos saben cuáles casas están verdes y cuáles maduras.

Lo fundamental de un análisis comparativo del mercado

La mejor manera de determinar con exactitud el valor justo de mercado de una vivienda, es preparar un *análisis comparativo del mercado* (*CMA,* por sus siglas en inglés). Un agente inmobiliario competente puede y debe preparar un *CMA* para la propiedad que le interesa a usted, antes de hacer su oferta de compra. Todas las oficinas de bienes raíces residenciales tienen su propio formato de *CMA*. De cualquier manera que se le presente la información, las Tablas 10-1 y 10-2 le muestran lo que un buen *CMA* contiene.

Tabla 10-1   Muestra de un Análisis Comparativo de Mercado — Sección de "Ventas Recientes"

Dirección	Fecha de Venta	Precio de Venta	Dormit/ Baño	Estaciona- miento	Condición	Comentarios
210 Oak	30/04/06	$390.000	3/3	2 autos	Muy buena	Mejor comp. Aprox. mismo tamaño que la casa de sus sueños; lote un poco más pequeño. 1867 pies cuadra-dos, $209/pie cuadrado
335 Elm	14/02/06	$368.500	3/2	2 autos	Es justo	Calle con mucho tráfico, baños viejos. 1.805 pies cuadrados, $204/pie cuadrado

Dirección	Fecha de Venta	Precio de Venta	Dormit/ Baño	Estaciona- miento	Condición	Comentarios
307 Ash	15/03/06	$385.000	3/3	2 autos	Buena	Más grande que casa soñada, buen comp. 1.850 pies cuadrados, $208/pie cuadrado
555 Ash	12/01/06	$382.500	3/2.5	+2 autos	Excelente	Más pequeña que casa soñada. 1.740 pies cuadrados, $220/pie cuadrado
75 Birch	20/04/06	$393.000	3/3	3 autos	Muy buena	Más grande que casa soñada, ubicación no muy buena, hermoso diseño de jardín. 1.910 pies cuadrados, $206/pie cuadrado

Éstos son los hechos. La sección de "Ventas recientes" del *CMA* ayuda a establecer el valor justo de mercado de 220 Oak —su *vivienda soñada* que está en el mercado ahora— comparándola con *todas* las otras propiedades que:

↙ Están ubicadas en el mismo vecindario

↙ Tienen aproximadamente la misma edad, tamaño y condición

↙ Se han vendido en los seis meses previos

Estas casas son llamadas *comps,* que es la abreviatura de *comparables*. Depende de cuándo comenzó la búsqueda de su vivienda, probablemente no ha visitado todas las propiedades similares que se vendieron. No importa. Un buen agente inmobiliario puede mostrarle la documentación del listado sobre las viviendas que no ha visto, llevarlo por un recorrido verbal de las propiedades, y explicarle cómo cada una se compara con la vivienda de sus sueños.

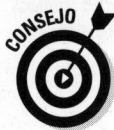

Una buena comunicación con su agente acerca del significado de términos subjetivos como *grande, con mucha luz, cerca de la escuela,* y otras, es extremadamente importante. Debe comprender con exactitud lo que el agente quiere decir cuando usa tales términos. Y al contrario, su agente tiene que comprender exactamente lo que usted quiere, lo que necesita y lo que puede pagar.

Si usted y su agente van a analizar la venta de viviendas similares del ejemplo, encontrarán que las viviendas comparables a la que desea comprar — 220 Oak, en la Tabla 10-2 — se están vendiendo por un poco más de $200 por pie cuadrado. Al expresar los precios de venta en la forma de costo por pie cuadrado, la comparación se hace mucho más fácil. Como puede ver en la Tabla 10-2, cualquiera que está muy por arriba o muy por debajo de la norma, le salta a la vista.

Tabla 10-2	Muestra de un Análisis Comparativo de Mercado — Sección "En Venta Actualmente"					
Dirección	*Fecha en que Fue Listada*	*Precio Inicial*	*Dormit/ Baño*	*Estaciona- miento*	*Condición*	*Comentarios*
220 Oak (ésta es la vivienda soñada)	25/04/06	$395.000	3/3	2 autos	Muy buena	Ubicación más tranquila que 123 Oak, detalles buenos, cocina vieja. 1.880 pies cuadrados, $210/pie cuadrado
123 Oak	01/05/06	$399.500	3/2	2 autos	Excelente	De lujo, reno- vada & precio apropiado, hecho, hecho, hecho. 1.855 pies cuadra- dos, $215/pie cuadrado
360 Oak	10/02/06	$375.000	3/2	1 auto	Es justo	Cocina & baño necesitan renov. no chimenea. 1.695 pies cuadrados, $221/pie cuadrado

Dirección	Fecha en que Fue Listada	Precio Inicial	Dormit/ Baño	Estaciona- miento	Condición	Comentarios
140 Elm	01/04/06	$379.500	3/3	2 autos	Buena	Calle mucho tráfico, cuartos y jardín pequeños. 1.725 pies cuadrados, $220/pie cuadrado
505 Elm	31/10/06	$425.000	2/2	1 auto	Es justo	Ilusiones de grandeza, precio muy excesivo. 1.580 pies cuadrados, $269/pie cuadrado
104 Ash	17/04/06	$389.500	3/2.5	2 autos	Muy buena	¡Gran comp! Buen plano, cuartos grandes, sorpresa, no se vendió. 1.860 pies cuadrados, $209/pie cuadrado
222 Ash	01/02/06	$419.500	3/2	1 auto	Es justo	Muy buena. Comp. a 505 Elm, no se venderá este a este precio. 1.610 pies cuadrados, $261/pie cuadrado

(continúa)

Tabla 10-2 *(continuación)*

Dirección	Fecha en que Fue Listada	Precio Inicial	Dormit/ Baño	Estaciona- miento	Condición	Comentarios
47 Birch	15/03/06	$409.000	4/3.5	2 autos	Buena	Linda casa, demasiada renovac. para el vecindario. 2.005 pies cuadrados, $204/pie cuadrado
111 Birch	25/04/06	$389.500	3/3	2 autos	Muy buena	Cocina hermosa, no chimenea. 1.870 pies cuadrados, $208/pie cuadrado

La sección "En venta actualmente" del *CMA* compara la casa de sus sueños (en este caso, 220 Oak) con las similares del vecindario que están *actualmente en venta*. Estas propiedades similares están incluidas en el análisis a fin de monitorear las tendencias de los precios:

✔ **Si los precios están bajando:** el valor inicial de las viviendas en el mercado hoy día será más bajo que los precios de venta de propiedades comparables.

✔ **Si los precios están subiendo:** verá precios iniciales más altos en la actualidad que los de propiedades similares vendidas hace tres o seis meses.

Si ha estado por algún tiempo mirando viviendas en una zona específica, probablemente ya ha visitado todas las comparables que están ahora en el mercado de esa zona. No necesita que nadie le diga lo que ha visto con sus propios ojos. Sin embargo, usted necesita la ayuda de un agente para poder comparar las viviendas similares que ha visto con las que no ha logrado ver, porque algunas de ellas se vendieron antes de que usted comenzara la búsqueda de su vivienda.

Como muestra la Tabla 10-2, la casa de sus sueños parece tener un precio muy cerca del valor justo de mercado basado en el precio de venta actual de la casa en 210 Oak (en la Tabla 10-1). Dado que la propiedad en 220 Oak tiene

1.880 pies cuadrados, a $209 por pie cuadrado, su precio es de $392.920. Basado en los hechos, es fácil establecer el valor de una propiedad una vez que sabe cómo hacerlo.

Su *CMA* debe ser completo. Debe incluir *todas* las ventas de viviendas similares en los seis meses previos, y *todas* las que están actualmente en el mercado. Es más difícil obtener una idea exacta del valor justo de mercado si faltan partes del rompecabezas, especialmente, en un vecindario donde las viviendas no están en venta con frecuencia.

Como la leche en su refrigeradora, las propiedades similares tienen una fecha de vencimiento. Las entidades crediticias no van a aceptar viviendas que se vendieron hace más de seis meses como comparación. Sus precios de venta no reflejan la confianza actual del consumidor, las condiciones de los negocios, o las tasas de interés hipotecarias. Como regla general, cuanto más viejas sean las casas similares, más probable es que no representen el valor justo del mercado actual.

Generalmente se acepta que seis meses es un período suficientemente largo para obtener una muestra representativa de la venta de las propiedades similares, pero es demasiado corto para mantener condiciones del mercado consistentes. El valor no está esculpido en piedra. Si una calamidad de proporciones gigantescas ocurrió hace tres meses, por ejemplo, seis meses es demasiado tiempo para una comparación válida. Por el contrario, si las viviendas en cierta zona raramente se venden, necesita examinar las ventas comparables que ocurrieron hace más de seis meses.

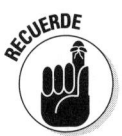

Los precios de venta siempre tienen más peso que los precios iniciales cuando se trata de determinar el valor justo del mercado. Los vendedores pueden pedir el precio que quieran por sus propiedades, pero estos precios, a veces, son una fantasía. Los precios de venta siempre son hechos —indican el valor justo de mercado. La mejor prueba de lo que vale una casa es su precio de venta. No trate de adivinar. Analice la venta de propiedades similares. Asegúrese de que incluye la información sobre los factores por los que se redujo el precio, o grandes créditos que se dieron para ejecutar trabajos de reparación (por ejemplo, $5.000 de crédito de los vendedores a los compradores para reemplazar una caldera).

Los defectos de los análisis comparativos del mercado

Los *CMA* son mucho mejores que las estadísticas de la mediana de los precios para establecer los valores equitativos de mercado, pero no son perfectos. Hemos visto gente que usa exactamente las mismas comparaciones y llegan a opiniones muy diferentes del valor justo de mercado. Las discrepancias surgen del mismo proceso del *CMA* si se comparan ciegamente las propiedades similares sin conocer los siguientes detalles de tales propiedades:

- **Desgaste por el uso:** no hay dos viviendas iguales después que han sido habitadas. Imagine que hay dos viviendas idénticas ubicadas una al lado de la otra. Una, cuyos dueños son una pareja mayor sin niños ni animales domésticos, está en condición perfecta. La otra, cuyos dueños son una familia con varios niños pequeños y varios perros grandes, parece una zona de desastre federal. Su idea es tan buena como la nuestra cuando se trata de determinar cuánto dinero se necesitará para hacer las reparaciones en la segunda casa debidas al daño causado por el uso, y el abuso. Un buen análisis comparativo hace el ajuste por la diferencia entre estas dos casas.

- **Diferencias de lugar dentro de un mismo vecindario:** aun cuando todas las propiedades similares están en el mismo vecindario, no están ubicadas precisamente en el mismo terreno. ¿Cuánto vale estar ubicados cerca del parque bonito? ¿Cuánto pagará usted por estar siete minutos más cerca de la parada del tren suburbano? Estos ajustes de valor son un poquito menos precisos que una operación del cerebro.

- **Propiedades similares fuera del vecindario:** imagine que en los últimos seis meses, no se vendieron propiedades en el vecindario de su elección. Al ir a otro vecindario para encontrar viviendas comparables, usted y su agente deben hacer ajustes de valor entre las conveniencias de los dos vecindarios (escuelas, centros comerciales, transporte y otros). La comparación entre vecindarios diferentes es mucho más difícil de hacer que los ajustes de valor dentro del mismo vecindario.

- **Ventas de viviendas no similares:** ¿Qué hacer si se vendieron cinco propiedades en el vecindario en los seis meses previos, pero ninguna de ellas era ni remotamente comparable en edad, tamaño, estilo, o condición a la vivienda que usted quiere comprar? Usted y su agente deben estimar el valor de las diferencias entre propiedades con tres dormitorios respecto a otras de cuatro, de unas con cocinas viejas con otras cuyas cocinas son nuevas, y deben hacer lo mismo con respecto a jardines pequeños o grandes, con garajes en lugar de cocheras abiertas, etc. Si la vivienda que quiere tiene una vista panorámica, y ninguna de las otras casas tiene una vista deseable, ¿cuánto aumenta el valor de la casa la vista que quiere? Cálculos como éstos no ponen a los astronautas en la luna.

Estas variables no son obstáculos infranqueables para establecer el valor justo de mercado de la casa de sus sueños. Sin embargo, aumentan enormemente el margen de error cuando se trata de determinar el monto de una oferta realista. Puede minimizar los problemas de determinación de precios creados por estas variables, si usted o su agente recorren personalmente las viviendas similares por dentro y por fuera.

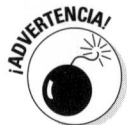

Es imposible lograr una comparación válida de la casa de sus sueños con las otras viviendas, si usted y su agente solamente han leído información acerca de las casas comparables en las descripciones de los listados, o simplemente las han visto en un sitio de la Web. He aquí el porqué:

- ✔ **La mayoría de las descripciones de los listados son exageradas en mayor o menor grado.** No sabe el grado de exageración de las descripciones si no ha visto la propiedad personalmente. Puede considerar el "gran" dormitorio principal como pequeñísimo. La única distinción de esa cocina "gourmet" puede ser solo una rejilla para asar. La vista increíble desde la sala puede existir solamente si usted es tan alto como Michael Jordan. Por supuesto, no va a saber ninguna de estas cosas si sólo leyó sus hojas de propaganda, en lugar de recorrerlas en persona.

- ✔ **Los planos de una vivienda influencian mucho su valor.** Dos casas, por ejemplo, pueden tener el mismo tamaño, edad y condición, y sin embargo, su valor puede ser totalmente diferente. Por ejemplo, el plano de una casa fluye suavemente de una habitación a otra, las habitaciones son de buen tamaño, con techos altos. Por el contrario, la otra casa no ofrece el mismo ambiente porque su plano no puede recorrerse de la misma manera y los techos son bajos. No es posible saber la diferencia leyendo las descripciones de las dos en el listado.

- ✔ **Quienquiera que controle la cámara, controla lo que usted ve.** Cuando mire esas fotos o videos de una casa publicados en un sitio de la Web, recuerde que se le permite ver solamente lo que la persona que tomó las fotos o filmó el video quiere que vea. Ciertamente no podrá darle una mirada a las cosas menos atractivas, como las partes desgastadas de la alfombra de la sala, o el graffiti pintado en la puerta del garaje en la casa de al lado.

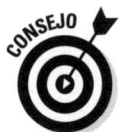

Mire con sus ojos bien abiertos. Mire de arriba para abajo. *Abra los ojos* — recorra personalmente las propiedades y note los detalles importantes adentro y afuera, con sus propios ojos, y decida cuáles viviendas se comparan realmente a la casa de sus sueños.

Obtenga una Segunda Opinión: Tasación y CMA

Si no tiene mucha prisa en presentar su oferta, y usted es una persona poco confiada, puede obtener una segunda opinión acerca del valor de la vivienda al que usted y su agente llegaron, antes de hacer una oferta por la casa de sus sueños. Puede pagar unos cuantos cientos de dólares para que un profesional haga la tasación de la propiedad.

Buscar una segunda opinión *objetiva,* siempre tiene un efecto tranquilizador. Un tasador no le dirá lo que usted quiere oír sólo para hacer una venta. El tasador no trata de venderle nada. Ya sea que compre o no la propiedad, el tasador recibe sus honorarios.

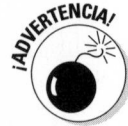

Desgraciadamente, el hecho de que el tasador cobre por su trabajo sin importar que usted compre la vivienda, beneficia a ambas partes. Imagine que usted y los vendedores no puedan llegar a un acuerdo en cuanto al precio y a los términos de la venta porque los vendedores creen ingenuamente en su precio. Aun si su oferta es rechazada, recibirá la factura del tasador. El pagar por las tasaciones o por los inspectores de propiedad antes de hacer la oferta, generalmente es considerado una buena inversión.

Si cree que la tasación de un profesional es ampliamente superior a la opinión de valor de su agente, piénselo de nuevo. El análisis comparativo de mercado (CMA) de su agente es usualmente tan meritorio como una tasación. Por el contrario, si la tasación de un profesional es muy superior porque su agente no es muy buen analista de los valores de la propiedad, debería buscar a un mejor agente.

En cualquier región geográfica, los tasadores generalmente no miran en persona tantas viviendas como los agentes que se concentran en esa zona. Los tasadores no son holgazanes, es simplemente que ellos usan su tiempo de otra manera.

Las tasaciones formales llevan mucho tiempo. Un tasador inspecciona la propiedad desde los cimientos hasta el ático, mide cuántos pies cuadrados tiene, toma notas detalladas sobre la calidad de la construcción y la cantidad de desgaste natural, saca fotografías interiores y exteriores de la vivienda, toma fotos de viviendas similares a la que está tasando, escribe su tasación, y otras cosas. Los agentes pueden visitar de 15 a 20 viviendas en el tiempo que le lleva a un tasador completar una evaluación.

Como la visita a las propiedades lleva tanto tiempo, los buenos agentes están ya haciendo el trabajo de campo, y como usualmente es imposible visitar una vivienda después de que se completa la venta, los tasadores, con frecuencia, llaman a los agentes para obtener información sobre las propiedades que ellos incluyen en sus listados, o sobre las vendidas que pueden compararse. Aunque la descripción de la vivienda de un buen agente es buena, nada es mejor que recorrer personalmente la propiedad. La exactitud de cualquier tasación disminuye algo cada vez que la tasación está basada en otras casas similares que el tasador no ha visto.

También, los agentes se llaman mutuamente para obtener información de casas que ellos no han visto, por eso, no piense que los tasadores son los únicos que llaman pidiendo información. Sin embargo, recuerde que usted está confiando en el conocimiento de su agente para ayudarle a determinar el valor de una propiedad. Si su agente no ha visto la mayoría de las viviendas similares usadas en su CMA, busque a un agente que conozca el mercado.

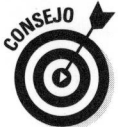

Excepto en casos en que usted esté totalmente inseguro del valor de una propiedad y desea gastar dinero aunque se haga o no el negocio, no gaste dinero en una tasación antes del contrato.

Por Qué Vendedores y Compradores Suelen Comenzar desde Posiciones Tan Distanciadas

El comprador promedio puede ser mas listo que el vendedor promedio. ¿De qué otra manera puede explicar el hecho de que los compradores son generalmente mucho más realistas acerca de los precios de la propiedad?

No es porque haya dos mercados de bienes raíces diferentes, uno más caro para los vendedores y otro más barato para los compradores. Los vendedores tienen acceso a exactamente las mismas viviendas similares que los compradores. Sin embargo, los precios de oferta de los compradores son mucho más realistas que los precios iniciales establecidos por los vendedores ¿Por qué? La Figura 10-1 le ofrece algunas ideas para responder a esa pregunta.

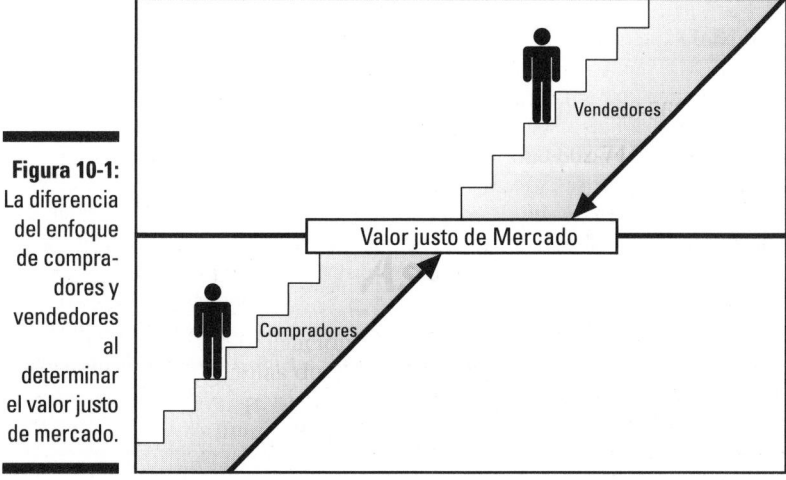

Figura 10-1: La diferencia del enfoque de compradores y vendedores al determinar el valor justo de mercado.

Algunas personas creen que el egoísmo de los compradores y de los vendedores los lleva a juzgar el valor justo de mercado desde posiciones opuestas. Los compradores hacen su oferta basados en el valor justo de mercado porque no quieren pagar más que eso. Los vendedores ajustan sus precios al valor justo de mercado porque odian la idea de perder cualquier dinero en la transacción.

Guerras de ofertas

Cuando los vendedores de una vivienda eligen a un agente, el proceso de la entrevista puede fracasar. Las guerras de ofertas con frecuencia se desarrollan entre los agentes que compiten para listar la propiedad en venta. El concepto del valor justo de mercado es la primera víctima de la guerra. Si usted trata de comprar dicha vivienda, puede convertirse en la segunda víctima. Esto es lo que pasa cuando los vendedores entrevistan a los agentes:

"Gracias por darme la oportunidad de listar su linda vivienda, Sr. y Sra. Vendedor," dice el primer agente. "Como puede ver al leer el CMA, mi análisis del valor justo de mercado indica que se vendieron ocho casas en su vecindario en los seis meses anteriores. Tres de ellas eran significativamente más grandes que la suya, y por eso no se pueden comparar con la suya. Las otras cinco casas comparables a la suya en tamaño, edad, ubicación y condición se vendieron entre $350.000 y $370.000. Basados en esos precios de ventas, le recomiendo que establezca un precio inicial de $375.000.

Ahora el segundo agente ataca. ¿A quién le importan los precios de las propiedades similares? Su casa está pintada de un tono atractivo de color turquesa, y su césped es más verde que los de cualquiera de las otras viviendas. Le sugiero comenzar con un buen precio inicial de $400.000.

El tercer agente sabe que probablemente no va a ganar el derecho a listar la casa, salvo que ofrezca más que los otros dos agentes. "El programa de mercadeo de Internet de nuestra firma tiene un éxito increíble", dice él, irradiando confianza. "A través de nuestro servicio de reubicación y referencias por Internet, sin duda seremos capaces de encontrar a un comprador que esté dispuesto a pagar $425.000".

Esta técnica de los sucesivos agentes valuando a más alto precio la propiedad es conocida como *la compra de un listado*. Los vendedores, al enfrentarse con la selección de la realidad del mercado en oposición a la fantasía, a menudo se rinden a la fantasía. Racionalizan su decisión diciéndose a sí mismos que el agente que valuó la propiedad con el precio más alto, es el que tiene más fe en su vivienda.

Esas son tonterías. Si los vendedores eligen al agente que hizo la valuación más alta, es porque ese agente los sedujo con los extras $50.000 que recibirían seleccionándolo a él para que venda su casa. Él les dijo lo que querían oír. La avaricia venció a la razón.

¿Entonces, quién gana la guerra de las ofertas? No los dueños de la propiedad. Si el precio que piden no tiene fundamento en el mundo real, usted no comprará. Tampoco lo hará ningún otro comprador instruido.

¿Como puede usted evitar convertirse en víctima de una guerra de ofertas? Bien, ya sabe lo que vamos a decir. Confíe en que las propiedades similares le dirán cuál es el valor de la vivienda. Si los vendedores no escuchan la voz de la razón, continúe con su búsqueda. Las comparaciones de viviendas similares no son fantasía. Usted tampoco debería fantasear.

Esto es lógico, pero simplista. Este razonamiento no explica por qué muchos vendedores tienden inicialmente a ser mucho más irrealistas que los compradores.

Cuanto mejor comprenda los procesos distorsionados del pensamiento de estos vendedores, mejor podrá manejar las objeciones irracionales a su perfectamente justa oferta. A tal fin, aquí les presentamos las causas comunes de precios iniciales absurdamente excesivos.

Agentes incompetentes

Sólo porque *usted* usó la información del Capítulo 9 para seleccionar a un agente fantástico, no quiere decir que todos lo harán. De hecho, mucha gente hace un trabajo horrible cuando elige a un agente.

Quizás el agente de los vendedores es un tonto incompetente que no sabe nada de los precios de la propiedad. Esos pobres vendedores desorientados no pusieron un precio realista a su vivienda porque sus agentes le dieron un consejo pésimo.

Cuando su agente descubra que el otro agente es incompetente —ya sea por la selección equivocada de las propiedades similares que el agente usó para establecer el precio inicial, o por su reputación (estas noticias viajan rápido dentro de la comunidad del corretaje inmobiliario)— ¿qué puede hacer usted? Eso depende.

Si la casa ha estado en el mercado por un mes o dos, y los vendedores están abiertos a razonar, las comparaciones de su brillante agente van a prevalecer sobre los precios de fantasía del otro agente. Los vendedores van a entender el concepto del valor justo de mercado, y aceptan agradecidamente su oferta, o hacen una modesta contraoferta, porque lo que usted ofrece es lógico, realista y justo.

Sin embargo, si la vivienda recién salió al mercado, usted tiene un problema. Probablemente los vendedores no van a creer nada de lo que usted y su agente les digan acerca del precio inicial. Obviarán su opinión del valor justo de mercado de su propiedad porque sospechan que está tratando de robarles su casa. También tendrán sospechas de una tasación formal hecha por un tasador que usted eligió.

El tiempo cura los precios excesivos de los agentes incompetentes. Cuanto más tiempo la vivienda permanece en el mercado sin venderse, más van a dudar los vendedores de su opinión del valor, y de la de su agente.

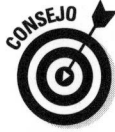

Si la vivienda de los vendedores tiene un precio que impide su venta, y los dueños no escuchan razones, abandone esa propiedad y vaya a la siguiente en su lista. Quién sabe cuanto tiempo les llevará a los vendedores entrar en razón. No ponga su vida en suspenso esperando que ellos cambien. Quizás ellos aprenden muy lentamente.

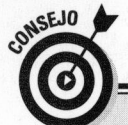
CONSEJO

Descubra que no es oro todo lo que brilla

Muchos agentes les muestran a los compradores casas con precios exagerados, pero su intención no es vendérselas. Una de las tácticas que los buenos agentes adoptan al principio de sus carreras es usar propiedades con precios muy altos para demostrar el valor de propiedades con precios verdaderamente justos.

Imagine que un agente le muestra una vivienda de tres dormitorios y dos baños a un precio de $299.500, y lo lleva luego a otra aún más atractiva de cuatro dormitorios y tres baños en el mismo vecindario y *con el mismo precio inicial*. El agente no necesita decir otra palabra —la diferencia entre el precio y el valor es claramente obvia. La vivienda más grande se vendió.

Otra manera de descubrir las propiedades con precios exagerados: éstas son muy visitadas, pero no atraen ofertas.

Vendedores irrealistas

Algunos vendedores reciben consejos excelentes acerca de precios de sus agentes —y deciden no prestarles atención. Los vendedores que intentan vender sin un agente, a menudo cometen el mismo error —optan por el método siempre popular de basar el precio en su necesidad personal (descrito anteriormente en este capítulo) para fijar el precio de venta.

Los vendedores necesitan tiempo para aceptar que los compradores no están interesados en saber cuánto pagaron por su propiedad, ni cuánto gastaron en renovación, ni cuánto dinero necesitan para comprar su próxima vivienda. Los vendedores deben resolver sus problemas. El comprador no es responsable de nada de esto.

A menos que una propiedad con un precio exagerado haya estado en el mercado por mucho tiempo, y esto haya hecho cambiar la posición de los dueños, déjela y vaya a otra de su lista. La mayoría de los vendedores no tienen la mente abierta a escuchar razones antes que hayan probado con su precio inicial por al menos un par de meses, o hasta encontrarse bajo presión para vender. Tratar de razonar con ese tipo de vendedores prematuramente es como tratar de enseñar a un cerdo a silbar. Es un mal uso de su tiempo, y el cerdo va a reaccionar negativamente.

Capítulo 11

Cómo Usar los Mejores Recursos del Internet

· ·

En Este Capítulo

▶ Obtención de información útil

▶ Investigación preliminar para comprar

▶ Prudencia al examinar información

· ·

No hay otra transacción monetaria que provoque más ansiedad financiera y emocional que comprar una casa. La mayoría de nosotros sentimos un gran miedo cuando tenemos que comprar algo que cuesta más de seis cifras. Hay que enfrentarse a decisiones como: cuánto gastar, con qué agente de bienes raíces tratar, la negociación de la propiedad, qué hipoteca escoger y los miles de detalles del cierre —los cuales son misteriosos, llenos de términos de la jerga de la industria y atestados de agentes de ventas, hambrientos por cobrar sus comisiones. (Lo mismo sucederá, y los dolores de cabeza también, a la hora de vender.) A eso, agréguele una fecha límite para mudarse a otra ciudad por cuestiones del trabajo o el nacimiento inminente de un bebé (o de dos) y tiene la receta segura para el estrés psicológico.

Aquí entra el Internet. En este capítulo, enfatizamos cómo puede usar el Internet para ser un consumidor con más conocimientos y que su búsqueda sea más eficaz. Le damos nombres de sitios o páginas Web y le recomendamos los mejores que hemos encontrado y, también, le avisamos sobre los obstáculos comunes que pueden presentarse cuando esté en línea.

Cómo Obtener Información Útil

El número de sitios de bienes raíces en la red excede a la cantidad de sitios dignos de ser marcados como favoritos. En esta sección le damos consejos para que pueda ir rápidamente a la dirección correcta al comienzo de su búsqueda.

Evite los buscadores tradicionales

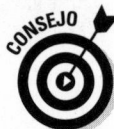

No pierda su tiempo usando buscadores tradicionales —un método en el que usted explora (busca por) el Internet tratando de encontrar sitios Web que contienen información que coincide con palabras o frases claves que usted escribe en la ventanilla del buscador. En un buscador popular, por ejemplo, escribimos "Santa Rosa California bienes raíces" en la ventanilla y, ¡los resultados aparecieron con más de 2 millones de sitios Web!

Los dueños de los sitios Web hacen todo lo que pueden para conseguir que sus sitios Web aparezcan entre los primeros de los resultados en una búsqueda específica. Digamos simplemente que no necesariamente encontrará los mejores sitios o las mejores compañías entre los primeros de la lista de una búsqueda en la red. A menos que esté buscando un sitio específico —como por ejemplo, el sitio de las escuelas públicas de Santa Rosa— le aconsejamos que no se moleste usando estos buscadores.

Empiece por sondear el tema en el sitio "Realtor.com"

Dada la inmensa cantidad de sitios para escoger, el mejor lugar para empezar a navegar la red en busca de propiedades es un sitio completo que incluya tanto recursos útiles de inmuebles residenciales como muchas listas de casas en ventas.

Nuestro sitio preferido para los mejores inmuebles residenciales en la red es `www.realtor.com`, patrocinado por la asociación nacional de agentes inmobiliarios (*National Association of Realtors* [*NAR,* por sus siglas en inglés]). En ediciones previas de este libro, este sitio no era digno de tanto halago, pero ahora sí lo es —gracias a los mejoramientos que le han hecho.

El sitio *Realtor.com* tiene más de 2 millones de listas de casas en venta de cientos de servicios de listados múltiples (*MLS,* por sus siglas en inglés) a través de todo el país. La mayoría de los listados están bastante detallados y normalmente incluyen mapas para que usted pueda ver aproximadamente dónde está ubicada la propiedad. Muchos listados también incluyen varias fotos y otros incluyen un "tour virtual". Claro, como es el sitio oficial de la *NAR,* no espere ver listados de propiedades marcadas "Venta directa por el propietario". Obviamente, el objetivo de este sitio es proporcionar recursos a compradores potenciales de casas (y a vendedores) con la esperanza de ponerlos en contacto con un agente de bienes raíces. Sin embargo, usted puede navegar este sitio de la manera que guste, sin proporcionar detalles personales o comprometerse con un agente.

El sitio también tiene recursos útiles para una búsqueda dentro de un poblado o vecindario específico porque puede obtener información de una comunidad como: estadísticas demográficas, información sobre las escuelas públicas, estadísticas de delincuencia y, también, le ayuda a comenzar el proceso de búsqueda de una entidad hipotecaria.

Nuestra queja mayor de este sitio Web es la inmensa cantidad de anuncios publicitarios que tiene. Sin embargo, lo bueno es que usted puede explorar los extensos recursos de este sitio sin tener que comprometerse a comprar nada ni a trabajar con ningún promotor de servicios.

Lea noticias excelentes sobre inmuebles

Generalmente, tiene que tener cuidado al navegar por la red y, en especial, al buscar información sobre bienes raíces que sea útil, objetiva y de buena calidad. A continuación le damos un par de sitios que recomendamos para que se mantenga al tanto con los últimos acontecimientos en bienes raíces y, al mismo tiempo, ir aumentando su conocimiento sobre bienes raíces:

✔ **DeadlineNews.com** (`www.deadlinenews.com`): el excelente escritor sobre temas de bienes raíces Broderick Perkins, quien escribió para el periódico "The San Jose Mercury News" por 16 años, maneja este sitio. Además de artículos sobre temas de bienes raíces regionales y nacionales, *DeadlineNews.com* incluye cobertura extensa de los mercados a veces locos y siempre fascinantes del estado de California.

✔ **InmanNews.com** (`www.inman.com`): aunque este sitio tiene algunos artículos de interés para personas involucradas en bienes raíces, la mayor parte de su contenido atrae a personas activamente involucradas en otras áreas de bienes raíces. Sin embargo, usted encontrará aquí numerosos columnistas sobre bienes raíces, entre ellos el experto columnista nacional Robert Bruss.

Descubra más información en estos sitios

Otras excelentes organizaciones en bienes raíces y gubernamentales, nos ofrecen información útil por medio de sus sitios Web. Entonces, ¿cómo puede saber dónde y qué buscar? ¡Nosotros se lo diremos! Aquí tiene nuestras opciones predilectas:

✔ **La Agencia Federal para el Manejo de Emergencias** (`www.fema.gov`) (*Federal Emergency Management Agency* [*FEMA,* por sus siglas en inglés]): este sitio le puede ayudar a ver dónde probablemente ocurran los distintos desastres naturales (como terremotos, tornados e inundaciones), y, además, le proporciona recursos educacionales útiles sobre temas como el seguro de riesgo de inundaciones y el de preparación y prevención de desastres. Este sitio también le proporciona otros recursos útiles en caso de que usted o sus seres queridos necesiten ayuda algún día.

✔ **La Sociedad Americana de Inspectores de Viviendas** (www.ashi.org) (*The American Society of Home Inspectors* [*ASHI*, por sus siglas en inglés]): este sitio le puede ayudar a encontrar un inspector con certificación *ASHI* y enseñarle más sobre el proceso de inspección de la vivienda (que cubrimos en el Capítulo 13). También encontrará información y enlaces a una variedad de temas relacionados con la protección al consumidor, tales como productos retirados del mercado por la Comisión para la Seguridad de los Productos de Consumo (Consumer Product Safety Comisión [*CPSC*, por sus siglas en inglés]) y también información sobre análisis del agua y sistemas sépticos.

✔ **El Departamento de Vivienda y Desarrollo Urbano de los EE.UU.** (www.hud.gov) (*The U.S. Department of Housing and Urban Development Housing* [*HUD*, por sus siglas en inglés]): este sitio es muy extenso e incluye listas de viviendas en venta de este departamento y de otras agencias gubernamentales. También tiene una sección excelente para personas con discapacidades y sus necesidades de vivienda. Las quejas de discriminación (ya sea como comprador o inquilino) se pueden presentar ante el *HUD*. Pero le recomendamos que traiga sus mejores lentes de aumento porque la letra en este sitio es ¡microscópica! en muchas partes.

✔ **La Oficina de Análisis Económico del Departamento de Comercio de los EE.UU** (www.bea.doc.gov) (*The U.S. Department of Commerce's Bureau of Economic Analysis* [*BEA*, por sus siglas en inglés]): este sitio contiene un tesoro de información estatal y local. Si quiere obtener información para sentirse más tranquilo sobre el estado de la economía de las comunidades en las que tal vez quiera comprar casa, ¡este sitio es para usted!

Cómo Hacer Compras Preliminares

Lo que más nos gusta sobre el uso del Internet, como herramienta para buscar viviendas, es que puede lograr rápidamente una noción general sobre lo que está pasando. Cuando sea conveniente para usted, según su horario, puede navegar de un sitio Web a otro sin la presión de los vendedores. Los compradores pueden usar el Internet para comparar datos de una comunidad con otra, como los resultados de las pruebas de las escuelas, el clima y las estadísticas de delincuencia. Puede investigar muchos aspectos del proceso de compra como, precios de casas, agentes de bienes raíces, inspectores de propiedades, hipotecas y servicios de mudanza, sin dejar su cómodo sillón. Con un simple clic del ratón, el Internet puede instantáneamente transportarlo a cualquier parte del mundo y a cualquier hora del día o de la noche. Y puede también ahorrar dinero porque la Web, supuestamente, elimina al hombre intermediario y sus costos adicionales.

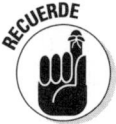

Una cosa que queremos que recuerde sobre el Internet es lo siguiente: "Ver para creer". Estar sentado frente a la pantalla de su computadora en su hogar no reemplaza una visita en persona para ver los vecindarios y las propiedades, ya que usted no puede hablar personalmente con la gente que se encuentra en la calle, conversar con el personal de la escuela ni ver la calidad y amabilidad de los dueños de los pequeños comercios locales.

Cómo seleccionar entre las casas en venta

Quizás la contribución más grande que ha aportado el Internet al proceso de compra ha sido la habilidad que le da de ver muchas listas de casas en venta cuando a usted le convenga hacerlo. El tener acceso a listados en línea es especialmente valioso cuando está contemplando mudarse de un estado a otro y quiere tener una idea general de lo que puede comprar. La opción de filtro, que tienen muchos de los sitios, le da una opción más cómoda que, por ejemplo, leer anuncios clasificados para una comunidad en particular cuando busca una casa con al menos tres habitaciones y aire acondicionado por menos de $300.000.

La mayoría de los agentes de bienes raíces de hoy día coordinan con usted para que reciba correo electrónico con información actualizada de listas de nuevas casas en venta que cumplen un criterio específico (por ejemplo, que tenga al menos tres dormitorios, que sea de 2.000 pies cuadrados o menos, etcétera). Solamente tenga cuidado de los agentes que estén usando este medio, por flojera, en lugar de ir personalmente a ver las propiedades y luego comunicarle a usted las que cumplen con sus requerimientos.

Si no está listo para trabajar con un agente, comience su búsqueda en `www.realtor.com`, que le permite buscar viviendas que cumplen con un criterio específico.

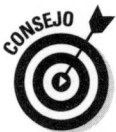

Para comunidades más pequeñas que no aparezcan en las listas de esos sitios Web, trate de localizar un periódico local; esto lo puede hacer por medio del sitio Web de la asociación periodística de América (*Newspaper Association of America,* `www.newsvoyager.com`). Un periódico local de un pueblo puede ser un recurso excelente para enterarse de lo que está sucediendo en el lugar que usted está considerando comprar su casa.

Si realmente quiere comprar una vivienda que ve anunciada en línea, por favor recuerde que no todo lo que ve es cierto. A pesar de que una de las supuestas virtudes del Internet es que la información es de último minuto, frecuentemente, eso *no* es el caso con sitios que muestran casas en venta. Como dijo el columnista Robert Bruss en una de sus columnas: "Mi experiencia ha sido que la mayoría de las listas de casas en los sitios Web contienen listados vencidos o incompletos, lo cual puede ser una gran pérdida de tiempo".

Obtenga información sobre las escuelas

Aunque no tenga niños en edad escolar, debe investigar lo que está pasando en las escuelas locales del vecindario donde está considerando comprar su casa. Si tiene hijos en la escuela, debería estar aún más motivado en obtener información sobre ellas para que le ayude con la importantísima decisión de escoger el sitio donde va a vivir.

Los sitios en el Internet con información escolar que nos gustan son `www.greatschools.net`, `www.schoolmatch.com`, `www.psk12.com` y `www.schoolmatters.com`. Estos sitios pueden ser útiles como punto de partida para obtener información básica sobre las escuelas públicas de una zona en particular. Ellos ofrecen información gratuita, pero también otro tipo de información y datos si paga una cuota. También puede ver cómo una determinada escuela o distrito están clasificados en relación a los demás del país. Además, frecuentemente los departamentos de educación estatales tienen información útil (aunque con difícil acceso) sobre las escuelas públicas. (Asimismo, visite `www.neighborhoodscout.com` para obtener información valiosa sobre las escuelas u otra información de la comunidad.)

Por supuesto, recuerde que la información que consigue de una escuela, por medio del Internet, no reemplaza una visita a la misma, o de hablar personalmente con los padres, administradores y maestros. Estos últimos pasos toman tiempo y energía, pero frecuentemente ayudan a las personas a tomar decisiones importantes basándose en una información más completa y verdadera.

Cómo examinar "los mejores lugares" para vivir

Cuando una transferencia de trabajo o un cambio en la familia motivan una mudanza, puede aparecer la pregunta: ¿dónde será el mejor lugar para vivir? Lo mejor, desde luego, varía porque sobre gustos y colores no han escrito los autores. Por ejemplo, una revista financiera alega que la ciudad *Moorestown* en *New Jersey*, es el mejor lugar para vivir. Con todo el respeto que se merecen esa bella ciudad y sus residentes, que tienen allí su hogar y gozan viviendo en ella, le hacemos hincapié en que no acepte el juicio de ninguna publicación ni de ninguna otra persona sobre cuál es el mejor lugar para vivir usted.

El Internet es una herramienta para vender

Quizás le parezca extraño que incluyamos un consejo sobre cómo vender una casa que aún no ha comprado, pero tarde o temprano la mayoría de las personas acaban vendiendo su vivienda por una razón u otra.

Cuando llega el momento de vender la casa, muchos vendedores están tentados a excluir a los agentes de bienes raíces — y su comisión típica del 6 por ciento — del proceso. Aunque parezca increíble, los sitios Web han avanzado muy poco en cuanto a ayudarles a los consumidores a eliminar a los agentes por medio del proceso llamado "Venta directa por el propietario" (*For Sale by Owner* [FSBO, por sus siglas en inglés]).

Algunos sitios ofrecen servicios limitados de agentes de bienes raíces por una comisión menor. Las comunidades que típicamente utilizan estos servicios tienden a tener casas más costosas. Piense en estos agentes de inmuebles como corredores de descuentos. Con el nivel reducido de servicio viene un precio reducido. Un sitio anuncia: "Venda con nosotros y pague solamente el 4,5 por ciento". Nuestra respuesta a eso es que cuando llegue la hora de vender su casa, contrate al mejor agente de bienes raíces que pueda y negocie la comisión. Puede tener un agente maravilloso y, por si fuera poco, una comisión menor que pagar. Compre la última edición de nuestro libro *House Selling For Dummies* para ver cómo hacerlo.

A pesar de que el Internet supuestamente amenaza con eliminar a los intermediarios y sus márgenes de ganancia, hasta ahora no parece ser que esto es lo que está pasando en el proceso de compra y venta de bienes raíces residenciales. El hecho de que los sitios *FSBO* no hayan tenido un éxito enorme es de notarse. Recuerde — nada puede reemplazar las visitas en persona. Nada, incluso el Internet, supera la experiencia de ver una casa y sus alrededores personalmente.

El sitio Web *Neighborhood Scout* (www.neighborhoodscout.com) es un sitio sensacional que le permite seleccionar criterios específicos bajo el cual puede buscar los mejores lugares que pueden satisfacer sus deseos. Si no quiere comenzar la búsqueda de este modo, puede comenzarla con los criterios preseleccionados del sitio (y que usted puede modificar después), como "Familias con niños" o "Comunidades paradisíacas para jubilarse". Estos criterios están diseñados para satisfacer grupos grandes de la población que comúnmente están buscando comprar casa.

Familiarícese con las opciones de financiamiento

Un número creciente de corredores y prestamistas hipotecarios en línea, proporcionan cotizaciones de tarifas y le ayudan a encontrar un préstamo a bajo costo. Las características interactivas de algunos de los sitios le permiten comparar el costo total de los préstamos, incluso los puntos y cuotas, simulando situaciones distintas como: el tiempo del préstamo y lo que le sucede al interés en hipotecas de tasa ajustable. Sin embargo, la interpretación de estas comparaciones requiere de un entendimiento pleno del vocabulario hipotecario y de los precios. Los peores sitios son aquellos que no son más que propagandas glorificadas de listas de prestamistas hipotecarios que han pagado por el anuncio publicitario en el sitio.

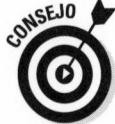

Entre los sitios Web hipotecarios, *E-Loan* (www.eloan.com) es nuestro favorito. *E-Loan* ofrece préstamos de docenas de prestamistas hipotecarios y otras herramientas útiles para comparar el costo de los diferentes préstamos. Para compradores de hipoteca que no están seguros del tipo de hipoteca que quieren, hay asesores hipotecarios disponibles por medio de una línea telefónica gratuita. A través del sitio, usted puede revisar el estatus de un préstamo solicitado. Una advertencia sobre este sitio: así como la mayoría de las entidades hipotecarias, este sitio tiene una calculadora muy sencilla que usa criterios tradicionales de los prestamistas (como, cantidad de la cuota inicial, sus ingresos, sus pagos mensuales de deudas y tasas de interés hipotecario) para determinar la cantidad de la hipoteca que usted posiblemente pueda pagar.

Este sitio, como la mayoría de los demás sitios, es más bien útil para aprender sobre el mercado hipotecario vigente y no para solicitar un préstamo. La razón es: el negocio de los préstamos hipotecarios es todavía un negocio que funciona localmente y que varía de acuerdo a las condiciones de los mercados de bienes raíces locales. Lynnea Key de la compañía de bienes raíces *Lynnea Key Realty*, en San Francisco, dice, "He pasado por situaciones casi desastrosas con sitios del Internet localizados fuera de esta zona, que no entienden el mercado local de aquí, donde hemos tenido ofertas múltiples y por encima de los precios. He tenido clientes que han tenido que correr como locos para encontrar un prestamista local a último minuto. En casos de ofertas múltiples de compra, cuando represento a un comprador potencial, algunos agentes se sienten incómodos cuando se les presentan cartas de préstamos hipotecarios que han sido previamente aprobadas pero de un sitio de Internet". (Hablamos sobre la aprobación previa de un préstamo hipotecario en el Capítulo 6.)

La compañía *HSH Associates* (www.hsh.com) es una rastreadora de datos de hipotecas y, además, editora que proporciona muchísima información y datos sobre hipotecas y otros tipos de préstamos a través de su sitio Web. Si está buscando una hipoteca con interés ajustable (*ARM*), puede revisar el historial de las variaciones de las tasas de interés de varios índices de interés ajustable que se usan, para que vea cuán rápido o lento se ajusta cada índice a cambios generales en las tasas de interés. El sitio también presume de ofrecer varios artículos útiles y enlaces con una variedad de hipotecas y de temas sobre la vivienda, tales como los peligros ambientales en el hogar.

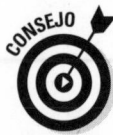

Fannie Mae también tiene información para el consumidor en su sitio www.homepath.com. Esta compañía respalda a la mayoría de los prestamistas hipotecarios, garantizándoles los préstamos que cumplen con sus estrictos criterios de crédito. Por ejemplo, puede buscar prestamistas que ofrecen préstamos hipotecarios específicos, tales como la Fannie 97, una hipoteca que sólo requiere de un 3 por ciento de cuota inicial y que le permite reunir los requisitos del préstamo con ingresos menores. También encontrará información excelente de los programas de hipoteca revertida de Fannie Mae — que ayudan a propietarios mayores a tener acceso al capital que tienen de la propiedad—, e información de las listas de casas en venta que han sido embargadas.

Las Desventajas de Buscar Casa en el Ciberespacio

Con frecuencia, la realidad de los sitios Web de bienes raíces decepciona las expectativas. Esté atento a lo que se presenta en las siguientes secciones.

Conflicto de intereses

Lamentablemente, la mayoría de los sitios Web no son templos de objetividad ni libres de comercialismo. Al contrario, los sitios del Internet frecuentemente tienen un interés o algo que promover. Generalmente la mayoría de sus ingresos, si no todos, provienen de propagandas publicitarias en el sitio. Por lo tanto, cuando esté en línea, manténgase alerta para ver si algo publicado o promovido es porque es realmente lo mejor o porque alguna compañía o persona le pagó al dueño del sitio Web para que lo promoviera.

Fíjese lo que hizo la compañía Yahoo! en su sección de bienes raíces desde que se publicó la edición previa de este libro. Antes, cuando los usuarios buscaban propiedades en Yahoo!, generalmente podían obtener listas de propiedades que cumplían con sus criterios personales de búsqueda. Ahora, desgraciadamente, los listados escasamente dan información —tanto en cantidad como en contenido—, gracias a la "relación comercial" que hay entre Yahoo! y la compañía de bienes raíces *Prudential Real Estate*. Para poder ver más listas de viviendas, los usuarios tienen que aceptar los largos acuerdos de uso que incluyen las siguientes perlitas. Por ejemplo: "Por la presente otorgo al dueño y administrador de la franquicia *Prudential Real Estate* ("Prudential Real Estate") mi permiso expreso, por escrito, para enviarme información no solicitada por mí por un período de hasta 18 meses".

Si usted cree que aceptando los términos de este acuerdo le permitirá ver todas las propiedades que cumplen con sus criterios de búsqueda personal, se equivoca. El acuerdo declara: "Es de mi conocimiento que *Prudential Real Estate* limitará el número de propiedades que me mostrará, de acuerdo a mi petición, en base a la exclusiva decisión de *Prudential Real Estate* del número de propiedades que estime prudente mostrar bajo un solo criterio solicitado. Esto es, según las condiciones actuales del mercado, el número total de los listados que coincidan en la compilación de la base de datos del *MLS* y otras restricciones "de uso prudente" que *Prudential Real Estate* considere apropiadas, y que pueden variar de un mercado a otro y de un periodo a otro".

Y si quiere ver una propiedad, los términos de uso declaran: "Acepto que no intentaré contactar personalmente a los vendedores de alguna propiedad que he seleccionado a través del sitio Web de *Prudential Real Estate*, y que no intentaré entrar a ninguna de esas propiedades a menos de que sea por medio de una cita concertada por medio de un agente o empleado de *Prudential Real Estate*".

Bancarrota

La mayoría de los sitios en la Web administrados por razones comerciales, terminan en bancarrota (como es en general, el caso de la mayoría de las pequeñas empresas). Debe tener cuidado al decidir hacer tratos con cualquier compañía en la Internet, especialmente las pequeñas o las nuevas en el campo de bienes raíces o las que estén a punto de quedarse sin capital.

Herramientas engañosas de avalúo de propiedades

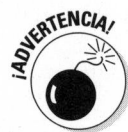

Tenga cuidado al usar las herramientas de avalúo de propiedades de los sitios Web que dan a entender que le ayudarán a determinar el valor justo de mercado de una casa o a examinar si los impuestos sobre su propiedad son los verdaderos. Usted puede encontrar muchas de estas herramientas en sitios Web de bienes raíces de interés general al público y en sitios como *Domania.com*. Como regla general, estos sitios no le dan el tipo de información que usted realmente necesita para encontrar propiedades similares y evaluarlas. Estos sitios casi siempre están en enlace con agentes de bienes raíces quienes le pagan una cuota al sitio por las referencias comerciales que reciben.

Ahora con sólo hacer clic con el ratón de su computadora, puede visitar una multitud de sitios Web que ofrecen direcciones, fechas de venta y precios de ventas de casas que se vendieron en años recientes. Puede realizar búsquedas — por una propiedad en particular, calle o por precios — en poblados donde quizás quiera vivir. (***Nota:*** no todas las ventas de propiedades de las comunidades se pueden encontrar en tales sitios —de hecho, en ciertas áreas se prohíbe la divulgación pública de esa información.)

Estos sitios Web animan a los compradores potenciales a usar su información de precios para encontrar zonas donde pueden comprar y para determinar lo que vale una casa específica. Los propietarios actuales supuestamente pueden usar la información para apelar avalúos de impuestos sobre su propiedad injustamente altos.

Si esto le suena demasiado bueno para ser verdad, ¡lea el Capítulo 10 inmediatamente para ver la forma correcta de valuar una casa! ¿A quién le importa si la casa número 123 Main Street se vendió a $275.000 en abril del año pasado? Usted necesita mucho más que la dirección, el precio y la fecha de venta para valuar correctamente una casa. ¿Y qué de los pequeños detalles como tamaño, edad, condiciones, área del jardín y otros más?

Calculadoras de hipotecas poco confiables

Normalmente hay una diferencia importante entre la cantidad que las muchísimas calculadoras hipotecarias en línea dicen que usted puede tomar prestado y cuánto realmente le *conviene* tomar prestado. La cantidad en dólares que le da una calculadora en línea se basa únicamente en la relación entre los pagos hipotecarios anticipados y sus ingresos. Aunque quizás esto satisfaga la preocupación de un prestamista sobre la probabilidad de que pague el préstamo, una calculadora tan sencilla ignora su condición financiera total: qué tanto (o qué tan poco) ha ahorrado para sus metas financieras a largo plazo —como su jubilación o la educación universitaria de sus hijos.

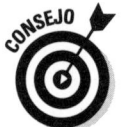

Fíjese muy bien en su presupuesto y en sus metas antes de decidir cuánto puede gastar en una casa; no permita que una calculadora vistosa, basada en programación Java, decida por usted.

Navegación lenta

La rapidez de su conexión en línea determina muchísimo la eficacia y satisfacción de su experiencia al navegar la red. En muchas comunidades, entre las más rápidas conexiones están las de línea digital de subscriptores (*Digital Subscriber Line* [*DSL,* por sus siglas en inglés]), y las de módem por cable (ofrecidas por una compañía de cablevisión local). Al comparar éstos con la conexión tradicional telefónica de módem de 56K, ellos descargan las páginas Web muchísimo más rápido, algo que es especialmente importante con sitios Web de bienes raíces ya que normalmente están llenos de propagandas. Otro beneficio de estas conexiones de Internet más rápidas es que, como siempre están conectadas, no tiene el problema del proceso tedioso y lento de establecer la conexión (ni de problemas con líneas ocupadas) cada vez que quiera revisar su correo electrónico o navegar por el Internet. Claro, estas conexiones rápidas no son gratis, así que tiene que considerar si los $40 al mes —más o menos— valen la pena. Pero, para los dueños de empresas pequeñas, para quienes el tiempo es oro, y para usuarios en sus casas que pasan mucho tiempo en el Internet, los servicios de Internet de alta velocidad sí que lo valen.

Parte IV
Cómo Cerrar el Contrato

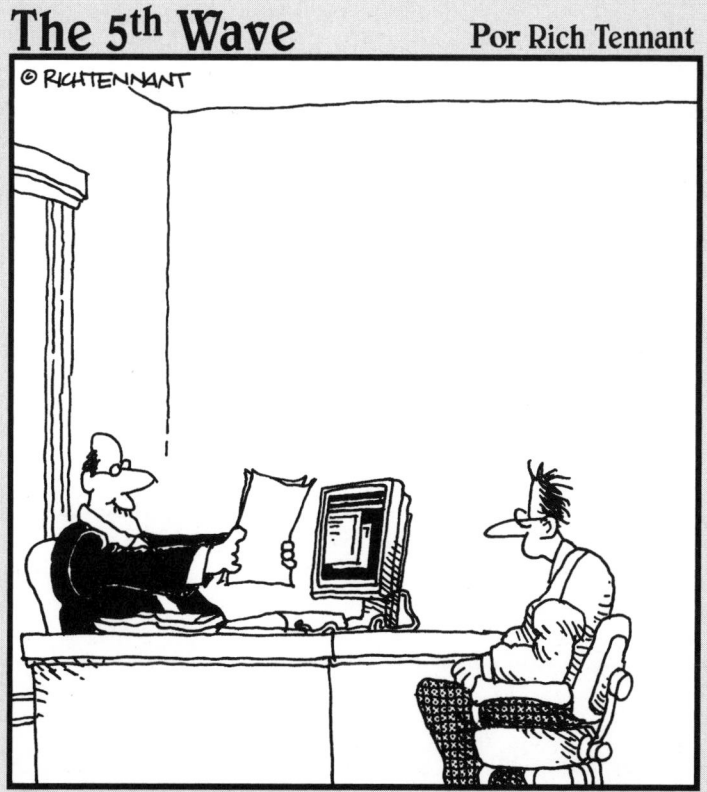

The 5th Wave — Por Rich Tennant

"El papeleo para el préstamo está listo. Ahora sólo falta sacarle un poquito de sangre para su firma, y habremos terminado con todo esto".

En esta parte . . .

¡Listos para empezar! Cuando usted haya hecho todo el trabajo preliminar, estará preparado para esta parte. Aquí es donde le enseñamos cómo negociar un excelente contrato y qué hacer para que su casa sea inspeccionada desde los cimientos hasta el techo, y así saber si está en perfectas condiciones o si está llena de defectos costosos.

Ya que no puede cerrar el contrato hasta que tenga su seguro de propiedad, le explicamos dónde, cuándo, cómo y qué tipo de seguro comprar que se ajuste a sus necesidades. Finalmente, describimos algunos aspectos legales y de impuestos de su compra, junto con otros consejos para que se asegure de que el cierre del contrato de compraventa se haga sin problemas y sin costos extras innecesarios.

Capítulo 12

Cómo Negociar el Mejor Precio

. . . .

En Este Capítulo

▶ Cómo controlar sus emociones

▶ Cómo probar los límites —si no es ilegal, es negociable.

▶ Cómo comprender las características de una buena oferta

▶ Cómo estructurar una oferta que el vendedor no puede rechazar

▶ Cómo considerar contingencias —cláusulas que lo protejan financiera y estructuralmente

▶ Cómo descubrir a los falsos vendedores

▶ Cómo detectar los beneficios y las desventajas

▶ Cómo manejar los créditos del depósito en garantía

. . . .

*E*n lo que respecta a la compra de cosas, los norteamericanos somos negociadores malos. La negociación no es parte de nuestra cultura. Nos hemos acostumbrados por generaciones a ser compradores dóciles, que pagamos cualquier precio marcado en una lata de frijoles o un aparato de TV. En vez de negociar con alguien cara a cara para rebajar el precio, lo más que hacemos es comparar precios entre diferentes tiendas para encontrar la que tiene el precio más bajo. (Y mucha gente muy ocupada ni siquiera hace eso.)

Ciertamente, podemos negociar cuando estamos entre la espada y la pared. Regateamos sobre los precios de cosas caras, como los automóviles, y hacemos lo mismo con el jefe cuando pedimos un aumento, pero nos incomoda hacerlo. Salimos de estos encuentros con la molesta sospecha de que perdimos en la negociación —que alguien podría haberlo hecho mejor.

Al darse cuenta de la incomodidad de nuestra nación frente a las negociaciones, algunos vendedores de autos han eliminado el regateo en la compra de los vehículos. En vez de usar tácticas de venta de alta presión, estos concesionarios ponen el precio del vehículo en el auto —*no se regatea con una etiqueta.* Ése es el precio, acéptelo o déjelo. Si usted lo acepta, probablemente no logrará el precio más bajo, pero algunas personas piensan que es una transacción justa, a fin de evitar lo desagradable de una negociación.

Un "buen" precio depende de la perspectiva

Prepárese. Puede sorprenderse de la respuesta de los vendedores a su oferta para la compra de su vivienda. Desde su perspectiva, usted hizo realmente una oferta muy buena. Ellos, por otro lado, pueden pensar que su oferta es un insulto.

La siguiente propuesta es, por ejemplo, la perspectiva de compradores de su primera vivienda, quienes destruyeron su prepuesto con una oferta de $210.000 por una propiedad con un precio de $239.000. "Mi amor, ¡estoy tan nerviosa! ¿Crees que los vendedores aceptarán nuestra oferta? Sé que la vivienda cuesta mucho más de lo que planeábamos gastar, pero tú sabes tanto como yo, que es el mejor lugar que hemos visto en los cuatro meses de nuestra búsqueda. ¿Por qué tardan tanto en contestarnos? El suspenso me está matando."

Y aquí está la perspectiva de la pareja jubilada que recibió la oferta por $210.000. "Cálmate, querida. Tu cara está roja como una remolacha; recuerda tu presión arterial. Estoy seguro que esa linda pareja joven no quiso insultarnos. Y no importa lo que tú digas, no puedo creer que ellos piensen que somos viejos chochos y tontos, que no sabemos cuál es el valor de nuestra propiedad. Probablemente ellos hicieron la mejor oferta que pudieron. Por favor, no la tires".

Dos interpretaciones completamente diferentes sobre exactamente la misma oferta. Los compradores piensan que están pagando demasiado. Los vendedores piensan que están regalando su casa. Cuando hay dinero real de por medio, estas percepciones conflictivas alimentan fuegos emocionales que calientan el proceso de negociación.

Pero usted no encontrará etiquetas para no regatear en las viviendas. Al contrario, generalmente todo, desde el precio de compra hasta la fecha de cierre de la cuenta de depósito en garantía, es negociable. Dados los altos precios vigentes de la propiedad en la mayoría de las poblaciones más densamente pobladas de los EE.UU., la compra de una vivienda es la que requiere una gran capacidad para negociar. Los buenos negociadores terminan sonriendo después de la compra de la vivienda. Los malos negociadores son castigados en sus bolsillos.

Si sigue los consejos en este capítulo estará en una posición ventajosa, que usted tanto merece, para negociar confiadamente a través de todo el proceso de compra. Y por supuesto, estos consejos le facilitarán la obtención de las llaves de su vivienda soñada, mucho más rápido, más fácilmente y a un precio más bajo.

Cómo Comprender y Enfrentar Sus Emociones

La emoción es una parte integral del proceso de compra de una vivienda. Las transacciones de bienes raíces son como las vueltas en la montaña rusa para todos los involucrados en el proceso.

A veces, como la niebla de San Francisco, las emociones se desvían sin rumbo en las transacciones, tan silenciosamente que usted apenas las nota. Sin embargo, con más frecuencia, truenan en los negocios como una manada de elefantes.

Cómo reconocer las fuerzas violentas en el proceso

Piense en las fuerzas violentas que actúan durante el proceso de compra de una vivienda:

- ✓ **Está en contacto con la más poderosa reacción instintiva de la gente.** Refugio, alimentos y seguridad son las tres necesidades más básicas de la vida. El hogar es donde está el corazón. Su vivienda es su castillo. La gente se torna violenta cuando sus viviendas están en peligro. Y hablando de impulsos instintivos, ahora usted sabe el porqué la búsqueda de un hogar es como ir de caza.

- ✓ **Usted pone en juego mucho dinero verdadero.** Aunque ésta sea su primera vivienda o la última, probablemente es la compra más grande de su vida. Cuánto paga por una vivienda no es lo importante. Cuando cantidades grandes de dinero están a riesgo, la intensidad emocional es inmensa para usted y para los vendedores, aunque la propiedad se venda por $250.000 o por $2.500.000.

- ✓ **Probablemente usted está pasando por un período de cambio en su vida.** El comprar una casa puede ser bastante estresante aun si tuviera que ocuparse solamente de buscar refugio y gastar montones de dinero. Agregue un cambio en la vida (como casamiento, divorcio, nacimiento, muerte, cambio de empleo, o jubilación) que generalmente es motivación suficiente para la compra de una vivienda, y usted ha creado una explosión de emociones.

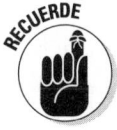

Como es imposible eliminar las emociones del proceso de compra, la mejor actitud para hacerles frente es reconocerlas y controlarlas. Por favor, comparta sus preocupaciones y frustraciones de manera productiva con su cónyuge, o con un amigo que haya comprado una casa, o mejor aún, con un buen terapeuta. No es saludable ni posible tragarse todas las emociones — cuanto más las esconda por dentro, peor será la explosión. Pero lo peor que puede hacer es descargar sus frustraciones y temores en otra gente, participantes en la transacción, especialmente en los vendedores. Las personas que mejor controlan y dirigen adecuadamente sus emociones, generalmente terminan concretando los mejores negocios.

Cómo controlarse a sí mismo

Aquí le presentamos cinco técnicas que puede usar para controlar sus emociones durante las negociaciones del proceso de compra de la vivienda.

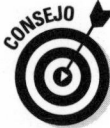

✔ **Ponga la transacción en perspectiva.** ¿Qué es peor: una compra que fracasa, o una operación del corazón? No importa cuán mal las cosas estén con su transacción inmobiliaria, recuerde constantemente que no es una situación de vida o muerte. Mañana será otro día. El sol brillará otra vez, los rosales florecerán de nuevo, los pájaros cantarán otra vez y los niños se reirán de nuevo. La vida continúa. Lo peor que puede ocurrir es que el negocio muera, pero usted vivirá y buscará otro lugar al que va a llamar hogar.

✔ **No deje que el tiempo lo intimide.** La mayoría de los cambios de vida tienen una duración predecible. Usted tiene notificación anticipada de los casamientos, nacimientos, jubilaciones, y otras por el estilo. No se ponga bajo innecesaria presión postergando cosas, o creando sin necesidad sus propias fechas de vencimiento. Disponga de tiempo suficiente para la compra de una vivienda. Distribuya adecuadamente el tiempo, y así será su propio amigo, en vez de su enemigo.

✔ **Mantenga las emociones lo más distantes posible.** Mantenga sus opciones abiertas. Esté listo para abandonar la compra de una vivienda, si no puede llegar a un acuerdo satisfactorio con los vendedores sobre los precios y las condiciones. Prepárese mentalmente con la idea de que el negocio puede fracasar. Las casas son como los autobuses: si pierde uno, otro vendrá tarde o temprano.

✔ **Acepte la incertidumbre como parte integral de la transacción.** Así como quiere saber todo acerca de la propiedad antes de hacer una oferta, hay que jugar el partido sin la información completa. Usted siempre tiene muchas más preguntas que respuestas al principio de una transacción. No se preocupe, todo saldrá bien siempre que sepa lo que necesita saber, y que obtenga las respuestas en un período de tiempo aceptable durante su transacción.

✔ **Sea objetivo.** Utilice un análisis comparativo del mercado (*CMA*, por sus siglas en inglés) para establecer objetivamente el valor justo de mercado de la vivienda que quiere comprar (vea el Capítulo 10). Un buen agente de bienes raíces puede ayudarle a usar la información para preparar una oferta equitativa. Si un agente no entra en sus planes, piense trabajar con un abogado en bienes raíces. Es aconsejable tener a alguien que sirva de apoyo en momentos inevitables de estados emocionales, cuando pierda su calma. Asegúrese de que trabaja con profesionales que tienen paciencia, que no lo presionan, y que están comprometidos a lograr el mejor negocio para usted.

Primero lo principal

Al principio de su carrera en bienes raíces, Ray trabajó con un comprador que insistió en tener todas las respuestas a las preguntas sobre una vivienda antes de presentar una oferta de compra. Él quería estructurar una oferta absolutamente perfecta. Como Ray no tenía mucha experiencia, aceptó ese plan. Se pasaron varias semanas perfeccionando el precio de la oferta usando información sobre propiedades comparables, y solicitando estimados de contratistas para determinar el costo de las reparaciones necesarias, que habían sido identificadas durante las inspecciones, ordenadas por un comprador anterior.

Desgraciadamente, Ray y el comprador recibieron una dura lección por no aceptar la incertidumbre, porque mientras ellos verificaban los más mínimos detalles, el comprador de Ray no hizo una oferta oficial para la vivienda. El vendedor se cansó de las idas y venidas, y de la constante recolección de información, y vendió su propiedad a otra persona.

Si usted es inteligente, hará lo que hizo un comprador de vivienda exitoso: llegue primero a un acuerdo. Condicione su oferta al logro de las respuestas a todas sus preguntas mientras la vivienda está atada a un contrato.

De esa manera, si todo va bien, se convertirá en el orgulloso dueño de una vivienda hermosa. Sin embargo, si no puede conseguir un préstamo, o no le gustan los resultados de los informes de la inspección, puede renegociar el arreglo, o salirse de la transacción y continuar la búsqueda de otra vivienda más promisoria. Mientras tanto, sin embargo, ha sacado la propiedad de la competencia al obtener la aceptación de su oferta.

No pierda tiempo en lograr las respuestas a preguntas secundarias hasta que usted conteste la pregunta principal: ¿Pueden llegar a un acuerdo usted y el vendedor acerca de las condiciones de la venta? Si fracasan en llegar a un consentimiento, pierde tiempo y dinero, y puede perder esa propiedad.

El Arte de la Negociación

¿Es la negociación semejante al agua o al hielo? Si usted dice "agua", colóquese una estrellita en la frente.

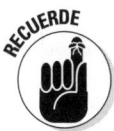

La negociación es fluida, no rígida. No hay una estrategia de negociación que sea la mejor de todas, y que usted pueda usar en cada situación de compra de una vivienda. Los buenos negociadores adaptan sus estrategias basadas en una variedad de factores, como:

- ✔ Cuán justo es el precio de la propiedad
- ✔ Cuánto tiempo hace que está en el mercado
- ✔ Qué motivación tienen los vendedores

> ✔ Cuán motivado está usted
>
> ✔ Si está negociando desde una posición muy buena (un mercado del comprador) o débil (un mercado de vendedores)

Los negociadores buenos, sin embargo, usan algunos principios básicos para cada situación. Si usted entiende estos principios, puede realmente aumentar las posibilidades de obtener lo que quiere.

Cómo ser realista

Los buenos negociadores comprenden que los hechos son la base de una negociación exitosa. Si quiere convertirse en un buen negociador, debe ver las cosas tal como son, y no como usted quiere que sean. El tener la ilusión de que todo será como lo desea, es el comienzo de una mala negociación.

¿Qué significa tener una ilusión? Un ilusión común en un mercado de bienes raíces, por ejemplo, con precios en aumento, es que usted quiera pagar los precios de ayer por una vivienda en el mercado de hoy. Quizás vio una casa similar en venta a un precio más bajo hace seis meses. Usted ignora el hecho de que los precios han aumentado desde entonces, lo cual elimina la oportunidad de comprar hoy día una vivienda al precio anterior. Otra ilusión común (y generalmente irrealista) es que tiene los medios para comprar una propiedad similar respecto a la que vivió en su niñez.

¿Cómo puede eliminar esa forma ilusionada de pensar? Reemplazando la fantasía por los hechos. Desdichadamente, eso es más fácil decirlo que hacerlo, porque es inevitable emocionarnos cuando participamos en la negociación de algo que deseamos de todo corazón. Aun cuando esa reacción emocional es parte de la naturaleza humana, permitir que la emoción se filtre en una negociación puede resultarle muy caro.

La importancia de la objetividad

A diferencia de usted y del vendedor, un buen agente inmobiliario no toma las cosas personalmente. El agente del vendedor, por ejemplo, no se ofenderá si su agente le dice a ella que usted odia la pintura verde esmeralda de la cocina y las paredes empapeladas con papel salpicado en rojo en la sala de la familia. Su agente, por otra parte, no se enfurecerá si el agente del vendedor le dice que su oferta es ridículamente baja.

Es fácil para los agentes ser objetivos. Después de todo, ellos no son los que pasaron tres largos fines de semana pintando la cocina o meses buscando el papel perfecto para empapelar la sala familiar. Tampoco es de ellos el dinero ahorrado durante toda una vida, lo que se está negociando.

Los buenos agentes escuchan lo que el mercado dice acerca del valor de una vivienda. No permiten que detalles que desvían la atención (como cuánto pagó el vendedor por la casa hace diez años, o cuán poco puede usted pagar por ella hoy) confundan las negociaciones. Como usted ya sabe, si leyó el Capítulo 10, no hay una correlación entre estos temas basados en necesidad y el valor justo del mercado actual.

Algunas personas piensan que los agentes tienen calculadoras por corazón. Pero, no es así. Los buenos agentes saben que si no son fríamente realistas acerca de los valores de la propiedad, la vivienda no se venderá, y ellos no ganarán nada.

Las señales de peligro en las negociaciones del agente

Si sigue nuestro consejo en el Capítulo 9 para elegir a su agente de bienes raíces, usted elegirá a uno que es un buen negociador.

Hacer un trabajo pobre en la selección del agente, le puede costar un dineral. Los malos agentes no saben cómo determinar los valores justos de mercado y, como resultado, puede ser que usted pague demasiado por su vivienda. ¿Y qué les importa a ellos? ¡Nada! Después de todo, cuanto más pague usted, más gana su agente, porque las comisiones de los agentes, típicamente, son un porcentaje del precio de compra. Si su agente le presiona para que compre, y no puede justificar el precio de la oferta usando la venta de viviendas similares, despida a su agente, y consiga uno bueno.

Los buenos negociadores evitan hacer juicios morales. Mientras que la posición del vendedor no sea ilegal, entonces no es ni inmoral ni injusta. Es, sencillamente, una posición para negociar. Naturalmente, los agentes son seres humanos. A veces, aún los mejores agentes pueden perder temporalmente su objetividad en la intensidad de la batalla. Usted sabe si esto ocurre cuando la cara de su agente se torna roja y comienza a acusar a la otra parte de ser injusta.

Si su agente pierde la calma y se recobra rápidamente, no es problema. Pero, si su agente no puede calmarse, usted perdió su amortiguador emocional. Los agentes que pierden su objetividad profesional son incapaces de negociar bien a su favor.

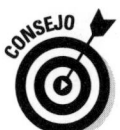

No importa la satisfacción que su agente y usted sientan después de desahogarse emocionalmente acerca de la increíble falta de gusto del vendedor, de su falta de conocimiento del mercado, o de sus escrúpulos, enojarse no le facilitará la compra de la vivienda. Si su agente no puede mantener una actitud profesional, pídale al corredor del agente (vea el Capítulo 9) que negocie por usted, o busque a otro agente.

Hechos y opiniones

Usted y los vendedores pueden usar exactamente los mismos hechos (es decir, los precios de viviendas similares vendidas recientemente) y aún así, llegar a opiniones totalmente diferentes del valor justo de mercado. Como lo señalamos en el Capítulo 10, aunque las casas pueden ser similares en cuanto a edad, tamaño y condición, no existen dos viviendas idénticas después que las personas han vivido en ellas.

Además, aun cuando todas las casas usadas en el análisis comparativo del mercado están en el mismo vecindario, *la ubicación diferente* (es decir, la proximidad a escuelas, una vista mejor, un jardín más grande, etc.) normalmente influye en el valor individual de las propiedades. Finalmente, aun cuando todas las casas comparables se vendieron durante los previos seis meses, los valores de la propiedad pueden ser influenciados por cambios en las tasas de interés de las hipotecas y por la confianza del consumidor.

Por ejemplo, su agente piensa que la casa número 123 en Main Street, que se vendió hace dos meses por $280.000, es la que se compara mejor con la casa que usted está tratando de comprar. El agente del vendedor está de acuerdo en que es una buena comparación, pero señala que esta casa tiene un garaje para dos autos, mientras que la de 123 Main Street tiene un garaje para sólo un auto. Su agente dice que la

de 123 Main Street tiene una cocina más grande con un rincón para desayunar y está dos cuadras más cerca del parque. El agente del vendedor dice que la propiedad que usted considera tiene gabinetes de cocina de más alta calidad y un refrigerador nuevo, y está tres cuadras más cerca de la parada del autobús.

Y así sigue el argumento. Todos están de acuerdo sobre el precio y la fecha de venta de la propiedad en 123 Main Street. Éstos son *hechos.* Son iguales para cualquiera que los mire.

Pero, ¿en cuánto aumenta el valor de la vivienda que quiere comprar si tiene un segundo espacio en el garaje? ¿El estar más cerca de la parada del autobús tiene más valor que la proximidad al parque? ¿Es una cocina donde se puede comer, más o menos valiosa para usted que los lujosos gabinetes y un refrigerador nuevo? Las respuestas a estas preguntas son *opiniones* basadas en sus juicios de valor. Otra persona probablemente podría asignarle un valor diferente a las conveniencias.

Los precios no son un 100 por ciento científicos en este nivel de comparación. No hay dos compradores iguales. Cada comprador tiene diferentes necesidades y debido a estas diferencias, llegarán a conclusiones distintas en cuanto a opiniones sobre el valor.

Cómo examinar su estilo como negociador

Encontrar a dos personas que tengan el mismo estilo como negociadores es muy difícil, lo mismo que encontrar dos casas idénticas construidas hace 200 años. Todos los estilos de negociación, sin embargo, se reducen a variaciones de uno de esos dos temas básicos:

✔ **Luchador (yo gano, usted pierde):** estos negociadores miran el ganar solamente en el contexto de derrotar a la otra parte. Para ellos, la negociación es una guerra. No toman prisioneros.

✔ **Cooperador (los dos ganamos):** estos negociadores tratan de resolver problemas, en vez de derrotar a los oponentes. Todos los involucrados en la transacción trabajan juntos para encontrar soluciones que sean satisfactorias para ambas parte.

¿Cuál estilo de negociación es mejor? Depende del tipo de persona que usted es, cuáles son sus objetivos, y de cuánto tiempo dispone.

La mayoría de las personas optan por la cooperación porque saben que el mundo es redondo —la manera en que actúa hoy casi siempre le regresa a usted para ayudarlo, o bien para perturbarlo. ¿De qué sirve luchar batallas en un juego extraño de segura destrucción mutua, si pueden trabajar juntos pacíficamente como aliados para resolver los problemas comunes?

La negociación agresiva se tolera en un mercado del comprador, o del vendedor. Esta forma de trabajar es *tolerada.* La gente juega un partido de "yo gano, usted pierde", a regañadientes, cuando no tiene otra alternativa. Sin embargo, en un mercado equilibrado, que no favorece ni a los vendedores ni a los compradores, normalmente se les dice a los negociadores agresivos "no voy a jugar su juego estúpido porque no me gusta su estilo".

La negociación cooperativa, por otro lado, funciona bien ante cualquier condición del mercado porque su meta es un apretón de manos para todos. A todos nos gusta ganar y odiamos perder. La gente a veces llora cuando es derrotada. Pero, los problemas nunca lloran cuando son resueltos.

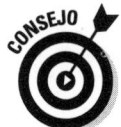

Por desgracia, algunas personas ya nacen siendo competitivas. La única cooperación que comprenden es la cooperación de un equipo que trabaja bien en grupo para derrotar a sus oponentes. Si usted es un negociador cooperativo, aquí le indicamos dos formas de protección ante los negociadores agresivos.

✔ **Trate de cambiar a los agresivos en cooperativos buscando maneras en las que ambos puedan ganar.** Cambie su énfasis de derrotarlo a usted a resolver el problema. "Usted quiere vender. Yo quiero comprar. ¿Cómo podemos hacerlo?"

✔ **Si fracasa, tire a la basura ese negocio.** Si continúa negociando, los competidores por naturaleza le sacarán su dinero de la cuenta de banco y la carne de sus huesos. Ellos confunden concesiones con debilidad. Si, por ejemplo, usted ofrece dividir la diferencia, ellos tomarán el 50 por ciento que les da como parte del precio justo, y entonces esperan el resto. No van a estar conformes hasta que gocen de una victoria que es aumentada por la derrota incondicional suya. La vida es demasiada corta para someterse a esta clase de castigo. No importa que el mercado de los vendedores que usted enfrenta sea muy fuerte, es posible encontrar vendedores que son cooperativos —si usted lo intenta.

Fuerza bruta o estilo

Ray conoce a un agente inmobiliario que es un técnico extraordinario. Es brillante cuando determina el valor justo de mercado de una vivienda, escribe contratos sin errores, comprende el financiamiento, y está actualizado con respecto a las leyes de bienes raíces, las reglas, y los reglamentos. Como técnico, es perfecto.

Desgraciadamente, él no tiene compasión. Es fríamente perfecto y espera la misma perfección de todo el mundo. Es un negociador muy despiadado, que no da ni espera misericordia de sus oponentes. Aún algunos de sus mismos clientes están disgustados por su estilo, pero todos lo respetan porque saben que luchará implacablemente a favor de ellos.

Otros agentes odian trabajar con este agente porque es un negociador feroz. Ellos trabajan con él solamente cuando no tienen otra alternativa. Si representa a un comprador en una situación de múltiples ofertas, por ejemplo, la oferta de su comprador no será elegida si el agente del vendedor puede encontrar la forma de salir del paso y trabajar con un comprador cuyo agente es menos agresivo.

Ray Jones, un agente de San Francisco que falleció hace varios años, era exactamente lo opuesto de ese agente. Jones carecía de un estilo elegante, pero era amable, justo y generoso, y hacía que las personas sonrieran de corazón. Sus clientes y otros agentes lo adoraban. En una situación de ofertas múltiples, la oferta de su comprador era aceptada o recibía una contra oferta, si era posible. Él hacía que comprar una vivienda fuera divertido.

Piénselo cuidadosamente cuando seleccione a un agente para que lo represente. La gente hace negocios con usted solamente por dos razones: porque ellos tienen que hacerlo o quieren hacerlo. El agente apropiado puede darle ventajas al negociar. El negociador implacable puede tener sentido para compradores que no tienen apuro en comprar y que desean encontrar un buen negocio. Para otros, esa piraña puede significar malas noticias.

Cómo negociar con diplomacia

Los negociadores capaces obtienen lo que quieren por acuerdo mutuo —no por fuerza bruta. La fuerza bruta es grosera, ruda, desagradable y decididamente nada amistosa. He aquí algunos conceptos que pueden serle útiles para negociar con diplomacia:

- ✔ **Los teléfonos son para hacer citas.** Nunca, nunca, nunca deje que su agente o abogado presente una oferta, o trate de negociar asuntos importantes por teléfono. Decir que no por teléfono es muy fácil para los vendedores; aun si están de acuerdo con todo lo que usted quiere, pueden cambiar de opinión hasta que llegue el momento de firmar el contrato.

- ✔ **Los acuerdos verbales son inútiles.** En nuestra sociedad, tenemos contratos escritos porque las personas tienen memorias notoriamente selectivas. Si quiere que su negocio tenga valor legal en un tribunal, ponga todo los detalles por escrito. Acostúmbrese a escribir memorandos cortos, con fecha (*Memos for Record* [*MFR*, por sus siglas en inglés]), para registrar conversaciones importantes (como "el 2 de junio —el prestamista dijo que obtendremos una hipoteca al 7,5 por ciento de interés"; "el 12 de junio —los vendedores quieren extender el cierre del depósito en garantía por una semana", etc.) Ponga estas notas en su archivo de la transacción, en caso de que las necesite para refrescar su memoria. Considere las palabras inmortales de Samuel Goldwyn: "Un acuerdo verbal no tiene el valor ni del papel en que está escrito".

✔ **La administración de las fechas de vencimiento es esencial.** Los contratos de bienes raíces están llenos de vencimientos de cosas como la remoción de los imprevistos, aumentos del depósito, y por supuesto, el cierre del depósito en garantía. Si se falla en cumplir con estos vencimientos es posible que resulten funestas consecuencias. Su negocio puede fracasar —usted puede hasta ser enjuiciado. La mayoría de los vencimientos, sin embargo, son flexibles— si usted los maneja correctamente. Imagine que recién se entera de que las inspecciones de la propiedad llevarán más tiempo para completarse que lo anticipado. *De inmediato* contacte a los vendedores para explicarles la razón de la tardanza y entonces obtenga una extensión por escrito de la fecha de vencimiento. Las postergaciones generalmente pueden acomodarse si son explicadas adecuadamente y de inmediato.

El Proceso de Negociación

La negociación es un proceso continuo —una serie de pasos sin un principio o fin nítidamente definido. Piense en el agua en movimiento.

Cada paso en el proceso de negociación comienza con la recolección de información. Cuando termine de leer este libro, comprenderá los varios aspectos de la compra de una vivienda. Entonces usted podrá convertir su información en acción que generará más información, y que le llevará a más acción. Y así continúa, hasta que usted se convierta en el propietario orgulloso de la casa de sus sueños.

Una forma de comenzar la primera fase de acción es poner sus finanzas en orden, obtener la aprobación previa de un crédito y seleccionar a un agente para trabajar con usted a lo largo de la fase siguiente de recolección de información. Usted y su agente luego investigan varios vecindarios y visitan casas para que así conozcan lo que hay en el mercado. También descubrirá la diferencia entre el precio inicial y el valor justo de mercado. Una vez que sepa el valor real de las viviendas, usted estará listo para enfocar su atención en el vecindario específico en el que desea vivir, y comenzará la búsqueda seria del hogar de sus sueños.

Cómo hacer una oferta de compra

Una vez que encuentre la vivienda de sus sueños, está listo para el siguiente paso de acción en el proceso de negociación: cómo hacer una oferta de compra. No hay un contrato de compra de bienes raíces estándar y universalmente aceptado en todo el país. Por el contrario, los contratos de compra varían en extensión y condiciones de estado a estado, y dentro de un mismo estado, de una localidad a otra.

Cuando usted esté listo para redactar una oferta, su agente de bienes raíces o su abogado le entregará un contrato que se usa en su localidad.

Los contratos de bienes raíces se revisan muy frecuentemente debido a cosas tales como cambios de las leyes de bienes raíces y a los requisitos obligatorios de declaración del vendedor. Un buen agente o abogado usa la versión más corriente del contrato. Verifique la fecha de revisión del contrato (generalmente aparece al pie, en la esquina izquierda o derecha de cada página) para asegurarse de que no está usando una versión apenas más nueva que la *Declaración de la Independencia*.

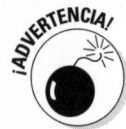

Una oferta escrita con un vocabulario pobre y no bien redactada, puede convertir lo que debería ser una negociación productiva en una lucha entre usted y los vendedores. En vez de trabajar juntos para resolver el problema común (es decir, "usted quiere comprar, y ellos quieren vender —¿cómo podemos *los dos*, obtener lo que *ambos* queremos?)", usted se desvía de los temas importantes que no se pueden resolver en esta fase del proceso de negociación.

Aunque la compra de una vivienda puede ser una experiencia extremadamente emocional, ofertas buenas calman esta situación potencialmente explosiva al reemplazar emociones por hechos. Los compradores y los vendedores tienen sentimientos que se pueden herir. Los hechos no. Por eso, los hechos son la base de negociaciones exitosas.

Todas las ofertas buenas tienen tres cosas en común:

- ✔ **Las buenas ofertas están basadas en las más importantes inquietudes de los vendedores: una oferta con un precio realista.** Usted no debe inventar el precio por arte de magia. En cambio, use los precios de las viviendas como base de su oferta (similares a la casa del vendedor en edad, tamaño, condición y ubicación) considerando las que se hayan vendido durante los seis meses anteriores. Como se explica en el Capítulo 10, el precio que piden los vendedores es a menudo una fantasía. Los precios reales de viviendas comparables son hechos. *Enfóquese en los hechos.*

- ✔ **Las buenas ofertas tienen condiciones de financiamiento realistas.** La tasa de interés de su hipoteca, costo de iniciar un préstamo, y período permitido para obtener financiamiento (se explica en la sección siguiente sobre contingencias) debe basarse en las condiciones actuales de los préstamos. Algunas ofertas se extinguen porque las condiciones del préstamo del comprador son irrealistas. *Enfóquese en los hechos.*

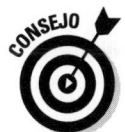

Si usted ha reunido los requisitos para obtener un préstamo, o mejor aún, tiene aprobación previa para un préstamo (vea el Capítulo 6), usted o su agente deben enfatizar esta ventaja cuando presenta su oferta. Esto les demuestra a los vendedores que usted es un comprador digno de crédito, que está listo, tiene el deseo y tiene la capacidad financiera para comprar la vivienda.

✔ **Las buenas ofertas no esperan un cheque en blanco de los vendedores.** Excepto cuando los defectos de la propiedad están claramente a la vista, ni usted ni los vendedores sabrán si son necesarios trabajos de reparación cuando la oferta es presentada inicialmente. Bajo estas circunstancias, es recomendable usar cláusulas sobre la inspección de la propiedad (lo que se explica en la sección siguiente) que le permitan reanudar las negociaciones relativas a cualquier trabajo de reparación necesario *después* que reciba los informes de las inspecciones.

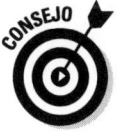

Recuerde que las negociaciones son un proceso continuo. Después de la *aceptación* de su oferta, sus inspectores de la propiedad recogen *información.* Después que ellos determinen qué trabajos de reparación son realmente necesarios, usted y los vendedores pueden reanudar las negociaciones *(la acción)* armados con los hechos *(la información)*. Esta secuencia permite evitar el tiempo y la energía de argüir con los vendedores sobre el costo total del trabajo de reparación, antes de que ninguno de ustedes sepa la cantidad precisa en dólares que se necesitarán para hacer las reparaciones necesarias. *Enfóquese en los hechos.*

Si los vendedores están de acuerdo con el precio y las condiciones incluidas en su oferta, ellos la firmarán. Su agente debe darle a usted inmediatamente una copia firmada de la oferta. Cuando tenga en sus manos una copia de la oferta firmada por los vendedores, usted tiene lo que se llama una *oferta ratificada* (es decir, una oferta firmada o aceptada). Esto no significa que es dueño de la propiedad o que ésta ha sido vendida. Todo lo que indica por ahora es que la venta está pendiente.

Prepare la posibilidad de escape: Contingencias

Aunque los vendedores han aceptado su oferta, ésta debe contener las muy importantes cláusulas de escape conocidas como contingencias, las cuales deben estar incluidas en su contrato para protegerlo. Una contingencia es una cosa que puede suceder o no suceder en el futuro, pero que debe satisfacerse para que se realice la venta. Le da a usted el derecho de salirse del negocio si ese acontecimiento no ocurre. Si usted no remueve la contingencia, la venta no se realiza, y su dinero de depósito es usualmente devuelto.

Estas dos contingencias aparecen en casi todas las ofertas:

- **Financiamiento:** usted puede terminar el negocio si el préstamo especificado en su contrato no es aprobado.

- **Inspecciones de la propiedad:** usted puede terminar el negocio si no aprueba los informes de las inspecciones, o si no puede llegar a un acuerdo con los vendedores acerca de la forma de manejar las reparaciones necesarias.

Otras contingencias estándares le dan el derecho de revisar y aprobar cosas como la escritura principal de la unidad del condominio, los estatutos, el presupuesto y, también, el informe del título de propiedad. Si quiere, puede hacer la transacción sujeto a la aprobación de su abogado, o a la inspección de la vivienda por sus padres. Como regla, ninguna contingencia *justa* será rechazada por el vendedor.

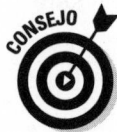

No exagere las contingencias si está compitiendo con varios compradores por la misma propiedad. A los vendedores, especialmente en mercados activos de bienes raíces, no les gustan las ofertas con muchas contingencias. Desde el punto de ellos, cuantas más contingencias hay en una oferta, mayor es la probabilidad de que la transacción no se lleve a efecto. Se debe equilibrar la necesidad de protegerse, con la imperiosa necesidad de que se acepte su oferta. Mantenga sus contingencias en un plazo de tiempo prudente, pero corto. Resuelva el mayor número posible de preguntas antes de presentar la oferta. Por ejemplo, si sus padres insisten en ver la propiedad que usted quiere comprar antes de prestarle el dinero para el depósito inicial, llévelos a visitar la vivienda antes de presentar su oferta a fin de eliminar esa contingencia.

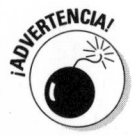

Si considera hacer que su oferta esté sujeta a la venta de otra vivienda (tal como en la que está viviendo ahora), no lo haga si está en una guerra competitiva con otros compradores. Consulte la sección "La negociación desde una posición de desventaja", que aparece más adelante en este capítulo, porque incluir esta contingencia puede resultar en la pérdida de la vivienda que usted está tratando de comprar.

Ésta es una contingencia típica:

> *Bajo la condición* (la palabra mágica) de que el comprador consiga una hipoteca a pagar en 30 años, con una tasa de interés fija garantizado por la propiedad, en la cantidad del 80 por ciento del precio de compra. Digamos que la tasa de interés no pase del 7,5 por ciento. Los puntos o costos no serán más del 2 por ciento del monto del préstamo. Si el comprador no puede conseguir ese financiamiento dentro de los 30 días de la aceptación de su oferta, el comprador le debe notificar, por escrito, al vendedor de que opta por la cancelación de este contrato, y por el reembolso de los depósitos que haya realizado.

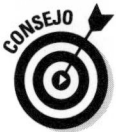

El acuerdo de compra que usted firma es un contrato por el que contrae una obligación legal. Como decimos en el Capítulo 9, es conveniente incluir de inmediato a un abogado en su equipo si tiene cualquier inquietud acerca de la legalidad de su contrato. Aun si no tiene un abogado cuando firma el contrato, puede ser prudente incluir la siguiente cláusula en su oferta, en caso de tener preguntas legales:

> Este contrato está sujeto a la aprobación de mi abogado en un período no mayor de cinco días a partir de su aceptación.

El uso de esta cláusula no significa que en realidad usted tenga que contratar a un abogado. Sin embargo, si lo hace, le da la opción de que un abogado suyo revise el contrato si usted lo desea. Además, un buen contrato provee un espacio en blanco para agregar términos y condiciones.

Incluya una condición en su contrato que específicamente diga que esas contingencias deben ser eliminadas por escrito. El hacerlo debería eliminar la confusión entre usted y los vendedores en relación a si la contingencia fue cumplida.

¿De qué sirve una oferta ratificada si está llena de cláusulas de escape? Bueno, una oferta ratificada (plagada de cláusulas de escape o no) retiene la propiedad. No tiene que preocuparse de que el dueño venda la propiedad a alguien mientras usted está gastando dinero y tiempo inspeccionándola.

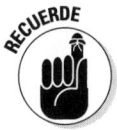

Primero obtenga un acuerdo sobre el precio y los términos de la venta — *luego* haga todas las otras preguntas que quiera.

Cómo obtener una contraoferta

Es muy difícil que los vendedores acepten su oferta como fue escrita originalmente. Aun cuando les guste el precio que ofrece, probablemente la cambiarán aquí y allá para hacerla más aceptable para ellos. Los vendedores usan *contraofertas* para refinar el precio, los términos y condiciones de las ofertas que reciben.

Le encantará saber que los formularios para las contraofertas son mucho menos complicados que los de las ofertas.

Imagine que ofrece $275.000 por una vivienda que le gusta, y pide que se cierre el depósito en garantía 30 días después de que los vendedores acepten su oferta. Como ellos tienen la propiedad listada por $289.000, los vendedores piensan que su oferta es un poquitito baja. Además, ellos necesitan seis semanas para trasladarse.

En vez de escribir otra vez la oferta completa, le dan a usted una contraoferta. Ésta declara que están dispuestos a aceptar todos los términos y condiciones de su oferta, excepto que quieren $285.000 y seis semanas después de ser aceptada para cerrar el depósito en garantía.

La pelota está otra vez en su lado de la cancha. A usted no le importan las seis semanas para cerrar el depósito en garantía, pero no quiere pagar más de los $280.000, entonces les da a los vendedores una contraoferta a su contraoferta para informarlos.

Ahora queda sólo una cosa por discutir: el precio. Los vendedores vuelven con un precio firme de $284.000. Rezongando, usted les responde que lo acepta por $281.000 e instruye a su agente a que les aclare que no subirá de esa suma. Los dos pueden jugar un partido *firme*. Ahora las negociaciones se parecen a la guerra de trincheras de la Primera Guerra Mundial.

Si usted realmente quiere la vivienda, esta fase del juego puede romperle los nervios. Se inquieta pensando que otro comprador les haga una mejor oferta a los vendedores y le roben la vivienda, mientras usted está tratando de bajar el precio $3.000 más. Los vendedores también están preocupados de que lo pueden perder si siguen presionándolo con insistencia por esos $3.000 finales. Usted no quiere pagar ni un centavo más de lo que debe. Los vendedores no quieren dejar ningún dinero en la mesa.

Usted y el vendedor están tentadoramente cerca de llegar a un acuerdo del precio. El precio de su oferta y el precio inicial de los vendedores están basados en los datos sobre las ventas recientes de casas similares en el vecindario. Entonces, ¿por qué el estancamiento? Porque a veces, los mismos hechos pueden conducir a conclusiones diferentes (vea el subtítulo "Hechos y opiniones", previamente en este capítulo).

Una forma equitativa de resolver este tipo de estancamiento es dividir la diferencia en partes iguales. Si los vendedores en nuestro ejemplo usan esta técnica, regresarán a usted con una oferta de $282.500 —rebaja de $1.500 de su precio inicial *firme* de $284.000, y subirán a $1.500 su oferta *firme* de $281.000. Las concesiones mutuas de $1.500 son iguales a menos del 1 por ciento del valor justo de mercado de la vivienda, a un precio de venta de $282.500. Esto se considera exactitud en una transacción de bienes raíces.

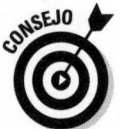

El compartir la diferencia no funciona en todas las situaciones. Sin embargo, es una manera justa de resolver rápidamente pequeñas diferencias de opinión (un pequeño porcentaje o menos, del precio de la propiedad) para que pueda cerrar la transacción y continuar con su vida normal.

Los Aspectos Más Delicados de la Negociación

Un mercado perfectamente equilibrado que no favorece ni al comprador ni al vendedor es raro. El mercado está casi siempre en un estado de cambio. Como resultado, el campo del juego normalmente se inclina hacia el comprador o el vendedor.

Cómo negociar cuando el campo de juego no está equilibrado

El presidente Lyndon Johnson era un político consumado. Él engatusó, prometió, torció el brazo, halagó, presionó, amenazó, mordió, aduló, atacó, o prometió favores, a otros políticos para que apoyaran sus legislaciones.

Los talentos de negociador del difunto presidente eran legendarios. Una vez, cuando fue acusado de usar tácticas no del todo éticas para obtener los votos necesarios para pasar uno de sus programas de la Gran Sociedad *(Great Society programs)*, LBJ solamente se encogió de hombros. "'Siento mucho que sientas de esa manera, hijo', se dice que él respondió, *'Todo lo que quería era mi injusta ventaja'*".

En un mundo perfecto, usted siempre tendría una ventaja injusta. Desgraciadamente, el mundo es imperfecto. No interesa lo bueno que usted sea como negociador, tarde o temprano tendrá que negociar desde una posición de desventaja. El truco en estas circunstancias es darse a sí mismo todas las ventajas posibles.

Los mercados del comprador y del vendedor

Al final de la década de los 80, muchos compradores de vivienda se quejaban amargamente de que los vendedores se estaban aprovechando injustamente de ellos. Dado el mercado desenfrenado del vendedor en esa época, no era difícil que los dueños de una propiedad de buen precio, recibieran múltiples ofertas por ella, mientras que sus agentes estaban aún clavando el cartel de "Se vende". (Un poco exagerado, pero usted entiende la idea.) Cinco años más tarde la bota con tachuelas estaba en el otro pie. En vez de un desequilibrio de la oferta y la demanda, hubo un desequilibrio de la demanda y la oferta. Los gritos angustiados ahora venían de los vendedores, que se quejaban de que los compradores se estaban aprovechando de *ellos*.

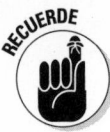

La parte en la posición desventajosa siempre caracteriza el mercado como "malo". Porque usted es un buscador de sabiduría y verdad, no se engañe. El mercado es en realidad, ni bueno ni malo; es impersonal. El mercado es el mercado. Quejarse y gemir por la injusta dinámica del mercado no le ayudará si está atrapado en un mercado del vendedor, lo mismo que las quejas de los vendedores no los ayudarán si están atrapados en las garras viciosas de un mercado del comprador.

La negociación desde una posición de desventaja

Las propiedades recientemente puestas en listas, que tienen el precio para venderse, a menudo reciben ofertas múltiples en un mercado del vendedor. Pero aun cuando el mercado no es de los vendedores, una vivienda con buen precio y un tentador listado nuevo, atrae muchas ofertas.

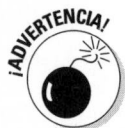

A menos que usted absolutamente tenga que tener una vivienda en particular, y el precio no es un obstáculo, tenga cuidado si entra en una guerra de competencia. Esas subastas pueden subir el precio de una vivienda muy por arriba del valor justo de mercado. Esa situación es excelente para el vendedor, pero es financieramente mala para usted. No queremos que usted pague demás.

Si realmente quiere una vivienda, y sabe que se harán otras ofertas, he aquí cómo puede mejorar sus posibilidades de ganar en una situación de ofertas múltiples.

- **Use información sobre ventas similares para predeterminar el precio más alto que pagará.** No se deje atrapar por el entusiasmo de una guerra de ofertas y no deje que las emociones anulen su sentido común. Asegúrese de haber leído el Capítulo 10, y aprenda cómo determinar el valor justo de mercado. Es necesario que fije el límite tope de la cantidad que ofrecerá. De otra manera, puede que pague mucho, en exceso.

- **Póngase en la posición del vendedor.** A los vendedores no les importa cuánto tiempo ha estado buscando una vivienda, o lo poco que puede pagar. Cuando reciben varias ofertas, los vendedores seleccionan la oferta que les da la mejor combinación de precio, términos y contingencias para la venta. Descubra cuáles son las necesidades de los vendedores antes de hacer una oferta. Los intereses personales de ellos siempre prevalecen.

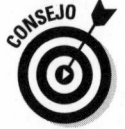

Un precio de compra alto no es la única forma de endulzar la transacción. Si tiene el dinero, haga un depósito muy grande (25 o 30 por ciento o más, del precio de la compra), así los vendedores saben que su préstamo seguramente va a ser aprobado. O usted puede ofrecerle al vendedor alquilarle su vivienda por un mes o dos después de cerrar el depósito en garantía (vea el Capítulo 14) o déle a los vendedores un tiempo largo para cerrar el depósito en garantía así ellos tienen bastante tiempo para encontrar otro hogar. También puede ofrecer comprarles la propiedad "como está" para que los vendedores no tengan que pagar ningún trabajo de reparación. Si hace esto, sin embargo, haga su oferta contingente con su aprobación de los informes de inspección para que pueda salirse de la transacción si la vivienda necesita demasiadas reparaciones.

✔ **Haga su mejor oferta al principio.** Los compradores que ganan la competencia de las ofertas, en las palabras del General Nathan Bedford Forrest, de la Guerra Civil, "los primeros con los más". Si quiere la casa, no se quede atrás en una situación de ofertas múltiples: quizás nunca tenga una segunda oportunidad para presentar la mejor oferta.

✔ **Consiga la aprobación previa de un préstamo.** Los vendedores informados se preocupan de la solidez financiera de los compradores potenciales. No quieren perder el tiempo con compradores que no reúnen los requisitos para obtener un préstamo. En igualdad de circunstancias, si usted ha sido previamente aprobado para un préstamo, (vea Capítulo 6), su oferta prevalecerá sobre las de otros compradores cuyo estatus financiero está en duda. Y si usted ya tiene la aprobación para un crédito, sabrá que usted no está perdiendo su tiempo ni dinero en una vivienda para la que, a lo mejor, no reúne los requisitos.

✔ **No haga su oferta sujeta a la venta de otra propiedad.** Como lo indicamos antes en este capítulo, en la sección de contingencias, si usted es dueño de una vivienda que *debe* vender para hacer un depósito para su nuevo hogar, es un problema. Probablemente estará compitiendo con otros compradores que no tienen esa limitación. Los vendedores tienen suficientes problemas vendiendo su propiedad como para preocuparse de la venta de su casa. ¿Por qué deberían ellos aceptar su oferta si pueden aceptar una sin la contingencia de una venta en ella? Las ofertas sujetas a la venta de otra propiedad no reciben respeto en una situación de ofertas múltiples.

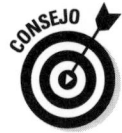

✔ **Si usted debe vender a fin de comprar, ponga su propiedad vieja en el mercado antes de hacer una búsqueda seria por otra vivienda.** Idealmente, usted tendría una oferta ratificada en su vieja vivienda antes de hacer una oferta para comprar una propiedad nueva. Entonces, aun con una cláusula estipulando que está sujeta a una venta, su posición será más fuerte en la negociación. Y no perderá tiempo preocupándose sobre cuánto dinero tendrá cuando se venda su casa y si se vende. Estipule el cierre del depósito en garantía a un plazo largo en la vivienda vieja y el derecho de alquilarla por varios meses después de la venta, así usted tendrá un tiempo adecuado para comprar la nueva propiedad.

Cómo descubrir a falsos vendedores

¿Por qué alguien querrá ser un vendedor falso? Es absurdo que algunas personas, sabiéndolo, malgasten tiempo y dinero en algo inútil como esto.

La palabra clave es *sabiéndolo*. Todos los vendedores comienzan el proceso de venta pensando que son sinceros. Sin embargo, a medida que la búsqueda de un comprador continúa, las circunstancias prueban que algunos vendedores son falsos.

Los falsos vendedores inteligentemente imitan a los genuinos. Al igual que los vendedores verdaderos, los vendedores falsos firman acuerdos para listar su propiedad, tienen carteles de "En venta" en sus jardines, lo publican en los periódicos, y abren sus viviendas al público los domingos. Exteriormente parecen ser el verdadero "ron". Si no sabe cómo detectar a los vendedores falsos, perderá su tiempo, energía y dinero con negociaciones infructuosas para comprar una vivienda que, en realidad, no está en venta.

La identificación de los vendedores que fingen serlo, es fácil una vez que aprende cómo se hace. Aquí le presentamos cinco pruebas simples que usted puede usar para detectar a vendedores falsos.

A veces, las viviendas se venden por un precio más bajo que el inicial

Amy era una compradora que sabía exactamente lo que quería. La vivienda de sus sueños no tenía que ser grande. Sin embargo, tenía que tener mucha luz y un ambiente espacioso, una cocina con aparatos para preparaciones de comida *"gourmet"*, vistas bonitas, un hermoso jardín y un garaje. Ella había estado buscando una casa por mucho tiempo porque se negaba a aceptar nada menos que la casa de sus sueños.

Amy tenía un buen agente. Cuando fue puesta a la venta una casa que reunía todos los requisitos de Amy por $295.000, ella y su agente estuvieron esperando en la puerta del frente el primer día que se abrió la vivienda para ser vista.

No estuvieron solas. Una muchedumbre de deseosos compradores y sus agentes estaban al frente de la casa también. Todos los aspectos de la propiedad, incluso su precio preciso y exacto, eran perfectos. La casa, definitivamente, tenía un precio para ser vendida.

El agente que hizo el listado les dijo a todos que se iban a aceptar las ofertas en dos días. Dado el alto interés de los compradores, la agente de Amy supo que habría múltiples ofertas. Ella sugirió que Amy podría quizás ganarle a los competidores si ofrecía $5.000 por encima del precio original. Basados en los precios de venta de propiedades similares en el vecindario, la agente dijo que la vivienda tenía un precio justo de mercado (o quizás era un poco inferior). Si todas las otras ofertas pagaban exactamente el precio original, los $300.000 ofrecidos por Amy se destacarían entre las de la muchedumbre.

Amy se negó. ¿Por qué gastar, razonó ella, $5.000 extra si no era necesario? Una oferta al precio total ciertamente no insultaría a los vendedores. Si no era suficiente dinero, Amy estaba segura de que los vendedores le darían una contraoferta.

Ella se equivocó. Los vendedores no hicieron contraofertas a ninguna de las ofertas recibidas, sino que, sencillamente aceptaron la oferta más alta, que no era la de Amy.

Amy tomó un riesgo calculado. Podría haber acertado. De hecho, hemos visto situaciones de múltiples ofertas en las cuales ninguna oferta fue igual al precio inicial. Las ofertas múltiples no garantizan que una vivienda se venderá al precio original o a uno más alto.

Cada situación es diferente y debe ser evaluada por sus propias características. Y no se olvide de mirar la información de las ventas de viviendas similares.

¿Son reales los vendedores?

La razón principal de que las viviendas no se vendan es que tienen precios irreales. Cuando la gente declara categóricamente que "no puede" vender una propiedad con un precio extremadamente alto, ellos se presentan a sí mismos como falsos compradores. Lo que en realidad dicen, es que se niegan a aceptar la opinión del mercado acerca del precio de su propiedad. Las personas que no escuchan razones no son vendedores —son propietarios que se disfrazan de vendedores.

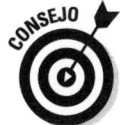

Los verdaderos vendedores pueden a veces poner un precio excesivo al principio. Sin embargo, a diferencia de los falsos, inevitablemente se dan cuenta de la realidad. Saben que tienen un problema si no reciben ofertas (o solamente unas ofertas muy bajas). Los vendedores auténticos aceptan la importancia de conocer los precios de ventas recientes de propiedades similares en el vecindario, para establecer el valor justo de mercado a la suya. Los vendedores genuinos son realistas.

¿Están motivados los vendedores?

La mayoría de los dueños no venden sus propiedades para generar comisiones para los agentes de bienes raíces. Generalmente están motivados por cambios en sus vidas, como las campanas que anuncian una boda, una transferencia de su empleo, un nacimiento o una muerte en sus familias. Quizás tienen un contrato para comprar otra vivienda, pero no pueden completar la compra hasta que se venda la suya. O su casa puede estar bajo embargo hipotecaria. Los auténticos vendedores siempre tienen la motivación de vender.

En situaciones desesperadas, como un embargo hipotecario o un divorcio, los vendedores a menudo instruyen a sus agentes a que no informen a nadie la razón de la venta. Sin embargo, si es posible, trate de saber por qué se vende la vivienda *antes* de hacer su oferta. El conocer la motivación de los vendedores le permite saber los términos de su oferta (es decir, cierre rápido del depósito en garantía, permitirle a los vendedores que alquilen la casa después de completar la transacción, y otros términos semejantes) a fin de acomodarse a las circunstancias de los vendedores.

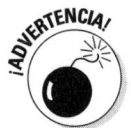

La falta de motivación es una gigantesca señal de peligro. Si los vendedores o sus agentes dicen que están examinando el mercado, escápese tan rápido como pueda en la dirección opuesta. Los vendedores sin motivación, no son vendedores.

¿Tienen los vendedores un plazo determinado?

Las fechas de vencimiento hacen que las cosas ocurran. Las fechas de vencimiento del vendedor son frecuentemente establecidas por cosas tales como: cuando los mellizos estén por nacer, cuando comience el año escolar, cuando tiene que comenzar un trabajo nuevo en otra ciudad, y otros más. Los vendedores genuinos siempre tienen una fecha fija en la que deben completar su venta.

El tiempo es una herramienta excelente para la negociación. Si usted no tiene prisa para comprar, y los vendedores deben vender de inmediato, (si no antes) el tiempo es su amigo y su enemigo. Por el contrario, si usted tiene menos de cuatro semanas para encontrar un lugar donde vivir antes de que los chicos comiencen la escuela, el reloj está en el otro lado. Idealmente, usted conoce la fecha de vencimiento de los vendedores, pero ellos no conocen la suya. La mayoría de las negociaciones ocurren a las 11.00 horas, 59 minutos y 59 segundos antes de las 12.00 horas, del vencimiento del plazo.

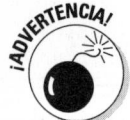

Puede verse en problemas serios si tiene una fecha fija y los vendedores no tienen ninguna. Si usted revela esta información a los vendedores, pueden usarla para presionarlo sin misericordia. Esté alerta a los retrasos. No deje que el tiempo lo intimide —y guarde sus plazos en su memoria.

¿Son sinceros los vendedores?

Los vendedores auténticos tienen una franqueza extraordinaria acerca de la parte estructural de la propiedad, de su estado financiero y legal. Saben que esconder información vital pone en peligro la venta y puede conducir a un juicio legal. La declaración de los problemas posibles hecha al principio, por otra parte, les da a todos el tiempo necesario para resolverlos. Los vendedores verdaderos no piensan que deben mantenerse "alertas al comprador."

Si continuamente se encuentra con sorpresas desagradables, es porque está tratando con vendedores falsos. Las personas francas tienen sólo una defensa contra los vendedores astutos que están participando en un juego caro, y posiblemente devastador de "Tengo un secreto" (*I've Got a Secret*): cancele la transacción.

¿Son los vendedores cooperativos?

Los auténticos vendedores buscan las maneras de hacer que las transacciones se deslicen sin problemas. Trabajan con usted para resolver problemas, en lugar de perder tiempo tratando de determinar quién tiene la culpa si algo no sale bien. Los vendedores genuinos tienen la actitud de que juntos podemos hacer que esto suceda. Ellos son buenos para cerrar las transacciones y no para destruirlas.

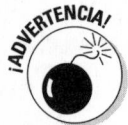

El comportamiento errático es una señal de peligro. Si los vendedores de pronto empiezan a no cumplir con los vencimientos del contrato, o niegan su cooperación, es posible que hayan perdido su motivación de vender. Quizás se pospuso la boda, o no se concretó el trabajo nuevo. Cualquiera que sea la razón, la gente a veces se convierte de vendedor de bienes raíces a falso vendedor, a mitad de camino. Vea por qué los vendedores están actuando de manera extraña tan pronto como note el cambio, y quizás pueda hacerle frente al problema. Si ignora las señales de peligro, nunca sabrá lo qué pasó cuando todo explote al final.

Haga una oferta baja

Una oferta baja es la que es muy inferior al precio real de la propiedad según el valor justo de mercado. Un ejemplo de este tipo es la oferta de $150.000 para una vivienda que vale hasta el último centavo $200.000.

¿Quién hace ofertas bajas? A veces, es alguien que se graduó de uno de eso seminarios de dudosa reputación, que prometen enseñarle el método para hacerse rico rápidamente en la industria inmobiliaria. Otra oferta baja puede llegar de alguien que está buscando a vendedores en situaciones financieras desesperadas. Con más frecuencia, sin embargo, es una táctica de nego-ciación usada por gente que categóricamente dice: "Nadie paga nunca el precio original. Usted siempre tiene que empezar con una oferta baja para terminar con un precio justo".

Por supuesto, esas declaraciones no son ciertas. Cuando investiga los pre-cios, usted aprende cuál es la diferencia entre una propiedad con un precio realista y las que tienen precios excesivos y engañosos. (Vea el Capítulo 10 para refrescar su memoria.)

¿Por qué, generalmente, no es buena idea presentar una oferta baja?

Como lo dijimos antes en este capítulo, ofrecer poco por una casa con un buen precio de venta, rompe la primera regla de una buena oferta: ofrezca un precio justo basado en los precios de venta de casas similares. Como los buenos negociadores entienden ambos lados del asunto, imagine que usted es el vendedor de una vivienda que está valuada a un precio tan cerca como es humanamente posible, al valor justo de mercado.

Después de varios días de que su casa sale al mercado, recibe una oferta con un precio de compra absurdamente bajo. Una vez que las venas de su cuello se normalicen, ¿qué conclusión puede formarse de los compradores que intencionalmente ofrecen precios bajos?

- ✔ **Tómelo con calma, los compradores, obviamente, no han investigado los precios de venta de las propiedades similares.** Porque son exage-radamente ignorantes acerca del precio justo de mercado, ¿por qué tratar de educarlos?

- ✔ **A lo mejor, los compradores piensan que usted no sabe realmente cuánto vale su propiedad, y están tratando de explotar su ignorancia.** (Esas venas del cuello comienzan a hincharse y a latir otra vez.)

- ✔ **Quizás los compradores están tratando de robarle su casa, basados en la impresión equivocada de que usted está desesperado por venderla.** Hay un nombre para los mal intencionados que se aprovechan de su desgracia: *buitres.*

Ninguna de estas conclusiones es de alguna forma favorable. Como vendedor, probablemente usted da una de las siguientes respuestas a los compradores que ofrecen un precio bajo a su propiedad bien valuada:

- **Hágales saber a los compradores que sus ofertas son inaceptables, y dígale a su agente que les conteste con un mensaje diciendo que no les vendería la vivienda a ellos así fueran los últimos compradores de este planeta.** ¿Por qué hacerle una contraoferta a gente que es estúpida o sinvergüenza?

- **Haga una contraoferta con el precio original.** Para demostrar su desprecio por los compradores, usted les despreciará todos y cada uno de los términos y condiciones de sus ofertas. (Dos pueden participar en este juego.)

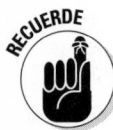

Los compradores que ofrecen un precio más bajo por propiedades que tienen un precio justo de venta —por vendedores que pueden esperar una oferta mejor— destruyen cualquier posibilidad de desarrollar una confianza mutua, y el sentido de relación equitativa sobre la que sea posible conducir una negociación cooperativa. Está bien buscar una propiedad a bajo precio, pero usted debe encontrar a un vendedor motivado y además, no apunte muy bajo. El comenzar al 25 por ciento por debajo del valor de la vivienda generalmente no funciona, excepto cuando el vendedor está desesperado.

Cuándo se justifican las ofertas bajas

Hay una gran diferencia entre presentar una oferta que es la mínima posible del valor justo de mercado, y una que es más baja que el valor real. Imagine que usted ofrece $280.000 por una vivienda en venta por $299.500. Usted basa el precio de su oferta en el hecho de que otras viviendas similares en el vecindario se vendieron recientemente en una gama de precios de $280.000 a $295.000. Usted está en la serie más baja de precios según el valor justo de mercado. Los vendedores están del lado de los más altos. Ambos son realistas.

Si su oferta está basada en las ventas reales de casas similares, no va a insultar al vendedor. Sin embargo, una oferta tan baja despertará un vivo debate porque los dos van a intentar defender su perspectiva. Entrando al proceso por el lado bajo del valor justo de mercado de la propiedad está bien mientras usted tenga mucho tiempo para negociar, y una razón para creer que el vendedor está motivado.

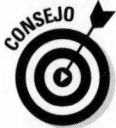

En situaciones como la precedente, su mayor posibilidad de éxito está en un análisis enciclopédico del mercado de las viviendas similares, y en un agente que *personalmente* verificó los precios más bajos de las viviendas similares. Siga las instrucciones que presentamos en el Capítulo 10.

Una oferta baja se justifica solamente cuando *no es más baja* que el precio justo. Paradójicamente, algunos vendedores provocan ofertas bajas por la forma poco inteligente de poner el precio. Estos vendedores insisten en dejar la puerta abierta para negociar sus precios porque ellos "saben" que los compradores nunca pagan el precio original.

¿Le parece haberlo oído antes? Desgraciadamente, esta profecía se hace realidad. Cuando los compradores que conocen los valores de la propiedad hacen una oferta para una vivienda con un precio excesivamente alto, su oferta inicial normalmente está del lado más bajo de los precios, a fin de guardar espacio para negociar. Puede ver que lo que se siembra se cosecha.

Imagínese que el valor justo de mercado de una vivienda es de $300.000. Si los vendedores ponen esta propiedad en el mercado a $360.000, para tener 20 por ciento disponibles para negociar, y usted ofrece $240.000 por la misma razón, usted y el vendedor comienzan con una diferencia de $120.000. Se necesita una montaña de negociaciones para llegar al otro lado cuando hay una diferencia tan grande.

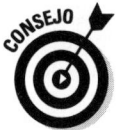

No participe en ese juego tonto de ellos, excepto si tiene tiempo para desperdiciar. Haga una oferta inicial al precio más bajo del valor justo de mercado, y vea cómo responden los vendedores. Si ellos se niegan a aceptar la evidencia real de la venta reciente de propiedades similares en el vecindario, no pierda su valioso tiempo tratando de educarlos. Ellos no son vendedores todavía —son propietarios disfrazados de vendedores. Si quiere la vivienda, espere el momento oportuno. No proceda hasta que ellos se eduquen y bajen su precio, o hasta que el agente de ellos le haga saber que son vendedores motivados y que no rechazarán ninguna oferta sensata.

Cómo negociar los créditos del depósito en garantía

El ponerle un precio bajo "para que se venda" a una vivienda, no es siempre lo suficiente para que ella se venda, especialmente si es un mercado de compradores flojo. Los vendedores a menudo descubren que tienen que darles a los compradores dinero en la forma de concesiones financieras pagadas para cerrar la transacción. Las dos concesiones más comunes son los costos de cierre que no se repiten, y los costos para el trabajo de las reparaciones.

Costos de cierre que no se repiten

Desde el comienzo, algunos vendedores son muy francos y le dicen que ellos pagarán los costos que no se repiten si el hacerlo ayuda a cerrar la transacción. *Los costos que no se repiten* son cargos que se pagan sólo una vez por cosas como su valuación, puntos del préstamo, informe del crédito, e inspecciones de la propiedad. Si ha leído el Capítulo 3, sabe que aquí estamos hablando de mucho dinero. Los costos de cierre son del 3 al 5 por ciento del precio de compra.

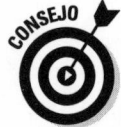

Aun si los vendedores no ofrecen pagar los costos de cierre que no se repiten, pedir estas concesiones como uno de los términos de su oferta, normalmente no daña la transacción. Hay dos excepciones generales a esta regla, una es cuando existe un mercado fuerte para los vendedores, o cuando está en una situación de ofertas múltiples.

He aquí cómo funcionan los créditos. Digamos que usted ha firmado un contrato para comprar una vivienda por $250.000. Tiene $55.000 en efectivo, y el oficial de custodia de la garantía le acaba de decir que tendrá gastos que no se repiten, equivalentes al 4 por ciento ($10.000) del precio de compra.

A esta altura, usted estará preguntándose "¿Por qué no reducir el precio de compra a $240.000 en vez de pedirles un crédito de $10.000 a los vendedores?" Después de todo, el beneficio neto de la venta para los vendedores es el mismo de cualquier manera, y la reducción del precio de compra es sencillamente menos complicado. Además, como los impuestos de la propiedad se basan con frecuencia en el precio de compra, un precio de compra más bajo probablemente disminuirá un poco sus impuestos anuales.

La razón es: si no tiene mucho dinero en efectivo, como la gran mayoría de los compradores, un crédito es una ayuda más grande que la reducción del precio. Si tiene que pagar $10.000 en costos de cierre, no tendrá suficiente dinero de sobra para hacer un depósito inicial del 20 por ciento ($48.000) para su hogar de $240.000. Con menos del 20 por ciento de depósito inicial, el costo mensual de su préstamo aumentará porque tendrá que pagar un interés más alto en su hipoteca, además del costo de un seguro privado de la hipoteca. Tampoco tendrá dinero de sobra en efectivo para emergencias. En estas circunstancias, probablemente decidirá comprar una propiedad más barata.

Compare ese escenario con el pago de $250.000 por la vivienda y lograr un crédito de los vendedores por costos de cierre que no se repiten. Después de poner el 20 por ciento en efectivo de depósito ($50.000) para obtener el préstamo con la tasa de interés más baja, todavía tiene $5.000 en el banco gracias al crédito de $10.000. El crédito sirve para sellar el negocio.

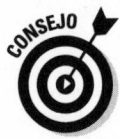

Si usted tiene mucho dinero en efectivo, le conviene más obtener una reducción del precio en vez de un crédito. En la mayoría de las zonas, cuanto más bajo sea su precio de compra, más bajo será su impuesto anual a la propiedad. Pero sepa que casi todos los agentes van a tratar de convencerlo de que es mejor el crédito, porque la reducción del precio de compra disminuye su comisión.

Trabajos de reparación

Típicamente, ni usted ni los vendedores saben cuánto trabajo de reparación puede ser necesario, cuando presenta su oferta. Por eso, los contratos de compra tienen provisiones para permitir negociaciones adicionales con relación al crédito para los trabajos de reparación, después que se hayan hecho todas las inspecciones necesarias.

Si los inspectores de la propiedad encuentran que es necesaria muy poca o ninguna reparación, tiene poco o nada que negociar. Sin embargo, imagine que los inspectores descubren que la vivienda que usted quiere necesita $25.000 de trabajos de reparación a causa de las termitas y porque la madera seca se ha podrido y está desintegrándose, reparación de los cimientos y un techo nuevo. Trabajos de reparación a alto costo pueden matar la transacción.

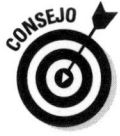

Ver para creer. Le recomendamos seriamente que usted y el agente del vendedor estén presentes, si es posible, durante las inspecciones de la propiedad para que ambos vean personalmente el daño real. Y cuando reciba los informes de la inspección, úselos como herramientas de negociación. Déles copias de los informes a los vendedores para que los revisen, antes de reunirse con ellos para negociar un crédito por el costo de las reparaciones.

Éste es el momento de la verdad en la mayoría de las ventas inmobiliarias. Los vendedores generalmente no quieren pagar por los trabajos de reparación. Usted tampoco quiere. El negocio no se realizará si este impasse no se puede resolver.

En este punto de las negociaciones, es crítico que el vendedor se dé cuenta que el valor de su propiedad se ha reducido por el monto de las reparaciones necesarias. Si las casas similares sin termitas o daños en la madera, con cimientos sólidos, y con buenos techos se venden por $250.000, esta vivienda vale solamente $225.000 en su condición presente. Dado su valor reducido, un 80 por ciento del préstamo es $180.000 —no $200.000 basado en un valor justo de mercado de $250.000. Si usted puede solicitar un préstamo de solamente $180.000, y los vendedores se niegan a reducir el precio de venta de $250.000 a $225.000, usted tiene que anular la compra.

Los vendedores pueden negarse a pagar por las reparaciones encontradas por los inspectores que usted empleó. Los vendedores pueden discutir sobre la imparcialidad o validez de la información de sus inspecciones y ordenar sus propias inspecciones para verificar o refutar las suyas. Los vendedores pueden también amenazar con quebrar el contrato si usted no retira sus condiciones.

Quienes tratan de castigar al mensajero, están normalmente cometiendo un gran error. Usted no trajo el daño consigo cuando llegó, y (por suerte para usted) no se lo llevará consigo cuando se vaya. Le guste o no, el vendedor está enterrado con la propiedad. Si hacen que usted se retire, pueden aún tener una obligación legal de decirles a otros compradores lo que usted ha descubierto. Esta declaración probablemente disminuirá el precio que cualquier comprador futuro pagará por su casa. Teniendo todo esto en cuenta, solucionar los problemas con usted será probablemente más rápido (y no más caro) para el vendedor que esperar a otro comprador.

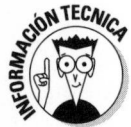

Los prestamistas también participan en los problemas de reparaciones necesarias. Ellos reciben copias de los informes de las inspecciones cuando los prestatarios les dicen que existen serios problemas, cuando su tasación indica una propiedad con obvios problemas que requieren reparaciones mayores, o cuando el contrato de compra contiene un crédito por reparaciones de mayor cuantía. Cuando la proporción entre el préstamo sobre la propiedad y el valor de la misma excede el 80 por ciento, los prestamistas ayudan activamente a los compradores a resolver los problemas de reparaciones.

Se pueden resolver problemas de varias maneras:

✔ **Idealmente, los vendedores depositan suficiente dinero en el depósito en garantía para cubrir reparaciones, con instrucciones para que el oficial de custodia pague a los contratistas cuando el trabajo esté terminado.** Esta estrategia tiene varias ventajas. Usted puede supervisar el trabajo para asegurarse de que los contratistas de su elección estén haciendo el trabajo satisfactoriamente. Los vendedores no tienen que sufrir mientras el trabajo se hace cuando todavía viven en la vivienda, y ellos no tienen ninguna responsabilidad por la calidad del trabajo. Por último, el prestamista sabe que el trabajo se hará.

✔ **Por otro lado, el prestamista retiene una porción del monto total del préstamo en la libreta de una cuenta de ahorros hasta que el trabajo de reparación se complete.** En casos en que el trabajo de reparaciones sea de mayor importancia, el prestamista puede negarse a proveer los fondos del préstamo hasta que se corrijan los problemas.

✔ **Los vendedores pueden dar un crédito por el trabajo de reparación directamente a los compradores cuando se cierra el depósito en garantía.** Normalmente, las entidades prestamistas no aprueban esta forma de proceder porque crea la incertidumbre de si realmente las reparaciones serán finalizadas. Si no lo son, el prestamista ve en peligro la seguridad de su préstamo.

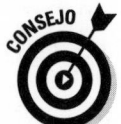

Usted puede hacer que los vendedores se sientan mejor ofreciéndoles pedir licitaciones del trabajo a varios contratistas licenciados y de buena reputación. Mientras que el licitador con la oferta más baja haga un trabajo de buena calidad en un tiempo definido, usted y los vendedores se benefician. Este esfuerzo adicional de su parte les muestra a los vendedores que no quiere hacerse rico a costa de ellos, y que todo lo que quiere es obtener lo que usted creyó que compraba al principio: una vivienda bien mantenida, con buenos cimientos y un techo sin goteras. La empatía es una táctica de negociación excelente.

Capítulo 13

Cómo Inspeccionar y Proteger Su Vivienda

Dado el alto precio de las viviendas hoy en día, sería tonto no inspeccionar cuidadosamente la vivienda que usted planifica comprar, antes de comprarla. Omitir la inspección para ahorrarse, relativamente, unos pocos dólares podría ser el error más grande que usted cometa. Piense en el fracaso más grande que usted haya sufrido, y multiplíquelo por cien. Esto le da una idea de la magnitud del error que usted puede cometer si compra una casa sin haberla inspeccionado *minuciosamente* primero, desde los cimientos hasta el techo.

¿Por qué estamos tan obsesionados con la inspección de la propiedad? Bueno, de acuerdo a un estudio auspiciado por el periódico *The Wall Street Journal* y conducido por el economista de bienes raíces Robert Sheehan, aproximadamente dos de cada cinco viviendas tienen al menos un defecto grande. Si la próxima vez que usted camina por la calle, las probabilidades de que fuese golpeado por un carro fuesen dos de cada cinco, ¡seguramente usted sería más cuidadoso de notar el tráfico que pasa antes de cruzar la calle!

Cómo Llevar a Cabo una Buena Inspección

Las condiciones físicas de una vivienda afectan muchísimo su valor. Usted se sentiría terrible si pagara una cantidad muy alta por una vivienda que pensó que estaba en las mejores condiciones, y que descubrió después de comprarla que estaba llena de defectos que van a costarle un montón de dinero.

Sin embargo, a menos que usted sea un profesional en inspección de propiedades, probablemente usted no tendrá ni la más remota idea de cuántos trabajos de reparación necesitará la casa con solo mirarla.

Créalo o no, comprar viviendas era aún más arriesgado hace una generación. La actitud que prevalecía en aquel entonces era simplemente: "Comprador, tenga cuidado".

Hoy en día, afortunadamente, la situación ha mejorado. La mayoría de los estados (aunque no todos) requieren que los vendedores y los agentes de bienes raíces, revelen a los compradores potenciales, de manera total e inmediata, todos los problemas o fallas mecánicas, estructurales y legales *conocidos* que estén asociados con la propiedad residencial ocupada por el propietario. Si esta tendencia continúa, llegará el momento cuando la advertencia diga: "Vendedores y agentes de bienes raíces, tengan cuidado". (Los agentes de bienes raíces también son responsables si no ponen al descubierto un problema conocido de la propiedad.)

No baje la guardia. A pesar de que el mercado de bienes raíces está más orientado hacia el consumidor en estos días comparado a como solía estarlo hace un tiempo, no se deje llevar por un falso sentido de confianza. Los *defectos latentes* —problemas escondidos en la vivienda que usted esté comprando y que los vendedores o agentes de bienes raíces no conocen— pueden meterlo en un montón de dificultades presupuestarias después que usted lleve a cabo la compra.

Si usted no ha leído aún el Capítulo 12, déle un vistazo a la sección sobre cómo negociar, ya sea un crédito para una reparación que tendrá que realizar, o una reducción en el precio. También, usted puede aprender cómo usar la inspección de modo que pueda recuperar el costo de ella varias veces.

Todas las propiedades deberían ser inspeccionadas

Inspeccionar una vivienda muchas veces es mucho mejor que inspeccionarla pocas veces. Suponga que usted gasta $350 para que un inspector profesional lleve a cabo una inspección completa de la vivienda que usted quiere comprar, y usted se da cuenta que no hay ningún problema con la casa. ¿Malgastó usted su dinero? Realmente no. Ahora usted puede dormir tranquilo sabiendo que su casa no necesita ninguna reparación.

Si por el contrario, usted omite la inspección para ahorrarse $350 y más tarde descubre que su casa necesita reparaciones por el monto de $35.000, usted termina gastando $100 en reparaciones por cada dólar que usted supuestamente se "ahorró". Muy bueno, ¿verdad? Asimismo, puede "ahorrarse" dinero no poniendo monedas en los parquímetros y pensar que las costosas multas por estacionamiento son parte de la experiencia normal de estacionar.

La siguiente es una lista de propiedades que *tienen* que ser inspeccionadas antes de la compra:

- ✔ **Casas usadas:** es más probable que usted desee que se hagan las inspecciones si su "nueva" casa es la casa que alguien más ha usado. Obviamente, mientras más vieja sea la casa, más grande es la probabilidad de que usted encontrará defectos en sus sistemas mecánicos y estructurales.

- ✔ **Casas nuevas:** aun si usted está comprando una casa recientemente construida en la que nadie ha vivido, es prudente hacer que la inspeccionen totalmente. Sólo porque la construcción es nueva, no significa que la vivienda fue construida adecuadamente. Créalo o no, las viviendas nuevas a menudo tienen fallas de construcción, y a veces bien grandes. Esto ocurre porque algunas compañías constructoras no son competentes, o hacen trabajos de menos calidad para ahorrarse dinero y aumentar sus ganancias.

- ✔ **Condominios (propiedad horizontal):** usted necesita realizar una inspección antes de comprar una unidad en un condominio. No se olvide que cuando usted compra este tipo de propiedad, usted también está comprando de alguna manera el edificio completo donde la propiedad está ubicada (vea el Capítulo 8). Como copropietario del edificio, usted tiene que pagar una cuota proporcional al costo de los trabajos de reparación de las áreas comunes, tales como el techo, el sistema de calentamiento o la fundación.

- ✔ **Casas tipo "Townhouse", apartamentos cooperativos, y todas las otras formas de propiedades compartidas:** mire el punto anterior acerca de los apartamentos. Una propiedad compartida no lo excluye de lo que hemos hablado. Usted aún necesita inspeccionar la propiedad.

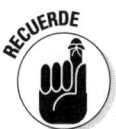

Todas las propiedades necesitan ser inspeccionadas. ¡Punto! Inspeccione residencias que tengan garaje separados o garajes incluidos, viviendas unifamiliares separadas, multifamiliares, edificios de apartamentos, cooperativas, casas tipo "townhouse" y cualquier otra cosa que tenga un cimiento y un techo. Si usted está gastando una gran suma de dinero en comprar una propiedad, proteja su inversión mandándola a inspeccionar.

Los dos tipos de defectos que puede tener una vivienda: Evidente y latente

Los defectos de las viviendas son de dos tipos generales: evidente y latente. Los *defectos evidentes* son aquellos que están a la vista para cualquiera que los note. Usted no necesita un inspector profesional para que le señale algunas cosas muy obvias, a la vista, como manchas de agua en el techo, grietas en las paredes o un sótano inundado. En cambio, usted sí necesita un profesional que le diga si estos problemas son consecuencias de defectos más graves o son simplemente problemas circunstanciales.

Los defectos latentes pueden ser más catastróficos financieramente hablando que los defectos evidentes, porque están escondidos. Como en un juego a las escondidas, usted debe encontrar los defectos latentes o, literalmente, pagar las consecuencias costosas.

Los defectos latentes están fuera de nuestra vista —detrás de las paredes o confinados en áreas inaccesibles debajo de la casa y arriba en el ático, lejos del campo visual de la persona. Algunos ejemplos de fallas físicas latentes son: un cableado defectuoso, daño por termitas, un intercambiador de calor roto en la calefacción, y problemas relacionados con la salud y seguridad, tales como plomo en las tuberías de agua y asbesto en el aislante térmico.

Los problemas legales, tales como violación de las normas de zonificación, y reclamos de títulos fraudulentos, ilustran otra clase de fallas latentes que solamente los expertos pueden detectar.

Señales de peligro de defectos evidentes

No tiene que ser un inspector profesional para poder darle a la vivienda un vistazo por encima. Aún el más novato puede verificar la presión de agua y abrir las llaves de agua para ver si gotean. También son pruebas fáciles, pero efectivas, el apagar y prender los interruptores de la luz y bajar el agua de los inodoros para fijarse si trabajan adecuadamente. Abra el refrigerador para ver si está frío por dentro. Prenda la estufa para ver si las hornillas calientan. Usted podría sorprenderse de cuántos defectos puede descubrir con estas pruebas tan sencillas.

De la misma manera, usted puede reconocer las señales de posibles problemas estructurales serios, aun si usted nunca ha tenido entrenamiento formal para ello; todo lo que tiene que saber es qué buscar mientras recorre la propiedad. Aunque nosotros le aconsejamos que contrate un inspector profesional, aquí le presentamos una lista de posibles señales de peligro que aun un comprador con conocimientos limitados, de cómo funcionan los sistemas en una vivienda, debería ser capaz de notar:

- ✔ **Grietas:** revise la fundación de la propiedad, las paredes internas y externas, la chimenea, los pisos de concreto (sótano, garaje y otros pisos), y la acera para detectar cualquier grieta grande. Cualquier grieta en la cual cabe un lápiz es una grieta grande. Busque grietas verticales en cualquier pared, y grietas largas horizontales o diagonales en las paredes exteriores.

✔ **Humedad:** busque manchas de agua en techos, paredes y pisos. Toque las paredes del sótano para sentir alguna humedad. Si percibe algún olor mohoso, encuentre de dónde sale dicho olor. Trate de detectar problemas de drenaje adentro y afuera viendo si hay agua estancada. Una bomba de achique en el sótano o garaje es un hecho que debe llamar su atención.

✔ **Adherencia:** todas las puertas del exterior, interior, del garaje y gabinetes deben abrir y cerrar fácilmente.

✔ **Holgura:** usted no debería poder ver luz alrededor de los sellos de las ventanas, puertas o tragaluces.

✔ **Desniveles o desigualdades:** los pisos no deben tener pendiente, y las paredes no deben tener protuberancias.

✔ **Insectos:** si la vivienda que usted está comprando está hecha de madera o de madera y estuco, podría tener problemas con insectos que comen madera ú otros animales. Túneles de barro a lo largo de la fundación de la vivienda o en el sótano, son una señal de infestación de termitas. Mire cuidadosamente aquellas áreas de la propiedad que tienen contacto con la tierra —como la fundación, porches, garajes y la cerca— a ver si nota la madera descompuesta o podrida.

✔ **Deslizamientos de tierra:** revise las laderas que están pegadas a la parte posterior de la vivienda para ver si tienen redes protectoras o muestran evidencia de deslizamientos de tierra o barro recientes.

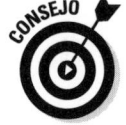

Antes de que su vivienda sea inspeccionada, infórmele al inspector de cualquier falla que usted descubrió. Deje que sea este profesional quien los revise y determine si son defectos grandes o simplemente defectos pequeños que usted puede corregir rápidamente, y sin incurrir en gastos altos. Una puerta que no abre suavemente, por ejemplo, puede indicar ya sea que la vivienda tiene un problema costoso relacionado con la fundación, o simplemente que la puerta absorbió humedad porque no fue sellada debidamente.

Los tipos de inspecciones de propiedad

¿Qué inspecciones debe realizar para proteger su inversión? Eso depende del lugar en el que vive en el país, de cómo la vivienda es construida, y qué planifica hacer usted con la propiedad después de comprarla. Aquí le vamos a presentar los tres tipos más comunes de inspección que se realizan —los cuales nosotros recomendamos que se hagan *después* que el vendedor ha aceptado su oferta de compra, pero *antes* de que se eliminen las condiciones relacionadas con la inspección. De esta manera, usted puede negociar la reparación de los problemas que se descubran con la inspección, como recomendamos en el Capítulo 12:

✔ **Inspección de componentes interiores y exteriores antes a la compra:** no importa si usted está comprando una cabaña de madera en el campo, o un apartamento en un edificio de 20 pisos construido de concreto y acero en una zona urbana, usted necesita una inspección completa del interior y el exterior de la propiedad. Dicha inspección debe cubrir áreas tales como el techo y los canales recolectores de agua de lluvia, la plomería, los sistemas eléctricos, los sistemas de aire acondicionado y calentamiento, el aislamiento, detectores de humo, cocina, baños, y la fundación. La inspección también debe señalar cualquier peligro de salud, de seguridad y del ambiente. Este tipo de inspección generalmente toma varias horas para ser realizada, y cuesta entre $300 y $600, dependiendo de cuan grande es la propiedad, y el nivel de detalle que ella cubra.

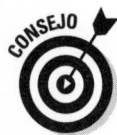

No se sorprenda si el inspector le sugiere que se realicen inspecciones adicionales. Los inspectores buenos son inspectores generales y están entrenados para identificar todas las áreas problemáticas. De la misma manera como lo hacen los doctores que son médicos generales, los inspectores recomiendan a sus clientes consultar con los especialistas, tales como los especialistas en techos, ingenieros civiles (para la estructura), e inspectores de control de plagas, si ellos descubren un problema que va más allá de su área de experticia. Los inspectores de propiedad saben que usted no puede tomar buenas decisiones a menos que usted tenga la mejor información posible.

✔ **Inspección para detectar plagas:** los climas cálidos, tales como los de las zonas del sur y el oeste, son una bendición a medias porque a usted no es el único a quién le encanta un clima cálido y suave. También le agrada a las termitas, a las hormigas carpinteras, a los escarabajos come-madera, a los hongos, y a otras infestaciones e infecciones relacionadas con la madera. Si éste es un problema en su zona, usted también necesita una inspección de plagas, la cual generalmente cuesta entre $150 y $400.

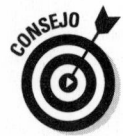

Las inspecciones para detectar plagas son muy limitadas en su alcance — los inspectores revisan si existen daños a la propiedad causados solo por los insectos que destruyen madera (infestaciones) y otros organismos (como las infecciones de madera podrida y hongos). Aunque algunas viviendas hechas de madera o madera y estuco son el objeto principal de destrucción de estas plagas, también las viviendas de adobe se encuentran expuestas a este riesgo. Si usted va a ordenar una inspección de plagas, ésta debe ser hecha además de la inspección de los componentes internos y externos que ya hablamos, y no ser un reemplazo de esta última.

✔ **Inspección del arquitecto o del contratista:** si está comprando una casa que requiere muchas reparaciones, usted necesita un contratista en el equipo de trabajo o un arquitecto. Estas personas pueden ayudarlo a llevar a cabo el trabajo de reparación, y ayudarlo en la planificación de una renovación grande en la vivienda, tal como agregar una habitación o instalar un nuevo baño. El arquitecto o el contratista pueden decirle si lo que usted quiere hacer es estructuralmente viable y si cumple con los códigos de planificación local, como las restricciones de altura y cobertura de terrenos. El inspector también puede darle un estimado del costo y del tiempo que puede tomar el proyecto.

Arquitectos y contratistas normalmente no cobran por las inspecciones iniciales de la propiedad porque quieren ser contratados por usted para los trabajos requeridos. Aunque estos profesionales proveen un servicio muy valioso, tome sus opiniones con cierta reserva. No espere que ellos le den una evaluación totalmente objetiva respecto a si usted debe comprar la propiedad, porque ciertamente ellos estarían encantados de hacerle los trabajos respectivos.

Cómo inspeccionar a los inspectores

Desafortunadamente, algunas personas que se llaman a sí mismos "inspectores de viviendas" no tienen ni la experiencia ni el entrenamiento para hacer inspecciones antes de la compra. Para empeorar esta situación, la mayoría de los estados no certifican, o dan permisos o regulan a los inspectores de vivienda. Si usted tiene una tabla para sujetar papeles, una camioneta, y una actitud de "familiaridad" cuando visita las propiedades, usted también puede ser un inspector en casi cualquier parte del país.

Lo que es peor, algunos contratistas inspeccionan su vivienda y luego llevan a cabo los trabajos de reparación que descubren durante sus propias inspecciones. Esto debe ser una señal para saber que algo no anda bien. Los contratistas sin ningún escrúpulo pueden —y de hecho lo hacen— manejar este conflicto para su provecho, "encontrando defectos" para ellos mismos repararlos.

Una manera de resolver este problema es contratar a alguien que únicamente haga inspecciones. De hecho, un número creciente de inspectores de propiedad son exactamente eso: inspectores profesionales de propiedad, y no contratistas. Pero esta distinción va más allá de la semántica. Hacer inspecciones requiere una habilidad especial que no todos los contratistas, ingenieros y arquitectos tienen.

Los inspectores profesionales están específicamente entrenados para hacer inspecciones y, solamente inspecciones; sólo trabajan y viven de sus honorarios como inspectores. Ellos no hacen trabajos de reparación, lo que elimina la tentación de encontrar problemas que no existen durante sus inspecciones.

Cómo seleccionar un inspector

¿Cómo puede encontrar un inspector de vivienda competente? Pregúnteles, a amigos y colegas que hayan comprado recientemente viviendas, a quién contrataron para la inspección de su propiedad. También, pídale a su agente de bienes raíces que le dé una lista de inspectores de propiedad. Sin embargo, tenga cuidado con inspectores que son muy populares entre los agentes, ya que esa popularidad *podría* venir de su actitud de ser muy complacientes en sus inspecciones, y no echar a perder el negocio de la compra. Consulte también las páginas amarillas de la guía telefónica local, bajo el título "Servicios de inspección de propiedades" o "Servicios de inspección de viviendas". Si varias fuentes recomiendan la misma persona, entonces probablemente usted ha encontrado un buen inspector.

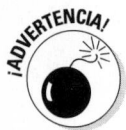

Solo porque una persona tiene un título emitido por una organización con un nombre llamativo, no significa que ese individuo sea un inspector de propiedad competente. Desafortunadamente, el criterio que algunas asociaciones "profesionales" utilizan para aceptar a sus miembros, es que éstos puedan pagar la cuota de membresía anual y otros gastos iniciales. No importa cuán impresionante sea el título, no se deje engañar por lo que podría ser un pedazo de papel sin valor alguno.

La *Asociación americana de inspectores de vivienda* (*American Society of Home Inspectors* [*ASHI,* por sus siglas en inglés]) es una asociación profesional de inspectores independientes. Sólo porque un inspector es miembro de *ASHI* no garantiza que le hará una buena inspección, pero ciertamente aumenta las probabilidades de que usted esté trabajando con una persona competente. Usted no puede ser parte de la asociación con sólo pagar la cuota. Todos los miembros certificados por la *ASHI* han realizado al menos 250 inspecciones de propiedad, y han pasado dos exámenes escritos de conocimiento en la materia, como requisito previo para ser miembro. Los miembros de la *ASHI* tienen que cumplir con los estándares de trabajo de la asociación, y con los requerimientos de educación continua y de ética. Para información sobre miembros en su zona, llame a la asociación al 800-743-2744 o visite su sitio Web www.ashi.org.

Nosotros le recomendamos que entreviste a varios inspectores antes de contratar uno. He aquí algunas preguntas que pueden ayudarlo a seleccionar el mejor inspector:

✔ **¿Es usted un inspector profesional a tiempo completo?** Sólo una respuesta es aceptable: sí.

✔ **¿Qué puede decirme acerca de su compañía?** Converse sobre el tamaño de la compañía, y cuánto tiempo lleva en el negocio.

✔ **¿Tiene usted un seguro contra errores y omisiones?** Un seguro de errores y omisiones cubre la posibilidad de que una inspección de propiedad haya pasado por alto algunos problemas. Si un inspector comete un error que le cuesta bastante dinero, un seguro de este tipo puede ayudar a subsanar esta situación.

✔ **¿Cuántas inspecciones hace usted personalmente cada año?** Aunque el número promedio de inspecciones varía de zona a zona, inspectores activos normalmente llevan a cabo entre 150 y 400 inspecciones por año. Averigüe si el inspector trabaja principalmente en la zona en la cual está ubicada la propiedad que usted desea adquirir, y por lo tanto está familiarizado con códigos de trabajo *locales* y regulaciones y problemas *locales* (tales como inundaciones, deslizamientos de tierra, terremotos, tornados y otros como esos).

✔ **¿Tiene usted algún título o certificación especial?** Los inspectores de propiedad generalmente tienen experiencia en algún área relacionada con la inspección, tal como construcción, ingeniería, arquitectura, electricidad, plomería o ajuste de reclamos de seguro. Esta diversidad le aporta conocimientos a sus inspecciones. De igual manera, ser miembro de *ASHI* u otra asociación comercial para inspectores de vivienda, indica al menos un conocimiento mínimo de los procedimientos de inspección.

✔ **¿Cuál es la importancia de una inspección previa a la compra?** Asegúrese de que la inspección cubra *todos* los sistemas mecánicos y estructurales principales de la propiedad, por dentro y por fuera, desde los cimientos hasta el techo. Menos de eso no se debe aceptar.

✔ **¿Cuánto tiempo va a tomar su inspección?** El tiempo que él o ella pasan en la propiedad es un punto muy importante. La inspección no es una carrera, y generalmente toma entre dos o tres horas para hacer una inspección completa y detallada de un apartamento o una casa de tamaño promedio.

✔ **¿Qué tipo de reporte me va a dar?** Reportes orales, como los contratos verbales, no tienen validez alguna. Un reporte estandarizado, tipo lista, con términos marcados es escasamente mejor que uno oral. Usted debe recibir una descripción detallada de la condición estructural y mecánica de la propiedad en cuestión. Usted necesita un reporte narrado, escrito de una manera directa, que explique claramente las consecuencias de las observaciones.

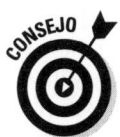

Solicite de cada inspector que consulte, un modelo de reporte. La mejor manera de ver si una compañía escribe un buen reporte es leer uno de tal modo que usted pueda sacar su propia conclusión.

✔ **¿Le importaría si lo acompaño durante su inspección?** ¿Debe importarle esto al inspector? Al contrario, los buenos inspectores insisten que usted esté presente durante la inspección de la propiedad.

✔ **¿Va a incluir su reporte un estimado del costo de las reparaciones que usted está recomendando?** Ésta es una pregunta engañosa. Si la respuesta del inspector es sí, no lo contrate. Inspectores profesionales y responsables sólo hacen inspecciones, y no hacen los trabajos de reparación. Tampoco promocionan este negocio para sus amigos. Los inspectores responsables lo ayudan a establecer sus costos de reparación recomendándole tres o cuatro contratistas de buena reputación, especialistas en techos, electricidad y otras compañías que usted puede llamar para que le den una cotización de los costos del trabajo. Como generalmente existe más de una manera de arreglar una falla o defecto, usted tiene que decidir cuál es la mejor forma de resolver este problema después que ha consultado la gente apropiada.

✔ **¿Cuánto cuesta la inspección?** Desafortunadamente, ésta es, generalmente, la primera pregunta que los compradores le formulan al inspector. Éste no es el momento de ahorrarse unos centavitos para luego tener que gastar una fortuna. Tenga cuidado con inspectores nuevos que le ofrezcan honorarios muy bajos y poco realistas, y promociones de "por esta semana solamente". No deje que estos inspectores novatos practiquen con usted. Las inspecciones que son de calidad cuestan más que una inspección que contiene una rápida lista de puntos generales, porque valen más la pena. En última instancia, como los honorarios que cobran los inspectores buenos son generalmente los mismos (por la presión de la competencia), usted probablemente terminará utilizando los criterios correctos para seleccionar su inspector: compatibilidad y conocimiento.

✔ **¿Le importaría si llamo a alguno de sus clientes más recientes para que me dé referencias?** A los inspectores buenos les gusta dar los nombres y teléfonos de sus clientes satisfechos. Los inspectores malos, en cambio, podrían poner obstáculos a tal requerimiento, o indicarle la gente que sabe que va a darle una opinión positiva de ellos. Asegúrese de revisar al menos tres referencias por cada inspector en la ciudad dónde está ubicada la propiedad. Pregúnteles a esas personas si, después de cerrada la compra, ellos descubrieron algún defecto grande que el inspector no vio y si utilizarían a ese inspector nuevamente.

Cómo optimizar su inspección

Aquí presentamos una guía para que le saque el máximo provecho al dinero que está invirtiendo en la inspección de la propiedad:

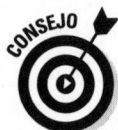

✔ **Haga siempre una oferta de compra sujeta a la revisión y aprobación, por su parte, de los reportes de inspección.** Hacerlo de esta manera, le da la oportunidad de negociar un crédito o una reducción del precio por concepto de trabajos de reparación que son descubiertos durante la inspección, o si usted lo desea, poder salirse del negocio. Este tema lo explicamos extensamente en el Capítulo 12.

✔ **Pregúnteles a los vendedores si tienen alguna inspección que hayan hecho, previa a la venta, o copia de reportes de inspección generados por previos compradores potenciales.** Si los obtiene, déselos a su inspector para que vea con detalle posibles áreas problemáticas. Pídale a su agente que ordene una investigación de permisos otorgados a la propiedad para ver si se han hecho trabajos eléctricos, de plomería, u otras reparaciones o mejoras en la misma.

Suponga que los vendedores le dan un reporte de inspección, el cual ellos ordenaron justo antes de poner la vivienda a la venta y que dice que la vivienda está en perfectas condiciones. Usted puede ahorrarse dinero si confía en tal reporte en lugar de ordenar el suyo propio.

¿Debería usted confiar? De ninguna manera. Nunca deje que el zorro le diga cómo están las cosas en el gallinero. Siempre pague por su propia inspección con un inspector que usted escoja.

✔ **Lea cuidadosamente el reporte generado por su inspector.** Si usted no ve algún defecto en el reporte, el cual el inspector le había específicamente mencionado durante la inspección, llame al inspector y averigüe por qué. Asimismo, no tenga miedo de llamar al inspector y obtener una explicación detallada de *cualquier cosa* que usted no entienda muy bien en el reporte.

✔ **No le reste importancia al costo de las reparaciones, y busque cotizaciones de varias contratistas autorizadas y de buena reputación.** Nunca intente ahorrar dinero usando contratistas no autorizadas que hacen el trabajo sin los permisos requeridos. Hacerlo es normalmente ilegal y puede crear problemas de salud y seguridad, y afectar negativamente el precio de reventa de la propiedad. Muchos estados requieren que los vendedores de la propiedad revelen el hecho de que se hicieron trabajos en la vivienda sin los permisos necesarios. Si por los momentos en su estado no es obligatorio este tipo de divulgación, probablemente lo será para el momento en que vaya a vender su casa.

✔ **Involucre al inspector de la propiedad en el proceso de ofertas de los contratistas.** Si los contratistas tienen preguntas concernientes a los problemas señalados en el reporte de inspección, indíqueles que le pregunten al inspector para que les aclare el problema. Por otra parte, por un honorario extra, algunos inspectores pueden ayudarlo a evaluar las ofertas que reciba para hacer el trabajo necesario.

Las inspecciones previas a la compra tienen la intención de darle a usted una idea de los hechos para negociar la corrección de trabajos costosos — no para que usted trate de sacarles unos centavos a los vendedores, logrando créditos por alfombras manchadas y cortinas desgastadas. Si su nueva casa es la casa usada de alguien más, deje que su precio de oferta refleje el valor reducido de la vivienda debido al desgaste normal.

Si su agente o el vendedor le ofrecen pagar un *plan de garantía de la vivienda*, o *plan de protección de la vivienda* (esto es, un contrato de servicio que cubre algunos de los sistemas y aparatos eléctricos más grandes de la casa), sería muy descortés de su parte decir que no a esta oferta. Sin embargo, nunca acepte ese plan como substituto de una inspección, y no compre ese tipo de plan para usted. Después que usted gasta $250 más o menos por el plan, usted paga un deducible adicional de $25 a $50 cada vez que necesita que alguien vaya a darle un vistazo al problema. Más aun, estos planes limitan significativamente cuánto pagarán ellos para resolver los problemas más grandes que se puedan presentar. Una mejor forma de gastar su dinero es contratar un inspector profesional para que inspeccione muy bien la casa y descubra todos los problemas existentes, de modo que usted pueda negociar la reparación con los propietarios.

Ver y leer es mucho mejor que solamente leer

Usted, su agente y el agente del vendedor deberían acompañar al inspector durante la inspección. Leer un reporte de inspección —aun el más completo— no es un buen sustituto de estar en la propiedad y ver los defectos con sus propios ojos. Ésta puede ser la mejor oportunidad para hacerle preguntas al inspector acerca de las consecuencias de un problema y de estudiar las varias formas de corregirlo. Al ver los defectos y hablar de ellos, usted entiende mejor por qué arreglar algunos de ellos no representa un gran problema, mientras otros son muy costosos para reparar.

Desde el punto de vista de negociación, los vendedores están más dispuestos a aceptar los resultados de una inspección si el agente de venta de ellos estuvo presente cuando la inspección fue hecha. Los vendedores sabrán que los defectos son reales, ya que su agente los vio y puede indicárselos antes de que ellos obtengan la copia del reporte. También reconocerán que un profesional especializado inspeccionó su casa —no un lunático que usted contrató para difamar la propiedad de modo que pudiera estafarles su dinero duramente ganado. Los compradores también se darán cuenta de que aunque lo hicieran huir por resistirse a pagar por los trabajos de reparación, todavía estarán atascados con el problema de vender una casa defectuosa.

Incluso si la casa está en perfectas condiciones, usted debería saber dónde están ciertas cosas. Si usted está presente durante la inspección, su inspector puede mostrarle dónde encontrar las cosas importantes como la caldera, el calentador de agua, y los protectores de circuitos. El inspector debe también mostrarle dónde se encuentran las válvulas de cierre de emergencia para el gas, la electricidad y los sistemas de agua. Al estar presente durante la inspección, usted aprenderá mucho más acerca del cuidado de la misma y del mantenimiento, que lo que aprendería al leer el reporte de inspección solamente.

Si le resulta absolutamente imposible estar durante la inspección porque está en otra ciudad o en una reunión importantísima de negocios, asegúrese que alguien de toda su confianza asista a la inspección (puede ser su agente, un familiar o amigo, o alguien más) para actuar como sus ojos y oídos. Pídale a su representante que haga una grabación o un video de toda la inspección, la cual usted puede usar para completar el reporte de inspección. Ver el video no es lo mismo que estar personalmente allí, pero seguro es mucho mejor que solamente leer el reporte. Usted también puede llamar al inspector si tiene preguntas acerca del reporte.

Por último, preste atención. No traiga a la inspección una pandilla de niños, familiares, amigos, colegas, pintores, suplidores de alfombras, plomeros, electricistas o contratistas que lo distraerán del trabajo que tiene que hacer: aprender todo lo que usted pueda de la propiedad que desea comprar. Enfóquese en la inspección.

No piense que con las inspecciones se eliminan todos los problemas de mantenimiento futuros. Con el transcurso del tiempo, el triturador de desperdicios puede romperse y todos los techos gotean alguna vez. Cuando estas cosas pasen, entienda que no son parte de un terrible plan para estafarlo.

Tarde o temprano, cualquier cosa en su vivienda que se pueda romper o pueda botar agua, se romperá y botará agua. Las reparaciones son parte de la experiencia de ser propietario. Después de cerrar la compra de su vivienda, el mantenimiento normal es su responsabilidad, y no la del vendedor. Después de todo, él tendrá sus propias reparaciones que hacer a su nueva casa.

Cómo Asegurar Su Casa

A nadie le gusta gastar dinero en seguros. Pero si algo puede causarle una catástrofe financiera, es necesario que se asegure contra ese riesgo. El objeto del seguro, es que usted gasta una cantidad relativamente pequeña de dinero para protegerse contra una pérdida de una gran cantidad. Por ejemplo, si su casa se destruye completamente en un incendio y no estaba asegurada, usted tendría que sacar miles (si no son cientos de miles) de dólares para reconstruirla.

Usted no debería desperdiciar dinero asegurando pérdidas potenciales muy pequeñas. Por ejemplo, si envía por correo un paquete que contiene un regalo que vale $50, y el servicio postal lo pierde, seguro que se sentirá mal, pero la pérdida no representará una catástrofe financiera para usted. Usted no debe desperdiciar dinero en ese seguro.

He aquí los tipos de seguros que usted necesita tener *antes* de comprar la casa de sus sueños.

Seguro de propietario

Cuando usted compra una casa, la mayoría de las entidades crediticias exigen que usted compre un seguro de propiedad. Aun si usted es uno de esos excepcionales casos de personas que pueden comprar una vivienda con efectivo sin necesidad de prestar dinero, usted debe tener un seguro con cobertura de la propiedad. ¿Y por qué? En primer lugar, le costaría una pequeña fortuna reemplazar su vivienda y su propiedad personal en la casa (muebles, alfombras, equipo de sonido, computadoras, vajilla, y otros), si usa dinero de su propio bolsillo.

Segundo, su casa puede ser la causa de una demanda, si alguien resulta herido o matan a alguien en ella; usted podría ser demandado por miles o cientos de miles de dólares, quizás hasta un millón de dólares o más.

Las secciones que siguen explican cómo obtener la cobertura de seguro de propiedad que usted necesita.

El costo de reconstrucción

Si su casa es destruida, lo cual muy frecuentemente resulta con los incendios, su póliza de seguro debe pagar por el costo de reconstrucción de su vivienda. La porción de la póliza que cubre esta pérdida es la sección de *cobertura del domicilio*. El monto de esta cobertura debe ser igual al costo de reconstruir la vivienda que usted posee, y debe estar basado en el área de su propiedad, medida en pies cuadrados. El monto de la cobertura del domicilio, no debe estar en función de lo que usted pagó por la vivienda o del monto de la hipoteca. Si usted está comprando un apartamento en un edificio de apartamentos, o uno de una cooperativa, analice qué cobertura tiene a través de la asociación de propietarios del edificio.

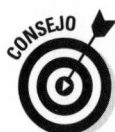

Obtenga una póliza que contenga una cláusula de *costo de reemplazo garantizado*. Esta cláusula asegura que la compañía reconstruirá la propiedad aun si el costo de construcción es mayor que el monto de la cobertura de la póliza. Si la compañía de seguros subestima la cobertura de domicilio, ella tiene la obligación de cubrir la diferencia.

Pregúnteles a los aseguradores cómo definen ellos la cobertura de *costo de reemplazo garantizado* —ya que cada compañía podría definirlo en forma diferente. Las pólizas más generosas en este sentido, por ejemplo, pagan por el costo total de reemplazo, sin importar cuánto termine costando éste. Otras compañías establecen límites —por ejemplo, acuerdan pagar hasta un 120 por ciento del total de la póliza de cobertura del domicilio.

Protección contra demandas

El seguro de *responsabilidad contra terceros,* lo protege contra demandas o juicios legales que provengan de daños a terceras personas que ocurran mientras están en su propiedad. Imagínese que un peatón conflictivo por casualidad se resbala con una concha de banana que dejaron en el camino de entrada a su casa. O, quizás, que el balcón del segundo piso de su vivienda se cae durante una divertida fiesta, y alguien se rompe una pierna o, quizás, dos.

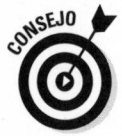

Compre un seguro que cubra al menos dos veces el valor de sus activos. Aunque las posibilidades de ser demandado son remotas, recuerde que si lo demandan, las consecuencias financieras pueden ser catastróficas. De hecho, si usted tiene una cantidad de activos considerables que proteger (cuyo valor es más de doscientos mil dólares, por ejemplo), usted debería considerar una *póliza a todo riesgo* adicional —llamada en inglés *umbrella*. Pregunte a las compañías aseguradoras de su vivienda y automóvil(es) acerca de esta cobertura adicional.

Protección de la propiedad personal

En un seguro de propiedad típico, la cobertura para propiedad personal generalmente está establecida alrededor de un 50 a un 75 por ciento del monto de la propiedad. Si usted es dueño de un apartamento en un edificio o residencia cooperativa, generalmente tendrá que determinar un monto específico para la cobertura de propiedad personal que usted quiera.

Algunas pólizas vienen con una *garantía de reemplazo de la propiedad personal*, que le paga por el costo de reemplazo de ese elemento específico en lugar del valor real de él en el momento en que fue dañado o robado. Si esta protección no es parte de la póliza estándar que vende su compañía de seguro, quizás usted pueda comprarla por medio de una cláusula o póliza adicional por una estipulación extra, siempre y cuando la ofrezcan.

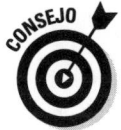

Si alguna vez usted necesita someter un reclamo, tener la documentación de su propiedad personal puede ser de gran ayuda. La manera más fácil y rápida de documentar sus efectos personales, es grabar un video de todas sus pertenencias. También puede tener un archivo con los recibos de las compras más grandes, y hacer un inventario por escrito de los objetos. No importa cómo documente usted sus pertenencias, asegúrese de colocar esta información en algún lugar fuera de su casa (y por favor, que no sea en el jardín). Una lista o un video no va a hacerle de mucha utilidad si está en su casa y se desaparece con el incendio o si es dañado irreparablemente en una horrible inundación.

Dónde encontrar una buena cobertura que no cueste mucho

Como con otros tipos de seguro y otros productos financieros, usted necesita salir a buscar las mejores opciones. Pero sabemos que usted tiene mejores cosas que hacer con su tiempo y, por eso, aquí le presentamos una lista de compañías que son conocidas por ofrecer pólizas de alta calidad y bajo costo:

- ✔ **AMICA:** para más información llame a la compañía al 800-242-6422. Aunque los clientes de AMICA generalmente le dan a la compañía una alta evaluación, los precios de AMICA son algunas veces un poco altos.

- ✔ **Erie Insurance:** esta compañía tiene negocios principalmente en los estados centro-occidentales y del Atlántico. Revise la guía telefónica de su localidad para ver agentes que venden pólizas de Erie Insurance, o llame al 800-458-0811 para que le informen dónde conseguir un agente en su localidad.

- ✔ **GEICO:** llame a la compañía al 800-841-3000, para pedir detalles.

- ✔ **Liberty Mutual:** busque en la guía telefónica de su localidad para ver agentes que venden pólizas de esta compañía.

- ✔ **Nationwide Mutual:** busque en la guía telefónica de su localidad para ver agentes que venden pólizas de esta aseguradora.

- ✔ **State Farm:** busque en la guía telefónica de su localidad para ver agentes que venden pólizas de esta compañía.

- ✔ **USAA:** las pólizas de esta compañía están disponible para los militares y sus familias. Llame a esta compañía para obtener más detalles y para determinar si usted reúne los requisitos que exigen (800-531-8080).

Otras catástrofes contra las cuáles protegerse

Dependiendo de donde esté localizada su vivienda, ésta puede estar expuesta a terremotos, inundaciones, huracanes, deslizamientos de tierra, tornados, incendios forestales u otros desastres. Las pólizas estándar de seguro de la propiedad no protegen contra todas estas catástrofes, así que usted debe contar con cláusulas adicionales para estos efectos.

Miles de comunidades en el país, están expuestas al riesgo de inundaciones. Por eso, si usted vive en una zona con peligro de inundación, necesita comprar un seguro adicional contra inundaciones. Consulte con compañías de seguro con las que potencialmente puede comprar el seguro de propietario. El programa de seguro contra inundación del gobierno federal (800-638-6620; www.fema.gov/nfip) puede ofrecerle información acerca de los tipos de pólizas disponibles a través de compañías de seguro privadas.

Los terremotos son otro riesgo contra el cual hay que protegerse. Además de California, algunas zonas de la parte central-occidental (y aún partes de la costa oriental) tienen fallas sísmicas activas.

Pregúnteles a las personas del lugar donde usted piensa vivir cuáles son los peligros del área. El departamento de los Estados Unidos *U.S. Geological Survey* (consulte la guía telefónica local para encontrar el teléfono; www.usgs.gov) y la Agencia Federal para el Manejo de Emergencias (*FEMA*, 800-358-9616; www.fema.gov) tienen mapas que muestran las zonas con riesgos de terremotos e inundaciones respectivamente. Tenga cuidado y manténgase informado.

Debido a que el costo de la cobertura de terremoto e inundación está basado en las evaluaciones de las compañías de seguros sobre los riesgos de acuerdo a la zona y al tipo de propiedad, usted *no* debe decidir de si comprar estas protecciones extras basándose solamente en su percepción de cuán pequeño es el riesgo de que ocurra alguno de estos eventos. El riesgo ya está incluido en el precio.

Si usted aumenta los deducibles en las partes principales de su seguro de propietario y de otras pólizas de seguro que tiene, quizás pueda pagar por una buena parte del costo de los seguros de terremotos y de inundación. Recuerde, usted puede pagar más fácilmente los reclamos más pequeños que los grandes. Si cree que el seguro de terremoto y el de inundación son muy costosos, compare estos costos de la cobertura con el gasto que usted tendría que hacer para reemplazar su vivienda y su propiedad personal. Compre estos seguros si vive en una zona que pueda verse afectada por estas catástrofes.

Usted puede que tenga acceso a información más específica del estado donde vive. Muchos departamentos de seguro estatales —los cuales usted puede encontrar en las listas del gobierno estatal en su guía telefónica— llevan a cabo encuestas de los precios de las compañías aseguradoras y, también, registran las quejas recibidas. En el Capítulo 11 también damos información de algunas páginas Web que le pueden ser muy útiles.

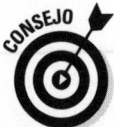

Mientras busca cotizaciones de seguros, pregunte acerca de descuentos especiales para viviendas con sistemas de seguridad, o sistemas de detección de incendios, descuentos para personas que tienen varias pólizas con la misma compañía aseguradora y descuentos para personas de la tercera edad.

Seguro de título de propiedad

Ahora, adelante la película de su vida varios meses en el futuro después que usted cierra el negocio de la compra de la vivienda de sus sueños. Ahora, en ese momento, imagínese que le pidamos que nos demuestre que usted es en realidad el dueño de la casa.

"Eso no es problema", piensa usted. Va a la caja de seguridad donde guarda todos sus documentos importantes y saca su documento de propiedad que la oficina del registro le envió por correo un par de semanas después que usted llevó a cabo la compra.

Lo sentimos mucho, pero este documento no es una prueba suficiente.

Déjenos contarle el siguiente caso. Un caballero y su "esposa" firmaron un documento que transfería el título de su casa a otra pareja. Unas semanas más tarde, los compradores estaban escandalizados al enterarse de que su título de propiedad no era válido porque la firma de la esposa verdadera había sido falsificada. De hecho, la verdadera esposa ni siquiera sabía que su esposo había vendido la propiedad.

Riesgos asociados con el título

En teoría, usted puede ir hasta la oficina de registro local del condado y averiguar quién es el dueño de una propiedad específica con solo revisar el registro público. Pero en realidad, toda clase de irregularidades en la historia de las diferentes personas que han sido dueños de la propiedad desde que fue construida originalmente, puede afectar el título de dicha propiedad. Estas irregularidades son difíciles o imposibles de encontrar, no importa con cuanto detenimiento investigue los registros públicos.

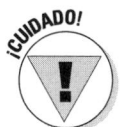

He aquí algunas de las causas de estos riesgos escondidos relacionados con el título:

- ✔ **Cónyuges secretos:** un vendedor puede indicar que es soltero(a), cuando en realidad, él o ella está casado secretamente en otro estado. O, quizás, el vendedor(a) se divorció en un estado que tiene un acuerdo de propiedad comunal, según el cual, a través del matrimonio, uno de los cónyuges obtiene una participación legal en la propiedad personal del otro cónyuge. Cualquiera que sea la razón, algunas veces el cónyuge actual o un ex cónyuge, del cual nadie sabía que existía, aparece de la nada y presenta una demanda contra la propiedad. Ésta es la razón por la cual los representantes de las compañías de títulos están curiosos de saber su estado civil. Ellos tienen que saber si usted es soltero, casado, divorciado, o viudo para poder tener los registros correctos.

- ✔ **Herederos secretos:** si los dueños de la propiedad fallecen y no hicieron un testamento, un tribunal de sucesiones o testamentos debe decidir quiénes son los legítimos herederos. Las decisiones del tribunal pueden no ser válidas o legales para herederos que no fueron notificados del proceso. Aun cuando exista un testamento, los juzgados de testamentos tienen, en algunas ocasiones, que resolver problemas en relación a la interpretación de los mismos. Herederos desconocidos aparecen a veces mágicamente y reclaman que ellos son los dueños de la propiedad en juicio.

✔ **Capacidad dudosa:** algunos menores de edad y personas declaradas incapacitadas mentalmente, no pueden formar parte de contratos a menos que sus custodios o representantes, designados por el juzgado o tribunal, manejen la transacción. Si, por ejemplo, el vendedor era menor de edad o incapacitado mentalmente cuando un documento de propiedad fue firmado, la transacción puede ser anulable o inválida.

✔ **Equivocaciones:** ésta es una categoría general, altamente técnica, donde se incluyen toda clase de errores humanos. Incluye de todo, desde empleados que pasaron por alto embargos registrados contra la propiedad —embargos por impuestos estatales y federales o impuestos locales a la propiedad que no fueron pagados—, y de otros documentos importantes mientras hacían la investigación del título, hasta técnicos que establecieron incorrectamente los límites de la propiedad. Estos simples errores crean muchos problemas en los títulos.

✔ **Falsificación y fraude:** así como ocurrió con el caso de la esposa falsa, muchas personas se pueden hacer pasar ilegalmente por los vende-dores. De la misma manera, las firmas pueden ser falsificadas en los documentos. Los oficiales o agentes en custodia de los depósitos en garantía para la compra, exigen identificación (esto es, una identifi-cación con fotografía, tal como una licencia para conducir emitida en los últimos cinco años, o un pasaporte actualizado) para poder establecer sin lugar a dudas *que usted es la persona que dice ser.*

✔ **Confusión de nombres:** muchos de los problemas de los títulos resultan porque la gente tiene nombres similares (o idénticos) al nombre del comprador o del vendedor. Aunque usted pruebe que usted es quien dice ser, también tiene que probar quién *no es* usted. Si usted tiene un apellido muy común, usted probablemente tendrá que llenar una declaración de información para ayudar a la compañía de título a distin-guirlo a usted de otras personas con nombres como el suyo. Si usted tiene un nombre común, como Brown, Chen, García, González, Johnson, Jones, Lee, Miller, Nguyen, Williams, o el siempre popular Smith, anticipe que le pidan completar una declaración de información.

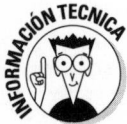

¿Qué tipo de información es solicitada en una declaración de informa-ción? Usted y su cónyuge, si está casado(a), tendrán que dar su nombre completo, número del seguro social, fecha y año de nacimiento, lugar de nacimiento, fecha y lugar del matrimonio (si es pertinente), información de su lugar de residencia y empleo, matrimonios anteriores, y otros como esos. Esta información será utilizada para diferenciarlo a usted, el siempre bueno y honrado, de los montones de otras personas con nom-bres similares al suyo.

Para qué sirve el seguro de título

Muchas personas que compran vivienda gastan cientos de dólares en seguro de título sin haber entendido realmente qué es lo que están obteniendo a cambio de ese dinero. El *seguro de título* le asegura a los propietarios y a las entidades crediticias que una propiedad tiene un título vendible (*válido*). Si alguien hace un reclamo que pone en duda su propiedad de la vivienda, la compañía de seguro de titulo de propiedad lo protege a usted y a su entidad crediticia contra pérdidas o daños, de acuerdo a las condiciones y estipulaciones de sus respectivas pólizas de seguro de título.

La mayor parte de la prima de su seguro de título, se destina a la investigación para determinar quién posee legalmente la propiedad que usted quiere comprar, y si hay algún embargo impositivo o juicios registrados contra ésta. Como las compañías de títulos de propiedad hacen un buen trabajo al eliminar los riesgos del título *antes* que la gente compre la propiedad, solamente cerca del 10 por ciento de la prima de seguro se destina a indemnizar a los propietarios contra reclamos del título después del cierre del depósito en garantía.

La prima de seguro de título que usted paga al cierre del depósito en garantía es la única prima de este seguro que usted tendrá que pagar *a menos que refinancie su hipoteca.*

El seguro de título de propiedad tiene que ver con su riesgo de pérdida por problemas *pasados* (tales como embargos por impuestos de propiedad no pagados, o falsificación en la historia del título) que *pudieran* existir en el momento en que su póliza es emitida. Como su póliza cubre el pasado, el cuál es un evento fijo, usted solamente paga una prima del seguro de título *mientras usted mantenga su hipoteca original.*

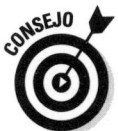

Si usted refinancia su préstamo, usted tendrá que obtener una nueva póliza de seguro de título para proteger a la entidad acreedora de los riesgos asociados al mismo (tales como embargos por impuesto sobre la renta o por impuestos a la propiedad) que puedan haber sido registrados contra su propiedad, desde el momento en que su póliza previa fue emitida, y la fecha de refinanciamiento. Si usted refinancia su préstamo, pregúntele a la compañía de título de propiedad si usted reúne los requisitos para una *prima de refinanciamiento* en su nueva póliza. La mayoría de las compañías de título, ofrecen una gran reducción de la prima —a veces hasta el 30 por ciento de sus primas normales— si su póliza anterior ha sido emitida cinco años o menos antes de la emisión de la nueva póliza.

Dos clases de seguro de título

Como propietario, usted puede escoger entre dos tipos de seguro de título de propietarios. Dependiendo de la cobertura que desee, usted puede obtener una póliza con cobertura estándar o una de cobertura amplia.

Ejemplos reales de problemas del seguro de título

La gente normalmente no presta mucha atención al seguro de título cuando está comprando una vivienda. La mayoría de las personas, compran este seguro sólo porque la entidad hipotecaria no les otorgará una hipoteca si no lo tienen. Pero los compradores de vivienda están contentísimos cuando un problema de título asoma su horrible nariz, y allí está la póliza para protegerlos.

Por ejemplo, una mujer gastó cerca de $10.000 para remodelar un garaje con techo y para construir una cerca a lo largo de la línea de la propiedad después de obtener el permiso del vecino. Todo iba muy bien hasta que su vecino vendió su casa varios años más tarde. Cuando los nuevos dueños hicieron el estudio de su propiedad, descubrieron que el garaje con techo y la cerca de la vecina se extendían cerca de 2 pies sobre su terreno. En lugar de deshacer todo el trabajo y demolerlo, lo cual fue el primer impulso de la mujer después de enterarse de la mala noticia, ella decidió presentar un reclamo a la compañía de seguro de título.

La compañía de título descubrió que ella había sido víctima de un cálculo defectuoso de los límites del terreno, y resolvió el problema comprándole a sus nuevos vecinos un *derecho de servidumbre perpetuo* para usar el terreno que ella había mejorado, de modo que podía dejar todo (cochera, cobertizo y cerca) exactamente donde estaba.

Otro ejemplo es el de una pareja cuya cocina fue destruida por un incendio. El departamento de construcción del condado dijo que para reconstruirla, la pareja tendría que quitar un garaje techado que se extendía 5 pies más allá en un terreno. Los dueños anteriores habían obtenido todos los permisos necesarios que se requerían para construir el garaje techado, pero las leyes de zonificación locales habían cambiado después que el mismo fue construido en 1970.

La pareja sabía lo que tenía que hacer. Llamaron al representante de la compañía de título, y después de las investigaciones necesarias, la compañía le pagó a una contratista $5.000 para retirar el garaje techado. La compañía también le pagó a la pareja $19.000 para indemnizarlos por la reducción del valor de la propiedad debido a que ya no tenía estacionamiento cubierto.

Como es de esperarse, una *póliza de seguro de título de cobertura estándar* es menos costosa que una amplia porque su cobertura es más limitada. Las pólizas estándar están limitadas a ciertos riesgos no registrados —tales como fraude en la historia del título, errores de registro, y capacidad—, más otros embargos *registrados* (en la oficina de registro del condado local) por una contratista a la cual no se le han pagado por trabajos hechos en la propiedad, estimación de impuestos, fallos, y otros defectos de la propiedad que puedan ser descubiertos durante una indagación en los registros públicos.

Las *pólizas de seguro de título de cobertura amplia* cubren todo lo que las estándares cubren, pero además proveen una cobertura mayor para los riesgos no registrados, que podrían ser descubiertos a través de una inspección de la propiedad, o investigando personas que han estado en posesión de la misma; también cubre defectos *no registrados* (nunca registrados en la oficina de registro del condado), tales como embargos hechos por una contratista a la cual no se le han pagado por trabajos realizados, o arrendamientos o contratos de ventas. Sólo una póliza amplia de seguro de título pudo haber protegido a los propietarios de los casos que mencionamos en la sección "Ejemplos reales de problemas del seguro de título", de los errores en las mediciones de la propiedad e incendio en la cocina.

Los costos del seguro de título varían muchísimo, dependiendo del área geográfica en la cual su vivienda esté ubicada, del precio de compra de la misma y del tipo de cobertura que usted obtenga. Además de la póliza de propietario que le recomendamos obtener para proteger su inversión, usted necesitará comprar una póliza para proteger a la entidad crediticia frente a la pérdida del monto del préstamo.

En algunos estados del este, las compañías de títulos tienen prohibido hacer investigaciones sobre los mismos. Si esa prohibición existe en su localidad, usted tendrá que contratar un abogado para que investigue el titulo de propiedad y el depósito de la garantía. En cualquier caso, investigue para determinar quién ofrece la mejor combinación de primas competitivas y una buena cobertura.

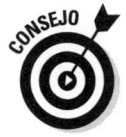

Las costumbres y usos locales determinan generalmente quién paga por el seguro de título. En algunas partes del país, la costumbre establece que el comprador paga por este concepto. En otros lugares, el vendedor podría pagar la prima del seguro, o compradores y vendedores pagan cada uno la mitad del costo. Como señalamos en el Capítulo 12, el pago del seguro de título es un punto negociable. Independientemente de la costumbre local, si usted está comprando en un momento en el cual el mercado de bienes raíces favorece a los compradores, los vendedores podrían ofrecer (o usted podría pedirles) pagar el costo del seguro de título para poder cerrar el negocio. Y al contrario, si usted está compitiendo con otros compradores por una vivienda en particular, usted podría hacer más atractiva su oferta, ofreciendo pagar por el seguro de título, aun cuando las costumbres locales indican que los vendedores son quienes pagan por él.

Capítulo 14

Esto No Termina Hasta que el Gordito que Administra el Depósito en Garantía Diga que Cerró

· ·

En Este Capítulo

▶ Qué son los depósitos en garantía y cómo funcionan

▶ Cómo revisar los costos del cierre y el estado de cuenta del cierre

▶ Por qué los depósitos en garantía al final del año pueden ser engañosos

▶ Cómo tomar posesión de su vivienda

▶ Cómo sobrellevar el remordimiento que acompaña a la compra

· ·

*E*l gran día se acerca. Muy pronto, si todo va bien, paga el resto del dinero correspondiente a la cuota inicial de la casa, firma en la línea punteada, y recoge las llaves de la casa de sus sueños.

Para la mayoría de las personas, la agonía final de comprar una casa representa una incertidumbre inmensa, mucha ansiedad y sudoración extrema. Usted, sin embargo, *no* es como la mayoría de las personas. Los consejos que usted encontrará en este capítulo calmarán su ansiedad, pulirán su camino de piedras al éxito, y harán el final de este juego placentero y agradable.

Un Depósito en Garantía Es Algo Bueno

Tan pronto como sea posible, después que usted y el vendedor tengan una *oferta ratificada* (o sea, han firmado un contrato), todos los fondos, documentos e instrucciones relacionados con su transacción deben ser entregados a un tercero, quien además es neutral: el *administrador del depósito en garantía* designado en el contrato de compra. La acción de entregar estos fondos, documentos e instrucciones al administrador del depósito en garantía se denomina *garantía*. Dependiendo del uso y la costumbre en su zona, la administración del depósito en garantía podrá hacerla un abogado, una compañía especializada en depósitos en garantía, o una compañía de títulos hipotecarios. Compradores y vendedores generalmente seleccionan un administrador basado en las recomendaciones de sus agentes. Sin embargo, como con otras compañías con quienes hace negocio en el proceso de compra, sepa que los gastos relacionados con el depósito en garantía y la calidad del servicio, varían.

Los negocios de bienes raíces casi siempre están caracterizados por una desconfianza mutua de las partes involucradas. Usted y el vendedor necesitan a alguien en quien ambos puedan confiar y que custodie los intereses de cada uno de ustedes, mientras ambos se reúnen a trabajar con los asuntos del contrato que están pendientes y sin resolver. El administrador del depósito en garantía (también conocido como el *agente del depósito en garantía o agente de cierre*) es su árbitro —una tercera persona neutral que no deberá mostrar ningún favoritismo por usted o por el vendedor.

Conozca a su agente de cierre

El administrador del depósito en garantía es responsable de preparar y revisar los documentos relacionados con la transferencia del *título* de propiedad —el documento legal que estipula la propiedad de la vivienda. Esto incluye, que los documentos estén apropiadamente firmados, entregarlos y registrarlos en un registro público, cumplir con las instrucciones de transferencia de fondos de la entidad hipotecaria, ordenar la investigación del título (explicada en el Capítulo 13), y entregarle a usted y al comprador los detalles financieros de la venta. El agente de la garantía lleva a cabo todo el papeleo esencial de la transacción y los detalles del dinero.

Cuando el proceso de depósito en garantía se abre, su contrato probablemente estará lleno de algunos vacíos, conocidos como *contingencias o condiciones de la venta*. Por ejemplo, su contrato debería estar escrito de tal forma que pueda anular la transacción de compra si usted no aprueba los resultados del reporte de inspección, o si el vendedor no puede traspasarle un título de propiedad limpio, o si usted no puede obtener un préstamo. El trabajo del agente de cierre es recibir y cumplir sus instrucciones. No le diga que le entregue su dinero al vendedor sino hasta que usted esté *totalmente* satisfecho de que el vendedor haya cumplido completamente con todo lo estipulado en el contrato. El Capítulo 12 explica con suficientes detalles estas contingencias y condiciones.

Idealmente, este proceso de garantía transcurrirá sin problemas desde el principio hasta el final. Sin embargo, si el administrador de la garantía recibe en algún momento instrucciones contradictorias de usted y del vendedor, o de la entidad hipotecaria, el proceso se detendrá súbitamente hasta que el conflicto se resuelva. ¿Qué tipo de instrucciones pueden ser instrucciones contradictorias? Bien, conflictos de si el precio de compra incluye algo específico (por ejemplo, un refrigerador, una lámpara, el protector de la chimenea, u otros) son siempre comunes. También son populares los desacuerdos acerca de si los trabajos de reparación deben ser ejecutados antes o después del cierre de la garantía.

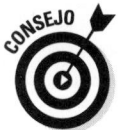

Nuestro amigo Kip Oxman, un excelente abogado y agente de bienes raíces, tiene un dicho que funciona a las mil maravillas para resolver situaciones conflictivas: "Cuando todo lo demás falla, **LEA EL C**ONTRATO" (LEC). Usted puede encontrar la respuesta a la mayoría de las controversias cuando lee el contrato.

Los agentes buenos de depósitos en garantía valen su peso en oro en momentos de crisis cuando los gritos, lágrimas y amenazas de demandas comienzan. En momentos como éstos, a menudo sólo la increíble paciencia del agente del cierre y sus habilidades para mediar en una crisis, mantienen el negocio a flote.

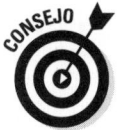

Provéase a sí mismo una ventaja personalizando su proceso de garantía. Llame o visite a su agente de garantía en su oficina para que lo conozca. Pregúntele si necesita alguna información adicional que usted pueda proveerle para que el proceso vaya más rápido y con menos problemas. Algunas preguntas que su agente de depósito en garantía puede hacerle son las siguientes: ¿Cuál es su segundo nombre?, ¿Dónde podemos comunicarnos con usted durante el día?, ¿Cuál es el nombre y número de teléfono de su agente de seguro?, y ¿Cuál es su número de seguro social? (De modo que su depósito pueda ser colocado en una cuenta que gane intereses.) Un poquito de atención personal y respeto ahora harán maravillas por usted más adelante, si el proceso de garantía llega a tomar un camino tortuoso.

Revise todos los detalles

Para evitar sorpresas desagradables preste especial atención a los tres aspectos siguientes:

Costos del cierre

Si usted tiene una mente ordenada y secuencial, sin duda ha leído los 13 capítulos anteriores, y sabe que hemos detallado punto por punto los costos de cierre en el Capítulo 3. Si usted es del tipo de persona que le encanta saltar de capítulo en capítulo, de acuerdo a como éstos llaman su atención, le sugerimos que lea esa sección acerca de los costos de cierre ahora, o los consejos que siguen no tendrán mucho sentido para usted.

Tan pronto como le sea posible, calcule aproximadamente cuánto dinero tendrá que tener al momento del cierre de la garantía. Inmediatamente después de abrir el proceso de la garantía, pídale al agente que le prepare una relación de los costos estimados del cierre. Aun cuando puede tomar varias semanas obtener los costos reales por honorarios de inspección, créditos por trabajos de reparación, de primas de seguro de la propiedad, y otros más, al menos dispondrá de un número preliminar que usted puede ajustar cuando tenga disponible el resto de la información. Tener conocimiento preliminar de estos costos es mucho mejor que ser martillado por costos de cierre inesperados un par de días antes del cierre de la compraventa.

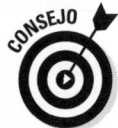

Estime los gastos del cierre un poco por encima de lo normal. Lo ideal es sobre estimarlos y luego, darse cuenta cuando los costos reales vengan, de que no necesitará tanto dinero para el cierre como inicialmente esperaba. Cuanto más pronto usted determine sus costos de cierre, mucho mejor es. No espere a que se presente el problema para resolverlo, contrólelo.

Si usted tiene que depositar dinero adicional en la garantía antes del cierre de la transacción —como la gran mayoría de las personas lo hacen—, utilice un cheque de gerencia, o un giro bancario u orden de pago, o haga que los fondos sean directamente transferidos electrónicamente a la entidad del depósito de garantía para prevenir retrasos. Asegúrese de estar pendiente de su banco para que la transferencia se haga a tiempo, porque a veces el banco puede retrasar el proceso. Los cheques personales toman tiempo para ser procesados, y las tarjetas de crédito no pueden ser usadas para los depósitos en garantía. Si tiene dudas de cuál es la *mejor forma* de hacer llegar los fondos, pregúntele a su agente con bastante anticipación al cierre. Si su dinero se encuentra en otra ciudad, por ejemplo, en una cuenta de mercado monetario de alto rendimiento (como lo recomendamos en el Capítulo 3), hable con la compañía de inversión para saber cómo hacer llegar su dinero hasta la cuenta del depósito en garantía fácilmente.

Reporte preliminar del título

Poco tiempo después que el proceso de la garantía ha sido abierto, usted debería recibir un documento sumamente importante de su compañía de título: el *reporte preliminar del título* (o *prelim,* como se le dice en inglés). Este reporte muestra quién es el dueño vigente de la propiedad que usted desea comprar, así como también cualquier reclamo o embargos relacionados con dinero que afecten la misma; por ejemplo, embargos por hipotecas, sentencia de impuestos sobre la renta, y tasaciones de impuestos a la propiedad. Asimismo, este reporte preliminar muestra restricciones e intereses de terceros sobre la propiedad, tales como convenios, condiciones y restricciones del condominio (*CC&R,* por sus siglas en inglés), y derechos de servidumbre de compañías de servicios públicos o privadas, que pueden limitar el uso de la misma.

Su contrato debe tener como condición para el cierre, la revisión y aprobación por su parte del reporte preliminar de título. Revíselo cuidadosamente, y pídale a su agente inmobiliario, al agente del cierre, a un abogado o representante de la compañía de título, que le expliquen alguna parte del reporte que no entienda. Y no sea tímido —las preguntas tontas no existen.

En lo que se refiere al contrato de compra, usted debe tener el derecho de *justificadamente* desaprobar ciertos reclamos o restricciones impuestos sobre la propiedad, que usted no quiera y el derecho de pedirle al dueño que los resuelva antes del cierre de la garantía. Por ejemplo, pedirle al vendedor que pague todas las deudas impuestas de embargos, gravámenes o diferentes acciones legales en contra de la propiedad, es sensato y justo. Por otra parte, pedirle al vendedor de un apartamento que elimine los convenios, condiciones y restricciones del condominio no sería sensato, porque como lo mencionamos en el Capítulo 8, las mismas son una parte integral de la propiedad.

Un reporte preliminar de título *no* es un seguro de título. Usted puede aprender más acerca de la diferencia entre ambos en la sección de seguro de título en el Capítulo 13.

Estado de cuenta final de los costos de cierre

Puede que crea que el documento más importante que va a recibir en el momento del cierre de la garantía es el título de propiedad. Pero, desde el punto de vista de la contabilidad, el documento más importante es el estado de cuenta con los costos de cierre finales que le entrega el agente de depósito en garantía, el día que la venta efectivamente se cierra.

Si piensa que el depósito de garantía es como si fuese una cuenta corriente, entonces, el estado final del cierre es como su chequera o registro de cheques. Este documento, registra todo el movimiento de dinero relacionado con la compra de la casa que se hizo a través de la garantía, ya sea como un crédito o como un débito:

- **Créditos:** cualquier dinero que contribuyó o depositó en la garantía aparecen como un crédito a su cuenta, tales como su depósito inicial para garantizar la compra, o la cuota inicial de la propiedad. También puede recibir créditos de parte del vendedor por cosas tales como costos por reparaciones e impuestos a la propiedad. Y por supuesto, el dinero del préstamo también es un crédito.

- **Débitos:** son los fondos pagados en su nombre con el depósito en garantía. Incluyen ciertos gastos módicos y no tan módicos, tales como lo que pagó gentilmente al vendedor por la casa de sus sueños, costos del préstamo, las primas del seguro de propiedad, y honorarios por la inspección de la vivienda.

Usted se reúne con el agente de depósito en garantía varios días antes del cierre para firmar los documentos del préstamo y otros papeles relacionados con la compra de la casa. En ese momento, usted recibirá un estado de cuenta de los costos de cierre estimado, el cual detalla los costos si la compraventa cierra en la fecha que se ha acordado. Revise este estado de cuenta con *muchísimo* cuidado, línea por línea, y de arriba a abajo, para estar absolutamente seguro que refleja en forma exacta sus créditos y débitos.

Los agentes del cierre son humanos también y a veces cometen errores. Igualmente, otras personas que participan en la transacción pueden haberle dado al agente la información equivocada. Cuando los errores aparecen, adivine, ¿a favor de quién cree usted que están? ¡Probablemente no a favor de usted! Es su dinero el que está sobre la mesa, así que preste atención a los detalles. Revise el documento de cierre, y cuestione cualquier aspecto que no sea correcto o no esté claro. No necesita analizar el estado del cierre en el momento en que firma los documentos del préstamo. Lléveselos a su casa, y continúe revisándolos y pídales a las diferentes partes involucradas en la transacción, que le clarifiquen lo que no entiende al respecto.

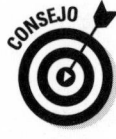

El documento final de cierre es sumamente importante. Quédese con una copia para sus archivos —podría serle de mucha utilidad cuando llegue el momento de hacer su declaración de impuestos sobre la renta. Como explicamos en el Capítulo 3, algunos gastos (tales como los de la solicitud del préstamo, y pagos de impuestos a la propiedad) son deducibles del impuesto. Además, el documento de cierre establece la base de costos inicial de impuestos a la propiedad. Cuando esté listo para vender su vivienda, podría deber impuestos a la ganancia de capital sobre cualquier ganancia que haya obtenido por venta de la propiedad a un precio mayor que lo señalado en la base de costos (vea el Capítulo 17 para más detalles).

Ésta es la época: Cierres en diciembre

Como regla general, diciembre es un mes lento para las ventas de viviendas. Una o dos semanas antes del Día de Acción de Gracias, la mayoría de los compradores cambian su atención de las casas a las fiestas y a las reuniones familiares, y ellos no piensan en comprar sino hasta después del domingo del *Super Bowl* a finales de enero.

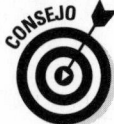

Aquí le damos dos razones para que decida ir en contra de la corriente:

- ✔ **Buscar las ofertas:** cuando los otros compradores se retiran del mercado, usted es el único en la ciudad para los vendedores que tienen que mudarse pronto o para aquellos muy testarudos que tontamente esperaron mucho para darse cuenta que el precio de su casa estaba muy alto.

Si ellos necesitan vender, entonces les dicen a sus agentes que informen que están dispuestos a negociar. La frase mágica aquí es: "Háganos una oferta". Si usted está buscando una buena oportunidad, esta época es el momento de dar el paso.

✔ **Deducciones de impuestos:** lo que usted consiga no es lo más importante —lo importante es con lo que se pueda quedar. Comprar una casa en diciembre le da las deducciones impositivas que puede usar para reducir sus impuestos federales y estatales en ese año. Como decimos en el Capítulo 3, ser dueño de una casa le da un techo físico y una ventaja impositiva. En sus impuestos sobre la renta, por ejemplo, puede deducir los costos de iniciación del préstamo (puntos), los intereses sobre la hipoteca y los impuestos a la propiedad que pague antes del 31 de diciembre.

Los cierres de compraventa son diablillos malvados aun bajo las mejores circunstancias. Son una prueba fehaciente de la Ley de Murphy, la cual establece que en una situación dada, lo que sea que pueda ir mal, irá mal —y *siempre* en el peor momento posible. Los agentes de depósitos en garantía que tienen experiencia, saben que los duendillos desagradables pueden asomar sus horrorosas narices en el momento menos esperado.

La lista de sorpresas potenciales es sumamente larga: fechas que no se cumplen, fallas en el título, problemas para pagar los préstamos existentes, cambios en las condiciones del préstamo, fondos insuficientes para cerrar la venta, fondos no transferidos como se habían prometido, y muchos otros.

Los cierres de garantías hechos en el mes de diciembre son particularmente caprichosos. Estar de fiesta en fiesta disminuye su energía y reduce su efectividad, y a muchas personas se les olvida firmar los papeles antes de irse de vacaciones. El 31 de diciembre es una fecha límite —y no se mueve— si usted quiere cerrar ese año por razones de impuesto. Si llegan los días finales de diciembre y su garantía aún no ha cerrado, aquí están algunas cosas que usted y su agente de bienes raíces podrían hacer para asegurarse que se haga el cierre antes de la fecha tope:

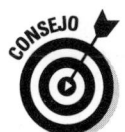

✔ **Manténganse en contacto con la entidad crediticia.** Las entidades financieras necesitan una documentación voluminosa para respaldar las solicitudes de préstamo. Asegúrese de que la entidad crediticia tiene todos los documentos requeridos tan pronto como sea posible. Las entidades dicen que la falta de seguimiento en la verificación de documentos del préstamo, es la causa principal de retrasos en las garantías. En el Capítulo 7, presentamos una lista completa de documentos que la entidad podría necesitar que usted les dé para verificar la información de su solicitud de préstamo, tales como los formularios W-2 para el impuesto, la declaración de impuestos, los estados de cuentas bancarios, y otros.

✔ **No deje ningún espacio en blanco en el formulario de solicitud de préstamo.** Trace una línea en cualquier sección cuya información no sea pertinente a usted. Si deja una sección en blanco, la entidad podría pensar que olvidó completarla. Igualmente, haga una copia de todos los documentos que presente por si acaso los originales se pierden, o si necesita consultarlos cuando la entidad de préstamo pregunte sobre algo que escribió en la solicitud.

✔ **Manténgase en contacto con su agente de depósito en garantía.** No deje que su caso quede enterrado en un montón de papeles y garantías pendientes en la esquina del escritorio de su agente del cierre. Usted o su agente de bienes raíces deben hablar con el agente de la garantía periódicamente para asegurarse que el proceso sigue su curso sin problemas.

✔ **Esté disponible al momento de firmar los documentos del préstamo.** Usted podría tener solamente 24 ó 48 horas después que su paquete del préstamo llegue a la entidad del depósito de la garantía, para firmar los documentos y devolvérselos a la entidad crediticia. Un retraso en este paso podría costarle el préstamo.

✔ **Si va a salir de la ciudad durante los días de fiestas, infórmeles, con suficiente antelación, a su agente inmobiliario, a la entidad crediticia y al agente de garantía.** Normalmente, usted puede hacer arreglos especiales para cerrar la garantía dónde sea que se encuentre, siempre y cuando las personas lo sepan de antemano y sepan cómo comunicarse con usted. La clave para el éxito es mantener a todos bien informados.

✔ **Revise el horario.** Muchas oficinas están abiertas solamente hasta el mediodía el día de Navidad y de Año Nuevo. Cuando estas fechas caen en sábado o en domingo, las horas de oficina pueden ser realmente anormales. Algunos negocios y oficinas públicas cierran el viernes anterior, otros el lunes siguiente, e incluso otros cierran el viernes y el lunes para darle a sus empleados cuatro días de fiesta. Durante estos días, asegúrese de revisar las horas de oficina de su agente inmobiliario, de la entidad crediticia, del agente de garantía y de las demás personas. No deje que el cierre de una oficina durante estas fiestas arruine su plan.

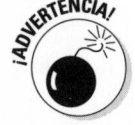

✔ **Permita un espacio de tiempo entre el momento que usted quiere cerrar y el momento cuando tiene que cerrar.** Regálese a sí mismo un espacio de tiempo para poder maniobrar y resolver problemas de último minuto que inevitablemente aparecen cuando menos los espera. No programe el cierre de la garantía para el último día de trabajo del año, ya que en ese caso no tendría margen para corregir algún error.

Haga un seguimiento

Las fiestas de compromisos son para las bodas, lo que los procesos de depósitos de garantías son para la compra de las casas. Al igual que las campanas no siempre repican para aquellos que se comprometen, igualmente, no todos los procesos de garantías empezados terminan siempre en la compra de la vivienda.

Muchos cierres de garantías podrían haber sido realizados si se hubiese usado el principio fundamental que se utiliza en tenis: haga un seguimiento. Los profesionales del tenis, por ejemplo, saben que en el juego es necesario algo más que simplemente pegarle a la pelota. Así que cuando golpean la pelota con un giro especial, continúan haciendo dicho giro aun después de haberla golpeado, porque saben que el último contacto con la pelota es tan importante como el contacto inicial. Si no completan su acción, la pelota no irá hacia donde ellos quieren que vaya.

Lo mismo ocurre con los negocios en bienes raíces. Los compradores, vendedores y agentes a menudo dicen que la casa ha sido *vendida* cuando el contrato de compra ha sido firmado. *¡Pero eso no es verdad!* Nada fue vendido. El comprador y el vendedor simplemente ratificaron una oferta. *¡Hay una gran diferencia!*

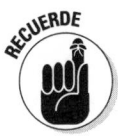

Si de verdad usted quiere comprar y mudarse a una vivienda —esto es, hacer el cierre de la garantía— todas las personas involucradas en su transacción tienen que completar todos los detalles que les corresponden. Usted no será el orgulloso propietario de la casa de sus sueños, ¡hasta que el gordito de la compañía de depósito en garantía diga que la garantía cerró!

La Forma Cómo Toma Posesión de la Vivienda Es Importante

Una de las decisiones más importantes que hace cuando compra una vivienda es en qué forma toma posesión de la propiedad. Si no está casado, sus alternativas son más simples porque toma posesión como único dueño. Sin embargo, cuando dos o más personas son copropietarias de la vivienda, el número de formas de propiedad de la vivienda aumenta astronómicamente.

La forma en que está titulada la propiedad es un asunto muy importante. Cada forma de copropiedad tiene su propia gama de ventajas y desventajas, de consecuencias impositivas y de repercusiones legales. Usted no debería tomar esta decisión precipitadamente en la oficina de la compañía de depósito en garantía mientras firma sus papeles del cierre; pero, desafortunadamente, eso es lo que normalmente ocurre.

¿Cuál es la mejor forma de copropiedad para usted? Eso realmente depende de las circunstancias. Aquí les presentamos algunas formas de copropiedad y las ventajas de cada una de ellas.

Tenencia conjunta

Suponga que usted y su cónyuge compran una casa bajo la forma de tenencia conjunta. Si su cónyuge fallece dentro de 20 años, la propiedad de la casa se transfiere directamente a usted sin tener que pasar a través de un tribunal de sucesiones o testamentos. Esta característica de la tenencia en conjunto se conoce como *derecho de supervivencia*.

Los beneficios de la tenencia conjunta no terminan allí. También tiene una *base gradual de valor de mercado* sobre el valor de la mitad de la propiedad de su cónyuge para efectos impositivos. Estas condiciones pueden ahorrarle una buena cantidad de dinero en los impuestos sobre las ganancias de capital, que tendrá que pagar si alguna vez vende su casa.

Veamos el siguiente ejemplo de cómo funciona la base gradual de valor de mercado. Digamos que usted y su cónyuge pagaron $180.000 por la casa cuando la compraron. Inmediatamente después de la muerte de su cónyuge, la casa fue valorada en $300.000.

Para efectos del impuesto, el nuevo costo de la casa es $240.000 ($90.000 correspondiente a la mitad del precio original de compra, más $150.000 por la mitad del valor de la casa de su cónyuge a la fecha de su fallecimiento) porque no se grava impuestos de ganancias de capital a los $60.000 de la plusvalía de la propiedad que le corresponde a su cónyuge.

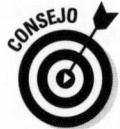

Aun cuando usamos una pareja casada en nuestro ejemplo, usted no necesita estar casado para usar esta forma de copropiedad. Sin embargo, un mínimo de dos personas deben ser copropietarias.

Propiedad comunal

Solamente parejas casadas pueden optar a este tipo de título de propiedad. La ventaja de la propiedad comunal, comparada con la tenencia conjunta, es que ambas partes o mitades de la vivienda son tratadas con una base gradual de valor de mercado al momento de la muerte de su cónyuge. Esto le permite ahorros impositivos aun mayores.

Usando las mismas cifras que en el ejemplo de tenencia conjunta, como cónyuge sobreviviente, la base gradual de costo es la cantidad completa de $300.000. El impuesto a las ganancias de capital no es cobrado en ninguna cantidad de la plusvalía del valor de la vivienda, desde la fecha de compra hasta la fecha de fallecimiento del cónyuge.

Otra ventaja de la propiedad comunal es el poder dejar, por medio de un testamento, su parte de la casa a quien usted quiera. Debido al derecho de supervivencia, esta alternativa no es posible cuando el título se tiene como tenencia conjunta.

Propietarios en tenencia en común

Tener el título como propietarios de tenencia en común o en sociedad no le permite usar una base gradual de valor de mercado al momento de la muerte de uno de los copropietarios. Ésta es una desventaja muy obvia desde el punto de vista impositivo.

Sin embargo, existen ciertas ventajas legales que compensan este aspecto negativo para personas copropietarias que no estén relacionadas, pero que adoptan esta forma de propiedad en convivencia o sociedad. Bajo esta forma de copropiedad, generalmente usted tiene el derecho de dejarle a alguien su parte en un testamento o de vender su parte de la propiedad sin permiso de los otros copropietarios. Además, los dueños no tienen que tener igual participación en la propiedad —una característica muy buena para aquellas personas que solo quieren disfrutar la propiedad pero con una participación financiera menor.

Cómo buscar ayuda para esbozar un acuerdo

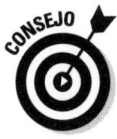

Si es listo —y sabemos que lo es porque de lo contrario no estaría leyendo este libro— usted y los otros copropietarios deberían tener un acuerdo o contrato legal por escrito, preparado por un abogado de bienes raíces, para resolver las posibles diferencias que aparezcan mientras comparten la propiedad (*Nota:* estos acuerdos son generalmente usados, y es aconsejable tenerlos cuando los socios que compran la propiedad no son una pareja casada.) He aquí unas cláusulas importantes que deben incluirse en los acuerdos escritos (usted puede obtener más información sobre estos asuntos en la sección de sociedades del Capítulo 8):

- Cláusulas que permitan comprarle a un copropietario que desea vender cuando los otros propietarios quieren mantener la propiedad.
- Cláusulas o condiciones para el prorrateo de los costos de reparación y mantenimiento entre los copropietarios con partes desiguales de la propiedad.
- Cláusulas para resolver conflictos relacionados con asuntos tales como de qué color pintar la casa.
- Cláusulas con penalizaciones si un copropietario no puede cumplir con su cuota de pagos del préstamo o de los impuestos a la propiedad

La información anterior no tiene la intención de ser su guía completa para los problemas reales de tenencia del título. Este capítulo simplemente indica los puntos más importantes que debe considerar. No tome una decisión de tanta importancia apresuradamente, especialmente si su situación es complicada y no muy normal. Además de decidir qué tipo legal de propiedad escogerá para su título de propiedad, también debería considerar la planificación de la disposición final de sus propiedades, tales como testamentos y fideicomisos potenciales (vea el Capítulo 2 para aprender un poco más acerca de la planificación de la propiedad).

La Posesión de Su Vivienda

El día que la compra cierra es, legalmente, muy complicado. Usted no es dueño de la vivienda cuando el día comienza a las 12:01 a.m., pero es el dueño en el registro cuando el día termina a la medianoche. En algún momento durante el día, el agente del depósito en garantía le entrega al vendedor su dinero, le notifica a usted que el documento ha sido registrado y oficialmente le anuncia que usted es el orgulloso dueño de la casa de sus sueños. ¡Felicitaciones!

El día de la mudanza

¿Cuándo puede tomar posesión de su casa y mudarse a ella? Eso depende de las condiciones del contrato. A continuación le mostramos las opciones que normalmente se tienen:

- **Mudarse el mismo día del cierre de la compraventa.** Esto está bien si los vendedores se han mudado ya. Sin embargo, si los vendedores aún no han salido de la casa —y no quieren entregar la vivienda hasta que estén absolutamente, 100 por ciento seguros que la garantía se ha cerrado—, entonces usted tiene un problema de logística, ya que es casi imposible que dos camiones de mudanza ocupen la entrada de la vivienda al mismo tiempo. Mudarse a una casa justo en el momento en que alguien más está desocupándola es algo que no intentará hacer más de una vez en su vida. Existen formas más fáciles de volverse loco.

- **Mudarse el día después que cierra la compraventa.** Le recomendamos esta alternativa si los vendedores no están dispuestos a entregar la vivienda hasta que la garantía cierre. Permita que los vendedores tengan el día que cierra la garantía como día de mudanza para ellos. Después de todo, los vendedores son todavía los dueños hasta que el título se transfiera. El día de mudanza es muy estresante, aun bajo las mejores circunstancias. ¿Para qué crear estrés innecesario al tratar de mudarse cuando los vendedores están saliendo?

Después que los vendedores se vayan, pero antes que la compañía de mudanza traiga sus cosas dentro de la casa, revise su nueva casa cuidadosamente por daños que la compañía de mudanza del vendedor pueda haber causado. Cuando estas compañías están involucradas, algunos accidentes pueden pasar. Hablamos de este tipo de problema en la sección siguiente.

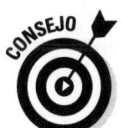

Sea que se mude a su casa el día del cierre de garantía o al día siguiente, usted empieza a pagar los servicios públicos y el seguro de propietario efectivamente desde ese día del cierre. No se olvide de coordinar la instalación del teléfono y el restablecimiento de los servicios públicos con las correspondientes compañías; es mejor hacerlo un par de semanas antes del cierre de garantía previsto.

✔ **Mudarse después de un retro alquiler del vendedor.** Los vendedores pueden permanecer en la casa por varias semanas después del cierre de la garantía mientras esperan mudarse a su nueva vivienda. En ese caso, el comprador firma separadamente un *contrato de retro alquiler* con los vendedores; este contrato entonces forma parte del contrato de compra. El acuerdo de retro alquiler cubre aspectos tales como quién paga por los servicios y mantenimiento, qué pasa si ocurre un daño a la propiedad, cuánto alquiler le deben pagar los vendedores a usted, y qué penalizaciones existen si el vendedor no desocupa la propiedad en la fecha especificada en el acuerdo de retro alquiler.

Es frecuente para los vendedores pagar un alquiler igual a lo que usted está pagando por capital e intereses en su hipoteca, más impuestos a la propiedad y seguros, de modo que usted no tenga gastos extras de lo que paga por ser dueño de la casa durante el tiempo del alquiler. El monto total correspondiente a *capital, intereses, impuestos y seguros* (conocido como *PITI,* por sus siglas en inglés) es prorrateado por día desde el cierre de la garantía hasta el día que el vendedor desocupe la vivienda. Suponga que el *PITI* es de $50 diarios, y los vendedores anticipan estar tres semanas después del cierre de la garantía. Ambas partes le piden al agente del depósito en garantía que retenga *cuatro* semanas de *PITI* en garantía para darles un pequeño colchón a los vendedores, en caso de que ellos tengan algún retraso en la mudanza a su nueva vivienda. Cuando finalmente los vendedores desocupen la vivienda, usted y ellos, conjuntamente, instruyen al agente de garantía a pagarle a usted el *PITI* correspondiente al tiempo real del alquiler, y a rembolsarles a los vendedores la parte de los fondos retenida en garantía que no fue usada.

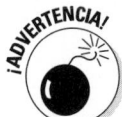

Si la casa que está comprando está vacante, puede sentirse tentado a pedir permiso para empezar a arreglarla antes del cierre de la garantía. Después de todo, pintar o pulir los pisos, por ejemplo, es mucho más fácil y más rápido cuando la casa está vacía. Pues bien, le recomendamos que *no lo haga.* Si el negocio no se cierra, usted habrá gastado tiempo y dinero arreglando la casa de alguien más. O si la casa se incendia, no tiene seguro para cubrir esas pérdidas. Aquí el riesgo es mayor que la recompensa. En lugar de hacer eso, permítase un tiempo para hacer estos trabajos *después* que cierre la garantía y *antes* de mudarse.

Verificación final de la condición de la vivienda

Si el contrato de su estado no contiene una cláusula de verificación final de la condición de la vivienda, pídale a su agente o abogado que le escriba una en su contrato. Casi todos los acuerdos tienen algo similar bajo "Otros términos y condiciones", que sirve para este tipo de inclusiones en el contrato.

Le recomendamos que inspeccione la propiedad unos días antes que la garantía cierre —sería ideal el mismo día del cierre de garantía—, para estar seguro que la propiedad está aún en las mismas condiciones generales que estaba cuando usted firmó el contrato inicial para comprarla. ¿Qué pasa si los vendedores hicieron un hueco en la pared de la cocina durante una fiesta? ¿Qué pasa si se les olvidó regar el césped y éste se convirtió en un jardín rocoso? ¿Qué pasa si un desagüe aparece de la nada en medio de la entrada de la cochera? La lista de "Qué pasas" es interminable.

Probablemente se dé cuenta que todo está bien. Pero si no lo está, puede pedirle al agente de garantía que detenga el proceso mientras resuelve el problema. Este hecho, siempre llama la atención del vendedor y del agente inmobiliario. Si no puede lograr una solución mutuamente satisfactoria con el vendedor, quizás tenga que deshacer el negocio; a veces esto es mejor que comprar un problema.

Cómo Sobrellevar el Remordimiento del Comprador

Muchos vendedores de vivienda están convencidos de que dejaron las joyas de la familia en la mesa cuando vendieron sus viviendas. Esta idea de que "regalaron la casa" es llamada *remordimiento del vendedor*. Este remordimiento es doloroso, pero generalmente desaparece en un mes o dos después de la venta. Los vendedores tienen mucha suerte de padecer de una demencia poco complicada.

Si usted es como la mayoría de los compradores, también sentirá lo opuesto de esa horrible psicosis. El *remordimiento del comprador* es ese sentimiento de vacío en el estómago de que pagó mucho, muchísimo, por su nueva casa.

Desafortunadamente, el remordimiento del comprador es mucho más complicado que el del vendedor. El del comprador va acompañado de muchas otras ansiedades —que obtuvo el peor de todos los préstamos, que el valor de la propiedad va a bajar en los años siguientes a la compra, que puede perder el trabajo, que su salud podría fallar y que su fiel perrito va a fallecer.

Estamos aquí para ayudarlo a enfrentarse a su miedo de pagar demás. Esas otras ansiedades son reacciones absolutamente normales a la incertidumbre que la mayoría de nosotros sentimos *inicialmente*. Dichas ansiedades desaparecerán y, por si esto lo hace sentir mejor, casi todos los compradores de vivienda están traumatizados por las mismas preocupaciones cuando llevan a cabo una compra.

Con el tiempo, descubrirá (como nosotros y millones de otras personas que lo hicieron antes que usted) que tiene una buena hipoteca, que los valores de la propiedad son estables, que su empleo es seguro, su salud está muy bien y su perrito también. Pero no nos crea así por así. Haga algunas llamadas telefónicas para verificar que realmente obtuvo un buen préstamo, lea los avisos clasificados para trabajos como el suyo, hable del valor de las propiedades con los vecinos, hágase un examen físico y lleve su perrito al veterinario.

Ahora bien, ¿y qué acerca de la duda de que pagó mucho, muchísimo? Si los dioses de bienes raíces lo aman, tendrá un caso poco grave de remordimiento de comprador, el cual puede curarlo tomando dos aspirinas. Sin embargo, algunos compradores, están tan desolados por este sentimiento, que tratan de romper el contrato.

Usted no puede enfrentar este sentimiento de arrepentimiento hasta que lo acepte por lo que es: miedo, simple y llanamente. Tiene miedo de haber pagado demás por la vivienda. Ese miedo acaba con muchos compradores. Los síntomas típicos del remordimiento de comprador son fáciles de notar. Por ejemplo, después que ha firmado el contrato para comprar la casa de sus sueños, usted hace una o algunas de las siguientes cosas:

- ✔ **Lee los avisos en la sección de bienes raíces de su periódico local con aún mayor atención que antes de firmar el contrato.** Busca viviendas similares a la suya, o más bonitas, con precios menores. (Se olvida que la mayoría de las casas lucen mejor en papel que cuando las ve con sus propios ojos en la visita respectiva.)

- ✔ **Pasa sábados y domingos recorriendo casas abiertas al público.** Leer los avisos no es suficiente para usted. Siente la necesitad de ir a la calle, a buscar una mejor compra que la que usted realizó. Después de todo, ver *es* creer. (Y hablando de ver, puede que vea a sus vendedores con remordimientos dando vueltas a las mismas casas que usted está mirando, tratando de encontrar propiedades menos bonitas con precios más altos que la que le vendieron.)

- ✔ **Habla de la compra con sus amigos, vecinos, colegas, y el tipo parado detrás de usted en la línea para comprar las entradas al cine.** Le pregunta a cualquiera, si piensa que usted pagó mucho, aunque el 99,9 por ciento de las personas con quienes hable no tienen ni idea de los valores de propiedades para casas similares a las suyas. (Acepta como absoluta verdad cualquier número que se les ocurra y que confirme sus sospechas.)

Después de hacer esas cosas *durante* el cierre de garantía y por un par de meses *después* de la compra (hasta que está emocional y físicamente exhausto), probablemente descubrirá que sus temores son infundados. Sus preocupaciones no son raras o anormales. Lo que está mal es dejar que estos miedos lo corroan secretamente por dentro, en lugar de afrontarlos abiertamente.

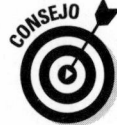

Los hechos conquistan el miedo. Mientras más rápido obtenga los datos reales, menos sufrirá.

Como explicamos en el Capítulo 10, una vivienda puede tener más de un precio correcto. Establecer precios y negociar es un arte y no una ciencia exacta. No se mortifique por los precios *iniciales* que piden por las casas. Usted está bien siempre y cuando el precio de *compra* de su vivienda está al mismo nivel que los precios de *venta* de viviendas similares.

Si usted sigue los principios que exponemos en este libro, ¡va a estar muy bien! A diferencia de muchos otros compradores, usted conoce cómo poner sus finanzas en orden antes de comprar, y también cómo determinar lo que realmente puede pagar por una casa. Además sabe cómo encontrar un buen vecindario, una excelente propiedad, una buena hipoteca, y un inspector de propiedad eficiente. Usted puede diferenciar entre una casa cuyo precio está sobre valorado, y una excelente oportunidad de compra. Ya sabe de inspecciones de propiedad y cómo negociar reparaciones de los defectos de la propiedad y, además, sabe cómo evitar gente odiosa y sorpresas desagradables.

El saber es poder. Después que haya asimilado los consejos ofrecidos en este libro, será sumamente poderoso. No tiene nada que temer. ¡Vaya y busque la casa de sus sueños!

Parte V
La Parte
de los Diez

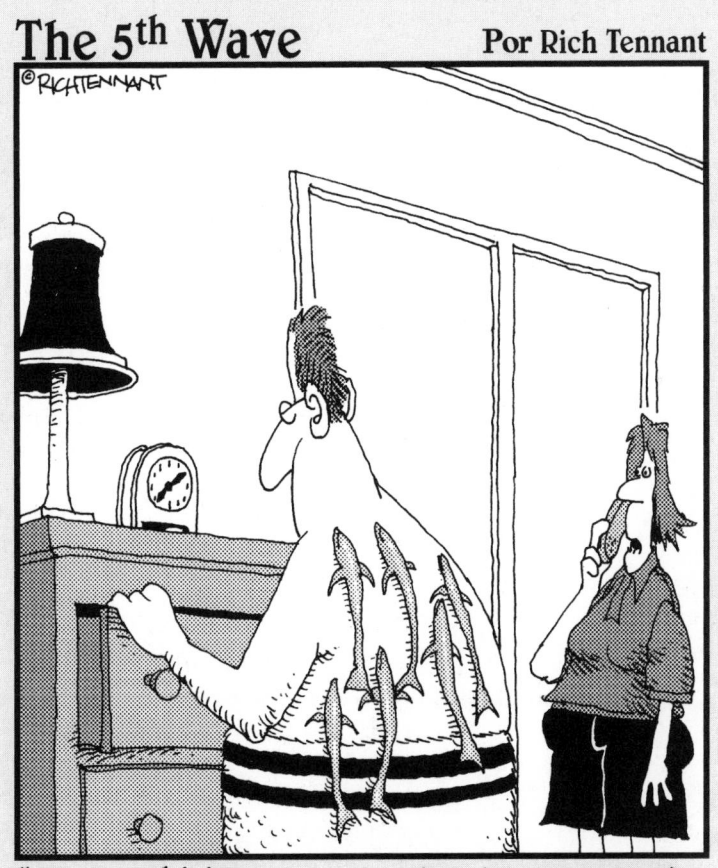

The 5th Wave   Por Rich Tennant

"Creo que hicimos lo correcto al comprar esta casa, pero Francisco tiene un caso muy grave de 'rémoradimiento' de comprador por todos los gastos".

En esta parte . . .

Esta parte presenta información sobre las diez estrategias financieras que debería tomar después de comprar, las diez cosas que debe saber cuando invierte en bienes raíces y diez puntos que debe considerar antes de vender su casa.

Capítulo 15

Diez Estrategias Financieras que Debería Tener en Cuenta Después de Comprar

A pesar de que pudo haber parecido que el día nunca llegaría, ¡pues finalmente llegó! ¡Usted es el propietario de una vivienda! Un propietario . . . ¿Puede creerlo? ¡Pues vaya y pínchese usted mismo!

Tal vez ya esté comentándoles a sus amigos que le han preguntado qué se siente ser propietario de una vivienda. La mayoría de los nuevos propietarios dicen: "Bueno, el banco tiene más casas que yo". De hecho, usted posee el 100 por ciento de la propiedad, ¡sólo que usted le debe a la entidad hipotecaria un montón de dinero! Confíe en nosotros cuando le decimos que aunque en estos momentos parezca mucho dinero, no lo parecerá a la vuelta de unas décadas. En ese momento agradecerá el haber decidido comprar en vez de seguir alquilando. Lo que debe hoy será suyo, sin condiciones, en 30 años —si no antes— al menos teóricamente.

Si piensa que la peor parte termina con la firma del contrato de compra, puede que se sorprenda saber que no es así. La mudanza probablemente no sea un picnic pero es justo donde comienza el hecho de que usted quiera transformar su nueva adquisición en una hermosa casa.

Como nuevo propietario, usted debe desechar muchas ofertas que estarán revoloteando a su alrededor. Desafortunadamente, cuando compra una casa, usted termina en una lista kilométrica de correos ya que la compra de su vivienda es un asunto que se registra públicamente. Incluso, algunas comunidades publican los avisos de ventas de casas (con los nombres completos del vendedor, del comprador y el precio de compraventa, ¡aunque no lo crea!).

Este capítulo puede ayudarlo a ser un propietario nuevo con unas finanzas buenas y, además, ayudarlo a evitar las trampas en las que muchos propietarios novatos han caído antes que usted.

Vigile Sus Gastos y Ahorros

Si usted es como la mayoría de los nuevos propietarios, luego de adquirir su nueva casa y mudarse, sus muebles y otras posesiones parecieran volverse más viejos y desteñidos que antes. Y debido a que ya está viviendo en la propiedad, pronto descubre aspectos y detalles que no le gustan mucho y que no vio antes cuando estaba buscando vivienda. Éste es un pequeño regaño del *remordimiento del comprador,* una congoja común de los nuevos compradores y que presentamos en el Capítulo 14.

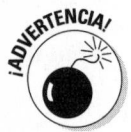

La mayoría de los compradores de vivienda pueden encontrar infinidades de proyectos de remodelación, así como también, muebles y aparatos electrodomésticos por comprar —que rápidamente acaban los ingresos de cualquiera, aun los de los ricos y famosos. Debido a estas tentaciones de gasto, la mayoría de los compradores terminan gastando sus ingresos duramente ganados. Algunos hasta recurren a tarjetas de crédito y a deudas de consumidor con altas tasas de interés porque sus gastos sobrepasan sus ingresos.

Es completamente normal sentir el presupuesto oprimido cuando se compra una casa. Después de todo, sus gastos de vivienda son más altos que cuando vivía alquilado. Y ésa es la mejor razón para que usted ajuste el resto del presupuesto y otros gastos (vea el Capítulo 2). Uno de ellos es hacer que su vivienda sea más eficiente en cuanto al consumo de energía, poniendo en práctica algunas cosas simples como incluir aislamiento e instalar controladores de agua en la grifería y ducha. Además, utilice su reporte de inspección de la vivienda para detectar áreas que pueda mejorar.

No descuide el ahorro en otras áreas importantes de sus metas financieras, como la jubilación. Tómese su tiempo en convertir su nuevo hogar en un auténtico palacio, y regocíjese y consuélese en el hecho de que tiene un techo sobre su cabeza, un lugar cálido y cómodo para dormir y un espacio adecuado para vivir —cosas que muchas personas en el mundo sólo pueden soñar en tener.

Haga Pagos Hipotecarios Electrónicamente

Los agentes hipotecarios desean que se les pague a tiempo y usted también desea pagarles a tiempo. El retraso en los pagos le puede salir caro — muchas hipotecas tienen penalizaciones del 5 por ciento de la cuota a pagar si su pago se retrasa. Si su pago se retrasa un mes, un recargo del 5 por ciento que le hagan ¡equivale a más del 60 por ciento con respecto a la tasa de interés anual! Incluso, el retraso de un día puede dar comienzo a una penalización. ¡Y pensar que usted creía que un 18 por ciento en la tarjeta de crédito era alto, ¿no?! Además, los pagos retrasados se muestran como *faltas* o *manchas* en su reporte crediticio.

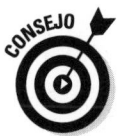

Subscríbase al servicio de pago automático de su agencia crediticia para efectuar el pago electrónicamente desde su cuenta bancaria a la de la agencia, el mismo día de cada mes. Si su agente hipotecario no ofrece este servicio, hágalo usted mismo a través de uno de los muchos servicios bancarios, tales como CheckFree (800-297-3180; www.checkfree.com), o a través de programas electrónicos como *Quicken* o *Microsoft Money*.

Aumente Su Reserva de Emergencia

La mayoría de las personas agotan su reserva de emergencia para poder reunir suficiente dinero en efectivo y así completar la compra de la vivienda. Teóricamente usted debería tener listo y disponible una reserva de emergencia en efectivo equivalente a al menos tres meses de sus gastos mensuales. Si su empleo es inestable y no cuenta con el apoyo financiero inmediato de su familia, opte por una reserva de emergencia de seis meses. Mantenga el dinero de emergencia en un fondo de inversión en activos del mercado monetario a alto rendimiento (vea el Capítulo 3).

Debido a que está ahorrando dinero para cumplir con otras metas financieras, la reposición de su reserva de emergencia le requiere hacer un plan financiero en donde usted gaste menos de lo que gana. Sabemos que es más fácil decirlo que hacerlo, especialmente con todas las cosas tentadoras que hay para gastar el dinero en la casa. Evite los centros comerciales, los catálogos para ordenar por correo y las tiendas para mejorar su hogar, ¡hasta que su estabilidad monetaria sea real!

Pase por Alto las Ofertas de Seguros Hipotecarios

Tan pronto como se mude a su nuevo hogar —a menudo en cuestión de pocas semanas o meses— su buzón de correos estará inundado con solicitudes ofreciéndole seguros hipotecarios de vida y de incapacidad. La mayoría de las solicitudes vienen de su agente hipotecario, pero otras pueden venir de compañías de seguros que lo escogieron de la información pública disponible que revela que usted recientemente compró su casa.

El problema fundamental con estas pólizas de seguros es que dada la cantidad de protección que ofrecen, son generalmente costosas y no proveen el número apropiado de beneficios. El monto de su hipoteca no necesariamente debería determinar el costo de su seguro de vida ni el de incapacidad. Si necesita la protección de un seguro de vida porque tiene personas que dependen de sus ingresos, generalmente es conveniente comprar una póliza de seguro a término, a bajo costo y de alta calidad. Asimismo, si usted depende de sus ingresos, asegúrese de tener un seguro de incapacidad a largo plazo apropiado. Vea el Capítulo 2 para leer más acerca de cómo solucionar sus necesidades de seguro.

Pase por Alto las Ofertas para Saldar Su Deuda Más Rápido

Otro tipo de ofertas que puede recibir es la que ensalza las virtudes —ahorros de miles de dólares en intereses— de liberar su hipoteca más rápidamente. Por una tarifa mensual, estas compañías ofrecen convertir su pago anual de hipoteca de 12 meses en 26 pagos bisemanales, cada uno de los cuales es la mitad de su cuota mensual. De esta manera, usted estará cancelando 13 cuotas de la hipoteca cada año en vez de 12. Haciéndolo así, esto generalmente le ahorrará cerca de 8 años del plan de repago en una hipoteca de 30 años.

Estas ofertas tienen dos problemas: primero, usted está pagando por liberar su hipoteca más rápido, que es algo que usted mismo puede hacer sin usar ese servicio y sin las tarifas que le cobran. Segundo, puede ser que liberar la hipoteca lo más pronto posible no sea su prioridad.

La pregunta que usted debe hacerse es, ¿qué haría con ese dinero extra mensual que estaría pagando si no estuviera cancelando la hipoteca más rápidamente? Si lo gastara en cosas frívolas o superfluas, entonces amortizar la deuda es probablemente una mejor opción para usar ese dinero. Asimismo, si usted es un inversionista de cierta edad (o que no le gustan los riesgos), entonces es poco probable que al invertir su dinero, gane una tasa de retorno lo suficientemente alta como para que valga la pena no cancelar la hipoteca más rápido.

Por otro lado, si usted pudiera ahorrar ese dinero en una cuenta de jubilación deducible de impuestos, el tratar de cancelar su hipoteca más rápido puede hacerle gastar dinero en lugar de ahorrarlo. Tampoco es bueno pagar sus deudas si esto lo deja sin dinero en efectivo. Suponga que pierde su trabajo y le toma varios meses conseguir otro; o, suponga que su casa necesita un techo nuevo y no tiene suficiente dinero para pagarlo. Sería conveniente que tuviera al menos una reserva equivalente de tres a seis meses de gastos mensuales en alguna inversión de fácil acceso como un fondo en el mercado monetario. Si no la tiene, puede que tenga que usar tarjetas de créditos con altas tasas de interés (no deducibles de impuestos) para pagar gastos inesperados.

Estudie la Posibilidad de Apelar Su Gravamen de Impuesto

En la mayoría de las comunidades, los impuestos de propiedad de bienes raíces están basados en un estimado del valor de su vivienda. Si el valor de las propiedades ha bajado desde que adquirió la vivienda, usted puede apelar su gravamen y disfrutar de una reducción en los impuestos de propiedad que debe pagar.

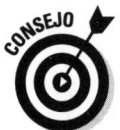

Hable con el asesor de impuestos de su localidad acerca de los trámites que debe hacer para apelar los impuestos de su propiedad. Generalmente, el procedimiento se basa en proveerle al asesor, por escrito, datos de ventas similares que prueben la reducción del valor de su vivienda. Si necesita ayuda con esto, llame al agente inmobiliario que le vendió la casa. Pero, tenga cuidado, ya que su agente inmobiliario puede tratar de hacerlo sentir como si su vivienda no hubiera bajado tanto en valor, sólo para que usted no se sienta mal (y hasta para él mismo no sentirse mal). Explíquele que usted está tratando de ahorrar dinero en sus impuestos de propiedad y que necesita comprobar que otras viviendas en el vecindario fueron vendidas por menos de lo que usted pagó por la suya. Vea el Capítulo 10 si necesita una rápida actualización en el cálculo de valores de propiedades.

Refinancie Si las Tasas de Interés Bajan

En los Capítulos 6 y 7 explicamos cómo seleccionar una magnífica hipoteca y damos varios consejos para obtener la mejor que pueda. Pero, si usted es como la mayoría de las personas, después de que se embarca en la rutina del pago de su hipoteca es probable que mantenga tan alta prioridad en permanecer atento a las estrategias para reducir al mínimo los costos de la misma, como la limpieza de sus dientes con el hilo dental tres veces al día.

Esté pendiente de las tasas de interés. Por favor, vea los recursos para la búsqueda de préstamos hipotecarios que recomendamos en el Capítulo 6 y, también, las páginas Web que recomendamos en el Capítulo 11 para ayudarlo de manera más eficiente en esta tarea. A lo mejor ya lo sabe, pero recuerde que las tasas de interés cambian como el clima. Si las tasas de interés disminuyen en comparación a como estaban cuando usted adquirió su hipoteca, usted puede refinanciar su hipoteca y ahorrarse algo de dinero. *El refinanciamiento* (como se describió en el Capítulo 6) significa simplemente que usted reemplaza su hipoteca de alto costo con una nueva de menor costo.

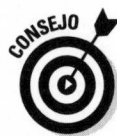

Si las tasas han bajado por lo menos un punto porcentual completo desde que usted adquirió el préstamo, comience a pensar en el refinanciamiento. El punto clave a calcular es cuántos meses le tomará recuperar los costos del refinanciamiento (gastos del préstamo más de títulos, seguros y otros). Suponga que su agente hipotecario favorito le dice que usted puede ahorrarse $150 de su pago mensual mediante el refinanciamiento. Suena bien, ¿verdad? Bueno, no tan rápido. ¡Espere! Primero, eso no significa que usted ahorrará esos $150 mensuales sólo porque su pago baje esa cantidad —no se olvide que usted perderá algunos desgravámenes del impuesto si deduce menos por concepto de hipoteca.

Para tener una mejor idea en cuánto realmente se reducirá el costo de su hipoteca, luego de deducir los impuestos, tome su tasa impositiva (como está explicado en el Capítulo 3) y réstele a esa cantidad los ahorros mensuales que usted estima obtener por el refinanciamiento. Si usted tiene un salario moderado, lo más probable es que esté en la categoría impositiva del 28 por ciento. Si su pago mensual de hipoteca disminuye en $150, y si reduce esos $150 por el 28 por ciento (para tomar en cuenta la pérdida por impuestos), su ahorro (después de los impuestos) sería en realidad $108 por mes.

Ahora bien, $108 mensuales no es nada malo, pero todavía debe considerar cuánto le costará el refinanciamiento de la deuda. Si el costo total del refinanciamiento, por ejemplo, es de $6.000, esto le tomará cerca de 56 meses ($6.000 dividido por $108) para recuperar estos costos. Si usted piensa mudarse en cinco años, el refinanciamiento no le ahorrará ningún dinero — al contrario, le costará dinero. Por otro lado, si el refinanciamiento le cuesta $3.000, usted puede recuperar estos costos en tres años. Si usted espera permanecer en su casa al menos por ese tiempo, probablemente el refinanciamiento es una buena inversión.

Guarde las Facturas de Todas las Mejoras

Tarde o temprano, usted invertirá dinero en su hogar. Usted debe documentar parte del dinero que gasta con el fin de minimizar la ganancia de capital que debe declarar al impuesto en el futuro. *La ganancia de capital* simplemente significa la diferencia de lo que recibe por la casa cuando la vende menos lo que le costó cuando la compró —con una importante modificación. El *IRS* le permite a usted agregar el costo de las mejoras al costo original de la casa para el cálculo de lo que se conoce como su *base de costo ajustado*.

Ganancia de capital = Precio de venta neto – (Precio de compra + Capital de mejoras)

Por ejemplo, si usted compra su casa por $225.000 y con el tiempo se revaloriza de manera que (después de pagar los costos de venta) su precio de venta neto es de $350.000, su ganancia de capital es de $125.000. Recuerde que el *IRS* le permite agregar a su precio de compra, el valor del capital de mejoras que le haga a su hogar.

El capital de mejoras es el dinero que usted gasta en su casa y que incrementa de forma permanente su valor y su vida útil —por ejemplo, instalar un nuevo techo a la casa en vez de colocar parches al techo existente. Así que si usted hizo mejoras por un valor de $10.000 a la casa que compró por $225.000, su ganancia de capital se verá reducida a $115.000. El dinero que se gasta en trabajos de mantenimiento, como arreglar una gotera en una tubería o reemplazar ventanas rotas, no se pueden agregar a su base de costo (vea el Capítulo 3 para más detalles).

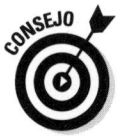

Antes de vender su casa, asegúrese, por favor, de entender los efectos económicos de impuestos que la venta ocasiona. Como lo explicamos en el Capítulo 17, muchos propietarios —que reúnen los requisitos—, tienen el derecho a sustraer de los impuestos una gran cantidad del capital ganado cuando les llegue el momento de vender la vivienda.

Pase por Alto las Ofertas para Proteger Su Propiedad

Otra oferta que usted como nuevo propietario puede conseguir en su buzón, es el de compañías "amistosas" que le ofrecen proteger su residencia contra embargos si les paga una cantidad entre $50 y $100. *La inembargabilidad de la vivienda* significa la protección de parte de su patrimonio contra embargos. Una compañía puede ofrecerle registrar el documento legal pertinente —y es muy sencillo— para proteger una porción del capital de su patrimonio contra embargos y reclamos judiciales.

Si usted vive en un estado donde necesite asegurar su vivienda contra embargos, no dude en hacerlo. Llame a la oficina de registros y pregunte cómo hacerlo. El proceso es sencillo —y en algunos estados es innecesario— y no vale la pena pagarle a una compañía para que lo haga por usted.

Relájese y Disfrute la Vida

Bueno, suena como un disco rayado, pero a menudo la gente trabaja, trabaja y trabaja para lograr su casa y se olvida de disfrutar la vida, la familia y los amigos (y aún su propia casa). Si usted adquiere una vivienda que encaja en su presupuesto y usted es de los que ahorran mientras vive allí, su vivienda no controlará sus finanzas ni su trabajo. Usted poseerá su casa y no la casa a usted.

Nadie (que nosotros sepamos) ha dicho alguna vez en su lecho de muerte que hubiese deseado haberse dedicado más al trabajo para tener más dinero para gastar en su casa (y por lo tanto, tener menos tiempo para él o para pasarlo con la familia o los amigos).

Capítulo 16

Diez Cosas que Debe Saber Cuando Invierta en Bienes Raíces

En Este Capítulo

▶ Cómo superar obstáculos en las inversiones

▶ Haga su tarea antes de invertir

▶ Cómo capitalizar las mejores opciones en bienes raíces

La propiedad de su casa y el pago de la hipoteca con el correr de los años deben originar *el capital,* esto es, la diferencia entre el valor de su vivienda y la porción que usted debe de ella. Aún si lo improbable ocurriera, y su vivienda no se revalorizara, usted iría erigiendo su capital en la medida en que iría pagando la hipoteca. Sin embargo, es mucho más probable que su vivienda se revalorice a medida que pase el tiempo y usted se va convirtiendo en su dueño.

Por lo tanto, su vivienda es una inversión. Usted puede utilizar en los años venideros el capital de su vivienda para una variedad de propósitos importantes como ayudar a financiar su jubilación, pagar costos de educación y a invertir en cosas frívolas y divertidas como viajar, entre otras. Además de ser propietario de su vivienda, usted puede invertir en bienes raíces en otras formas. En este capítulo le damos nuestros diez mejores consejos y cosas que debe saber si va a invertir en bienes raíces.

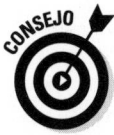

Si usted desea invertir en bienes raíces, o en la bolsa de valores, en bonos, fondos mutuales, en pequeños negocios u otros similares, primero, invierta tiempo investigando cómo funcionan, y aprenda cómo tomar decisiones bien fundamentadas de manera que se ajusten a su situación y metas financieras personales. Busque una copia de las ediciones más recientes de *Investing For Dummies, Real Estate Investing For Dummies* y *Mutual Funds For Dummies* de Eric, para aprender más acerca del tema.

Los Bienes Raíces Son una Inversión Sólida a Largo Plazo

Durante los años 90, muchas personas fueron arrastradas por la euforia de un auge en el mercado de valores estadounidense. Año tras año el mercado devolvía fácilmente ganancias de dos cifras a los inversionistas. Algunas veces escuchamos historias de personas que hicieron pequeñas fortunas al invertir en las acciones apropiadas en el momento apropiado. Mientras tanto, en muchas partes del país, los precios de los bienes raíces aumentaron muy poco en comparación con las acciones. Así que a mucha gente le pareció — incluso a los expertos de los medios de comunicación— que la inversión en bienes raíces era una cosa del pasado.

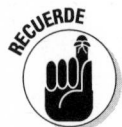

El valor de las viviendas en todas partes siempre ha tenido sus altos y bajos. Sin embargo, la tendencia a largo plazo es a subir y, generalmente, los aumentos son mucho más altos que las disminuciones que le siguen. (La bolsa de valores, como usted sabe, pasan por ciclos similares y en muchos casos más fuertes, como la gran depresión a principios del año 2000). De manera que si usted tiene en la mira un tiempo de inversión de largo plazo (una década o más sería ideal), usted estaría haciendo lo correcto si invierte en bienes raíces. El promedio anual de retorno es similar a los obtenidos por inversionistas de la bolsa de valores a largo plazo. El mejor momento para comprar una casa es siempre una década antes. Dentro de una década, los precios de hoy parecerán estar por el suelo.

La Inversión en Bienes Raíces No Es para Todos

Si usted es una persona impaciente y ocupada, es probable que la inversión en bienes raíces no sea la mejor opción para usted. ¿La razón? La ubicación, negociación y cierre del trato pueden tomar una porción bastante considerable de su tiempo si quiere comprar una buena propiedad a un buen precio. Luego está la tarea de administrar la propiedad (y el sumidero por donde se va el tiempo), ya que usted es responsable de todo, desde conseguir los inquilinos hasta mantener la edificación limpia y en buen estado. Sus inversiones en fondos mutuales y en la bolsa de valores no lo llamarán en medio de la noche para arreglar un problema de plomería, ¡pero puede que sus inquilinos sí!

Aún si usted tiene tiempo para invertir en bienes raíces, examine también otros aspectos importantes de su situación financiera. Como lo presentamos en el Capítulo 2, el tomar ventaja de las cuentas de jubilación deducibles del impuesto es vital para su bienestar financiero a largo plazo y para poder jubilarse. El comprar inversiones en bienes raíces le puede impedir ahorrar en las cuentas de jubilación; el ahorrar para la cuota inicial puede obstaculizar su capacidad de pasar fondos a estas cuentas de jubilación. Además, la mayoría de las propiedades que usted compre requerirán desembolsar dinero en los primeros años.

Los REIT Son Buenos Si No le Gusta Ser un Administrador

Si usted desea invertir algo de dinero en bienes raíces pero no le gusta la idea de ser el administrador, tenga en cuenta a los Consorcios de inversiones en Bienes Raíces (*Real Estate Investment Trusts* [*REIT*, por sus siglas en inglés]). Los *REIT* son manejados por una compañía que junta su dinero con el de otros inversionistas para comprar una variedad de propiedades de inversión en bienes raíces y que ellos administran.

Los *REIT* hacen inversiones en las grandes bolsas de valores, pero algunos fondos mutuales también invierten en los *REIT*. Entre los mejores fondos mutuales que invierten en *REIT* se pueden considerar los siguientes:

- ✔ **CGM Realty:** 800-345-4048; www.cgmfunds.com
- ✔ **Cohen & Steers Realty Shares:** 800-437-9912; www.cohenandsteers.com
- ✔ **Fidelity Real Estate Investment Portfolio:** 800-544-8888; www.fidelity.com
- ✔ **T. Rowe Price Real Estate Fund:** 800-638-5660; www.troweprice.com
- ✔ **Vanguard REIT Index Fund:** 800-662-7447; www.vanguard.com

No Invierta en Asociaciones Limitadas

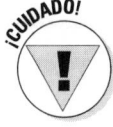

Evite las asociaciones limitadas de bienes raíces que son vendidas a través de compañías de corretajes de seguros. Los corredores de seguros, que a menudo operan bajo el engañoso seudónimo de *consultores financieros* o *consejeros financieros*, gustan de vender asociaciones limitadas debido a las abultadas comisiones que ellas pagan a los corredores. La comisión del corredor puede ser del 10 por ciento o más. Y, ¿adivine de dónde sale ese dinero? Si responde, "de los dólares que invertí", ¡usted se lleva el premio!

Además del gran defecto de que solo 90 centavos del dólar que usted invierte van a trabajar para usted, las inversiones que el corredor hace generalmente tienen una considerable tarifa anual operativa entre el 2 y el 3 por ciento. De manera que cuando usted suma todo (o mejor dicho, después que todas estas comisiones y tarifas son sustraídas de sus bien ganados dólares) las asociaciones limitadas están destinadas a convertirse en una pobre inversión para usted.

Evite los Condominios y Viviendas Vacacionales

Otra manera en la que gente inteligente pierde grandes cantidades de dinero cuando invierte en bienes raíces es a través de la inversión en condominios y viviendas vacacionales. El atractivo de estas inversiones es el tener un lugar donde escapar para divertirse y relajarse.

Con un condominio vacacional usted está comprando básicamente el uso por una semana del mismo. Suponga que por este privilegio usted paga una tarifa de $7.000 una sola vez. Aunque parezca que $7.000 no sean mucho, si una semana cuesta esa cantidad, el comprar los derechos de todo un año para utilizar el condominio vacacional viene a costar más de $350.000. ¡Sin embargo, el comprar un condominio similar en esa misma zona puede costarle aproximadamente $125.000! De manera que usted está pagando una *gran* cantidad por la membresía de una semana debido a los costos que se generan por vender todas esas semanas y la necesidad del administrador del condominio de sacarle un beneficio a la transacción. (Y, además, usted también estará pagando un par de cientos de dólares o más de la cuota anual de mantenimiento.)

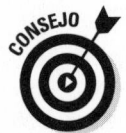

Una posibilidad mejor sería alquilar un condominio que otra persona posea; esto es más barato que ser propietario. Usted puede ir a diferentes condominios y en distintos lugares cada año (esquiar, playa, lo que guste) sin tener el dolor de cabeza de administrar la propiedad. O, usted puede comprar un reconocido condominio, alquilarlo a otros en el transcurso del año y, luego alquilar otro condominio que no sea el suyo, por una, dos o las semanas que usted quiera cada año, para el disfrute de sus vacaciones.

Otra idea escalofriante: los condominios vacacionales son casi imposibles de vender. Como lo decimos en el Capítulo 8, el mejor momento de pensar en vender una propiedad es *antes* de comprarla. En todo caso, los bienes raíces son una forma de inversión relativamente sólida; ¿por qué congelar su sólido dinero en un condominio vacacional?

Las viviendas vacacionales presentan un problema diferente. La mayoría de las personas que compran las viviendas vacacionales las usan sólo por unas semanas al año. El resto del tiempo la propiedad permanece vacante creando un desagüe de dinero. Ahora bien, si usted está lo suficientemente solvente como para darse estos lujos, no nos vamos a interponer en su camino para disuadirlo de poseer más de una propiedad. Pero muchas personas que compran viviendas vacacionales no tienen suficiente dinero como para poderlas mantener.

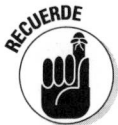

Antes de comprar una propiedad vacacional, examine sus finanzas para determinar si usted todavía puede ahorrar lo suficiente cada mes, una vez que realice la compra, como para lograr sus metas financieras importantes, tales como pagar la educación superior de sus hijos o cimentar el nidito para su jubilación. Si usted compra una vivienda vacacional, tome en cuenta comprar una propiedad que pueda alquilar el tiempo que no la ocupe.

Las Propiedades Residenciales Son Su Mejor Inversión

Si usted va a invertir en bienes raíces, la propiedad residencial es generalmente la inversión más segura y confiable:

- ✔ Primero, porque probablemente usted está más familiarizado con este tipo de propiedades debido a que ya ha vivido en una (y quizás hasta comprado).

- ✔ Segundo, la propiedad residencial pudiera ser más fácil para usted de manejar y administrar día a día. (Asegúrese de conocer todo lo concerniente a las leyes vigentes que rigen los alquileres, si las hay, en su comunidad y cómo afectarían a la propiedad que pueda comprar.)

No se olvide que con la administración de un condominio vienen también las responsabilidades y, ocasionalmente, las situaciones delicadas. Es por eso que insistimos que consulte a un buen abogado en bienes raíces de la localidad si tiene *cualquier* duda acerca de la parte legal de comprar y administrar su propiedad para alquiler. Hablamos sobre los sabuesos legales en el Capítulo 9.

Los bienes raíces comerciales tienen muchos matices legales y financieros con los que usted probablemente no ha lidiado ni querrá lidiar. El negocio de bienes raíces comerciales tiende también a ser más volátil en su valor debido a que es más fácil aumentar la construcción y el número de negocios, a diferencia del número de personas en una localidad, puede reducirse más rápidamente durante unas condiciones económicas precarias. No estamos diciendo que usted nunca debería tratar de invertir en este tipo de propiedades más complicadas, sino que es mejor que aprenda a nadar en la piscina del patio de atrás de su casa antes de dar el salto a un mar infestado de tiburones.

Considere los Ingresos por Propiedades con Defectos Corregibles

La propiedad residencial que presenta defectos corregibles (Vea el Capítulo 8), o sea que se pueden reparar, puede ser una buena inversión para las personas que pueden dedicarse a la reparación y mejoramiento de la misma. Usted debe comprar esta propiedad al más bajo precio posible. Para un inversionista, estas propiedades pueden proporcionarle un flujo de ingreso proveniente del alquiler, así como también la revalorización del inmueble debido a las mejoras realizadas para devolverle su aspecto y uso original.

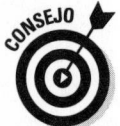

Antes de tratar de comprar y reparar un inmueble, hable con las personas en su localidad que ya han tenido esta experiencia. Los agentes de bienes raíces y tasadores de impuestos probablemente puedan darle los nombres de otros inversionistas que piensan como usted. Pídale a ellos que le expliquen todo el trabajo que eso abarca, las sorpresas que enfrentaron y si harían adquisiciones similares si ellos hubieran sabido lo que saben ahora.

Piense en Convertir Edificios de Apartamentos en Condominios

En los mercados de bienes raíces, como aquéllos ubicados en zonas densamente pobladas, comprar un edificio multifamiliar y convertirlo en un condominio puede resultar extremadamente rentable. Para hacer esta transformación exitosa, usted necesita de un agente inmobiliario que sepa del valor del inmueble al convertirlo de apartamentos a condominios y de un buen abogado en bienes raíces. Además, también necesita un contratista que sepa y le ayude a estimar los costos del trabajo, y que lo ayude en la obtención de los permisos pertinentes a la construcción.

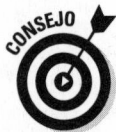

Así como le recomendamos a aquéllos que están contemplando comprar propiedades corregibles, le recomendamos a usted que antes de comprar un edificio multifamiliar y convertirlo en un condominio, hable con otros inversionistas que ya lo han hecho. También visite la oficina de permisos del departamento de planificación y construcción de su ciudad para ver qué tipo de normas tiene que cumplir. Si la propiedad se encuentra bajo control del alquiler, asegúrese de que su abogado investigue las ramificaciones que se deriven de la obtención del permiso para la conversión a condominio; una de las ramificaciones puede incluir ciertos requerimientos de tener que dar un arrendamiento de por vida a minusválidos y a personas de la tercera edad que viven en el edificio.

Considere el Flujo de Caja de la Propiedad

Cuando esté considerando la compra de bienes raíces como inversión, usted debe hacer ciertas cuentas. De todas maneras no necesita recordar Cálculo (ni siquiera el álgebra del bachillerato) para hacer estos cálculos: basta con las operaciones básicas de suma, resta, multiplicación y división.

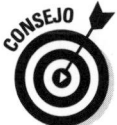

Para decidir cuánto vale una propiedad en particular (como comprador potencial) y entender las consecuencias financieras de poseer esa propiedad, calcule lo que se ha llamado *el flujo de caja* de la propiedad. Éste se calcula sumando el ingreso mensual por alquiler que una propiedad genera y luego réstele todos los gastos mensuales, como la cuota de la hipoteca, impuestos de propiedad, seguro, gastos de servicios públicos que usted, como administrador, paga, costos de reparación y mantenimiento, gastos de publicidad, el 5 por ciento (o más) como factor de desocupación, y otros. Sea realista y tome en cuenta todos los costos. Si los dueños actuales de la propiedad que usted está comprando la tienen como una inversión de bienes raíces, pídales una copia del Anexo E (*Schedule E*) de su declaración de impuestos (Ingresos y Pérdidas Suplementarias).

Sus Pérdidas por Alquiler Son Limitadas para Propósitos de Impuestos

Si usted adquiere una propiedad alquilada que produce un flujo de caja negativo, debería saber, antes de comprar, si puede declarar esa pérdida en su declaración de impuestos. Si sus ingresos son altos (más de $100.000 al año), la deducción de estas pérdidas puede verse limitada. Y, si sus ingresos son aún más altos (más de $150.000 al año) puede que no se le permita efectuar estas deducciones.

Capítulo 17

Diez Puntos que Debe Tener en Cuenta Cuando Venda Su Casa

....

En Este Capítulo

▶ ¿Vender o no vender?

▶ ¿Cuál es el valor?

▶ Cómo escoger un agente

▶ Planificación para después de la venta

....

*U*na vez que usted posee una vivienda, las probabilidades de que algún día la venda son extraordinariamente altas. Es rara la gente que vive toda su vida en la primera casa. (Los abuelos maternos de Eric lograron esta extraordinaria hazaña: ¡Vivieron más de seis décadas en la misma casa!)

Generalmente vender una vivienda es algo menos complicado que comprarla. Pero solo porque venderla puede resultar más fácil que comprarla no significa que la mayoría de la gente lo haga de manera apropiada.

Si se le ocurre comentar que está pensando en vender su casa, los agentes inmobiliarios se sentirán atraídos a usted como moscas a la miel. Y cuando usted vende una casa, el *IRS* y los funcionarios de los impuestos estatales pueden estar esperándolo con las alforjas abiertas listos para tomar una por-ción de sus ganancias, especialmente si no toma tiempo para entender las leyes de impuestos y qué hacer para que ellas le beneficien antes de vender. En este capítulo le aconsejamos algunos puntos importantes que usted debería ponderar antes de vender. Y si decide vender, queremos que haga la mejor venta posible y que evite al hombre de los impuestos (legalmente, por supuesto). Además de leer este capítulo, cuando llegue el momento de vender lea el libro compañero de éste: *House Selling For Dummies* (Wiley).

¿Por Qué Quiere Vender?

Comience con lo básico. Si está pensando en vender, piense si sus razones para hacerlo son buenas. Por ejemplo, ¿a quién no le gustaría vivir en una casa más grande con más comodidades y lujos? Pero si usted de manera apresurada pone a la venta su casa con el fin de comprar una más grande, puede que esté cometiendo un gran error. Si su próxima vivienda más cara asfixia sus finanzas, usted podría terminar arruinado.

Cuando usted necesita mudarse por cuestiones de trabajo o porque ha tenido un cambio en su estilo de vida, la mudanza puede llegar a ser una necesidad. Aún así, usted debe sopesar lo positivo y lo negativo de quedarse con su vivienda o de venderla. Comience este análisis leyendo el resto de este capítulo.

¿Puede Darse el Lujo de Comprar una Nueva Casa?

Si usted desea adquirir una propiedad más cara, este paso se llama *"vender para mejorar"* en el ámbito de los bienes raíces. Es apremiante hacer un análisis sincero de si puede darse el lujo de adquirir una propiedad de mayor valor. Como lo decimos en el Capítulo 3, ninguna entidad hipotecaria o agente hipotecario pueden contestar de manera objetiva esa pregunta por usted. Basado en sus ingresos y egresos, el agente hipotecario le puede decir lo máximo que le pueden prestar, pero no la cantidad que usted puede gastar y, todavía, poder lograr sus metas financieras personales.

Uno de los mayores errores que cometen los compradores de vivienda al vender para mejorar, es meterse en una deuda muy grande para adquirir una propiedad más costosa. El impacto de esto en sus presupuestos puede ser considerablemente grave: tal vez no quede dinero para los ahorros de jubilación, los gastos de educación o simplemente para diversión. En el peor de los casos, la gente ha terminado perdiendo sus viviendas por embargos y bancarrota al pasar por eventos inesperados, como la pérdida de un empleo o el fallecimiento de uno de los cónyuges que no tenía un seguro apropiado.

Antes de comprar su próxima vivienda, le recomendamos que repase los ejercicios financieros descritos en los Capítulos 2 y 3. Conozca los gastos de una casa que usted realmente puede afrontar. A menos que su ingreso o activos se hayan incrementado considerablemente desde el tiempo en que usted compró su última casa, probablemente no puede darse el lujo de adquirir una más costosa. El punto más importante a ser examinado por las personas es cómo el aumento del gasto mensual de la casa afectará su capacidad de ahorro para la jubilación.

¿Cuál Es el Valor?

Cuando esté listo para vender su casa, es mejor que tenga claro el valor de ella. Usted (y su agente, si es que está usando uno para vender su casa) debe analizar cómo se están vendiendo otras propiedades comparativamente similares a la suya en su vecindario. Vea el Capítulo 10 para un análisis de comparación de mercados.

Si necesita vender su casa sin perder mucho tiempo y energía, haga lo que hacen los vendedores inteligentes: póngale un precio justo de venta. No estamos recomendando que regale su propiedad, por así decirlo, pero sí le sugerimos que evite inflar el precio que usted está pidiendo hasta un punto muy por encima de lo que las ventas de casas similares sugieren que es el valor de su casa.

Usted puede estar tentado, especialmente si no está apurado por vender, a aumentar el valor de su casa de una manera exagerada con la esperanza de que un comprador inexperto le dé más de lo que la propiedad realmente vale. El peligro de esta estrategia es que no encontrará un tonto que se desprenda de esa cantidad de dinero para pagarle su súper cara propiedad, y, como consecuencia, nadie más tratará de comprarla. Luego, a medida que empieza a bajarle el precio —más cerca a lo que la casa realmente vale— compradores potenciales pueden ver con recelo el adquirir una propiedad que ha estado tanto tiempo en el mercado. Al final, puede que le sea muy difícil obtener 100 por ciento del valor real de su casa.

¿Ha Hecho Su Tarea para Conseguir un Buen Agente de Bienes Raíces?

Cuando la mayoría de las personas están preparadas para vender su casa, generalmente, contratan los servicios de un agente de bienes raíces. Los buenos pueden merecer su comisión si saben cómo preparar la propiedad para venderla, poner anuncios y avisos de venta y venderla a un buen precio. A diferencia de cuando usted va a comprar una casa, sus intereses como vendedor están alineados con los de un buen agente: el mejor precio que usted logre por su casa representa una mejor ganancia neta para usted y una mejor comisión para él.

Dado que las casas cuestan mucho —y lo que cuesta venderlas y comprarlas—, usted se debe a sí mismo la responsabilidad de conseguir un buen agente que lo represente en la venta de su casa. Asegúrese de que el agente que escogió no tenga en lista tantas propiedades para vender que no vaya a tener el tiempo necesario para trabajar apropiadamente en su caso. Por otro lado, el agente con quien usted trabajó cuando compró la casa no necesariamente es el mejor para venderla. Para vender una casa (más que para comprarla) se requieren diferentes estrategias y conocimientos.

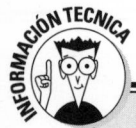

El acuerdo de listado cubre el servicio y no la venta

Un *acuerdo de listado no* es un contrato entre usted y un agente de bienes raíces para vender su casa. Tampoco es un contrato de venta; es simplemente un contrato personal de servicio. No tiene nada que ver con la transferencia de su propiedad a los compradores y, únicamente, autoriza a un agente a actuar como su agente para encontrar personas que deseen comprar su casa.

En el acuerdo aparecen dos requisitos básicos: su agente acuerda en hacer lo mejor que puede en conseguir compradores para su casa y usted acuerda pagarle una comisión si consigue compradores que estén dispuestos y sean capaces de comprar su casa al precio y en los términos convenidos en el acuerdo de listado.

Aquí es donde la cosa se pone delicada: aunque registrar la casa para la venta, técnicamente hablando, no lo obliga a usted a venderla, en ciertas ocasiones usted tendrá que pagarle al agente su comisión si él consigue un comprador dispuesto a comprar al precio y los términos acordados, pero usted repentinamente

decide no venderla —por alguna razón trivial, como que no le cae bien la mascota malcriada del comprador. Pero, si usted decide no vender porque el trabajo que le ofrecieron ya no está disponible, es muy poco probable que tenga que pagar esa comisión.

Sin embargo, si el agente le presenta una oferta que no cumple con el precio y los términos del acuerdo, usted no tiene que aceptarla y, por lo tanto, no debe ninguna comisión —no importa el tiempo, la energía y el dinero que el agente haya gastado en su nombre. El vender una casa no es como jugar a las bochas en donde el que está más cerca gana. En el mercado de bienes raíces la cercanía no cuenta: el que está más cerca no gana.

Evite firmar un acuerdo de listado que lo obligue a trabajar con un solo agente por más de tres meses. Si éste hace un buen trabajo y necesita renovar la lista porque su casa no se ha vendido todavía, usted puede renovarla o extenderla. Si por el contrario, el agente hace un pésimo trabajo, usted solo sufrirá por tres meses.

¿Tiene Usted las Destrezas Necesarias para Vender Su Propia Vivienda?

Aunque algunos propietarios tienen el tiempo y las destrezas necesarias para vender su propia vivienda, la gran mayoría no las tienen. El anzuelo que lo puede atraer para vender usted mismo su vivienda es el evitar pagar la comisión que los agentes exigen antes de iniciar el proceso de venta de la propiedad, la cual es del 5 al 7 por ciento del precio de la misma. Sin embargo, no se olvide que la mitad de esta comisión es para el agente del comprador. Debido a que la mayoría de los compradores trabajan con agentes (en parte porque sus servicios parecen no costarle a ellos), teóricamente usted ahorrará entre un 2,5 al 3,5 por ciento sobre el precio final de venta si la vende usted mismo, esto es, sin la ayuda de ningún agente.

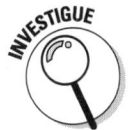

Venda usted mismo su casa o no, entreviste a varios agentes que hayan demostrado que conocen su vecindario porque han registrado y vendido propiedades en él, y pídales que le preparen un análisis comparativo de mercado de su casa. Base su precio de venta de acuerdo al precio de las propiedades comparativamente similares que se hayan vendido en los últimos seis meses. Si usted está buscando un agente, pídale a cada uno una lista de todas las casas que han vendido en los últimos 12 meses, de esta manera usted obtiene los nombres de los propietarios que han vendido sus casas con ellos como referencia.

¿Ha Preparado Usted Apropiadamente Su Casa para la Venta?

El verdadero trabajo de vender una propiedad comienza mucho antes de ponerla oficialmente en el mercado para su venta o de permitirle al primer posible comprador que entre por la puerta principal de su casa. Prepare su casa para la venta por dentro y por fuera. Como mínimo, usted debería realizar una limpieza como la que hace antes de que sus padres lo visiten (o tal vez los suegros); usted sabe: recorriendo toda la casa, *limpiando y acomodando todo* (¡o al menos echar todo debajo de las camas y en los clósets!).

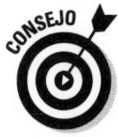

Pero usted tiene que hacer algo más que simplemente pasar la aspiradora (luego de recoger la ropa sucia del piso) y lavar los platos. Consígase unos buenos amigos, bien sinceros, y algunos agentes que examinen la casa con usted y le señalen los defectos e imperfecciones que no le costarán un mundo arreglar (por ejemplo, reparar goteras en griferías o pintar paredes que necesitan ser retocadas). No se ponga a la defensiva; ¡tome nota! Evite las reparaciones grandes como la remodelación de la cocina, construir otra habitación, u otras cosas. Muy pocas veces usted ganará más dinero en la venta que compensen estos gastos (y dolores de cabeza) extras que ocasionan estos proyectos —y esto, sin mencionar el tiempo que usted invierte en coordinar o hacer el trabajo.

¿Conoce Usted los "Puntos Atrayentes" de Su Casa?

La gente no compra casas; compra un *punto atrayente,* y el resto de la casa se vende con éste. Los puntos atrayentes varían de una casa a otra. Las cocinas despampanantes o baños bien decorados, las chimeneas, las vistas y jardinería ornamental son frecuentemente puntos que atraen o venden la vivienda. Por ejemplo, la ubicación es un punto atrayente para la gente que *desea* vivir en un cierto vecindario.

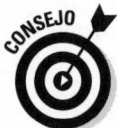

¿Cómo puede usted determinar los "puntos atrayentes" de su vivienda? Retroceda en el tiempo y piense en lo que lo atrajo a usted cuando la adquirió. Probablemente ésos sigan siendo los mismos puntos que atraigan al próximo comprador también. Luego que identifique esos atractivos, destáquelos en la lista descriptiva de la vivienda, en las listas múltiples y en los avisos de periódicos. Los vendedores con éxito saben lo que los compradores adquirirán antes de comenzar el proceso de venta.

¿Cuáles Son las Consecuencias Financieras de una Venta?

Antes de vender su casa, usted debe saber las consecuencias financieras de la venta. Por ejemplo, ¿cuánto dinero gastará en los trabajos para arreglar la casa para poder venderla? ¿Cuánto debiera de ganarle para poder adquirir su nueva vivienda?

A menos que desee y pueda darse el lujo de ser el orgulloso propietario de dos viviendas, le recomendamos vender su vivienda actual antes de emprender la compra de una nueva. Si es necesario, usted puede pedir ciertas condiciones como posponer la fecha de cierre de la venta o que le permitan alquilarla, de manera que usted tenga tiempo de cerrar la compra de su próxima casa sin tener que "quedarse en la calle" por un tiempo. Asegúrese de que estas condiciones estén claras desde el principio, para evitarse sorpresas desagradables en el camino o después de la venta.

¿Conoce las Leyes Impositivas sobre las Ganancias del Capital en la Venta de una Casa?

De acuerdo con las leyes impositivas vigentes, la mayoría de los propietarios disfrutan de una considerable deducción de los impuestos al vender sus casas. Específicamente, una gran cantidad de la *ganancia del capital* o beneficios, en la venta de una casa, se excluyen del impuesto: hasta $250.000 para contribuyentes solteros y $500.000 para casados que declaren en conjunto. (Vea el Capítulo 15 para obtener información sobre cómo calcular sus ganancias.)

Para tener derecho a estas exoneraciones de las ganancias del capital, el propietario ha debido usar la vivienda como residencia principal por lo menos durante dos de los cinco años previos, y puede usar la exoneración solamente una vez cada dos años.

Las nuevas leyes vigentes de compraventa de viviendas reemplazaron a las anteriores en relación a las ganancias del capital obtenidas por la venta de una casa. Por lo tanto, los propietarios no pueden ahora usar las ganancias de la venta de su casa para comprarse una más cara para evitar pagar impuestos sobre esas ganancias. Tampoco existe el requisito de tener un mínimo de 55 años de edad para tener derecho a la deducción de $125.000 de las ganancias.

Para la gran mayoría de propietarios con casas en venta, las nuevas leyes son una bendición. Para muchos de ellos, las ganancias del capital por venta de sus casas ni siquiera llegan cerca de los nuevos límites de exoneración, y muchos se beneficiarán por la eliminación del requisito de edad. Sin embargo, hay algunos propietarios —especialmente los que viven en vecindarios de alto precio y que han vivido en sus casas por muchos años— cuyas ganancias exceden los límites de $250.000 o $500.000, que han perdido el privilegio de usar estas ganancias en la adquisición de una vivienda de mayor precio. Si ellos venden, deberán impuestos sobre las ganancias que exceden sus límites de exoneración.

Parte VI
Apéndices

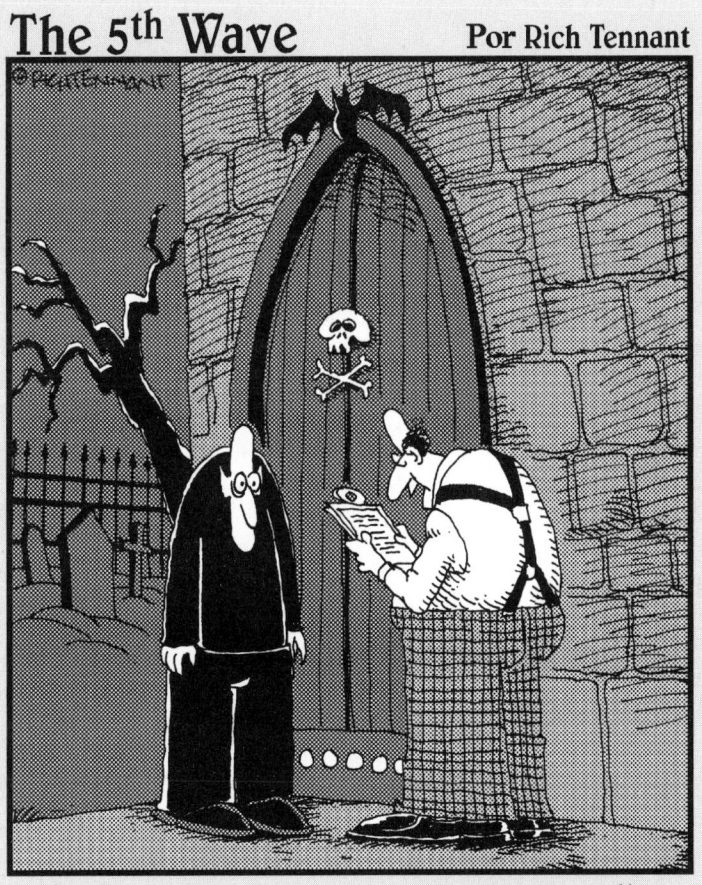

The 5th Wave — Por Rich Tennant

"¡Ya inspeccioné la casa! Las puertas movedizas, los pasadizos secretos y las mazmorras están bien, pero yo me aseguraría de poner pegamento alrededor del criadero de serpientes".

En esta parte . . .

No tenga miedo cuando vea la palabra *apéndices*. Esta sección tiene dos grandes regalos: un modelo de un excelente reporte de inspección y un glosario repleto de términos que no son tan fáciles de adivinar y que se usan en la jerga de bienes raíces.

Apéndice A

Ejemplo de un Buen Informe de Inspección

*E*ste apéndice le muestra un ejemplo de lo que usted debería ver en un buen informe de inspección.

Como podrá ver en nuestro modelo, su informe de inspección debe describir vívidamente, en palabras, la casa que usted vaya a comprar. El informe debe estar lleno de explicaciones y no debe ser simplemente una planilla estándar, con una lista con marcas de verificación y con notas escritas rápida y descuidadamente.

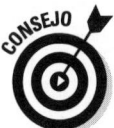

Obtenga el máximo provecho del dinero invertido en la inspección. Busque una compañía de inspección profesional que inspeccione cuidadosamente, por dentro y por fuera, los sistemas mecánicos y los componentes estructurales de la propiedad, desde los cimientos hasta el techo. Y que además, le entregue un informe completo en el cual usted pueda basarse para tomar una decisión con confianza. (Vea el Capítulo 13 para obtener información sobre cómo conseguir un buen inspector de vivienda.)

Warren Camp Inspection Services
P.O. Box 986, Arnold, CA 95223
(209) 795-1661

- **Fecha de inspección:** _____ ___, 2006
- **Número de informe:** 06 - _____
- **Fecha del informe:** _____ ___, 2006
- **Inspector:** Warren Camp, ASHI®
  - Miembro acreditado: #732
- **Informe:** Inspección previa a la compra de la propiedad ubicada en la calle _____, en San Francisco.
- **Tipo de vivienda:** Vivienda unifamiliar separada
- **Clima:** No ha llovido en los últimos 10 días
- **Presentes durante la inspección:**
  - **Comprador:** Red E. Toobuy
  - **Agente del comprador:** Ken B. Elpful / Manny Elpful y Asociados
  - **Agente del vendedor:** A. Frank Lister / Frank y Asociados, SRL
  - **Otros:** Bugzie O. Bliterate / Nuke'em, Treat'em, Treat'em Compañía de Control de Plagas
- **La vivienda estaba amoblada cuando se realizó la inspección.**
- **Los informes de inspección estructural, control de plagas no fueron suministrados.**
- **La declaración de la condición de la propiedad no fue suministrada por el vendedor.**

Este informe se hace a petición del comprador o de su agente, para uso exclusivo del mismo, y para ser usado junto con la presentación oral hecha en la propiedad. Este informe no es para ser usado por terceras personas, ni nosotros estamos en la obligación de analizarlo con ellas. Dado que un representante de Warren Camp no ha hablado personalmente con nadie sobre la extensión y el tipo de problemas descubiertos durante la inspección, sino solamente con las personas presentes durante la misma, prohíbe terminantemente a otras personas utilizar partes de este informe. Las personas interesadas deben concertar una cita con un representante de Warren Camp para realizar una inspección que llene los requisitos individuales de cada una de ellas.

Este informe ofrece la opinión profesional de las condiciones generales de la propiedad (presentes en el momento de la inspección) y de las fallas más importantes encontradas en ella y en sus sistemas. Este informe no analiza necesariamente las propiedades circunvecinas ni da información de ellas; tampoco cubre problemas del medio ambiente ni del vecindario, y solamente presenta las observaciones hechas de los elementos inspeccionados de acuerdo a los estándares normales de inspección de propiedad. Esta inspección está limitada a los elementos presentados aquí y no es técnicamente un reporte minucioso ya que ciertos problemas varían (la longitud de las separaciones y grietas se agrandan con el tiempo; las lecturas de las nivelaciones y de plomería pueden cambiar con el tiempo; los niveles de erosión y corrosión no son estáticos y muchas más cosas más), nadie debe confiar en ninguno de los hechos reportados aquí después de un lapso de 60 días.

Éste no es un informe para verificar si la vivienda cumple con los códigos locales, ni es un producto o garantía de un sistema de ningún tipo; tampoco es una evaluación para verificar la facilidad de su comercialización. Incluye solamente las áreas que tengan acceso a una inspección visual y en donde no se han movido muebles, o desmantelado o destruido físicamente algún sistema en preparación para este informe. Este reporte no llena los requisitos establecidos en la sección 1102 del Código Civil de California en relación a los requerimientos de declaración de la condición de la propiedad por el cedente de la misma.

El inspector de Warren Camp le explicó al cliente los dos tipos de reportes disponibles. El cliente escogió este informe estándar en lugar del informe narrado, completo y con extensas recomendaciones. Ciertos hechos y recomendaciones que generalmente se incluyen en el informe narrado, no serán incluidos en este informe estándar.

Por favor, llámenos si tiene preguntas.

ÍNDICE

Sociedad Americana de Inspectores de Viviendas
(ASHI, por sus siglas en inglés)

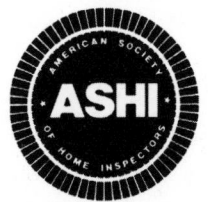

MIEMBRO AUTORIZADO

• Informe de inspección previa a la compra
Calle _____ , San Francisco, California   _____ __, 2006

INTRODUCCIÓN

La vivienda inspeccionada es una vivienda unifamiliar separada y la mayor parte de su interior se encontraba desamoblada. El cableado de bajo voltaje, los intercambiadores de calor, jardines, cercas, muros de contención, tubería subterránea, tanques de almacenamiento y aspersores de jardines, no están incluidos en este tipo de informe.

Las inspecciones de la compañía Warren Camp Inspection Service (WCIS, por sus siglas en inglés) están diseñadas para cumplir y exceder las "Normas de Práctica Profesional" establecidas por la Sociedad Americana de Inspectores de Viviendas (American Society of Home Inspectors®, [ASHI®, por sus siglas en inglés]) de la cual la compañía Warren Camp es un miembro autorizado. Hay ejemplares disponibles de las Normas estándar, si los solicita.

Esta propiedad es de un piso, con una estructura construida sobre un espacio con acceso entre el piso y la superficie que se encuentra debajo del piso. La armazón original de madera de esta vivienda, construida alrededor de 1955, parece de fabricación común. Aparentemente no se ven daños grandes o fuera de lo común; sin embargo, varios elementos necesitan ser reparados.

Partes de esta vivienda unifamiliar han sido renovadas recientemente. Los cambios en los sistemas de plomería y eléctrico, así como también en varias partes del sistema estructural en la parte posterior adicionada, fueron realizados de una manera no profesional. Estas fallas se indican de nuevo en otras secciones de este informe. Dado que muchas de las paredes y techos interiores estaban cerrados, no fue posible determinar el alcance total de la remodelación. Si se requiere más información sobre estas áreas, entonces: (a) consulte con un ingeniero de estructuras, (b) revise copias de permisos y contratos de remodelación que se hayan otorgados, y (c) examine la declaración de la condición de la propiedad del vendedor.

En su mayor parte, las partes interior y exterior de la vivienda han tenido un mantenimiento adecuado. Pero, por supuesto, todas las construcciones tienen fallas. Mostraremos varias de esas fallas, pero no podemos presentar y analizar cada una de ellas. Esta inspección e informe no son técnicamente minuciosos, y WCIS no provee un análisis completo o en detalle de las áreas con problemas. Dado que solamente hay un número limitado de horas para inspeccionar toda la propiedad, WCIS proporciona, en lo que cabe, una opinión sobre la condición de la vivienda basándose en su experiencia. El inspector de Warren Camp no es un ingeniero profesional ni un experto en todas las materias o profesiones. Solamente muestras representativas de varios segmentos expuestos visualmente en esta propiedad fueron analizadas. Si otros elementos adicionales o condiciones se descubren cuando las reparaciones o arreglos se estén llevando a cabo, llame a WCIS inmediatamente antes de continuar con el trabajo de reparación.

Todas las secciones importantes de este informe fueron presentadas a E. Toobuy y a su agente Ken B. Elpful, en el momento de la inspección. Las siguientes secciones describen los puntos presentados.

Reparaciones, correcciones y otros puntos a considerar (Nota: Los puntos señalados con una marca (✓) son simplemente cosas importantes de lo que el inspector encontró. Lea todo el reporte para realmente apreciar la magnitud de su cobertura. Donde a usted le interese, siga éstas y las siguientes recomendaciones y hable con los especialistas en los diferentes campos para solucionar esos puntos presentados que pueden no haber sido incluidos en esta inspección o en el informe.)

✓ *Verifique con el departamento de inspección de construcciones, los permisos e inspecciones solicitados para una construcción, reedificación o adición.*

PARTE EXTERIOR DE LA VIVIENDA

La parte exterior de la vivienda

Esta vivienda, con paredes de tablas enlistonadas verticalmente en la fachada y frisadas en la base, necesita mantenimiento en la parte de la construcción anexa. Las superficies deben ser protegidas contra la intemperie en un futuro no muy lejano para impedir la entrada de humedad. Cuando se haga referencia a la parte del frente, a la parte posterior o a los lados derecho e izquierdo de la propiedad, éstas se hacen mirando el frente de la misma desde la calle _____.

Se encontraron otros elementos sin pintura y sin protección contra el agua: cinco rejillas de ventilación en las paredes, la puerta del garaje, una puerta de entrada nueva, y varias partes de las molduras de las ventanas.

En la parte posterior del garaje, la tierra o el pavimento se encuentran cerca o a nivel de la parte superior de la fundación. Esta condición puede causar la descomposición de la madera y su deterioro. Dado que Warren Camp no está autorizado para realizar inspecciones estructurales o de plagas, vea un reporte vigente para examinar los problemas y las recomendaciones sugeridas.

• Informe de inspección previa a la compra
Calle _____ , San Francisco, California   _____ __, 2006

Fueron detectados contactos entre la madera y la tierra en las columnas de la escalera y en el umbral de las puertas. Estos contactos favorecen la putrefacción de la madera, la entrada de plaga y la retención de humedad. Ellos deben ser reparados de manera apropiada y los niveles adecuados de pendientes deben ser mantenidos.

Se encontraron varios clavos oxidados, por estar expuestos a la intemperie, en la moldura del alero del techo de la construcción anexa. Esas superficies deben ser preparadas debidamente o deben cambiarse antes de ser pintadas.

Se notó la presencia de varias grietas pequeñas en el frisado o estuco que cubre las paredes. Probablemente esas grietas se deban al estiramiento o encogimiento del material, a la sequía, a movimientos sísmicos o a los movimientos normales de la construcción. Esas grietas deben ser rellenadas con macilla y selladas contra la intemperie. Contrate a un especialista en impermeabilización y pintura para proteger y sellar las superficies exteriores y así prevenir la entrada de agua.

El friso en la pared posterior y en la del lado del patio se extiende hacia abajo sobre la fundación y hace contacto con la tierra (el césped o vegetación). Esto puede ocasionar la entrada de insectos u organismos que destruyen la madera por detrás del friso. Como solución, suba varias pulgadas la base del friso que cubre la madera hasta hacer visible la fundación o baje el nivel de la pendiente.

Puertas y ventanas
Las ventanas de aluminio en la edificación anexa a la vivienda lucen bien. WCIS sugiere que las superficies expuestas a la intemperie de los marcos de madera, del alféizar de las ventanas y de los adornos adyacentes a las armazones de metal de las ventanas se les den mantenimiento frecuentemente para prevenir la posible entrada de agua. Varias ventanas fueron abiertas durante la inspección y un número de ellas abrió a un nivel aceptable.

Muchas de las ventanas originales de la vivienda, selladas con la pintura cuando fueron pintadas, y con el alféizar de madera no se pudieron abrir, impidiendo la ventilación adecuada en algunas habitaciones. Además, en una situación de emergencia o incendio, sería sumamente difícil y peligroso tratar de salir a través de esas ventanas cerradas ya que son difíciles de maniobrar. *Esta falla debe ser solucionada inmediatamente.* Asimismo, se recomienda el mantenimiento rutinario de los dispositivos de madera de subida y bajada de las ventanas, del acabado de madera y de la masilla de vidrio para eliminar la potencial filtración del agua y así poder extender la vida útil de las mismas.

La puerta de entrada al garaje es del tipo de subida y bajada sin ventanillas que se puedan abrir.

Los resortes de balance no están equipados con un dispositivo de seguridad que prevenga el disparo del resorte si éste se llegara a romper cuando se encuentre bajo presión. Llame a un técnico en instalación de puertas de garaje para corregir este problema.

El pavimento y drenaje
Las diferentes alturas del pavimento en el camino de entrada pueden ser peligrosas y ocasionar caídas. Hay que tener cuidado en esta área.

Esta construcción se encuentra ubicada en la empinada ladera de una colina. Hay visibles grietas de erosión del suelo en diferentes partes. Como no somos ingenieros de ningún tipo, WCIS no puede evaluar o emitir una opinión sobre esta condición. El comprador potencial, Red E. Toobuy, puede consultar con ingenieros profesionales en relación a la estabilidad de la construcción, de la colina y también sobre pasados, presentes o futuros terraplenes del suelo o movimientos del mismo o de la construcción.

Es importante que haya un buen drenaje del suelo en las viviendas de la zona Bay Area ya que el tipo de suelo en esta área se esponja cuando se encuentra saturado y puede dañar los cimientos de la construcción. El suelo al frente tiene una inclinación notable lo cual provee un drenaje adecuado de los cimientos durante las tormentas de lluvia.

El drenaje del área posterior y de los lados no fue tan fácil de predecir. Probablemente haya entrada de agua a los espacios reducidos debajo de la construcción y, posiblemente se deba a que el suelo y el pavimento no tienen un declive apreciable desde la fundación hacia afuera. El drenaje y sus niveles deben ser monitoreados regularmente ya que se consiguieron muestras de calcificación y manchas en algunas partes de la fundación. Esto debe ser arreglado.

Las condiciones de humedad y de drenaje varían de acuerdo a los tipos de suelos, a los diseños ornamentales de jardinería y a los cambios climáticos. Por lo tanto, esta compañía de inspección no puede opinar sobre la estabilidad del suelo ni reportar problemas de filtraciones o acumulación de agua. Lea la declaración de la condición de la propiedad del vendedor o un informe de un ingeniero especialista en suelos o geólogo, y vea la posibilidad de la existencia de un sistema de drenaje subterráneo tipo "French" y para comprender la realidad de la posible entrada de agua, sea ésta causada por lloviznas, arroyos naturales o lluvias fuertes prolongadas, u otras causas. Como regla general, mantenga los desagües de agua, patios y vías de accesos limpios y bien cuidados.

Instalaciones subterráneas

Como se puede ver, la inspección de sistemas subterráneos de drenaje sin acceso no se pudo realizar. WCIS tampoco pudo inspeccionar otros sistemas subterráneos como conductos de sistemas de suministro de gas y agua, conductos de desagüe y ventilación u otros más, ni tampoco los componentes debajo de la placa de cimientos. WCIS no hace pruebas de las tuberías de desagüe.

    WCIS no detectó indicios externos de la existencia actual o previa de un tanque de almacenamiento subterráneo (UST, por sus siglas en inglés) en las áreas inspeccionadas (por ejemplo, una toma para llenar el tanque, tubo de ventilación, conductos de tubería y líneas de retorno, o un tablero de fusibles identificado "quemador de aceite"—que son indicadores típicos de la existencia de un UST). Las personas interesadas en este tipo de inspección pueden investigar más a fondo ya que éste no se encuentra dentro de las normas estándar de inspección profesional de la ASHI®.

✓ Libere las ventanas y hágales mantenimiento, así como también a los acabados y a la ferretería.
✓ Vea un reporte vigente de inspección de estructura o control de plagas para ver los problemas y las recomendaciones dadas.
✓ Pinte e impermeabilice todos los materiales en bruto.
✓ Repare los problemas indicados.
✓ Restituya la pendiente necesaria y restablezca el diseño de la jardinería, paredes y caminos de entrada donde sea necesario.
✓ Busque un ingeniero especialista en suelos o geólogo para investigar la erosión y estabilidad de la ladera de la colina.

LOS CIMIENTOS

Solamente hay acceso parcial a los cimientos o fundación ya que el espacio es muy reducido entre el piso y los cimientos. No hay una malla metálica que impida la entrada de ratas debajo de la sala de estar, la cual puede ser un buen detalle de protección.

    Las paredes desde la base hasta el piso, vistas desde la puerta de entrada y del exterior de la vivienda, han sido instaladas de acuerdo a las normas estándar usadas.

    El garaje y el espacio reducido bajo el piso fueron construidos con cemento en una sola placa; éste, generalmente, es reforzado con vigas de acero inoxidable pero no pudo ser examinado o comprobado.

    Hay una pequeña grieta en el cimiento correspondiente a la sala construida. Esta grieta, en una edificación de este tipo y edad, es muy común y debe ser monitoreada periódicamente. Si ella aumenta de tamaño o aparecen nuevas grietas, busque a un ingeniero para realizar una evaluación. No se detectaron señales externas de movimiento de la fundación, o transferencia de esos movimientos a paredes contiguas, techos o pisos. No fue posible determinar si esa grieta es un problema reciente. En las normas de inspección de la ASHI® no se encuentran el diagnosticar si hay movimiento, rotación o asentamiento de la fundación, ni tampoco decir si aparecerán más grietas o si las existentes se extenderán o agrandarán. WCIS tampoco puede predecir la probabilidad de que una falla, movimiento o asentamiento de la fundación ocurra en el futuro. Si necesita más información, por favor, busque un ingeniero de estructuras o geólogo, con experiencia en estructuras similares, para que inspeccione y evalúe los problemas indicados y resuelva otros problemas estructurales como medidas de prevención para movimientos sísmicos.

✓ Monitorear la fundación con frecuencia.

ARMAZÓN ESTRUCTURAL

Subestructura

Se vio la armazón original y nueva en la construcción anexa. Las partes bajas de la armazón parcialmente accesibles y visibles estaban limitadas a los espacios reducidos por debajo del piso. La armazón, casi en su totalidad, es estándar y no tiene señales visibles de pandeo, grietas, deterioro o movimiento.

    Los postes de madera en el espacio reducido bajo el piso debajo de la sala de estar se encuentran en malas condiciones. La parte inferior de los postes de soporte debajo de la viga central no están conectados a los pilares enterrados de cemento.

No se ven sujetadores de unión como tornillos, clavos o pernos. Se debe corregir este problema y es fácil de hacerlo bajo la asesoría de un ingeniero de estructuras.

El travesaño sosteniendo la entrada del garaje es un poco preocupante porque los sujetadores usados en los dos extremos no tienen el tamaño adecuado. Este travesaño también ha comenzado a moverse haciendo que los sujetadores no fijen bien las conexiones. Desde el punto de vista estructural, las conexiones entre una parte estructural y otra son sumamente importantes. Las conexiones en la base y parte superior del poste y las conexiones de las vigas entre sí y a las vigas de anclaje son muy pocas pero pueden ser colocadas fácilmente.

Las columnas de carga crítica en la pared del garaje y en los espacios reducidos por debajo del piso están conectadas de manera estándar. Sin embargo, ellas no tienen pernos extras ni paneles de madera contrachapada de cobertura que se sabe que ofrecen una mayor protección a las construcciones de madera ubicadas en zonas sísmicas.

Muchas de las columnas estructurales, vigas y pernos no han sido preparados para posibles movimientos sísmicos. Es recomendable preparar estos elementos para un movimiento sísmico eventual y los trabajos deben ser realizados por un ingeniero en estructuras.

Se encontraron manchas de humedad en las paredes interiores del garaje. Estas manchas lucen y se sienten secas, y cuando se probaron con el medidor bipolar eléctrico de humedad, las manchas accesibles estaban secas. Dado que la causa de estas manchas de agua y la determinación de cuán viejas o nuevas son es muy difícil de hacer, vea la declaración de la condición de la vivienda del vendedor para ver qué se ha hecho para solucionar estos problemas.

Se encontró excremento de roedores en el espacio reducido bajo el piso. Consulte con una compañía de control de plagas para efectuar una evaluación.

Partes de la parte superior del espacio reducido bajo el piso fueron instaladas con aislante térmico; sin embargo, una "inspección de cálculo de energía" no es algo que se hace en este tipo de inspección. Varias partes estaban sueltas y otras cayeron en la tierra en el espacio reducido bajo el piso. Estas áreas necesitan ser reparadas.

La armadura principal

No se encontraron evidencias de movimiento estructural durante la inspección de un número representativo de puertas, ventanas, pisos, paredes y del techo interior. La parte superior de algunas puertas estaban cortadas en forma cónica para permitir el movimiento de las paredes con el paso de los años. Las separaciones entre las paredes, las molduras o los techos interiores, o el pandeo o desnivel de los pisos parecen ser el resultado del movimiento estructural normal o de la expansión entre la armazón y el soporte del suelo. La opinión de WCIS es que estas cosas no representan movimientos vigentes de importancia.

El ático

El ático tiene la puerta de acceso en el techo del pasillo. No hay tablas de piso entre las vigas transversales por lo que esta área es peligrosa para caminar. Además, el aislante térmico cubre las vigas de la mayor parte del techo interior. Por consiguiente, se hizo solamente una inspección visual del área cerca de la entrada de acceso.

Sobre y a través de las vigas del piso del ático pasan cables eléctricos. Hay que tener cuidado cuando se necesite tener acceso al mismo.

El aislante térmico se encuentra instalado en casi todo el piso del ático. El reportar fallas en la instalación del aislante térmico no es parte de los estándares de la industria de inspección. Tampoco hubiese sido posible examinar o ver fallas o peligros, debajo de o entre el material de aislamiento térmico. Un electricista autorizado podría inspeccionar el cableado empotrado como medida de seguridad y otorgar un certificado de seguridad.

Los deflectores del aislante térmico, los cuales son necesarios alrededor de elementos productores de calor (tales como artefactos de alumbrado y conductos de salida de humo), no eran visibles fácilmente y debieran ser instalados en donde sea necesario.

Los soportes del techo, visualmente accesibles en la parte principal de la construcción, fueron construidos de acuerdo a las normas. Se encontró un número significativo de correas (partes de soporte) y aros de unión (partes que unen dos secciones del techo). Desafortunadamente, el acceso al ático que está encima de la nueva parte construida es imposible, por lo tanto no se pudo realizar la inspección de esa área.

Hay buenas entradas de ventilación en el alero del techo exterior. La ventilación fue instalada de acuerdo a las normas y se le ha hecho mantenimiento.

✓ Contrate los servicios de un ingeniero de estructuras para revisar la estructura de la sala de estar.
✓ Actualice desde el punto de vista sísmico, las columnas estructurales, vigas, láminas y vigas verticales para protección contra el viento y terremotos.
✓ Arregle el travesaño y asegúrelo como debe ser.
✓ Vea un reporte vigente de inspección de estructura o control de plagas para ver los problemas y las recomendaciones dadas.
✓ Coloque los deflectores del aislante donde sea necesario y sujete el material aislante desprendido en el espacio reducido bajo el piso.

PREVENCIÓN DE INCENDIOS Y SEGURIDAD DE LA VIVIENDA
Prevención de incendios

WCIS tiene algunas dudas en relación a la protección contra incendios en esta propiedad. La superficie de las paredes del garaje, contiguas a las habitaciones, no son cien por ciento a prueba de fuego. Actualmente, hay un riesgo de esparcimiento de llamas y también de fuga de radón hacia las áreas habitables. Aísle completamente las áreas con sistemas mecánicos de las áreas habitables (por ejemplo, selle todas las entradas y separaciones con yeso resistente al fuego, coloque láminas metálicas, o ponga elementos de construcción resistentes al fuego donde sea necesario). WCIS no consiguió detectores de humo o rociadores en esta área. Se debe instalar un sistema de alarma monitoreado, con detectores de humo y de calor.

Algunos detectores de humo fueron instalados en esta edificación: en las paredes de tres habitaciones y en el techo interior del pasillo central. Dado que los códigos estadales y locales cambian con frecuencia, consulte con el departamento de construcciones para saber el número adecuado, el tipo y la ubicación de los mismos. Recuerde cambiar las baterías cada año. El colocar apagafuegos o extinguidores de incendio apropiados también aumenta la seguridad de la vivienda contra incendios.

La seguridad

La puerta principal de la vivienda está equipada con una cerradura con llave, un cerrojo del tipo dormido y un panel grande de cristal. El cristal no tiene un sello que identifique de qué tipo es (por ejemplo, vidrio templado o de seguridad). Las lunas de las puertas y ventanas con cristales que no son certificados como seguros pueden ser peligrosas cuando se quiebran, por eso los códigos de construcción vigentes requieren vidrios identificados como seguros para minimizar posibles lesiones. No es un requisito cambiar estos vidrios; sin embargo, tenga cuidado y mucho sentido común cuando se encuentre en esta área para prevenir roturas accidentales del vidrio y lesiones personales.

La cerradura de la puerta principal necesita un ajuste pequeño para su seguridad y para un fácil manejo.

La puerta es maciza, la cual la hace más resistente a los golpes y al fuego que una puerta hueca o lisa. (No todas las puertas huecas son ignífugas, a menos que sean identificadas como tal.)

La puerta de cristal y panel que da acceso del garaje a la entrada contigua de al lado no es una puerta fuerte y no proporciona mucha seguridad.

Las puertas del frente y posterior del garaje no tienen una cerradura de seguridad con un pestillo y pasador de por lo menos una pulgada. Para todas las puertas con acceso al exterior, se recomiendan las cerraduras con pestillos de golpe que ofrecen más seguridad.

La cerradura de la puerta que da a la cocina es del tipo de doble llave, una llave por dentro y otra por fuera. Esto trae como consecuencia que en caso de emergencia si esas llaves no se encuentran accesibles, sería imposible salir, ocasionando terribles consecuencias. El cambiar las cerraduras a una cerradura sencilla de una sola llave no es costoso y debería ser considerado. Consulte con un cerrajero.

Ventanas de vidrio y salidas de emergencia en caso de incendio

Las ventanas de la sala de estar fueron instaladas cerca del piso. Desafortunadamente, ninguna lámina de vidrio está identificada con un sello de seguridad (por ejemplo, vidrio templado o de seguridad). El reemplazar esos vidrios, el recubrimiento plástico o las instalaciones de protección no es necesario ahora, pero tenga cuidado cuando se encuentre en estas áreas hasta que se mejoren esas condiciones.

Las salidas de la casa en caso de emergencia presentan un problema de seguridad. Cuando se trataron de abrir las ventanas de los dormitorios, con acceso hacia el exterior, se encontró que las partes de madera y los mecanismos de metal están pintados por encima, sellándolas, y no se pueden abrir.

La iluminación exterior e interior debe ser aumentada para acrecentar la protección y seguridad.

También queremos recordarle que antes de que se instale en su nueva casa, le haga un nuevo fresado a las llaves para aumentar su protección y tranquilidad.

✓ Instale las protecciones contra incendios en las áreas donde se necesiten, y también los deflectores del aislante térmico, de los dispositivos y del sistema de alarma.

✓ Aumente la protección y seguridad de su casa con cerraduras protectoras.

✓ Arregle las ventanas con acceso al exterior para que sean fáciles de abrir en caso de incendio.

PLOMERÍA

Sistema de suministro de agua

La válvula principal que cierra el suministro de agua a la vivienda se encuentra en la pared del frente. Se puede abrir y cerrar y no hay huellas de goteo o filtración. La tubería es de cobre de 3/4 de pulgada y va desde la tubería principal hasta la vivienda. Los sistemas internos de suministros de agua fría y caliente son casi todos de cobre.

El inspector de WCIS encontró que algunas de las tuberías de suministro de agua al frente de la vivienda son de hierro galvanizado y otras de cobre. A lo mejor el vendedor puede darle información sobre hasta dónde se ha hecho el reemplazo con la tubería de cobre. Las tuberías de hierro galvanizado se corroen con el tiempo debido a la acumulación de minerales en las paredes de las mismas, restringiendo así el flujo de agua. La corrosión puede que sea extensa o no; el inspector de WCIS no puede predecir la velocidad en la cual ella ocurre.

La presión estática en la tubería de agua, tomada en la válvula principal, fue de 89 libras por pulgada cuadrada (PSI, por sus siglas en inglés), la cual indica un nivel bueno, de moderado a alto. Las presiones de agua se encuentran establecidas entre un 55 a un 65 libras por pulgada cuadrada para prevenir goteos o derramamientos debido al exceso de presión. Se recomienda colocar un regulador de la presión del agua o manómetro en la entrada de la línea principal para comprobar la presión del agua regularmente.

Parte de la tubería de agua caliente en el espacio bajo el piso no tiene un aislante térmico. Una instalación completa de material de aislamiento térmico disminuirá el gasto de energía y mejorará la velocidad a la cual el agua caliente llega a cada grifo de agua.

La tubería de agua en esta área tampoco tiene las correas apropiadas ni los sujetadores o soportes que la aseguren a la parte inferior del piso. Esta falla puede ocasionar goteo o ruidos estridentes en estas tuberías, como los que el inspector escuchó en los dos baños.

Sistemas de ventilación, de drenaje y colectores

A lo largo de esta construcción, los conductos visibles de eliminación de desechos y de ventilación son de hierro fundido. Una tubería de eliminación de desechos de hierro fundido o de ventilación, de 2 pulgadas de ancho, que se encuentra en el espacio reducido bajo el piso está quebrada y deteriorada. Necesita ser sustituida en un futuro cercano.

En el garaje, un tubo de eliminación de desechos o de ventilación está incompleto; le falta la tapa o tapón de protección. Como se encuentra ubicado a la derecha del equipo de calefacción, un plomero puede instalar la tapa o tapón adecuada sin problemas.

Varios conductos de drenaje fueron inspeccionados y tienen un buen sello hidráulico.

Los sifones de los dos lavabos preocupan al inspector de WCIS porque gotean y no están sujetos a una pieza de cola. Es importante colocar conexiones de tubería apropiadas. Los sifones son fáciles de cambiar y no son caros.

Abastecimiento de gas natural

La válvula de gas principal, ubicada en la pared exterior del frente de la vivienda, estaba herméticamente cerrada. Si esta válvula no es accesible o no se puede maniobrar con facilidad, o en caso de una emergencia, la compañía PG&E (por sus siglas en inglés) puede ser contactada para corregir este problema.

✓ Instale un regulador de la presión del agua o manómetro en la entrada de la tubería principal de suministro de agua.

✓ Sujete firmemente las tuberías de agua y de desechos a la estructura.

✓ Substituya la tubería de desecho de hierro fundido que se encuentra agrietada.

✓ Cubra o coloque una tapa o tapón sobre los tubos de ventilación de desechos.
✓ Reemplace los colectores de agua de los lavabos.

CALENTADOR DE AGUA

El calentador de agua es del tipo de gas natural y se encontraba en funcionamiento en el momento de la inspección. No tiene un protector de aislamiento térmico de fibra de vidrio. Debe ser recubierto con esa cobertura aislante térmica la cual debe tener un corte o ventanilla en donde se encuentra la placa de identificación del calentador, permitiendo ver esa información.

El calentador no tiene correas sujetadoras ni bloques empotrados diseñados para sostenerlo y resistir movimientos sísmicos.

Se puede ver que es un modelo instalado recientemente. Es un tanque de fibra de vidrio, con una placa informativa de marca A. O. Smith, con una capacidad de 40 galones, de 38.000 BTU y una tasa de recuperación de 40,4 galones por hora.

La base del tanque se encuentra libre de óxido. No hay evidencias de goteos o derrames.

Una válvula de seguridad en la parte superior del tanque, llamada "válvula de liberación de la presión y temperatura", es necesaria para el funcionamiento seguro de este aparato. Esta válvula de liberación de la presión y temperatura (T&PR, por sus siglas en ingles) se encuentra bien ubicada y el tubo de desagüe del agua estaba conectado a la válvula de acuerdo a las normas estándares.

La válvula de cierre de suministro de agua fría está en buenas condiciones. No hay evidencias de goteos o derrames.

La tubería del agua caliente contigua al calentador de agua tiene una cubierta de protección térmica; sin embargo, una "inspección de la eficacia energética" no está dentro de las normas de práctica profesional de esta inspección.

Cuando se abrió la válvula de desagüe en la base del tanque, se observó muy poca sedimentación.

Fue difícil maniobrar la válvula de cierre del gas por lo que debe ser arreglada.

El aire fresco necesario para una combustión completa es mínimo en este lugar. Se recomienda tener más ventilación continua de aire fresco. Ventanas y ventanillas abiertas pueden proveer esa ventilación necesaria.

Los calentadores de gas natural siempre deben tener acceso a ventilación adecuada. Las porciones visibles del conducto de salida de humos fueron instaladas de una manera insegura, y partes inaccesibles de la tubería no fueron inspeccionadas. Las conexiones de la salida de humos fueron inadecuadamente cubiertas con un material que parece ser asbesto. La simple presencia de asbesto en un material de construcción no necesariamente implica un problema de seguridad para la salud. Muchos factores deben ser considerados antes de dar una opinión o dictamen (por ejemplo, el porcentaje de asbesto en el material, el tipo exacto de asbesto y la condición actual del material). Dada la edad de esta edificación, puede que se encuentren presentes otros materiales que contienen asbesto que pueden no ser visibles o detectables, y que no se puedan identificar en este informe. Busque a contratistas especialistas en este campo para que realicen pruebas y análisis de laboratorio para detectar la presencia de asbesto y, si es positiva, darles un estimado para su retiro o aislamiento de acuerdo a las normas de la Agencia de Protección Ambiental de los Estados Unidos (EPA, por sus siglas en inglés).

El conducto de humos estaba manchado sugiriendo una filtración de agua a nivel del techo o de condensación debida a la carencia de aire fresco en este lugar. Sin embargo, no se notó la presencia de humedad cuando la inspección fue realizada.

Como una precaución estándar de protección contra posibles movimientos sísmicos, algunas o todas de las siguientes recomendaciones deben realizarse si es que no se encuentran ya instaladas:

a. Las tuberías de suministro de agua al calentador deben ser flexibles.
b. Las correas de interconexión cruzada para protección sísmica deben funcionar.
c. La tubería de suministro de gas natural al calentador y a los aparatos electrodomésticos que usan gas debe ser flexible.

    ✓ Proporcionar circulación continua de aire fresco.

CUARTO DE LAVANDERÍA

El área de la lavandería localizada en el garaje ya no funciona y no se encontraron aparatos electrodomésticos aquí.

Las cámaras de aire en las tuberías de agua localizadas arriba del lavadero no han sido instaladas todavía. Ya que ellas ayudan a la circulación del agua caliente y fría en esas tuberías, deben ser instaladas por un plomero profesional antes de que el lavadero pueda ser utilizado.

El lavadero de hierro y cemento estaba asegurado de manera adecuada a la pared posterior del garaje. No ha sido instalado en este lavadero un sifón, ni tampoco una tubería de ventilación de desagüe arriba del mismo. Contrate a un plomero profesional para que realice las debidas instalaciones.

La válvula de cierre del gas estaba apretada y requerirá de un ajuste cuando estén conectando las tuberías de gas.

"El flujo de aire fresco" es mínimo en esta área. El abrir las ventanas con regularidad ayuda a su ventilación.

Es preocupante un enchufe flojo de corriente de 120 voltios que se encuentra junto al lavadero. Este es un trabajo de reparación menor y, como el enchufe flojo puede afectar la conexión a tierra, debe ser realizado muy pronto por *un electricista autorizado para que examine y asegure el enchufe a su receptáculo.*

✓ Haga las mejoras de plomería cuando arregle el área del lavadero.

✓ Instale un conducto de ventilación y un sifón en el lavadero, y asegure la caja del enchufe.

SISTEMA ELÉCTRICO

Conductores del servicio de electricidad e interruptor principal de desconexión

El servicio de energía eléctrica a esta edificación es por medio de cables elevados que proveen aproximadamente 240 voltios de corriente al medidor.

El interruptor principal de desconexión y el tablero se encuentran situados en la pared derecha exterior y tienen un dispositivo de protección de sobrecargas eléctricas de 60 amperios para la edificación. Las identificaciones del calibre de los cables están tapadas con cinta adhesiva pero sus tamaños sugieren que son conductores de alambre #8. La impedancia (la capacidad del conductor de entrada) era insignificante, tomando en cuenta la demanda actual de electricidad de la vivienda. Para asegurarse de tener la cantidad necesaria de electricidad, o para aumentarla, contrate a un electricista autorizado para que haga un cálculo del factor de utilización y una evaluación.

El tablero eléctrico principal está asegurado a la parte exterior de la vivienda pero no está protegido contra la intemperie. Hay corrosión dentro del tablero y del conducto para los cables. Estas partes se deben cambiar ya que se sabe que el óxido causa cortocircuitos.

El tablero está sumamente sucio por dentro y por fuera, por lo tanto hay que tener cuidado alrededor de esta área porque algún elemento externo puede ocasionar un arco voltaico y por consiguiente un cortocircuito.

Tableros auxiliares de distribución eléctrica

El interruptor principal de desconexión de esta vivienda se encuentra en un tablero junto con otros circuitos. Ningún otro tablero auxiliar estaba a la vista ni se inspeccionó.

La combinación del tablero principal con el tablero de distribución (protegido por interruptores de cortocircuitos) tiene el siguiente esquema de circuitos:

> 1 circuito de 120 voltios de 15 amperios
> 4 circuitos de 120 voltios de 20 amperios

Este tablero auxiliar no tiene todos los circuitos identificados con etiquetas, pero deberían estar. Sin embargo, estaba protegido por el frente por una cubierta protectora.

Hay "una toma o cometida doble" (esto es, la conexión de dos conductores a un interruptor) en este tablero. *Esta conexión debe ser corregida inmediatamente* porque una toma doble aumenta la posibilidad y frecuencia de activar el dispositivo de protección contra sobrecargas eléctricas.

Parte de un programa regular de mantenimiento de la propiedad es comprobar que todos los interruptores de corriente sean probados anualmente para asegurarse de que estén bien y de que continuarán en esas condiciones.

La conexión a tierra y la polaridad

Por supuesto, todas las conexiones eléctricas deben estar conectadas a tierra de una manera adecuada y segura. El conector a tierra que se encuentra debajo del tablero principal no fue fácil de localizar. Algunos de los toma corrientes e interruptores que se probaron tenían muy poca o ninguna protección a tierra.

Hay conexiones sin puesta a tierra en la sala, en las tres habitaciones y en la sala de estar, lo cual puede ser peligroso. *Esta falla debe ser corregida inmediatamente para más seguridad personal.*

Al probar varios toma corrientes al azar, se encontró "polaridad invertida" en varios de ellos (en los dos baños y a los dos lados del lavaplatos en la cocina). Esta condición, peligrosa en ciertas circunstancias, se puede corregir fácilmente y

Este informe ha sido preparado para el uso exclusivo de Red E. Toobuy.
Se prohíbe el uso de esta información a otras personas.

• Página 8

debe hacerse. Lo que es más, el enchufe en el baño principal no está protegido con el dispositivo protector de descarga a tierra como debe ser.

El cableado

El cableado eléctrico en esta vivienda está compuesto del original más otro cableado.

La mayoría de los cables rotos son del tipo Romex®.

Las siguientes observaciones son ejemplos de problemas en el sistema eléctrico. Éstas no deben sustituir una inspección hecha por un electricista autorizado, la cual es necesaria:

a. Se necesita reemplazar un interruptor defectuoso del dispositivo de iluminación que alumbra el área del lavaplatos en la cocina.

b. Los accesorios de iluminación en los dos baños se encuentran sumamente flojos. Esto puede comprometer la protección contra descargas a tierra. Asegure cada accesorio inmediatamente.

c. Parte de los cables, de tipo Romex, en las paredes del garaje tienen una altura de menos de 8 pies y no están protegidos; esto puede causar daño a los cables. Los cables expuestos deben ser colocados en conductos de metal o cubiertos con un material protector como láminas de yeso.

d. En la habitación principal hay un cable de extensión usado incorrectamente como substituto de un cable permanente. Él debe ser conectado en forma apropiada si se va a continuar usando.

e. Los accesorios de iluminación en el garaje y en el baño principal no tienen bombillas. Puesto que el contacto accidental con esas áreas expuestas puede ser peligroso, se deben poner bombillas en cada uno de esos accesorios.

En resumen, hay problemas de seguridad tanto en el cableado interno como en los cables proveedores del servicio de electricidad en la entrada. Recomendamos que contrate a un electricista autorizado lo más pronto posible para que examine todo el sistema eléctrico y haga las correcciones necesarias.

La compañía Warren Camp siempre recomienda la instalación de interruptores de circuito con conexión a tierra en la cocina, en los baños y en otras áreas donde haya humedad como medidas de precaución y seguridad. Deben ser colocados bajo la recomendación de un electricista autorizado.

✓ Se debe limpiar el tablero principal, reemplazar los componentes deteriorados en su interior, identificar todas las partes de los circuitos y proteger el tablero de la intemperie.

✓ Se deben solucionar inmediatamente todos los problemas relacionados con los cables, la polaridad, la iluminación y las conexiones a tierra.

✓ Sujetar bien los enchufes, receptáculos y los accesorios de iluminación.

SISTEMA DE CALEFACCIÓN

Fuente de energía de calefacción y sus condiciones

El sistema de calefacción de la marca Borg Warner es a base de gas y tiene una capacidad de entrada de 64.000 BTU, y está ubicado en la parte posterior del garaje. Como fue instalado hace muchos años, debe estar muy cerca a la última etapa de su "vida útil" de funcionamiento. Si se quiere saber cuántos años más de funcionamiento tendrá, hay que contratar a un especialista en sistemas de calefacción. Se encontraron los siguientes problemas:

a. La válvula de cierre del gas está muy apretada y necesita un pequeño ajuste.

b. Hay una fuga de gas natural en la parte del frente del horno de calefacción. Esta fuga podría ser sumamente peligrosa y debe ser arreglada de inmediato. Consulte con un plomero autorizado o llame a la compañía PG&E para que revisen y realicen un análisis completo.

c. No se vio un historial de servicio durante esta inspección. Una lista vigente de chequeos realizados daría información sobre el mantenimiento de este sistema de calefacción.

d. Este equipo no tiene la ventaja de un encendido automático. Un conector termopar, el cual puede cerrar la entrada de gas si el piloto no está encendido, sería una gran medida de protección.

e. En el lado izquierdo del horno se encuentra montado un interruptor de corriente eléctrica para facilitar la interrupción de electricidad hacia este aparato durante su mantenimiento y reparación.

f. No hay instalada una cubierta aislante térmica en el conducto de retorno de aire arriba del horno. Ya que este conducto se encuentra en un área sin aire acondicionado o fría, este falla origina más consumo de energía que los conductos protegidos térmicamente.

g. Los conductos de aire caliente y la cámara de sobrepresión se encuentran recubiertos con un material parecido al asbesto que se está desintegrando. Busque a contratistas especialistas en este campo para que realicen pruebas y análisis de laboratorio para detectar la presencia de asbesto y, si es positiva, darles un estimado para su retiro o aislamiento de acuerdo a las normas de la Agencia de Protección Ambiental de los Estados Unidos (EPA, por sus siglas en inglés).

Movimiento del aire y ventilación

El conducto de retorno de aire, los quemadores, la cámara y la base del horno están sucios. En el piso del pasillo, el dispositivo de entrada de aire caliente y su interior están sumamente sucios. Estas partes deben limpiarse inmediatamente, y con regularidad, con una aspiradora.

El receptáculo del filtro tiene capacidad para un filtro de 14 x 25 x 1 pulgadas. El filtro está limpio y bien instalado. Los filtros deben cambiarse cada dos a cuatro meses. En realidad, los filtros sucios impiden la circulación de aire al intercambiador de calor causando su recalentamiento. El mantenimiento inadecuado de los filtros es la primera causa del agrietamiento prematuro del intercambiador de calor.

Las fuentes de oxígeno necesarias para la combustión completa en el horno son muy pocas. Las entradas de aire fresco se encuentran obstaculizadas por cajas de uso personal que bloquean las rejillas de ventilación de la pared. Quite las cajas y permita que haya una corriente continua de aire fresco al intercambiador de calor.

Conductos de ventilación y de salida de humos

Se encontró un conducto de salida de humos del tipo de asbestos y concreto (Transite®). (Vea la nota sobre asbesto en otras secciones de este informe.)

El conducto de salida de humos está ubicado en una parte no recomendada y puede ser peligroso para la vivienda y sus moradores. Las salidas de humos que no sobrepasan el nivel del techo exterior deben ser extendidas hacia arriba o deben ser reinstaladas.

Intercambiador de calor

Los quemadores de gas parecen que no están equilibrados produciendo llamas oscilantes. Este desequilibrio es difícil de solucionar pero un especialista en calefacción o un técnico de la compañía de gas natural pueden hacer un análisis y equilibrarla. Esta reparación debe ser hecha tan pronto como sea posible.

Hay una pequeña oxidación y perforaciones debido a la corrosión en la parte frontal del área del intercambiador de calor.

La cámara de combustión (del intercambiador) separa el aire caliente del medio ambiente y lo transmite de nuevo, el cual también calienta y mueve. No es posible realizar una inspección completa de la unidad de calefacción sin desmantelarla completamente; esta compañía de inspección no realiza este tipo de trabajo. Tampoco hay una apertura para usar un espejo de inspección. Pídale a la compañía PG&E o a un especialista en calefacción que haga ahora una inspección de seguridad en este aparato y en todos los aparatos que usan gas, en las líneas de suministro del mismo y en los conductos de humo; y también que se haga esta inspección cuando hayan nuevos ocupantes en la vivienda.

✓ Repare la fuga de gas inmediatamente.
✓ Afloje la válvula de cierre de gas para que se pueda maniobrar con facilidad.
✓ Investigue la composición del material que parece ser asbesto.
✓ Limpie las partes de ventilación y circulación del aire.
✓ Proporcione circulación continua de aire fresco.
✓ Alargue la parte superior del conducto de humo más allá del nivel del techo exterior.
✓ Pídale a la compañía PG&E o a un especialista en calefacción que prenda la unidad y que haga una inspección de seguridad en todos los aparatos que usan gas, en las líneas de suministro del mismo y en los conductos de humo.

PARTE INTERIOR DE LA VIVIENDA

Condición general

En su gran mayoría, a las paredes, los techos y pisos se les ha dado el mantenimiento adecuado. La industria de la inspección no cubre detalles de enlucidos.

Ventanas, puertas y escaleras

Debido a que el manejo de la mayoría de las ventanas ha sido afectado por la pintura, la disponibilidad de aire fresco ha disminuido; éste debe ser incrementado mediante la apertura regular de las mismas. La reparación debe hacerse según se necesite.

Las ventanas de ciertas habitaciones requieren más atención. Se necesita ajustar algunas cerraduras de ventanas y otros dispositivos mecánicos de las mismas. Además, al menos tres marcos de ventanas en la habitación principal tiene rotos varios cables. Y una ventana del garaje tiene un panel de vidrio roto que debe ser reparado. Generalmente, cualquier ventana, puerta, cerradura u otros componentes de ellas que se encuentren deteriorados, rotos o que falten, deben ser reparados o reemplazados aún cuando no estén especificados en este informe.

Pisos y paredes

La mayor parte del piso de la sala de estar se encuentra alfombrada. El piso de madera de la sala, que estaba al descubierto, está en buenas condiciones y se le ha dado el mantenimiento adecuado.

Hay un hueco en la pared del vestíbulo. Aparentemente la falta de un tope de puerta es la causa de este daño, el cual debe ser reparado antes de ser pintado.

✓ Repare o ajuste las ventanas, puertas y sus componentes según se necesite.
✓ Instale el tope de puerta y repare el hueco en el vestíbulo.

CHIMENEA

La chimenea de la sala está en buenas condiciones. Se observaron muy pocas grietas en los ladrillos o en las juntas de mortero. El fogón estaba vacío.

Un punto de atención es la limpieza del fogón, del conducto de humo y de toda la chimenea en general. La Asociación Nacional de Prevención de Incendios (The National Fire Prevention Association) recomienda que se haga una inspección a fondo de toda la chimenea cuando hay un cambio de dueño en una vivienda y ésta tenga una chimenea que utiliza combustible sólido. Por lo tanto, contacte a un fontanero profesional para examinar, reparar y limpiar de manera regular las áreas que lo necesiten, así como también aquellas áreas a las cuales no se tuvo acceso durante la inspección de hoy. Esto asegurará el funcionamiento adecuado, eficiente y seguro de la chimenea.

El conducto de salida de humo tiene un tope tipo atrapa-chispas. Este dispositivo protector contra las brasas está en buenas condiciones.

La puerta del amortiguador se encuentra en buenas condiciones y bien instalada. Sin embargo, no hay una pantalla protectora contra las brasas ni una puerta de vidrio instalada en la entrada del acceso al fogón. Coloque algún tipo de protección antes de prender la chimenea nuevamente.

La repisa de madera en la parte superior de la chimenea, la coraza protectora y el enlozado de la parte exterior del fogón están en buenas condiciones, y se les ha dado buen mantenimiento.

✓ Instale un protector contra las brasas o una puerta de vidrio en la entrada del acceso al fogón.
✓ Contrate a un fontanero o inspector de chimeneas antes de usarla.

COCINA

La cocina se ve cuidada. El fregadero, el grifo, el sifón y las válvulas de cierre funcionaron cuando se probaron. La presión de agua era adecuada.

El goteo en la unión de la grifería se debe reparar inmediatamente.

El triturador de desperdicios eléctrico funciona bien. No se notaron ruidos extraños o exceso de vibración.

Las superficies internas del lavaplatos automático se encontraron vacías y limpias. No tiene un dispositivo contrasifonaje, pero está bien asegurado a la parte superior del interior del mueble. Este dispositivo instalado por encima del borde del fregadero previene el retorno de desperdicios o desechos al lavaplatos automático en caso de que el sistema de drenaje se tape. Para la instalación de este dispositivo contrate un plomero profesional.

• Informe de inspección previa a la compra
Calle _____ , San Francisco, California   _____ __, 2006

Los gabinetes de madera satinados están en buenas condiciones; sin embargo, sólo se inspeccionó una muestra de las puertas, conexiones y gavetas de la cocina.

Los mostradores de plástico laminado están en buenas condiciones, aunque el área de salpicaduras, a la derecha de la estufa, está floja. Es necesario ajustar e impermeabilizar las juntas en todo el gabinete, en el área de salpicaduras y del fregadero; ellas deben ser selladas frecuentemente con un impermeabilizante flexible y de buena calidad que ayude a prevenir la penetración del agua o de la humedad.

El conducto del extractor de aire, ubicado en la parte superior del horno de microondas, funciona. El filtro del extractor está grasoso y el motor del ventilador extrae aire sin fuerzas; esto puede que se deba al exceso de grasa acumulada. Para un funcionamiento adecuado, limpie, repare o reemplace las partes componentes según se necesiten.

El piso de vinilo resistente fue instalado recientemente y está en buenas condiciones.
- ✓ Instale el dispositivo contrasifonaje para el lavaplatos automático.
- ✓ Asegure el área de salpicaduras floja y aplique impermeabilizante flexible donde sea necesario.
- ✓ Limpie, repare o reemplace los componentes del extractor de aire.

BAÑOS

Esta edificación tiene dos baños que fueron remodelados recientemente. Los lavabos, los grifos, los sifones y drenajes funcionaron bien cuando se les probó.

La presión de agua es adecuada, sin embargo, la medición es solo una apreciación relativa. Los nuevos propietarios deben personalmente poner a prueba cada dispositivo para familiarizarse con cada uno de ellos y efectuar las modificaciones que deseen.

Al probar "el flujo de agua dinámico" (esto es, cuando se abren dos o más grifos de agua fría al mismo tiempo) se observó una disminución notable en el volumen de agua. Se les mostró a Red F. Toobuy y a su agente de bienes raíces cómo realizar una "prueba de flujo de agua dinámico y de temperatura para el propietario", en cada dispositivo, para establecer el riesgo de quemaduras por agua caliente cuando alguien esté tomando una ducha y otra persona abre los grifos de agua fría.

No se encontraron evidencias de deterioros significativos o anormales en las tuberías de desagüe visibles. Los drenajes que se pusieron a prueba drenaron fácilmente; sin embargo, se encontró una fuga de agua en el lavabo del baño de visitas que debe ser reparado inmediatamente.

Los dos inodoros están bien asegurados al piso y bien sellados e impermeabilizados. El asiento del inodoro del baño de visitas está sumamente flojo y debe ser ajustado.

El vidrio de la ducha del baño principal tiene el sello que identifica de qué tipo es (vidrio templado o de seguridad). Tanto la tina como la ducha tienen asideros bien fijados.

El extractor de techo del baño de visitas extrae el aire sin fuerza y parece que necesita una limpieza o servicio, o hay que reemplazarlo.

El piso de vinilo del baño de visitas tiene una junta despegada que necesita pegarse y sellarse.
- ✓ Arregle la fuga en el drenaje del lavabo del baño de visitas.
- ✓ Ajuste el asiento del inodoro del baño de visitas.
- ✓ Limpie, repare o reemplace los componentes del extractor de aire.
- ✓ Pegue la junta en el piso de vinilo del baño de visitas y séllelo con un impermeabilizante.

TECHO
Acceso
El techo exterior tiene acceso por medio de escaleras. El inspector de Warren Camp efectuó personalmente una inspección completa del techo y solo se observaron las condiciones generales visibles del mismo. Generalmente, las pruebas de agua, de las membranas impermeabilizantes de techo, de la chimenea, de las cunetas, tapajuntas metálicas y otras no son hechas por los inspectores de viviendas.

Tipo de membrana impermeabilizante y condición
Parece que se han colocados múltiples capas de tejas de aglomerado. No se puede determinar el número de tejas instaladas ni el peso combinado de ellas sobre la armazón de la vivienda. Las capas múltiples de tejas preocupan a los instaladores de techo y a los inspectores por varias razones: ellas crean una superficie irregular y retienen la humedad y los vapores entre las

---

Este informe ha sido preparado para el uso exclusivo de Red E. Toobuy.
Se prohíbe el uso de esta información a otras personas.

• Página 12

membranas impermeabilizantes de techo; además, pueden ocasionar la degradación de las partes estructurales y agregan un peso excesivo a la estructura. Cuando se vayan a colocar nuevas membranas impermeabilizantes de techo en un techo con múltiples capas, todo el material existente en el techo debe ser sacado y desechado. Considere la posibilidad de instalar nuevos paneles de madera contrachapada apropiada en ese momento.

A pesar de que no se ven muy nuevas, y muestran señales de uso debido a la intemperie, las tejas de aglomerado en cada pendiente del techo se ven bien. No hay evidencia, o tal vez muy poca, de deterioro significativo o fuera de lo común aunque había a la vista musgo creciendo en la parte inferior de la parte norte del techo. Consulte con un instalador de techos para determinar las maneras de eliminar ese musgo.

Se consiguieron escombros en la parte frontal del techo donde un árbol alto ha estado desprendiendo hojas y ramas con el tiempo. El techo se debe limpiar y darle mantenimiento con regularidad.

Chimeneas, cunetas y tapajuntas

El tapajuntas de metal de las tejas es una medida de la calidad. Se pudo ver en la base de la chimenea. Se observó óxido en una parte de este tapajuntas, por lo que se sugiere una investigación más detallada por un experto en hojas metálicas.

Los conductos de ventilación y los tapajuntas metálicos perimetrales se encuentran en buenas condiciones.

En el valle del techo se observaron partes de los tapajuntas rotos. Pero en general, la condición del techo es buena.

Tres de las juntas de las cunetas están notoriamente oxidadas, especialmente en la parte interior. Además, se encontraron dos extremos de cunetas que estaban perdidos o separados y que deben ser reinstalados. Contrate a un experto en hojas metálicas para hacer las reparaciones o reemplazos necesarios.

Las cunetas presentan desechos orgánicos provenientes de los árboles altos. Mantenga las cunetas, bajantes y otros drenajes limpios de escombros para mantener el funcionamiento adecuado de los mismos durante el año.

El sistema de bajantes está, en su mayor parte, instalado de la manera estándar. Desafortunadamente, un número de bajantes probablemente desagüen directamente en el área de la fundación lo que puede ocasionar erosión y el asentamiento de la vivienda con el tiempo. Se pueden instalar disipadores o placas extendidas en la base de estos bajantes para desviar el agua recaudada. Como una opción investigue si un plomero profesional puede conectar los bajantes a una línea de desagüe existente.

Otros problemas

Los techos son inspeccionados muy raras veces, si es que se hace. Aunque la compañía Warren Camp Inspection Services haya hecho la inspección del techo, los problemas de techos generalmente están ocultos y son difíciles de evaluar. Debido a que los inspectores de propiedades a menudo no tienen la experticia y accesibilidad que los expertos en techo tienen, cualquier pregunta acerca de las condiciones del techo se debe consultar con un especialista de techos quien puede hacer una inspección y evaluación completa.

Cada dos años, antes de la estación de lluvias, los techos deben ser examinados por un especialista en techos y hacerles un mantenimiento de rutina.

    ✓ Limpie el techo del crecimiento de musgo y del sucio de los árboles.
    ✓ Haga que un experto en hojas metálicas analice la corrosión en las juntas de las tejas.
    ✓ Repare o remplace las cunetas oxidadas y las piezas terminales que se encuentran separadas o perdidas.
    ✓ Instale extensiones o cambie la dirección de la parte inferior de los bajantes para que drenen el agua de lluvia lejos de la fundación de la edificación.

Notas del análisis de los mapas sísmicos (evaluación opcional ordenada por Red B. Toobuy)

    Mapa #1 — **Intensidad del temblor del suelo durante un fuerte terremoto (con una intensidad de 8 ó más en la escala de Richter)** . . . Desde "A" hasta "E," la ubicación de esta propiedad es clasificada "E" (la clasificación menos intensa en la ciudad)

    Mapa #2 — **Ubicación en un zona de deslizamiento potencial del terreno** . . . Esta edificación está dentro de esta ubicación. y se encuentra aproximadamente a tres cuadras de una zona de deslizamiento activa.

• Informe de inspección previa a la compra
Calle _____ , San Francisco, California   _____ __, 2006

Mapa #3 — **Daños estimados a la edificación ocasionados por un fuerte terremoto** . . . Se estiman daños mínimos a esta edificación y a las contiguas.

Mapa #4 — **Fallo potencial de reservorios de agua** . . . La edificación está fuera de esta ubicación.

Mapa #5 — **Composición geológica del suelo debajo de la edificación** . . . La edificación se encuentra en un sustrato rocoso tipo Franciscano (KJU, por sus siglas en inglés), el cual está clasificado como el de **mayor estabilidad** en la ciudad.

Mapa #6 — **Licuefacción potencial** . . . La edificación está fuera de esta ubicación.

Mapa #7 — **Hundimiento potencial** . . . Esta edificación está fuera de esta ubicación.

Mapa #8 — **Tsunami potencial** . . . Esta edificación está fuera de esta ubicación.

Gracias por usar los servicios de Warren Camp, su inspector de viviendas certificado por ASHI.

Material de lectura adicional y folletos entregados:
Folleto All-Points: Un folleto que habla sobre remodelación y reparación de la vivienda de la compañía PG&E. Artículos publicados por la compañía Warren Camp sobre detectores de humo, asbesto, filtraciones de agua, y sobre receptáculos eléctricos GFCI (por sus siglas en inglés); y también una lista de verificación con todos los elementos de inspección que deben hacerse durante el año.

Se entregaron copias a:	entrega	enviado por correo	entregado personalmente	fax	correo electrónico
Comprador:	[ ]	[ ]	[ ]	[ ]	[ ]
Agente del comprador:	[ ]	[ ]	[ ]	[ ]	[ ]
Agente del vendedor:	[ ]	[ ]	[ ]	[ ]	[ ]

Apéndice B

Glosario

· ·

*L*os términos que aparecen en letra cursiva en los diferentes párrafos están definidos en este glosario.

Administración Federal para la Vivienda (*Federal Housing Administration* **[***FHA,* **por sus siglas en inglés]):** las *hipotecas FHA* son otorgadas a personas de modestos recursos. La principal ventaja de estas hipotecas es que requieren de una pequeña *cuota inicial,* normalmente del 3 al 5 por ciento. Las hipotecas de la *FHA* también ofrecen una *tasa de interés* competitiva, generalmente de un 0,5 a un 1 por ciento por debajo de la tasa de interés en otras hipotecas. La desventaja es que con una hipoteca de la *FHA,* el comprador debe adquirir un seguro de *incumplimiento de pago* de la hipoteca. (Vea *seguro hipotecario privado.*)

agente de bienes raíces o agente inmobiliario: un *agente de bienes raíces* es la hormiguita de las ventas de bienes raíces. También llamados "los vendedores", los agentes son supervisados por un corredor de bienes raíces. El estado concede títulos o licencias a los agentes para ejercer su profesión; sus honorarios se basan totalmente en las *comisiones* generadas por la venta de la propiedad.

agente de bienes raíces agremiado: un agente de bienes raíces *agremiado* es un agente de bienes raíces o un *corredor* que pertenecen a la Asociación Nacional de Agentes Inmobiliarios (*National Association of Realtors*). Ésta es una asociación profesional cuyos miembros acuerdan regirse por ordenanzas o estatutos especiales bajo los cuales llevan a cabo los negocios inmobiliarios y su código de ética. La Asociación Nacional de Agentes Inmobiliarios ofrece a sus miembros seminarios y cursos relacionados con temas de bienes raíces.

alquiler con opción a compra: un *alquiler con opción a compra* es algo de lo que es fanático Robert J. Bruss, columnista de bienes raíces con difusión nacional. Una propiedad que usted puede alquilar con la opción a comprar en una fecha posterior, tiene una cláusula en el contrato de este tipo. Estos contratos generalmente requieren un pago por adelantado (llamado "consideración para la opción") para asegurar la opción a compra. Este pago generalmente se deposita como un crédito en la *cuota inicial* cuando usted ejerce su opción a comprar la casa. Un factor importante en un alquiler con opción a compra es saber cuál es la porción de los pagos mensuales (generalmente un tercio) que se asignan al precio de compra si finalmente efectúa la compra. Usted generalmente pagará un alquiler un poco más alto por el privilegio de la opción a compra.

amortización negativa: aunque le parezca lenguaje de ciencia ficción, la *amortización negativa* ocurre cuando su saldo de hipoteca pendiente se incrementa a pesar de que usted cumple con los pagos mensuales puntualmente. La amortización negativa ocurre con las *hipotecas con tasa de interés variables* que ponen un tope a los incrementos en las cuotas mensuales pero no a la *tasa de interés*. Por lo tanto, sus cuotas mensuales no cubren todo el interés que usted actualmente debe. Si alguna vez se ha fijado en el efecto "bola de nieve" en el balance de su tarjeta de crédito cuando sólo paga la cuota mínima, entonces ya tiene experiencia con este tipo de fenómeno. ¡Evite los préstamos con estas características!

análisis comparativo de mercado (*CMA*, por sus siglas en inglés): comprar un *Ford Taurus* en el primer concesionario que visite sería impulsivo y tonto. Usted necesita ir a varios concesionarios para saber cuál le ofrece el mejor negocio para este tipo de carro. Lo mismo ocurre con las viviendas; si está interesado en comprar una casa, necesita saber por cuánto se han vendido otras casas del vecindario. Debe identificar casas "parecidas" que se hayan vendido en los últimos seis meses y que se encuentren en el mismo sector en el cual desea comprar, y que sean similares a la que usted desea en términos de tamaño, años de construcción y condiciones. Debe hacer lo mismo con las casas similares que se encuentran en el mercado para saber si los precios están aumentando, o se han mantenido o disminuido. Un *análisis comparativo de mercado* (*CMA*) es un reporte escrito de la venta real de viviendas similares a la que usted desea, en comparación con la venta de viviendas similares en los últimos seis meses.

arbitraje de conflictos: es un método para resolver conflictos contractuales, pero generalmente menos costoso y más rápido que llevar el caso a un tribunal. En el *arbitraje,* los compradores y vendedores presentan sus diferencias a un árbitro neutral que, de acuerdo a los argumentos que exponen las partes, toma una decisión que resuelve el conflicto. La decisión del árbitro es final y debe ser cumplida como si fuera hecha por un juzgado o tribunal. Consulte con un abogado en bienes raíces si alguna vez tiene que usar un arbitraje. (Vea también *mediación de disputas.*)

Asociación Nacional Federal de Hipotecas (*Federal National Mortgage Association* [*FNMA*, por sus siglas en inglés]): la *FNMA* (o *Fannie Mae,* nombre popular de la asociación en inglés) es una de las instituciones más conocidas en el mercado hipotecario secundario. Fannie Mae compra las hipotecas a los bancos y otras instituciones hipotecarias y vende estas hipotecas a inversionistas. Estas inversiones sobre préstamos se consideran seguras ya que Fannie Mae compra hipotecas sólo de compañías que cumplen sus estrictas regulaciones acerca de hipotecas y garantiza el pago del capital e intereses sobre el préstamo que vende.

aval: si tiene un pasado no muy bueno en el mundo de los créditos, puede que necesite ayuda para obtener un préstamo hipotecario aún cuando usted se encuentre financieramente estable. Un amigo o familiar puede venir en su rescate convirtiéndose en aval o fiador de su hipoteca (lo que significa literalmente que adquiere su deuda). Un *aval* no puede mejorar su *reporte crediticio* pero sí ayuda a la posibilidad de obtener una hipoteca. Sin embargo, los avales deben estar conscientes de que esta acción afectará de manera adversa su futuro crediticio también, ya que el préstamo se convierte en una obligación contra su capacidad de obtener financiamiento.

avalúo: usted debe pagarle a la entidad crediticia la contratación de un técnico o agente para que dé una "opinión del valor" (es decir, el agente da un precio de acuerdo al valor del mercado) de la casa que desea comprar. Esta opinión profesional previene a la entidad crediticia de prestarle dinero para comprar una casa que está valorada en menos de lo que usted aceptó pagar. Para viviendas típicas, la tasa de *avalúo* es normalmente unos cientos de dólares.

base de costos: vea *base de costos ajustados.*

base de costos ajustados: para propósitos del impuesto, la *base de costos ajustados* es importante cuando vende su propiedad ya que le permite determinar cuál es la ganancia o pérdida de la venta. Usted puede obtener la base de costos ajustados sumando el costo del capital invertido en las mejoras que le ha hecho a la casa, y el precio al que compró la vivienda. El capital para las mejoras incrementa el valor de su propiedad y la vida útil de la misma.

buydown o *compra a la baja*: un *buydown* o *compra a la baja,* es un plan de préstamo de la Administración de Asuntos de los Veteranos (*Veterans Affairs,* [*VA,* por sus siglas en inglés]) disponible sólo en algunos desarrollos habitacionales nuevos para personal militar o veteranos con bajos o modestos ingresos. *Buydown* significa simplemente que el constructor acuerda pagar parte de la hipoteca del comprador durante los primeros años. Los vendedores algunas veces también efectúan *buydowns* de la tasa de interés para crear un financiamiento atractivo para los compradores de sus casas, pagándole a la entidad crediticia una cantidad predeterminada de dinero de manera que ellas reduzcan sus tasas de interés en la hipoteca.

capital de un préstamo hipotecario: es la cantidad de dinero que usted pide prestada. Si usted pide $100.000 prestado, su capital es de $100.000. Cada cuota de la hipoteca consta de una porción de capital que debe ser pagada más los intereses que el prestamista le está cargando por el uso del dinero. Durante los primeros años de su hipoteca, el pago del préstamo es principalmente para los intereses.

capital propio en la propiedad o activo: en el mundo de bienes raíces, el *capital propio en la propiedad* (o capital) es la diferencia entre el valor de mercado de su casa y el saldo de su deuda pendiente por pagar. Por ejemplo, si su casa está valorada en $250.000, y usted tiene un saldo pendiente de $170.000, su capital en la propiedad es de $80.000.

cláusula de las 72 horas: también llamada cláusula de liberación, normalmente es insertada en las ofertas de compra de bienes raíces, cuando la adquisición de una vivienda está sujeta a la venta de la casa actual del comprador. El vendedor acepta la oferta del comprador pero se reserva el derecho de aceptar una mejor si aparece durante la negociación. Sin embargo, el vendedor no puede hacer esto de manera arbitraria. Si él recibe una oferta que desea aceptar, debe notificar por escrito su decisión al comprador, quien dispone de 72 horas (aunque el tiempo asignado puede variar) desde la notificación del vendedor para anular la cláusula de contingencia de venta y proceder con la compra, o su oferta es cancelada.

cláusula de pago anticipado: tenga cuidado con algunas *cláusulas de pago anticipado* en el contrato hipotecario. Esta provisión da el derecho a la entidad crediticia a demandar el pago de todo el saldo pendiente del préstamo si usted deja de pagar un mes, vende la propiedad o falla en hacer los pagos de acuerdo a lo estipulado en el contrato hipotecario. (Vea también la *cláusula de vencimiento a la venta*.) ¡Uy!

cláusula de vencimiento a la venta: una *cláusula de vencimiento a la venta* contenida en la hipoteca autoriza a la entidad crediticia a demandar el pago completo de la deuda remanente del préstamo, si usted vende o transfiere el título de propiedad.

comisión: la *comisión* es el porcentaje sobre el precio de compra de la casa que se le paga al *agente de bienes raíces* y al *corredor*. Para los compradores es importante entender cómo la comisión influye en la forma en que los agentes y corredores trabajan, ya que éstos cobran sus servicios de acuerdo a esa cantidad. Los agentes y corredores ganan dinero únicamente cuando usted efectúa la compra, y ganan más dinero cuando el precio es mayor. Escoja cuidadosamente su agente y sopese su consejo con mucho cuidado, ya que un conflicto de intereses, subyacente a menudo, puede hacer que la visión y las metas del agente difieran de las suyas.

condiciones: ver *contingencias*.

condominios: los *condominios* son desarrollos habitacionales en los cuales usted posee una unidad o apartamento y una parte del resto del desarrollo habitacional (entrada, estacionamientos, terrenos y otros, conocidos como áreas comunes). Los condominios son un tipo de vivienda pero menos costosos que las unifamiliares separadas. Por esta razón, algunas personas los ven erróneamente como una buena forma de comenzar a adquirir vivienda. Desafortunadamente, los condominios en general no incrementan su valor tan rápido como las viviendas unifamiliares, debido a que su demanda es menor que la de las casas. Y además, como los condominios son más fáciles de construir que las viviendas unifamiliares separadas, por lo general, su oferta supera a la demanda.

consorcios de inversiones en bienes raíces (*Real Estates Investment Trust* [*REIT*, por sus siglas en inglés]): un *consorcio de inversión en bienes raíces* es como un fondo mutual de inversiones de bienes raíces. Estos consorcios invierten en una variedad de propiedades (desde centros comerciales hasta edificios de apartamentos). Los *REIT* comercian en las grandes bolsas de valores. Si usted desea invertir en bienes raíces sin meterse en los líos inherentes al manejo de una propiedad, los consorcios o fondos de inversión de bienes raíces son quizás la mejor opción para usted.

contingencias: las *contingencias* son condiciones contenidas en casi todas las ofertas de compraventa de vivienda. El vendedor o comprador deben satisfacer todas las contingencias antes de cerrar el trato. Estas condiciones están relacionadas con asuntos tales como la revisión y aprobación por parte del comprador de la inspección de la propiedad, o la posibilidad de que al comprador se le otorgue el financiamiento hipotecario planteado en el contrato.

convenios, condiciones y restricciones (*CC&Rs,* por sus siglas en inglés): los *CCR* establecen un condominio al crear una asociación de propietarios, estipulan cómo se manejarán el mantenimiento y las reparaciones del *condominio,* y regulan lo que se puede o no hacer a las viviendas y áreas comunes. Estas restricciones afectan el mantenimiento de las áreas verdes, colores de cortinas en las ventanas y otros semejantes. Algunos *CCR* ponen los derechos de decisión de la comunidad en las manos de una asociación de propietarios.

cooperativas (*co-ops en inglés*): las *cooperativas* son edificios de apartamentos cuya propiedad usted comparte con una corporación cuyo principal activo es el edificio que usted habita. En zonas de alto costo, las cooperativas (como sus primos, los *condominios* y las *viviendas en serie o tipo «townhouses»*) son alternativas más económicas que adquirir viviendas unifamiliares. Desafortunadamente, las cooperativas también tienen una semejanza a sus primos, los condominios, en que generalmente no se revalorizan como las viviendas unifamiliares. Por regla general, las cooperativas son también, más difíciles que los condominios para obtener préstamos y para venderlas.

Corporación Federal de Préstamos Hipotecarios a la Vivienda (Federal Home Loan Mortgage Corporation [*FHLMC,* por sus siglas en inglés]): el *FHLMC* (o *Freddie Mac,* nombre popular de la corporación en inglés) es una de las instituciones más conocidas en el mercado hipotecario secundario. Freddie Mac compra las hipotecas a los bancos y a otras instituciones hipotecarias o crediticias, y las vende a inversionistas. Estas inversiones sobre préstamos se consideran seguras, ya que Freddie Mac compra hipotecas sólo de compañías que cumplen sus estrictas regulaciones acerca de hipotecas, y además garantiza el pago del *capital* e intereses sobre las hipotecas que vende.

corredor: un *corredor* de bienes raíces está en un nivel superior al *agente de bienes raíces* (o vendedor) en el escalafón profesional de los bienes inmuebles. Legalmente, los agentes no pueden trabajar por su cuenta, sino que deben ser supervisados por un corredor. Para llegar a ser un corredor, en la mayoría de los estados, un vendedor de bienes raíces debe tener una determinada cantidad de años de experiencia dedicados a este campo, y también cumplir con requisitos educativos especiales y aprobar el examen para obtener una licencia o autorización estatal. Vea también *agente de bienes raíces* y *agente de bienes raíces asociado.*

corredores del comprador: históricamente, los *agentes de bienes raíces* y *corredores* trabajaban sólo para los vendedores. El *corredor del comprador* le debe lealtad sólo al comprador y no debe tener ninguna relación con el vendedor. Aunque esto aparentemente es una mejora para todos los compradores del mundo, no se entusiasme demasiado. Los corredores de compradores todavía cobran por comisión cuando usted hace la compra, así que no espere a que salgan en su ayuda si usted no mueve un dedo para llevarla a cabo. También tenga en cuenta que a mayor precio de compra de la casa, mayor es la cantidad que gana el corredor del comprador.

corredor de hipotecas: un *corredor de hipotecas* es una persona que puede ayudarlo a conseguir una hipoteca. Los corredores de hipoteca compran hipotecas al por mayor a los prestamistas, les hacen un recargo (generalmente del 0,5 al 1 por ciento) y luego las revenden a los compradores. Un corredor de hipoteca es una buena opción para aquellas personas que no les gusta buscar por sí mismas o que tengan problemas en su *reporte crediticio*.

costos de cierre: luego de vencer todos los obstáculos y alcanzar la meta de adquirir su vivienda, aparece una última piedra en el camino con la figura de *costos de cierre*. Estos costos generalmente representan del 2 al 5 por ciento del precio de compra de la casa y son completamente independientes de (y adicionales a) la *cuota o pago inicial*. Los costos de cierre incluyen los *puntos* (es decir, los *gastos de solicitud* del préstamo que cubren los costos administrativos de la entidad financiera), el costo del *avalúo* y del *reporte de crédito,* el interés de la hipoteca que cubre el período entre la fecha del contrato de compra y el pago de la primera cuota, la prima del *seguro de propietario*, *seguro sobre el título de propiedad*, *impuestos a la propiedad* prorrateados y cargos por registro y transferencias. De manera que cuando ya está listo para comprar, necesita disponer del efectivo suficiente para cubrir todos estos gastos y poder adquirir la casa de sus sueños.

costos de origen o iniciación: vea *puntos*.

cuota inicial: la *cuota o pago inicial* es la porción del precio de compra que el comprador paga en efectivo, por adelantado y no financiada por la hipoteca. En general, mientras mayor sea la cuota inicial, mejor serán las condiciones de financiamiento que puede obtener en la hipoteca. Generalmente, puede tener acceso a mejores financiamientos hipotecarios, si tiene una cuota inicial del 20 por ciento del valor de compra de su casa.

daños liquidados: en la mayoría de los contratos de bienes raíces, los compradores y vendedores pueden acordar al comienzo de la transacción qué cantidad de dinero, por indemnización, recibiría una de las partes si la otra no cumple con los términos del contrato sin una causa justificada. Los *daños liquidados* confinan y definen la cantidad que puede recuperar la parte agraviada. Los compradores, por ejemplo, generalmente limitan sus pérdidas a la cantidad de su depósito. Hable con un abogado o un *agente de bienes raíces* acerca de si es conveniente o no utilizar la provisión de los daños liquidados.

deducible de impuestos: el *deducible de impuestos* se refiere a los pagos que usted puede deducir de sus impuestos federales y estatales. La porción del interés, los *puntos* de préstamo y los *impuestos sobre la propiedad* son deducibles de impuestos, ¡su ingreso no!

depósito de garantía: el depósito de *garantía* es la custodia de documentos importantes y de dinero (relacionados con la compraventa de una propiedad) llevada a cabo por una tercera parte neutral (el agente o administrador de garantía) antes del cierre de la transacción. Después que el vendedor acepta la oferta del comprador, éste no se muda inmediatamente a la casa. Existe un período durante el cual las *contingencias* deben ser cumplidas o eliminadas. Durante este período, la compañía que custodia la garantía retiene la *cuota inicial* del comprador y los documentos del comprador y del vendedor relacionados con la venta. "Cerrar la garantía" significa que el trato o negocio ha sido hecho. Entre otros deberes del agente de garantía están asegurarse que la hipoteca anterior esté pagada en su totalidad, que los fondos del préstamo estén disponibles y que se les haya pagado a los *agentes de bienes raíces*.

depreciación: vea *valorización*.

embargo hipotecario: el *embargo* hipotecario o simplemente *embargo* es el proceso legal por medio del cual la entidad hipotecaria se apodera de la propiedad y la vende para saldar la deuda pendiente. Cuando usted *incumple el pago* de una hipoteca y la entidad crediticia estima que no es capaz de pagar la deuda, usted puede perder su vivienda por embargo. No obstante, el incumplimiento del pago no necesariamente conlleva al embargo. Algunas entidades financieras son indulgentes y le ayudan a solventar la situación si consideran que es pasajera. El embargo es traumático para el propietario y costoso para las entidades crediticias.

escritura: vea *título de propiedad*.

Fannie Mae: vea Asociación Nacional Federal de Hipotecas (*Federal National Mortgage Association*).

fiador: vea *aval*.

fórmula: no estamos hablando en este caso de la bebida para bebés. En el jerga de bienes raíces, la fórmula es la forma en que usted calcula la *tasa de interés* para una *hipoteca con tasa de interés variable*. Sume el margen al índice para obtener la tasa de interés (margen + índice = tasa de interés).

frecuencia de ajuste: vea *periodo de ajuste*.

Freddie Mac: vea Corporación Federal de Préstamos Hipotecarios a la Vivienda *(Federal Home Loan Mortgage Corporation)*.

ganancias de capital: para propósitos del impuesto, una *ganancia de capital* es aquella que usted genera cuando compra una casa. Si usted adquiere una vivienda por $175.000 y luego (años más tarde) la vende por $325.000, su ganancia de capital es de $150.000. Del impuesto federal se excluye una considerable cantidad de la ganancia de capital sobre la venta de una casa: hasta $250.000 para contribuyentes solteros y $500.000 para casados que declaren en conjunto.

gastos de iniciación del préstamo: vea *puntos.*

gravamen: un *gravamen* es un embargo preventivo sobre la propiedad con el propósito de asegurar el pago por trabajos efectuados o por préstamos que se han hechos, por fallos legales o reclamos. Los gravámenes son cargos y necesitan ser cancelados antes de que la propiedad sea vendida o se pueda transferir el título a otro comprador. Los gravámenes sobre una propiedad a la venta aparecen en un reporte preliminar del título de la propiedad.

hipoteca "asumible": algunas hipotecas permiten que los futuros compradores de su casa se encarguen del resto del préstamo que usted todavía debe. Si necesita vender su casa pero la *tasa de interés* está alta, obtener una *hipoteca asumible* puede resultar útil, ya que puede ofrecerle al comprador su préstamo a una tasa de interés más baja que la vigente. La mayoría de las hipotecas asumibles son *hipotecas con tasa de interés variable* —las *hipotecas asumibles de tasa fija* casi no existen ya que las entidades crediticias calcularon que pierden una gran cantidad de dinero con este tipo de hipotecas cuando los intereses suben mucho.

hipoteca con tasa de interés variable convertible: a diferencia de una *hipoteca con tasa de interés variable* convencional, una *hipoteca con tasa de interés variable convertible* le da la oportunidad de convertir la hipoteca en una de *tasa fija* generalmente entre los 13 y 60 meses de la concesión del préstamo. Por este privilegio, la hipoteca con tasa de interés variable convertible tiene una tasa más alta que la de una hipoteca con tasa de interés variable convencional. Además se debe cancelar un honorario por conversión que puede variar entre varios cientos de dólares, o más o menos el 1 por ciento de la cantidad del préstamo pendiente por pagar. Si escoge llevar a cabo la conversión a tasa fija, usted pagará una tasa un poco más alta que la que pudiera obtener si busca en el mercado las mejores tasas disponibles en el momento que proceda a la conversión.

hipoteca con tasa de interés variable o ajustable (*ARM,* por sus siglas en inglés): una hipoteca con tasa de interés variable o ajustable es aquella cuya tasa varía durante la vigencia de la hipoteca. Las *ARM* comienzan generalmente con una tasa de interés generalmente baja (ver *tasa de enganche*) y que aumenta gradualmente con el tiempo. Si, en general, los niveles de las tasas de interés caen (medidos por una variedad de índices, ver *índice*), la tasa de interés de su *ARM* generalmente hace lo mismo. De igual manera, si las tasas suben, así mismo lo harán las tasas de interés de su hipoteca y su mensualidad. Los topes (ver también *tope periódico* y *tope constante*) limitan la escala en la cual la tasa de interés puede fluctuar. Antes de que acepte una hipoteca con tasa de interés variable, asegúrese que puede pagar las cuotas más altas que pudieran resultar si las tasas de interés de su hipoteca se incrementaran al máximo permitido.

hipoteca de pago gradual: una especie rara en estos días, la hipoteca de pago gradual le da la oportunidad de disminuir los costos de interés totales. Con este tipo de hipoteca, sus pagos mensuales son incrementados mediante una fórmula predeterminada (por ejemplo, un incremento del 3 por ciento cada año durante siete años, período después del cual los pagos no fluctúan más). Si estima tener un trabajo que le permita cubrir estas mensualidades más altas, quizás quiera considerar esta opción.

hipoteca de sólo interés: es una hipoteca en la cual en sus primeros años el prestatario sólo paga los intereses. Generalmente, varios años después que se inicia, la cuota sube típicamente en la medida que el prestatario comienza a hacer pagos al capital y al interés.

hipoteca de tasa fija: la hipoteca de tasa fija es la abuelita de todas las hipotecas. Usted se garantiza una tasa de interés (por ejemplo, 7,5 por ciento) y ésta nunca cambiará durante la vigencia de su hipoteca a 15 ó 30 años. Su pago mensual será el mismo cada mes. Compare las hipotecas de tasa fija con las *hipotecas de tasa variable.*

hipoteca revertida: una *hipoteca revertida* le permite a los propietarios de la tercera edad, que generalmente no disponen de mucho dinero en efectivo, disponer del *capital en la propiedad* sin vender su casa o mudarse. Específicamente, una institución crediticia emite un cheque mensual el cual usted puede usar como lo desee. Este dinero es realmente un préstamo contra el valor de su vivienda; debido a que el dinero que usted recibe es un préstamo, este dinero está libre de impuestos cuando lo recibe. El lado malo de estos préstamos es que reducen el capital de su patrimonio, los honorarios y *tasas de interés* tienden a ser altos y algunos requieren repagos en un cierto número de años.

hipoteca secundaria: una *hipoteca secundaria* es la que se registra después de una primera hipoteca. En el caso de un *embargo*, el procedimiento de vender la casa pasa por la cancelación de los préstamos en el orden en el cual fueron adquiridos. Usted puede tener una tercera hipoteca (incluso una cuarta), pero mientras más lejos se encuentre la hipoteca en el orden de cancelación de préstamos, mayor es el riesgo de *incumplimiento del pago* de la misma —y por lo tanto, mayor la tasa de interés que pagará. Vea también *préstamo sobre el capital en la propiedad.*

impuesto a la propiedad: usted debe pagar el *impuesto a la propiedad* por la casa que posee. Anualmente, el impuesto sobre la propiedad promedia del 1 al 2 por ciento del valor de la casa, pero las tasas del impuesto a la propiedad varían ampliamente en esta gran nación.

incumplimiento del pago: el *incumplimiento de pago* ocurre cuando no se pagan a tiempo las cuotas o mensualidades de la hipoteca. Oficialmente, está incumpliendo el pago cuando se retrasa en dos o más cuotas mensuales. El incumplimiento también se refiere a otras fallas en el cumplimiento de las condiciones de la hipoteca. El incumplimiento de pago puede llevarlo a un *embargo hipotecario* de su casa.

índice: el *índice* es la medida calculada del total de las tasas de interés que el prestamista utiliza como referencia para calcular la tasa de interés específica para un préstamo de tasa variable. El *índice* más el *margen* es la *fórmula* para determinar la tasa de interés en una *hipoteca con tasa de interés variable*. Un índice utilizado en algunas hipotecas es una letra del Tesoro a seis meses. Si la tasa vigente para estas letras del Tesoro es del 5,5 por ciento, y el margen es de 2,5 por ciento, su tasa de interés sería del 8 por ciento. Otros índices comúnmente utilizados son los de certificados de depósito, el índice del Costo de Fondos del Distrito 11 y el índice LIBOR.

informe crediticio: vea *reporte crediticio*.

inspección de vivienda: al igual que el *seguro de propiedad*, creemos que es necesaria la *inspección de la vivienda*. A continuación sugerimos una lista de partes que se deben inspeccionar: condiciones generales de la propiedad, tanto por dentro como por fuera, los sistemas de electricidad, de calefacción y plomería, fundaciones, techo, control de plaga y pudrición seca de la madera, y riesgos de desplazamientos de tierra o sísmicos. Una buena inspección de vivienda puede ahorrarle dinero mediante el descubrimiento de los problemas. Con el reporte de inspección en la mano, usted puede pedirle al vendedor que efectúe la reparación o que las deduzca del precio de venta. Contrate su propio inspector. Nunca se sienta satisfecho con los reportes de inspección del vendedor.

la propiedad como inversión: los bienes raíces son una buena inversión a largo plazo que ha producido retornos similares a aquéllos provenientes de un portafolio diversificado de la bolsa de valores durante años. En la práctica, la inversión en bienes raíces es diferente a la inversión en la bolsa. Usted también puede *manipular* su inversión en bienes raíces, es decir, puede sacarle provecho a la inversión así como también al préstamo de dinero. La inversión en bienes raíces es muy difícil (aunque invertir en la bolsa también puede serlo si no cuenta con un administrador profesional de dinero). También debe tener aptitud para dirigir y administrar dinero si desea verle los frutos a las inversiones en bienes raíces. Un inconveniente de la *propiedad de inversión* es que usted no puede proteger los beneficios de este tipo de inversión en una cuenta de jubilación en la forma en que lo puede hacer con los beneficios obtenidos en una inversión en la bolsa.

Listado Múltiple de Casas en Venta (*MLS,* por sus siglas en inglés): es un servicio cooperativo de los *agentes de bienes raíces* que contiene las descripciones de la mayoría de las casas en venta. Los agentes de bienes raíces utilizan sus servicios computarizados para mantenerse actualizados acerca de las propiedades en venta, con miembros del MLS en sus áreas.

margen: el *margen* es la cantidad que es sumada al *índice* para calcular su *tasa de interés* en una *hipoteca con tasa de interés variable*. La mayoría de los préstamos tienen márgenes de alrededor del 2,5 por ciento. A diferencia del índice (el cual constantemente sube o baja), el margen nunca cambia durante la vida del préstamo.

mediación de conflictos: es una rápida y económica manera de resolver simples diferencias de contratos. En la mediación, los compradores y vendedores presentan sus diferencias a un mediador neutral quien no tiene la potestad de imponer una decisión a ninguno de los dos grupos. En vez de eso, el mediador ayuda a los compradores y vendedores a alcanzar una solución aceptable para ambas partes. Es probable que sea mejor para usted mediar su problema antes que llevarlo a un árbitro o a una demanda en un tribunal. (Vea también *arbitraje de conflictos*).

mora en el pago: primero usted se encuentra en *mora en el pago* y luego en la situación de *incumplimiento de pago*. La mora en el pago ocurre cuando éste no se recibe en la fecha establecida en las condiciones de la hipoteca.

multa por pago anticipado: una de las ventajas de la mayoría de las hipotecas es que usted puede hacer pagos por adelantado para cancelar rápidamente el préstamo si tiene la decisión y el dinero para hacerlo. Una *multa por pago anticipado* lo disuade a usted de hacer estos anticipos utilizando la penalización por pagos anticipados. Algunos estados prohíben este tipo de penalizaciones. ¡Evite las hipotecas que penalizan los anticipos!

pago inicial: vea *cuota inicial*.

palanca financiera: vea *ventaja financiera*.

período de ajuste o **frecuencia de ajuste:** este término no tiene nada que ver con las primeras semanas después que ha terminado con su pareja; se refiere a cuantas veces la *tasa de interés* cambia a causa de la *hipoteca con tasa de interés variable*. Algunas tasas hipotecarias variables cambian mensualmente, pero es más común tener uno o dos ajustes por año. En la medida que sean menos frecuentes los cambios de tasas de su préstamo, menor es la incertidumbre financiera que usted pueda tener. Pero en la medida que la frecuencia de los ajustes en su tasa hipotecaria sea menor, en esa medida obtendrá una tasa de interés inicial o tasa de enganche superior. (La tasa de interés inicial o de enganche es llamada también "tasa de inicio").

plan de garantía de la vivienda: un *plan de garantía de la vivienda* es un tipo de seguro que cubre las reparaciones de partes específicas de la casa por un período predeterminado de tiempo. Debido a que estos planes usualmente cubren sólo pequeñas reparaciones, no vale la pena adquirirlos. Es preferible gastar el dinero en una buena *inspección de la casa* antes de comprarla, para así identificar cualquier problema grande (eléctrico, plomería o estructural).

porcentaje de deuda respecto al ingreso o razón deuda-ingreso: antes de salir a comprar casa, usted debería determinar cuál es el margen de precios que usted puede pagar. Las entidades crediticias generalmente estiman que usted no debería gastar más del 33 al 40 por ciento de sus ingresos mensuales en costos de vivienda. El *porcentaje de deuda respecto al ingreso* mide sus gastos mensuales futuros, que incluyen el pago de la hipoteca, el impuesto a la propiedad y el seguro, en relación con su ingreso mensual.

préstamo "puente": si se encuentra en la nada envidiable situación de haber hecho el negocio de adquirir su casa nueva antes de vender la anterior, probablemente necesite un *préstamo puente* de corto plazo. Este tipo de préstamo le permite obtener una hipoteca contra la ganancia acumulada de capital que tenga su casa anterior hasta que sea vendida. Le decimos "puente" porque este préstamo es lo único que lo mantendrá "a flote" durante el tiempo que usted sea dueño de dos viviendas. Los préstamos puente son costosos en comparación con otras alternativas, tales como utilizar la *reserva de efectivo,* o pedir préstamos a familiares y amigos o utilizar las ganancias de la venta de su vivienda anterior para comprar la nueva. En la mayoría de los casos, usted necesitará el préstamo puente por solamente unos pocos meses para respaldarlo hasta que venda su casa. Por tanto, los costos de trámite del préstamo pueden ser altos (cerca del 10 por ciento de la cantidad a prestar) para un préstamo de corto plazo.

préstamo sobre el capital en la propiedad: el *préstamo sobre el capital en la propiedad* en la jerga técnica es lo que se llamaba una *segunda hipoteca*. Con este tipo de préstamo, usted presta contra el *capital en la propiedad* de su casa. Si se utiliza sabiamente, este tipo de préstamo puede ayudar a las personas a cancelar deudas con una tasa generalmente más alta que los préstamos sobre el capital en la propiedad y que no son deducibles del impuesto. O también puede ser utilizado para otras necesidades a corto plazo como el pago de un proyecto de remodelación.

préstamos híbridos: los préstamos híbridos combinan las características de las *hipotecas con tasa de interés variable* y las de *tasa fija*. La *tasa de interés inicial* de un préstamo híbrido puede ser mantenida durante los primeros tres a diez años del préstamo (en oposición a sólo 6 a 12 meses para una hipoteca con tasa de interés variable convencional); a partir de allí la tasa de interés se ajusta cada uno o dos años. Recuerde que cuanto mayor sea el tiempo en que se mantenga la tasa inicial, más alta será luego la tasa de interés. Estos préstamos híbridos son buenos para personas que piensan ser dueños de la casa por un corto plazo (menos de diez años) y no quieren la volatilidad de una típica hipoteca con tasa de interés variable.

préstamos reembolsables al vencimiento o balón: estos préstamos establecen niveles de pago como los de una *hipoteca de tasa fija* de 15 o 30 años. Pero con bastante anticipación a la fecha de vencimiento (la fecha en la que termina de saldar la deuda), generalmente entre tres y diez años después del inicio de la misma, el monto restante del préstamo se vence y tiene que pagarse en su totalidad. Aunque los *préstamos balón* pueden ahorrarle dinero ya que se hacen con una tasa de interés menor en comparación a la de los préstamos a tasa fija, éstos pueden resultar muy peligrosos. La capacidad de *refinanciar* una deuda nunca es segura. ¡Tenga cuidado con los préstamos balón!

préstamos VA (préstamos de vivienda para los soldados de la guerra) (*Department of Veterans Affairs* [*VA,* por sus siglas en inglés]): el Congreso de los Estados Unidos aprobó la ley de reinserción del soldado (*Serviceman's Readjustmente Act*), comúnmente conocida como Derechos de los soldados (*GI Bill of Rights*), en 1944. Una de sus provisiones permite al *VA* ayudar a las personas que reúnen los requisitos y que se encuentran activos en el servicio y a ex combatientes o veteranos de la guerra a obtener hipotecas en términos favorables (generalmente, del 0,5 al 1 por ciento por debajo de la *tasa de interés* vigente en préstamos convencionales) para adquirir viviendas principales. Al igual que la *FHA,* el *VA* no maneja dinero propio. Garantiza préstamos con instituciones crediticias convencionales que participan en los programas de hipotecas para el *VA.*

propiedad comunal: junto con la *tenencia conjunta* y la *tenencia en común*, la *propiedad comunal* es una manera en que parejas casadas pueden obtener el título o tomar posesión de la propiedad. La propiedad comunal ofrece dos grandes ventajas con respecto a la tenencia conjunta y a la tenencia en común. Primero, la propiedad comunal le permite a los esposos transferir sus participaciones mediante un testamento u otro medio, a quienes ellos deseen. La segunda ventaja de poseer una vivienda como propiedad comunal es que el cónyuge sobreviviente obtiene ciertas ventajas impositivas. Para efectos de calcular la ganancia gravable, se utiliza el valor de mercado de la casa al momento de la fecha de fallecimiento del cónyuge (este valor es conocido también como "base de valor de mercado") en lugar de su costo original, lo que reduce la ganancia gravable (asumiendo que el inmueble se ha revalorizado) cuando se vende la casa.

propiedad horizontal: vea *condominios.*

prorrateos: ciertos conceptos como los *impuestos sobre la propiedad* y las cuotas de las asociaciones de propietarios son gastos constantes que deben ser prorrateados (distribuidos) entre los compradores y vendedores al cierre del *depósito en garantía.* Si los compradores, por ejemplo, deben dinero a los vendedores por impuestos a la propiedad que estos últimos han pagado por adelantado, la cantidad prorrateada de dinero que se le debe a los vendedores al cierre del depósito de garantía aparece como un débito (cargo) a los compradores y como un crédito a los vendedores.

puntos: también conocido como los *costos de origen* del prestamista, los puntos son cargos de intereses pagados por adelantado cuando solicita un préstamo. De hecho, los puntos son un porcentaje del total de su préstamo (un punto es equivalente al 1 por ciento del total del préstamo). Para un préstamo de $100.000, un punto le cuesta $1.000. Hablando en forma general, a mayor número de puntos que tenga un préstamo, menor será la *tasa de interés*. Todos los puntos que usted paga en la compra de una hipoteca son deducibles del impuesto en el año que usted los paga. Sin embargo, si usted *refinancia* su hipoteca, los puntos que usted paga al momento del refinanciamiento deben ser amortizados durante la vida del préstamo. Si usted obtiene una hipoteca de 30 años cuando refinancia, por ejemplo, usted puede deducir sólo la treintava parte de los puntos de sus impuestos cada año.

recargo por mora: un *recargo por mora* es una multa que se cobra si se recibe con retraso un pago de la hipoteca. Un recargo por mora puede ser alto, tanto como el 5 por ciento del pago. ¡Más le vale hacer los pagos a tiempo!

refinanciamiento: el *refinanciamiento,* o "refi," es una palabra elegante para definir un nuevo préstamo hipotecario (normalmente a una *tasa de interés* más baja) para cancelar una hipoteca existente (generalmente a un interés más alto). El refinanciamiento no es automático ni está garantizado y puede ser también problemático y costoso. Sopese cuidadosamente los costos y beneficios de esta transacción.

reporte crediticio: un *reporte o informe crediticio o de crédito* es el reporte principal que una entidad crediticia utiliza para determinar si usted tiene capacidad de pago. Usted le paga a la entidad por este reporte, el cual ella utilizará para determinar su capacidad de administrar sus gastos y cancelar préstamos en el tiempo establecido.

reserva de efectivo: la mayoría de las entidades crediticias requieren que los compradores tengan disponible suficiente dinero en efectivo al momento de la compra como para cancelar las dos primeras cuotas de la hipoteca o cubrir una emergencia financiera.

retorno de inversión: el *retorno de inversión* es el porcentaje de beneficio que usted recibe al efectuar una inversión. Si usted invierte $1.000 y en un año tiene en su cuenta $1.100, usted ha obtenido un beneficio de $100. Su retorno es el beneficio ($100) dividido por la inversión inicial ($1.000) —esto es, el 10 por ciento. Vea también *ventaja o palanca financiera.*

seguro contra inundación: "Cuando las aguas de la inundación retroceden, el pobre pueblo comienza de la nada". (Richard Wright, autor). Usted comienza de la nada si no tiene un *seguro contra inundación.* En las zonas de inundación designadas por el gobierno, se requiere de un seguro como éste. Es prudente tener un seguro contra inundación aún si la posibilidad de una catástrofe como ésta en su área sea remota.

seguro contra terremotos: aunque la costa oeste del país está asociada a menudo con los terremotos, hay otras áreas propensas a ellos también. Una cláusula adicional de *seguro contra terremotos* en su póliza de seguro de propietario, paga la reparación de los daños o la reconstrucción de la casa en caso de que ese evento ocurra. Si usted vive en un área con riesgo de terremoto, ¡adquiera un seguro contra terremotos!

seguro de propietario: estos se requieren y son necesarios. Nada de "si" o "pero" con respecto a esto: usted necesita una "cobertura de vivienda" que pueda cubrir el costo de reconstruir su casa. La porción de responsabilidad civil de esta póliza lo protege contra accidentes que ocurran en su propiedad. Otra parte esencial es la cobertura de la propiedad personal que paga el reemplazo de sus objetos personales y que normalmente es del 50 al 75 por ciento de la cobertura de la vivienda. Finalmente, obtenga un *seguro contra inundaciones* o un *seguro contra terremotos* si vive en áreas susceptible a estos desastres naturales. Al igual que otros tipos de seguros, obtenga los deducibles más altos que pueda de acuerdo a su situación financiera.

seguro de título: el *seguro de título* cubre los honorarios y gastos legales necesarios para defender su título de reclamos que pueden ser hechos contra su propiedad. La extensión de su cobertura depende de si usted tiene una cobertura de propietario estándar o un seguro de título de cobertura amplia (*umbrella*). Para obtener una hipoteca, usted también tiene que comprar un seguro de título del prestamista para proteger a su prestamista contra los riesgos de títulos.

seguro de vida hipotecario: el seguro de vida hipotecario garantiza que el prestamista recibirá su dinero en el caso de que usted muera. Muchas personas pueden tratar de convencerlo de que usted necesita este seguro para proteger a sus seres queridos. ¡Le recomendamos que no pierda ni tiempo ni dinero adquiriendo este seguro! El seguro de vida hipotecario es costoso. Si necesita un seguro de vida, mejor compre uno a término, de alta calidad y a bajo costo.

seguro hipotecario privado (*PMI*, por sus siglas en inglés): si su *cuota inicial* es menos del 20 por ciento del monto de la compra de su casa, usted probablemente necesite comprar un *seguro hipotecario privado* (también conocido como "seguro de incumplimiento del pago de la hipoteca"). Cuanto menor sea la cuota inicial, mayor probabilidad tiene el comprador de *incumplir el pago* del préstamo. El seguro hipotecario privado puede agregarle unos cientos de dólares por año a sus costos de préstamo. Luego de que el *capital en su propiedad* se incremente al 20 por ciento, no necesitará más el seguro. No confunda este seguro con el *seguro de vida hipotecario*.

sociedades residenciales: las sociedades residenciales son una manera en la que personas que no estén casadas puedan tomar posesión de una propiedad. Las sociedades ocurren más a menudo entre las personas que tienen una relación de negocios y que adquieren la propiedad bien sea como un activo o como una inversión. Si estima adquirir una propiedad con otros socios, asegúrese de que un abogado en bienes raíces prepare un contrato por escrito de la sociedad y que todos los socios lo firmen antes de efectuar la compra.

tenencia conjunta o en conjunto: es una forma de ser propietario, que le da a cada persona intereses y derechos en la propiedad, incluso el derecho de supervivencia. Si uno de los copropietarios muere, automáticamente la propiedad pasa al copropietario sobreviviente de la tenencia. Este tipo de posesión de la propiedad es la más apropiada para parejas no casadas pero que tienen una relación sentimental de largo tiempo. Algunas limitaciones de la tenencia conjunta son que cada persona debe poseer partes iguales de la propiedad, y que el derecho de supervivencia se invalida si uno de los copropietarios cambia su parte de tenencia conjunta a *tenencia en común*.

tenencia en común: es un tipo de sociedad residencial que es probablemente la mejor manera en que copropietarios sin estar casados obtengan la propiedad de una casa (excepto aquellos copropietarios que tienen una relación de pareja fuerte y duradera —vea *tenencia conjunta*). Los copropietarios no necesitan poseer partes iguales de la propiedad. Una tenencia en común no da tampoco derecho a la supervivencia que automáticamente concede la propiedad del socio fallecido al sobreviviente sin *venta de sucesión*. La parte de la propiedad de un fallecido, tenida como tenencia en común, pasa a la persona designada por él o ella a través de un testamento o un fideicomiso en vida del fallecido.

súper vendedores: la gente comenta que el 20 por ciento de todos los *agentes de bienes raíces* son los que ganan el 80 por ciento de todas las ventas. Tenga cuidado. ¿Por qué estos agentes son *súper vendedores o "productores"* (como se les conoce también)? Algunos vendedores llegan a ser súper vendedores porque presionan a sus compradores y porque venden una gran cantidad de propiedades sin educar a los mismos pacientemente. ¡Que no sea ése el tipo de agente que usted desea! Sin embargo, si el agente es un súper vendedor por que trabaja duro para satisfacer las necesidades de sus clientes, entonces ser súper vendedor es algo bueno.

tasa de interés garantizada: una *tasa de interés garantizada* es un compromiso por escrito del prestamista hipotecario para garantizarle al comprador una *tasa de interés* específica de la vivienda siempre y cuando la compraventa se haga en el lapso de tiempo estipulado. Esta garantía normalmente especifica también el número de *puntos* que se deben pagar en el momento del cierre. La mayoría de los prestamistas no garantizarán la *tasa de interés* de su hipoteca a menos que usted haya hecho una oferta de compra de la propiedad y que la misma haya sido valuada. Usted deberá pagar una pequeña tasa de interés adicional por el privilegio de garantizar por adelantado la tasa de interés del cierre de un préstamo.

tasa de interés: el interés es lo que los prestamistas le cobran a usted por utilizar el dinero de ellos. Los prestamistas generalmente cargan las tasas más altas en préstamos de alto riesgo. Para *hipotecas de tasa fija* recuerde que la *tasa de interés* tiene una relación de "sube y baja" con los *puntos*. Normalmente se asocia un alto número de puntos con una tasa de interés baja y viceversa. Para una *hipoteca con tasa de interés variable,* asegúrese de entender la *fórmula* (el *índice* más el *margen*) que determina cómo se calcula la tasa de interés después de que la tasa inicial o enganche se vence.

tasa inicial o de enganche: conocida también como la *tasa de interés* inicial, la *tasa inicial o de enganche* es la atractiva tasa con la que la mayoría de las hipotecas con tasa de interés variable comienzan. No se sienta atraído por una hipoteca sólo porque tiene una baja tasa inicial. Observe la *fórmula* de hipoteca (*índice + margen = tasa de interés*) para estimar con este método confiable la futura tasa de interés del préstamo — la que será una vez que el préstamo sea "completamente indexado".

tasa porcentual anual (*APR*, por sus siglas en inglés): este porcentaje representa el costo anual total de una hipoteca expresada según la tasa de interés real cancelada. La *APR* incluye la *tasa de interés* base, los *puntos* u otros honorarios y costos agregados al préstamo. Por lo tanto, la *APR* es invariablemente superior a la tasa de interés que la entidad crediticia cotiza para la hipoteca.

tenencia en conjunto: la *tenencia en conjunto* o *tenencia conjunta* es una forma de copropiedad que le da a todos los beneficiarios iguales derechos e intereses sobre la propiedad, incluso el derecho de supervivencia. A la muerte de uno de los beneficiarios, la propiedad automáticamente se transfiere al otro que le sobrevive. Esta forma de propiedad es más apropiada para gente que no está casada pero que tienen una relación por mucho tiempo. Algunas de las limitaciones de la tenencia en conjunto son: primero, cada beneficiario debe poseer la vivienda en partes iguales y segundo, el derecho de supervivencia se anula si una persona cambia su título de propiedad de tenencia en conjunto a *sociedad residencial*.

título de propiedad o escritura: un *título* o *escritura* es el documento que convierte la propiedad en algo real. Antes de recibir el título, la compañía del *seguro del título* debe recibir el pago de la entidad hipotecaria y sus pagos por concepto de *cuota inicial* y *costos de cierre*. Por su parte, la compañía de *seguro del título* debe demostrar que el vendedor posee el título legal y sin ningún gravamen a la propiedad que se esté transfiriendo.

topes: los *topes* en bienes raíces no tienen nada que ver con los topes de las casas. Hay dos tipos de topes para las *hipotecas con tasas de interés variables*. El *tope constante* limita la *tasa de interés* más alta y la *más baja* permitidas para su hipoteca durante la vigencia de la misma. El *tope variable* limita la cantidad que la tasa de interés puede variar en un *período de ajuste*. Una *ARM* de un año, por ejemplo, puede tener una tasa inicial del 7,5 por ciento con un tope de ajuste periódico de más o menos un 2 por ciento y un tope máximo durante la vigencia del préstamo del 6 por ciento. En el peor de los casos, la tasa de interés del préstamo pudiera ser del 9,5 por ciento en el segundo año, 11,5 en el tercero y 13,5 en el cuarto año y el resto del tiempo (7,5 por ciento de tasa de inicio más el 6 por ciento del tope constante).

tope de por vida: el *tope de por vida* o simplemente tope determina la cantidad *máxima* o *mínima* que la tasa de interés ajustable de su hipoteca y la cuota mensual pueden fluctuar durante la vigencia del préstamo. El tope de por vida es diferente del *tope periódico*, el cual limita los límites superior e inferior entre los cuales la tasa de interés puede cambiar en cualquier *período de ajuste*.

tope periódico: este tope limita la cantidad que la *tasa de interés* de una *hipoteca con tasa de interés variable* puede subir o bajar en un período de ajuste. Vea también *topes*.

townhouses: la *vivienda en serie o townhouses* es un nombre decorativo para una hilera de casas adyacentes. Este tipo de viviendas es más económico que las individuales separadas ya que utilizan paredes y techos comunes y por lo tanto, ahorran espacio y terreno. En términos de una inversión por su potencial de revalorización, las viviendas townhouses se encuentran entre las viviendas unifamiliares separadas y los *condominios*.

transacción de capital en la propiedad compartida: en una *transacción de capital en la propiedad compartida,* un inversionista privado contribuye con dinero a la compra de una vivienda para luego compartir el *capital de la propiedad* como copropietario. Cuando se vende una vivienda, el inversionista toma una parte del beneficio o pérdida. Estos tipos de transacciones suelen ser un poco complicadas cuando se desarrollan conflictos entre los intereses del inversionista y del residente. Por ejemplo, el inversionista puede que desee vender la propiedad para sacarle beneficio, pero puede que el residente no esté de acuerdo y quiera seguir como está. Si usted intenta participar en una transacción de este tipo, haga que un abogado que trabaje con *sociedades* de bienes raíces residenciales le prepare un acuerdo escrito de sociedad para que todas las partes firmen antes de efectuar la compra de la propiedad.

valor prorrateado: el *valor prorrateado* es el valor de la propiedad (de acuerdo al valor del asesor de impuestos de su localidad) con el propósito de determinar el *impuesto a la propiedad.*

valorización/depreciación: la *valorización* se refiere al incremento del valor de una propiedad. La *depreciación* (lo contrario de la valorización) es cuando la propiedad pierde valor.

venta de sucesiones: una *venta de sucesiones* es la venta de una vivienda que ocurre cuando el dueño de una casa muere y la propiedad se divide entre los herederos o es vendida para pagar deudas. El ejecutor de los bienes organiza la venta de la sucesión y un juez de un tribunal o juzgado de sucesiones supervisa el proceso. El participante que ofrece más recibe la propiedad.

ventaja o palanca financiera: se refiere a la gran influencia o ventaja que se puede lograr sin mucho esfuerzo. Comprar una casa le permite aumentar su dinero de dos maneras: Suponga que usted da una *cuota inicial* del 20 por ciento para una casa de $100.000 —es decir, invierte $20.000. La primera ventaja o palanca es que usted controla una propiedad de $100.000 con solamente $20.000. Si su casa se revaloriza en $120.000, usted ha generado una ganancia de $20.000 con una inversión de $20.000 —un retorno del 100 por ciento gracias a la ventaja. Sin embargo, el apalancamiento o ventaja trabaja en ambas direcciones, así que si su casa se deprecia. . .

viviendas en serie: vea *townhouses*.

Índice

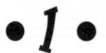

Notas

Notas

Notas

Libros en Español

Disponibles en cualquier lugar donde vendan libros, o través de dummies.com

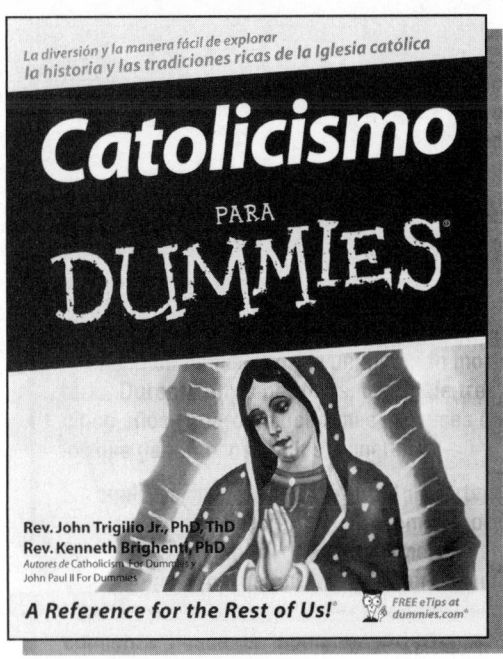

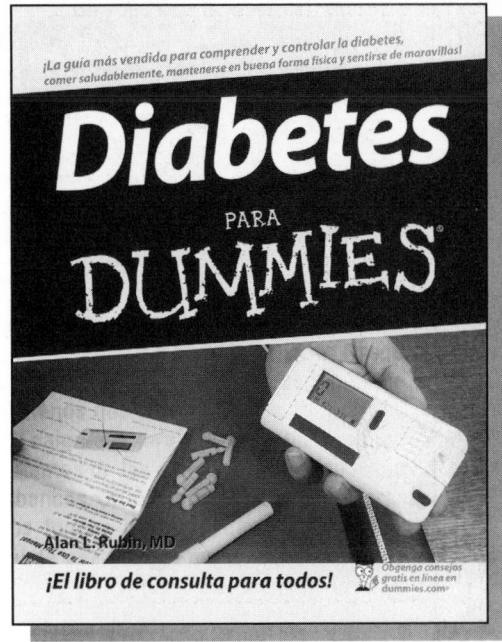

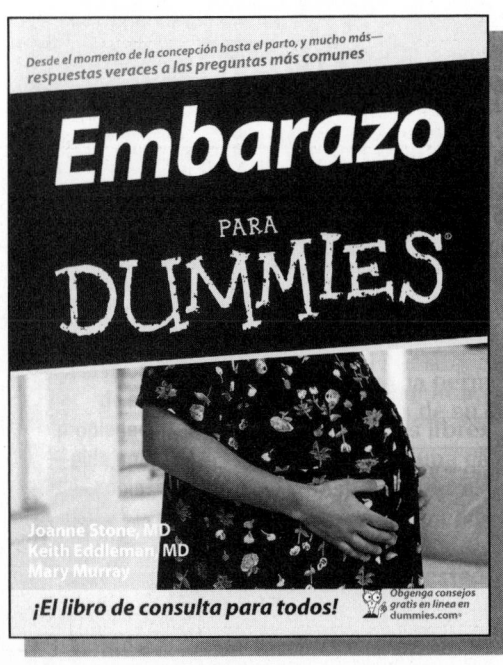

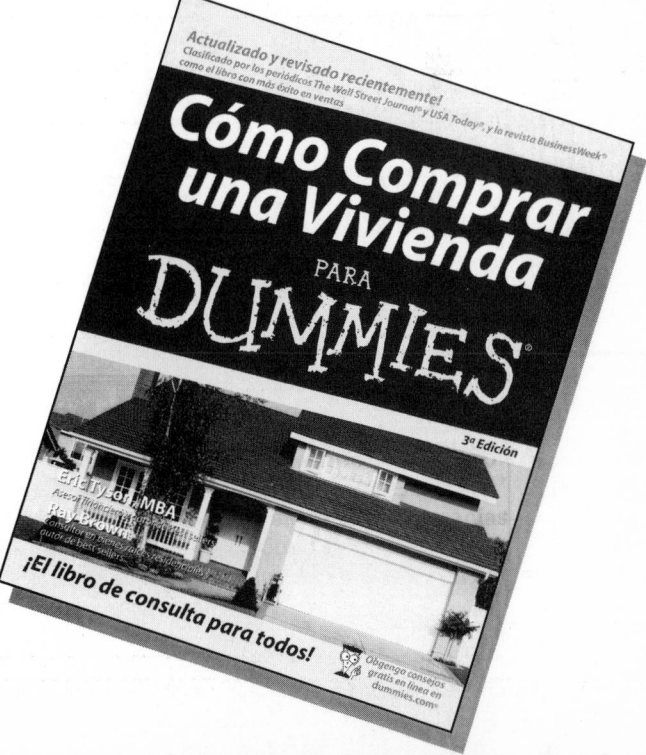

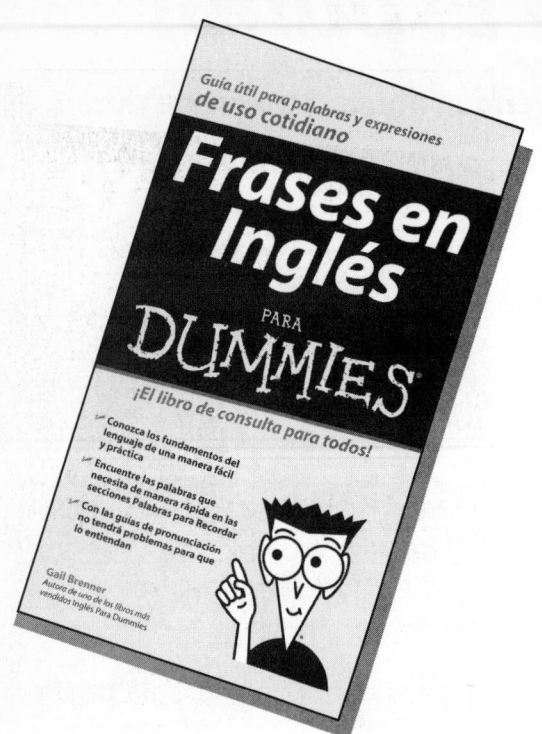

Guía útil para palabras y expresiones de uso cotidiano

Frases en Inglés

PARA

DUMMIES

¡El libro de consulta para todos!

- Conozca los fundamentos del lenguaje de una manera fácil y práctica
- Encuentre las palabras que necesita de manera rápida en las secciones Palabras para Recordar
- Con las guías de pronunciación no tendrá problemas para que lo entiendan

Gail Brenner
Autora de uno de los libros más vendidos Inglés Para Dummies

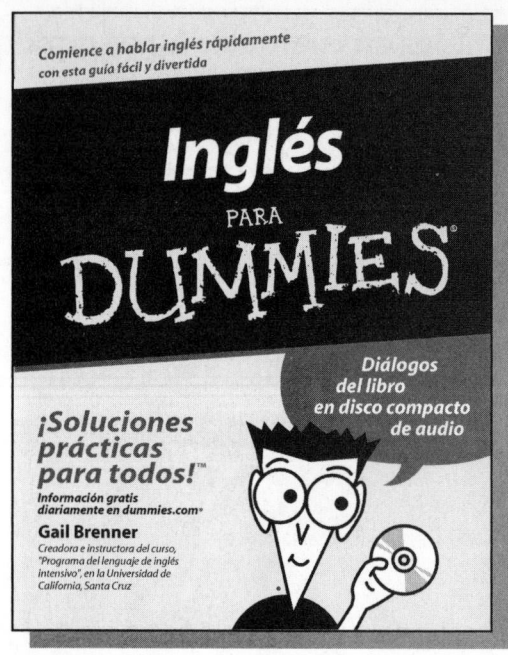

Comience a hablar inglés rápidamente con esta guía fácil y divertida

Inglés

PARA

DUMMIES

Diálogos del libro en disco compacto de audio

¡Soluciones prácticas para todos!

Información gratis diariamente en dummies.com

Gail Brenner
Creadora e instructora del curso, "Programa del lenguaje de inglés intensivo", en la Universidad de California, Santa Cruz

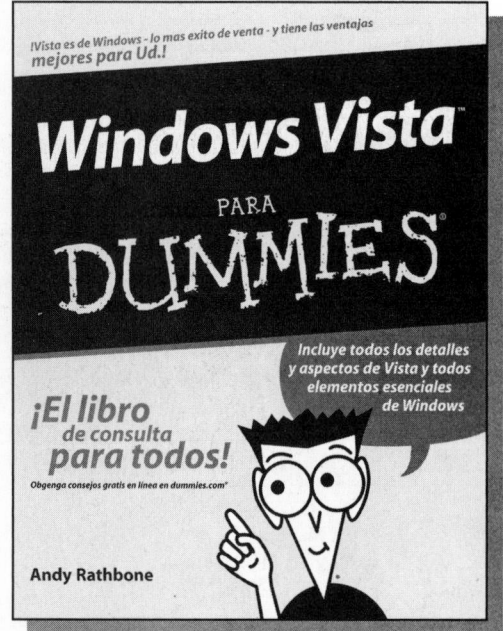

¡Vista es de Windows - lo mas exito de venta - y tiene las ventajas mejores para Ud.!

Windows Vista

PARA

DUMMIES

Incluye todos los detalles y aspectos de Vista y todos elementos esenciales de Windows

¡El libro de consulta para todos!

Obgenga consejos gratis en linea en dummies.com

Andy Rathbone

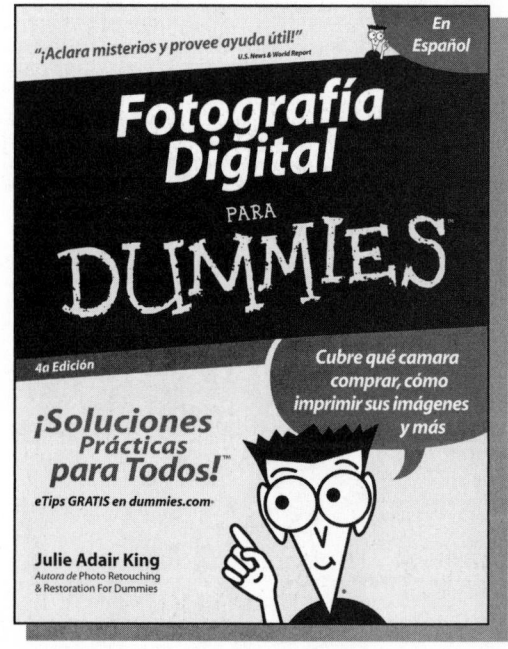

"¡Aclara misterios y provee ayuda útil!"
U.S. News & World Report

En Español

Fotografía Digital

PARA

DUMMIES

4a Edición

Cubre qué camara comprar, cómo imprimir sus imágenes y más

¡Soluciones Prácticas para Todos!

eTips GRATIS en dummies.com

Julie Adair King
Autora de Photo Retouching & Restoration For Dummies

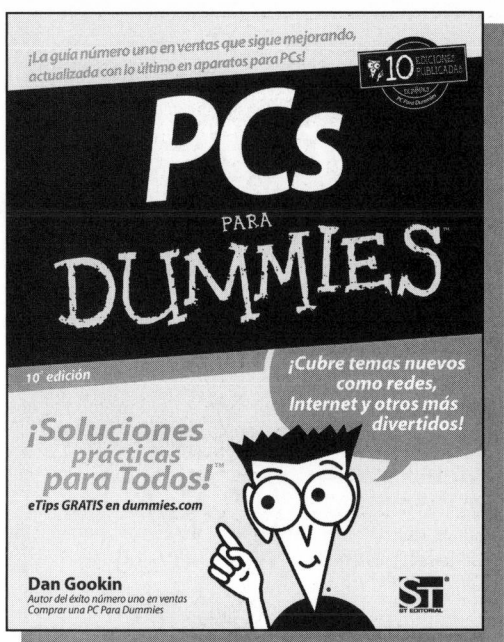

¡La guía número uno en ventas que sigue mejorando, actualizada con lo último en aparatos para PCs!

10 EDICIONES PUBLICADAS

PCs

PARA

DUMMIES

10° edición

¡Cubre temas nuevos como redes, Internet y otros más divertidos!

¡Soluciones prácticas para Todos!™

eTips GRATIS en dummies.com

Dan Gookin
Autor del éxito número uno en ventas
Comprar una PC Para Dummies

ST EDITORIAL

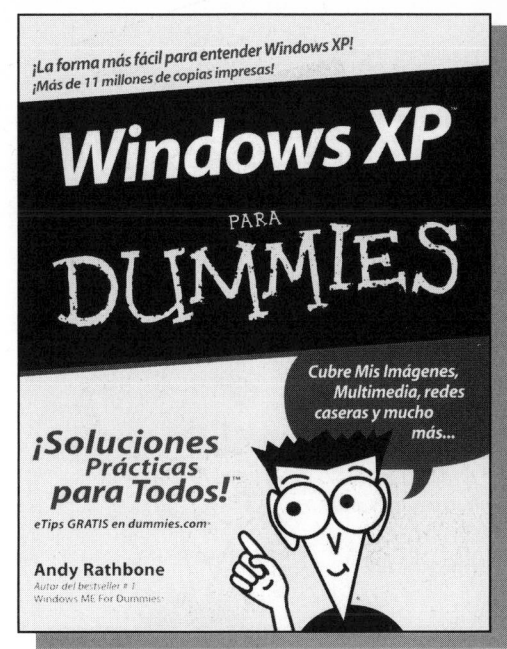

¡La forma más fácil para entender Windows XP!
¡Más de 11 millones de copias impresas!

Windows XP

PARA

DUMMIES

Cubre Mis Imágenes, Multimedia, redes caseras y mucho más...

¡Soluciones Prácticas para Todos!™

eTips GRATIS en dummies.com

Andy Rathbone
Autor del bestseller # 1
Windows ME For Dummies

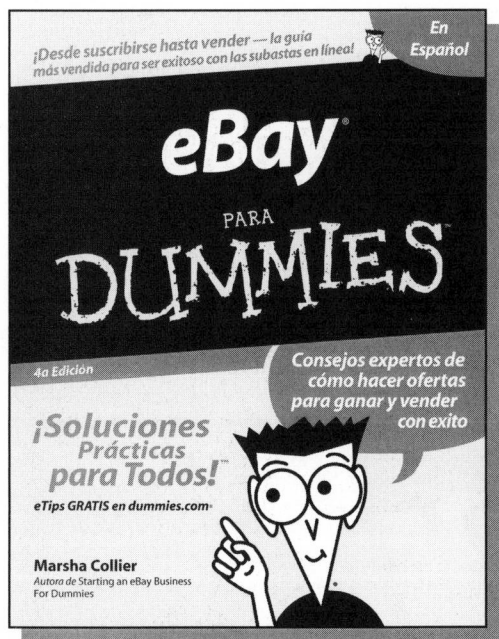

En Español

¡Desde suscribirse hasta vender — la guía más vendida para ser exitoso con las subastas en línea!

eBay

PARA

DUMMIES

4a Edición

Consejos expertos de cómo hacer ofertas para ganar y vender con éxito

¡Soluciones Prácticas para Todos!™

eTips GRATIS en dummies.com

Marsha Collier
Autora de Starting an eBay Business For Dummies

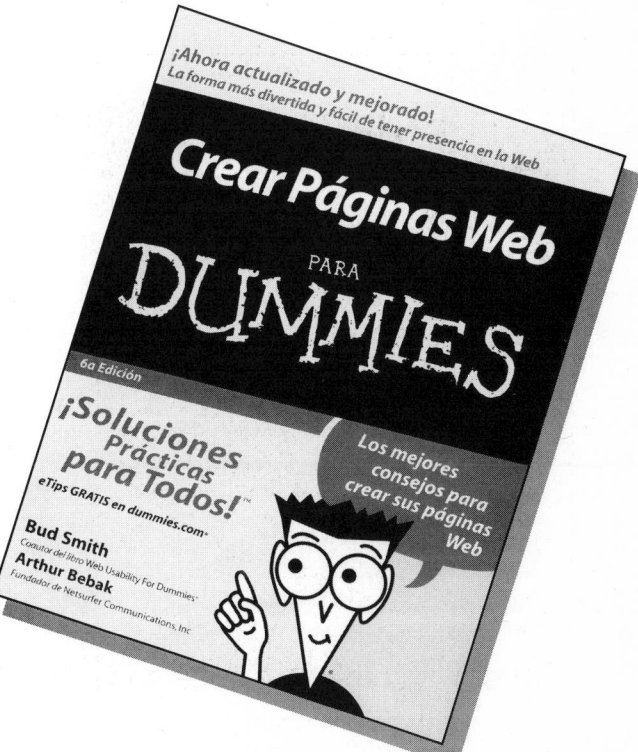

¡Ahora actualizado y mejorado!
La forma más divertida y fácil de tener presencia en la Web

Crear Páginas Web

PARA

DUMMIES

6a Edición

¡Soluciones Prácticas para Todos!™

eTips GRATIS en dummies.com

Los mejores consejos para crear sus páginas Web

Bud Smith
Coautor del libro Web Usability For Dummies
Arthur Bebak
Fundador de Netsurfer Communications, Inc.

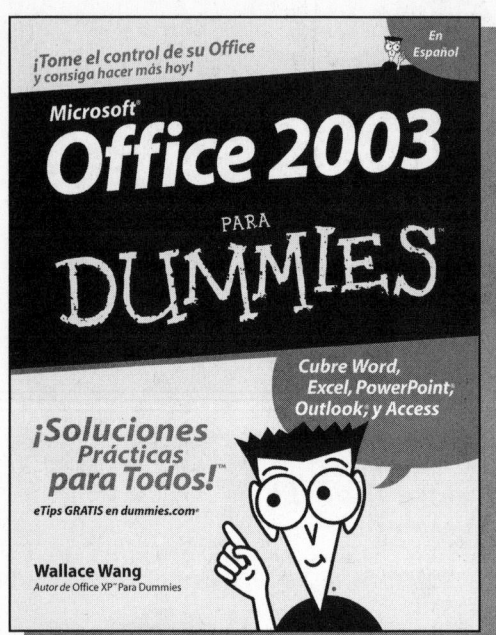

¡Tome el control de su Office
y consiga hacer más hoy!

En Español

Microsoft®

Office 2003

PARA

DUMMIES

Cubre Word,
Excel, PowerPoint;
Outlook; y Access

¡Soluciones
Prácticas
para Todos!
eTips GRATIS en dummies.com®

Wallace Wang
Autor de Office XP™ Para Dummies

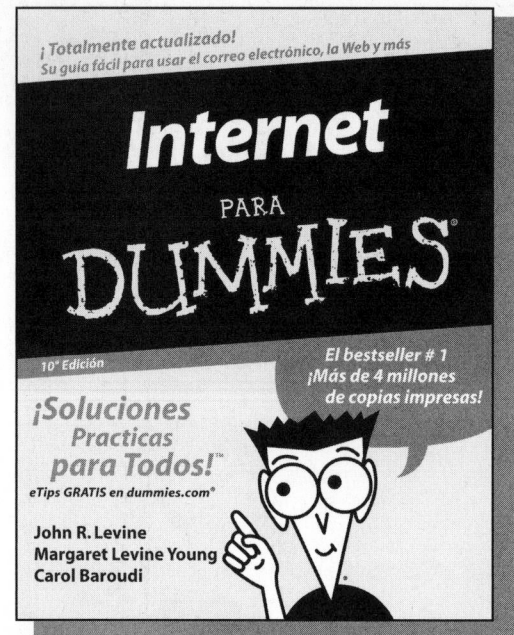

¡ Totalmente actualizado!
Su guía fácil para usar el correo electrónico, la Web y más

Internet

PARA

DUMMIES

10ª Edición

El bestseller # 1
¡Más de 4 millones
de copias impresas!

¡Soluciones
Practicas
para Todos!
eTips GRATIS en dummies.com®

John R. Levine
Margaret Levine Young
Carol Baroudi

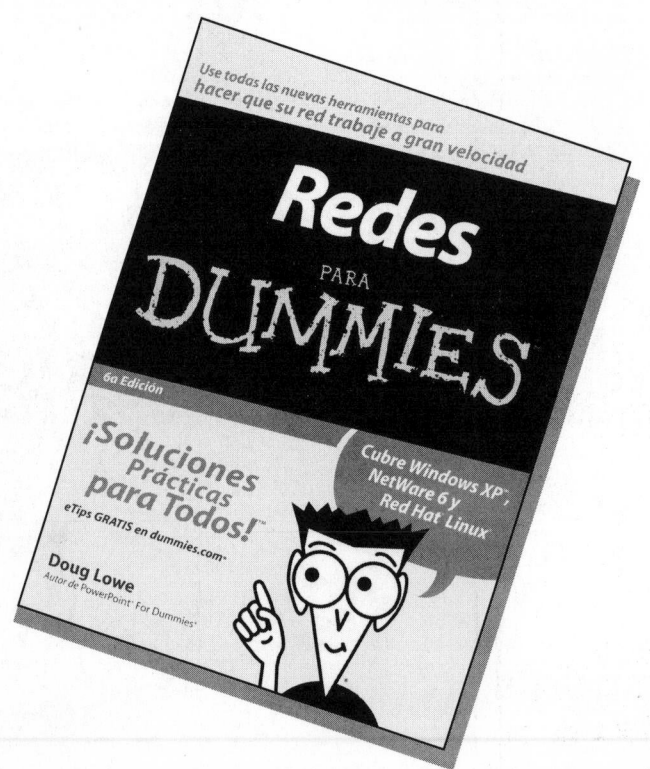

Use todas las nuevas herramientas para
hacer que su red trabaje a gran velocidad

Redes

PARA

DUMMIES

6a Edición

¡Soluciones
Prácticas
para Todos!
eTips GRATIS en dummies.com®

Doug Lowe
Autor de PowerPoint® For Dummies®

Cubre Windows XP®,
NetWare 6 y
Red Hat Linux